Medicode's 2000 Publications & Software For Coders

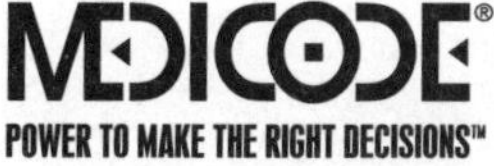

Medicode, Inc. 5225 Wiley Post Way, Suite 500, Salt Lake City, UT 84116 • 801.536.1000 • FAX 801.536.1011

ORDER TOLL FREE OR CALL FOR A FREE CATALOG 800.999.4600

AVAILABLE FROM YOUR MEDICAL BOOKSTORE OR DISTRIBUTOR.

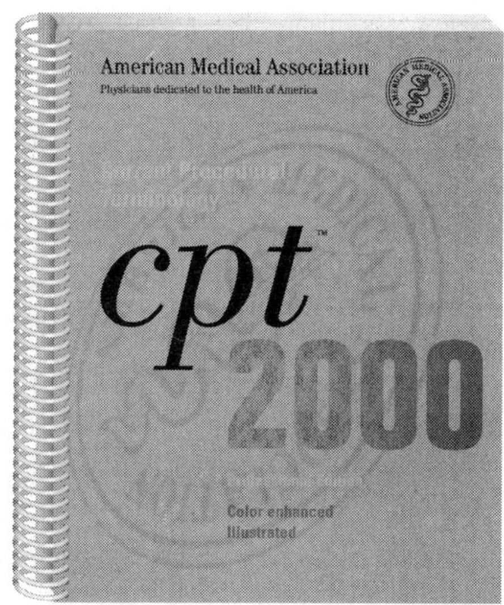

Don't Risk Filing with Obsolete CPT™ Codes

Available November 1999

Hundreds of CPT code changes will soon be in effect. Make sure you have a current CPT code book in your office — or risk rejected claims, delayed payments, and even charges of fraud and abuse!

CPT Professional Binder Version
Binder offers flexibility, color keys and illustrations.
ISBN 1-57947-019-X
(Item #2516) **$74.95**

CPT Professional Spiralbound Version
Durable and easy-to-use with color coding and illustrations.
ISBN 1-57947-018-1
(Item #2515) **$66.95**

CPT Standard Spiralbound
Economical, easy-to-use and durable
ISBN 1-57947-017-3
(Item #2518) **$51.95**

CPT Standard Softbound
AMA's economical classic
ISBN 1-57947-016-5
(Item #2517) **$47.95**

Medicodes Relative Values & CPT ASCII File*
(Item #3902) **$249.95**
Available January 2000

2000 CPT Minibooks
You can now order AMA Minibooks individually. Eight specialties to choose from for just **$29.95**

- **Dermatology, Plastic & Reconstructive Surgery**
  ISBN 1-57947-020-3
  (Item #3267)
- **General Surgery**
  ISBN 1-57947-021-1
  (Item #3264)
- **Gynecology, Obstetrics & Urology**
  ISBN 1-57947-022-X
  (Item #3261)
- **Head & Neck Surgery, Oral & Maxillofacial Surgery, Ophthalmology & Otorhinolaryngology**
  ISBN 1-57947-023-8
  (Item #3265)
- **Medical Specialties**
  ISBN 1-57947-024-6
  (Item #3266)
- **Neurological & Orthopaedic Surgery**
  ISBN 1-57947-025-4
  (Item #3262)
- **Pathology & Laboratory Medicine**
  ISBN 1-57947-026-2
  (Item #3260)
- **Radiology**
  ISBN 1-57947-027-0
  (Item #3263)

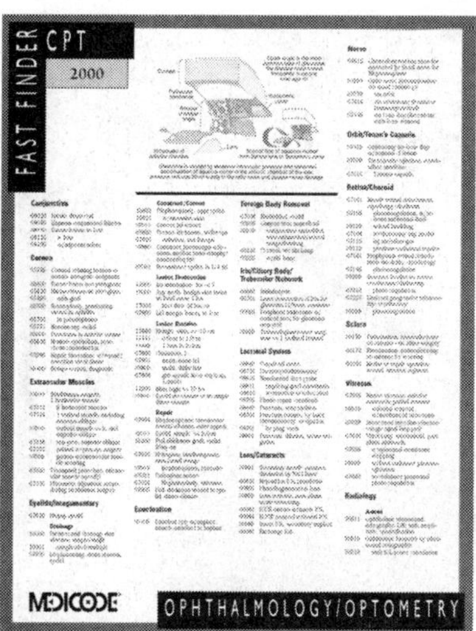

Shortcuts to Precision Coding

2000 CPT Specialty Fast Finders

Available November 1999

Each double-sided, laminated sheet provides a quick reference list of the most common CPT codes for each specialty.

- NEW! **Updated for 2000.** Prevents use of invalid codes. Only current codes are included.
- **Specialized and complete.** Includes 21 specialties on separate and laminated sheets.
- **Quick-Reference to CPT descriptions.** Condenses CPT descriptions in a format that ensures accurate coding.
- **All-inclusive code sets.** Covers the spectrum of CPT, including surgery, laboratory, radiology, medicine, E/M, and anesthesia.

$24.95 per sheet

Allergy and Immunology (Item #3150)
Cardiology (Item #3151)
Cardiovascular and Thoracic Surgery (Item #3152)
Dental/OMS (Item #3153)
Dermatology (Item #3154)
ENT (Item #3155)
Gastroenterology (Item #3156)
General Surgery (Item #3157)
Hematology/Oncology (Item #3158)
Laboratory and Pathology (Item #3159)
Neurology (Item #3160)
Obstetrics, Gynecology and Infertility (Item #3161)
Ophthalmology (Item #3162)
Orthopaedic Surgery (Item #3163)
Pediatrics (Item #3164)
Physical Medicine/Rehab/PT (Item #3165)
Plastic and Reconstructive Surgery (Item #3166)
Primary Care and Internal Medicine (Item #3167)
Psychiatry (Item #3168)
Radiology (Item #3169)
Urology and Nephrology (Item #3170)

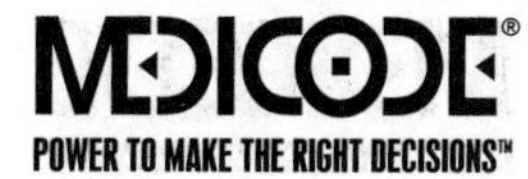

Medicode, Inc. 5225 Wiley Post Way, Suite 500, Salt Lake City, UT 84116 • 801.536.1000 • FAX 801.536.1011

LARGEST NATIONWIDE HEALTH INSURANCE BILLING DIRECTORY

Insurance Directory

MEDICODE®

First printing, August 1999

First edition published 1989
Second edition published 1990
Third edition published 1991
Fourth edition published 1992
Fifth edition published 1993
Sixth edition published 1994
Seventh edition published 1995
Eighth edition published 1996
Ninth edition published 1997
Tenth edition published 1998

The Medicode *2000 Insurance Directory* is designed to be an accurate and authoritative source of information about the insurance industry. Every effort has been made to verify the accuracy of the listings and all information is believed reliable at the time of publication. Absolute accuracy cannot be guaranteed, however. This publication is made available with the understanding that the publisher is not engaged in rendering legal or other services that require a professional license.

ISBN 1-56337-329-7

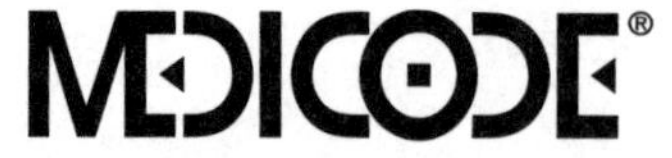

5225 Wiley Post Way, Suite 500
Salt Lake City, UT 84116-2889

Medicode Publishing Staff

Publisher	Susan P. Seare
Associate Medical Director	Thomas G. Darr, MD, FACEP
Editorial Director	Lynn Speirs
Product Manager	Brad Ericson, MPC
Project Editor	Chris B. Fraizer, MA, CPC
Contributing Editor	Jennifer Spetsas
Typesetter	Kerrie Hornsby
Editorial Assistance	Camille Durfee Brittney Harkness Allie Lawrence Darius McCormick Traci Millward Tracy Overstreet Kristen Owens Becky Workman Jodi Workman Melissa Workman

Contents

1 Introduction

The *2000 Insurance Directory* is a comprehensive reference of more than 5,000 listings for all United States, Puerto Rico, and Guam insurance companies processing medical claims. Medicode structures this publication to offer providers, payers, and employers a ready reference of insurance companies' addresses, phone and fax numbers, and the types of claims they process. Each listing in the *2000 Insurance Directory* provides the user with easily identifiable icons to identify the types of claims processed by individual insurance companies (e.g., medical, dental, vision, HCPCS Level II codes, and Medigap policies). Medicode makes every effort to assure the validity and accuracy of the *2000 Insurance Directory* by personally calling each insurance company listed to verify and update the information published.

In addition to specific company information the *2000 Insurance Directory* is updated with an extensive introduction explaining insurance claims policies and procedures that are new for the year. For example, the *2000 Insurance Directory* outlines the steps for completing the form required for Medicare Part B reimbursement (HCFA-1500) in compliance with Y2K requirements and provides a copy of the standard Electronic Data Interchange (EDI) enrollment form that must be completed prior to submitting electronic media claims to Medicare. Medicode also gives you the most current information regarding national identification programs for health care providers and health care organizations.

The *2000 Insurance Directory* introduces new features, as described later in this introduction, and continues popular standard features such as the state-by-state listing of private payers, the addresses and phone numbers of individual state insurance commissioners, and a listing of companies that process HCPCS Level II claims.

New For 2000

The *2000 Insurance Directory* enhances standard features, such as the identification of companies offering Medigap policies, and adds information that may expedite claims processing. The *2000 Insurance Directory* gives you the latest about the merger and consolidation of businesses operated on multistate, regional, and national levels. We also teach you the language used by the health care industry in an expanded reference section that defines and explains terms such as HMOs, IPAs, PPOs, and MSOs.

Places of Operation

Whether it's a consolidation, merger, or centralized office, the *2000 Insurance Directory* provides the information you need for getting claims to the right place. New indexes list companies with centralized claims offices and the companies that have gone through mergers or acquisitions over the past year. The *2000 Insurance Directory* also directs you to the electronic addresses of third-party administrators (TPAs) for quick "on-line" assistance with your claims questions.

HCPCS and Medigap Identifiers

The *2000 Insurance Directory* identifies a greater number of companies that accept HCPCS Level II codes and a greater number of payers offering Medigap policies. HCPCS and Medigap can be defined as follows:

- HCPCS (pronounced "hick-picks") is an acronym for Health Care Financing Administration (the "H") Common Procedure Coding System. These codes are used to report medical services and supplies not specifically identified in the *Physicians' Current Procedural Terminology* (CPT) manual, published by the American Medical Association, including drugs administered by injection and durable medical equipment. HCPCS codes are required for reporting most medical services and supplies provided to Medicare and Medicaid patients, and are often required for private payer reimbursement. Payers that require HCPCS codes are identified with the icon ( ).
- A Medigap policy, as defined by HCFA, is a health insurance policy or other health benefit plan offered by a private company to those entitled to Medicare benefits. The policy provides payment for Medicare charges not payable due to deductibles, coinsurance amounts, or other Medicare and Medicaid imposed limitations. Payers offering Medigap policies are identified with the icon (Ⓜ).

Electronic Claims Capability

The *2000 Insurance Directory* continues to identify the payers accepting claims filed electronically. The Health Insurance Portability and Accountability Act (HIPAA) requires that payers have the capability to receive claims electronically by the year 2000 to reduce the costs and administrative functions of health care tracking and reimbursement. The Administrative Simplification provision of HIPAA applies to all payers and providers and affects all health claims and equivalent encounter information (professional, institutional, and dental).

Electronic Data Interchange (EDI)
HCFA estimates that Medicare claims transmitted electronically are paid usually within 13 days while paper claims can take up to 27 days. The *2000 Insurance Directory* contains a copy of HCFA's Standard EDI enrollment form that must be completed prior to submitting electronic media claims to Medicare. The agreement is required from each provider of health care services, physician, or supplier that intends to submit electronic media claims (EMC). New and existing EMC billers must complete and sign the form and submit it to their local carrier or fiscal intermediary.

Expanded Reference Section
The *2000 Insurance Directory* provides a reference of health care terms that will help you keep pace with the language that changes as rapidly as the modes of service delivery. The expanded reference found in the introduction gives the acronyms and definitions of the most commonly used terms in the managed health care environment.

National Provider Identifier (NPI)
The Department of Health and Human Services (HHS) published a Notice of Proposed Rulemaking (NPRM) in the May 8, 1998 Federal Register that recommended the adoption of the NPI. The public comment period closed on July 6, 1998 and the HHS will publish a Final Rule for the NPI in December 1999. The rule will stipulate the effective date, though HHS expects a July 2000 date.

For more information about NPI:
http://www.hcfa.gov/stats/npi/overview.htm

The effective date marks the start of a two-year period, during which all health plans, except small health plans, all health clearinghouses, and those providers that conduct the standard health care transactions electronically must implement NPI. Small health plans have three years to comply.

The NPI is an 8-position alphanumeric identifier that will be assigned to each individual, organization, and group provider. The NPI contains no embedded intelligence (i.e., information about the health care provider, such as the type of health care provider or state where the health care provider is located). The eighth digit is a numeric check to identify erroneous or invalid NPIs. HCFA has been developing a national provider identifier program since 1993. In 1996, the administrative simplification provision of HIPAA mandated an identifier system for use in electronic transactions of health claims, health encounter information, health plan eligibility, health care payment and remittance advice, health plan premium payments, first report of injury, health claim status, and referral certification and authorization.

Plan ID
HIPAA requires the HHS to adopt a standard, unique identifier for each health plan. HHS expects to issue a Notice of Proposed Rule Making in December 1999, proposing the Plan ID as the standard. Plan ID is a new name for the program formerly identified as PAYERID. The plan ID will identify health plans, and is not limited to payers. The publication of the proposed rule begins a 60-day public comment period. HHS anticipates publishing a final rule in May 2001 and an effective date of July 2001 for Plan ID.

> Note insurance information changes rapidly, and while Medicode attempts to provide the latest information possible, there will be new information Medicode must hold until the next printing or edition of the *Insurance Directory*.

Electronic Data Interchange (EDI) Enrollment Form

The provider agrees to the following provisions for submitting Medicare claims electronically to HCFA or to HCFA's contractors.

A. The Provider Agrees:

1. That it will be responsible for all Medicare claims submitted to HCFA by itself, its employees, or its agents.
2. That it will not disclose any information concerning a Medicare beneficiary to any other person or organization, except HCFA and/or its contractors, without the express written permission of the Medicare beneficiary or his/her parent or legal guardian, or where required for the care and treatment of a beneficiary who is unable to provide written consent, or to bill insurance primary or supplementary, to Medicare, or as required by State or Federal law.
3. That it will submit claims only on behalf of those Medicare beneficiaries who have given their written authorization to do so, and to certify that required beneficiary signatures, or legally authorized signatures on behalf of beneficiaries, are on file.
4. That it will ensure that every electronic entry can be readily associated and identified with an original source document. Each source document must reflect the following information:
   - Beneficiary's name,
   - Beneficiary's health insurance claim number,
   - Date(s) of service,
   - Diagnosis/nature of illness, and
   - Procedure/service performed.
5. That the Secretary of Health and Human Services or his/her designee and/or the contractor has the right to audit and confirm information submitted by the provider and shall have access to all original source documents and medical records related to the provider's submissions, including the beneficiary's authorization and signature. All incorrect payments that are discovered as a result of such an audit shall be adjusted according to the applicable provisions of the Social Security Act, Federal Regulations, and HCFA guidelines.
6. That it will ensure that all claims for Medicare primary payment have been developed for other insurance involvement and that Medicare is the primary payor.
7. That it will submit claims that are accurate, complete, and truthful.
8. That it will retain all original source documentation and medical records pertaining to any such particular Medicare claim for a period of at least 6 years, 3 months after the bill is paid.
9. That it will affix the HCFA-assigned unique identifier number of the provider on each claim electronically transmitted to the contractor.
10. That the HCFA-assigned unique identifier number constitutes the provider's legal electronic signature and an assurance by the provider that services were performed as billed.
11. That it will use sufficient security procedures to ensure that all transmissions of documents are authorized and protect all beneficiary-specific data from improper access.
12. That it will acknowledge that all claims will be paid from Federal funds, that the submission of such claims is a claim for payment under the Medicare program, and that anyone who misrepresents or falsifies or causes to be misrepresented or falsified any record or other information relating to that claim that is required pursuant to this Agreement may, upon conviction, be subject to a fine and/or imprisonment under applicable Federal law.

13. That it will establish and maintain procedures and controls so that information concerning Medicare beneficiaries, or any information obtained from HCFA or it contractor, shall not be used by agents, officers, or employees of the billing service except as provided by the contractor (in accordance with §11106(a) of the Act).
14. That it will research and correct claim discrepancies.
15. That it will notify the contractor or HCFA within 2 business days if any transmitted data are received in an unintelligible or garbled form.

B. The Health Care Financing Administration Agrees To:

1. Transmit to the provider an acknowledgement of claim receipt.
2. Affix the intermediary/carrier number, as its electronic signature, on each remittance advice sent to the provider.
3. Ensure that payments to providers are timely in accordance with HCFA's policies.
4. Ensure that no contractor may require the provider to purchase any or all electronic services from the contractor or from any subsidiary of the contractor or from any company for which the contractor has an interest. The contractor will make alternative means available to any electronic biller to obtain such services.
5. Ensure that all Medicare electronic billers have equal access to any services that HCFA requires Medicare contractors to make available to providers or their billing services, regardless of the contractor sells directly, indirectly, or by arrangement.
6. Notify the provider within 2 business days if any transmitted data are received in an unintelligible or garbled form.

NOTICE:

Federal law shall govern both the interpretation of this document and the appropriate jurisdiction and venue for appealing any final decision made by HCFA under this document.

This document shall become effective when signed by the provider. The responsibilities and obligations contained in this document will remain in effect as long as Medicare claims are submitted to HCFA or the contractor. Either party may terminate this arrangement by giving the other party (30) days of written notice of its intent to terminate. In the event that the notice is mailed, the written notice of termination shall be deemed to have been given upon the date of mailing, as established by the postmark or other appropriate evidence of transmittal.

C. Signature:

I am authorized to sign this document on behalf of the indicated party and I have read and agree to the foregoing provisions and acknowledge same by signing below.

Provider's Name ______________________________

____

____

Title ______________________________

Address ______________________________

City/State/Zip ______________________________

By______________________________

Title ______________________________

Date ______________________________

2 Claims Processing

The term *claims processing* describes the course of submitting a claim to the payer and subsequent adjudication. Understanding how this process works allows physicians and staff members to file claims properly and leads to maximum and timely reimbursement. In addition, this knowledge will allow you and your staff to serve as a resource to patients in understanding this process.

Patient Information

Before filing any claim you need to obtain clear, accurate information from your patients. A good patient information (PI) form is the key to this aspect of claims submission. The PI form should include such basic items as the policy name and number, insured's name, dates of coverage, and secondary insurance information. While this information is a good place to start, it is by no means all of the information required by most insurers. Providing as much information as possible will reduce the insurance company's need to contact your office. Avoiding unnecessary contact will reduce the costs of claims processing and hasten your payment.

You may also wish to preregister new patients over the phone or, if time permits, through the mail. Having a shortened version of your PI form for phone registrations could be valuable.

Patient information must be updated regularly. Most offices verify the information at each visit. If you work in a multiple physician office or clinic, establishing a uniform information policy makes everyone accountable for current and correct patient data.

Patient information forms follow the same basic pattern, but each differs by the type of patient your office might encounter. Each form is titled with the targeted group's name. If your office has some special information needs or you wish to include additional instructions, consider using the back of the form. If your practice has a high volume of Medicare patients, you may want to consider two separate forms — one for Medicare patients and another for non-Medicare patients. These forms could be printed on different colored paper for easy identification.

Primary Vs. Secondary Coverage

Households with dual incomes often have more than one insurer. You must determine which is the primary and which is the secondary insurance company. For commercial plans the subscriber's or insured's insurance company is always primary for the subscriber. In other words, the husband's insurance company is primary for him and the wife's insurance company is primary for her. However, the primary insurance company for any dependents is determined by the insureds' birthdays, the primary insured being the individual whose birthday is first during the year. This is often referred to as the "birthday rule." For example, if the husband's birthday is October 15, 1965 and the wife's birthday is March 1, 1967, the wife is primary for their dependents because her birthday is first during the year (year of birth is ignored). Therefore, obtaining a date of birth for both subscribers is important.

Assignment of Benefits and Release of Information

If you haven't already done so, consider adding an *assignment of benefits* statement to your patient information form. It should state that the patient has agreed to have insurance payments sent directly to the physician and that medical information can be released to the patient's insurance company. A signed copy of this assignment submitted with a claim helps ensure at least partial payment from most commercial insurers. Assignments also reduce collection expenses. An alternative, *lifetime assignment of benefits*, should nearly eliminate the need to obtain a signature after each date of service; however, there are a few payers who require a current signature with each claim.

If your office participates with Medicare, remember that an assignment of benefits and release of billing are still necessary. To avoid the hassle of obtaining updated signatures, you may want to obtain lifetime assignment agreements and a commercial insurer's yearly signature agreement. The yearly signature agreement form is accepted by most commercial payers, but it is not applicable to the Medicare patient.

Determining Coverage

Ideally, a patient's insurance coverage should be verified ***before*** any service is rendered with the common sense exception of emergency treatment. This policy shouldn't apply exclusively to new patients. Established patients may have changed employers, married or divorced, or are no longer covered by the policy that was in effect during their last visit.

When a new patient appointment is made, stress that the patient must present a current insurance identification card. However, a copy of the card does not guarantee eligibility. You may want to take the pertinent information over the phone to verify benefits before the patient arrives. The law requires Medicaid patients to provide current proof of eligibility with each visit, and requesting this information from all patients can be done in a pleasant manner without alienating anyone.

During the visit, photocopy insurance cards and place the copies in the patient's record. Always check and highlight the eligibility dates as well as coverage information. Many offices have a policy that the first visit is always paid at the time of service, with the exception of Medicare, Medicaid, and any contractual arrangement your office may have with an individual payer. Payment for the first service allows you time to verify coverage prior to additional treatment.

The Claim

The most important document for correct reimbursement is the insurance claim form. Other information, such as operative reports, chart notes, and cover letters may establish medical necessity, but the claim itself "sets the stage."

With commercial insurance companies, you may submit the claim directly to the payer or provide your patient with the necessary information to submit the claim. If you've signed an agreement with Blue Cross/Blue Shield or with an HMO or PPO, you are probably required to send the claim directly to them. Medicare now requires that you submit all Medicare claims directly to the carrier, whether you participate or not.

If patients pay at the time of service, you may wish to provide an itemized statement or superbill attached to a claim form that they can submit to their insurance company. This arrangement works well for office services, but surgical services are usually more accurately reimbursed if you bill your hospital and surgical services directly to the payer.

Use a standard claim form (HCFA-1500) when submitting your charges, and be sure to complete the form neatly and accurately. In the past, offices were given a great deal of latitude with claims submission, but today the insurance industry (both government and private) demands greater uniformity, making it even more important to understand how to complete the fields of the claim form accurately.

The HCFA-1500

The following information is a step-by-step guide through the HCFA-1500 claim form. These guidelines reflect the latest changes. You'll find that we've combined the explanations of fields or "items" with related information to show the importance of those relationships.

For complete instructions:
http://www.hcfa.gov/medicare/edi/1500mast.pdf

The Health Care Financing Administration (HCFA) regularly updates the 1500 form. The item-by-item changes are reflected in the following text. In addition, there are changes in the form due to Y2K, electronic transmission, and related provisions of the Health Insurance Portability and Accountability Act (HIPAA). A summary of revisions for this year are noted below:

- Since the use of National Provider Identifiers (NPIs) has been delayed as a result of HIPPA, the HCFA instructions include UPINs and PINs to eliminate confusion.
- Use your data requirements and HCFA-1500 instructions for completing items 3, 9b, and 11a. Y2K guidelines specify an eight-digit when completed by a provider of service or supplier.
- Providers of services and suppliers may enter either a six- or an eight-digit date in items 11b, 14, 16, 18, 19, or 24a. However, the use of either a six- or an eight-digit date must be consistent for all these fields. Do not mix the application of six- and eight-digit dates. For example, do not enter an eight-digit date for item 24a if you have entered a six-digit date for items 11b, 14, 16, 18, and 19. Items 12 and 31 are exempt from this requirement since providers of service and suppliers often report alphanumeric dates (e.g., October 1, 1998) in these fields. HCFA was concerned that subjecting these fields to this requirement may result, at some future date, in unnecessary returns, rejects, or denials.
- Items 19 and 23 of Form HCFA-1500 instructions have been revised to express a new reporting policy. Due to the increase in the usage of these items, it is necessary to set a limit on the amount and type of information reported in these fields. Only information listed in the specific instructions for items 19 and 23 can be reported in items 19 and 23 of Form HCFA-1500. Item 19 can contain up to three conditions per claim, item 23 can contain only one condition. If a claim meets more than three of the stated conditions in item 19, additional conditions must be reported on a separate Form HCFA-1500. For item 23, any additional conditions must be reported on a separate Form HCFA-1500.
- The billing "absentee" physician's Provider Identification Number (PIN) must continue to be reported in item 33 under solo practice arrangements and in item 24k under group practice arrangements.

Item 1

The information in this item identifies the patient's insurers. You may need to check more than one box. Correctly complete item 9 for information regarding other benefits.

Item 1a
Enter the patient's Medicare Health Insurance Claim Number (HICN) whether Medicare is the primary or secondary payer. Follow individual payer rules for completing this item. Generally, list the insured's identification (I.D.) number here. Verify that the I.D. number corresponds to the insured listed in item 4. The patient and the insured aren't always the same person. Some payers assign unique I.D. numbers to each enrollee or dependent and require the number of the enrollee or dependent receiving services (the patient) instead of the insured's number in this item.

Items 2 and 5
The patient's name and demographic information are extremely important. Instructions tell you to list the patient's last name first, then first name and middle initial. With electronic claims processing, claims listing the first name first may be delayed.

Another important detail is to check your spelling. Simple transposition of letters or misspelled names can result in denial or suspension of your claim. Also, verify the demographic information about your patient. The patient's address may not be the same as the insured's – a common cause of delayed payments.

Item 3
The patient's date of birth and sex are required by most insurance companies. Enter the patient's sex and eight-digit birth date (MM/DD/CCYY). Insurer's use the birthdate as verification of the patient as well as an indication of Medicare eligibility.

Item 4
If Medicare is primary, leave blank.

Item 6
This item describing the patient's relationship to the insured verifies eligibility. Remember the patient's relationship to the insured is not always "self." Complete item 4 before item 6.

Items 7, and 11
Demographic information continues with the item asking for the insured's name. As a rule of thumb for Medicare, the patient and insured are the same. For private payers, some insurers assign a unique number to each enrollee. List the name of the insured if the patient's primary insurance is other than Medicare. Enter "same" when the insured is the patient.

Additionally, the subscriber's demographics are important. Assuming that the address of the subscriber and your patient are the same may cost you time and result in an unpaid claim. Supplying all information, including phone numbers with area codes, may avoid delays when an insurance company must contact the insured for additional information. Enter "same" in item 7 when the insured is the patient.

Keep each patient's insurance information up-to-date. With dual coverage becoming more common, confusion easily arises over which insurer is primary and which is secondary. Understanding the "birthday rule" (explained previously) is critical for commercial payers. Carefully follow your carrier's guidelines for Medicare Secondary Payor (MSP) situations and make it a specific employee's responsibility to verify each patient's insurance data at the time of each office visit.

Note: For a paper claim to be considered for Medicare secondary payer benefits a copy of the primary payers explanation of benefits (EOB) notice must be forwarded along with the claim form.

Items 11a–11c expand on the insured's information. Beginning with the policy or group number, you must also list the insured's birthdate, sex, and employer's name or school name. Data from these fields help the payer determine primary and secondary coverage. For Medicare claims, enter "None" and do not complete items 11a–11c if no insurance is primary to Medicare and proceed to item 12. Item 11d is not required by Medicare. Leave blank.

Item 8
This field indicates the patient's marital and employment or student status. This information relates to item 6. If you check "spouse" as the relationship to the insured and then mark "single" under patient status, a good edit system will suspend your claim.

Item 9
Physicians and suppliers must complete this section when assigned Medigap benefits by the beneficiary. (See the reference of Medicare and health care terms in the Introduction to the *2000 Insurance Directory*.) If no Medigap benefits are assigned, leave blank. The field may be used in the future for supplemental insurance plans. However, do not list other supplemental coverage in this section at the time a Medicare claim is filed. Other supplemental claims are forwarded automatically to the private payer contracted with the carrier to send Medicare claim information electronically.

Item 10
This multiple choice item determines whether the patient's condition is related to employment or an accident. Note that auto accident has its own line and a field exists for the state in which the accident occurred. Item 10 is important to the payer because it indicates liability. Incorrect completion of this item will cause your claim to be suspended or denied.

Item 10d is exclusively for Medicaid (MCD) information.

Item 12
Item 12 authorizes the release of information, allowing you to provide any medical information required to file the claim.

The patient or authorized representative must sign and enter either a six- or an eight-digit or an alphanumeric dates unless the signature is on file. In lieu of signing the claim, the patient may sign a statement that must be kept in the appropriate file. An authorization is effective indefinitely unless revoked.

Item 13
The signature authorizes payment of mandated Medigap benefits to the participating physician or supplier. See item 9 for information regarding Medigap benefits.

Items 14 and 15
The remainder of the information on the form defines the patient's medical problem and provides information for treatment provided. Most insurance companies require information on the patient's illness, such as when the symptoms first appeared and if the patient has had the same or similar problems. Enter either a six- or an eight-digit date for the onset of the current illness, injury, or pregnancy. For chiropractic services, enter either the six- or an eight-digit date when treatment was provided or initiated. Medicare does not require that item 15 be completed.

Item 16
This field indicates the days a patient may be unable to work in his or her current occupation. While these dates may not be important to Medicare and private payers, they are very important to a workers compensation claim. Your state workers compensation carrier may require additional forms explaining when the patient can return to work or forms providing disability information. Become familiar with these forms when treating an employment-related injury or disease.

Items 17 and 17a
Medicare requires the referring or ordering provider's name. The National Provider number regulations regarding electronic transmission have delayed NPI and HCFA has instructed providers to use their Unique Physician Identification Number (UPIN) until such time as the NPI is implemented. The rule recommending the NPI as the standard healthcare provider identifier was publised in the Federal Register on May 7, 1998. Providers will be notified of NPI numbers, and physicians who are not assigned an NPI must contact their Medicare carriers prior to submitting a claim.

Item 18
Enter either a six-digit or an eight-digit code when a medical service is furnished as a result of, or subsequent to, a related hospitalization. The dates of admission and discharge are necessary for hospital care. The dates you list must match the hospital's dates because payers often use these records to verify billed services.

Item 19
Use this field to enter additional information, including:

- Eight-digit date the patient was last seen and the National Provider ID (NPI) or UPIN of the patient's attending physician for physical and occupational therapists. (Due to the delay of NPI, use the UPIN.)
- Eight-digit x-ray date for chiropractor services.
- Drug name and dosage when submitting a claim for not otherwise classified (NOC) drugs.
- A clear description of "unlisted procedure codes."
- Applicable modifiers when -99 is listed in the line items window.
- The statement "Homebound" when a homebound/institutionalized patient has an EKG tracing or specimen obtained from an independent lab.
- Enter the statement "testing for hearing aid" for intentional denial when other payers are involved.
- When dental exams are billed, enter the specific surgery that required the exam.
- The specific name and dosage are required when low osmolar contrast material is billed and not covered by a HCPCS Level II code.
- Enter the six- or eight-digit assumed or relinquished date for a global surgery claim when providers share post-operative care.
- The statement "attending physician, not hospice employee" should be entered when the attending physician rendering services to a hospice patient is not employed by the hospice.
- Demonstration identification number 30 should be applied to all emphysema treatment trial claims.

Item 20
Complete item 20 when billing diagnostic tests subject to purchase price limitations. Enter "no" if no purchase tests are indicated on the claim. Enter "yes" and complete item 32 if the diagnostic test was performed outside of the entity billing for the service. When billing for multiple purchased diagnostic tests, each test must be submitted on a separate claim.

Item 21
Item 21 has four slots for diagnostic codes, numbered 1 through 4. Enter the numeric codes from ICD-9-CM *(International Classification of Diseases, 9th Edition, Clinical Modification)*.

The following are common diagnostic coding problems that are likely to cause payment delays:

- The diagnosis doesn't establish the medical necessity of the treatment. When a problem or illness is acute, your diagnostic code must convey the emergent nature of the patient encounter.

- A patient's chronic diagnosis, which is not the reason for this visit, is incorrectly billed as the primary diagnosis.
- The ICD-9-CM code is incomplete or inaccurate. Always code to the highest specificity, adding appropriate 4th and 5th digits when available. Never "create" codes not actually found in ICD-9-CM.
- Occasionally, the code does not correspond to the treatment provided, e.g., coding treatment of a femoral fracture as a fracture of the tibia.
- Errors can also occur when italicized ICD-9-CM codes are used as primary diagnoses. Never use these codes alone or as the primary diagnosis. Code first the etiology of the disease, then its manifestations.
- E codes report external causes of injury or poisoning, including place of occurrence, and are never used alone or as primary diagnoses.

Item 22
Not required by Medicare. Leave blank.

Item 23
List the prior authorization number in this field. It is required by Medicare, Medicaid, and many managed care organizations.

Medicare requires the 10-digit Clinical Laboratory Improvement Act (CLIA) certification number for laboratory services billed by a physician office laboratory. Enter the six-digit Medicare provider number of the home health agency or hospice when billing CPT code 99375 or 99376 or HCPCS code G0064, G0065, or G0066.

The investigational device exemption (IDE) number must be entered when such a device is used in an FDA-approved clinical trial.

Item 24
Be sure to complete these fields accurately, including date(s) of service, place of service, procedure codes and modifiers, charges, days/units, and type of service.

List the actual date of service, not the date you file the claim. If you provided a service for several consecutive days, list the beginning and ending dates, and place the number of days of service in column G.

CPT codes are keyed to place of service (POS), so column B has become even more important. These codes are required by government payers and listed next. However, check with private payers to determine whether they use these POS codes or have developed their own.

There is a new place of service code for an adult living center, which took effect January 1, 1999. The new POS (35) is used when billing services rendered at a residential care facility which houses beneficiaries who cannot live alone but do not need around-the-clock skilled medical services. The facility provides room, board, and other personal assistance services. The facility services do not include a medical component.

Place of Service Codes

Code	Description
G	Suppliers must furnish the units of oxygen contents
11	Office
12	Patient's home
21	Inpatient hospital
22	Outpatient hospital
23	Emergency room – hospital
24	Ambulatory surgical center
25	Birthing center
26	Military treatment facility
31	Skilled nursing facility
32	Nursing facility
33	Custodial care facility
34	Hospice
35	Adult living care facility
41	Ambulance – land
42	Ambulance – air or water
50	Federally Qualified Health Center
51	Inpatient psychiatric facility
52	Psychiatric facility – partial hospitalization
53	Community mental health center
54	Intermediate care facility – mentally retarded
55	Residential substance abuse treatment facility
56	Psychiatric residential treatment center
60	Mass immunization center
61	Comprehensive inpatient rehabilitation facility
62	Comprehensive outpatient rehabilitation facility
65	End stage renal disease treatment facility
71	State or local public health clinic
72	Rural health clinic
81	Independent laboratory
99	Other unlisted facility

Type of service (TOS) codes also appeared on the back of the previous form, but have been deleted from the current one. Even though this field remains on the form (column C), not all government and private payers require this information. For your convenience in providing information for all payers, the following are HCFA's standard TOS codes:

Code	Description
0	Whole blood or packed red cells
1	Medical care
2	Surgery
3	Consultation
4	Diagnostic x-ray
5	Diagnostic laboratory
6	Radiation therapy
7	Anesthesia
8	Assistance at surgery
9	Other medical service

- A Used DME
- B High risk screening mammography
- C Low risk screening mammography
- F Ambulatory surgical center (facility usage)
- I Installment purchase DME
- L Renal supplies
- M Monthly capitation payment for dialysis
- N Kidney donor
- P Lump sum purchase of DME
- R Rental of DME
- T Psychological therapy
- U Occupational therapy
- V Pneumococcal vaccine
- W Physical therapy
- Y Second opinion on elective surgery
- Z Third opinion on elective surgery

Column D is the place for procedure codes (CPT and HCPCS). Include any applicable modifiers.

To establish medical necessity for the services provided, use column E to reference the appropriate diagnoses from item 21 to each procedure. List the diagnoses by item numbers 1, 2, 3, or 4 rather than by ICD-9-CM code.

Charges in column F are important since you're telling the payer how much you want to be paid. Each service or line item should have a separate fee with the total charges noted in item 28. Unless there are unusual circumstances surrounding the service (e.g., additional time and effort) or if the service is reduced, the fees you charge should be consistent on a code-by-code basis. Exceptions are noted by adding a modifier to the affected procedure code.

List days or units in column G. This information is essential for payment of multiple days in the hospital or multiple units of the same code, such as drugs. For anesthesia, show the total minutes required for the procedure. Suppliers must furnish the units of oxygen contents.

Column H indicates Early Periodic Screening and Developmental Testing (EPSDT) and family planning.

Column I identifies treatment provided in an emergency department. Remember that emergency services must also be indicated with the appropriate place of service code in column B. Medicare no longer requires this field.

Column J is used for coordination of benefits.

Any special use for column K is determined by individual payers. For Medicare claims, enter the carrier-assigned provider number when the performing physician/supplier belongs to a group practice. When more than one physician/supplier within a group bills on the same form, enter the individual provider number for the corresponding line items.

Item 25

Place your Federal Tax I.D. or Social Security number in this field. Use either your employer or tax I.D. number consistently to avoid confusion on the 1099 forms you receive from third-party payers. Always verify the tax I.D. numbers on your 1099 forms because an error in unreported income may trigger an IRS audit.

Item 26

The patient account number field is optional. Many payers list your patient's account number on the EOB which saves you the time it takes to research which "Mrs. Jones's" account should be credited with this payment.

Item 27

This item generally applies to government claims but may apply to other payers with whom you have a contractual agreement. If your office participates with Medicare, this item must always be checked "yes."

Nonparticipating physicians may decide on a claim-by-claim basis whether to accept assignment and check "yes" or "no." Medicare assumes the claim is unassigned if this item is left blank and sends the check to the patient. If a participating physician leaves this blank, it could be viewed as a violation of the participation agreement with Medicare.

Items 28, 29, and 30

Many claims are submitted with multiple pages that can be confusing to payers when only the grand total is listed for all services on the final page. Instead, each page of the claim should list the total charges, amount paid, and balance due for that page. Also, report only the services and procedures actually provided.

The amount charged (item 28) is the total of all charges in item 24f. The amount paid area (item 29) indicates payment by the patient or by another insurance company. Failure to indicate payment by the primary insurer may result in claims denial or overpayment by the secondary payer.

The balance due (item 30) is left blank for Medicare.

Item 31

The physician's signature, stamped signature (if acceptable), or an authorized signature must appear in this item. Most payers return unsigned claims. This signature affirms that the information on the claim is correct. For electronic claims, the HCFA-assigned identifier number serves as the provider's electronic signature.

Item 32

Enter the name and address of the facility if the services were furnished in a hospital, clinic, laboratory, or facility other than the patient's home or physician's office. When the name and address of the facility where the services were furnished are the same as the biller's name and address shown in item 33, enter the word "same." Providers of services (namely physicians) must identify the supplier's name, address, and NPI when billing for purchased diagnostic tests. When more than one supplier is used, a separate HCFA–1500 should be used to bill for each supplier.

This item is completed whether the supplier performs the work at the physician's office or at another location.

If a QB or QU modifier is billed, indicating the service was rendered in a Health Professional Shortage Area (HPSA), the physical location where the service was rendered must be entered if other than home. However, if the address shown in item 33 is in a HPSA and is the same as where the services were rendered, enter the word "SAME."

If the supplier is a certified mammography screening center, enter the six-digit FDA approved certification number. Complete this item for all laboratory work performed outside a physician's office. If an independent laboratory is billing, enter the place where the test was performed.

Item 33

The information for this item further identifies your practice to the insurer. Enter the appropriate, payer-specific provider number as well as your group name, address, and phone number. For Medicare claims, enter the provider number, for a performing physician/supplier who is not a member of a group practice. Enter the group number for a performing physician/supplier who is a member of a group practice.

Note

The HCFA-1500 form is also available in a scannable red-ink version for carriers using Optical Character Recognition (OCR) equipment to process claims. The red ink used to print this form cannot be duplicated by your PC, so do not attempt to print red-ink versions of the HCFA-1500 form from your printer. Carriers are not able to process any form but the official HCFA-1500 red-ink version. If a Medicare carrier is not currently using OCR equipment to process claims, they may accept a facsimile of the HCFA-1500 form generated by dot matrix or laser jet printers, as long as the originals are submitted for payment. Contact your carrier to ask which type of claim form is being accepted for processing.

Clean Claims

Claims submitted with all of the information necessary for processing are referred to as "clean" and are usually paid in a timely manner. Paying careful attention to what should appear on your claim form helps produce these clean claims. Now we'll discuss some of the common reasons that claims are denied. Being aware of common mistakes helps you avoid them. It's extremely important to read the communications you receive from insurers. Their information will often put you on the right track to correct your errors through resubmission.

Common Errors

- The patient's I.D. number is incorrect.
- The patient's name and address don't match the insurer's records.
- The physician's tax I.D. number, provider number, or Social Security number is missing.
- There is little or no information regarding primary or secondary coverage.
- The physician's or authorized person's signature is missing.
- Dates of service are incorrect or don't relate to the claims information from other providers (hospital, nursing homes, etc.).
- Dates are not six or eight digits as required.
- The fee column is blank or not itemized and totaled.
- The patient information is incomplete.
- The CPT and ICD-9 codes are invalid, or the diagnostic codes aren't linked to the correct services or procedures.
- The claim is illegible.

Standardized Claims Processing

The turn of the millennium will change the way claims are processed. According to recent legislation (the Health Insurance Portability and Accountability Act of 1996, or HIPAA), payers must have the capability to receive claims electronically by the year 2000. Those who must comply include all health plans, all payers (TPAs included), and all clearinghouses that process health data. Small health plans and workers compensation are exempt, at this time. The provision is intended to reduce the costs and administrative chores of healthcare by standardizing electronic transmission of certain administrative and financial transactions currently carried out on paper. The following transactions will be affected: health claims and equivalent encounter information (such as dental), coordination of benefits (COB), enrollment in a health plan, terminating participation in a health plan, healthcare payment and remittance advice, health plan premium payments, first report of injury, health claim status, and referral certification and authorization.

Preauthorization

A preauthorization should supply and organize the information regarding a procedure's insurance coverage. Determining in advance the benefits and allowables provides you with reimbursement figures in advance. Under most circumstances you'll be able to discuss the deductible, copayment, and balance over and above the allowable with the patient prior to providing costly surgical services. Asking a few pointed questions of the patient and insurer will provide you with additional information regarding allowables, for example:

- How much is the deductible and has it been met for the current year?
- What are the allowables for the quoted procedures?
- What percentage of the allowables will be paid?

Be prepared to answer questions regarding any proposed procedures and the diagnosis for each. In other words, have your CPT and ICD-9-CM codes ready.

When an insurer won't give you exact information, involve your patient. Most patients don't like surprises in the form of a large unpaid balance after the insurance company has determined its benefits.

Submitting your claim is the next (though not final) step toward receiving payment. Verify the insurance company's name and address before mailing the claim and you may save the time and aggravation of having it returned.

PLEASE DO NOT STAPLE IN THIS AREA

BAR CODE AREA

(APPROVED OMB-0938-0008)

HEALTH INSURANCE CLAIM FORM

PICA

PICA

Carrier

1. MEDICARE (Medicare No.) MEDICAID (Medicaid No.) CHAMPUS (Sponser's SSN) CHAMPVA (VA File No.) GROUP HEALTH PLAN (SSN or ID) FECA BLK LUNG (SSN) OTHER (ID)

1a. INSURED'S I.D. NUMBER (FOR PROGRAM IN ITEM 1)

2. PATIENT'S NAME (Last Name , First Name, Middle Initial)

3. PATIENT'S BIRTH DATE MM DD YY SEX M F

4. INSURED'S NAME (Last Name, First Name, Middle Initial)

5. PATIENT'S ADDRESS (No., Street)

6. PATIENT RELATIONSHIP TO INSURED Self Spouse Child Other

7. INSURED'S ADDRESS (No. Street)

CITY STATE

8. PATIENT STATUS Single Married Other Employed Full-time Student Part-time Student

CITY STATE

ZIP CODE TELEPHONE (Include Area Code) ( )

ZIP CODE TELEPHONE (Include Area Code) ( )

9. OTHER INSURED'S NAME (Last Name, First Name, Middle Intial)

10. IS PATIENT'S CONDITION RELATED TO:

11. INSURED'S POLICY, GROUP OR FECA NUMBER

a. OTHER INSURED'S POLICY OR GROUP NUMBER

a. EMPLOYMENT? (CURRENT OR PREVIOUS) YES NO

a. INSURED'S DATE OF BIRTH MM DD YY SEX M F

b. OTHER INSURED'S DATE OF BIRTH MM DD YY SEX M F

b. AUTO ACCIDENT? PLACE (State) YES NO

b. EMPLOYER'S NAME OR SCHOOL NAME

c. EMPLOYER'S NAME OR SCHOOL NAME

c. OTHER ACCIDENT? YES NO

c. INSURANCE PLAN NAME OR PROGRAM NAME

d. INSURANCE PLAN NAME OR PROGRAM NAME

10d. RESERVED FOR LOCAL USE

d. IS THERE ANOTHER HEALTH BENEFIT PLAN? YES NO If yes, return to and complete item 9 a-d

READ BACK OF FORM BEFORE COMPLETING & SIGNING THIS FORM

12. PATIENT'S OR AUTHORIZED PERSON'S SIGNATURE I authorize the release of any medical information necessary to process this claim. I also request payment of government benefits either to myself or to the party who accepts assignment below.

SIGNED ____ DATE ____

13. INSURED'S OR AUTHORIZED PERSON'S SIGNATURE I authorize payment of medical benefits to undersigned physician or supplier for services described below.

SIGNED ____

Patient and Insured Information

14. DATE OF CURRENT MM DD YY ILLNESS (First symptom) OR INJURY (Accident) OR PREGNANCY (LMP)

15. IF PATIENT HAS HAD SAME OR SIMILAR ILLNESS GIVE FIRST DATE MM DD YY

16. DATES PATIENT UNABLE TO WORK IN CURRENT OCCUPATION FROM MM DD YY TO MM DD YY

17. NAME OF REFERRING PHYSICIAN OR OTHER SOURCE

17a. I.D. NUMBER OF REFERRING PHYSICIAN

18. HOSPITALIZATION DATES RELATED TO CURRENT SERVICES FROM MM DD YY TO MM DD YY

19. RESERVED FOR LOCAL USE

20. OUTSIDE LAB ? YES NO $ CHARGES

21. DIAGNOSIS OR NATURE OF ILLNESS OR INJURY (RELATE ITEMS 1, 2, 3 OR 4 TO ITEM 24E BY LINE)

1 ___ . ___ 3 ___ . ___

2 ___ . ___ 4 ___ . ___

22. MEDICAID RESUBMISSION CODE ORIGINAL REF. NO.

23. PRIOR AUTHORIZATION NUMBER

24. A DATE(S) OF SERVICE From MM DD YY To MM DD YY	B Place of Service	C Type of Service	D PROCEDURES, SERVICES, OR SUPPLIES (Explain Unusual Circumstances) CPT/HCPCS MODIFIER	E DIAGNOSIS CODE	F $ CHARGES	G DAYS OR UNITS	H EPSDT Family Planning	I	J	K RESERVED FOR LOCAL USE

25. FEDERAL TAX I.D. NUMBER SSN EIN

26. PATIENT'S ACCOUNT NO.

27. ACCEPT ASSIGNMENT? (For govt. claims, see back) YES NO

28. TOTAL CHARGE $

29. AMOUNT PAID $

30. BALANCE DUE $

31. SIGNATURE OF PHYSICIAN OR SUPPLIER INCLUDING DEGREES OR CREDENTIALS (I certify that the statements on the reverse apply to this bill and are made a part thereof.)

SIGNED ____ DATE ____

32. NAME AND ADDRESS OF FACILITY WHERE SERVICES RENDERED (If other than home or office)

33. PHYSICIAN'S, SUPPLIER'S BILLING NAME, ADDRESS, ZIP CODE & PHONE #

PIN # GRP#

Physician or Supplier Information

Approved by AMA Council on Medical Services

Please Print or Type

FORM HCFA - 1500 (12-90) FORM OWCP-1500 FORM RRB-1500

3 Monitoring Claims

A Day in the Life of a Claim

Once a claim has been received by the payer, the process of adjudication follows a well-established path. Hopefully, the claim will proceed unimpeded toward reimbursement, but along the way the claim may be stopped and returned to your office for lack of information. Let's look at this adjudication process so you know what to expect and how to speed up your payment.

The Claim Arrives

Upon receipt, each claim is dated and possibly microfilmed or photocopied. If the payer uses an optical recognition scanner (OCR), any attachments such as operative reports, cover letters, pathology reports, etc., are separated from the claim. Save a few headaches by stamping your practice name, provider number, address, and phone number on all forms and attachments. This helps the payer avoid losing the documentation necessary to pay the claim.

The Claims Adjudicator

The data are entered into the payer's computer system, and if the claim is "clean" (no problems) it's paid. But first, claims must pass through a series of edits to verify the patient's coverage and eligibility as well as check for medical necessity and noncovered services. If the claim requires additional information, also known as development, the insurer contacts either you or your patient. Let your patients know you're available to help them with questions. This contact for development is usually by mail, but it can also be by phone. Many problem claims are denied immediately or placed at the bottom of the pile due to lack of information. The best way to receive prompt and correct payment is to submit a clean claim. This is definitely a case where time well spent is money earned.

Occasionally, your office will submit a claim that contains all pertinent information needed for payment but requires examination by the payer's medical review department. This will delay your payment. However, if your office has a program for monitoring claims, you'll not only be watching your claims for timely payment, you'll also know where your claim is in the processing system when payment is delayed. Carefully tracking the progress of your claims will alert you to those unpaid claims which have been "lost" and need to be resubmitted.

Why Monitor?

Monitoring insurance submissions can significantly improve an office's cash and profit position because, as you track specific claims, you assure timely and appropriate payment. Leaving your claims to chance can cause problems that can easily be solved if brought to the processor's attention at first submission. Since some insurance companies have been found to commit errors on as many as 25 percent of all claims, monitoring should be an ongoing process. The payer may have neither the information nor the incentive to catch mistakes made in payment. When an incorrect payment is received by the patient, who is generally uninformed about insurance billing, errors again go unnoticed. An alert insurance clerk carefully monitoring reimbursement is the best safeguard against insurance company errors.

Once you've sent a claim, either on paper or electronically, you need a mechanism for following it through to reimbursement. Commonly, this takes four to six weeks, but it may vary geographically or by payer. If your office uses computers, the software package should include a reporting system for tracking claims. You need to define "prompt payment" for the computer system. In other words, you have to tell the computer what you feel is a reasonable time delay before the computer alerts you that no payment has been received. Optimally, your computerized system allows you to set this parameter for individual payers.

One downfall of most computer systems is found in payment posting. Do you relate portions of a payment to each individual service or to the original service date? The former is generally referred to as "open item billing" and is considered a more accurate tracking method. Unfortunately, many offices don't use this capability, ultimately reducing the accuracy of claims tracking. If you lack the ability to track your claims via the computer, you will want to use a manual tracking system.

Tracking Systems

The Suspension File System

For non-automated offices filing paper claims, it's wise to create a suspension file. Simply set up a series of files for a month at a time. Usually it's better not to mix claims that are current (under 30 days) with claims over 30 days. Depending on your practice, you may find it necessary to have a current file, a 30 day file, and a 60+ day file.

A practical method for creating your suspension file is to use three separate hanging files, each with four separate folders marked Week 1, Week 2, etc.—one folder for each week of the month. Mark the hanging files Month 1, Month 2, and Month 3. Place the current month's claims in the hanging file marked Month 1. Place the claims over one month old in the file for Month 2 and claims 60+ days old in Month 3. As each week goes by, roll the outstanding claims to the next file. Keep the claims in each file in alphabetic order to eliminate the time and energy spent looking for them when the payment is received.

Claims review should be given a high priority and a regularly scheduled part of your work week. Insurance claims that are current, or have been filed in the current month, generally require no additional work until the EOB and payment is received. Claims over 30 days old should be reviewed for possible inquiries to the payer.

Make it a rule in your office that most inquiries are written. Notably, this rule applies to Medicare and Medicaid carriers, many of whom require their own forms. Some inquiries are most efficiently made by phone. For example, if a claim has been denied for a simple reason, without notification, a quick phone call is time well spent. If resubmission is the solution, always attach a note with the date, contact person's name, and a description of the conversation. This provides you with the documentation needed if you have to repeat this process.

Your office computer software program may provide you with a comment field or area for "collection" notes. If you don't have this luxury, keep hard copy files of your claims inquiries.

The Log System

An alternative to the suspension file is to record your claims information on a log sheet (see figure 2-1). When a claim is submitted, record the filing date, patient's name and chart number, account number, name and address of the payer, and the amount billed. The claim itself can be filed temporarily in either the patient's chart or an unpaid insurance file.

After all of the day's or week's claims have been recorded, leave a blank space to tag the claims submitted during that time frame. You may want to highlight those dates in a specific color for review in about three to four weeks.

As payments come in, pull the original claim form and compare it to the EOB. Record the amount paid along with any difference on your log sheet. Any notations such as "claim sent to review" or "claim denied for additional information" should be recorded in the status column.

Understanding Explanation Of Benefits (EOB)

The EOB is the key to knowing what you were paid and why, but understanding what this document really means is sometimes not as easy as it sounds. EOBs have their own language: "applied to deductible," "above usual and customary," "patient co-pay," "allowable," and so on. Often hidden in this language is the explanation of what the patient is responsible for paying. Too many offices write off thousands of dollars of earned income each year because the EOBs are misunderstood or not carefully read.

Each EOB has its own format. Some are very confusing and may even lead the patient to believe he or she is not responsible for a balance. Knowing how to read EOBs can help you collect full reimbursement, including any balance owed by the patient.

It's frustrating, but payers sometimes change your CPT codes and pay you based on a CPT code different from the one you submitted. Watch these changes carefully, as many payment mistakes occur from simple data entry errors by the insurer. Read and learn from your EOBs; you may be the one making a common coding error that could be easily corrected.

A wise tactic is to "volunteer" to review the EOBs sent to your patients. Your help accomplishes two things: Assures that your office receives the payment, and you show your patients that you take an interest in their financial well-being.

Monitoring EOBs and comparing payments allow you to track your claims and tells you which claims have been sent for medical review. There's also the benefit of understanding why insurance companies pay the way they do.

Medicare Summary Notice

The Explanation of Medicare Benefits (EOMB) shares the same problem as the EOB: they are both confusing to the provider and the beneficiary. To resolve the problem, at least for Medicare beneficiaries, HCFA has developed the Medicare Summary Notice (MSN). The MSN lists all claims filed during each month for each beneficiary. One type covers inpatient and outpatient facility services, another type includes all Part B physician and other services, and a third type covers durable medical equipment (DME). Each periodically carries messages pertinent to the beneficiary, such as the hotline for reporting fraud and abuse.

The MSN will replace the Part A Medicare Benefits Notice, the Explanation of Your Medicare Part B Benefits (EOMB) forms that are sent out individually for every claim filed by every single Part B provider who filed a claim, and benefit denial letters (HCFA 1954, Benefit Denial Letter sent for partially denied claims, and HCFA 1955 sent for totally denied claims). The new notices are being phased in over the next several years, though some Medicare contractors are already sending them to beneficiaries.

For more information regarding the Medicare Summary Notice, contact Michelle Sanders at (410) 786-0808 or Michelle Hochberg at (410) 786-6955.

INSURANCE CLAIM REGISTER							
Filing Date	Chart Number	Patient's Name	Name & Address Where Claim Submitted	Amount Billed	Amount Paid	Difference	Status or Comment
7/30/99	1221	Matthew Kramer	First Insurance 1st Avenue, Newark, NJ 12345	$525.00			9/26 busy 9/27 busy 9/28 " "
8/30/99	1032	Mark Lane	Fine Insurance 2nd Avenue New Haven, CT 12346	$50.00	$40.00	$10.00	Pd. at 80% Pt. owes balance
8/30/99	1350	Luke Myers	Better Insurance 3rd Avenue New York City, NY 02111	$1,200.00	$700.00	$500.00	Requested review 9/23
8/30/99	1118	John Jacobs	Gold Insurance 4th Avenue Newton, WI 12456	$50.00			9/23 claim being processed today
8/30/99	1179	Mary Byer	Transaccident Insurance 5th Avenue New Hill, NC 24567	$50.00			9/23 no record of claim-resubmit
8/30/99	1098	Christi Wilson	County Farm Insurance 6th Avenue New Era, IA 45678	$125.00	$50.00	$75.00	$75.00 deductible; bill patient
8/30/99	1352	Rose Larsen	Last Insurance 7th Avenue New Hope, MS 56789	$1,500.00	0		Sent to medical review 9/10/99

Figure 2-1

Common Payment Errors

There will be times when your diligent monitoring shows claim problems that are difficult to resolve. The following chart may help you determine what caused an incorrect payment.

Result	Why?
✓ *A service is reduced.*	✓ *The adjudicator may have downcoded the claim for lack of documentation.*
✓ *Reimbursement is made at a much reduced rate.*	✓ *Possibly a data entry error. Compare the CPT code submitted to the code paid.*
✓ *Low or no reimbursement.*	✓ *Precertification was not completed.*
✓ *Low or no reimbursement.*	✓ *Insufficient documentation to establish medical necessity.*
✓ *Multiple units are paid as one unit.*	✓ *The insurer "missed" your number in the units column.*
✓ *The reimbursement for a procedure or service suddenly drops.*	✓ *This could mean a recalculation of allowables or an error. Phone the payor.*
✓ *Payment is not received.*	✓ *Claim is lost or "caught in the system." Begin your inquiry.*
✓ *Multiple procedures were not paid.*	✓ *The insurance company either ignored the additional procedures or lumped them in with the primary procedure.*

Gathering Information

Most physicians' offices have contractual arrangements with government or private third-party payers. Many of these payers provide your office with a "fee schedule" or other type of payment information. In the past, Medicare provided prevailing data for your locality and specialty, but current Medicare payment is based on the Medicare Fee Schedule, also known as Resource Based Relative Value Scale or RBRVS.

Another good source of information is available in those states that have developed a Relative Value Study (RVS) for their state workers compensation payers. These states usually pay at a set rate based on the relative value of a procedure multiplied by a dollar conversion factor.

As a rule, commercial insurers don't readily provide fee information, but it can be obtained. When a payment is received, record the amount in a payment log, such as shown in figure 2-2 (fees are for illustration purposes only). For frequently billed payers, devote a column to each payer. List all procedures performed and be conscientious in keeping this information up-to-date. This helps you develop a UCR (usual, customary, and reasonable) reimbursement amount by payer for each procedure and service performed by your practice.

Information from a variety of sources helps you develop a fee schedule that is "in-step" with accepted relative values. It also helps you identify reimbursement errors. If you know your fee for a service is fair, low reimbursement indicates an error may have occurred in processing the claim.

When it's apparent an error has been made, don't hesitate to challenge the payment. Medicare and private payers will correct proven mistakes, when brought to their attention. Errors such as billing the wrong procedure code, omitting a procedure code usually billed with that service, or omitting a standard supply are acceptable reasons for resubmission. Payers usually require this resubmission in a timely manner.

Payment Rationales

Contrary to popular belief, most payers do follow logical mechanisms for reimbursing claims. Many insurers base payments on UCR amounts adjusted for specific geographic areas. Payers acquire this information from several sources, then adjust it to fit their needs in written policies. This UCR information is gathered within specific geographic boundaries though is not broken down by specialty. Other payers gather their own data for the regions they service and base their payment on a percentage of the UCR charge they've established for your area.

Workers compensation payers often use a straightforward relative value study chosen by that state. Payments are determined by multiplying a conversion factor, usually established by the state's industrial commission, against the relative value for the service.

HMO and PPO fee schedules are usually developed internally by each organization and are often published on request for their participants. These fee schedules are generally updated on a yearly basis.

Downcoding

Downcoding or recoding by an insurance company is another possible cause of reduced payments. When claims are submitted with deleted or nonexistent CPT codes, the payer may assign one. Obviously, you may not like the choice. Similar problems occur when an insurer's payment system is based on CPT codes and you submit an RVS code that does not directly translate to CPT. These claims are reviewed by a claims adjustor who assigns a valid CPT code. The opposite may occur in billing workers compensation. Many workers compensation payers are RVS-based, and if your CPT code doesn't match the RVS code, your code will be reassigned. Knowing which coding systems your payers use helps you avoid these problems.

Inquiries, Reviews, and Appeals

Inquiries, reviews, and appeals are the final essential component to monitoring your payments whether you choose the suspension file or log system, or create your own method of tracking claims.

When your claims and EOB monitoring turns up an error (yours or the payer's), correct the claim and resubmit it for appropriate reimbursement. If this doesn't solve the problem, immediately appeal.

Claims Correction

When a claims error is discovered that could result, or already has resulted, in inaccurate reimbursement, send a corrected claim. Clearly mark this claim as a "CORRECTED BILLING—NOT A DUPLICATE CLAIM." Include a note describing the error, plus any additional documentation necessary to support your position. Don't be tempted to keep overpayments; bring it to the attention of the insurance company with a refund. Medicare does not look favorably on practices holding claim overpayments and will prosecute.

Appealing Incorrect Payments

Before appealing a claim, whether with Medicare or a private insurer, notify the insurer in writing that an error has occurred. Many payers have a set time allowance for claims appeals and often print it on their EOBs. Don't let appeals slide. Actively monitor your claims and stay current with any appeals in progress.

One of the basic rules for appealing a claim is to always include a copy of the original claim, EOB or EOMB, (or MSN) and any additional documentation necessary to provide evidence for the appeal. Cover letters are also effective for appeals and will "set the stage" with the claims reviewer. If you feel the payer has not responded to your complaint, don't give up — there are alternatives. Contact your state's insurance commissioner and send a clear, well-documented account of your dissatisfaction. Your argument carries greater weight if you have several examples of the problem from the same insurance company.

Appealing a Medicare Claim

Medicare claims appeals have several levels supported by numerous regulations. This complex journey starts when either the physician or beneficiary disagrees with the carrier's determination as explained on the EOMB (or MSN). If the claim was assigned, only the physician can initiate the review. If the claim was unassigned, the beneficiary usually initiates the review or can stipulate in writing that the physician is authorized to act on his or her behalf.

The review request must come within six months of the date the original determination was made. The request needs to be submitted in writing or on the HCFA-1964 Request for Review form. Forward the request to your carrier, prominently marked as a "review" to avoid denial as a duplicate claim. As with any review, always include a copy of the claim, the EOMB (or MSN), and any information that will make the review determination possible, i.e., a statement that the low payment was due to a clerical error, or documentation to support payment at the appropriate level (chart notes, operative report, hospital records, etc.).

Insurance Payment Log

CPT Code	Payment	Payment	Payment	Payment	Payment
47600	$1,832	$1,600			
	$1,950				
	$1,250				
	$2,150				
47605	$2,000	$1,900			
	$2,460	$2,158			
	$2,833				
	$2,112				
47610	$2,150	$2,066			
	$2,380				
	$2,740				
	$2,950				

Figure 2-2

Fair Hearing
If you've gone through the basic review steps and still disagree with the payer's determination, you may want to request a Fair Hearing with a HCFA-1965 form. To qualify, the amount in question must be at least $100. However, Medicare will allow you to batch claims with the same problem and procedure to equal the required $100 base. You must request the hearing within six months of the date the informal review decision was made. Make your request in writing and send it to your Medicare hearing officer or coordinator. Your request for a Fair Hearing will be pursued in one of three ways:

Hearing on Record
In a hearing on record, a hearing officer investigates all aspects of the claim. The physician does not testify unless oral testimony is deemed necessary. A hearing on record is often the most productive Fair Hearing procedure. The physician is advised of the officer's decision and a copy of the decision is forwarded to the local Medicare carrier for appropriate action.

Telephone Hearing
In a telephone hearing the physician presents the case by phone to a hearing office. Prior to the scheduled hearing, the physician is provided with information in the hearing officer's file. A careful study of this information may help avoid surprises. The physician is advised of the decision and a copy is forwarded to the Medicare carrier for action.

Personal Hearing
When the physician wants an in-person hearing the Medicare hearing officer may agree to schedule a meeting to discuss the case. Complete and well-organized records help present the best case possible.

Administrative Law Judge Review
Prior to January 1987, a Fair Hearing was the final appeal effort a physician could make. Legislation enacted through the Omnibus Budget Reconciliation Act (OBRA 87) provided an additional level, the Administrative Law Judge (ALJ). In order to pursue this next level of appeal, the claim must have completed the Fair Hearing process, the dollar amount in question must be at least $500, and the appeal must be requested within 60 days of the Fair Hearing judgment.

The Provider Reimbursement Review Board (PRRB)
The PRRB is an independent panel that offers another avenue for appealing a final determination of a fiscal intermediary of HCFA. A decision by the PRRB may be affirmed, modified, reversed, or vacated and remanded by a HCFA administrator within 60 days of notification of the provider of that decision.

Fostering a Spirit of Cooperation
Whether the appeal is to a government carrier or commercial payer, you're bound to be frustrated by the whole affair. However, be cooperative; combative behavior toward a claims reviewer never works in your favor. Concentrate instead on developing a respectful working relationship with one person in each frequently billed insurance company. If you've worked with a particularly good reviewer, send your review requests to that individual's attention. Using the fax numbers found in the *2000 Insurance Directory,* you'll be able to send your request directly to that individual.

Measuring Your Success

One way of viewing the financial health of a practice is with an accounts receivable report. The age (30, 60, 90 days, etc.) of each unpaid balance should be calculated every month. Offices that develop good monitoring systems and collection plans find their outstanding accounts are more current. Receivables can also be influenced by the physician's specialty, type of practice, and participation agreements with insurance companies.

Periodically review your billing, monitoring, and collection policies. Don't hesitate to adjust them if necessary. Set goals for your accounts receivable and track them very carefully. This will help you develop greater efficiency in your claims monitoring habits.

Collecting the remainder (co-insurance, deductible, and unpaid amounts) after the insurer has paid is also important. If you don't already have a good plan for collecting these balances, you should: (1) predetermine insurance coverage while patients are in your office and have them pay the anticipated remainder at the time of the service, and (2) regularly bill and follow up on all unpaid balances.

Summary

- Label all attachments to claims with identifying information.
- Actively monitor claims payments by comparing the EOB to the original claim.
- Gather reimbursement data to help evaluate your fee schedule.
- Resubmit claims if necessary to correct errors.
- Avoid payer downcoding or coding changes by using current CPT and ICD-9 codes.
- Follow the correct steps when appealing claims.
- Frequently evaluate your office's billing and monitoring patterns.

4 The Payers

Today's health insurance industry is comprised of many companies each with its own policies, rules, and regulations. The benefits available to groups or individuals vary and the definitions for medical exclusions and pre-existing conditions are almost certain to differ among comparable policies. This variability makes it difficult for a billing staff to predict an insurance company's response to a particular claim submission.

There are ways around the problem. First, get as much information as possible. The policyholder may be the best place to start. The policyholder should be aware of how his or her insurance plan works. But you might have to prod his or her memory with the following questions:

- Are you aware of any exclusions?
- Is there an annual or lifetime maximum allowed under your policy?
- Is there a waiting period for the policy to take effect?
- Are there any coverage limitations based on a specific illness, such as mental disorders?

These variables and a policy's deductible and copayment create an endless number of problems in preparing a claim.

Patients with dual coverage (more than one policy) present a special billing challenge. Generally, the primary payer will pay the full benefit (allowable less copayments and deductible) on an individual's plan. The secondary payer and payers providing supplemental coverage will pay an additional amount up to the allowable or contracted rate or the difference between the actual (billed) charge and the amount paid by the primary payer. The total of the combined payments from the primary and secondary payers should not exceed the total billed charges. When an overpayment occurs, contact the payers.

When setting standards for dealing with payers, a rule of thumb is to contact them directly for certain basic facts regarding claims submission. Record the information on 3x5 cards indexed alphabetically for quick reference (see Figure 3-1). Try to get the answers from a supervisor or provider relations person to help ensure accuracy of the claim processing information.

Company name________________ Date________________
Contestable (Pre-existing) period________________
Coverage limitations________________
Exclusions ________________
Precertification requirements ________________
RVS or CPT codes________________ Form required ________________
HCPCS ________________
How to appeal________________

Figure 3-1

Payer Comparisons

The following sections discuss the common ground between Blue Cross/Blue Shield and the government payers. Compare this with the information on the bulletins you receive from your local carriers. There may be some variations specific to your state.

Blue Cross/Blue Shield Plans

Blue Cross is a nonprofit health organization providing hospital benefits. In most states, this plan has merged with its counterpart, Blue Shield, which offers physician services benefits to provide total healthcare coverage for its subscribers. Although all of the plans in the United States, Canada, and Puerto Rico are separate entities, they are coordinated through the national Blue Cross and Blue Shield Plan Association headquartered in Chicago.

Like Medicare, Blue Cross and Blue Shield plans have provider I.D. numbers and participating and nonparticipating provider arrangements. Most plans pay participating providers directly, and the providers agree not to bill the patient for the difference between the allowable and the fee.

Blue Cross and Blue Shield payments are subject to deductibles and copayments which vary according to the patient's plan. A tip: Your office should request a recent provider manual for your state's Blue Cross and Blue Shield plans. It is a good idea to obtain a current provider manual from all participating major health plans. This will be valuable to understanding how and why you are paid.

Healthcare Service Plans (HSPs)
Healthcare service plans, typically operated by Blue Cross and Blue Shield Plans throughout the country, have provided healthcare coverage for many years. Although initially they acted like indemnity carriers, merely paying claims, many HSPs began to develop managed care products to compete with companies offering HMO, PPO, and EPO products. The products were not necessarily offered through the same organizations which operate the healthcare service plans.

CHAMPUS
The Civilian Health and Medical Program for the Uniformed Services (CHAMPUS) provides health insurance benefits to military personnel (active and retired) and their dependents. CHAMPUS patients can seek medical care from nonmilitary providers, but it's advisable to check with the carrier for eligibility and coverage of the proposed treatment.

Unfortunately, some CHAMPUS carriers require providers to bill services on a special CHAMPUS claim form rather than the HCFA-1500. Check with your patient and ask for the correct form.

Health Maintenance Organizations (HMOs)
HMOs are the most common form of managed care. Generally, they incorporate all of the techniques listed above in varying degrees to manage care. HMOs must follow the requirements of P.L. 1301 of the Publich Health Service Act and 42 CFR 417.100–417.109.

Staff model plans, also called group models, are HMOs that own the facilities and employ personnel to provide care to their enrollees.

Capitation
By the year 2000, it is estimated that one of two individuals will be covered by managed care organizations operating under capitated contracts. The *2000 Insurance Directory* provides a summary of capitation, and terms related to the capitated contract.

Capitation places a cap on the number of dollars spent on health care. Capitation contracts emphasize high volume practices and/or primary care, and generally where one provider is the gatekeeper for the patient's overall management. Payment is based on certain amount of dollars per member, and the amount does not vary according to the actual number of patients in the member population seen by the provider. Subsequently, health care in a capitated system depends on shared risk, or the ability to successfully manage a practice or a specialty clinic according to fees paid on a "per capita" basis. This varies significantly from fee-for-service (FFS) health plans. Under capitation, incentive depends upon providing quality care in the most appropriate and lowest cost setting, whereas incentives in a FFS depend on volume and number of procedures actually performed. Terms important to capitation contracts include the following:

- Risk Pool — a portion of the capitated payment set aside to cover certain expenses, such as a portion a primary physician may set aside to pay for laboratory diagnostic services.
- Stop-Loss Provision — a member's age, sex, co-payment, use patterns, and the scope of services covered by the plan are factors influencing the dollar amount in a capitated contract. The provider's financial risk increases with the number of services offered in the contract since reimbursement is set in advance and does not vary despite the intensity of services provided. The "stop-loss" provision of a capitated contract pays for the patient whose needs exceed the capitated rate.
- Withholds — the portion of the capitation rate that a health plan retains and repays to the physician if the health plan does not exceed its budget. Under this arrangement, the financial risk becomes a shared responsibility between the health plan and provider.

Point-of-Service Plan (POS)
A point-of-service health plan allows the covered person to choose to receive a service from participating or a non-participating provider, with different benefit levels associated with the use of participating providers. If a POS is purchased, a non-participating provider may cost the subscriber the deductibles and 30 percent of the remaining costs up to a set limit. When the costs exceed the limit, the HMO assumes the remaining expenses.

Point-of-service can be provided in several ways (and in various combinations):

- An HMO may allow members to obtain limited services from non-participating providers.
- An HMO may provide non-participating benefits through a supplemental major medical policy.
- A PPO may be used to provide both participating and non-participating levels of coverage and access.

Facts About Managed Care Organizations

- Who owns the managed care organization?
- Who is already participating with the plan?
- Are there restrictions regarding ancillary services?
- Are covered services, noncovered services, prior approvals, and medical necessity clearly defined?
- How are appeals and denials handled?
- What is the payment process?
- Is there an amount withheld from provider payments?
- How many "covered lives" are there?

Independent Practice Association (IPA)
An Independent Practice Association (IPA) consists of physicians who have not combined their assets and liabilities and are not practicing in a truly integrated

fashion. They maintain their separate practices and participate in the IPA as a means to contract with HMOs or other health plans. Providers may also see patients who are not enrolled in HMO plans. Where IPAs primarily contract with the HMO to provide services to the HMO's members, the HMO model typically is called the IPA model HMO.

IPAs are developed in two ways. Providers may market themselves as an IPA group and perform their own administrative functions, or payers may develop an IPA from a panel of contracted providers. Whether developed by the providers or a payer, provider members of the IPA should appoint a committee to meet with payer representatives to negotiate contracts, review financial performance of the plan, and settle payer-provider or provider-enrollee disputes. In addition, the committee should be responsible for sanctioning IPA providers, and adding/deleting providers from the panel.

Preferred Provider Organizations (PPOs)
A Preferred Provider Organization (PPO) typically contracts on behalf of employer groups or other plans with hospital and physician providers at reduced rates. The hospitals and physicians participating in the preferred provider network generally are called either preferred or participating providers. Usually, there is an incentive to the patient to use a preferred provider. A patient who visits a physician who is not a preferred provider likely will have to pay a higher copayment or deductible. Providers offer discounts to PPOs in anticipation of achieving additional patient volumes, or to minimize the chances that their patient volume will go to another provider.

Exclusive Provider Organizations (EPOs)
An Exclusive Provider Oganization (EPO) is a variation of a PPO. EPOs contract with providers on a discounted basis, but enrollees must receive care within the network. EPOs, like PPOs, provide no penalties to providers if the patient opts to obtain care outside the network. Instead, the enrollee assumes responsibility for out-of-network costs.

Third-Party Administrators (TPAs) and Administrative Services Organizations (ASOs)
TPAs and ASOs are neither health plans nor insurers, but organizations that provide claims-paying functions for the clients which they service. Many self-insured groups, such as employers and union trusts use Third-Party Administrators (TPAs) or Administrative Services Organizations (ASOs) to manage and pay their claims. In lieu of paying premiums to health insurers who would charge group premiums, these self-insured groups assume the risk of the provision of such services on their own, usually with some stop loss insurance. The self-insured group may contract directly with providers, and it may use the services of a PPO. Although historically such TPAs and ASOs merely paid claims, their functions have expanded. Many have some function in the management of care. In addition, many self-insured groups were pioneers in PPO development, and thus a TPA or ASO may be paying claims based on discounted rates negotiated by a PPO on behalf of a self-insured group.

Single or Specialty Service Plans
There also are single or specialty service plans, such as health plans which provide services only in the mental health area, or vision and dental plans. Plans for mental health were developed to slow the rising costs of care. Employer groups can contract with these specialty health plans for services which focus on mental health. Vision and dental plans often have been add-on or supplemental coverage to health plans. They vary greatly in the benefits services that they offer, and represent another example of single specialty service plans.

Medicaid
The Medicaid program is jointly administered by the federal and state governments and may have a different name in your state, such as Welfare, Title XIX, or Medi-Cal. Medicaid payers do have some common characteristics: they're all subject to the same federal guidelines; they have unique, individual guidelines for claims submission; and each publishes a handbook that outlines and updates the Medicaid rules for that state.

The program issues each recipient an eligibility card that indicates coverage dates. Examine this card carefully to confirm coverage on the date of service. Coverage can change monthly so verify coverage frequently. This card also contains the I.D. number, which must be included on your claim. A photocopy of the Medicaid card should be placed in the patient's file.

Medicaid, Blue Cross/Blue Shield, and Medicare assign each physician and supplier a local provider number that must be printed in the appropriate box on the claim form. An obvious difficulty arises when a physician provides care to a patient residing in a different state. When this happens, make it a priority to apply immediately for a provider number in that state before submitting the claim. If your office is in a border town or close to a state line, apply for a provider number in both states.

Medicare
The Medicare program, created in 1966, was originally intended to provide health insurance benefits (both hospital and nonhospital) to people over age 65. The program was expanded in July 1973 to include persons of any age who are entitled to monthly disability benefits for 24 consecutive months under Social Security or the Railroad Retirement program. Additionally, end-stage renal disease (ESRD) patients requiring hemodialysis or kidney transplant are eligible. HCFA was established in 1977 to administer this growing program and is headquartered in Baltimore with 10 regional offices.

As with Medicaid, each Medicare patient is issued an identification card listing a Medicare number and letter combination. The letter suffix identifies the patient's status, e.g., A (wage earner), B (wife of wage earner), D (widow). A complete listing is available from your local Social Security office.

The Medicare program is divided into two components, somewhat like Blue Cross/Blue Shield. Part A covers hospital facility services (operating suites, hospital rooms, and supplies) skilled nursing facilites, home health services and hospice care. Part B covers medical or nonhospital services such as office visits, outpatient surgery and supplies, etc. Part B is voluntary, with premiums deducted from the beneficiary's social security check, allowing the beneficiary to refuse this portion of the Medicare program and maintain only Part A coverage.

Both Part A and Part B have deductibles, but they're handled in different ways. Part A's deductible is based on benefit periods and may have to be satisfied for each hospitalization. The deductible for Part B is met yearly and renews each January 1st. Under most circumstances, Medicare benefits are paid at 80 percent of the allowable, and the patient is responsible for the remaining 20 percent if the claim is assigned. When a claim is unassigned, the patient is responsible for the entire amount remaining after Medicare makes its payment. Remember, participating physicians can only submit assigned claims and always check "yes" in Box 27 on the HCFA-1500 form.

When a claim is unassigned, the beneficiary is responsible for the entire amount in excess of Medicare's payment, though there are limits that physicians and suppliers can charge "in excess" of Medicare. When assignment is accepted the supplier or physician cannot seek additional payment — beyond the Medicare reimbursement — from the beneficiary or co-insurer.

Medicare HMOs

Medicare risk plans are relatively new Medicare benefit plans introduced in recent years in an effort to control Medicare costs. Managed care organizations must apply with HCFA for approval to offer this type of plan to Medicare beneficiaries. Once approved, the managed care organization receives a monthly premium payment based on the Adjusted Average Per Capita Cost (AAPCC) from HCFA for each beneficiary enrolled under the Medicare risk plan. In return for these monthly premiums, the managed care organization assumes full financial responsibility for all covered services. All services normally covered by Medicare are included in the benefit plan, but the managed care organization has the option of enhancing these benefits to include items such as pharmacy and vision coverage. Generally, the managed care organization provides both basic Medicare coverage (80 percent of allowed charges) and supplemental coverage. When filing claims on Medicare beneficiaries enrolled in Medicare risk plans, the claim should be sent directly to the managed care organization. The managed care organization then adjudicates the claim at 100 percent of allowed charges, based on contract rates, thereby eliminating a step in the Medicare claims adjudication process. The allowed charges may be different rates negotiated with physicians and other providers specifically for Medicare HMO beneficiaries. Because the managed care organization has assumed full financial risk for all care provided to Medicare risk beneficiaries, the MCO strictly monitors all care provided. Therefore, it is crucial to follow all prior approval requirements mandated by the managed care organization to assure that claims will be paid.

Medicare+Choice Program

The Medicare+Choice or Part C of the Medicare program modifies the method the federal government uses to establish capitation rates for Medicare beneficiaries enrolled in managed care plans. Under this program, eligible individuals may elect to receive Medicare benefits through enrollment in one of many private health plans choices beyond the original Medicare programs or plans not available through MCOs. Among these alternatives are M+C coordinated care plans (including plans offered by HMOs, PPOs, and PSOs); Medical Saving Account (MSA) plans, which combine a high deductible M+C health insurance plan and a contribution to an M+C MSA, and M+C private fee-for-service plans. HCFA has allowed other arrangements, such as social health maintenance organizations (SHMOs) and the Program of All-inclusive Care for the Elderly (PACE), which cover acute and long-term care services and are jointly financed with Medicaid.

Following are five points to remember when choosing Medicare+Choice or Part C plans:

1. A health plan's Medicare revenue is based on the highest of three capitation rates rather than the single rate computed under the old method.
2. Medicare payments for medical education costs are increasingly no longer included in the capitation rates.
3. The annual update to Medicare capitation rates is no longer solely dependent on Medicare spending for fee-for-service beneficiaries.
4. States are now permitted to reconfigure their Medicare payment areas into geographic areas larger than the traditional counties.
5. Health status is to be added to the demographic factors used to risk adjust the capitation rates by January 1, 2000.

Indemnity Plans

Although many indemnity plans continue to exist, they are not viewed as managed care organizations. Usually, the indemnity carrier will pay the provider directly where the patient has assigned his or her benefits to the indemnity carrier. Many of the indemnity carriers have attempted to include PPO like characteristics to reduce their costs.

Physician Hospital Organizations (PHOs)

A Physician Hospital Organization (PHO) is created by a hospital and a physician organization, or physicians and physician groups, to assist in managed care contracting on behalf of the parties. The best PHOs include a physician organization that has its own structure, providing a means for reviewing pertinent issues both internal and external, such as contracts, payer disputes, or physician monitoring.

Management Services Organizations (MSOs)

A Management (or Medical) Services Organization (MSO) provides services to physicians and physician groups. It also may provide services to a hospital or hospitals. A MSO may acquire physicians' tangible assets and certain intangible assets, as with the PHO. A MSO, like a PHO, is generally not a provider or supplier of hospital or medical services for Medicare purposes. Goods and services provided by the MSO should be provided to the physicians and not patients, unless the MSO can practice medicine.

MSOs which are unable to employ physicians contract with them. MSOs might provide office space, equipment, furnishings, management information systems, nonprofessional and certain professional personnel, and services to physicians on a turnkey basis.

MSOs generally are good vehicles for physician recruitment because physicians can contract with the MSO to run their practices. The costs of opening and operating a practice can be offered by the MSO to the physicians on a flat fee, percentage, or hybrid basis.

Workers Compensation

All states require workers compensation benefits to provide medical and disability coverage for employees who are injured, contract an illness or disease, or become disabled as a result of their employment. In most states, employers voluntarily provide these benefits, but the criteria for mandatory coverage varies. Some states require employers to carry workers compensation coverage only if they hire a certain number of people.

The requirements for filing a claim also vary from state to state. In some states the claim is sent directly to a court or the workers compensation office, while others want it sent to the employer or directly to the insurance carrier.

There does seem to be a common denominator for claims payment. The amount paid is based on an allowable for that service, and the physician doesn't bill the patient for an unpaid balance. When your practice accepts a workers compensation case, you've essentially agreed to accept the allowable as payment in full.

Most programs do require an initial accident or medical report, a periodic progress report, and a final report if the patient is temporarily disabled and unable to return to work.

Other Helpful Terms

Adjusted Average Per Capita Cost (AAPCC)

AAPCC is the estimated average cost of Medicare benefits for an individual, based on the following criteria: age, sex, institutional status, Medicaid, disability, and end stage renal failure. HCFA uses AAPCC as a guide to make monthly payments to risk and cost contractors.

Alternative Delivery System (ADS)

This is a phrase indicating any healthcare delivery system other than traditional fee-for-service.

Average Length of Stay (ALOS)

The hospital establishes an average number of days stay for each type of admission. The number is derived from the simple formula: the total number of patient days divided by the total number of admissions for a determined period.

Coordination of Benefits (COB)

COB is a contract that applies when an individual is covered by more than one healthcare plan. This contract requires that the payment of benefits be coordinated by all insurers to eliminate the possibility of duplication and overpayment of benefits.

Consolidated Omnibus Budget Reconciliation Act (COBRA)

COBRA is a federal law that allows and requires past employees to be covered under company health insurance plans for a set premium. This program gives individuals the opportunity to remain insured when their current plan or position has been terminated.

Certificate of Coverage (COC)

The COC describes the benefits included in an individual's health plan. State law requires that all individuals insured under a health plan must receive a COC, as well as any employer offering a healthcare plan.

Duplicate Coverage Inquiry (DCI)

DCIs are requests made to insurance companies or medical providers to determine whether other medical coverage exists under another plan.

Durable Medical Equipment (DME)

DME is any equipment that usually can withstand repeated use, is useable at home, and is not beneficial to a person without an illness or injury. Splinting, orthopedic bracing, and wheelchairs are good examples of DME.

Date of Service (DOS)

This is the date on which a healthcare service was provided to an individual under a particular health plan.

Health Employer Data and Information Set (HEDIS)
HEDIS provides a set of performance measures for employers and other purchasers of health plans to understand and evaluate a health plan's performance.

Health Insurance Purchasing Cooperatives (HIPC)
A HIPC is a pool of purchasers that uses its large numbers of participants as leverage for negotiating with healthcare providers and insurers. Small employers and communities of individuals lacking large numbers of healthcare purchasers pursue HIPCs to minimize costs and increase negotiating power with providers and purchasers.

Independent Medical Evaluation (IME)
IMEs are independent examinations of a patient by an unbiased provider, to resolve a dispute over an illness or injury incurred by the patient.

Length of Stay (LOS)
This is the length of stay or number of days that an individual stays in an inpatient setting.

Ordering Physician
Physician who orders non-physician services for the patient, such as diagnostic laboratory tests, clinical laboratory tests, pharmaceutical services, or durable medical equipment.

Out-of-Area (OOA)
OOA indicates services obtained by a covered individual outside the area where the individual is insured.

Participating Provider (Par)
A hospital, pharmacy, physician, or ancillary services provider who has contracted with a health plan to provide medical services for a determined fee or payment.

Peer Review Organization (PRO)
A PRO is usually instituted by a physician group or insurance company to determine if the services provided are medically necessary, in the proper setting, and following professional norms and standards.

Referring Physician
Physician who requests an item or service for the beneficiary. Payment may be made under the Medicare program.

Usual, Customary, and Reasonable (UCR)
UCR is a term indicating fees charged for medical services that are considered normal, common, and in line with the prevailing fees in the provider's area.

5 Supplemental Insurance

Supplemental Insurance for Medicare

It is common for Medicare patients to buy another insurance policy to pay for expenses not covered by the government's plan. Though a benefit for the patient, supplemental insurance is added paperwork for your practice. Since the September 1, 1990 law requiring physicians to file all primary Medicare claims, many practices have felt the need to analyze their stance on filing supplemental insurance claims.

Your Medicare patients may subscribe to an additional policy with an automatic coordination of benefits. Your only requirement is to list the secondary coverage in the appropriate space on the HCFA-1500 and Medicare does the rest of the work.

Medigap

The term Medigap was coined by Medicare to fit this supplemental coverage concept. As defined by HCFA, Medigap is a health insurance plan or policy purchased by the Medicare beneficiary from a private company, such as the American Association of Retired Persons (AARP). The two exclusions noted in the Omnibus Budget Reconciliation Act of 1987 (OBRA 87) are:

- A policy or plan offered by an employer to current or former employees.
- A policy or plan offered by a labor organization to current or former members.

Only the supplemental insurance coverage that has been privately purchased directly by the beneficiary meets the definition of a Medigap policy. This policy or plan provides reimbursement to the beneficiary for charges such as a deductible, co-insurance, or other benefits Medicare has limited.

To facilitate this process, OBRA created a mechanism to pay participating physicians directly for supplemental benefits. This process allows your Medicare carrier to send an EOMB directly to the Medigap carrier. HCFA requires Medigap carriers to accept the EOMB (or MSN) as a replacement for the HCFA-1500 form, eliminating the need for an additional claim. The Medigap carrier issues the payment for coinsurance, deductible, or other charges directly to participating physicians.

Conveying the Correct Information

When completing the HCFA-1500, provide your Medicare carrier with the appropriate information. Refer to the *2000 Insurance Directory* section describing the HCFA-1500 form for further instructions.

Your local carrier may have special instructions regarding addresses, so watch for this information in carrier newsletters. It's also noted if a patient has more than one Medigap policy. Medicare will send this payment information to only one of the carriers.

For participating physicians, the assignment of benefits on the claim form must authorize the payment to be made directly to your practice. In addition to the Medicare assignment of benefits, you must have a Medigap assignment of benefits.

Medigap carriers may require the assignment of benefits for this supplemental insurance to be carrier specific. You could add a statement to your current Medicare assignment of benefits stating:

> I authorize payment of all medical benefits to apply to all occasions for primary and supplemental (Medigap) coverage to be paid to (physician's name). This assignment will remain in effect until revoked by me in writing.

A photocopy of this assignment is considered as valid as the original.

Once the claim has been processed, Medicare has 30 days to forward the EOMB (or MSN) to the Medigap carrier.

Participating physicians receive notification on the EOMB (or MSN) stating that a copy has been sent to the Medigap carrier. Medicare will not forward an EOMB (or MSN) to a Medigap carrier if the charges are denied as noncovered.

If you don't accept assignment on Medicare claims, either you or your patients need to submit claims directly to the supplemental insurance carrier to receive benefits. To assist your patients, present them with an itemized statement (at the time of service) and instructions, such as the following:

> As of September 1, 1990, Dr.______________is required by law to submit your claim to Medicare. You will still receive the payment from Medicare that is subject to coinsurance and deductible in most cases. An exception to this is laboratory services, which have been billed separately to Medicare. When you receive your explanation of Medicare benefits (EOMB) or Medicare Summary Notice (MSN), attach it to this itemized statement and forward both to your supplemental carrier. If we can assist you in billing your supplemental carrier, please notify our billing and insurance department.

These instructions may be preprinted on a separate sheet or on the back of your itemized statement. Stamp or print the following phrase on your statement: "Medicare has been billed for these charges." This prevents your patient from sending a duplicate bill to Medicare.

Nonparticipating physicians treating Medicare patients who have secondary coverage through Medicaid must accept assignment on these claims. In most states the Medicare carrier automatically transmits the forms to Medicaid for payment.

American Association of Retired Persons (AARP)

The AARP offers supplemental coverage for its members. This coverage may be for both hospital and nonhospital charges. The AARP does not require an insurance form, only a copy of the benefits summary.

The national headquarters for the AARP is in Philadelphia, PA. Inquiries are handled at this single location for claims and the insurance program itself. Send claims to the following address:

AARP Health Insurance Plan
PO Box 13999
Philadelphia, PA 19187-0216
1-800-523-5880

6 Insurance Commissioners

The following is a list of state insurance commissioners. They function as a source of appeal against commercial insurers just as the Medicare appeals process is set up to ensure fair treatment from Medicare payers (see Chapter 2). To appeal to an insurance commissioner, carefully document the problems you are experiencing, particularly repeated problems with an individual payer. Forward this information to the appropriate office as listed on the following pages.

Alabama Insurance Commissioner
Monroe St, Ste 1700
Montgomery, AL 36104
(334) 269-3550
(334) 241-4192 FAX

Alaska Division of Insurance
PO Box 110805
Juneau, AK 99811-0805
(907) 465-2515
(907) 465-3422 FAX

American Samoa
Pago Pago, Am. Samoa 96799
(011-684) 633-4116
(011-684) 633-2269 FAX

Arizona Director of Insurance
2910 N 44th St, Ste 210
Phoenix, AZ 85018-7256
(602) 912-8400
(602) 912-8452 FAX

Arkansas Insurance Commissioner
1200 W 3rd St
Little Rock, AR 72201-1904
(501) 371-2600
(501) 371-2618 FAX

California Insurance Commissioner
300 Capitol Mall, Ste 1500
Sacramento, CA 95814
(916) 492-3500
(916) 445-5280 FAX

Colorado Division of Insurance
1560 Broadway, Ste 850
Denver, CO 80202
(303) 894-7499
(303) 894-7455 FAX

Connecticut Insurance Commissioner
PO Box 816
153 Market St, 11th Fl
Hartford, CT 06142-0816
(860) 297-3800
(860) 566-7410 FAX

Delaware Department of Insurance
PO Box 7007
Rodney Bldg
841 Silver Lake Blvd
Dover, DE 19903-1507
(302) 739-4251
(302) 739-5280 FAX

District of Columbia Superintendent of Insurance
One Judiciary Sq
441 4th St, Ste 870 N
Washington, DC 20001
(202) 727-8000
(202) 727-8055 FAX

Florida Insurance Commissioner
200 E Gaines St
Larsen Bldg
Tallahassee, FL 32399-0300
(904) 922-3100
(904) 488-3334 FAX

Georgia Department of Insurance
Attn: Consumer Services
704 West Tower
Floyd Memorial Bldg
Two Martin Luther King Jr. Drive
Atlanta, GA 30334
(404) 656-2056
(404) 656-4030 FAX

Government of Guam, Department of Revenue & Taxation Commissioner
Bldg 13-1, 2nd Fl
Mariner Ave
Tiyan Barrigada, Guam 96913
(671) 475-1817
(671) 472-2643 FAX

Hawaii Insurance Division
Department of Commerce and Consumer Affairs
250 S King St
Fifth Fl
Honolulu, HI 96813
(808) 586-2790
(808) 586-2806 FAX

Idaho Department of Insurance
700 W State St
Third Fl
Boise, ID 83720-0043
(208) 334-4250
(208) 334-4398 FAX

Illinois Department of Insurance
320 W Washington St
Fourth Fl
Springfield, IL 62767
(217) 785-0116
(217) 524-6500 FAX

Indiana Department of Insurance
311 W Washington St, Ste 300
Indianapolis, IN 46204-2787
(317) 232-2385
(317) 232-5251 FAX

Iowa Division of Insurance
Lucas State Office Bldg
Sixth Fl
Des Moines, IA 50319
(515) 281-5705
(515) 281-3059 FAX

Kansas Department of Insurance
420 S W 9th St
Topeka, KS 66612-1678
(785) 296-7801
(785) 296-2283 FAX

Kentucky Department of Insurance
215 West Main St
PO Box 517
Frankfort, KY 40602-0517
(502) 564-6027
(502) 564-6090 FAX

Louisiana Department of Insurance
950 N 5th St
Baton Rouge, LA 70802
(504) 342-5423
(504) 342-8622 FAX

Maine Bureau of Insurance
Department of Professional & Financial Regulation
State Office Bldg
Station 34
Augusta, ME 04333-0034
(207) 624-8475
(207) 624-8599 FAX

Maryland Insurance Administration
525 Saint Paul Place
Stanbalt Bldg, Seventh Fl S
Baltimore, MD 21202-2272
(410) 468-2090
(410) 468-2020 FAX

Division of Insurance Commonwealth of Massachusetts
Division of Insurance
470 Atlantic Ave, Sixth Fl
Boston, MA 02210-2223
(617) 521-7794
(617) 521-7770 FAX

Michigan Insurance Bureau
Department of Commerce
611 W Ottawa St, 2nd Fl N
Lansing, MI 48933-1020
(517) 373-9273
(517) 335-4978 FAX

Minnesota Department of Commerce
133 E 7th St
Saint Paul, MN 55101
(612) 296-6848
(612) 296-4328 FAX

Mississippi Department of Insurance
550 High St
Jackson, MS 39201
(601) 359-3569
(601) 359-2474 FAX

Missouri Director of Insurance
PO Box 690
Jefferson City, MO 65102
(573) 751-4126
(573) 751-1165 FAX

Montana Department of Insurance
126 North Sanders
Mitchell Bldg, Rm 270
Helena, MT 59601
(406) 444-2040
(406) 444-3497 FAX

Nebraska Department of Insurance
Terminal Bldg
941 "O" St, Ste 400
Lincoln, NE 68508
(402) 471-2201
(402) 471-4610 FAX

Nevada Division of Insurance
1665 Hotsprings Rd, Ste 152
Carson City, NV 89710
(702) 687-4270
(702) 687-3937 FAX

New Hampshire Department of Insurance
169 Manchester St
Concord, NH 03301
(603) 271-2261
(603) 271-1406 FAX

New Jersey Department of Insurance
20 W State St
CN325
Trenton, NJ 08625
(609) 292-5363
(609) 292-3144 FAX

New Mexico Department of Insurance
PO Drawer 1269
Sante Fe, NM 87504-1269
(505) 827-4601
(505) 827-4734 FAX

New York Department of Insurance
State of New York
25 Beaver St
New York, NY 10004-2319
(212) 480-2287
(212) 480-2310 FAX

North Carolina Department of Insurance
PO Box 26387
Raleigh, NC 27611
(919) 733-7349
(919) 733-6495 FAX

North Dakota Department of Insurance
600 E Blvd Avenue
Bismarck, ND 58505-0302
(701) 328-2440
(701) 328-4880 FAX

Ohio Department of Insurance
2100 Stella Ct
Columbus, OH 43215-1067
(614) 644-2658
(614) 644-3743 FAX

Oklahoma Department of Insurance
3814 North Santa Fe
Oklahoma City, OK 73118
(405) 521-2686
(405) 521-6635 FAX

Oregon Division of Insurance
Department of Consumer & Business Services
350 Winter St NE, Rm 200
Salem, OR 97310-0700
(503) 378-4271
(503) 378-6444 FAX

Pennsylvania Insurance Department
1326 Strawberry Sq, 13th Fl
Harrisburg, PA 17120
(717) 783-0442
(717) 772-1969 FAX

Puerto Rico Department of Insurance
Cobian's Plaza Bldg
1607 Ponce de Leon Avenue
Santurce, PR 00909
(787) 722-8686
(787) 722-4400 FAX

Rhode Island Insurance
Department of Business Regulation
233 Richmond St, Ste 233
Providence, RI 02903-4233
(401) 277-2223
(401) 751-4887 FAX

South Carolina Department of Insurance
1612 Marion St
PO Box 100105
Columbia, SC 29201
(803) 737-6160
(803) 737-6229 FAX

South Dakota Division of Insurance
Department of Commerce & Regulation
118 West Capitol Ave
Pierre, SD 57501-2000
(605) 773-3563
(605) 773-5369 FAX

Tennessee Department of Commerce & Insurance
Volunteer Plaza
500 James Robertson Pky
Nashville, TN 37243-0565
(615) 741-2241
(615) 532-6934 FAX

Texas Department of Insurance
333 Guadalupe St
PO Box 149104
Austin, TX 78714-9104
(512) 463-6464
(512) 475-2005 FAX

Utah Department of Insurance
State Office Bldg, Ste 3110
Salt Lake City, UT 84114-1201
(801) 538-3800
(801) 538-3829 FAX

Vermont Division of Insurance
Department of Banking Insurance & Securities
89 Main St
Drawer 20
Montpelier, VT 05620-3101
(802) 828-3301
(802) 828-3306 FAX

Virginia Bureau of Insurance
State Corp Com
1300 E Main St
Richmond, VA 23219
(804) 371-9694
(804) 371-9873 FAX

Virgin Islands Division of Banking & Insurance
1131 King St
Christiansted
St. Croix, VI 00820
(809) 773-6449
(809) 773-4052 FAX

Washington Office of the Insurance Commissioner
14th Avenue & Water St
PO Box 40255
Olympia, WA 98504-0255
(360) 753-7301
(360) 586-3535 FAX

West Virginia Department of Insurance
PO Box 50540
Charleston, WV 25305-0540
(304) 558-3354
(304) 558-0412 FAX

State of Wisconsin
Office of the Commissioner of Insurance
121 E Wilson
Madison, WI 53702
(608) 266-0102
(608) 261-8579 FAX

Wyoming Insurance Commission
Herschler Bldg 3E
122 W 25th St, 3rd E
Cheyenne, WY 82002-0440
(307) 777-7401
(307) 777-5895 FAX

7 Using the Directory

Formatting

With more than 5,000 entries, the directory is formatted in a four-column-per-page style for easy reference. The entries are read alphabetically down the first column, down the second, third, and fourth columns, rather than across the page.

All listings are alphabetized by company name, and are printed in large, bold type. The address immediately following the company name is either the only claims office or, in the case of companies with branch offices, the home office. Additional offices are listed alphabetically by state under an italicized heading such as Alaska Claims Office. Just as each company name appears only once before all of its offices, the italicized heading appears once before the first entry falling within that state.

The addresses are printed in capital letters with no punctuation. This follows guidelines set by the U.S. Postal Service to facilitate more efficient electronic scanning. See appendix B for acceptable abbreviations. We've also included the post office's recommendations for addressing envelopes.

Icons

To make the *2000 Insurance Directory* even more valuable, we verified the types of claims processed by each office and identified them with an icon. These icons represent the types of claims processed, and the key is printed across the bottom of facing pages.

If no icon is given, the office is either a corporate office or an office that did not verify claims information when contacted.

- Casualty/Liability
- Dental
- Disability
- EMC–Electronic Media Claims
- HCPCS*
- H HMO
- Home Health
- Medical
- Medigap
- ℞ Pharmaceutical
- ☆ Reassurance/Reinsurance
- Self-Insured
- 3 TPA–Third Party Corporation Administrator
- Vision
- Workers Compensation

*Note: Although companies within the *2000 Insurance Directory* have indicated that they process HCPCS Level II codes, it is important to check that the particular plan being billed processes these claims.

State-By-State Index

For your convenience, we've sorted all entries in the directory into a state-by-state index. The company name is listed once though there may be more than one office in that state.

8 The Directory

20TH CENTURY INSURANCE CO

CALIFORNIA CLAIMS OFFICE
6301 OWENSMOUTH AVE
WOODLAND HILLS, CA 91367-2286
TEL: (818) 704-3700
FAX: (818) 704-3796
TOLL FREE: (800) 443-3100
WWW.20THCENTINS.COM

A & I BENEFIT PLAN ADMINISTRATORS

OREGON CLAIMS OFFICE
1220 SW MORRISON, STE 300
PORTLAND, OR 97205-2222
TEL: (503) 224-0048
FAX: (503) 228-0149
TOLL FREE: (800) 547-4457
IN-STATE: (800) 547-4457

A-1 LIFE INSURANCE CO

NEW YORK CLAIMS OFFICE
70 PINE ST- 5TH FL
NEW YORK, NY 10270
TEL: (212) 770-7000
FAX: (212) 943-1125
TOLL FREE: (888) 244-3200

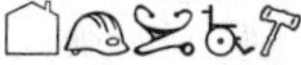

AAA LIFE INSURANCE CO

FLORIDA CLAIMS OFFICE
1000 AAA DR
PO BOX 45
HEATHROW, FL 32746-5063
TEL: (407) 444-8550
FAX: (407) 444-8567
TOLL FREE: (800) 222-4805

SOUTH CAROLINA CLAIMS OFFICE
1000 AAA DR
PO BOX 1000
HEATHROW, FL 32746-5063
TEL: (407) 444-8550
FAX: (407) 444-8567
TOLL FREE: (800) 222-4805

AARP CLAIMS UNIT

PENNSYLVANIA CLAIMS OFFICE
CLAIMS UNIT PRUDENTIAL INSURANCE
PO BOX 13999
PHILADELPHIA, PA 19187-0216
TOLL FREE: (800) 523-5800
WWW.AARPHEALTHCARE.COM

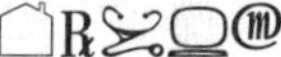

AB CHANCE WELFARE BENEFIT TRUST

MISSOURI CLAIMS OFFICE
210 N ALLEN ST
CENTRALIA, MO 65240-1302
TEL: (573) 682-5521
FAX: (573) 682-8648

ACACIA MUTUAL LIFE INSURANCE CO

DISTRICT OF COLUMBIA CLAIMS OFFICE
AMERITAS LIFE INSURANCE
51 LOUISIANA AVE NW
PO BOX 81889
LINCOLN, NE 68501-1889
TOLL FREE: (800) 745-6665

AMERITAS LIFE INSURANCE
7315 WISCONSIN AVE
BETHESDA, MD 20814
TEL: (301) 280-1000
FAX: (301) 280-1261
TOLL FREE: (800) 444-1889
WWW.ACACIAGROUP.COM

MARYLAND CLAIMS OFFICE
AMERITAS LIFE INSURANCE
7315 WISCONSIN AVE
BETHESDA, MD 20814
TEL: (301) 280-1000
FAX: (301) 280-1261
TOLL FREE: (800) 444-1889
WWW.ACACIAGROUP.COM

SOUTH CAROLINA CLAIMS OFFICE
AMERITAS LIFE INSURANCE
7315 WISCONSIN AVE
BETHESDA, MD 20814
TEL: (301) 280-1000
FAX: (301) 280-1261
TOLL FREE: (800) 444-1889
WWW.ACACIAGROUP.COM

AMERITAS LIFE INSURANCE
51 LOUISIANA AVE NW
WASHINGTON, DC 20001-2105
TEL: (202) 628-4506
TOLL FREE: (800) 444-1889

ACADEMY LIFE INSURANCE GROUP

PENNSYLVANIA CLAIMS OFFICE
PO BOX 650
TAYLOR, PA 18517
FAX: (570) 969-4030
TOLL FREE: (800) 345-6352

ACCESS ADMINISTRATORS INC

TEXAS CLAIMS OFFICE
7100 WESTWIND DR, STE 115
PO BOX 12609
EL PASO, TX 79912-1799
TEL: (915) 581-8182
FAX: (915) 581-7537
TOLL FREE: (800) 854-2339

ACMG, INC

OHIO CLAIMS OFFICE
2570 TECHNICAL DR
MIAMISBURG, OH 45342
TEL: (937) 866-6660
FAX: (937) 866-8083
TOLL FREE: (800) 848-2264

ACORDIA NATIONAL

WEST VIRGINIA CLAIMS OFFICE
602 VIRGINIA ST E
PO BOX 3262
CHARLESTON, WV 25332-3262
TEL: (304) 340-0253
FAX: (304) 353-8773
TOLL FREE: (800) 624-8605
WWW.ACORDIA.COM

ACS CLAIMS SERVICE

TEXAS CLAIMS OFFICE
PO BOX 296
DALLAS, TX 75221
TEL: (214) 826-8148
FAX: (214) 826-8239
TOLL FREE: (800) 456-9653

ACS NORTH AMERICAN

GEORGIA CLAIMS OFFICE
411 A GORDON AVE
PO BOX 1478
THOMASVILLE, GA 31799-1478
TEL: (912) 228-7026
FAX: (912) 228-7464
TOLL FREE: (888) 298-5959

AD CON SERVICES, INC

TENNESSEE CLAIMS OFFICE
RR 1- BOX 63 B5
STEWART, TN 37175
TEL: (931) 721-4448
FAX: (931) 721-4449

ADMAR CORP

ARIZONA CLAIMS OFFICE
1551 N TUSTIN AVE, STE 300
PO BOX 478
SANTA ANA, CA 92701-3055
TEL: (714) 953-9600
FAX: (714) 953-9060
TOLL FREE: (800) 422-0294
WWW.ADMARINC.COM

ARKANSAS CLAIMS OFFICE
1551 N TUSTIN AVE, STE 300
PO BOX 478
SANTA ANA, CA 92701-3055
TEL: (714) 953-9600
FAX: (714) 953-9060
TOLL FREE: (800) 422-0294
WWW.ADMARINC.COM

CALIFORNIA CLAIMS OFFICE
1551 N TUSTIN AVE, STE 300
PO BOX 478
SANTA ANA, CA 92701-3055
TEL: (714) 953-9600
FAX: (714) 953-9060
TOLL FREE: (800) 422-0294
WWW.ADMARINC.COM

LOUISIANA CLAIMS OFFICE
1551 N TUSTIN AVE, STE 300
PO BOX 478
SANTA ANA, CA 92701-3055
TEL: (714) 953-9600
FAX: (714) 953-9060
TOLL FREE: (800) 422-0294
WWW.ADMARINC.COM

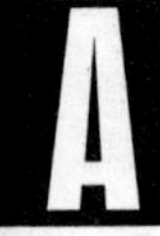

MISSISSIPPI CLAIMS OFFICE
1551 N TUSTIN AVE, STE 300
PO BOX 478
SANTA ANA, CA 92701-3055
TEL: (714) 953-9600
FAX: (714) 953-9060
TOLL FREE: (800) 422-0294
WWW.ADMARINC.COM

NEVADA CLAIMS OFFICE
1551 N TUSTIN AVE, STE 300
PO BOX 478
SANTA ANA, CA 92701-3055
TEL: (714) 953-9600
FAX: (714) 953-9060
TOLL FREE: (800) 422-0294
WWW.ADMARINC.COM

NEW MEXICO CLAIMS OFFICE
1551 N TUSTIN AVE, STE 300
PO BOX 478
SANTA ANA, CA 92701-3055
TEL: (714) 953-9600
FAX: (714) 953-9060
TOLL FREE: (800) 422-0294
WWW.ADMARINC.COM

TENNESSEE CLAIMS OFFICE
1551 N TUSTIN AVE, STE 300
PO BOX 478
SANTA ANA, CA 92701-3055
TEL: (714) 953-9600
FAX: (714) 953-9060
TOLL FREE: (800) 422-0294
WWW.ADMARINC.COM

TEXAS CLAIMS OFFICE
1551 N TUSTIN AVE, STE 300
PO BOX 478
SANTA ANA, CA 92701-3055
TEL: (714) 953-9600
FAX: (714) 953-9060
TOLL FREE: (800) 422-0294
WWW.ADMARINC.COM

ADMINISTAR

INDIANA CLAIMS OFFICE
PO BOX 7073
INDIANAPOLIS, IN 46207-7073
TEL: (317) 845-2992
FAX: (317) 841-4691

ADMINISTRATION SERVICES, INC

WASHINGTON CLAIMS OFFICE
WEST 111 CATALDO, STE 110
PO BOX 5434
SPOKANE, WA 99205
TEL: (509) 328-0300
FAX: (509) 328-8623
TOLL FREE: (800) 716-0300
E-MAIL: ASI@ADMIN-SERV.COM

ADMINISTRATION SYSTEMS RESEARCH CORP

MICHIGAN CLAIMS OFFICE
3033 ORCHARD VISTA DR SE
GRAND RAPIDS, MI 49546-7000
TEL: (616) 957-1751
FAX: (616) 957-8986
TOLL FREE: (800) 968-2449
WWW.ASRCORP.COM, WWW.PHYSICIANSCARE.COM

ADMINISTRATIVE CONCEPTS, INC

NEW YORK CLAIMS OFFICE
6250 S BAY RD
PO BOX 3580
SYRACUSE, NY 13220
TEL: (315) 699-5809
FAX: (315) 699-8357

ADMINISTRATIVE CONSULTANTS, INC

CONNECTICUT CLAIMS OFFICE
92 BROOKSIDE RD
PO BOX 1471
WATERBURY, CT 06721
TEL: (203) 756-8061
FAX: (203) 754-3941

ADMINISTRATIVE ENTERPRISES, INC

ARIZONA CLAIMS OFFICE
3404 W CHERYL DR, STE 280
PHOENIX, AZ 85051-9588
TEL: (602) 789-1170
FAX: (602) 789-9369
TOLL FREE: (800) 762-2234

NEVADA CLAIMS OFFICE
3404 W CHERYL DR, STE 280
PHOENIX, AZ 85051-9588
TEL: (602) 789-1170
FAX: (602) 789-9369
TOLL FREE: (800) 762-2234

ADMINISTRATIVE PROCEDURES

INDIANA CLAIMS OFFICE
2111 W LINCOLN HWY
MERRILLVILLE, IN 46410-5334
TEL: (219) 769-6944
FAX: (219) 769-4834
TOLL FREE: (800) 759-6944

ADMINISTRATIVE SERVICE CONSULTANTS

NATIONAL CLAIMS OFFICE
3301 E ROYALTON RD
BROADVIEW HEIGHTS, OH 44147
TEL: (440) 526-2730
FAX: (440) 526-1608
TOLL FREE: (800) 634-8816
WWW.ASCOFOHIO.COM

OHIO CLAIMS OFFICE
215 STANFORD PKY
PO BOX 928
FINDLAY, OH 45840
TEL: (419) 423-3823
FAX: (419) 423-7097
TOLL FREE: (800) 523-5789
IN-STATE: (800) 472-6630

ADMINISTRATIVE SERVICES, INC

FLORIDA CLAIMS OFFICE
7990 SW 117TH AVE
PO BOX 839000
MIAMI, FL 33283
TEL: (305) 595-4040
FAX: (305) 596-6820
TOLL FREE: (800) 749-1858
E-MAIL: INFO@ADMINSERV.COM
WWW.ADMINSERV.COM

ADMINITRON, INC

NATIONAL CLAIMS OFFICE
214 CENTERVIEW DR, STE 250
PO BOX 5095
BRENTWOOD, TN 37027
TEL: (615) 373-3537
FAX: (615) 373-2214
TOLL FREE: (800) 735-7340

ADMIRAL INSURANCE CO

NEW JERSEY CLAIMS OFFICE
1255 CALDWELL RD
PO BOX 5725
CHERRY HILL, NJ 08034-3220
TEL: (609) 429-9200
FAX: (609) 428-3390
WWW.ADMIRALINS.COM

ADVANCED BENEFIT ADMINISTRATORS

IDAHO CLAIMS OFFICE
6420 SW MACADAM AVE, STE 380
PORTLAND, OR 97201-3519
TEL: (503) 245-3770
FAX: (503) 245-4122
TOLL FREE: (800) 443-6531

OREGON CLAIMS OFFICE
6420 SW MACADAM AVE, STE 380
PORTLAND, OR 97201-3519
TEL: (503) 245-3770
FAX: (503) 245-4122
TOLL FREE: (800) 443-6531

WASHINGTON CLAIMS OFFICE
6420 SW MACADAM AVE, STE 380
PORTLAND, OR 97201-3519
TEL: (503) 245-3770
FAX: (503) 245-4122
TOLL FREE: (800) 443-6531

ADVANCED INSURANCE SERVICES

TENNESSEE CLAIMS OFFICE
600 JEFFERSON AVE
PO BOX 19
MEMPHIS, TN 38101-0019
TEL: (901) 544-2344
FAX: (901) 544-2328
TOLL FREE: (800) 772-1352

ADVANTAGE HEALTH

PENNSYLVANIA CLAIMS OFFICE
121 7TH ST
PITTSBURGH, PA 15222
TEL: (412) 391-9300
FAX: (412) 391-0377
TOLL FREE: (800) 333-3930

WEST VIRGINIA CLAIMS OFFICE
121 7TH ST
PITTSBURGH, PA 15222
TEL: (412) 391-9300
FAX: (412) 471-6893
TOLL FREE: (800) 333-3930

ADVANTAGE HEALTH QUALMED

OHIO CLAIMS OFFICE
137 WADDELS RUN RD
WHEELING, WV 26003-6155
TEL: (304) 243-1489
FAX: (304) 243-1975
TOLL FREE: (800) 477-0682

PENNSYLVANIA CLAIMS OFFICE
137 WADDELS RUN RD
WHEELING, WV 26003-6155
TEL: (304) 243-1489
FAX: (304) 243-1975
TOLL FREE: (800) 477-0682

WEST VIRGINIA CLAIMS OFFICE
137 WADDELS RUN RD
WHEELING, WV 26003-6155
TEL: (304) 243-1489
FAX: (304) 243-1975
TOLL FREE: (800) 477-0682

AEGIS SECURITY INSURANCE CO

PENNSYLVANIA CLAIMS OFFICE
2407 PARK DR, STE 200
HARRISBURG, PA 17110
TEL: (717) 657-9671
FAX: (717) 657-0340
TOLL FREE: (800) 233-2160

SOUTH CAROLINA CLAIMS OFFICE
2407 PARK DR, STE 200
HARRISBURG, PA 17110
TEL: (717) 657-9671
FAX: (717) 657-0340
TOLL FREE: (800) 233-2160

AEGON INSURANCE GROUP

NATIONAL CLAIMS OFFICE
COMMONWEALTH LIFE INSURANCE
400 W MARKET ST
PO BOX 32830
LOUISVILLE, KY 40232-2800
TEL: (502) 587-7371
TOLL FREE: (800) 693-3080
IN-STATE: (800) 638-3080
WWW.AEGON.COM

AETNA LIFE INSURANCE CO OF CANADA

ONTARIO CLAIMS OFFICE
AETNA CANADA CLAIMS
3080 YOUNG ST, STE 3040
PO BOX 120
TORONTO, ON M4N-3P2
TEL: (416) 864-8000
TOLL FREE: (800) 361-7979
WWW.AETNA.COM

AETNA CANADA HEADQUARTERS
79 WELLINGTON ST W- T. P. CTR
TORONTO, ON MSK-1N9
TEL: (416) 864-8575
FAX: (416) 864-1270
TOLL FREE: (800) 361-7979
WWW.AETNA.COM

AETNA / U.S. HEALTHCARE

CALIFORNIA CLAIMS OFFICE
6795 N PALM AVE
FRESNO, CA 93704
TEL: (209) 241-1000
FAX: (209) 241-1226
TOLL FREE: (800) 756-7039
WWW.AETNAUSHC.COM

CONNECTICUT CLAIMS OFFICE
151 FARMINGTON AVE
PO BOX 150417
HARTFORD, CT 06156
TEL: (860) 273-0123
TOLL FREE: (800) 872-3862
WWW.AETNAUSHEALTHCARE.COM

1000 MIDDLE ST
MIDDLETOWN, CT 06457-4621
TEL: (860) 636-8300
FAX: (860) 638-6599
TOLL FREE: (800) 445-3184
WWW.AETNAUSHC.COM

FLORIDA CLAIMS OFFICE
4300 W CYPRESS ST
PO BOX 31450
TAMPA, FL 33631-3450
TEL: (813) 870-6670
TOLL FREE: (800) 872-3862
WWW.AETNAUSHC.COM

PO BOX 30167
TAMPA, FL 33630-3167
TEL: (813) 870-7940
FAX: (813) 878-7839
TOLL FREE: (800) 323-9930
IN-STATE: (800) 282-3517
WWW.AETNAUSHC.COM

GEORGIA CLAIMS OFFICE
AETNA HEALTH PLANS OF GEORGIA
PIEDMONT RD NE, STE 300
ATLANTA, GA 30305-1565
TEL: (770) 346-1000
TOLL FREE: (800) 353-5980
WWW.AETNAUSHC.COM

LOUISIANA CLAIMS OFFICE
3900 N CSWY BLVD, STE 410
METAIRIE, LA 70002-7283
TEL: (504) 830-5600
FAX: (504) 837-6571
TOLL FREE: (800) 685-4857
WWW.AETNAUSHC.COM

MASSACHUSETTS CLAIMS OFFICE
400-1 TOTTEN POND RD
WALTHAM, MA 02154
TEL: (781) 273-5600
FAX: (781) 902-3871
TOLL FREE: (800) 448-8742
WWW.AETNAUSHC.COM

400-1 TOTTEN POND RD
WALTHAM, MA 02154
TEL: (781) 273-5600
FAX: (781) 902-3871
TOLL FREE: (800) 448-8742
WWW.AETNAUSHC.COM

NEW JERSEY CLAIMS OFFICE
55 LANE RD
FAIRFIELD, NJ 07004
TEL: (973) 575-5600
FAX: (973) 244-3911
TOLL FREE: (800) 852-0629
WWW.AETNAUSHC.COM

NEW YORK CLAIMS OFFICE
GREATER NEW YORK CLAIM SERVICE CENTER
100 BAYLIS RD
MELVILLE, NY 11747-5500
TEL: (516) 755-0822
TOLL FREE: (800) 872-3862
WWW.AETNAUSHC.COM

2700 WESTCHESTER AVE
PURCHASE, NY 10577-2554
TEL: (914) 251-0600
FAX: (914) 251-1537
TOLL FREE: (800) 722-7315
WWW.AETNAUSHC.COM

PENNSYLVANIA CLAIMS OFFICE
1425 UNION MEETING RD
PO BOX 1125
BLUE BELL, PA 19422
TEL: (215) 775-4800
TOLL FREE: (800) 233-3105
WWW.AETNAUSHC.COM

PO BOX 1125
BLUE BELL, PA 19422
TEL: (412) 788-0500
FAX: (412) 788-5067
TOLL FREE: (800) 323-9930
WWW.AETNAUSHC.COM

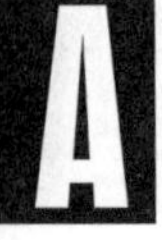

TEXAS CLAIMS OFFICE
2777 STEMMONS FWY
PO BOX 569440
DALLAS, TX 75356-9440
TEL: (214) 200-8000
WWW.HEALTHLINE.COM

4300 CENTURY WAY PL
ARLINGTON, TX 76018
TEL: (817) 417-2000
FAX: (817) 417-2599
TOLL FREE: (800) 428-6111
WWW.AETNAUSHC.COM

VIRGINIA CLAIMS OFFICE
AETNA HEALTH PLANS OF THE MID-ATLANTIC, INC
7600 A LEESBURG PIKE, STE 300
FALLS CHURCH, VA 22043-2413
TEL: (703) 903-7100
FAX: (703) 903-0316
TOLL FREE: (800) 231-8415
WWW.AETNAUSHC.COM

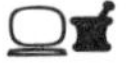

AETNA / U.S. HEALTHCARE CO

NATIONAL CLAIMS OFFICE
7601 ORA GLEN DR
GREENBELT, MD 20770-3647
TEL: (301) 441-1600
FAX: (301) 489-5284
TOLL FREE: (800) 635-3121
IN-STATE: (800) 635-3121

AETNA U.S. HEALTHCARE, INC

CONNECTICUT CLAIMS OFFICE
213 COURT ST- 7TH FL
MIDDLETOWN, CT 06457-3342
TEL: (860) 636-8300
TOLL FREE: (800) 872-3862

H

AETNA / U.S. HEALTHCARE OF THE CAROLINAS, INC

NORTH CAROLINA CLAIMS OFFICE
128 S TRYON ST, STE 2000
CHARLOTTE, NC 28202
TEL: (704) 379-6700
FAX: (704) 379-1729
TOLL FREE: (800) 278-0122
IN-STATE: (800) 545-7110
WWW.AETNAUSHC.COM

SOUTH CAROLINA CLAIMS OFFICE
128 S TRYON ST, STE 2000
CHARLOTTE, NC 28202
TEL: (704) 379-6700
FAX: (704) 379-1729
TOLL FREE: (800) 278-0122
IN-STATE: (800) 545-7110
WWW.AETNAUSHC.COM

AFFORDABLE BENEFIT ADMINISTRATORS INC

ARIZONA CLAIMS OFFICE
444 IRVING DR, STE 202
PO BOX 10787
BURBANK, CA 91510-0787
TEL: (818) 842-0147
FAX: (818) 842-0225
TOLL FREE: (800) 350-0148

CALIFORNIA CLAIMS OFFICE
444 IRVING DR, STE 202
PO BOX 10787
BURBANK, CA 91510-0787
TEL: (818) 842-0147
FAX: (818) 842-0225
TOLL FREE: (800) 350-0148

COLORADO CLAIMS OFFICE
444 IRVING DR, STE 202
PO BOX 10787
BURBANK, CA 91510-0787
TEL: (818) 842-0147
FAX: (818) 842-0225
TOLL FREE: (800) 350-0148

GEORGIA CLAIMS OFFICE
444 IRVING DR, STE 202
PO BOX 10787
BURBANK, CA 91510-0787
TEL: (818) 842-0147
FAX: (818) 842-0225
TOLL FREE: (800) 350-0148

MASSACHUSETTS CLAIMS OFFICE
444 IRVING DR, STE 202
PO BOX 10787
BURBANK, CA 91510-0787
TEL: (818) 842-0147
FAX: (818) 842-0225
TOLL FREE: (800) 350-0148

NEW YORK CLAIMS OFFICE
444 IRVING DR, STE 202
PO BOX 10787
BURBANK, CA 91510-0787
TEL: (818) 842-0147
FAX: (818) 842-0225
TOLL FREE: (800) 350-0148

TEXAS CLAIMS OFFICE
444 IRVING DR, STE 202
PO BOX 10787
BURBANK, CA 91510-0787
TEL: (818) 842-0147
FAX: (818) 842-0225
TOLL FREE: (800) 350-0148

WASHINGTON CLAIMS OFFICE
444 IRVING DR, STE 202
PO BOX 10787
BURBANK, CA 91510-0787
TEL: (818) 842-0147
FAX: (818) 842-0225
TOLL FREE: (800) 350-0148

AFLAC

GEORGIA CLAIMS OFFICE
1932 WYNNTON RD
COLUMBUS, GA 31999-7251
TEL: (706) 323-3431
FAX: (706) 596-3782
TOLL FREE: (800) 992-3522
WWW.AFLAC.COM

AFLAC NEW YORK

CONNECTICUT CLAIMS OFFICE
PO BOX 15087
ALBANY, NY 12212-5087
TEL: (518) 438-0764
FAX: (518) 438-0896
TOLL FREE: (800) 366-3436

MASSACHUSETTS CLAIMS OFFICE
PO BOX 15087
ALBANY, NY 12212-5087
TEL: (518) 438-0764
FAX: (518) 438-0896
TOLL FREE: (800) 366-3436

NEW JERSEY CLAIMS OFFICE
PO BOX 15087
ALBANY, NY 12212-5087
TEL: (518) 438-0764
FAX: (518) 438-0896
TOLL FREE: (800) 366-3436

NEW YORK CLAIMS OFFICE
PO BOX 15087
ALBANY, NY 12212-5087
TEL: (518) 438-0764
FAX: (518) 438-0896
TOLL FREE: (800) 366-3436

AGENCY SERVICES, INC

ALABAMA CLAIMS OFFICE
2250 RIDGEWAY
PO BOX 17237
MEMPHIS, TN 38187-0237
TEL: (901) 767-4271
FAX: (901) 685-9811
TOLL FREE: (800) 777-0988
WWW.AGENCYSERVICES.COM

ARKANSAS CLAIMS OFFICE
2250 RIDGEWAY
PO BOX 17237
MEMPHIS, TN 38187-0237
TEL: (901) 767-4271
FAX: (901) 685-9811
TOLL FREE: (800) 777-0988
WWW.AGENCYSERVICES.COM

Casualty/Liability · Dental · Disability · EMC · HCPCS · Home Health · H HMO · Medical

MISSISSIPPI CLAIMS OFFICE
2250 RIDGEWAY
PO BOX 17237
MEMPHIS, TN 38187-0237
TEL: (901) 767-4271
FAX: (901) 685-9811
TOLL FREE: (800) 777-0988
WWW.AGENCYSERVICES.COM

TENNESSEE CLAIMS OFFICE
2250 RIDGEWAY
PO BOX 17237
MEMPHIS, TN 38187-0237
TEL: (901) 767-4271
FAX: (901) 685-9811
TOLL FREE: (800) 777-0988
WWW.AGENCYSERVICES.COM

AGIA, INC

ARIZONA CLAIMS OFFICE
7878 N 16TH ST, STE 215
PO BOX 9060
PHOENIX, AZ 85068-9060
TEL: (602) 870-4121
FAX: (602) 870-3026
TOLL FREE: (800) 782-7267
WWW.AGIA.COM

AGRI-SERVICE AGENCIES

NEW YORK CLAIMS OFFICE
5001 BRITTONFIELD PKY
PO BOX 4910
EAST SYRACUSE, NY 13057
TEL: (315) 433-2332
FAX: (315) 433-2345
TOLL FREE: (800) 654-8840

AID ASSOCIATION FOR LUTHERANS

WISCONSIN CLAIMS OFFICE
4321 N BALLARD RD
APPLETON, WI 54919-0001
TEL: (920) 734-5721
FAX: (920) 730-4757
TOLL FREE: (800) 225-5225

AIG CLAIM SERVICES, INC

ALABAMA CLAIMS OFFICE
270 CARPENTER DR, STE 400
PO BOX 105180
ATLANTA, GA 30348
TEL: (404) 250-7000
TOLL FREE: (800) 448-9707

270 CARPENTER DR, STE 400
PO BOX 720551
ATLANTA, GA 30358
TEL: (404) 706-2200
TOLL FREE: (800) 242-2418

ALASKA CLAIMS OFFICE
222 SW COLUMBIA, STE 1000
PORTLAND, OR 97201
TEL: (503) 417-8300
FAX: (503) 224-6891
TOLL FREE: (800) 422-5132
IN-STATE: (800) 242-2923
WWW.AIG.COM

ARIZONA CLAIMS OFFICE
2201 CAMELBACK RD, STE 400 B
PHOENIX, AZ 85016
TEL: (602) 468-8700
FAX: (602) 957-1554
TOLL FREE: (800) 456-1547

ARKANSAS CLAIMS OFFICE
TCBY TOWER, 425 W CAPITAL, STE 1600
PO BOX 34130
LITTLE ROCK, AR 72201
TEL: (501) 375-5040
FAX: (501) 375-5066
TOLL FREE: (800) 955-6520

9401 INDIAN CREEK PKY- BLDG 40, STE 1300
PO BOX 25588
SHAWNEE MISSION, KS 66225
TEL: (913) 338-9200
FAX: (913) 338-9330
TOLL FREE: (800) 242-2987
WWW.AIG.COM

CALIFORNIA CLAIMS OFFICE
3090 BRISTOL ST, STE 450
PO DRAWER 1110
COSTA MESA, CA 92628-1110
TEL: (714) 435-6500
FAX: (714) 435-6428
TOLL FREE: (800) 242-2304
WWW.AIG.COM

222 SW COLUMBIA, STE 1000
PORTLAND, OR 97201
TEL: (503) 417-8300
FAX: (503) 224-6891
TOLL FREE: (800) 422-5132
IN-STATE: (800) 242-2923
WWW.AIG.COM

2 RINCON CTR- 121 SPEAR ST, 4TH FL
PO BOX 88-908
SAN FRANCISCO, CA 94188-0908
TEL: (415) 836-3300
FAX: (415) 836-3130
WWW.AIG.COM

COLORADO CLAIMS OFFICE
2201 CAMELBACK RD, STE 400 B
PHOENIX, AZ 85016
TEL: (602) 468-8700
FAX: (602) 957-1554
TOLL FREE: (800) 456-1547

222 SW COLUMBIA, STE 1000
PORTLAND, OR 97201
TEL: (503) 417-8300
FAX: (503) 224-6891
TOLL FREE: (800) 422-5132
IN-STATE: (800) 242-2923
WWW.AIG.COM

CONNECTICUT CLAIMS OFFICE
120 GREAT OAKS OFC PK- 2ND FL
ALBANY, NY 12203
TEL: (518) 464-3100
FAX: (518) 464-3200
TOLL FREE: (800) 242-2977

99 SUMMER ST- 7TH FL
BOSTON, MA 02110
TEL: (617) 790-9000
FAX: (617) 790-3023
TOLL FREE: (888) 239-0628
WWW.AIG.COM

120 GREAT OAKS OFC PK- 2ND FL
ALBANY, NY 12203
TEL: (518) 464-3100
FAX: (518) 464-3200
TOLL FREE: (800) 242-2977

DELAWARE CLAIMS OFFICE
11311 MCCORMICK RD
HUNT VALLEY, MD 21031
TEL: (410) 316-8700
FAX: (410) 316-8712
TOLL FREE: (800) 654-1204
IN-STATE: (800) 638-3394
WWW.AIG.COM

DISTRICT OF COLUMBIA CLAIMS OFFICE
11311 MCCORMICK RD
HUNT VALLEY, MD 21031
TEL: (410) 316-8700
FAX: (410) 316-8712
TOLL FREE: (800) 654-1204
IN-STATE: (800) 638-3394
WWW.AIG.COM

FLORIDA CLAIMS OFFICE
ATLANTA WORKERS' COMP CENTER
PO BOX 3030
ALPHARETTA, GA 30023-3030
TEL: (770) 870-2300
FAX: (770) 870-2305
TOLL FREE: (800) 242-2418
WWW.AIG.COM

PO BOX 25477
TAMPA, FL 33622-5477
TEL: (813) 218-3000
FAX: (813) 272-1122
IN-STATE: (800) 647-4767
WWW.AIG.COM

PROPERTY/CASUALTY CENTER
PO BOX 2970
ATLANTA, GA 30023-2970
TEL: (707) 870-2000
FAX: (707) 870-2003
TOLL FREE: (800) 242-2418
WWW.AIG.COM

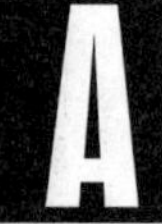

GEORGIA CLAIMS OFFICE
PROPERTY/CASUALTY CENTER
PO BOX 2970
ATLANTA, GA 30023-2970
TEL: (707) 870-2000
FAX: (707) 870-2003
TOLL FREE: (800) 242-2418
WWW.AIG.COM

ATLANTA WORKERS' COMP CENTER
PO BOX 3030
ALPHARETTA, GA 30023-3030
TEL: (770) 870-2300
FAX: (770) 870-2305
TOLL FREE: (800) 242-2418
WWW.AIG.COM

HAWAII CLAIMS OFFICE
222 SW COLUMBIA, STE 1000
PORTLAND, OR 97201
TEL: (503) 417-8300
FAX: (503) 224-6891
TOLL FREE: (800) 422-5132
IN-STATE: (800) 242-2923
WWW.AIG.COM

IDAHO CLAIMS OFFICE
200 N 4TH ST, STE 206
BOISE, ID 83702
TEL: (208) 384-0204
FAX: (208) 384-0248
IN-STATE: (800) 417-8300
WWW.AIG.COM

222 SW COLUMBIA, STE 1000
PORTLAND, OR 97201
TEL: (503) 417-8300
FAX: (503) 224-6891
TOLL FREE: (800) 422-5132
IN-STATE: (800) 242-2923
WWW.AIG.COM

ILLINOIS CLAIMS OFFICE
1230 E DIEHL RD, STE 200
NAPERVILLE, IL 60563
TEL: (630) 505-7400
FAX: (630) 505-7565
TOLL FREE: (800) 892-9779
WWW.AIG.COM

3201 W WHITE OAKS DR, STE 300A
PO BOX 5019
SPRINGFIELD, IL 62705
TEL: (217) 793-4666
FAX: (217) 793-6998
TOLL FREE: (800) 523-8653
WWW.AIG.COM

INDIANA CLAIMS OFFICE
1401 50TH STREET, BLDG 2, STE 200
PO BOX 5168
DES MOINES, IA 50306
TEL: (515) 221-6800
FAX: (515) 221-6810
TOLL FREE: (800) 242-2921
WWW.AIG.COM

400 S 4TH AVE, STE 400
LOUISVILLE, KY 40202-3442
TEL: (502) 561-8700
FAX: (502) 589-2657
TOLL FREE: (800) 428-2422
WWW.AIG.COM

1401 50TH STREET, BLDG 2, STE 200
PO BOX 5168
DES MOINES, IA 50306
TEL: (515) 221-6800
FAX: (515) 221-6810
TOLL FREE: (800) 242-2921
WWW.AIG.COM

IOWA CLAIMS OFFICE
1401 50TH STREET, BLDG 2, STE 200
PO BOX 5168
DES MOINES, IA 50306
TEL: (515) 221-6800
FAX: (515) 221-6810
TOLL FREE: (800) 242-2921
WWW.AIG.COM

3201 W WHITE OAKS DR, STE 300A
PO BOX 5019
SPRINGFIELD, IL 62705
TEL: (217) 793-4666
FAX: (217) 793-6889
TOLL FREE: (800) 523-8653

3201 W WHITE OAKS DR, STE 300A
PO BOX 5019
SPRINGFIELD, IL 62705
TEL: (217) 793-4666
FAX: (217) 793-6998
TOLL FREE: (800) 523-8653
WWW.AIG.COM

KANSAS CLAIMS OFFICE
9401 INDIAN CREEK PKY- BLDG 40, STE 1300
PO BOX 25588
SHAWNEE MISSION, KS 66225
TEL: (913) 338-9200
FAX: (913) 338-9336
TOLL FREE: (800) 242-2987

120 S CENTRAL AVE, STE 300
CLAYTON, MO 63105
TEL: (314) 719-4000
FAX: (314) 863-5939
TOLL FREE: (888) 745-7819
WWW.AIG.COM

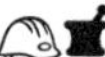

9401 INDIAN CREEK PKY- BLDG 40, STE 1300
PO BOX 25588
SHAWNEE MISSION, KS 66225
TEL: (913) 338-9200
FAX: (913) 338-9330
TOLL FREE: (800) 242-2987
WWW.AIG.COM

KENTUCKY CLAIMS OFFICE
1401 50TH STREET, BLDG 2, STE 200
PO BOX 5168
DES MOINES, IA 50306
TEL: (515) 221-6800
FAX: (515) 221-6810
TOLL FREE: (800) 242-2921
WWW.AIG.COM

400 S 4TH AVE, STE 400
LOUISVILLE, KY 40202-3442
TEL: (502) 561-8700
FAX: (502) 589-2657
TOLL FREE: (800) 428-2422
WWW.AIG.COM

1401 50TH STREET, BLDG 2, STE 200
PO BOX 5168
DES MOINES, IA 50266
TEL: (515) 221-6800
FAX: (515) 221-6810
TOLL FREE: (800) 242-2921
WWW.AIG.COM

1401 50TH STREET, BLDG 2, STE 200
PO BOX 5168
DES MOINES, IA 50266
TEL: (515) 221-6800
FAX: (515) 221-6810
TOLL FREE: (800) 242-2921
WWW.AIG.COM

LOUISIANA CLAIMS OFFICE
9401 INDIAN CREEK PKY- BLDG 40, STE 1300
PO BOX 25588
SHAWNEE MISSION, KS 66210
TEL: (913) 338-9200
FAX: (913) 338-9336
TOLL FREE: (800) 242-2987

LL&E TOWER, 11TH & 12TH FLOORS, 909 POVDRAS ST
NEW ORLEANS, LA 70112
TEL: (504) 524-5600
FAX: (504) 522-7096
TOLL FREE: (800) 225-6130
IN-STATE: (800) 737-5420
WWW.AIG.COM

9401 INDIAN CREEK PKY- BLDG 40, STE 1300
PO BOX 25588
SHAWNEE MISSION, KS 66225
TEL: (913) 338-9200
FAX: (913) 338-9330
TOLL FREE: (800) 242-2987
WWW.AIG.COM

MAINE CLAIMS OFFICE
99 SUMMER ST- 7TH FL
BOSTON, MA 02110
TEL: (617) 790-3030
FAX: (617) 790-3024
TOLL FREE: (888) 239-0628
WWW.AIG.COM

MARYLAND CLAIMS OFFICE
11311 MCCORMICK RD
HUNT VALLEY, MD 21031
TEL: (410) 316-8700
FAX: (410) 316-8712
TOLL FREE: (800) 654-1204
IN-STATE: (800) 638-3394
WWW.AIG.COM

MASSACHUSETTS CLAIMS OFFICE
99 SUMMER ST- 7TH FL
BOSTON, MA 02110
TEL: (617) 790-9000
FAX: (617) 790-3023
TOLL FREE: (888) 239-0628
WWW.AIG.COM

99 SUMMER ST- 7TH FL
BOSTON, MA 02110
TEL: (617) 790-9000
FAX: (617) 790-3023
TOLL FREE: (888) 239-0628
WWW.AIG.COM

MICHIGAN CLAIMS OFFICE
1401 50TH STREET, BLDG 2, STE 200
PO BOX 5168
DES MOINES, IA 50306
TEL: (515) 221-6800
FAX: (515) 221-6810
TOLL FREE: (800) 242-2921
WWW.AIG.COM

2601 COOLIDGE RD, STE 200
PO BOX 30098
EAST LANSING, MI 48909
TEL: (517) 336-2100
FAX: (517) 336-4258
TOLL FREE: (800) 875-5600
WWW.AIG.COM

1401 50TH STREET, BLDG 2, STE 200
PO BOX 5168
DES MOINES, IA 50306
TEL: (515) 221-6800
FAX: (515) 221-6810
TOLL FREE: (800) 242-2921
WWW.AIG.COM

MINNESOTA CLAIMS OFFICE
1401 50TH STREET, BLDG 2, STE 200
PO BOX 5168
DES MOINES, IA 50306
TEL: (515) 221-6800
FAX: (515) 221-6810
TOLL FREE: (800) 242-2921
WWW.AIG.COM

2601 COOLIDGE RD, STE 200
PO BOX 30098
EAST LANSING, MI 48909
TEL: (517) 336-2100
FAX: (517) 336-4258
TOLL FREE: (800) 875-5600
WWW.AIG.COM

1401 50TH STREET, BLDG 2, STE 200
PO BOX 5168
DES MOINES, IA 50306
TEL: (515) 221-6800
FAX: (515) 221-6810
TOLL FREE: (800) 242-2921
WWW.AIG.COM

MISSISSIPPI CLAIMS OFFICE
RIVER OAKS OFFICE PLAZA, 1080 RIVER OAKS DR, STE B200
PO BOX 4466
JACKSON, MS 39208
TEL: (601) 933-0100
FAX: (601) 936-7423
TOLL FREE: (800) 498-0443

ATLANTA WORKERS' COMP CENTER
PO BOX 3030
ALPHARETTA, GA 30023-3030
TEL: (770) 870-2300
FAX: (770) 870-2305
TOLL FREE: (800) 242-2418
WWW.AIG.COM

PROPERTY/CASUALTY CENTER
PO BOX 2970
ATLANTA, GA 30023-2970
TEL: (707) 870-2000
FAX: (707) 870-2003
TOLL FREE: (800) 242-2418
WWW.AIG.COM

MISSOURI CLAIMS OFFICE
9401 INDIAN CREEK PKY- BLDG 40, STE 1300
PO BOX 25588
SHAWNEE MISSION, KS 66225
TEL: (913) 338-9200
FAX: (913) 338-9336
TOLL FREE: (800) 242-2923

120 S CENTRAL AVE, STE 300
CLAYTON, MO 63105
TEL: (314) 719-4000
FAX: (314) 863-5939
TOLL FREE: (888) 745-7819

9401 INDIAN CREEK PKY- BLDG 40, STE 1300
PO BOX 25588
SHAWNEE MISSION, KS 66225
TEL: (913) 338-9200
FAX: (913) 338-9330
TOLL FREE: (800) 242-2987
WWW.AIG.COM

MONTANA CLAIMS OFFICE
222 SW COLUMBIA, STE 1000
PORTLAND, OR 97201
TEL: (503) 417-8300
FAX: (503) 224-6891
TOLL FREE: (800) 422-5132
IN-STATE: (800) 242-2923
WWW.AIG.COM

NEBRASKA CLAIMS OFFICE
1401 50TH STREET, BLDG 2, STE 200
PO BOX 5168
DES MOINES, IA 50306
TEL: (515) 221-6800
FAX: (515) 221-6810
TOLL FREE: (800) 242-2921
WWW.AIG.COM

1401 50TH STREET, BLDG 2, STE 200
PO BOX 5168
DES MOINES, IA 50306
TEL: (515) 221-6800
FAX: (515) 221-6810
TOLL FREE: (800) 242-2921
WWW.AIG.COM

3201 W WHITE OAKS DR, STE 300A
PO BOX 5019
SPRINGFIELD, IL 62705
TEL: (217) 793-4666
FAX: (217) 793-6998
TOLL FREE: (800) 523-8653

3201 W WHITE OAKS DR, STE 300A
PO BOX 5019
SPRINGFIELD, IL 62705
TEL: (217) 793-4666
FAX: (217) 793-6998
TOLL FREE: (800) 523-8653
WWW.AIG.COM

NEVADA CLAIMS OFFICE
101 CONVENTION CENTER DRIVE, #1100
LAS VEGAS, NV 89109
TEL: (702) 792-2848
FAX: (702) 792-3995
TOLL FREE: (800) 547-9475
WWW.AIG.COM

NEW HAMPSHIRE CLAIMS OFFICE
99 SUMMER ST- 7TH FL
BOSTON, MA 02110
TEL: (617) 790-9000
FAX: (617) 790-3023
TOLL FREE: (888) 239-0628
WWW.AIG.COM

99 SUMMER ST- 7TH FL
BOSTON, MA 02110
TEL: (617) 790-9000
FAX: (617) 790-3023
TOLL FREE: (888) 239-0628
WWW.AIG.COM

NEW JERSEY CLAIMS OFFICE
ONE INTERNATIONAL PLZ, STE 200
PO BOX 499
ESSINGTON, PA 19029-0499
TEL: (610) 362-3110
FAX: (610) 894-0853
TOLL FREE: (800) 222-4309
WWW.AIG.COM

120 GREAT OAKS OFC PK- 2ND FL
ALBANY, NY 12203
TEL: (518) 464-3100
FAX: (518) 464-3200
TOLL FREE: (800) 242-2977
WWW.AIG.COM

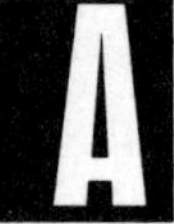

160 WATER ST- 21ST FL
NEW YORK, NY 10038
TEL: (212) 820-6200
FAX: (212) 425-2248
TOLL FREE: (800) 603-1785
WWW.AIG.COM

120 GREAT OAKS OFC PK- 2ND FL
ALBANY, NY 12203
TEL: (518) 464-3100
FAX: (518) 464-3200
TOLL FREE: (800) 242-2977

NEW MEXICO CLAIMS OFFICE
7510 MONTGOMERY NE, STE 204
ALBUQUERQUE, NM 87109
TEL: (505) 888-0073
FAX: (505) 888-0060
TOLL FREE: (800) 472-2109
WWW.AIG.COM

NEW YORK CLAIMS OFFICE
660 WHITE PLAINS RD- 2ND FL
PO BOX 8
TARRYTOWN, NY 10591
TEL: (914) 333-2800
FAX: (914) 332-8603
IN-STATE: (800) 443-0455
WWW.AIG.COM

70 PINE ST
NEW YORK, NY 10270-0002
TEL: (212) 770-7000
FAX: (212) 943-1125
WWW.AIG.COM

120 GREAT OAKS OFC PK- 2ND FL
ALBANY, NY 12203
TEL: (518) 464-3100
FAX: (518) 464-3200
TOLL FREE: (800) 242-2977

120 GREAT OAKS OFC PK- 2ND FL
ALBANY, NY 12203
TEL: (518) 464-3100
FAX: (518) 464-3200
TOLL FREE: (800) 242-2977

2 JERICHO PLZ- 2ND FL WNGB
PO BOX 9008
JERICHO, NY 11753-8908
TEL: (516) 949-4800
FAX: (516) 949-5227
TOLL FREE: (800) 242-2811

160 WATER ST- 21ST FL
NEW YORK, NY 10038
TEL: (212) 820-6200
FAX: (212) 425-2248
TOLL FREE: (800) 603-1785
WWW.AIG.COM

NORTH CAROLINA CLAIMS OFFICE
WORKERS' COMP OFFICE
4201 CONGRESS ST, STE 455
PO BOX 12985
CHARLOTTE, NC 28220-2985
TEL: (704) 553-5100
FAX: (704) 553-5220
TOLL FREE: (800) 644-6430
WWW.AIG.COM

ATLANTA WORKERS' COMP CENTER
PO BOX 3030
ALPHARETTA, GA 30023-3030
TEL: (770) 870-2300
FAX: (770) 870-2305
TOLL FREE: (800) 242-2418
WWW.AIG.COM

PROPERTY/CASUALTY CENTER
PO BOX 2970
ATLANTA, GA 30023-2970
TEL: (707) 870-2000
FAX: (707) 870-2003
TOLL FREE: (800) 242-2418
WWW.AIG.COM

NORTH DAKOTA CLAIMS OFFICE
1401 50TH STREET, BLDG 2, STE 200
PO BOX 5168
DES MOINES, IA 50306
TEL: (515) 221-6800
FAX: (515) 221-6810
TOLL FREE: (800) 242-2921
WWW.AIG.COM

1401 50TH STREET, BLDG 2, STE 200
PO BOX 5168
DES MOINES, IA 50306
TEL: (515) 221-6800
FAX: (515) 221-6810
TOLL FREE: (800) 242-2921
WWW.AIG.COM

1401 50TH STREET, BLDG 2, STE 200
PO BOX 5168
DES MOINES, IA 50306
TEL: (515) 221-6800
FAX: (515) 221-6810
TOLL FREE: (800) 242-2921
WWW.AIG.COM

OHIO CLAIMS OFFICE
120 GREAT OAKS OFC PK- 2ND FL
ALBANY, NY 12203
TEL: (518) 464-3100
FAX: (518) 464-3200
TOLL FREE: (800) 242-2977

120 GREAT OAKS OFC PK- 2ND FL
ALBANY, NY 12203
TEL: (518) 464-3100
FAX: (518) 464-3200
TOLL FREE: (800) 242-2977

1 CLEVELAND CTR- 1375 E 9TH ST
CLEVELAND, OH 44114
TEL: (216) 479-8977
FAX: (216) 479-8818
TOLL FREE: (800) 892-9779
WWW.AIG.COM

OKLAHOMA CLAIMS OFFICE
9401 INDIAN CREEK PKY- BLDG 40, STE 1300
SHAWNEE MISSION, KS 66225
TEL: (913) 338-9200
FAX: (913) 338-9330
TOLL FREE: (800) 242-2987

9401 INDIAN CREEK PKY- BLDG 40, STE 1300
PO BOX 25588
SHAWNEE MISSION, KS 66225
TEL: (913) 338-9200
FAX: (913) 338-9330
TOLL FREE: (800) 242-2987
WWW.AIG.COM

ONTARIO CLAIMS OFFICE
145 WELLINGTON ST W
TORONTO, ON M5J-1H8
TEL: (416) 596-3000
FAX: (416) 596-4197
TOLL FREE: (800) 387-4481
IN-STATE: (800) 387-4426
WWW.AIG.COM

OREGON CLAIMS OFFICE
222 SW COLUMBIA, STE 1000
PORTLAND, OR 97201
TEL: (503) 417-8300
FAX: (503) 224-6891
TOLL FREE: (800) 422-5132
IN-STATE: (800) 242-2923
WWW.AIG.COM

PENNSYLVANIA CLAIMS OFFICE
512 TOWNESHIP LINE RD- 1 VALLEY SQ, STE 200
PO BOX 3021
BLUE BELL, PA 19422
TEL: (215) 283-5600
FAX: (215) 283-5605
TOLL FREE: (800) 242-2733
WWW.AIG.COM

1700 CNG TWR, 625 LIBERTY AVE
PITTSBURGH, PA 15222
TEL: (412) 393-3960
FAX: (412) 288-5959
TOLL FREE: (800) 892-9779
IN-STATE: (800) 258-7152
WWW.AIG.COM

ONE INTERNATIONAL PLZ, STE 200
PO BOX 499
ESSINGTON, PA 19029-0499
TEL: (610) 362-3110
FAX: (610) 894-0853
TOLL FREE: (800) 222-4309
WWW.AIG.COM

PUERTO RICO CLAIMS OFFICE
AIG OF PUERTO RICO
PO BOX 9172
SAN JUAN, PR 00908-9172
TEL: (787) 764-6200
WWW.AIG.COM

RHODE ISLAND CLAIMS OFFICE
99 SUMMER ST- 7TH FL
BOSTON, MA 02110
TEL: (617) 790-9000
FAX: (617) 790-3023
TOLL FREE: (888) 239-0628
WWW.AIG.COM

SOUTH CAROLINA CLAIMS OFFICE
WORKERS' COMP OFFICE
4201 CONGRESS ST, STE 455
PO BOX 12985
CHARLOTTE, NC 28220-2985
TEL: (704) 553-5100
FAX: (704) 553-5220
TOLL FREE: (800) 644-6430
WWW.AIG.COM

ATLANTA WORKERS' COMP CENTER
PO BOX 3030
ALPHARETTA, GA 30023-3030
TEL: (770) 870-2300
FAX: (770) 870-2305
TOLL FREE: (800) 242-2418
WWW.AIG.COM

PROPERTY/CASUALTY CENTER
PO BOX 2970
ATLANTA, GA 30023-2970
TEL: (707) 870-2000
FAX: (707) 870-2003
TOLL FREE: (800) 242-2418
WWW.AIG.COM

SOUTH DAKOTA CLAIMS OFFICE
1401 50TH STREET, BLDG 2, STE 200
PO BOX 5168
DES MOINES, IA 50306
TEL: (515) 221-6800
FAX: (515) 221-6810
TOLL FREE: (800) 242-2921
WWW.AIG.COM

2601 COOLIDGE RD, STE 200
PO BOX 30098
EAST LANSING, MI 48823
TEL: (517) 336-2100
FAX: (517) 336-4258
TOLL FREE: (800) 875-5600
WWW.AIG.COM

1401 50TH STREET, BLDG 2, STE 200
PO BOX 5168
DES MOINES, IA 50306
TEL: (515) 221-6800
FAX: (515) 221-6810
TOLL FREE: (800) 242-2921
WWW.AIG.COM

2601 COOLIDGE RD, STE 200
PO BOX 30098
EAST LANSING, MI 48909
TEL: (517) 336-2100
FAX: (517) 336-4258
TOLL FREE: (800) 875-5600
WWW.AIG.COM

TENNESSEE CLAIMS OFFICE
ATLANTA WORKERS' COMP CENTER
PO BOX 3030
ALPHARETTA, GA 30023-3030
TEL: (770) 870-2300
FAX: (770) 870-2305
TOLL FREE: (800) 242-2418
WWW.AIG.COM

PROPERTY/CASUALTY CENTER
PO BOX 2970
ATLANTA, GA 30023-2970
TEL: (707) 870-2000
FAX: (707) 870-2003
TOLL FREE: (800) 242-2418
WWW.AIG.COM

TEXAS CLAIMS OFFICE
1999 BRYAN ST, 24TH FLOOR
PO BOX 219059
DALLAS, TX 75221
TEL: (214) 932-2600
FAX: (214) 932-2725
TOLL FREE: (800) 233-8541
WWW.AIG.COM

9401 INDIAN CREEK PKY- BLDG 40, STE 1300
PO BOX 25588
SHAWNEE MISSION, KS 66225
TEL: (913) 338-9200
FAX: (913) 338-9330
TOLL FREE: (800) 242-2987

9401 INDIAN CREEK PKY- BLDG 40, STE 1300
PO BOX 25588
SHAWNEE MISSION, KS 66225
TEL: (913) 338-9200
FAX: (913) 338-9330
TOLL FREE: (800) 242-2987
WWW.AIG.COM

UTAH CLAIMS OFFICE
101 CONVENTION CENTER DRIVE, #1100
LAS VEGAS, NV 89109
TEL: (702) 792-2848
FAX: (702) 792-3995
TOLL FREE: (800) 547-9475
WWW.AIG.COM

VERMONT CLAIMS OFFICE
99 SUMMER ST- 7TH FL
BOSTON, MA 02110
TEL: (617) 790-9000
FAX: (617) 790-3023
TOLL FREE: (888) 239-0628
WWW.AIG.COM

VIRGINIA CLAIMS OFFICE
ATLANTA WORKERS' COMP CENTER
PO BOX 3030
ALPHARETTA, GA 30023-3030
TEL: (770) 870-2300
FAX: (770) 870-2305
TOLL FREE: (800) 242-2418
WWW.AIG.COM

PROPERTY/CASUALTY CENTER
PO BOX 2970
ATLANTA, GA 30023-2970
TEL: (707) 870-2000
FAX: (707) 870-2003
TOLL FREE: (800) 242-2418
WWW.AIG.COM

WASHINGTON CLAIMS OFFICE
222 SW COLUMBIA, STE 1000
PORTLAND, OR 97201
TEL: (503) 417-8300
FAX: (503) 224-6891
TOLL FREE: (800) 422-5132
IN-STATE: (800) 242-2923
WWW.AIG.COM

WEST VIRGINIA CLAIMS OFFICE
ATLANTA WORKERS' COMP CENTER
PO BOX 3030
ALPHARETTA, GA 30023-3030
TEL: (770) 870-2300
FAX: (770) 870-2305
TOLL FREE: (800) 242-2418
WWW.AIG.COM

PROPERTY/CASUALTY CENTER
PO BOX 2970
ATLANTA, GA 30023-2970
TEL: (707) 870-2000
FAX: (707) 870-2003
TOLL FREE: (800) 242-2418
WWW.AIG.COM

WISCONSIN CLAIMS OFFICE
13400 BISHOPS LANE STE 290
BROOKFIELD, WI 53005
TEL: (414) 641-4999
FAX: (414) 641-9463
TOLL FREE: (800) 892-9779
WWW.AIG.COM

1401 50TH STREET, BLDG 2, STE 200
PO BOX 5168
DES MOINES, IA 50306
TEL: (515) 221-6800
FAX: (515) 221-6810
TOLL FREE: (800) 242-2921
WWW.AIG.COM

2601 COOLIDGE RD, STE 200
PO BOX 30098
EAST LANSING, MI 48823
TEL: (517) 336-2100
FAX: (517) 336-4258
TOLL FREE: (800) 875-5600
WWW.AIG.COM

WYOMING CLAIMS OFFICE
222 SW COLUMBIA, STE 1000
PORTLAND, OR 97201
TEL: (503) 417-8300
FAX: (503) 224-6891
TOLL FREE: (800) 422-5132
IN-STATE: (800) 242-2923
WWW.AIG.COM

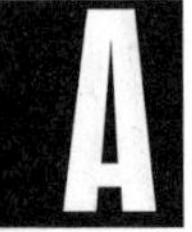

ALABAMA REASSURANCE CO
ALABAMA CLAIMS OFFICE
2330 UNIVERSITY BLVD
PO BOX 020152
TUSCALOOSA, AL 35402
TEL: (205) 345-5600
FAX: (205) 345-3937

ALASKA NATIONAL INSURANCE CO
NATIONAL CLAIMS OFFICE
7001 JEWEL LAKE RD
ANCHORAGE, AK 99502-2825
TEL: (907) 266-9227
FAX: (907) 266-9250
TOLL FREE: (800) 292-0588

ALASKA TIMBER INSURANCE EXCHANGE
ALASKA CLAIMS OFFICE
2555 1ST AVE
KETCHIKAN, AK 99901-5803
TEL: (907) 225-9451
FAX: (907) 225-9454

ALBANY INSURANCE CO
NEW JERSEY CLAIMS OFFICE
GRE INSURANCE GROUP
600 COLLEGE RD E
PRINCETON, NJ 08540
TEL: (800) 443-4000
FAX: (609) 275-2761
TOLL FREE: (800) 955-5513

ALBERT H. WOHLERS & CO
ILLINOIS CLAIMS OFFICE
SEAEURY SMITH
1440 N NORTHWEST HWY
PARK RIDGE, IL 60068-1400
TEL: (847) 803-3100
FAX: (847) 803-4649
TOLL FREE: (800) 323-2106

ALFA INSURANCE CORP
ALABAMA CLAIMS OFFICE
ALFA MUTUAL INSURANCE / ALFA MUTUAL GENERAL & FIRE INSURANCE / ALFA INSURANCE CORP.
2108 E SOUTH BLVD
PO BOX 11000
MONTGOMERY, AL 36191-0001
TEL: (334) 288-3900
FAX: (334) 613-4466
IN-STATE: (800) 392-5705
WWW.ALFAINS.COM

ALL AMERICA FINANCIAL
MASSACHUSETTS CLAIMS OFFICE
440 LINCOLN ST
PO BOX 1018
WORCESTER, MA 01653-0001
TEL: (508) 855-1000
FAX: (508) 853-6332
TOLL FREE: (800) 423-6011
WWW.ALLMERICA.COM

PUERTO RICO CLAIMS OFFICE
440 LINCOLN ST
PO BOX 1018
WORCESTER, MA 01653-0001
TEL: (508) 855-1000
FAX: (508) 853-6332
TOLL FREE: (800) 423-6011
WWW.ALLMERICA.COM

ALL NATION INSURANCE CO
MINNESOTA CLAIMS OFFICE
PO BOX 64697
SAINT PAUL, MN 55164
FAX: (612) 224-4918
TOLL FREE: (800) 869-1346

ALL RISK ADMINISTRATORS
FLORIDA CLAIMS OFFICE
PO BOX 66237
SAINT PETERSBURG BEACH, FL 33736-6210
TEL: (727) 367-3315
FAX: (727) 367-4510
TOLL FREE: (800) 338-4485

ALLEGIANCE INSURANCE CO
CALIFORNIA CLAIMS OFFICE
2151 E CONVENTION WAY
PO BOX 5011
UPLAND, CA 91785-5011
TEL: (909) 937-1755
FAX: (909) 937-1753
TOLL FREE: (800) 695-0624

ALLEN MEDICAL CLAIMS ADMINISTRATORS
GEORGIA CLAIMS OFFICE
302 MARTIN LUTHER KING, JR BLVD
PO BOX 978
FT VALLEY, GA 31030-0978
TEL: (912) 825-5406
FAX: (912) 825-5314
TOLL FREE: (800) 825-5406

ALLIANCE BLUE CROSS & BLUE SHIELD
MISSOURI CLAIMS OFFICE
RIGHTCHOICE
1831 CHESTNUT ST
PO BOX 66834
SAINT LOUIS, MO 63166-6834
TEL: (314) 923-4444
TOLL FREE: (800) 634-4395
IN-STATE: (800) 392-8740
WWW.BCBSMO.COM

ALLIANCE UNDERWRITERS, LLC
TENNESSEE CLAIMS OFFICE
FKA AMERICAN PROGRESSIVE BENEFITS
155 FRANKLIN RD, STE 250
PO BOX 908
BRENTWOOD, TN 37024-0908
TEL: (615) 377-2008
FAX: (615) 377-2025
TOLL FREE: (800) 899-2035
WWW.ALLIANCEU.COM

ALLIANZ LIFE INSURANCE CO OF NORTH AMERICA
MINNESOTA CLAIMS OFFICE
1750 HENNEPIN AVE
MINNEAPOLIS, MN 55403
TEL: (612) 347-6500
FAX: (612) 337-6227
TOLL FREE: (800) 328-5600
WWW.ALLIANZLIFE.COM

ALLIED ADMINISTRATORS, INC
CALIFORNIA CLAIMS OFFICE
777 DAVIS ST
SAN FRANCISCO, CA 94111
TEL: (415) 986-6276
FAX: (415) 439-5857

2831 CAMINO DEL RIO S, STE 311
SAN DIEGO, CA 92108-3829
TEL: (619) 297-8235
FAX: (619) 574-0645

ALLIED BENEFIT SYSTEMS, INC
ILLINOIS CLAIMS OFFICE
208 S LASALLE
CHICAGO, IL 60604
TEL: (312) 906-8080
FAX: (312) 906-8359
TOLL FREE: (800) 288-2078
WWW.ALLIEDBENEFIT.COM

ALLIED BENEFITS ADMINISTRATORS
WEST VIRGINIA CLAIMS OFFICE
422 9TH ST, STE 100
PO BOX 59
HUNTINGTON, WV 25706
TEL: (304) 529-2345
FAX: (304) 523-6319
TOLL FREE: (800) 869-2345

ALLIED GROUP
NEBRASKA CLAIMS OFFICE
700 N COTNER
PO BOX 80758
LINCOLN, NE 68505-0758
TEL: (402) 467-2381
FAX: (402) 465-7880
TOLL FREE: (800) 228-4011

ALLIED GROUP INSURANCE CO

COLORADO CLAIMS OFFICE
350 BLACK HAWK ST
PO BOX 5190
DENVER, CO 80217-5190
TEL: (303) 366-8998
FAX: (303) 343-2217
TOLL FREE: (800) 233-0394
WWW.ALLIEDGROUP.COM

MINNESOTA CLAIMS OFFICE
PO BOX 1420
MINNEAPOLIS, MN 55440-1420
TEL: (612) 896-1774
FAX: (612) 896-6640
TOLL FREE: (800) 862-6024

ALLIED INSURANCE CO

CALIFORNIA CLAIMS OFFICE
PO BOX 849
SANTA ROSA, CA 95402-0849
TEL: (707) 542-2502
FAX: (707) 579-3065
TOLL FREE: (800) 962-5140

IOWA CLAIMS OFFICE
3820 109TH ST
DES MOINES, IA 50391
TEL: (515) 280-4211
FAX: (515) 252-8389
TOLL FREE: (800) 532-1212
WWW.ALLIEDGROUP.COM

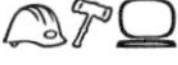

NEVADA CLAIMS OFFICE
PO BOX 849
SANTA ROSA, CA 95402-0849
TEL: (707) 542-2502
FAX: (707) 579-3065
TOLL FREE: (800) 962-5140

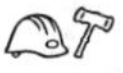

ALLINA

MINNESOTA CLAIMS OFFICE
PHYSICIANS HEALTH PLAN OF MINNESOTA, INC
5601 SMETANA DR
MINNETONKA, MN 55343
TEL: (612) 992-3200
FAX: (612) 992-3232

H

ALLMERICA FINANCIAL

MASSACHUSETTS CLAIMS OFFICE
440 LINCOLN ST
WORCESTER, MA 01653-0001
TEL: (508) 855-1000
FAX: (508) 853-6332
TOLL FREE: (800) 423-6011
WWW.ALLMERICA.COM

ALLSTATE INSURANCE CO

GEORGIA CLAIMS OFFICE
ATLANTA SUBROGATION CLAIMS CENTER
PO BOX 4264
ATLANTA, GA 30302-4264
TEL: (770) 984-4700
FAX: (770) 984-4763
TOLL FREE: (800) 726-1211
WWW.ALLSTATE.COM

5500 INTERSTATE N PKY, STE 300
PO BOX 105584
ATLANTA, GA 30348
TEL: (770) 984-3300
FAX: (770) 984-3327
TOLL FREE: (800) 729-7201
IN-STATE: (800) 366-7889
WWW.ALLSTATE.COM

ILLINOIS CLAIMS OFFICE
CORPORATE OFFICE
2775 SANDERS RD
NORTHBROOK, IL 60062
TEL: (847) 402-5000
FAX: (847) 402-0169
WWW.ALLSTATE.COM

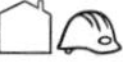

PO BOX 810
ARLINGTON HEIGHTS, IL 60006
TEL: (847) 413-8450
FAX: (847) 413-8461
TOLL FREE: (800) 877-2387
WWW.ALLSTATE.COM

NATIONAL CLAIMS OFFICE
740 CARILLON PKY
PO BOX 12189
SAINT PETERSBURG, FL 33733
TEL: (727) 571-5000
FAX: (727) 571-5099
TOLL FREE: (800) 877-4809
WWW.ALLSTATE.COM

HUDSON OFFICES
PO BOX 337
HUDSON NORTH, OH 44236
TEL: (330) 656-6100
FAX: (330) 656-6063
TOLL FREE: (800) 686-9990
WWW.ALLSTATEINS.COM

PO BOX 3578
AKRON, OH 44309
TEL: (610) 631-3400
TOLL FREE: (800) 729-3005

OREGON CLAIMS OFFICE
PORTLAND MCO
8905 SW NUMBUS, STE 400
BEAVERTON, OR 97008
TEL: (503) 672-7900
FAX: (503) 672-3932
TOLL FREE: (888) 442-6219
WWW.ALLSTATE.COM

CLACKAMAS MCO
10135 SE SUNNYSIDE RD, STE 200
CLACKAMAS, OR 97015
TEL: (503) 353-9271
FAX: (503) 353-2859
TOLL FREE: (800) 927-4970

TEXAS CLAIMS OFFICE
12331 A RIATA TRACE PKY- BLDG 2, STE 150
PO BOX 15326
AUSTIN, TX 78727
TEL: (512) 344-5700
FAX: (512) 344-5717
TOLL FREE: (800) 669-8579

UTAH CLAIMS OFFICE
6056 FASHION SQ DR
PO BOX 57995
MURRAY, UT 84107
TEL: (801) 264-2000
FAX: (801) 264-2140
IN-STATE: (800) 662-5366

WASHINGTON CLAIMS OFFICE
33801 FIRST WAY S, STE 111
FEDERAL WAY, WA 98003
TEL: (253) 952-0158
FAX: (253) 952-1912
TOLL FREE: (800) 733-7550

PO BOX 39
MARYSVILLE, WA 98270
TEL: (360) 658-2000
FAX: (360) 658-2002
TOLL FREE: (800) 726-8550
WWW.ALLSTATE.COM

18911 N CREEK PKY #201
PO BOX 24107
SEATTLE, WA 98124
TEL: (425) 489-2200
FAX: (800) 788-4997

ALPHA DATA SYSTEMS, INC

TEXAS CLAIMS OFFICE
1545 W MOCKINGBIRD LN, STE 6000
DALLAS, TX 75235
TEL: (214) 638-1485
TOLL FREE: (800) 342-5248

ALTERNATIVE HEALTH CARE

KENTUCKY CLAIMS OFFICE
BLUE CROSS & BLUE SHIELD
1901 CAMPUS PL
PO BOX 23705
LOUISVILLE, KY 40223
TEL: (502) 261-2100
FAX: (502) 261-2257
TOLL FREE: (800) 955-3035
WWW.AICI.COM

ALTERNATIVE RISK MANAGEMENT, INC

ILLINOIS CLAIMS OFFICE
ARM LTD
3275 N ARLINGTON HTS RD, STE 401
ARLINGTON HEIGHTS, IL 60004
TEL: (847) 394-1700
FAX: (847) 394-1770
TOLL FREE: (800) 392-1770

AM CASTLE & CO NON-BARGAINING

3400 N WOLF RD
FRANKLIN PARK, IL 60131-1319
TEL: (847) 455-7111
FAX: (847) 455-9320
WWW.AMCASTLE.COM

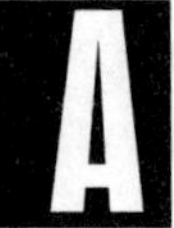

AMALGAMATED LIFE & HEALTH INSURANCE CO
333 S ASHLAND AVE
CHICAGO, IL 60607-2702
TEL: (312) 738-6150
FAX: (312) 738-0784

AMERAPLAN, INC
MICHIGAN CLAIMS OFFICE
22500 METROPOLITAN PKY, STE 100
CLINTON, MI 48035
TEL: (810) 792-4000
FAX: (810) 791-0537
TOLL FREE: (800) 221-4254
WWW.AMERIPLAN.COM

AMERICA LIFE & HEALTH
CALIFORNIA CLAIMS OFFICE
FIRST HEALTH GROUP CORP
PO BOX 3680
LAGUNA HILLS, CA 92654
TEL: (949) 380-0880
FAX: (949) 380-7403
TOLL FREE: (800) 338-7634

AMERICA RE-INSURANCE
NEW JERSEY CLAIMS OFFICE
555 COLLEGE RD E
PO BOX 5241
PRINCETON, NJ 08543-5241
TEL: (609) 243-4200
FAX: (609) 243-4257

AMERICAID AMERIGROUP CO
TEXAS CLAIMS OFFICE
617 7TH AVE- 2ND FL
FT WORTH, TX 76112
TEL: (817) 348-7800
FAX: (817) 870-3658
TOLL FREE: (800) 454-3730
IN-STATE: (800) 600-4441

AMERICAN ADMINISTRATIVE INSURANCE GROUP
FLORIDA CLAIMS OFFICE
IDEALIFE INSURANCE CO
2536 COUNTRYSIDE BLVD
PO BOX 9100
CLEARWATER, FL 33763
TEL: (727) 791-1369
FAX: (727) 725-4190
TOLL FREE: (800) 554-8744

AMERICAN AGRICULTURAL INSURANCE CO
ILLINOIS CLAIMS OFFICE
225 W TOUHY AVE
PO BOX 438
PARK RIDGE, IL 60047
TEL: (847) 685-8773
FAX: (847) 685-8965
WWW.AAIC.FB.COM

AMERICAN AMBASSADOR CASUALTY CO
1501 E WOODFIELD RD, STE 300 E
SCHAUMBURG, IL 60173-6000
TEL: (847) 330-3000
FAX: (847) 330-8135
TOLL FREE: (800) 323-6291

AMERICAN BANKERS INSURANCE GROUP
FLORIDA CLAIMS OFFICE
AMERICAN BANKERS ASSURANCE CO
11222 QUAIL ROOST DR
MIAMI, FL 33157-6543
TEL: (305) 253-2244
FAX: (305) 252-6987
TOLL FREE: (800) 852-2244

AMERICAN BENEFIT MANAGEMENT
OHIO CLAIMS OFFICE
6520 WHIPPLE AVE NW
PO BOX 35008
NORTH CANTON, OH 44735
TEL: (330) 966-5500
FAX: (330) 966-5506
TOLL FREE: (800) 456-4002

AMERICAN BENEFIT PLAN ADMINISTRATORS
COLORADO CLAIMS OFFICE
7000 N BROADWAY- BLDG 3, STE 300A
DENVER, CO 80221-2907
TEL: (303) 428-5141
FAX: (303) 429-4162
TOLL FREE: (800) 247-7876

AMERICAN CENTENNIAL INSURANCE CO
DELAWARE CLAIMS OFFICE
INTERNATIONAL AMERICAN MANAGEMENT CO
FOULKSTONE PLZ- 1415 FOULK RD, STE 202
WILMINGTON, DE 19803-2766
TEL: (302) 479-2100
FAX: (302) 479-2103
TOLL FREE: (800) 533-7628

AMERICAN COMMERCIAL LINES
INDIANA CLAIMS OFFICE
1701 E MARKET ST
PO BOX 610
JEFFERSONVILLE, IN 47131-0610
TEL: (812) 288-0100
FAX: (812) 288-1720
TOLL FREE: (800) 548-7689

AMERICAN COMMUNITY MUTUAL INSURANCE CO
MICHIGAN CLAIMS OFFICE
39201 SEVEN-MILE RD
LIVONIA, MI 48152-1056
TEL: (734) 591-9000
FAX: (734) 591-4628
TOLL FREE: (800) 991-2642
WWW.AMERICAN-COMMUNITY.COM

AMERICAN CREDITORS LIFE INSURANCE CO
CALIFORNIA CLAIMS OFFICE
PO BOX 17748
IRVINE, CA 92623
TEL: (714) 474-7600
FAX: (714) 474-7607

AMERICAN DENTAL EXAMINERS, INC
NEW YORK CLAIMS OFFICE
370 7TH AVE, STE 1206
NEW YORK, NY 10001-3907
TEL: (212) 465-0900
FAX: (212) 465-8784

AMERICAN EMPIRE SURPLUS LINES INSURANCE CO
OHIO CLAIMS OFFICE
515 MAIN ST
PO BOX 5370
CINCINNATI, OH 45201
TEL: (513) 369-3000
FAX: (513) 369-3062

AMERICAN FAMILY INSURANCE
ARIZONA CLAIMS OFFICE
PO BOX 6000
SCOTTSDALE, AZ 85261-6000
TEL: (602) 922-4930
FAX: (602) 905-8041
TOLL FREE: (800) 374-1111
WWW.AMFAM.COM

COLORADO CLAIMS OFFICE
9110 E NICHOLS AVE, STE 310
PO BOX 3328
ENGLEWOOD, CO 80155
TEL: (303) 799-3515
FAX: (303) 799-1630
TOLL FREE: (800) 374-1111

ILLINOIS CLAIMS OFFICE
PO BOX 3220
PEORIA, IL 61612-3220
TEL: (309) 688-0622
FAX: (309) 688-9718
TOLL FREE: (800) 374-1111

1946 DAIMLER RD
PO BOX 7747
ROCKFORD, IL 61126
TEL: (815) 398-3908
FAX: (815) 398-9813
IN-STATE: (800) 374-0008
WWW.AMFAM.COM

475 N MARTINGALE RD, STE 600
SCHAUMBURG, IL 60173
TEL: (847) 605-0660
FAX: (847) 605-9012
TOLL FREE: (800) 374-1111
WWW.AMFAM.COM

2201 W WHITE OAKS DR
PO BOX 1588
SPRINGFIELD, IL 62704
TEL: (217) 793-0870
FAX: (217) 793-3257
TOLL FREE: (800) 374-1111
WWW.AMFAM.COM

INDIANA CLAIMS OFFICE
HOME OFFICE
6000 AMERICAN PKY
MADISON, WI 53783-0001
FAX: (317) 842-3893
TOLL FREE: (800) 374-1111
WWW.AMFAM.COM

IOWA CLAIMS OFFICE
4009 W 49TH ST
PO BOX I
SIOUX FALLS, SD 57101-1924
TEL: (605) 361-5000
FAX: (605) 361-5005
TOLL FREE: (800) 374-0008

3737 WESTOWN PKY, STE 2A
PO BOX 65630
WEST DES MOINES, IA 50266
TEL: (515) 223-1145
FAX: (515) 224-1555
TOLL FREE: (800) 374-1111
WWW.AMFAM.COM

MINNESOTA CLAIMS OFFICE
PO BOX 59173
MINNEAPOLIS, MN 55459
TEL: (612) 933-4446
FAX: (612) 933-7268
TOLL FREE: (800) 374-1111
WWW.AMFAM.COM

4009 W 49TH ST
PO BOX I
SIOUX FALLS, SD 57101-1924
TEL: (605) 361-5000
FAX: (605) 361-5005
TOLL FREE: (800) 374-0008

MISSOURI CLAIMS OFFICE
3600 AMAZONAS
PO BOX 1786
JEFFERSON CITY, MO 65102-1786
TEL: (573) 893-5600
FAX: (573) 893-5728
TOLL FREE: (800) 374-1111

6301 JAMES A REED RD
KANSAS CITY, MO 64133-4775
TEL: (816) 356-2100
FAX: (816) 737-2172
TOLL FREE: (800) 374-1111
WWW.AMFAM.COM

4802 MITCHELL AVE
SAINT JOSEPH, MO 64507-2500
FAX: (816) 364-1541
TOLL FREE: (800) 374-1111

AMERICAN FAMILY MUTUAL INSURANCE
11789 BORMAN DR
PO BOX 28408
SAINT LOUIS, MO 63146-0908
TEL: (314) 991-0070
FAX: (314) 991-2935
TOLL FREE: (800) 374-0008
WWW.AMFAM.COM

NORTH DAKOTA CLAIMS OFFICE
2829 S UNIVERSITY DR
PO BOX 966
FARGO, ND 58107-0966
TEL: (701) 280-1100
FAX: (701) 280-1102
TOLL FREE: (800) 374-1111

SOUTH DAKOTA CLAIMS OFFICE
4009 W 49TH ST
PO BOX I
SIOUX FALLS, SD 57101-1924
TEL: (605) 361-5000
FAX: (605) 361-5005
TOLL FREE: (800) 374-0008

WISCONSIN CLAIMS OFFICE
3232 N BALLARD RD
PO BOX 2639
APPLETON, WI 54913-2639
TEL: (920) 739-5514
FAX: (920) 739-8407
TOLL FREE: (800) 374-1111
WWW.AMFAM.COM

3119 GOLF RD
PO BOX 1550
EAU CLAIRE, WI 54702-1550
TEL: (715) 834-6626
FAX: (715) 834-6175
TOLL FREE: (800) 374-1111
WWW.AMFAM.COM

PO BOX 899
JANESVILLE, WI 53547-0899
TEL: (608) 756-3671
FAX: (608) 756-1908
TOLL FREE: (800) 374-1111
WWW.AMFAM.COM

AMERICAN FAMILY MUTUAL INSURANCE
440 S EXECUTIVE DR
PO BOX 2927
MILWAUKEE, WI 53201-2927
TEL: (414) 784-9100
FAX: (414) 784-0684
TOLL FREE: (800) 374-1111
WWW.AMFAM.COM

PO BOX 69
ONALASKA, WI 54650-0069
TEL: (608) 781-2880
FAX: (608) 781-2868
TOLL FREE: (800) 374-1111
WWW.AMFAM.COM

AMERICAN FAMILY MUTUAL INSURANCE
5439 DURAND AVE, STE 100
RACINE, WI 53406-5008
TEL: (414) 552-8080
FAX: (414) 554-4659
TOLL FREE: (800) 374-1111
WWW.AMFAM.COM

AMERICAN FAMILY MUTUAL INSURANCE
PO BOX 530
SCHOFIELD, WI 54476-0530
TEL: (715) 359-9487
TOLL FREE: (800) 374-1111
WWW.AMFAM.COM

AMERICAN FAMILY LIFE ASSURANCE CO

GEORGIA CLAIMS OFFICE
AFLAC
1932 WYNNTON RD
COLUMBUS, GA 31999
TEL: (706) 323-3431
TOLL FREE: (800) 992-3522
WWW.AFLAC.COM

AMERICAN FAMILY MUTUAL INSURANCE

NEBRASKA CLAIMS OFFICE
AMERICAN STANDARD INSURANCE
10843 OLD MILL RD
OMAHA, NE 68154-2643
TEL: (402) 330-1010
FAX: (402) 330-6123
TOLL FREE: (800) 374-1111
WWW.AMFAM.COM

WISCONSIN CLAIMS OFFICE
6000 AMERICAN PKY
MADISON, WI 53783-0001
TEL: (608) 249-2111
FAX: (608) 243-4910
TOLL FREE: (800) 374-0008

AMERICAN FIDELITY ASSURANCE CO

NATIONAL CLAIMS OFFICE
2000 CLASSEN BLVD
PO BOX 25523
OKLAHOMA CITY, OK 73125-0523
TEL: (405) 523-2000
FAX: (405) 523-5762
TOLL FREE: (800) 955-0789
WWW.AF-GROUP.COM

2000 CLASSEN BLVD
PO BOX 25160
OKLAHOMA CITY, OK 73125-0160
TEL: (405) 523-5025
FAX: (405) 523-5762
TOLL FREE: (800) 662-1113
WWW.AF-GROUP.COM

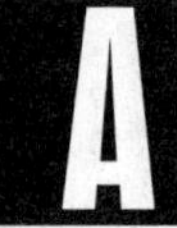

AMERICAN FREIGHTWAYS, INC
ARKANSAS CLAIMS OFFICE
2200 FORWARD DR
PO BOX 840
HARRISON, AR 72602-0840
TEL: (870) 741-9000
FAX: (870) 741-3003
TOLL FREE: (800) 874-4723

AMERICAN GENERAL LIFE & ACCIDENT INSURANCE CO
TENNESSEE CLAIMS OFFICE
AMERICAN GENERAL CTR
PO BOX 1500
NASHVILLE, TN 37202-1500
TEL: (615) 749-1000
FAX: (615) 749-2932
TOLL FREE: (800) 888-2452

AMERICAN GENERAL LIFE INSURANCE CO OF NEW YORK
NEW YORK CLAIMS OFFICE
300 S STATE ST
SYRACUSE, NY 13202
TEL: (315) 471-1121
FAX: (315) 471-4423
TOLL FREE: (800) 456-4441

AMERICAN GROUP ADMINISTRATORS
3010 WESTCHESTER AVE
PURCHASE, NY 10577
TEL: (914) 694-1200
FAX: (914) 694-2518
TOLL FREE: (800) 826-5722

AMERICAN GROUP ADMINISTRATORS, INC
TENNESSEE CLAIMS OFFICE
ASSOCIATED HEALTH SERVICES
260 W MAIN ST, STE 215
PO BOX 1349
HENDERSONVILLE, TN 37077-1349
TEL: (615) 824-7931
FAX: (615) 824-7257
TOLL FREE: (800) 346-6509
WWW.AGA+AHSA.COM

AMERICAN HARDWARE INSURANCE GROUP
MINNESOTA CLAIMS OFFICE
5995 OPUS PKY
PO BOX 435
MINNEAPOLIS, MN 55440-0435
TEL: (612) 935-1400
FAX: (612) 935-7823
TOLL FREE: (800) 544-8400

AMERICAN HEALTH CARE
NATIONAL CLAIMS OFFICE
PO BOX 7000
RICHTON, IL 60471
TEL: (630) 916-8400
FAX: (630) 261-7988
TOLL FREE: (800) 624-8568

AMERICAN HEALTH CARE PROVIDERS, INC
ARKANSAS CLAIMS OFFICE
900 S SHACKLEFORD RD, STE 110
LITTLE ROCK, AR 72211-3845
TEL: (501) 221-3534
FAX: (501) 221-3049
TOLL FREE: (800) 333-3534

AMERICAN OCCUPATIONAL HEALTH SERVICES
4601 SAUK TRAIL
PO BOX 7000
RICHTON PARK, IL 60471
TEL: (708) 503-5000
FAX: (708) 503-5001
TOLL FREE: (800) 242-7460

ILLINOIS CLAIMS OFFICE
AMERICAN OCCUPATIONAL HEALTH SERVICES
4601 SAUK TRAIL
PO BOX 7000
RICHTON PARK, IL 60471
TEL: (708) 503-5000
FAX: (708) 503-5001
TOLL FREE: (800) 242-7460

INDIANA CLAIMS OFFICE
AMERICAN OCCUPATIONAL HEALTH SERVICES
4601 SAUK TRAIL
PO BOX 7000
RICHTON PARK, IL 60471
TEL: (708) 503-5000
FAX: (708) 503-5001
TOLL FREE: (800) 242-7460

AMERICAN HEALTHCARE PROVIDERS
ILLINOIS CLAIMS OFFICE
MAXICARE ILLINOIS
4601 SAUX TRAIL
RICHTON PARK, IL 60471
TOLL FREE: (800) 688-6294

AMERICAN HERITAGE LIFE INSURANCE CO
FLORIDA CLAIMS OFFICE
1776 AMERICAN HERITAGE LIFE DR
JACKSONVILLE, FL 32224-3492
TEL: (904) 992-1776
FAX: (904) 992-2695
TOLL FREE: (800) 535-8086

AMERICAN HOME ASSURANCE CO
NEW YORK CLAIMS OFFICE
70 PINE ST
NEW YORK, NY 10270
TEL: (212) 770-7000
FAX: (212) 943-1125

AMERICAN INCOME LIFE INSURANCE CO
NATIONAL CLAIMS OFFICE
1200 WOODED ACRES
PO BOX 2608
WACO, TX 76797-0001
TEL: (254) 751-8600
FAX: (254) 751-8637
TOLL FREE: (800) 433-3405
WWW.AILINS.COM

AMERICAN INDUSTRIES
TEXAS CLAIMS OFFICE
6006 BELLAIRE BLVD
PO BOX 2952
HOUSTON, TX 77252-2952
TEL: (713) 667-7566
FAX: (713) 661-5659
TOLL FREE: (800) 881-4404

AMERICAN INSURANCE ADMINISTRATORS, INC
CALIFORNIA CLAIMS OFFICE
3415 S SEPULVEDA, STE 200
LOS ANGELES, CA 90034-6035
TEL: (310) 397-7220
FAX: (310) 398-6105
IN-STATE: (800) 654-7942

AMERICAN INVESTORS LIFE INSURANCE CO, INC
ARKANSAS CLAIMS OFFICE
SEWOLL ASSOCIATES
#10 SHACKLEFORD PLZ
PO BOX 8212
LITTLE ROCK, AR 72221-8212
TEL: (501) 227-6660
FAX: (501) 227-4430
TOLL FREE: (800) 467-0028

AMERICAN LIFE & HEALTH INSURANCE CO
CALIFORNIA CLAIMS OFFICE
23092 MILL CREEK RD
PO BOX 3680
LAGUNA HILLS, CA 92654
TEL: (949) 380-0880
FAX: (949) 859-2815
TOLL FREE: (800) 338-7634

AMERICAN LIFE INSURANCE CO
ILLINOIS CLAIMS OFFICE
208 S LA SALLE ST, STE 2070
CHICAGO, IL 60604
TEL: (312) 372-5722
FAX: (312) 372-5727

Casualty/Liability · Dental · Disability · EMC · HCPCS · Home Health · HMO · Medical

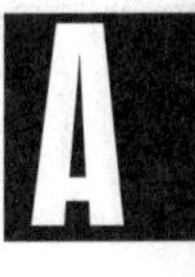

AMERICAN MAYFLOWER LIFE INSURANCE CO OF NEW YORK

NEW YORK CLAIMS OFFICE
GE FINANCIAL ASSURANCE COMPANY
125 PARK AVE- 6TH FL
PO BOX 3045
NEW YORK, NY 10163
TEL: (212) 672-4200
FAX: (212) 672-4299
TOLL FREE: (888) 265-5433

AMERICAN MEDICAL & LIFE INSURANCE CO

35 N BROADWAY
HICKSVILLE, NY 11801-4236
TEL: (516) 822-8700
FAX: (516) 931-1010
TOLL FREE: (800) 822-0004

AMERICAN MEDICAL SECURITY

ALABAMA CLAIMS OFFICE
3100 AMS BLVD
PO BOX 19032
GREEN BAY, WI 54307-9032
TEL: (920) 661-1111
FAX: (920) 661-6161
TOLL FREE: (800) 232-5432
WWW.AMSCHOICES.COM

ARIZONA CLAIMS OFFICE
3100 AMS BLVD
PO BOX 19032
GREEN BAY, WI 54307-9032
TEL: (920) 661-1111
FAX: (920) 661-6161
TOLL FREE: (800) 232-5432
WWW.AMSCHOICES.COM

ARKANSAS CLAIMS OFFICE
3100 AMS BLVD
PO BOX 19032
GREEN BAY, WI 54307-9032
TEL: (920) 661-1111
FAX: (920) 661-6161
TOLL FREE: (800) 232-5432
WWW.AMSCHOICES.COM

COLORADO CLAIMS OFFICE
3100 AMS BLVD
PO BOX 19032
GREEN BAY, WI 54307-9032
TEL: (920) 661-1111
FAX: (920) 661-6161
TOLL FREE: (800) 232-5432
WWW.AMSCHOICES.COM

DELAWARE CLAIMS OFFICE
3100 AMS BLVD
PO BOX 19032
GREEN BAY, WI 54307-9032
TEL: (920) 661-1111
FAX: (920) 661-6161
TOLL FREE: (800) 232-5432
WWW.AMSCHOICES.COM

DISTRICT OF COLUMBIA CLAIMS OFFICE
3100 AMS BLVD
PO BOX 19032
GREEN BAY, WI 54307-9032
TEL: (920) 661-1111
FAX: (920) 661-6161
TOLL FREE: (800) 232-5432
WWW.AMSCHOICES.COM

FLORIDA CLAIMS OFFICE
3100 AMS BLVD
PO BOX 19032
GREEN BAY, WI 54307-9032
TEL: (920) 661-1111
FAX: (920) 661-6161
TOLL FREE: (800) 232-5432
WWW.AMSCHOICES.COM

GEORGIA CLAIMS OFFICE
3100 AMS BLVD
PO BOX 19032
GREEN BAY, WI 54307-9032
TEL: (920) 661-1111
FAX: (920) 661-6161
TOLL FREE: (800) 232-5432
WWW.AMSCHOICES.COM

ILLINOIS CLAIMS OFFICE
3100 AMS BLVD
PO BOX 19032
GREEN BAY, WI 54307-9032
TEL: (920) 661-1111
FAX: (920) 661-6161
TOLL FREE: (800) 232-5432
WWW.AMSCHOICES.COM

INDIANA CLAIMS OFFICE
3100 AMS BLVD
PO BOX 19032
GREEN BAY, WI 54307-9032
TEL: (920) 661-1111
FAX: (920) 661-6161
TOLL FREE: (800) 232-5432
WWW.AMSCHOICES.COM

IOWA CLAIMS OFFICE
3100 AMS BLVD
PO BOX 19032
GREEN BAY, WI 54307-9032
TEL: (920) 661-1111
FAX: (920) 661-6161
TOLL FREE: (800) 232-5432
WWW.AMSCHOICES.COM

KANSAS CLAIMS OFFICE
3100 AMS BLVD
PO BOX 19032
GREEN BAY, WI 54307-9032
TEL: (920) 661-1111
FAX: (920) 661-6161
TOLL FREE: (800) 232-5432
WWW.AMSCHOICES.COM

LOUISIANA CLAIMS OFFICE
3100 AMS BLVD
PO BOX 19032
GREEN BAY, WI 54307-9032
TEL: (920) 661-1111
FAX: (920) 661-6161
TOLL FREE: (800) 232-5432
WWW.AMSCHOICES.COM

MARYLAND CLAIMS OFFICE
3100 AMS BLVD
PO BOX 19032
GREEN BAY, WI 54307-9032
TEL: (920) 661-1111
FAX: (920) 661-6161
TOLL FREE: (800) 232-5432
WWW.AMSCHOICES.COM

MICHIGAN CLAIMS OFFICE
3100 AMS BLVD
PO BOX 19032
GREEN BAY, WI 54307-9032
TEL: (920) 661-1111
FAX: (920) 661-6161
TOLL FREE: (800) 232-5432
WWW.AMSCHOICES.COM

MINNESOTA CLAIMS OFFICE
3100 AMS BLVD
PO BOX 19032
GREEN BAY, WI 54307-9032
TEL: (920) 661-1111
FAX: (920) 661-6161
TOLL FREE: (800) 232-5432
WWW.AMSCHOICES.COM

MISSISSIPPI CLAIMS OFFICE
3100 AMS BLVD
PO BOX 19032
GREEN BAY, WI 54307-9032
TEL: (920) 661-1111
FAX: (920) 661-6161
TOLL FREE: (800) 232-5432
WWW.AMSCHOICES.COM

MISSOURI CLAIMS OFFICE
3100 AMS BLVD
PO BOX 19032
GREEN BAY, WI 54307-9032
TEL: (920) 661-1111
FAX: (920) 661-6161
TOLL FREE: (800) 232-5432
WWW.AMSCHOICES.COM

NEBRASKA CLAIMS OFFICE
3100 AMS BLVD
PO BOX 19032
GREEN BAY, WI 54307-9032
TEL: (920) 661-1111
FAX: (920) 661-6161
TOLL FREE: (800) 232-5432
WWW.AMSCHOICES.COM

NEVADA CLAIMS OFFICE
3100 AMS BLVD
PO BOX 19032
GREEN BAY, WI 54307-9032
TEL: (920) 661-1111
FAX: (920) 661-6161
TOLL FREE: (800) 232-5432
WWW.AMSCHOICES.COM

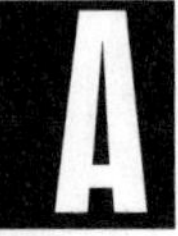

NEW MEXICO CLAIMS OFFICE
3100 AMS BLVD
PO BOX 19032
GREEN BAY, WI 54307-9032
TEL: (920) 661-1111
FAX: (920) 661-6161
TOLL FREE: (800) 232-5432
WWW.AMSCHOICES.COM

NORTH CAROLINA CLAIMS OFFICE
3100 AMS BLVD
PO BOX 19032
GREEN BAY, WI 54307-9032
TEL: (920) 661-1111
FAX: (920) 661-6161
TOLL FREE: (800) 232-5432
WWW.AMSCHOICES.COM

NORTH DAKOTA CLAIMS OFFICE
3100 AMS BLVD
PO BOX 19032
GREEN BAY, WI 54307-9032
TEL: (920) 661-1111
FAX: (920) 661-6161
TOLL FREE: (800) 232-5432
WWW.AMSCHOICES.COM

OHIO CLAIMS OFFICE
3100 AMS BLVD
PO BOX 19032
GREEN BAY, WI 54307-9032
TEL: (920) 661-1111
FAX: (920) 661-6161
TOLL FREE: (800) 232-5432
WWW.AMSCHOICES.COM

OKLAHOMA CLAIMS OFFICE
3100 AMS BLVD
PO BOX 19032
GREEN BAY, WI 54307-9032
TEL: (920) 661-1111
FAX: (920) 661-6161
TOLL FREE: (800) 232-5432
WWW.AMSCHOICES.COM

PENNSYLVANIA CLAIMS OFFICE
3100 AMS BLVD
PO BOX 19032
GREEN BAY, WI 54307-9032
TEL: (920) 661-1111
FAX: (920) 661-6161
TOLL FREE: (800) 232-5432
WWW.AMSCHOICES.COM

SOUTH CAROLINA CLAIMS OFFICE
3100 AMS BLVD
PO BOX 19032
GREEN BAY, WI 54307-9032
TEL: (920) 661-1111
FAX: (920) 661-6161
TOLL FREE: (800) 232-5432
WWW.AMSCHOICES.COM

SOUTH DAKOTA CLAIMS OFFICE
3100 AMS BLVD
PO BOX 19032
GREEN BAY, WI 54307-9032
TEL: (920) 661-1111
FAX: (920) 661-6161
TOLL FREE: (800) 232-5432
WWW.AMSCHOICES.COM

TENNESSEE CLAIMS OFFICE
3100 AMS BLVD
PO BOX 19032
GREEN BAY, WI 54307-9032
TEL: (920) 661-1111
FAX: (920) 661-6161
TOLL FREE: (800) 232-5432
WWW.AMSCHOICES.COM

TEXAS CLAIMS OFFICE
3100 AMS BLVD
PO BOX 19032
GREEN BAY, WI 54307-9032
TEL: (920) 661-1111
FAX: (920) 661-6161
TOLL FREE: (800) 232-5432
WWW.AMSCHOICES.COM

UTAH CLAIMS OFFICE
3100 AMS BLVD
PO BOX 19032
GREEN BAY, WI 54307-9032
TEL: (920) 661-1111
FAX: (920) 661-6161
TOLL FREE: (800) 232-5432
WWW.AMSCHOICES.COM

VIRGINIA CLAIMS OFFICE
3100 AMS BLVD
PO BOX 19032
GREEN BAY, WI 54307-9032
TEL: (920) 661-1111
FAX: (920) 661-6161
TOLL FREE: (800) 232-5432
WWW.AMSCHOICES.COM

WASHINGTON CLAIMS OFFICE
3100 AMS BLVD
PO BOX 19032
GREEN BAY, WI 54307-9032
TEL: (920) 661-1111
FAX: (920) 661-6161
TOLL FREE: (800) 232-5432
WWW.AMSCHOICES.COM

WEST VIRGINIA CLAIMS OFFICE
3100 AMS BLVD
PO BOX 19032
GREEN BAY, WI 54307-9032
TEL: (920) 661-1111
FAX: (920) 661-6161
TOLL FREE: (800) 232-5432
WWW.AMSCHOICES.COM

WISCONSIN CLAIMS OFFICE
3100 AMS BLVD
PO BOX 19032
GREEN BAY, WI 54307-9032
TEL: (920) 661-1111
FAX: (920) 661-6161
TOLL FREE: (800) 232-5432
WWW.AMSCHOICES.COM

AMERICAN MINING INSURANCE CO, INC

ALABAMA CLAIMS OFFICE
CGH INSURANCE GROUP
550 MONTGOMERY HWY
PO BOX 660847
BIRMINGHAM, AL 35266-0847
TEL: (205) 823-4496
FAX: (205) 823-6177
TOLL FREE: (800) 448-5621
WWW.CGHINSURANCE.COM

AMERICAN MODERN INSURANCE GROUP

OHIO CLAIMS OFFICE
7000 MIDLAND BLVD
PO BOX 5323
AMELIA, OH 45201-5323
TEL: (513) 943-7100
FAX: (513) 943-7363
TOLL FREE: (800) 543-2644
WWW.MIDLANDCOMPANY.COM

AMERICAN MUTUAL REINSURANCE CO

ILLINOIS CLAIMS OFFICE
222 MERCHANDISE MART PLZ, STE 1450
CHICAGO, IL 60654
TEL: (312) 836-9500
FAX: (312) 836-1944

AMERICAN NATIONAL INSURANCE CO

TEXAS CLAIMS OFFICE
1 MOODY PLZ
PO BOX 1520
GALVESTON, TX 77550-1520
TEL: (409) 763-4661
FAX: (409) 766-6694
TOLL FREE: (800) 899-6805
WWW.ANICO.COM

AMERICAN NATIONAL PROPERTY & CASUALTY CO

ALABAMA CLAIMS OFFICE
ATTN: CLAIMS
1949 E SUNSHINE ST
SPRINGFIELD, MO 65899-0001
TEL: (417) 887-0220
FAX: (417) 887-1801
TOLL FREE: (800) 333-2860
WWW.ANPAC.COM

ALASKA CLAIMS OFFICE
ATTN: CLAIMS
1949 E SUNSHINE ST
SPRINGFIELD, MO 65899-0001
TEL: (417) 887-0220
FAX: (417) 887-1801
TOLL FREE: (800) 333-2860
WWW.ANPAC.COM

ARIZONA CLAIMS OFFICE
ATTN: CLAIMS
1949 E SUNSHINE ST
SPRINGFIELD, MO 65899-0001
TEL: (417) 887-0220
FAX: (417) 887-1801
TOLL FREE: (800) 333-2860
WWW.ANPAC.COM

ARKANSAS CLAIMS OFFICE
ATTN: CLAIMS
1949 E SUNSHINE ST
SPRINGFIELD, MO 65899-0001
TEL: (417) 887-0220
FAX: (417) 887-1801
TOLL FREE: (800) 333-2860
WWW.ANPAC.COM

CALIFORNIA CLAIMS OFFICE
ATTN: CLAIMS
1949 E SUNSHINE ST
SPRINGFIELD, MO 65899-0001
TEL: (417) 887-0220
FAX: (417) 887-1801
TOLL FREE: (800) 333-2860
WWW.ANPAC.COM

COLORADO CLAIMS OFFICE
ATTN: CLAIMS
1949 E SUNSHINE ST
SPRINGFIELD, MO 65899-0001
TEL: (417) 887-0220
FAX: (417) 887-1801
TOLL FREE: (800) 333-2860
WWW.ANPAC.COM

FLORIDA CLAIMS OFFICE
ATTN: CLAIMS
1949 E SUNSHINE ST
SPRINGFIELD, MO 65899-0001
TEL: (417) 887-0220
FAX: (417) 887-1801
TOLL FREE: (800) 333-2860
WWW.ANPAC.COM

GEORGIA CLAIMS OFFICE
ATTN: CLAIMS
1949 E SUNSHINE ST
SPRINGFIELD, MO 65899-0001
TEL: (417) 887-0220
FAX: (417) 887-1801
TOLL FREE: (800) 333-2860
WWW.ANPAC.COM

IDAHO CLAIMS OFFICE
ATTN: CLAIMS
1949 E SUNSHINE ST
SPRINGFIELD, MO 65899-0001
TEL: (417) 887-0220
FAX: (417) 887-1801
TOLL FREE: (800) 333-2860
WWW.ANPAC.COM

ILLINOIS CLAIMS OFFICE
ATTN: CLAIMS
1949 E SUNSHINE ST
SPRINGFIELD, MO 65899-0001
TEL: (417) 887-0220
FAX: (417) 887-1801
TOLL FREE: (800) 333-2860
WWW.ANPAC.COM

INDIANA CLAIMS OFFICE
ATTN: CLAIMS
1949 E SUNSHINE ST
SPRINGFIELD, MO 65899-0001
TEL: (417) 887-0220
FAX: (417) 887-1801
TOLL FREE: (800) 333-2860
WWW.ANPAC.COM

IOWA CLAIMS OFFICE
ATTN: CLAIMS
1949 E SUNSHINE ST
SPRINGFIELD, MO 65899-0001
TEL: (417) 887-0220
FAX: (417) 887-1801
TOLL FREE: (800) 333-2860
WWW.ANPAC.COM

KANSAS CLAIMS OFFICE
ATTN: CLAIMS
1949 E SUNSHINE ST
SPRINGFIELD, MO 65899-0001
TEL: (417) 887-0220
FAX: (417) 887-1801
TOLL FREE: (800) 333-2860
WWW.ANPAC.COM

KENTUCKY CLAIMS OFFICE
ATTN: CLAIMS
1949 E SUNSHINE ST
SPRINGFIELD, MO 65899-0001
TEL: (417) 887-0220
FAX: (417) 887-1801
TOLL FREE: (800) 333-2860
WWW.ANPAC.COM

LOUISIANA CLAIMS OFFICE
ATTN: CLAIMS
1949 E SUNSHINE ST
SPRINGFIELD, MO 65899-0001
TEL: (417) 887-0220
FAX: (417) 887-1801
TOLL FREE: (800) 333-2860
WWW.ANPAC.COM

MISSISSIPPI CLAIMS OFFICE
ATTN: CLAIMS
1949 E SUNSHINE ST
SPRINGFIELD, MO 65899-0001
TEL: (417) 887-0220
FAX: (417) 887-1801
TOLL FREE: (800) 333-2860
WWW.ANPAC.COM

MISSOURI CLAIMS OFFICE
ATTN: CLAIMS
1949 E SUNSHINE ST
SPRINGFIELD, MO 65899-0001
TEL: (417) 887-0220
FAX: (417) 887-1801
TOLL FREE: (800) 333-2860
WWW.ANPAC.COM

MONTANA CLAIMS OFFICE
ATTN: CLAIMS
1949 E SUNSHINE ST
SPRINGFIELD, MO 65899-0001
TEL: (417) 887-0220
FAX: (417) 887-1801
TOLL FREE: (800) 333-2860
WWW.ANPAC.COM

NEBRASKA CLAIMS OFFICE
ATTN: CLAIMS
1949 E SUNSHINE ST
SPRINGFIELD, MO 65899-0001
TEL: (417) 887-0220
FAX: (417) 887-1801
TOLL FREE: (800) 333-2860
WWW.ANPAC.COM

NEVADA CLAIMS OFFICE
ATTN: CLAIMS
1949 E SUNSHINE ST
SPRINGFIELD, MO 65899-0001
TEL: (417) 887-0220
FAX: (417) 887-1801
TOLL FREE: (800) 333-2860
WWW.ANPAC.COM

NEW MEXICO CLAIMS OFFICE
ATTN: CLAIMS
1949 E SUNSHINE ST
SPRINGFIELD, MO 65899-0001
TEL: (417) 887-0220
FAX: (417) 887-1801
TOLL FREE: (800) 333-2860
WWW.ANPAC.COM

NORTH CAROLINA CLAIMS OFFICE
ATTN: CLAIMS
1949 E SUNSHINE ST
SPRINGFIELD, MO 65899-0001
TEL: (417) 887-0220
FAX: (417) 887-1801
TOLL FREE: (800) 333-2860
WWW.ANPAC.COM

NORTH DAKOTA CLAIMS OFFICE
ATTN: CLAIMS
1949 E SUNSHINE ST
SPRINGFIELD, MO 65899-0001
TEL: (417) 887-0220
FAX: (417) 887-1801
TOLL FREE: (800) 333-2860
WWW.ANPAC.COM

OKLAHOMA CLAIMS OFFICE
ATTN: CLAIMS
1949 E SUNSHINE ST
SPRINGFIELD, MO 65899-0001
TEL: (417) 887-0220
FAX: (417) 887-1801
TOLL FREE: (800) 333-2860
WWW.ANPAC.COM

OREGON CLAIMS OFFICE
ATTN: CLAIMS
1949 E SUNSHINE ST
SPRINGFIELD, MO 65899-0001
TEL: (417) 887-0220
FAX: (417) 887-1801
TOLL FREE: (800) 333-2860
WWW.ANPAC.COM

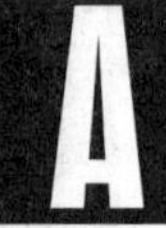

PENNSYLVANIA CLAIMS OFFICE
ATTN: CLAIMS
1949 E SUNSHINE ST
SPRINGFIELD, MO 65899-0001
TEL: (417) 887-0220
FAX: (417) 887-1801
TOLL FREE: (800) 333-2860
WWW.ANPAC.COM

SOUTH CAROLINA CLAIMS OFFICE
ATTN: CLAIMS
1949 E SUNSHINE ST
SPRINGFIELD, MO 65899-0001
TEL: (417) 887-0220
FAX: (417) 887-1801
TOLL FREE: (800) 333-2860
WWW.ANPAC.COM

SOUTH DAKOTA CLAIMS OFFICE
ATTN: CLAIMS
1949 E SUNSHINE ST
SPRINGFIELD, MO 65899-0001
TEL: (417) 887-0220
FAX: (417) 887-1801
TOLL FREE: (800) 333-2860
WWW.ANPAC.COM

TENNESSEE CLAIMS OFFICE
ATTN: CLAIMS
1949 E SUNSHINE ST
SPRINGFIELD, MO 65899-0001
TEL: (417) 887-0220
FAX: (417) 887-1801
TOLL FREE: (800) 333-2860
WWW.ANPAC.COM

TEXAS CLAIMS OFFICE
ATTN: CLAIMS
1949 E SUNSHINE ST
SPRINGFIELD, MO 65899-0001
TEL: (417) 887-0220
FAX: (417) 887-1801
TOLL FREE: (800) 333-2860
WWW.ANPAC.COM

UTAH CLAIMS OFFICE
ATTN: CLAIMS
1949 E SUNSHINE ST
SPRINGFIELD, MO 65899-0001
TEL: (417) 887-0220
FAX: (417) 887-1801
TOLL FREE: (800) 333-2860
WWW.ANPAC.COM

VIRGINIA CLAIMS OFFICE
ATTN: CLAIMS
1949 E SUNSHINE ST
SPRINGFIELD, MO 65899-0001
TEL: (417) 887-0220
FAX: (417) 887-1801
TOLL FREE: (800) 333-2860
WWW.ANPAC.COM

WASHINGTON CLAIMS OFFICE
ATTN: CLAIMS
1949 E SUNSHINE ST
SPRINGFIELD, MO 65899-0001
TEL: (417) 887-0220
FAX: (417) 887-1801
TOLL FREE: (800) 333-2860
WWW.ANPAC.COM

WEST VIRGINIA CLAIMS OFFICE
ATTN: CLAIMS
1949 E SUNSHINE ST
SPRINGFIELD, MO 65899-0001
TEL: (417) 887-0220
FAX: (417) 887-1801
TOLL FREE: (800) 333-2860
WWW.ANPAC.COM

WYOMING CLAIMS OFFICE
ATTN: CLAIMS
1949 E SUNSHINE ST
SPRINGFIELD, MO 65899-0001
TEL: (417) 887-0220
FAX: (417) 887-1801
TOLL FREE: (800) 333-2860
WWW.ANPAC.COM

AMERICAN PIONEER LIFE

FLORIDA CLAIMS OFFICE
11 N BAYLEN ST
PO BOX 130
PENSACOLA, FL 32591-0130
TEL: (850) 469-8220
FAX: (850) 433-1186
TOLL FREE: (800) 999-2224

AMERICAN PIONEER LIFE INSURANCE CO

600 COURTLAND ST, STE 600
PO BOX 3509
ORLANDO, FL 32802-3509
TEL: (407) 628-1776
FAX: (407) 628-3679
TOLL FREE: (800) 538-1053

NEW YORK CLAIMS OFFICE
600 COURTLAND ST, STE 600
PO BOX 3509
ORLANDO, FL 32802-3509
TEL: (407) 628-1776
FAX: (407) 628-3679
TOLL FREE: (800) 538-1053

AMERICAN POLICY HOLDERS LIQUIDATING TRUST

MASSACHUSETTS CLAIMS OFFICE
11 NORTH AVE
PO BOX 1620
BURLINGTON, MA 01803-3305
TEL: (781) 221-1600
FAX: (781) 270-9740
TOLL FREE: (800) 225-3646
IN-STATE: (800) 284-3571

AMERICAN POSTAL WORKERS UNION HEALTH PLAN

NATIONAL CLAIMS OFFICE
12345 NEW COLUMBIA PIKE
PO BOX 967
SILVER SPRING, MD 20910-0967
TEL: (301) 622-1700
FAX: (301) 622-6074
TOLL FREE: (800) 222-2798
IN-STATE: (800) 222-2798
WWW.APWUHP.COM

AMERICAN PROGRESSIVE LIFE & HEALTH INSURANCE CO

SENIOR HEALTH SERVICE CENTER
PO BOX 130
PENSACOLA, FL 32591-0130
TOLL FREE: (800) 645-4116

NEW YORK CLAIMS OFFICE
6 INTERNATIONAL DR
RYE BROOK, NY 10573
TEL: (914) 934-8300
FAX: (914) 934-9123
TOLL FREE: (800) 332-3377

AMERICAN PROTECTION INSURANCE CO

COLORADO CLAIMS OFFICE
KEMPER NATIONAL INSURANCE CO
10375 E HARVARD AVE
PO BOX 5347
DENVER, CO 80217
TEL: (303) 696-1441
FAX: (303) 752-5425
TOLL FREE: (800) 321-9515

AMERICAN PUBLIC LIFE INSURANCE CO

MISSISSIPPI CLAIMS OFFICE
2305 LAKELAND DR
PO BOX 925
JACKSON, MS 39208
TEL: (601) 936-6600
FAX: (601) 939-0655
TOLL FREE: (800) 256-8606

AMERICAN REPUBLIC INSURANCE CO

IOWA CLAIMS OFFICE
NATIONAL HEADQUARTERS
601 6TH AVE
PO BOX 10
DES MOINES, IA 50301-0001
TEL: (515) 245-2000
FAX: (515) 245-4282
TOLL FREE: (800) 247-2190

AMERICAN RESERVE LIFE INSURANCE CO

OKLAHOMA CLAIMS OFFICE
1722 S CARSON AVE, STE 3200
TULSA, OK 74119-4617
TEL: (918) 583-8585
FAX: (918) 583-2738
TOLL FREE: (800) 753-4243

AMERICAN RESOURCES INSURANCE CO

ALABAMA CLAIMS OFFICE
1111 HILLCREST RD
PO BOX 91149
MOBILE, AL 36691
TEL: (334) 639-0985
FAX: (334) 633-2944
TOLL FREE: (800) 826-6570

KENTUCKY CLAIMS OFFICE
1111 HILLCREST RD
PO BOX 91149
MOBILE, AL 36691
TEL: (334) 639-0985
FAX: (334) 633-2944
TOLL FREE: (800) 826-6570

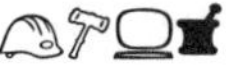

AMERICAN SECURITY INSURANCE CO

GEORGIA CLAIMS OFFICE
260 INTERSTATE NORTH CIRCLE SE
PO BOX 50355
ATLANTA, GA 30327
TEL: (707) 763-1000

AMERICAN SENTINEL INSURANCE CO

MARYLAND CLAIMS OFFICE
1800 LINGLESTOWN, STE 305
HARRISBURG, PA 17110-3343
TEL: (717) 238-4559
FAX: (717) 238-8531
TOLL FREE: (800) 692-7338

PENNSYLVANIA CLAIMS OFFICE
1800 LINGLESTOWN, STE 305
HARRISBURG, PA 17110-3343
TEL: (717) 238-4559
FAX: (717) 238-8531
TOLL FREE: (800) 692-7338

AMERICAN SERVICE LIFE INSURANCE CO

TEXAS CLAIMS OFFICE
9151 GRAPEVINE HWY
PO BOX 982017
NORTH RICHLAND HILLS, TX 76182
FAX: (817) 255-8101
TOLL FREE: (800) 733-8880
IN-STATE: (800) 733-1110

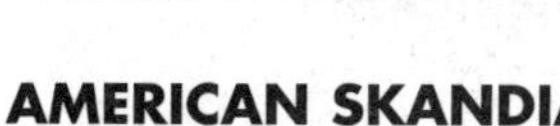

AMERICAN SKANDIA LIFE REINSURANCE CORP

CONNECTICUT CLAIMS OFFICE
1 CORPORATE DR
PO BOX 883
SHELTON, CT 06484-0883
TEL: (203) 926-1888
FAX: (203) 929-8071
TOLL FREE: (800) 752-6342
IN-STATE: (800) 704-6201
WWW.AMERICAN_SKANDIA.COM

AMERICAN SOUTHERN INSURANCE CO

NATIONAL CLAIMS OFFICE
3715 N SIDE PKY NW- BLDG 400- 8TH FL
PO BOX 723030
ATLANTA, GA 31139
TEL: (404) 266-9599
FAX: (404) 266-8327
TOLL FREE: (800) 241-1172

AMERICAN STATES INSURANCE CO

CONNECTICUT CLAIMS OFFICE
A SAFECO COMPANY
700 STANLEY DR
PO BOX 9010
NEW BRITAIN, CT 06050-9010
TEL: (860) 827-4200
FAX: (860) 827-4395
TOLL FREE: (800) 245-5365
WWW.SAFECO.COM

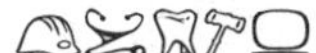

IOWA CLAIMS OFFICE
A SAFECO COMPANY
2001 52ND AVE, STE 1
PO BOX 8805
MOLINE, IL 61266
TEL: (309) 736-0502
FAX: (309) 736-1226

SOUTH DAKOTA CLAIMS OFFICE
A SAFECO COMPANY
PO BOX 84250
SIOUX FALLS, SD 57109-1002
TOLL FREE: (888) 557-5010
WWW.SAFECO.COM

AMERICAN TRAVEL, INC

INDIANA CLAIMS OFFICE
CONSECO
11815 N PENNSYLVANIA ST
CARMEL, IN 46082-1955
TEL: (317) 817-4200
FAX: (317) 817-3604
TOLL FREE: (800) 242-4852
WWW.CONSECO.COM

AMERICAN TRUST ADMINISTRATORS, INC

KANSAS CLAIMS OFFICE
CLAIMS DEPT
7101 COLLEGE BLVD, STE 1505
PO BOX 87
SHAWNEE MISSION, KS 66201
TEL: (913) 451-4900
FAX: (913) 451-0598
TOLL FREE: (800) 843-4121

AMERICAN UNDERWRITERS LIFE INSURANCE CO

1035 S 18300 ST W
PO BOX 9510
WICHITA, KS 67277-0510
TEL: (316) 794-2200
FAX: (316) 794-8470

AMERICAN UNION LIFE INSURANCE CO

ILLINOIS CLAIMS OFFICE
303 E WASHINGTON
PO BOX 2814
BLOOMINGTON, IL 61701-2814
TEL: (309) 829-1061
FAX: (309) 827-0303

AMERICAN UNITED LIFE INSURANCE CO

INDIANA CLAIMS OFFICE
1 AMERICAN SQ
PO BOX 368
INDIANAPOLIS, IN 46204
FAX: (317) 263-1033
TOLL FREE: (800) 553-3522

AMERICAN WEST INSURANCE CO

NORTH DAKOTA CLAIMS OFFICE
2100 LIBRARY CIR
PO BOX 13278
GRAND FORKS, ND 58208-3278
TEL: (701) 775-4226
FAX: (701) 780-1360
TOLL FREE: (800) 688-2942

AMERICAN YOUTH STUDENTS & SPORTS INSURANCE

ILLINOIS CLAIMS OFFICE
40 SHUMAN BLVD, STE 245
PO BOX 1390
WHEATON, IL 60189-1390
TEL: (630) 778-1900
FAX: (630) 778-1959
TOLL FREE: (800) 338-1938

AMERIHEALTH

FLORIDA CLAIMS OFFICE
10151 DEERWOOD PRK BLVD- BLDG 200, STE 400
PO BOX 40238
JACKSONVILLE, FL 32203
TEL: (904) 998-6700
FAX: (904) 998-5402
TOLL FREE: (800) 331-0017
IN-STATE: (800) 888-5256

PENNSYLVANIA CLAIMS OFFICE
720 BLAIR MILL RD
HORSHAM, PA 19044-2269
TEL: (215) 657-8900
FAX: (215) 784-0262
TOLL FREE: (800) 492-2385
WWW.AMERIHEALTHTPA.COM

TEXAS CLAIMS OFFICE
10151 DEERWOOD PRK BLVD- BLDG 200, STE 400
PO BOX 40238
JACKSONVILLE, FL 32203
TEL: (904) 998-6700
FAX: (904) 998-5411
TOLL FREE: (800) 274-5466

AMERIHEALTH ADMINISTRATORS

PENNSYLVANIA CLAIMS OFFICE
720 BLAIR MILL RD
HORSHAM, PA 19044
TEL: (610) 358-5711
FAX: (215) 241-0426
TOLL FREE: (800) 444-6282

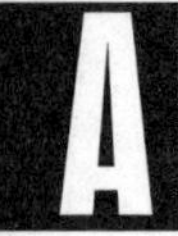

AMERIHEALTH HMO, INC

DELAWARE CLAIMS OFFICE
AMERIHEALTH INSURANCE CO
919 N MARKET ST
WILMINGTON, DE 19801-3021
FAX: (302) 777-6444
TOLL FREE: (800) 444-6282

NEW JERSEY CLAIMS OFFICE
AMERIHEALTH INSURANCE CO
919 N MARKET ST
WILMINGTON, DE 19801-3021
FAX: (302) 777-6444
TOLL FREE: (800) 444-6282

PENNSYLVANIA CLAIMS OFFICE
AMERIHEALTH INSURANCE CO
919 N MARKET ST
WILMINGTON, DE 19801-3021
FAX: (302) 777-6444
TOLL FREE: (800) 444-6282

AMERISURE COMPANIES

ALABAMA CLAIMS OFFICE
2100-A SOUTHBRIDGE PKY, STE 450
PO BOX 59867
BIRMINGHAM, AL 35259
TEL: (205) 879-3411
FAX: (205) 870-8768
IN-STATE: (800) 421-7656

FLORIDA CLAIMS OFFICE
6133 CENTRAL AVE
PO BOX 10790
SAINT PETERSBURG, FL 33733
TEL: (727) 381-6789
FAX: (727) 341-5403
TOLL FREE: (800) 282-2743

ILLINOIS CLAIMS OFFICE
701 EMERSON, STE 320
PO BOX 419058
SAINT LOUIS, MO 63141
TEL: (314) 994-3400
FAX: (314) 993-0791
TOLL FREE: (800) 325-1721

INDIANA CLAIMS OFFICE
3600 WOODVIEW TRACE
PO BOX 68876
INDIANAPOLIS, IN 46268-0876
TEL: (317) 872-8694
FAX: (800) 528-9187
TOLL FREE: (800) 752-5929
WWW.AMERISUE.COM

MICHIGAN CLAIMS OFFICE
26777 HALSTED
PO BOX 2060
FARMINGTON HILLS, MI 48333-2060
TEL: (248) 615-9000
FAX: (248) 615-8372
TOLL FREE: (800) 437-5735
IN-STATE: (800) 257-1900

207 E FULTON
PO BOX 116
GRAND RAPIDS, MI 49501-0116
TEL: (616) 451-2971
FAX: (616) 451-4579
TOLL FREE: (800) 632-4597

MISSOURI CLAIMS OFFICE
701 EMERSON, STE 320
PO BOX 419058
SAINT LOUIS, MO 63141
TEL: (314) 994-3400
FAX: (314) 993-0791
TOLL FREE: (800) 325-1721

NORTH CAROLINA CLAIMS OFFICE
PO BOX 560769
CHARLOTTE, NC 28256
TEL: (704) 510-1135
FAX: (704) 510-8327
TOLL FREE: (800) 532-6230

TENNESSEE CLAIMS OFFICE
57 GERMANTOWN CTR, STE 100
CORDOVA, TN 38018
TEL: (901) 682-3341
FAX: (901) 683-6001
IN-STATE: (800) 678-2637
WWW.AMERISURE.COM

TEXAS CLAIMS OFFICE
7610 STEMMONS FWY, STE 350
PO BOX 569680
DALLAS, TX 75356-9680
TEL: (214) 631-6370
FAX: (214) 634-9139
TOLL FREE: (800) 441-0293
WWW.AMERISURE.COM

AMERITAS LIFE INSURANCE CORP

NATIONAL CLAIMS OFFICE
5900 O ST
PO BOX 81889
LINCOLN, NE 68501
TEL: (402) 467-1122
FAX: (402) 467-7935
TOLL FREE: (800) 487-5553
E-MAIL: GROUP@AMERITAS.COM
WWW.AMERITAS.COM

AMERITECH CORP

ILLINOIS CLAIMS OFFICE
225 W RENDOLPH, STE 30B
CHICAGO, IL 60606
TEL: (312) 727-2993
FAX: (312) 845-3512
TOLL FREE: (888) 306-9288

INDIANA CLAIMS OFFICE
225 W RENDOLPH, STE 30B
CHICAGO, IL 60606
TEL: (312) 727-2993
FAX: (312) 845-3512
TOLL FREE: (888) 306-9288

MICHIGAN CLAIMS OFFICE
225 W RENDOLPH, STE 30B
CHICAGO, IL 60606
TEL: (312) 727-2993
FAX: (312) 845-3512
TOLL FREE: (888) 306-9288

OHIO CLAIMS OFFICE
225 W RENDOLPH, STE 30B
CHICAGO, IL 60606
TEL: (312) 727-2993
FAX: (312) 845-3512
TOLL FREE: (888) 306-9288

WISCONSIN CLAIMS OFFICE
225 W RENDOLPH, STE 30B
CHICAGO, IL 60606
TEL: (312) 727-2993
FAX: (312) 845-3512
TOLL FREE: (888) 306-9288

AMGUARD INSURANCE CO

DELAWARE CLAIMS OFFICE
NORGUARD OR EASTGUARD TITAN
16 S RIVER ST
PO BOX AH
WILKES-BARRE, PA 18703
TEL: (570) 829-5400
FAX: (570) 823-5930
TOLL FREE: (800) 673-2465

MAINE CLAIMS OFFICE
NORGUARD OR EASTGUARD TITAN
16 S RIVER ST
PO BOX AH
WILKES-BARRE, PA 18703
TEL: (570) 829-5400
FAX: (570) 823-5930
TOLL FREE: (800) 673-2465

MARYLAND CLAIMS OFFICE
NORGUARD OR EASTGUARD TITAN
16 S RIVER ST
PO BOX AH
WILKES-BARRE, PA 18703
TEL: (570) 829-5400
FAX: (570) 823-5930
TOLL FREE: (800) 673-2465

PENNSYLVANIA CLAIMS OFFICE
NORGUARD OR EASTGUARD TITAN
16 S RIVER ST
PO BOX AH
WILKES-BARRE, PA 18703
TEL: (570) 829-5400
FAX: (570) 823-5930
TOLL FREE: (800) 673-2465

AMICA MUTUAL INSURANCE

CALIFORNIA CLAIMS OFFICE
3200 PRK CTR DR, STE 300
COSTA MESA, CA 92626
TEL: (714) 444-1144
FAX: (714) 444-3166
TOLL FREE: (800) 242-6422

PO BOX 27717
SANTA ANA, CA 92799-7717
TEL: (714) 444-1144
FAX: (714) 978-0256
TOLL FREE: (800) 242-6422

RHODE ISLAND CLAIMS OFFICE
PO BOX 6008
PROVIDENCE, RI 02940-9986
TEL: (401) 334-6000
FAX: (401) 334-3672
TOLL FREE: (800) 99 AMICA (992-6422)

AMOCO INSURANCE PLANS

PENNSYLVANIA CLAIMS OFFICE
COMBINED INSURANCE COMPANY OF AMERICA
4850 STREET RD
TREVOSE, PA 19049-8000
TEL: (215) 953-3000
FAX: (215) 953-3156
TOLL FREE: (800) 626-0038

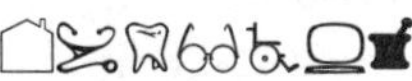

AMWAY CORP

MICHIGAN CLAIMS OFFICE
7575 E FULTON RD
ADA, MI 49355-0001
TEL: (616) 787-6000
FAX: (616) 787-6177
TOLL FREE: (800) 528-5748

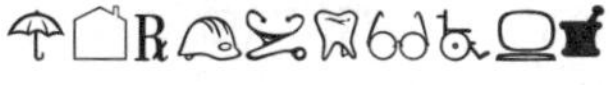

ANDERSON CO

NATIONAL CLAIMS OFFICE
USI
1250 WOODBRANCH PARK DR, STE 300
PO BOX 218060
HOUSTON, TX 77218-8060
TEL: (281) 496-3400
FAX: (281) 496-6729
TOLL FREE: (800) 583-0255

ANDREW JERGENS CO

OHIO CLAIMS OFFICE
2535 SPRING GROVE AVE
CINCINNATI, OH 45214-1729
TEL: (513) 421-1400
FAX: (513) 632-7759

ANTHEM BLUE CROSS & BLUE SHIELD

KENTUCKY CLAIMS OFFICE
ANTHEM BLUE CROSS & BLUE SHIELD OF SOUTHWEST OHIO
PO BOX 37180
LOUISVILLE, KY 40233
TEL: (513) 872-8100
FAX: (513) 872-8174
TOLL FREE: (800) 442-1832

OHIO CLAIMS OFFICE
30 MERCHANT ST, STE 350
CINCINNATI, OH 45246
TEL: (513) 326-9191
FAX: (513) 326-9192

2400 MARKET ST
YOUNGSTOWN, OH 44507
TEL: (330) 492-2151

ANTHEM BLUE CROSS BLUE SHIELD

1351 WILLIAM H TAFT RD
PO BOX 37180
CINCINNATI, OH 45206-7180
TEL: (513) 872-8100
TOLL FREE: (800) 442-1832

ANTHEM BLUE CROSS & BLUE SHIELD OF CONNECTICUT

CONNECTICUT CLAIMS OFFICE
370 BASSETT RD
HAVEN, CT 06473
TEL: (203) 239-4911
FAX: (203) 985-7834
TOLL FREE: (800) 922-4670
WWW.ANTHEMBCBSCT.COM

ANTHEM BLUE CROSS & BLUE SHIELD OF SOUTHWEST OHIO

OHIO CLAIMS OFFICE
PO BOX 37180
LOUISVILLE, KY 40233
TEL: (513) 872-8100
FAX: (513) 872-8174
TOLL FREE: (800) 442-1832

ANTHEM HEALTH

CALIFORNIA CLAIMS OFFICE
1188 FRANKLIN ST, STE 102
SAN FRANCISCO, CA 94109
TEL: (415) 928-4475
FAX: (415) 928-0361
TOLL FREE: (800) 955-7376

FLORIDA CLAIMS OFFICE
1188 FRANKLIN ST, STE 102
SAN FRANCISCO, CA 94109
TEL: (415) 928-4475
FAX: (415) 928-0361
TOLL FREE: (800) 955-7376

GEORGIA CLAIMS OFFICE
1188 FRANKLIN ST, STE 102
SAN FRANCISCO, CA 94109
TEL: (415) 928-4475
FAX: (415) 928-0361
TOLL FREE: (800) 955-7376

NEW JERSEY CLAIMS OFFICE
1188 FRANKLIN ST, STE 102
SAN FRANCISCO, CA 94109
TEL: (415) 928-4475
FAX: (415) 928-0361
TOLL FREE: (800) 955-7376

NEW YORK CLAIMS OFFICE
1188 FRANKLIN ST, STE 102
SAN FRANCISCO, CA 94109
TEL: (415) 928-4475
FAX: (415) 928-0361
TOLL FREE: (800) 955-7376

OHIO CLAIMS OFFICE
1188 FRANKLIN ST, STE 102
SAN FRANCISCO, CA 94109
TEL: (415) 928-4475
FAX: (415) 928-0361
TOLL FREE: (800) 955-7376

OREGON CLAIMS OFFICE
1188 FRANKLIN ST, STE 102
SAN FRANCISCO, CA 94109
TEL: (415) 928-4475
FAX: (415) 928-0361
TOLL FREE: (800) 955-7376

WASHINGTON CLAIMS OFFICE
1188 FRANKLIN ST, STE 102
SAN FRANCISCO, CA 94109
TEL: (415) 928-4475
FAX: (415) 928-0361
TOLL FREE: (800) 955-7376

ANTHEM HEALTH & LIFE INSURANCE AGENCY

GEORGIA CLAIMS OFFICE
3575 KOGER BLVD, STE 400
DULUTH, GA 30136
TEL: (770) 806-6300
FAX: (770) 806-6188
TOLL FREE: (800) 888-1966

ANTHEM, INC

INDIANA CLAIMS OFFICE
CORPORATE OFFICE
120 MONUMENT CIR
INDIANAPOLIS, IN 46204-4903
TEL: (317) 488-6000
TOLL FREE: (800) 331-1476
WWW.ANTHEM-INC.COM

ANTHEM INSURANCE

NEW JERSEY CLAIMS OFFICE
ONE CENTENNIAL AVE
PO BOX 1326
PISCATAWAY, NJ 08855-1326
TEL: (732) 980-4000
FAX: (732) 980-4138
TOLL FREE: (800) 221-3231
WWW.AHLIC.COM

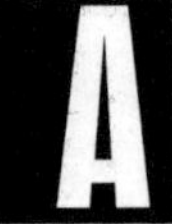

ANTHEM LIFE
OHIO CLAIMS OFFICE
6740 N HIGH ST, STE 200
PO BOX 10
WORTHINGTON, OH 43085-0010
TEL: (614) 436-0688
FAX: (614) 438-3959
TOLL FREE: (800) 551-7265
WWW.ANTHEM-INC.COM

ANTHEM SERVICES ADMINISTRATORS
1650 WATERMARK DR
PO BOX 528
COLUMBUS, OH 43216
TEL: (614) 481-8391
FAX: (614) 487-2427
TOLL FREE: (800) 824-6796

AON SELECT
NATIONAL CLAIMS OFFICE
310 W 4TH ST
PO BOX 15
WINSTON-SALEM, NC 27101-2839
TEL: (336) 728-2000
FAX: (336) 725-0040
TOLL FREE: (800) 368-3804

APPALACHIAN LIFE INSURANCE CO
WEST VIRGINIA CLAIMS OFFICE
1124 4TH AVE
PO BOX 299
HUNTINGTON, WV 25707-0299
TEL: (304) 529-4181
FAX: (304) 529-0491

ARCHDIOCESE OF MIAMI HEALTH PLAN
FLORIDA CLAIMS OFFICE
9401 BISCAYNE BLVD
MIAMI SHORES, FL 33138
TEL: (305) 893-0068
FAX: (305) 893-6433

ARCTIC ADJUSTERS, INC
ALASKA CLAIMS OFFICE
3701 E TUDOR RD, STE 206
ANCHORAGE, AK 99507
TEL: (907) 272-2595
FAX: (907) 277-2032

ARGONAUT GREAT CENTRAL INSURANCE CO
ILLINOIS CLAIMS OFFICE
3625 N SHERIDAN RD
PO BOX 807
PEORIA, IL 61652-0807
TEL: (309) 688-8571
FAX: (309) 688-1666
TOLL FREE: (800) 447-1972

ARGONAUT INSURANCE CO
CALIFORNIA CLAIMS OFFICE
250 MIDDLEFIELD RD
MENLO PARK, CA 94025-3500
TEL: (650) 858-6495
FAX: (650) 858-6631
TOLL FREE: (800) 222-7811

ILLINOIS CLAIMS OFFICE
8750 W BRYN MAWR AVE, STE 1300
CHICAGO, IL 60631
TEL: (773) 380-8000
FAX: (773) 380-2374
TOLL FREE: (800) 422-9120
WWW.CHI.ARGONAUTGROUP.COM

ARGUS SERVICES CORP
GEORGIA CLAIMS OFFICE
9500 FOREST LN, STE 300
DALLAS, TX 75243-5938
TEL: (972) 701-0595
FAX: (972) 701-0873

LOUISIANA CLAIMS OFFICE
9500 FOREST LN, STE 300
DALLAS, TX 75243-5938
TEL: (972) 701-0595
FAX: (972) 701-0873

TEXAS CLAIMS OFFICE
9500 FOREST LN, STE 300
DALLAS, TX 75243-5938
TEL: (972) 701-0595
FAX: (972) 701-0873

ARISTA INSURANCE CO
NEW YORK CLAIMS OFFICE
116 JOHN ST
NEW YORK, NY 10038
TEL: (212) 964-2150
FAX: (212) 608-6473
TOLL FREE: (800) 367-4420

ARIZONA FARM BUREAU MUTUAL INSURANCE CO
ARIZONA CLAIMS OFFICE
WESTERN AGRICULTURAL INSURANCE
3401 E ELWOOD ST
PO BOX 20180
PHOENIX, AZ 85036
TEL: (602) 470-0088
FAX: (602) 470-1137

ARIZONA PHYSICIANS, IPA, INC
3141 N 3RD AVE
PHOENIX, AZ 85013
TEL: (602) 274-6102
FAX: (602) 664-5466
IN-STATE: (800) 348-4058

ARIZONA PIPE TRADES
3109 N 24TH ST- BLDG B
PHOENIX, AZ 85016-7396
TEL: (602) 956-1894
FAX: (602) 956-1943

ARIZONA PREFERRED PROVIDER
NATIONAL CLAIMS OFFICE
6464 E GRANT RD
TUCSON, AZ 85715-3819
TEL: (520) 298-5297
FAX: (520) 296-7948

ARIZONA PUBLIC SERVICE CO
ARIZONA CLAIMS OFFICE
STA 8482
PO BOX 53970
PHOENIX, AZ 85072-3970
TEL: (602) 250-3578
FAX: (602) 250-2453

ARKANSAS BEST CORP
ARKANSAS CLAIMS OFFICE
BENEFIT DEPARTMENT
3801 OLD GREENWOOD RD
PO BOX 10048
FORT SMITH, AR 72917-0048
TEL: (501) 785-6178
FAX: (501) 785-6011

ARKANSAS FARM BUREAU MUTUAL INSURANCE
10720 KANIS RD
PO BOX 31
LITTLE ROCK, AR 72211-0031
TEL: (501) 224-4400
FAX: (501) 228-1458
WWW.ARFB.COM

ARNETT HMO
INDIANA CLAIMS OFFICE
ARNETT HEALTH PLANS
415 N 26TH ST
PO BOX 6108
LAFAYETTE, IN 47903-6108
FAX: (765) 448-7700
TOLL FREE: (888) 448-7440

ARNOT OGDEN MEDICAL CENTER
NEW YORK CLAIMS OFFICE
600 ROE AVE
ELMIRA, NY 14905
TEL: (607) 737-7734
FAX: (607) 737-7771

ARROW MUTUAL LIABILITY INSURANCE CO
MASSACHUSETTS CLAIMS OFFICE
23 COMMONWEALTH AVE
CHESTNUT HILL, MA 02167-1099
TEL: (617) 244-5730
FAX: (617) 244-4106
IN-STATE: (800) 457-9753

ARTHUR J. GALLAGAR & CO

NATIONAL CLAIMS OFFICE
A. J. GALLAGAR & CO
2345 GRAND BLVD, STE 800
KANSAS CITY, MO 64108
TEL: (816) 421-7788
FAX: (816) 472-5517
TOLL FREE: (800) 279-7500

ARTHUR J. GALLAGHER

MISSISSIPPI CLAIMS OFFICE
ROBINSON, JULIENNE & BAILEY, INC
750 WOODLANDS PKY, STE 200
PO BOX 14997
JACKSON, MS 39236-4997
TEL: (601) 949-4141
FAX: (601) 957-1347
TOLL FREE: (800) 866-4142

ASH GROVE CEMENT CO

KANSAS CLAIMS OFFICE
EMPLOYEE HEALTH CARE PLAN
8900 INDIAN CRK PKY
PO BOX 25900
OVERLAND PARK, KS 66225-5900
TEL: (913) 451-8900
FAX: (913) 451-8324
TOLL FREE: (800) 545-1822

ASO INDIANA

NATIONAL CLAIMS OFFICE
7222 ENGLE RD, STE 200
PO BOX 8311
FT WAYNE, IN 46804
TEL: (219) 459-2204
FAX: (219) 459-2502
TOLL FREE: (800) 407-5406
IN-STATE: (800) 678-4005

ASSOCIATED ADMINISTRATORS, INC

OREGON CLAIMS OFFICE
2929 NW 31ST AVE
PO BOX 5096
PORTLAND, OR 97210-1721
TEL: (503) 223-3185
FAX: (503) 727-7444
TOLL FREE: (800) 888-9603

ASSOCIATED PLAN ADMINISTRATORS

CONNECTICUT CLAIMS OFFICE
4133 WHITNEY AVE
PO BOX 9568
NEW HAVEN, CT 06518
TEL: (203) 287-1272
FAX: (203) 288-9428
TOLL FREE: (800) 626-3880

ASSOCIATES FINANCIAL LIFE

TEXAS CLAIMS OFFICE
290 E JOHN CARPENTER FWY
PO BOX 223727
DALLAS, TX 75222-3727
TEL: (972) 652-4000
FAX: (972) 652-7371
TOLL FREE: (800) 336-8913

ASSOCIATION PLAN ADMINISTRATORS, INC

FLORIDA CLAIMS OFFICE
9 MARKET ST
AMSTERDAM, NY 12010
TEL: (518) 843-6463
FAX: (518) 843-6989
TOLL FREE: (800) 510-7953

NEW YORK CLAIMS OFFICE
9 MARKET ST
AMSTERDAM, NY 12010
TEL: (518) 843-6463
FAX: (518) 843-6989
TOLL FREE: (800) 510-7953

VERMONT CLAIMS OFFICE
9 MARKET ST
AMSTERDAM, NY 12010
TEL: (518) 843-6463
FAX: (518) 843-6989
TOLL FREE: (800) 510-7953

ASSOCIATION RISK MANAGEMENT

TEXAS CLAIMS OFFICE
3420 EXECUTIVE CTR DR, STE 151
PO BOX 9728
AUSTIN, TX 78731
TEL: (512) 345-7500
FAX: (512) 345-1972
TOLL FREE: (800) 252-9641

ASSOCIATION & SOCIETY INSURANCE CORP

NATIONAL CLAIMS OFFICE
ASI
11300 ROCKVILLE PIKE, STE 500
PO BOX 2510
ROCKVILLE, MD 20852
TEL: (301) 816-0045
FAX: (301) 816-1125
TOLL FREE: (800) 638-2610
WWW.ASICORPORATION.COM

ASSUMPTION MUTUAL LIFE INSURANCE CO

NEW BRUNSWICK CLAIMS OFFICE
770 MAIN ST
PO BOX 160
MONCTON, NB E1C-8L1
TEL: (506) 853-6040
FAX: (506) 853-5459
TOLL FREE: (800) 455-7337

ASSURE CARE

ILLINOIS CLAIMS OFFICE
340 QUADRANGLE DR
BOLINGBROOK, IL 60440-3448
TEL: (630) 759-1311
FAX: (630) 759-5219
TOLL FREE: (800) 759-7422

MICHIGAN CLAIMS OFFICE
4660 S HAGADORN RD, STE 210
EAST LANSING, MI 48823
TEL: (517) 351-6616
FAX: (517) 351-6633
TOLL FREE: (800) 968-6616

ATLANTA CASUALTY CO

GEORGIA CLAIMS OFFICE
3169 HOLCOMB BRG
PO BOX 105436
ATLANTA, GA 30348-5436
TEL: (770) 447-8930
FAX: (770) 441-3572
TOLL FREE: (800) 225-8930
IN-STATE: (800) 263-1029

ATLANTIC AMERICAN CORP

BANKERS FIDELITY LIFE INSURANCE CO
4370 PEACHTREE RD NE
PO BOX 190240
ATLANTA, GA 31119-0240
TEL: (404) 266-5500
FAX: (404) 266-5596
TOLL FREE: (800) 241-1439

ATLANTIC COAST LIFE INSURANCE CO

SOUTH CAROLINA CLAIMS OFFICE
4500 LEEDS AVE
PO BOX 20010
CHARLESTON, SC 29413-1729
TEL: (843) 746-1400
FAX: (843) 746-1407

ATLANTIC MUTUAL / CENTENNIAL INSURANCE CO

ARIZONA CLAIMS OFFICE
PO BOX 14046
ORANGE, CA 92863
TEL: (714) 740-0888
FAX: (714) 740-0891
TOLL FREE: (800) 283-0064

CALIFORNIA CLAIMS OFFICE
PO BOX 14046
ORANGE, CA 92863
TEL: (714) 740-0888
FAX: (714) 740-0891
TOLL FREE: (800) 283-0064

601 UNION ST, STE 1700
SEATTLE, WA 98101-2371
TEL: (206) 464-0620
FAX: (206) 464-1025
TOLL FREE: (800) 283-2856

CONNECTICUT CLAIMS OFFICE
628 HEBORN AVE- BLDG 2
PO BOX 6510
GLASTONBURY, CT 06033-6510
TEL: (860) 657-9966
FAX: (860) 657-7962
TOLL FREE: (800) 289-2299
WWW.ATLANTICMUTUAL.COM

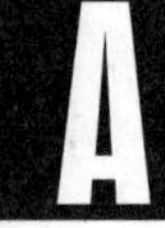

GEORGIA CLAIMS OFFICE
10 PIEDMONT CTR, STE 600
ATLANTA, GA 30305-1737
TEL: (404) 261-5582
FAX: (404) 364-3733
TOLL FREE: (800) 283-2876
WWW.ATLANTICMUTUAL.COM

ILLINOIS CLAIMS OFFICE
222 W ADAM ST, STE 2000
CHICAGO, IL 60606-5397
TEL: (312) 634-0700
FAX: (312) 634-0801
TOLL FREE: (800) 289-6548
WWW.ATLANTICMUTUAL.COM

701 EMERSON RD, STE 440
PO BOX 419063
CREVE COEUR, MO 63141-9063
TEL: (314) 872-3979
FAX: (314) 872-8573
TOLL FREE: (800) 937-3747
WWW.ATLANTICMUTUAL.COM

IOWA CLAIMS OFFICE
701 EMERSON RD, STE 440
PO BOX 419063
CREVE COEUR, MO 63141-9063
TEL: (314) 872-3979
FAX: (314) 872-8573
TOLL FREE: (800) 937-3747
WWW.ATLANTICMUTUAL..COM

KANSAS CLAIMS OFFICE
701 EMERSON RD, STE 440
PO BOX 419063
CREVE COEUR, MO 63141-9063
TEL: (314) 872-3979
FAX: (314) 872-8573
TOLL FREE: (800) 937-3747
WWW.ATLANTICMUTUAL.COM

MARYLAND CLAIMS OFFICE
303 INTERNATIONAL CIR, STE 305
HUNT VALLEY, MD 21031-1002
TEL: (410) 785-4880
FAX: (410) 527-1971
TOLL FREE: (800) 283-0054

MASSACHUSETTS CLAIMS OFFICE
628 HEBORN AVE- BLDG 2
PO BOX 6510
GLASTONBURY, CT 06033-6510
TEL: (860) 657-9966
FAX: (860) 657-7962
TOLL FREE: (800) 289-2299
WWW.ATLANTICMUTUAL.COM

MICHIGAN CLAIMS OFFICE
222 W ADAM ST, STE 2000
CHICAGO, IL 60606-5397
TEL: (312) 634-0700
FAX: (312) 634-0801
TOLL FREE: (800) 289-6548
WWW.ATLANTICMUTUAL.COM

MINNESOTA CLAIMS OFFICE
8400 NORMANDALE LK BLVD, STE 950
BLOOMINGTON, MN 55437
TEL: (612) 897-1480
FAX: (612) 897-1243
TOLL FREE: (800) 811-3080

MISSOURI CLAIMS OFFICE
701 EMERSON RD, STE 440
PO BOX 419063
CREVE COEUR, MO 63141-9063
TEL: (314) 872-3979
FAX: (314) 872-8573
TOLL FREE: (800) 937-3747
WWW.ATLANTICMUTUAL.COM

NEBRASKA CLAIMS OFFICE
701 EMERSON RD, STE 440
PO BOX 419063
CREVE COEUR, MO 63141-9063
TEL: (314) 872-3979
FAX: (314) 872-8573
TOLL FREE: (800) 937-3747
WWW.ATLANTICMUTUAL.COM

NEVADA CLAIMS OFFICE
PO BOX 14046
ORANGE, CA 92863
TEL: (714) 740-0888
FAX: (714) 740-0891
TOLL FREE: (800) 283-0064

NEW HAMPSHIRE CLAIMS OFFICE
628 HEBORN AVE- BLDG 2
PO BOX 6510
GLASTONBURY, CT 06033-6510
TEL: (860) 657-9966
FAX: (860) 657-7962
TOLL FREE: (800) 289-2299
WWW.ATLANTICMUTUAL.COM

NEW JERSEY CLAIMS OFFICE
THREE GIRALDA FARMS
PO BOX 821
MADISON, NJ 07940-1004
TEL: (973) 408-6000
FAX: (973) 408-6124
TOLL FREE: (800) 445-9075

NEW MEXICO CLAIMS OFFICE
PO BOX 14046
ORANGE, CA 92863
TEL: (714) 740-0888
FAX: (714) 740-0891
TOLL FREE: (800) 283-0064

NEW YORK CLAIMS OFFICE
48 S SERVICE RD
PO BOX 9090
MELVILLE, NY 11747-9090
TEL: (516) 454-0200
FAX: (516) 391-3160
TOLL FREE: (800) 888-5103
WWW.HOME.ATLANTICOS.COM

601 UNION ST, STE 1700
SEATTLE, WA 98101-2371
TEL: (206) 464-0620
FAX: (206) 464-1025
TOLL FREE: (800) 283-2856

OREGON CLAIMS OFFICE
601 UNION ST, STE 1700
SEATTLE, WA 98101-2371
TEL: (206) 464-0620
FAX: (206) 464-1025
TOLL FREE: (800) 283-2856

PENNSYLVANIA CLAIMS OFFICE
610 W GERMANTOWN PIKE
PO BOX 911
PLYMOUTH MEETING, PA 19462-0911
TEL: (610) 941-4000
FAX: (610) 941-9047
TOLL FREE: (800) 444-2856

RHODE ISLAND CLAIMS OFFICE
628 HEBORN AVE- BLDG 2
PO BOX 6510
GLASTONBURY, CT 06033-6510
TEL: (860) 657-9966
FAX: (860) 657-7962
TOLL FREE: (800) 289-2299
WWW.ATLANTICMUTUAL.COM

TEXAS CLAIMS OFFICE
7557 RAMBLER RD, STE 1000
DALLAS, TX 75231-2304
TEL: (214) 365-6700
FAX: (214) 696-5308
TOLL FREE: (800) 888-6090

VIRGINIA CLAIMS OFFICE
601 UNION ST, STE 1700
SEATTLE, WA 98101-2371
TEL: (206) 464-0620
FAX: (206) 464-1025
TOLL FREE: (800) 283-2856

WASHINGTON CLAIMS OFFICE
601 UNION ST, STE 1700
SEATTLE, WA 98101-2371
TEL: (206) 464-0620
FAX: (206) 464-1025
TOLL FREE: (800) 283-2856

ATLANTIC RISK MANAGERS, INC

NEW YORK CLAIMS OFFICE
AHRC USA
120 COMAC ST
RONKONKOMA, NY 11779
TEL: (516) 471-2747
FAX: (516) 471-2746

B

ATLANTIC SOUTHERN INSURANCE CO
PUERTO RICO CLAIMS OFFICE
1056 MUNOZ RIVERA ST
PO BOX 362889
SAN JUAN, PR 00936-2889
TEL: (787) 767-9750
FAX: (787) 764-6103
TOLL FREE: (800) 981-5564

ATRIUM HEALTH PLAN
WISCONSIN CLAIMS OFFICE
BLUE CROSS & BLUE SHIELD OF MINNESOTA
2215 VINE ST, STE E
HUDSON, WI 54016
TEL: (715) 386-6886
FAX: (715) 386-8326
TOLL FREE: (800) 535-4041
IN-STATE: (800) 535-4041

H

AULTCARE
OHIO CLAIMS OFFICE
2600 6TH ST SW
PO BOX 6910
CANTON, OH 44706-0910
TEL: (330) 438-6381
FAX: (330) 454-7845
TOLL FREE: (800) 344-8858

AUSTIN MUTUAL INSURANCE CO
MINNESOTA CLAIMS OFFICE
10 2ND ST NE, STE 300
PO BOX 401
MINNEAPOLIS, MN 55440-0401
TEL: (612) 378-8600
FAX: (612) 378-8696
TOLL FREE: (800) 328-4628

AUTO ALLIANCE INTERNATIONAL
MICHIGAN CLAIMS OFFICE
ATTN: HEALTH CENTER
1 INTERNATIONAL DR
FLAT ROCK, MI 48134-9498
TEL: (734) 782-7800
TOLL FREE: (800) 392-2889

AUTO OWNERS INSURANCE CO
NATIONAL CLAIMS OFFICE
6101 ANACAPRI BLVD
PO BOX 30660
LANSING, MI 48917
TEL: (517) 323-1200
FAX: (517) 323-8796
WWW.AUTO-OWNERS.COM

AUTOMATED BENEFITS SERVICES, INC
MICHIGAN CLAIMS OFFICE
8220 IRVING
PO BOX 37504
STERLING HEIGHTS, MI 48312
TEL: (810) 826-4380
FAX: (810) 826-4820
TOLL FREE: (800) 521-1321

AUTOMOBILE CLUB INSURANCE CO
CALIFORNIA CLAIMS OFFICE
2601 S FIGUEROA ST
LOS ANGELES, CA 90007
TEL: (213) 741-3403
FAX: (213) 741-3637

OHIO CLAIMS OFFICE
3590 TWIN CREEKS DR
PO BOX 182579
COLUMBUS, OH 43218-2579
TEL: (614) 272-6951
TOLL FREE: (800) 282-2913

AUTOMOBILE MECHANICS LOCAL NO 701
ILLINOIS CLAIMS OFFICE
HEALTH & WELFARE FUND
500 W PLAINFIELD RD
COUNTRYSIDE, IL 60525
TEL: (708) 482-0110
FAX: (708) 482-9140
TOLL FREE: (800) 704-6270

AUTOMOTIVE PETROLEUM & ALLIED
MISSOURI CLAIMS OFFICE
300 S GRAND AVE, RM 232
SAINT LOUIS, MO 63103-2430
TEL: (314) 531-3052
FAX: (314) 531-5285

AV-MED HEALTH PLAN
FLORIDA CLAIMS OFFICE
4300 NW 89TH BLVD
PO BOX 749
GAINSVILLE, FL 32606
TEL: (352) 372-8400
FAX: (352) 337-8726
TOLL FREE: (800) 346-0231
WWW.ABNET.COM

H

9400 S DADELAND BLVD
PO BOX 569000
MIAMI, FL 33256-9000
TEL: (305) 671-5437
FAX: (305) 671-6167
TOLL FREE: (800) 228-0660
WWW.AVMED.COM

H

AXA REINSURANCE CO
NEW YORK CLAIMS OFFICE
17 STATE ST
NEW YORK, NY 10004
TEL: (212) 493-9300
FAX: (212) 425-3799

BABB, INC
PENNSYLVANIA CLAIMS OFFICE
850 RIDGE AVE
PITTSBURGH, PA 15212
TEL: (412) 237-2020
FAX: (412) 322-1756
TOLL FREE: (800) 245-6102
IN-STATE: (800) 892-1015

BADGER MUTUAL INSURANCE CO
WISCONSIN CLAIMS OFFICE
1635 W NATIONAL AVE
PO BOX 2092
MILWAUKEE, WI 53201-2092
TEL: (414) 383-1234
FAX: (414) 383-1535
TOLL FREE: (800) 837-7833

BAKERY & CONFECTIONARY UNION
MARYLAND CLAIMS OFFICE
INDUSTRY INTERNATIONAL HEALTH BENEFITS FUND
10401 CONNECTICUT AVE
KENSINGTON, MD 20895
TEL: (301) 468-3700
FAX: (301) 468-3789

BALBOA INSURANCE
NATIONAL CLAIMS OFFICE
18581 TELLER AVE
PO BOX 19702
IRVINE, CA 92623-9702
TEL: (949) 553-0700
FAX: (949) 553-7788
TOLL FREE: (800) 854-6115
WWW.BALBOAINSURANCE.COM

BALBOA LIFE & CASUALTY
CALIFORNIA CLAIMS OFFICE
18581 TELLER AVE
PO BOX 19702
IRVINE, CA 92612-1627
TEL: (949) 553-0700
FAX: (949) 660-6580
TOLL FREE: (800) 854-6115
WWW.BALBOAINSURANCE.COM

BANC ONE KENTUCKY INSURANCE CO
KENTUCKY CLAIMS OFFICE
BANC ONE INSURANCE SERVICES CORPORATION
312 S FOUR ST, STE 402
PO BOX 32500
LOUISVILLE, KY 40232-2500
TEL: (502) 566-1610
FAX: (502) 566-2269
TOLL FREE: (800) 542-2265

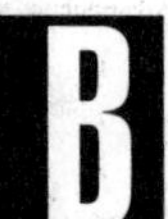

BANK OF AMERICA

ILLINOIS CLAIMS OFFICE
231 S LASALLE ST
CHICAGO, IL 60697-0001
TEL: (312) 828-2345

BANKERS COMMERCIAL LIFE INSURANCE CO

TEXAS CLAIMS OFFICE
5720 LBJ FWY, STE 200
PO BOX 809047
DALLAS, TX 75240-9699
TEL: (972) 980-1151
FAX: (972) 980-4310
TOLL FREE: (800) 980-2216

BANKERS FIDELITY LIFE INSURANCE

GEORGIA CLAIMS OFFICE
4370 PEACHTREE RD NE
PO BOX 190240
ATLANTA, GA 31119-0240
TEL: (404) 266-5500
FAX: (404) 266-5596
TOLL FREE: (800) 241-1439
IN-STATE: (800) 282-0480

BANKERS INSURANCE GROUP

NATIONAL CLAIMS OFFICE
360 CENTRAL AVE
PO BOX 15707
SAINT PETERSBURG, FL 33733-5707
TEL: (727) 823-4000
FAX: (727) 898-2317
TOLL FREE: (800) 765-9700
WWW.BANKERSINSURANCE.COM

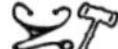

BANKERS LIFE & CASUALTY CO

ALABAMA CLAIMS OFFICE
CONSECO LLC
222 MERCHANDISE MART PLZ
PO BOX 66927
CHICAGO, IL 60654
TEL: (312) 396-6000
FAX: (312) 396-5951
TOLL FREE: (800) 621-3724
WWW.BANKLIFE.COM

ARIZONA CLAIMS OFFICE
CONSECO LLC
222 MERCHANDISE MART PLZ
PO BOX 66927
CHICAGO, IL 60654
TEL: (312) 396-6000
FAX: (312) 396-5951
TOLL FREE: (800) 621-3724
WWW.BANKLIFE.COM

CALIFORNIA CLAIMS OFFICE
CONSECO LLC
222 MERCHANDISE MART PLZ
PO BOX 66927
CHICAGO, IL 60654
TEL: (312) 396-6000
FAX: (312) 396-5951
TOLL FREE: (800) 621-3724
WWW.BANKLIFE.COM

COLORADO CLAIMS OFFICE
CONSECO LLC
222 MERCHANDISE MART PLZ
PO BOX 66927
CHICAGO, IL 60654
TEL: (312) 396-6000
FAX: (312) 396-5951
TOLL FREE: (800) 621-3724
WWW.BANKLIFE.COM

CONNECTICUT CLAIMS OFFICE
CONSECO LLC
222 MERCHANDISE MART PLZ
PO BOX 66927
CHICAGO, IL 60654
TEL: (312) 396-6000
FAX: (312) 396-5951
TOLL FREE: (800) 621-3724
WWW.BANKLIFE.COM

DELAWARE CLAIMS OFFICE
CONSECO LLC
222 MERCHANDISE MART PLZ
PO BOX 66927
CHICAGO, IL 60654
TEL: (312) 396-6000
FAX: (312) 396-5951
TOLL FREE: (800) 621-3724
WWW.BANKLIFE.COM

FLORIDA CLAIMS OFFICE
CONSECO LLC
222 MERCHANDISE MART PLZ
PO BOX 66927
CHICAGO, IL 60654
TEL: (312) 396-6000
FAX: (312) 396-5951
TOLL FREE: (800) 621-3724
WWW.BANKLIFE.COM

GEORGIA CLAIMS OFFICE
CONSECO LLC
222 MERCHANDISE MART PLZ
PO BOX 66927
CHICAGO, IL 60654
TEL: (312) 396-6000
FAX: (312) 396-5951
TOLL FREE: (800) 621-3724
WWW.BANKLIFE.COM

IDAHO CLAIMS OFFICE
CONSECO LLC
222 MERCHANDISE MART PLZ
PO BOX 66927
CHICAGO, IL 60654
TEL: (312) 396-6000
FAX: (312) 396-5951
TOLL FREE: (800) 621-3724
WWW.BANKLIFE.COM

ILLINOIS CLAIMS OFFICE
CONSECO LLC
222 MERCHANDISE MART PLZ
PO BOX 66927
CHICAGO, IL 60654
TEL: (312) 396-6000
FAX: (312) 396-5951
TOLL FREE: (800) 621-3724
WWW.BANKLIFE.COM

INDIANA CLAIMS OFFICE
CONSECO LLC
222 MERCHANDISE MART PLZ
PO BOX 66927
CHICAGO, IL 60654
TEL: (312) 396-6000
FAX: (312) 396-5951
TOLL FREE: (800) 621-3724
WWW.BANKLIFE.COM

IOWA CLAIMS OFFICE
CONSECO LLC
222 MERCHANDISE MART PLZ
PO BOX 66927
CHICAGO, IL 60654
TEL: (312) 396-6000
FAX: (312) 396-5951
TOLL FREE: (800) 621-3724
WWW.BANKLIFE.COM

KANSAS CLAIMS OFFICE
CONSECO LLC
222 MERCHANDISE MART PLZ
PO BOX 66927
CHICAGO, IL 60654
TEL: (312) 396-6000
FAX: (312) 396-5951
TOLL FREE: (800) 621-3724
WWW.BANKLIFE.COM

KENTUCKY CLAIMS OFFICE
CONSECO LLC
222 MERCHANDISE MART PLZ
PO BOX 66927
CHICAGO, IL 60654
TEL: (312) 396-6000
FAX: (312) 396-5951
TOLL FREE: (800) 621-3724
WWW.BANKLIFE.COM

LOUISIANA CLAIMS OFFICE
CONSECO LLC
222 MERCHANDISE MART PLZ
PO BOX 66927
CHICAGO, IL 60654
TEL: (312) 396-6000
FAX: (312) 396-5951
TOLL FREE: (800) 621-3724
WWW.BANKLIFE.COM

MAINE CLAIMS OFFICE
CONSECO LLC
222 MERCHANDISE MART PLZ
PO BOX 66927
CHICAGO, IL 60654
TEL: (312) 396-6000
FAX: (312) 396-5951
TOLL FREE: (800) 621-3724
WWW.BANKLIFE.COM

MARYLAND CLAIMS OFFICE
CONSECO LLC
222 MERCHANDISE MART PLZ
PO BOX 66927
CHICAGO, IL 60654
TEL: (312) 396-6000
FAX: (312) 396-5951
TOLL FREE: (800) 621-3724
WWW.BANKLIFE.COM

MICHIGAN CLAIMS OFFICE
CONSECO LLC
222 MERCHANDISE MART PLZ
PO BOX 66927
CHICAGO, IL 60654
TEL: (312) 396-6000
FAX: (312) 396-5951
TOLL FREE: (800) 621-3724
WWW.BANKLIFE.COM

MISSISSIPPI CLAIMS OFFICE
CONSECO LLC
222 MERCHANDISE MART PLZ
PO BOX 66927
CHICAGO, IL 60654
TEL: (312) 396-6000
FAX: (312) 396-5951
TOLL FREE: (800) 621-3724
WWW.BANKLIFE.COM

MONTANA CLAIMS OFFICE
CONSECO LLC
222 MERCHANDISE MART PLZ
PO BOX 66927
CHICAGO, IL 60654
TEL: (312) 396-6000
FAX: (312) 396-5951
TOLL FREE: (800) 621-3724
WWW.BANKLIFE.COM

NEVADA CLAIMS OFFICE
CONSECO LLC
222 MERCHANDISE MART PLZ
PO BOX 66927
CHICAGO, IL 60654
TEL: (312) 396-6000
FAX: (312) 396-5951
TOLL FREE: (800) 621-3724
WWW.BANKLIFE.COM

NEW HAMPSHIRE CLAIMS OFFICE
CONSECO LLC
222 MERCHANDISE MART PLZ
PO BOX 66927
CHICAGO, IL 60654
TEL: (312) 396-6000
FAX: (312) 396-5951
TOLL FREE: (800) 621-3724
WWW.BANKLIFE.COM

NEW JERSEY CLAIMS OFFICE
CONSECO LLC
222 MERCHANDISE MART PLZ
PO BOX 66927
CHICAGO, IL 60654
TEL: (312) 396-6000
FAX: (312) 396-5951
TOLL FREE: (800) 621-3724
WWW.BANKLIFE.COM

NEW MEXICO CLAIMS OFFICE
CONSECO LLC
222 MERCHANDISE MART PLZ
PO BOX 66927
CHICAGO, IL 60654
TEL: (312) 396-6000
FAX: (312) 396-5951
TOLL FREE: (800) 621-3724
WWW.BANKLIFE.COM

NORTH CAROLINA CLAIMS OFFICE
CONSECO LLC
222 MERCHANDISE MART PLZ
PO BOX 66927
CHICAGO, IL 60654
TEL: (312) 396-6000
FAX: (312) 396-5951
TOLL FREE: (800) 621-3724
WWW.BANKLIFE.COM

OHIO CLAIMS OFFICE
CONSECO LLC
222 MERCHANDISE MART PLZ
PO BOX 66927
CHICAGO, IL 60654
TEL: (312) 396-6000
FAX: (312) 396-5951
TOLL FREE: (800) 621-3724
WWW.BANKLIFE.COM

OREGON CLAIMS OFFICE
CONSECO LLC
222 MERCHANDISE MART PLZ
PO BOX 66927
CHICAGO, IL 60654
TEL: (312) 396-6000
FAX: (312) 396-5951
TOLL FREE: (800) 621-3724
WWW.BANKLIFE.COM

PENNSYLVANIA CLAIMS OFFICE
CONSECO LLC
222 MERCHANDISE MART PLZ
PO BOX 66927
CHICAGO, IL 60654
TEL: (312) 396-6000
FAX: (312) 396-5951
TOLL FREE: (800) 621-3724
WWW.BANKLIFE.COM

SOUTH CAROLINA CLAIMS OFFICE
CONSECO LLC
222 MERCHANDISE MART PLZ
PO BOX 66927
CHICAGO, IL 60654
TEL: (312) 396-6000
FAX: (312) 396-5951
TOLL FREE: (800) 621-3724
WWW.BANKLIFE.COM

SOUTH DAKOTA CLAIMS OFFICE
CONSECO LLC
222 MERCHANDISE MART PLZ
PO BOX 66927
CHICAGO, IL 60654
TEL: (312) 396-6000
FAX: (312) 396-5951
TOLL FREE: (800) 621-3724
WWW.BANKLIFE.COM

TENNESSEE CLAIMS OFFICE
CONSECO LLC
222 MERCHANDISE MART PLZ
PO BOX 66927
CHICAGO, IL 60654
TEL: (312) 396-6000
FAX: (312) 396-5951
TOLL FREE: (800) 621-3724
WWW.BANKLIFE.COM

TEXAS CLAIMS OFFICE
CONSECO LLC
222 MERCHANDISE MART PLZ
PO BOX 66927
CHICAGO, IL 60654
TEL: (312) 396-6000
FAX: (312) 396-5951
TOLL FREE: (800) 621-3724
WWW.BANKLIFE.COM

VERMONT CLAIMS OFFICE
CONSECO LLC
222 MERCHANDISE MART PLZ
PO BOX 66927
CHICAGO, IL 60654
TEL: (312) 396-6000
FAX: (312) 396-5951
TOLL FREE: (800) 621-3724
WWW.BANKLIFE.COM

VIRGINIA CLAIMS OFFICE
CONSECO LLC
222 MERCHANDISE MART PLZ
PO BOX 66927
CHICAGO, IL 60654
TEL: (312) 396-6000
FAX: (312) 396-5951
TOLL FREE: (800) 621-3724
WWW.BANKLIFE.COM

WASHINGTON CLAIMS OFFICE
CONSECO LLC
222 MERCHANDISE MART PLZ
PO BOX 66927
CHICAGO, IL 60654
TEL: (312) 396-6000
FAX: (312) 396-5951
TOLL FREE: (800) 621-3724
WWW.BANKLIFE.COM

WEST VIRGINIA CLAIMS OFFICE
CONSECO LLC
222 MERCHANDISE MART PLZ
PO BOX 66927
CHICAGO, IL 60654
TEL: (312) 396-6000
FAX: (312) 396-5951
TOLL FREE: (800) 621-3724
WWW.BANKLIFE.COM

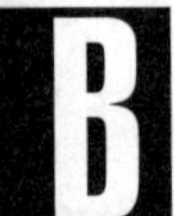

WISCONSIN CLAIMS OFFICE
CONSECO LLC
222 MERCHANDISE MART PLZ
PO BOX 66927
CHICAGO, IL 60654
TEL: (312) 396-6000
FAX: (312) 396-5951
TOLL FREE: (800) 621-3724
WWW.BANKLIFE.COM

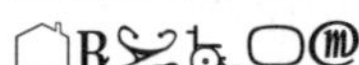

WYOMING CLAIMS OFFICE
CONSECO LLC
222 MERCHANDISE MART PLZ
PO BOX 66927
CHICAGO, IL 60654
TEL: (312) 396-6000
FAX: (312) 396-5951
TOLL FREE: (800) 621-3724
WWW.BANKLIFE.COM

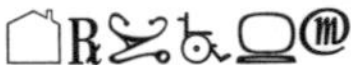

BANKERS SECURITY LIFE INSURANCE SOCIETY
VIRGINIA CLAIMS OFFICE
4601 N FAIRFAX DR
PO BOX 3700
ARLINGTON, VA 22203
TEL: (703) 875-3500
FAX: (703) 875-3616
TOLL FREE: (800) 537-5024

BASHAS', INC
ARIZONA CLAIMS OFFICE
FOOD CITY, A.J.'S MERCADO BARGAIN BASKET
22402 S BASHA RD
PO BOX 488
CHANDLER, AZ 85244
TEL: (602) 895-5247
FAX: (602) 802-5497
TOLL FREE: (800) 755-7292
WWW.BASHAS.COM

BASS PRO SHOPS INC EMPLOYEE BENEFIT PLAN
MISSOURI CLAIMS OFFICE
2500 E KEARNEY
SPRINGFIELD, MO 65898-0001
TEL: (417) 873-5000
FAX: (417) 865-9812

BASSETT FURNITURE INDUSTRIES, INC
VIRGINIA CLAIMS OFFICE
3525 SAIRYSTONE PRK HWY
PO BOX 626
BASSETT, VA 24055-0626
TEL: (540) 629-6000
FAX: (540) 629-6346

BCS LIFE INSURANCE CO
ILLINOIS CLAIMS OFFICE
676 N SAINT CLAIR ST
PO BOX 10939
CHICAGO, IL 60610
TEL: (312) 951-7700
FAX: (312) 951-7788
TOLL FREE: (800) 621-9215

BEAR RIVER MUTUAL INSURANCE CO
UTAH CLAIMS OFFICE
778 E WINCHESTER ST
PO BOX 571310
MURRAY, UT 84157
TEL: (801) 267-5000
FAX: (801) 267-5033
TOLL FREE: (800) 925-5177
IN-STATE: (800) 925-5177
E-MAIL: BRMUTUAL.COM
WWW.BRMUTUAL.COM

BEAULIEU OF AMERICA, INC
GEORGIA CLAIMS OFFICE
600 5TH AVE
PO BOX 4539
DALTON, GA 30719
TEL: (706) 275-4432
TOLL FREE: (800) 596-6622

BEECH STREET, INC
CALIFORNIA CLAIMS OFFICE
173 TECHNOLOGY
PO BOX 17719
IRVINE, CA 92618
TEL: (949) 727-9300
FAX: (949) 727-1793
TOLL FREE: (800) 877-1333

BEHAVIORAL HEALTHCARE OPTIONS
NEVADA CLAIMS OFFICE
2801 S VALLEY VIEW, STE 6
PO BOX 15645
LAS VEGAS, NV 89102
TEL: (702) 364-1484
FAX: (702) 364-0843
TOLL FREE: (800) 873-2246

BELIOT MEMORIAL HOSPITAL, INC
WISCONSIN CLAIMS OFFICE
(DRA) FIRST CHOICE BENEFITS MANAGEMENT
1969 W HART RD
BELOIT, WI 53511
TEL: (608) 364-5123
FAX: (608) 364-8585

BELLSOUTH ADMINISTRATORS
LOUISIANA CLAIMS OFFICE
3616 S I-10 SERVICE RD
PO BOX 8570
METAIRIE, LA 70011-8570
TEL: (504) 849-1459
FAX: (504) 849-1347
TOLL FREE: (800) 366-2475

BENEFICIAL LIFE INSURANCE CO
UTAH CLAIMS OFFICE
36 S STATE ST
SALT LAKE CITY, UT 84136-0001
TEL: (801) 531-7979
FAX: (801) 531-3397
TOLL FREE: (800) 233-7979

BENEFIT ACTUARIES
MICHIGAN CLAIMS OFFICE
4875 CASCADE RD SE
GRAND RAPIDS, MI 49506
TEL: (616) 940-1156
FAX: (616) 940-1450

BENEFIT ADMINISTRATION CORP
CALIFORNIA CLAIMS OFFICE
770 E SHAW AVE, STE 200
PO BOX 9800
FRESNO, CA 93794
TEL: (559) 225-3030
FAX: (559) 225-6837
TOLL FREE: (800) 282-5246

BENEFIT ADMINISTRATIVE SYSTEMS, LTD
ILLINOIS CLAIMS OFFICE
17475 JOVANNA DR, STE 1B
HOMEWOOD, IL 60430
TEL: (708) 799-7400
FAX: (708) 799-7533
TOLL FREE: (800) 523-0582
IN-STATE: (800) 843-3831
E-MAIL: ADMIN@BENADMINSYS.COM
WWW.BENADMINSYS.COM

BENEFIT ADMINISTRATORS, INC
NATIONAL CLAIMS OFFICE
1111 S GLENSTONE, STE 2-203
PO BOX 10868
SPRINGFIELD, MO 65808
TEL: (417) 866-8913
FAX: (417) 866-2103
TOLL FREE: (800) 375-8913
E-MAIL: CLAIMS@BATPA.COM
WWW.BATPA.COM

SOUTH CAROLINA CLAIMS OFFICE
JOHNSON INSURANCE
PO BOX 21308
COLUMBIA, SC 29221-1308
TEL: (803) 739-0001
FAX: (803) 739-2200

BENEFIT ASSISTANCE CORPORATION
WEST VIRGINIA CLAIMS OFFICE
305 E MAIN ST
PO BOX 99
MILTON, WV 25541
TEL: (304) 743-1455
FAX: (304) 743-1459
TOLL FREE: (800) 448-1131

BENEFIT CLAIMS PAYERS, INC

ARIZONA CLAIMS OFFICE
1717 W NORTHERN AVE, STE 200
PO BOX 37400
PHOENIX, AZ 85069
TEL: (602) 861-6868
FAX: (602) 861-6878
TOLL FREE: (800) 266-6868
WWW.DHSNYU.COM

BENEFIT CONSULTANTS, INC

ARKANSAS CLAIMS OFFICE
13515 BARRETT PKY DR, STE 265
BALLWIN, MO 63021-5870
TEL: (314) 822-7890
FAX: (314) 822-0992
TOLL FREE: (800) 434-4620

ILLINOIS CLAIMS OFFICE
13515 BARRETT PKY DR, STE 265
BALLWIN, MO 63021-5870
TEL: (314) 822-7890
FAX: (314) 822-0992
TOLL FREE: (800) 434-4620

MISSOURI CLAIMS OFFICE
13515 BARRETT PKY DR, STE 265
BALLWIN, MO 63021-5870
TEL: (314) 822-7890
FAX: (314) 822-0992
TOLL FREE: (800) 434-4620

BENEFIT COORDINATORS CORP

PENNSYLVANIA CLAIMS OFFICE
200 FLEET ST- 5TH FL
PITTSBURGH, PA 15220-2910
TEL: (412) 920-2200
FAX: (412) 920-2279
TOLL FREE: (800) 685-6100

BENEFIT MANAGEMENT CORP

FLORIDA CLAIMS OFFICE
1609 TOWNCENTER BLVD
WESTON, FL 33326
TEL: (954) 384-1000
FAX: (954) 384-6425
TOLL FREE: (800) 262-9175

BENEFIT MANAGEMENT, INC

ARKANSAS CLAIMS OFFICE
628 W BROADWAY, STE 100
PO BOX 5989
LITTLE ROCK, AR 72119
TEL: (501) 375-5500
FAX: (501) 375-4718

MISSOURI CLAIMS OFFICE
HERRINGTON BENEFITS
809 ILLINOIS
PO BOX 3810
JOPLIN, MO 64803-3810
TEL: (417) 623-3860
TOLL FREE: (800) 826-6912

BENEFIT PLAN ADMINISTRATION OF WI, INC

WISCONSIN CLAIMS OFFICE
11270 W PRK PL, STE 950
MILWAUKEE, WI 53224
TEL: (414) 577-3700
FAX: (414) 577-3710

BENEFIT PLAN ADMINISTRATORS, INC

KENTUCKY CLAIMS OFFICE
101 S JEFFERSON ST
PO BOX 11746
ROANOKE, VA 24022-1746
TEL: (540) 345-2721
FAX: (540) 342-0282
TOLL FREE: (800) 277-8973
WWW.BPATPA.COM

MARYLAND CLAIMS OFFICE
101 S JEFFERSON ST
PO BOX 11746
ROANOKE, VA 24022-1746
TEL: (540) 345-2721
FAX: (540) 342-0282
TOLL FREE: (800) 277-8973
WWW.BPATPA.COM

NEW YORK CLAIMS OFFICE
ONE HUNTINGTON QUANDRANGLE, STE 4N
PO BOX 8911
MELVILLE, NY 11747
TEL: (516) 694-4900
FAX: (516) 694-5650

NORTH CAROLINA CLAIMS OFFICE
101 S JEFFERSON ST
PO BOX 11746
ROANOKE, VA 24022-1746
TEL: (540) 345-2721
FAX: (540) 342-0282
TOLL FREE: (800) 277-8973
WWW.BPATPA.COM

SOUTH CAROLINA CLAIMS OFFICE
101 S JEFFERSON ST
PO BOX 11746
ROANOKE, VA 24022-1746
TEL: (540) 345-2721
FAX: (540) 342-0282
TOLL FREE: (800) 277-8973
WWW.BPATPA.COM

TENNESSEE CLAIMS OFFICE
101 S JEFFERSON ST
PO BOX 11746
ROANOKE, VA 24022-1746
TEL: (540) 345-2721
FAX: (540) 342-0282
TOLL FREE: (800) 277-8973
WWW.BPATPA.COM

VIRGINIA CLAIMS OFFICE
101 S JEFFERSON ST
PO BOX 11746
ROANOKE, VA 24022-1746
TEL: (540) 345-2721
FAX: (540) 342-0282
TOLL FREE: (800) 277-8973
WWW.BPATPA.COM

WEST VIRGINIA CLAIMS OFFICE
101 S JEFFERSON ST
PO BOX 11746
ROANOKE, VA 24022-1746
TEL: (540) 345-2721
FAX: (540) 342-0282
TOLL FREE: (800) 277-8973
WWW.BPATPA.COM

BENEFIT PLAN SERVICES, INC

NORTH CAROLINA CLAIMS OFFICE
131 W PARRIS AVE
PO BOX 2793
HIGH POINT, NC 27261
TEL: (336) 889-2003
FAX: (336) 841-2556

BENEFIT PLANNERS, INC

TEXAS CLAIMS OFFICE
PO BOX 690450
SAN ANTONIO, TX 78269-0450
TEL: (210) 699-1872
FAX: (210) 697-3108
TOLL FREE: (800) 292-5386
E-MAIL: SERVICE@BENPLAN.COM
WWW.BENPLAN.COM

194 S MAIN
BOERNE, TX 78006
TEL: (210) 699-1872
FAX: (210) 697-3108
TOLL FREE: (800) 292-5386
E-MAIL: SERVICE@BENPLAN.COM
WWW.BENPLAN.COM

BENEFIT PLANS

OHIO CLAIMS OFFICE
BANKERS FIDELITY
PO BOX 190240
ATLANTA, GA 31119-0240
TOLL FREE: (800) 282-0480

BENEFIT RESOURCES

NATIONAL CLAIMS OFFICE
HARDMAN & CO
15721 N GRNWY HAYDEN LOOP, STE 205
SCOTTSDALE, AZ 85260
TEL: (602) 607-6100
FAX: (602) 607-6199
TOLL FREE: (800) 658-5874

BENEFIT & RISK MANAGEMENT SERVICES

CALIFORNIA CLAIMS OFFICE
3610 AMERICAN RIVER DR, STE 150
SACRAMENTO, CA 95864
TEL: (916) 974-2626
FAX: (916) 974-2653
TOLL FREE: (800) 476-0218
WWW.BEST-ONLINE.COM

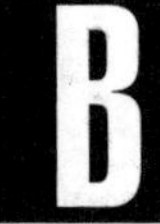

BENEFIT SUPPORT, INC

ALABAMA CLAIMS OFFICE
305 GREEN ST
PO BOX 2977
GAINESVILLE, GA 30503
TEL: (770) 532-2690
FAX: (770) 532-1514
IN-STATE: (800) 777-4782

FLORIDA CLAIMS OFFICE
305 GREEN ST
PO BOX 2977
GAINESVILLE, GA 30503
TEL: (770) 532-2690
FAX: (770) 532-1514
IN-STATE: (800) 777-4782

GEORGIA CLAIMS OFFICE
305 GREEN ST
PO BOX 2977
GAINESVILLE, GA 30503
TEL: (770) 532-2690
FAX: (770) 532-1514
IN-STATE: (800) 777-4782

INDIANA CLAIMS OFFICE
305 GREEN ST
PO BOX 2977
GAINESVILLE, GA 30503
TEL: (770) 532-2690
FAX: (770) 532-1514
IN-STATE: (800) 777-4782

KENTUCKY CLAIMS OFFICE
305 GREEN ST
PO BOX 2977
GAINESVILLE, GA 30503
TEL: (770) 532-2690
FAX: (770) 532-1514
IN-STATE: (800) 777-4782

MISSISSIPPI CLAIMS OFFICE
305 GREEN ST
PO BOX 2977
GAINESVILLE, GA 30503
TEL: (770) 532-2690
FAX: (770) 532-1514
IN-STATE: (800) 777-4782

NORTH CAROLINA CLAIMS OFFICE
305 GREEN ST
PO BOX 2977
GAINESVILLE, GA 30503
TEL: (770) 532-2690
FAX: (770) 532-1514
IN-STATE: (800) 777-4782

OHIO CLAIMS OFFICE
305 GREEN ST
PO BOX 2977
GAINESVILLE, GA 30503
TEL: (770) 532-2690
FAX: (770) 532-1514
IN-STATE: (800) 777-4782

SOUTH CAROLINA CLAIMS OFFICE
305 GREEN ST
PO BOX 2977
GAINESVILLE, GA 30503
TEL: (770) 532-2690
FAX: (770) 532-1514
IN-STATE: (800) 777-4782

TENNESSEE CLAIMS OFFICE
305 GREEN ST
PO BOX 2977
GAINESVILLE, GA 30503
TEL: (770) 532-2690
FAX: (770) 532-1514
IN-STATE: (800) 777-4782

VIRGINIA CLAIMS OFFICE
305 GREEN ST
PO BOX 2977
GAINESVILLE, GA 30503
TEL: (770) 532-2690
FAX: (770) 532-1514
IN-STATE: (800) 777-4782

WASHINGTON CLAIMS OFFICE
305 GREEN ST
PO BOX 2977
GAINESVILLE, GA 30503
TEL: (770) 532-2690
FAX: (770) 532-1514
IN-STATE: (800) 777-4782

BENEFIT SYSTEMS, INC

INDIANA CLAIMS OFFICE
9102 N MERIDIAN ST, STE 200
PO BOX 6001
INDIANAPOLIS, IN 46206-6001
TEL: (317) 573-2004
FAX: (317) 573-2016
TOLL FREE: (800) 842-3216
IN-STATE: (800) 624-8316

BENEFIT SYSTEMS & SERVICES, INC

ILLINOIS CLAIMS OFFICE
760 PASQUINELLI DR, STE 320
WESTMONT, IL 60559-5555
TEL: (630) 789-2082
FAX: (630) 789-2093
TOLL FREE: (800) 423-1841

BENEFITSOURCE, INC

MICHIGAN CLAIMS OFFICE
23 E FRONT, STE 201
PO BOX 240
MONROE, MI 48161
TEL: (734) 242-4443
FAX: (734) 242-4437
TOLL FREE: (800) 742-4441
WWW.BENEFITSOURCEINC.COM

BENICOMP, INC

INDIANA CLAIMS OFFICE
8310 CLINTON PK DR
FT WAYNE, IN 46825
TEL: (219) 482-7400
FAX: (219) 482-8991
TOLL FREE: (800) 837-7400
E-MAIL: BENICOMP@BENICOMP.COM
WWW.BENICOMP.COM

BENICORP INSURANCE CO

5285 W LAKEVIEW PKY S DR
PO BOX 68917
INDIANAPOLIS, IN 46268-4111
TEL: (317) 290-1205
FAX: (317) 216-7877
TOLL FREE: (800) 837-1205
E-MAIL: CLAIMS@BENICORP.COM
WWW.BENICORP.COM

BERKSHIRE LIFE INSURANCE CO

ALABAMA CLAIMS OFFICE
700 SOUTH ST
PITTSFIELD, MA 01201-8212
TEL: (413) 499-4321
FAX: (413) 499-4831

ARIZONA CLAIMS OFFICE
700 SOUTH ST
PITTSFIELD, MA 01201-8212
TEL: (413) 499-4321
FAX: (413) 499-4831

CALIFORNIA CLAIMS OFFICE
700 SOUTH ST
PITTSFIELD, MA 01201-8212
TEL: (413) 499-4321
FAX: (413) 499-4831

COLORADO CLAIMS OFFICE
700 SOUTH ST
PITTSFIELD, MA 01201-8212
TEL: (413) 499-4321
FAX: (413) 499-4831

CONNECTICUT CLAIMS OFFICE
700 SOUTH ST
PITTSFIELD, MA 01201-8212
TEL: (413) 499-4321
FAX: (413) 499-4831

DISTRICT OF COLUMBIA CLAIMS OFFICE
700 SOUTH ST
PITTSFIELD, MA 01201-8212
TEL: (413) 499-4321
FAX: (413) 499-4831

FLORIDA CLAIMS OFFICE
700 SOUTH ST
PITTSFIELD, MA 01201-8212
TEL: (413) 499-4321
FAX: (413) 499-4831

GEORGIA CLAIMS OFFICE
700 SOUTH ST
PITTSFIELD, MA 01201-8212
TEL: (413) 499-4321
FAX: (413) 499-4831

ILLINOIS CLAIMS OFFICE
700 SOUTH ST
PITTSFIELD, MA 01201-8212
TEL: (413) 499-4321
FAX: (413) 499-4831

INDIANA CLAIMS OFFICE
700 SOUTH ST
PITTSFIELD, MA 01201-8212
TEL: (413) 499-4321
FAX: (413) 499-4831

MAINE CLAIMS OFFICE
700 SOUTH ST
PITTSFIELD, MA 01201-8212
TEL: (413) 499-4321
FAX: (413) 499-4831

MARYLAND CLAIMS OFFICE
700 SOUTH ST
PITTSFIELD, MA 01201-8212
TEL: (413) 499-4321
FAX: (413) 499-4831

MASSACHUSETTS CLAIMS OFFICE
700 SOUTH ST
PITTSFIELD, MA 01201-8212
TEL: (413) 499-4321
FAX: (413) 499-4831

MICHIGAN CLAIMS OFFICE
700 SOUTH ST
PITTSFIELD, MA 01201-8212
TEL: (413) 499-4321
FAX: (413) 499-4831

MISSOURI CLAIMS OFFICE
700 SOUTH ST
PITTSFIELD, MA 01201-8212
TEL: (413) 499-4321
FAX: (413) 499-4831

NEW JERSEY CLAIMS OFFICE
700 SOUTH ST
PITTSFIELD, MA 01201-8212
TEL: (413) 499-4321
FAX: (413) 499-4831

NEW MEXICO CLAIMS OFFICE
700 SOUTH ST
PITTSFIELD, MA 01201-8212
TEL: (413) 499-4321
FAX: (413) 499-4831

NEW YORK CLAIMS OFFICE
700 SOUTH ST
PITTSFIELD, MA 01201-8212
TEL: (413) 499-4321
FAX: (413) 499-4831

NORTH CAROLINA CLAIMS OFFICE
700 SOUTH ST
PITTSFIELD, MA 01201-8212
TEL: (413) 499-4321
FAX: (413) 499-4831

OHIO CLAIMS OFFICE
700 SOUTH ST
PITTSFIELD, MA 01201-8212
TEL: (413) 499-4321
FAX: (413) 499-4831

PENNSYLVANIA CLAIMS OFFICE
700 SOUTH ST
PITTSFIELD, MA 01201-8212
TEL: (413) 499-4321
FAX: (413) 499-4831

RHODE ISLAND CLAIMS OFFICE
700 SOUTH ST
PITTSFIELD, MA 01201-8212
TEL: (413) 499-4321
FAX: (413) 499-4831

TEXAS CLAIMS OFFICE
700 SOUTH ST
PITTSFIELD, MA 01201-8212
TEL: (413) 499-4321
FAX: (413) 499-4831

VIRGINIA CLAIMS OFFICE
700 SOUTH ST
PITTSFIELD, MA 01201-8212
TEL: (413) 499-4321
FAX: (413) 499-4831

WASHINGTON CLAIMS OFFICE
700 SOUTH ST
PITTSFIELD, MA 01201-8212
TEL: (413) 499-4321
FAX: (413) 499-4831

BERKSHIRE MUTUAL INSURANCE CO

MASSACHUSETTS CLAIMS OFFICE
703 W HOUSATONIC
PO BOX 11640
PITTSFIELD, MA 01202
TEL: (413) 443-4461
FAX: (413) 499-8871
TOLL FREE: (800) 292-5026

BERTHALON-ROWLAND CORP

ILLINOIS CLAIMS OFFICE
600 W FULTON ST- 2ND FL
CHICAGO, IL 60661-1110
TEL: (312) 930-0020
FAX: (312) 930-0371
TOLL FREE: (800) 621-9903

BERWANGER OVERMYER ASSOCIATES

OHIO CLAIMS OFFICE
2245 NORTHBANK DR
PO BOX 20945
COLUMBUS, OH 43220
TEL: (614) 457-7000
FAX: (614) 457-1507
TOLL FREE: (800) 837-0503
IN-STATE: (800) 837-0503
E-MAIL: BOA@BOA-INS.COM
WWW.BOA-INS.COM

BEST LIFE ASSURANCE CO OF CALIFORNIA

CALIFORNIA CLAIMS OFFICE
2505 MCCABE WAY
PO BOX 19721
IRVINE, CA 92623-9721
TEL: (949) 253-4080
FAX: (949) 222-1005
TOLL FREE: (800) 433-0088
E-MAIL: BASSURANCE@EARTHLINK.NET

BETTER BRANDS & AFFILIATES

GEORGIA CLAIMS OFFICE
755 JEFFERSON ST NW
PO BOX 93707
ATLANTA, GA 30377
TEL: (404) 872-4731
FAX: (404) 870-9236

BILL'S DOLLAR STORES, INC

NATIONAL CLAIMS OFFICE
BILL'S MEDICAL PLAN
PO BOX 6019
RIDGELAND, MS 39158-6019
TEL: (601) 899-4659
FAX: (601) 899-4799

BIOMET, INC

INDIANA CLAIMS OFFICE
PO BOX 587
WARSAW, IN 46581-0587
TEL: (219) 267-6639
FAX: (219) 372-1783

BITUMINOUS CASUALTY CORP

ALABAMA CLAIMS OFFICE
600 VESTAVIA PKY, STE 121
PO BOX 360865
BIRMINGHAM, AL 35236-0865
TEL: (205) 822-6041
FAX: (205) 822-8772
TOLL FREE: (800) 356-8720

111 VETERANS BLVD, STE 1526
PO BOX 19994
NEW ORLEANS, LA 70179-0994
TEL: (504) 837-5480
FAX: (504) 831-0720
TOLL FREE: (800) 605-0311

ARKANSAS CLAIMS OFFICE
10800 FINANCIAL CTR PKY, STE 400
PO BOX 25326
LITTLE ROCK, AR 72221-5326
TEL: (501) 224-3080
FAX: (501) 224-8147
TOLL FREE: (800) 876-8147

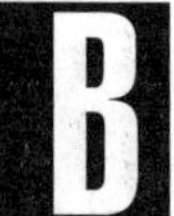

COLORADO CLAIMS OFFICE
PO BOX 412178
KANSAS CITY, MO 64141-2178
TEL: (816) 753-6808
FAX: (816) 753-3952
TOLL FREE: (800) 821-5354

GEORGIA CLAIMS OFFICE
2310 PARKLAKE DR NE, STE 550
ATLANTA, GA 30345-2904
TEL: (770) 934-9010
FAX: (770) 934-3734
TOLL FREE: (800) 822-2905

ILLINOIS CLAIMS OFFICE
OLD REPUBLIC INTERNATIONAL CORP
307 N MICHIGAN AVE
CHICAGO, IL 60601
TEL: (312) 346-8100
FAX: (312) 726-0309

234 MADISON AVE- BUS STE 102
PEORIA, IL 61602-8600
TEL: (309) 999-3720
FAX: (309) 999-3719

1600 4TH AVE- 3RD FL
ROCK ISLAND, IL 61201-8632
TEL: (309) 788-9361
FAX: (309) 788-9366
TOLL FREE: (800) 592-8991

INDIANA CLAIMS OFFICE
2601 FORTUNE CIR E, STE 201B
PO BOX 42608
INDIANAPOLIS, IN 46242-0608
TEL: (317) 243-6721
FAX: (317) 241-8922
TOLL FREE: (800) 382-9991

IOWA CLAIMS OFFICE
BITUMINOUS FIRE & MARINE INSURANCE CO
3737 WOODLAND, STE 240
PO BOX 65605
WEST DES MOINES, IA 50265-0605
TEL: (515) 223-1122
FAX: (515) 223-4315
TOLL FREE: (800) 383-1122

KANSAS CLAIMS OFFICE
PO BOX 718
SHAWNEE, MO 66201-0718
TEL: (913) 262-4664
FAX: (913) 262-0997
TOLL FREE: (800) 821-5354

KENTUCKY CLAIMS OFFICE
312 WHITTINGTON PKY
PO BOX 7567
LOUISVILLE, KY 40257-0567
TEL: (502) 426-9400
FAX: (502) 426-4787
TOLL FREE: (800) 633-0607

LOUISIANA CLAIMS OFFICE
111 VETERANS BLVD, STE 1526
PO BOX 19994
NEW ORLEANS, LA 70179-0994
TEL: (504) 837-5480
FAX: (504) 831-0720
TOLL FREE: (800) 605-0311

MARYLAND CLAIMS OFFICE
1301 YORK RD
PO BOX 509
LUTHERVILLE, MD 21094-0509
TEL: (410) 321-7670
FAX: (410) 296-7413
TOLL FREE: (800) 346-5108

MICHIGAN CLAIMS OFFICE
27777 FRANKLIN RD, STE 1160
SOUTHFIELD, MI 48034-2367
TEL: (248) 352-8052
FAX: (248) 352-8637
TOLL FREE: (800) 356-8727

MISSISSIPPI CLAIMS OFFICE
111 VETERANS BLVD, STE 1526
PO BOX 19994
NEW ORLEANS, LA 70179-0994
TEL: (504) 837-5480
FAX: (504) 831-0720
TOLL FREE: (800) 605-0311

MISSOURI CLAIMS OFFICE
PO BOX 718
SHAWNEE, MO 64141-2178
TEL: (913) 262-4664
FAX: (913) 262-0997
TOLL FREE: (800) 821-5354

10733 SUNSET OFFICE DR, STE 430
SAINT LOUIS, MO 63127-1033
TEL: (314) 822-4446
FAX: (314) 822-9850
TOLL FREE: (800) 723-8632

NEW MEXICO CLAIMS OFFICE
PO BOX 718
SHAWNEE, MO 66201-0718
TEL: (913) 262-4664
FAX: (913) 262-0997
TOLL FREE: (800) 821-5354

NORTH CAROLINA CLAIMS OFFICE
4801 E INDEPENDENCE BLVD, STE 505
CHARLOTTE, NC 28212-5400
TEL: (704) 341-3725
TOLL FREE: (800) 642-2507

NORTH DAKOTA CLAIMS OFFICE
BITUMINOUS FIRE & MARINE INSURANCE CO
3737 WOODLAND, STE 240
PO BOX 65605
WEST DES MOINES, IA 50265-0605
TEL: (515) 223-1122
FAX: (515) 223-4315
TOLL FREE: (800) 383-1122

OKLAHOMA CLAIMS OFFICE
GRAND CENTRE OFFICE BLDG
5400 NW GRAND BLVD, STE 545
OKLAHOMA CITY, OK 73112
TEL: (405) 947-0809
FAX: (405) 947-1006
TOLL FREE: (800) 947-0809

PENNSYLVANIA CLAIMS OFFICE
651 HOLIDAY DR- FOSTER PLZ 5
PITTSBURGH, PA 15220-2757
TEL: (412) 937-9000
FAX: (412) 937-1143
TOLL FREE: (800) 253-1232

SOUTH DAKOTA CLAIMS OFFICE
BITUMINOUS FIRE & MARINE INSURANCE CO
3737 WOODLAND, STE 240
PO BOX 65605
WEST DES MOINES, IA 50265-0605
TEL: (515) 223-1122
FAX: (515) 223-4315
TOLL FREE: (800) 383-1122

TENNESSEE CLAIMS OFFICE
5401 KINGSTON PIKE
PO BOX 10347
KNOXVILLE, TN 37939-0347
TEL: (423) 588-8157
FAX: (423) 558-8658
TOLL FREE: (800) 374-2318

2630 ELM HILL PIKE, STE 175
PO BOX 291689
NASHVILLE, TN 37229-1689
TEL: (615) 871-9042
FAX: (615) 871-0783
TOLL FREE: (800) 342-5786

TEXAS CLAIMS OFFICE
16225 PART TEN PLACE, STE 430
HOUSTON, TX 77084
TEL: (281) 398-2208
FAX: (281) 398-2211
TOLL FREE: (800) 462-8999

222 W LAS COLINAS BLVD, STE 1720
PO BOX 167968
IRVING, TX 75016-7968
TEL: (972) 506-9591
FAX: (972) 556-1539
TOLL FREE: (800) 683-9591

VIRGINIA CLAIMS OFFICE
7201 GLEN FOREST DR, STE 200
PO BOX 26503
RICHMOND, VA 23261
TEL: (804) 282-7641
FAX: (804) 282-2433
TOLL FREE: (800) 552-0101

WISCONSIN CLAIMS OFFICE
3333 N MAYFAIR RD, STE 104
MILWAUKEE, WI 53222-3226
TEL: (414) 476-5440
FAX: (414) 476-8887
TOLL FREE: (800) 242-6258

WYOMING CLAIMS OFFICE
PO BOX 412178
KANSAS CITY, MO 64141-2178
TEL: (816) 753-6808
FAX: (816) 753-3952
TOLL FREE: (800) 821-5354

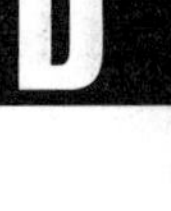

BITUMINOUS FIRE & MARINE INSURANCE CO

MONTANA CLAIMS OFFICE
3737 WOODLAND, STE 240
PO BOX 65605
WEST DES MOINES, IA 50265-0605
TEL: (515) 223-1122
FAX: (515) 223-4315
TOLL FREE: (800) 383-1122

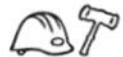

NATIONAL CLAIMS OFFICE
320 18TH ST
ROCK ISLAND, IL 61201-8744
TEL: (309) 786-5401
FAX: (309) 786-7073
TOLL FREE: (800) 475-4477
WWW.BITUMINOUSINSURANCE.COM

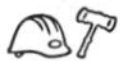

NEBRASKA CLAIMS OFFICE
3737 WOODLAND, STE 240
PO BOX 65605
WEST DES MOINES, IA 50265-0605
TEL: (515) 223-1122
FAX: (515) 223-4315
TOLL FREE: (800) 383-1122

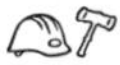

BITUMINOUS INSURANCE CO

TEXAS CLAIMS OFFICE
1031 ANDREWS HWY, STE 204
MIDLAND, TX 79701-3873
TEL: (915) 689-2114
FAX: (915) 697-3279
TOLL FREE: (800) 849-9305

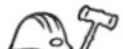

BLUE CARE NETWORK

MICHIGAN CLAIMS OFFICE
BLUE CARE NETWORK OF WEST MICHIGAN
611 CASCADE W PKY SE
GRAND RAPIDS, MI 49546-2107
TEL: (616) 957-5057
FAX: (616) 957-3476
TOLL FREE: (800) 968-2583

BLUE CARE NETWORK OF SOUTHEAST MICHIGAN
25925 TELEGRAPH RD
PO BOX 5043
SOUTHFIELD, MI 48086-5043
TEL: (248) 354-7450
FAX: (248) 799-6972
IN-STATE: (800) 821-6886
WWW.BCBSM.COM

BLUE CROSS & BLUE SHIELD

ALABAMA CLAIMS OFFICE
BLUE CROSS & BLUE SHIELD OF ALABAMA
450 RIVERCHASE PKY E
PO BOX 995
BIRMINGHAM, AL 35298-0001
TEL: (205) 988-2100
FAX: (205) 988-2949
E-MAIL: WEBINPUT@BCBSAL.ORG
WWW.BCBSAL

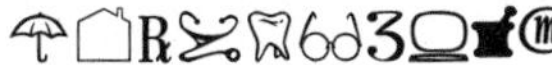

ARIZONA CLAIMS OFFICE
BLUE CROSS & BLUE SHIELD OF ARIZONA
PO BOX 2924
PHOENIX, AZ 85062-2924
TEL: (602) 864-4400
FAX: (602) 864-4242
TOLL FREE: (800) 232-2345

ARKANSAS CLAIMS OFFICE
BLUE CROSS & BLUE SHIELD OF ARKANSAS
601 GAINES ST
PO BOX 2181
LITTLE ROCK, AR 72203-2181
TEL: (501) 378-2000
FAX: (501) 378-2037
TOLL FREE: (800) 827-4814

CALIFORNIA CLAIMS OFFICE
BLUE CROSS & BLUE SHIELD OF CALIFORNIA
21555 OXNARD ST
PO BOX 70000
WOODLAND HILLS, CA 91470
TEL: (818) 703-2345
FAX: (818) 703-2563

BLUE CROSS & BLUE SHIELD OF CALIFORNIA
21555 OXNARD ST
PO BOX 70000
WOODLAND HILLS, CA 91367-4943
TEL: (818) 703-2345
FAX: (818) 703-2848
TOLL FREE: (800) 999-3643
WWW.BLUECROSSCA.COM

COLORADO CLAIMS OFFICE
BLUE CROSS & BLUE SHIELD OF COLORADO
700 BROADWAY
DENVER, CO 80273
TEL: (303) 831-2131
TOLL FREE: (800) 433-5447
WWW.BCBSCO.COM

DELAWARE CLAIMS OFFICE
BLUE CROSS & BLUE SHIELD OF DELAWARE
ONE BRANDYWINE GTWY
PO BOX 1991
WILMINGTON, DE 19899-1991
TEL: (302) 421-3000
FAX: (302) 421-2089
TOLL FREE: (800) 633-2563
IN-STATE: (800) 292-7865
WWW.BCBSDE.COM

DISTRICT OF COLUMBIA CLAIMS OFFICE
BLUE CROSS & BLUE SHIELD OF MARYLAND
550 12TH ST SW
WASHINGTON, DC 20065
TEL: (202) 479-8000
FAX: (202) 479-3520
TOLL FREE: (800) 424-7474

FLORIDA CLAIMS OFFICE
BLUE CROSS & BLUE SHIELD OF FLORIDA
532 RIVERSIDE AVE
PO BOX 1798
JACKSONVILLE, FL 32231-0014
TEL: (904) 791-6111
FAX: (904) 791-8738

3191 MAGUIRE BLVD, STE 125
ORLANDO, FL 32803-3723
TEL: (407) 894-3434
TOLL FREE: (800) 333-9797

GEORGIA CLAIMS OFFICE
BLUE CROSS & BLUE SHIELD OF GEORGIA
PO BOX 4445
ATLANTA, GA 30302-4445
TEL: (404) 842-8000
FAX: (404) 842-8010
TOLL FREE: (800) 441-2273
WWW.BCBSGA.COM

BLUE CROSS & BLUE SHIELD OF GEORGIA
2357 WARM SPRINGS RD
PO BOX 9907
COLUMBUS, GA 31908-9907
TEL: (706) 571-5371
FAX: (706) 571-5487
TOLL FREE: (800) 241-7475
WWW.BCBSGA.COM

HAWAII CLAIMS OFFICE
HAWAII MEDICAL SERVICE ASSOCIATION
818 KEEAUMOKU ST
PO BOX 860
HONOLULU, HI 96808-0860
TEL: (808) 948-5110
FAX: (808) 948-6555
IN-STATE: (800) 790-4672

ILLINOIS CLAIMS OFFICE
BLUE CROSS & BLUE SHIELD OF ILLINOIS
PO BOX 1364
CHICAGO, IL 60690-1364
TEL: (312) 653-6000
FAX: (312) 819-1220
WWW.BCBSIL.COM

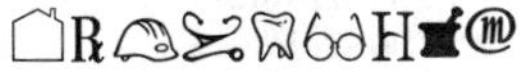

INDIANA CLAIMS OFFICE
5451 W LAKEVIEW PKY S DR
INDIANAPOLIS, IN 46268
TEL: (317) 921-7000
FAX: (317) 488-6477
TOLL FREE: (800) 331-1476
WWW.AICI.COM

IOWA CLAIMS OFFICE
BLUE CROSS OF WESTERN IOWA & SOUTH DAKOTA
PO BOX 1677
SIOUX CITY, IA 51102-1677
TEL: (712) 277-3081
FAX: (712) 279-8450
TOLL FREE: (800) 245-6105
WWW.WALMARK.COM

KANSAS CLAIMS OFFICE
BLUE CROSS & BLUE SHIELD OF KANSAS
1133 SW TOPEKA BLVD
PO BOX 239
TOPEKA, KS 66629-0001
TEL: (785) 291-7000
FAX: (785) 291-8465
TOLL FREE: (800) 332-0307
IN-STATE: (800) 234-0495

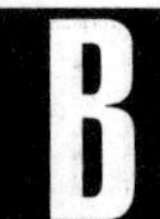

KENTUCKY CLAIMS OFFICE
ANTHEM BLUE CROSS & BLUE SHIELD- DELTA DENTAL
9901 LINN STATION RD
LOUISVILLE, KY 40223
TEL: (502) 423-2011
FAX: (502) 423-2627
TOLL FREE: (800) 880-2583
WWW.ANTHEM.COM

LOUISIANA CLAIMS OFFICE
BLUE CROSS & BLUE SHIELD OF LOUISIANA
PO BOX 98029, ATTN: CLAIMS PROCESSING
BATON ROUGE, LA 70898-9029
TEL: (225) 295-3307
TOLL FREE: (800) 599-2583
WWW.LABLUE.COM

MAINE CLAIMS OFFICE
BLUE CROSS & BLUE SHIELD OF MAINE
2 GANNETT DR
SOUTH PORTLAND, ME 04106-6911
TEL: (207) 822-7000
FAX: (207) 822-7375
TOLL FREE: (800) 482-0966
IN-STATE: (800) 482-0966
WWW.MAINEBLUE.COM

MARYLAND CLAIMS OFFICE
CARE FIRST BLUE CROSS & BLUE SHIELD
10455 MILL RUN CIR- ATTN:CLAIMS DEPT
OWINGS MILLS, MD 21117
TEL: (410) 581-3000
FAX: (410) 998-5576
TOLL FREE: (800) 524-4555
WWW.CAREFIRST.COM

MASSACHUSETTS CLAIMS OFFICE
BLUE CROSS & BLUE SHIELD OF MASSACHUSETTS, INC
100 SUMMER ST
BOSTON, MA 02110
TEL: (617) 832-5000

MICHIGAN CLAIMS OFFICE
BLUE CROSS & BLUE SHIELD OF MICHIGAN
600 E LAFAYETTE EAST
DETROIT, MI 48226-2998
TEL: (313) 225-9000
FAX: (313) 225-6239
TOLL FREE: (800) 637-2227

MINNESOTA CLAIMS OFFICE
BLUE CROSS & BLUE SHIELD OF MINNESOTA
PO BOX 64338
SAINT PAUL, MN 55164-0560
TEL: (651) 456-8000
FAX: (651) 456-6860
TOLL FREE: (800) 382-2000
WWW.BLUECROSSMN.COM

MISSISSIPPI CLAIMS OFFICE
BLUE CROSS & BLUE SHIELD OF MISSISSIPPI
PO BOX 1043
JACKSON, MS 39215-1043
TEL: (601) 932-3704
FAX: (601) 939-7035
TOLL FREE: (800) 222-8046
IN-STATE: (800) 222-8046

MISSOURI CLAIMS OFFICE
2301 MAIN ST
PO BOX 419169
KANSAS CITY, MO 64141-6169
TEL: (816) 395-2222
FAX: (816) 395-3959
TOLL FREE: (800) 892-6048
WWW.BCBSKC.COM

ALLIANCE BLUE CROSS & BLUE SHIELD OF MISSOURI
1831 CHESTNUT ST
SAINT LOUIS, MO 63103-2275
TEL: (314) 923-4444
FAX: (417) 888-9075
TOLL FREE: (800) 392-8740
WWW.ABCBS.COM

MONTANA CLAIMS OFFICE
BLUE CROSS & BLUE SHIELD OF MONTANA, INC
PO BOX 5004
GREAT FALLS, MT 59403-5004
TEL: (406) 791-4000
FAX: (406) 727-9355
TOLL FREE: (800) 447-7828
WWW.BCBSMT.COM

BLUE CROSS & BLUE SHIELD OF MONTANA, INC
404 FULLER
PO BOX 4309
HELENA, MT 59604-4309
TEL: (406) 444-8200
FAX: (406) 442-6946
TOLL FREE: (800) 447-7828
E-MAIL: GENERAL@BCBSMT.COM
WWW.BCBSMT.COM

NATIONAL CLAIMS OFFICE
BLUE CROSS & BLUE SHIELD OF NEBRASKA
7261 MERCY RD
PO BOX 3248
OMAHA, NE 68180
TEL: (402) 390-1820
FAX: (402) 392-2141
WWW.BCBSNE.COM

BLUE CROSS & BLUE SHIELD OF NORTH CAROLINA
PO BOX 2291
DURHAM, NC 27702-2291
TEL: (919) 489-7431
WWW.BCBSNC.COM

BLUE CROSS & BLUE SHIELD OF GEORGIA — COLUMBUS
PO BOX 7368
COLUMBUS, GA 31908-7368
TEL: (706) 571-5371
FAX: (706) 571-5487
TOLL FREE: (800) 441-2273
WWW.BCBSGA.COM

BLUE CROSS & BLUE SHIELD OF NEBRASKA
7261 MERCY RD
PO BOX 3248
OMAHA, NE 68180-0001
TEL: (402) 390-1800
FAX: (402) 392-2141
TOLL FREE: (800) 642-8980
WWW.BCBSNE.COM

BLUE CROSS & BLUE SHIELD OF NORTH DAKOTA
4510 13TH AVE SW
FARGO, ND 58121-0001
TEL: (701) 282-1100
FAX: (701) 277-2005
TOLL FREE: (800) 874-2656
IN-STATE: (800) 342-4718
WWW.BCBSND.COM

NEVADA CLAIMS OFFICE
BLUE CROSS & BLUE SHIELD OF NEVADA
PO BOX 173690
DENVER, CO 80217-3690
TOLL FREE: (800) 992-6907

NEW HAMPSHIRE CLAIMS OFFICE
BLUE CROSS & BLUE SHIELD OF NEW HAMPSHIRE
3000 GOFFS FALLS RD
MANCHESTER, NH 03111-0001
TEL: (603) 695-7000
FAX: (603) 695-7304
TOLL FREE: (800) 225-2666
WWW.BCBSNH.COM

NEW JERSEY CLAIMS OFFICE
HORIZON BLUE CROSS & BLUE SHIELD OF NEW JERSEY, INC
3 PENN PLZ E
NEWARK, NJ 07105
TEL: (973) 466-4000
TOLL FREE: (800) 355-2583
WWW.HORIZONBCBSNJ.COM

NEW MEXICO CLAIMS OFFICE
BLUE CROSS & BLUE SHIELD OF NEW MEXICO
PO BOX 27630
ALBUQUERQUE, NM 87125-7630
TEL: (505) 291-3500
FAX: (505) 291-3541
TOLL FREE: (800) 432-0750

NEW YORK CLAIMS OFFICE
BLUE CROSS OF WESTERN NEW YORK, INC
1901 MAIN ST
PO BOX 80
BUFFALO, NY 14240-0109
TEL: (716) 887-6900
FAX: (716) 887-8981
TOLL FREE: (800) 888-0757

EMPIRE BLUE CROSS & BLUE SHIELD
622 3RD AVE
PO BOX 345
NEW YORK, NY 10017
TEL: (212) 476-1000
TOLL FREE: (800) 261-5962
WWW.EMPIREBCBS.COM

Insurance Directory

BLUE CROSS & BLUE SHIELD OF CENTRAL NEW YORK, INC
344 S WARREN ST
PO BOX 4809
SYRACUSE, NY 13221-4809
TEL: (315) 448-3700
FAX: (315) 448-6950
TOLL FREE: (800) 633-6066
WWW.BCBSCNY.ORG

BLUE CROSS & BLUE SHIELD OF UTICA-WATERTOWN
12 RHOADS DR- UTICA BUSINESS PARK
UTICA, NY 13502-6398
TEL: (315) 798-4200
FAX: (315) 792-9752
TOLL FREE: (800) 765-5226

BLUE CROSS & BLUE SHIELD OF ROCHESTER
165 COURT ST
ROCHESTER, NY 14647-0001
TEL: (716) 454-1700
FAX: (716) 238-4400
TOLL FREE: (800) 847-1200

NORTH CAROLINA CLAIMS OFFICE
BLUE CROSS & BLUE SHIELD OF NORTH CAROLINA
800 S DUKE ST
PO BOX 2291
DURHAM, NC 27702
TEL: (919) 489-7431
FAX: (919) 765-4837
TOLL FREE: (800) 222-2783
IN-STATE: (800) 222-5028
WWW.BCBSNC.COM

OHIO CLAIMS OFFICE
ANTHEM BLUE CROSS & BLUE SHIELD OF OHIO- HOME OFFICE
1351 WILLIAM HOWARD TAFT RD
CINCINNATI, OH 45206
TEL: (513) 872-8100
FAX: (513) 872-8174
TOLL FREE: (800) 442-1832
WWW.AICI.COM

MEDICAL MUTUAL OF OHIO
2060 E 9TH ST
CLEVELAND, OH 44115-1355
TEL: (216) 687-7000
FAX: (216) 687-6044
WWW.MMOH.COM

MUTUAL MEDICAL OF OHIO
3737 W SALVANIA AVE
PO BOX 943
TOLEDO, OH 43656-0001
TEL: (419) 473-7100
FAX: (419) 473-6200
WWW.MMOH.COM

ANTHEM BLUE CROSS & BLUE SHIELD
6740 N HIGH ST
PO BOX 425
WORTHINGTON, OH 43085
TEL: (614) 438-3500
FAX: (513) 872-8174
WWW.AICI.COM

ANTHEM BLUE CROSS & BLUE SHIELD-CUSTOMER SERVICE OFFICE
3530 VELMONT
YOUNGSTOWN, OH 44505
TEL: (330) 759-0771
TOLL FREE: (800) 458-6813
WWW.MMOH.COM

OKLAHOMA CLAIMS OFFICE
BLUE CROSS & BLUE SHIELD OF OKLAHOMA
1215 S BOULDER
PO BOX 3283
TULSA, OK 74102-3283
TEL: (918) 560-3500
WWW.BCBSOK.COM

PENNSYLVANIA CLAIMS OFFICE
CAPITAL BLUE CROSS & PENNSYLVANIA BLUE SHIELD
1221 W HAMILTON ST
ALLENTOWN, PA 18102-4370
TEL: (610) 820-2700
FAX: (610) 820-2663
TOLL FREE: (800) 958-5558
WWW.CAPBLUECROSS.COM

PENNSYLVANIA BLUE SHIELD
1800 CENTER ST
PO BOX 890089
CAMP HILL, PA 17089-0089
TEL: (717) 763-3151

PENNSYLVANIA BLUE SHIELD
PO BOX 898200
CAMP HILL, PA 17089-8200
TEL: (717) 763-3151

INDEPENDENCE BLUE CROSS PENNSYLVANIA
1901 MARKET ST
PHILADELPHIA, PA 19103
TEL: (215) 241-2400
FAX: (215) 241-2133
TOLL FREE: (800) 358-0050
WWW.IBX.COM

HIGHMARK BLUE CROSS & BLUE SHIELD
120 FIFTH AVE
PITTSBURGH, PA 15222-3099
TEL: (412) 544-7000
IN-STATE: (800) 547-3627
WWW.HIGHMARK.COM

BLUE CROSS OF NORTHEASTERN PENNSYLVANIA FIRST PRIORITY HEALTH
70 N MAIN ST
WILKES-BARRE, PA 18711
TEL: (717) 829-6011
FAX: (717) 829-0188
TOLL FREE: (800) 829-8599
WWW.BCNEPA.COM

PUERTO RICO CLAIMS OFFICE
TRIPLE-S
PO BOX 363628
SAN JUAN, PR 00936-3628
TEL: (787) 749-4949
FAX: (787) 749-4190

RHODE ISLAND CLAIMS OFFICE
BLUE CROSS & BLUE SHIELD OF RHODE ISLAND
444 WESTMINSTER ST
PROVIDENCE, RI 02903-3279
TEL: (401) 459-1000
FAX: (401) 351-2050
TOLL FREE: (800) 637-3718
WWW.BCBSRI.COM

SOUTH CAROLINA CLAIMS OFFICE
BLUE CROSS & BLUE SHIELD OF SOUTH CAROLINA
I-20 E AT ALPINE RD
COLUMBIA, SC 29219-0001
TEL: (803) 788-3860
FAX: (803) 736-3420
TOLL FREE: (800) 868-2500
IN-STATE: (800) 288-2227
WWW.BCBSSC.COM

SOUTH DAKOTA CLAIMS OFFICE
WELLMARK BLUE CROSS & BLUE SHIELD OF SOUTH DAKOTA
1601 W MADISON ST
SIOUX FALLS, SD 57104-5710
TEL: (605) 361-5800
FAX: (605) 361-5897
TOLL FREE: (800) 831-4818
WWW.WELLMARK.COM

TENNESSEE CLAIMS OFFICE
BLUE CROSS & BLUE SHIELD OF TENNESSEE
801 PINE ST
CHATTANOOGA, TN 37402-2556
TEL: (423) 755-5600
FAX: (423) 755-2178

BLUE CROSS & BLUE SHIELD OF TENNESSEE
PO BOX 98
MEMPHIS, TN 38101
TEL: (901) 544-2111
FAX: (901) 544-2440
TOLL FREE: (800) 222-7212
WWW.BCBSTN.COM

TEXAS CLAIMS OFFICE
BLUE CROSS & BLUE SHIELD OF TEXAS
901 S CENTRAL EXPY
PO BOX 655730
RICHARDSON, TX 75080
TEL: (972) 766-6900
FAX: (972) 766-6060
TOLL FREE: (800) 521-2227
WWW.BCBS.COM

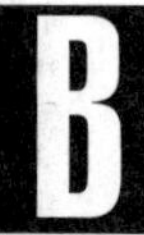

BLUE CROSS & BLUE SHIELD OF TEXAS HMO
BLUE EL PASO
4150 PINNACLE, STE 203
EL PASO, TX 79902-1035
TEL: (915) 542-1547
FAX: (915) 496-6719
TOLL FREE: (800) 831-0576
WWW.BCBSPX.COM

UTAH CLAIMS OFFICE
REGENTS BLUE CROSS & BLUE SHIELD OF UTAH
2890 E COTTONWOOD PKY
PO BOX 30270
SALT LAKE CITY, UT 84121-0270
TEL: (801) 333-2000
FAX: (801) 333-6523
TOLL FREE: (800) 624-6519
E-MAIL: UT.CUSTSERV@REGENTS.COM
WWW.BCBSUTAH.COM

VERMONT CLAIMS OFFICE
BLUE CROSS & BLUE SHIELD OF VERMONT
PO BOX 186
MONTPELIER, VT 05601-0186
TEL: (802) 223-6131
FAX: (802) 223-1077
TOLL FREE: (800) 457-6648
IN-STATE: (800) 247-2583
WWW.BCBSVT.COM

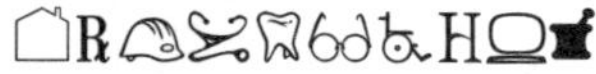

VIRGINIA CLAIMS OFFICE
TRIGON BLUE CROSS & BLUE SHIELD
PO BOX 27401
RICHMOND, VA 23279-7401
TEL: (804) 354-7000
FAX: (804) 354-7600
TOLL FREE: (800) 451-1527
WWW.TRIGON.COM

TRIGON BLUE CROSS & BLUE SHIELD
PO BOX 27401
RICHMOND, VA 23279
TEL: (804) 342-0010
TOLL FREE: (800) 533-1120
WWW.TRIGON.COM

WASHINGTON CLAIMS OFFICE
PREMERA BLUE CROSS & BLUE SHIELD OF ALASKA & WASHINGTON
PO BOX 327
SEATTLE, WA 98111-0327
TEL: (425) 670-4000
FAX: (425) 670-4900
TOLL FREE: (800) 213-5470
IN-STATE: (800) 345-6784
WWW.PREMERA.COM

REGENCE BLUE CROSS & BLUE SHIELD - KING COUNTY MEDICAL
1800 9TH AVE
PO BOX 21267
SEATTLE, WA 98111-3267
TEL: (206) 464-3600
FAX: (206) 389-6778
TOLL FREE: (800) 464-3663
IN-STATE: (800) 458-3523

MEDICAL SERVICE CORPORATION PREMERA BLUE CROSS
EAST 3900 SPRAGUE
PO BOX 3048
SPOKANE, WA 99220-3048
TEL: (509) 536-4700
TOLL FREE: (800) 835-3510
IN-STATE: (800) 572-0778
WWW.PREMERA.COM

PREMERA BLUE CROSS & BLUE SHIELD OF ALASKA & WASHINGTON
PO BOX 327
SEATTLE, WA 98111-0327
TEL: (425) 670-4000
FAX: (425) 670-4900
TOLL FREE: (800) 213-5470
IN-STATE: (800) 345-6784
WWW.PREMERA.COM

WISCONSIN CLAIMS OFFICE
BLUE CROSS & BLUE SHIELD UNITED OF WISCONSIN
401 W MICHIGAN ST
PO BOX 2025
MILWAUKEE, WI 53201-2025
TEL: (414) 226-5000
FAX: (414) 226-5040
TOLL FREE: (800) 558-1584
WWW.BCBSUW.ORG

WYOMING CLAIMS OFFICE
BLUE CROSS & BLUE SHIELD OF WYOMING
PO BOX 2266
CHEYENNE, WY 82003-2266
TEL: (307) 634-1393
FAX: (307) 778-8582
TOLL FREE: (800) 442-2376
IN-STATE: (800) 442-2376

BLUE CROSS & BLUE SHIELD OF MAINE

MAINE CLAIMS OFFICE
TWO GINNETT DR
SOUTH PORTLAND, ME 04106-6909
TEL: (207) 822-8282
FAX: (207) 822-7375
IN-STATE: (800) 822-6011
WWW.MAINEBLUECROSS.COM

BLUE CROSS OF IDAHO HEALTH SERVICE, INC

IDAHO CLAIMS OFFICE
3000 E PINE AVE
PO BOX 7408
BOISE, ID 83707
TEL: (208) 345-4550
FAX: (208) 331-7311
TOLL FREE: (800) 627-6655
WWW.BCIDAHO.COM

BLUE PLUS

MINNESOTA CLAIMS OFFICE
BLUE CROSS & BLUE SHIELD OF MINNESOTA BLUE PLUS & AFFILIATES
PO BOX 64179
SAINT PAUL, MN 55164-0179
TEL: (651) 456-8501
FAX: (651) 456-1004
TOLL FREE: (800) 382-2000
WWW.BCBSMN.COM

BLUE RIDGE ADMINISTRATORS

VIRGINIA CLAIMS OFFICE
COMMONWEALTH HEALTH ALLIANCE, INC
105 S PANTOPS DR, STE C3
PO BOX 1067
CHARLOTTESVILLE, VA 22902
TEL: (804) 977-3500
FAX: (804) 979-5626
TOLL FREE: (800) 677-1867
WWW.COMCLIN.NET

BLUE RIDGE INSURANCE CO

NEW YORK CLAIMS OFFICE
200 ELWOOD DAVIS RD
PO BOX 116
LIVERPOOL, NY 13088-0116
TEL: (315) 451-2246
FAX: (315) 457-4509
TOLL FREE: (800) 961-1121

TEXAS CLAIMS OFFICE
PO BOX 519
SIMSBURY, CT 06070-0519
TEL: (860) 651-1065
FAX: (860) 408-3268
TOLL FREE: (800) 961-1121
WWW.BLUERIDGEINS.COM

BLUE SHIELD OF CALIFORNIA

CALIFORNIA CLAIMS OFFICE
CARE AMERICA
103 WOOD MERE
PO BOX 272550
FOLSOM, CA 95630
TOLL FREE: (800) 424-6521
IN-STATE: (800) 424-6521
WWW.BLUESHIELDCA.COM

SENIOR PLANS
129 N GUILD AVE
PO BOX 241004
LODI, CA 95241-9504
TEL: (209) 367-2800
TOLL FREE: (800) 248-2341
WWW.BLUESHIELDCA.COM

PERS CARE SERVICE CENTER
129 N GUILD AVE
PO BOX 272530
CHICO, CA 95927-2530
TEL: (209) 367-2800
TOLL FREE: (800) 444-2595
WWW.BLUESHIELDCA.COM

Insurance Directory

HMO CLAIMS FOR LODI
129 N GUILD AVE
PO BOX 272540
CHICO, CA 95927-2540
TEL: (209) 367-2800
TOLL FREE: (800) 444-1409
WWW.BLUESHIELDCA.COM

H

HMO CLAIMS FOR SOUTHERN AREA
129 N GUILD AVE
PO BOX 272540
CHICO, CA 95927-2540
TEL: (209) 367-2800
TOLL FREE: (800) 535-8000
WWW.BLUESHIELDCA.COM

H

CLAIMS CENTER FOR GENERAL ELECTRIC
40 NE ST
PO BOX 769028
WOODLAND, CA 95776-9028
TEL: (530) 674-0504
FAX: (530) 668-2801
TOLL FREE: (800) 688-0327
WWW.GEOACCESS.COM

℞ 3 H

CLAIMS CENTER FOR BANK OF AMERICA
40 N EAST ST
PO BOX 769014
WOODLAND, CA 95776-9014
TEL: (209) 241-4896
TOLL FREE: (800) 995-2800
WWW.BLUESHIELDCA.COM

℞ 6d H

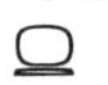

50 BEALE ST
PO BOX 7168
SAN FRANCISCO, CA 94105
TEL: (415) 229-5000
WWW.BCBSCA.COM

6d

BLUE SHIELD OF CALIFORNIA HEADQUARTERS

CALIFORNIA PHYSICIAN SERVICES
50 BEALE ST
PO BOX 7168
SAN FRANCISCO, CA 94120-7168
TEL: (415) 229-5000
TOLL FREE: (800) 640-1013
WWW.BLUESHIELOFCALIFORNIA.COM

℞ 6d 3 H

BLUE SHIELD OF NORTHEASTERN NEW YORK

NEW YORK CLAIMS OFFICE
187 WOLF RD
PO BOX 15013
ALBANY, NY 12212
TEL: (518) 453-5700
FAX: (518) 438-1837
TOLL FREE: (800) 888-1238
WWW.BLUECARES.COM/BLUECARD

℞ 6d 3 H ☆

BLUELINCS HMO

OKLAHOMA CLAIMS OFFICE
3401 NW 63RD ST
PO BOX 21128
TULSA, OK 74121-1128
TEL: (405) 841-9777
FAX: (405) 841-9629
TOLL FREE: (800) 722-5675
WWW.BCBSOK.COM

H

BOLLINGER FOWLER AGENCY

NATIONAL CLAIMS OFFICE
830 MORRIS TPKE
PO BOX 706
SHORT HILLS, NJ 07078-2620
TEL: (973) 467-0444
FAX: (973) 467-0190
TOLL FREE: (800) 526-1379

℞ 6d

BOON-CHAPMAN

TEXAS CLAIMS OFFICE
7600 CHEVY CHASE DR, STE 300
PO BOX 9201
AUSTIN, TX 78766-9201
TEL: (512) 454-2681
FAX: (512) 459-1552
TOLL FREE: (800) 252-9653
WWW.BOONCHAPMAN.COM

℞ 6d

BOSTON MUTUAL LIFE INSURANCE CO

MASSACHUSETTS CLAIMS OFFICE
120 ROYALL ST
CANTON, MA 02021-1098
TEL: (781) 828-7000
FAX: (781) 821-4976
TOLL FREE: (800) 669-2668
WWW.BOSTONMUTUAL.COM

BPS INC

NATIONAL CLAIMS OFFICE
145 N CHURCH ST, STE 300
PO BOX 1227
SPARTANBURG, SC 29304-1227
TEL: (864) 585-4338
FAX: (864) 573-7709
TOLL FREE: (800) 868-7526
WWW.BPSINC.COM

℞ 6d 3 ☆

BR ASSOCIATES INC

INDIANA CLAIMS OFFICE
4201A MANNHEIM RD
JASPER, IN 47546-9618
TEL: (812) 482-3212
FAX: (812) 482-4013

6d

BRADFORD FINANCIAL CENTER

IOWA CLAIMS OFFICE
215 N MAIN
PO BOX 540
CLARION, IA 50525-1439
TEL: (515) 532-6661
FAX: (515) 532-6547
TOLL FREE: (800) 348-4419
E-MAIL: BRADFORD@NETINS.NET

3

BREMEN FARMERS MUTUAL INSURANCE CO

KANSAS CLAIMS OFFICE
PO BOX 98
BREMEN, KS 66412
TEL: (785) 337-2203
FAX: (785) 337-2414
TOLL FREE: (800) 562-5712

BRETHREN MUTUAL INSURANCE CO

MARYLAND CLAIMS OFFICE
149 N EDGEWOOD DR
HAGERSTOWN, MD 21740-6599
TEL: (301) 739-0950
FAX: (301) 739-6301
TOLL FREE: (800) 621-4264
WWW.BMICONLINE.COM

BRICKLAYERS & STONE MASONS LOCAL 20

ILLINOIS CLAIMS OFFICE
FRINGE BENEFIT FUNDS
2751 W WASHINGTON ST
WAUKEGAN, IL 60085
TEL: (847) 244-3685
FAX: (847) 244-0556

6d

BRISTOL WEST INSURANCE SERVICES

FLORIDA CLAIMS OFFICE
SECURITY NATIONAL
6067 HOLLYWOOD BLVD
PO BOX 229080
HOLLYWOOD, FL 33022-9080
TEL: (954) 985-4262
FAX: (954) 963-7663
TOLL FREE: (800) 537-2133
WWW.BRISTOLWEST.COM

BRITISH AMERICAN INSURANCE CO

TEXAS CLAIMS OFFICE
3535 TRAVIS ST, STE 300
PO BOX 1590
DALLAS, TX 75221-1590
TEL: (214) 559-4887
FAX: (214) 443-5581
TOLL FREE: (800) 964-4242

6d H

8031 AIRPORT BLVD, STE 214
PO BOX 1590
DALLAS, TX 75221
TEL: (214) 559-4887
FAX: (214) 443-5581
TOLL FREE: (800) 964-4242

BRODART CO

CALIFORNIA CLAIMS OFFICE
500 ARCH ST
WILLIAMSPORT, PA 17705
TEL: (717) 326-2461
FAX: (717) 326-3039
TOLL FREE: (800) 233-8467

℞

OREGON CLAIMS OFFICE
500 ARCH ST
WILLIAMSPORT, PA 17705
TEL: (717) 326-2461
FAX: (717) 326-3039
TOLL FREE: (800) 233-8467

℞

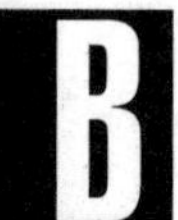

PENNSYLVANIA CLAIMS OFFICE
500 ARCH ST
WILLIAMSPORT, PA 17705
TEL: (717) 326-2461
FAX: (717) 326-3039
TOLL FREE: (800) 233-8467

WASHINGTON CLAIMS OFFICE
500 ARCH ST
WILLIAMSPORT, PA 17705
TEL: (717) 326-2461
FAX: (717) 326-3039
TOLL FREE: (800) 233-8467

BROKERAGE CONCEPTS, INC

PENNSYLVANIA CLAIMS OFFICE
BENEFIT CONCEPTS
651 ALLENDALE RD
PO BOX 60608
KING OF PRUSSIA, PA 19406-0608
TEL: (610) 337-2600
FAX: (610) 491-4992
TOLL FREE: (800) 220-2600

BROKERAGE SERVICES, INC

NEW MEXICO CLAIMS OFFICE
11200 LOOMAS BLVD NE
PO BOX 11020
ALBUQUERQUE, NM 87192-0020
TEL: (505) 292-5533
FAX: (505) 293-7725
TOLL FREE: (800) 274-5533

BRONX HEALTH PLAN

NEW YORK CLAIMS OFFICE
1 FORDHAM PLZ- 2ND FL, STE E-220
BRONX, NY 10458-5870
TEL: (718) 733-4747
FAX: (718) 733-4750

BROOKSHIRE BROTHERS, LTD

TEXAS CLAIMS OFFICE
1201 ELLEN TROUT DR
PO BOX 1688
LUFKIN, TX 75902-1688
TEL: (409) 634-8155
FAX: (409) 634-8646
IN-STATE: (800) 364-6690

BROTHERHOOD MUTUAL INSURANCE CO

INDIANA CLAIMS OFFICE
6400 BROTHERHOOD WY
PO BOX 2227
FT WAYNE, IN 46801-2227
TEL: (219) 482-8668
FAX: (219) 482-3589

BUEHLER FOOD MARKETS

OHIO CLAIMS OFFICE
1401 OLD MANSFIELD RD
PO BOX 196
WOOSTER, OH 44691-0196
TEL: (330) 264-4355

BUFFALO GENERAL HOSPITAL

NEW YORK CLAIMS OFFICE
HEALTH CARE SYSTEM
100 HIGH ST
BUFFALO, NY 14203-1154
TEL: (716) 859-5600
FAX: (716) 859-2650
TOLL FREE: (800) 242-0055

BUFFALO ROCK CO, INC

ALABAMA CLAIMS OFFICE
103 OXMOOR RD
PO BOX 10048
BIRMINGHAM, AL 35202-0048
TEL: (205) 942-3435
FAX: (205) 940-7768

BUILDERS TRANSPORT, INC

SOUTH CAROLINA CLAIMS OFFICE
PO BOX 24949
COLUMBIA, SC 29223
TEL: (803) 699-9940
FAX: (803) 699-6673

BUILDING LABORERS LOCAL #310 HEALTH & WELFARE

OHIO CLAIMS OFFICE
3250 EUCLID AVE, RM 150
CLEVELAND, OH 44115
TEL: (216) 431-2130
FAX: (216) 431-7707

BUNZL DISTRIBUTION USA, INC

MISSOURI CLAIMS OFFICE
701 EMERSON RD, STE 500
PO BOX 419111
SAINT LOUIS, MO 63141-9111
TEL: (314) 997-5959
FAX: (314) 997-0247

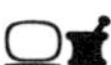

BURKLEY RISK SERVICES

COLORADO CLAIMS OFFICE
1873 S BEL AIR, STE 1010
DENVER, CO 80222
TEL: (303) 331-9942
FAX: (303) 331-4187
TOLL FREE: (800) 332-2089

BURLINGTON MOTOR CARRIERS

ALABAMA CLAIMS OFFICE
14611 W COMMERCE RD
DALEVILLE, IN 47334-9702
TEL: (765) 378-0261
FAX: (765) 378-4195
TOLL FREE: (800) 428-0461
WWW.BMTR.COM

ALBERTA CLAIMS OFFICE
14611 W COMMERCE RD
DALEVILLE, IN 47334-9702
TEL: (765) 378-0261
FAX: (765) 378-4195
TOLL FREE: (800) 428-0461
WWW.BMTR.COM

ARIZONA CLAIMS OFFICE
14611 W COMMERCE RD
DALEVILLE, IN 47334-9702
TEL: (765) 378-0261
FAX: (765) 378-4195
TOLL FREE: (800) 428-0461
WWW.BMTR.COM

ARKANSAS CLAIMS OFFICE
14611 W COMMERCE RD
DALEVILLE, IN 47334-9702
TEL: (765) 378-0261
FAX: (765) 378-4195
TOLL FREE: (800) 428-0461
WWW.BMTR.COM

BRITISH COLUMBIA CLAIMS OFFICE
14611 W COMMERCE RD
DALEVILLE, IN 47334-9702
TEL: (765) 378-0261
FAX: (765) 378-4195
TOLL FREE: (800) 428-0461
WWW.BMTR.COM

CALIFORNIA CLAIMS OFFICE
14611 W COMMERCE RD
DALEVILLE, IN 47334-9702
TEL: (765) 378-0261
FAX: (765) 378-4195
TOLL FREE: (800) 428-0461
WWW.BMTR.COM

COLORADO CLAIMS OFFICE
14611 W COMMERCE RD
DALEVILLE, IN 47334-9702
TEL: (765) 378-0261
FAX: (765) 378-4195
TOLL FREE: (800) 428-0461
WWW.BMTR.COM

CONNECTICUT CLAIMS OFFICE
14611 W COMMERCE RD
DALEVILLE, IN 47334-9702
TEL: (765) 378-0261
FAX: (765) 378-4195
TOLL FREE: (800) 428-0461
WWW.BMTR.COM

Insurance Directory

DELAWARE CLAIMS OFFICE
14611 W COMMERCE RD
DALEVILLE, IN 47334-9702
TEL: (765) 378-0261
FAX: (765) 378-4195
TOLL FREE: (800) 428-0461
WWW.BMTR.COM
☂

DISTRICT OF COLUMBIA CLAIMS OFFICE
14611 W COMMERCE RD
DALEVILLE, IN 47334-9702
TEL: (765) 378-0261
FAX: (765) 378-4195
TOLL FREE: (800) 428-0461
WWW.BMTR.COM
☂

FLORIDA CLAIMS OFFICE
14611 W COMMERCE RD
DALEVILLE, IN 47334-9702
TEL: (765) 378-0261
FAX: (765) 378-4195
TOLL FREE: (800) 428-0461
WWW.BMTR.COM
☂

GEORGIA CLAIMS OFFICE
14611 W COMMERCE RD
DALEVILLE, IN 47334-9702
TEL: (765) 378-0261
FAX: (765) 378-4195
TOLL FREE: (800) 428-0461
WWW.BMTR.COM
☂

IDAHO CLAIMS OFFICE
14611 W COMMERCE RD
DALEVILLE, IN 47334-9702
TEL: (765) 378-0261
FAX: (765) 378-4195
TOLL FREE: (800) 428-0461
WWW.BMTR.COM
☂

ILLINOIS CLAIMS OFFICE
14611 W COMMERCE RD
DALEVILLE, IN 47334-9702
TEL: (765) 378-0261
FAX: (765) 378-4195
TOLL FREE: (800) 428-0461
WWW.BMTR.COM
☂

INDIANA CLAIMS OFFICE
14611 W COMMERCE RD
DALEVILLE, IN 47334-9702
TEL: (765) 378-0261
FAX: (765) 378-4195
TOLL FREE: (800) 428-0461
WWW.BMTR.COM
☂

IOWA CLAIMS OFFICE
14611 W COMMERCE RD
DALEVILLE, IN 47334-9702
TEL: (765) 378-0261
FAX: (765) 378-4195
TOLL FREE: (800) 428-0461
WWW.BMTR.COM
☂

KANSAS CLAIMS OFFICE
14611 W COMMERCE RD
DALEVILLE, IN 47334-9702
TEL: (765) 378-0261
FAX: (765) 378-4195
TOLL FREE: (800) 428-0461
WWW.BMTR.COM
☂

KENTUCKY CLAIMS OFFICE
14611 W COMMERCE RD
DALEVILLE, IN 47334-9702
TEL: (765) 378-0261
FAX: (765) 378-4195
TOLL FREE: (800) 428-0461
WWW.BMTR.COM
☂

LOUISIANA CLAIMS OFFICE
14611 W COMMERCE RD
DALEVILLE, IN 47334-9702
TEL: (765) 378-0261
FAX: (765) 378-4195
TOLL FREE: (800) 428-0461
WWW.BMTR.COM
☂

MAINE CLAIMS OFFICE
14611 W COMMERCE RD
DALEVILLE, IN 47334-9702
TEL: (765) 378-0261
FAX: (765) 378-4195
TOLL FREE: (800) 428-0461
WWW.BMTR.COM
☂

MANITOBA CLAIMS OFFICE
14611 W COMMERCE RD
DALEVILLE, IN 47334-9702
TEL: (765) 378-0261
FAX: (765) 378-4195
TOLL FREE: (800) 428-0461
WWW.BMTR.COM
☂

MARYLAND CLAIMS OFFICE
14611 W COMMERCE RD
DALEVILLE, IN 47334-9702
TEL: (765) 378-0261
FAX: (765) 378-4195
TOLL FREE: (800) 428-0461
WWW.BMTR.COM
☂

MASSACHUSETTS CLAIMS OFFICE
14611 W COMMERCE RD
DALEVILLE, IN 47334-9702
TEL: (765) 378-0261
FAX: (765) 378-4195
TOLL FREE: (800) 428-0461
WWW.BMTR.COM
☂

MEXICO CLAIMS OFFICE
14611 W COMMERCE RD
DALEVILLE, IN 47334-9702
TEL: (765) 378-0261
FAX: (765) 378-4195
TOLL FREE: (800) 428-0461
WWW.BMTR.COM
☂

MICHIGAN CLAIMS OFFICE
14611 W COMMERCE RD
DALEVILLE, IN 47334-9702
TEL: (765) 378-0261
FAX: (765) 378-4195
TOLL FREE: (800) 428-0461
WWW.BMTR.COM
☂

MINNESOTA CLAIMS OFFICE
14611 W COMMERCE RD
DALEVILLE, IN 47334-9702
TEL: (765) 378-0261
FAX: (765) 378-4195
TOLL FREE: (800) 428-0461
WWW.BMTR.COM
☂

MISSISSIPPI CLAIMS OFFICE
14611 W COMMERCE RD
DALEVILLE, IN 47334-9702
TEL: (765) 378-0261
FAX: (765) 378-4195
TOLL FREE: (800) 428-0461
WWW.BMTR.COM
☂

MISSOURI CLAIMS OFFICE
14611 W COMMERCE RD
DALEVILLE, IN 47334-9702
TEL: (765) 378-0261
FAX: (765) 378-4195
TOLL FREE: (800) 428-0461
WWW.BMTR.COM
☂

MONTANA CLAIMS OFFICE
14611 W COMMERCE RD
DALEVILLE, IN 47334-9702
TEL: (765) 378-0261
FAX: (765) 378-4195
TOLL FREE: (800) 428-0461
WWW.BMTR.COM
☂

NEBRASKA CLAIMS OFFICE
14611 W COMMERCE RD
DALEVILLE, IN 47334-9702
TEL: (765) 378-0261
FAX: (765) 378-4195
TOLL FREE: (800) 428-0461
WWW.BMTR.COM
☂

NEVADA CLAIMS OFFICE
14611 W COMMERCE RD
DALEVILLE, IN 47334-9702
TEL: (765) 378-0261
FAX: (765) 378-4195
TOLL FREE: (800) 428-0461
WWW.BMTR.COM
☂

NEW BRUNSWICK CLAIMS OFFICE
14611 W COMMERCE RD
DALEVILLE, IN 47334-9702
TEL: (765) 378-0261
FAX: (765) 378-4195
TOLL FREE: (800) 428-0461
WWW.BMTR.COM
☂

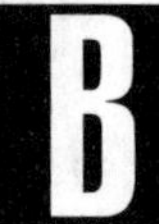

NEW HAMPSHIRE CLAIMS OFFICE
14611 W COMMERCE RD
DALEVILLE, IN 47334-9702
TEL: (765) 378-0261
FAX: (765) 378-4195
TOLL FREE: (800) 428-0461
WWW.BMTR.COM

NEW JERSEY CLAIMS OFFICE
14611 W COMMERCE RD
DALEVILLE, IN 47334-9702
TEL: (765) 378-0261
FAX: (765) 378-4195
TOLL FREE: (800) 428-0461
WWW.BMTR.COM

NEW MEXICO CLAIMS OFFICE
14611 W COMMERCE RD
DALEVILLE, IN 47334-9702
TEL: (765) 378-0261
FAX: (765) 378-4195
TOLL FREE: (800) 428-0461
WWW.BMTR.COM

NEW YORK CLAIMS OFFICE
14611 W COMMERCE RD
DALEVILLE, IN 47334-9702
TEL: (765) 378-0261
FAX: (765) 378-4195
TOLL FREE: (800) 428-0461
WWW.BMTR.COM

NEWFOUNDLAND CLAIMS OFFICE
14611 W COMMERCE RD
DALEVILLE, IN 47334-9702
TEL: (765) 378-0261
FAX: (765) 378-4195
TOLL FREE: (800) 428-0461
WWW.BMTR.COM

NORTH CAROLINA CLAIMS OFFICE
14611 W COMMERCE RD
DALEVILLE, IN 47334-9702
TEL: (765) 378-0261
FAX: (765) 378-4195
TOLL FREE: (800) 428-0461
WWW.BMTR.COM

NORTH DAKOTA CLAIMS OFFICE
14611 W COMMERCE RD
DALEVILLE, IN 47334-9702
TEL: (765) 378-0261
FAX: (765) 378-4195
TOLL FREE: (800) 428-0461
WWW.BMTR.COM

NOVA SCOTIA CLAIMS OFFICE
14611 W COMMERCE RD
DALEVILLE, IN 47334-9702
TEL: (765) 378-0261
FAX: (765) 378-4195
TOLL FREE: (800) 428-0461
WWW.BMTR.COM

OHIO CLAIMS OFFICE
14611 W COMMERCE RD
DALEVILLE, IN 47334-9702
TEL: (765) 378-0261
FAX: (765) 378-4195
TOLL FREE: (800) 428-0461
WWW.BMTR.COM

OKLAHOMA CLAIMS OFFICE
14611 W COMMERCE RD
DALEVILLE, IN 47334-9702
TEL: (765) 378-0261
FAX: (765) 378-4195
TOLL FREE: (800) 428-0461
WWW.BMTR.COM

ONTARIO CLAIMS OFFICE
14611 W COMMERCE RD
DALEVILLE, IN 47334-9702
TEL: (765) 378-0261
FAX: (765) 378-4195
TOLL FREE: (800) 428-0461
WWW.BMTR.COM

OREGON CLAIMS OFFICE
14611 W COMMERCE RD
DALEVILLE, IN 47334-9702
TEL: (765) 378-0261
FAX: (765) 378-4195
TOLL FREE: (800) 428-0461
WWW.BMTR.COM

PENNSYLVANIA CLAIMS OFFICE
14611 W COMMERCE RD
DALEVILLE, IN 47334-9702
TEL: (765) 378-0261
FAX: (765) 378-4195
TOLL FREE: (800) 428-0461
WWW.BMTR.COM

PRINCE EDWARD ISLAND CLAIMS OFFICE
14611 W COMMERCE RD
DALEVILLE, IN 47334-9702
TEL: (765) 378-0261
FAX: (765) 378-4195
TOLL FREE: (800) 428-0461
WWW.BMTR.COM

QUEBEC CLAIMS OFFICE
14611 W COMMERCE RD
DALEVILLE, IN 47334-9702
TEL: (765) 378-0261
FAX: (765) 378-4195
TOLL FREE: (800) 428-0461
WWW.BMTR.COM

RHODE ISLAND CLAIMS OFFICE
14611 W COMMERCE RD
DALEVILLE, IN 47334-9702
TEL: (765) 378-0261
FAX: (765) 378-4195
TOLL FREE: (800) 428-0461
WWW.BMTR.COM

SASKATCHEWAN CLAIMS OFFICE
14611 W COMMERCE RD
DALEVILLE, IN 47334-9702
TEL: (765) 378-0261
FAX: (765) 378-4195
TOLL FREE: (800) 428-0461
WWW.BMTR.COM

SOUTH CAROLINA CLAIMS OFFICE
14611 W COMMERCE RD
DALEVILLE, IN 47334-9702
TEL: (765) 378-0261
FAX: (765) 378-4195
TOLL FREE: (800) 428-0461
WWW.BMTR.COM

SOUTH DAKOTA CLAIMS OFFICE
14611 W COMMERCE RD
DALEVILLE, IN 47334-9702
TEL: (765) 378-0261
FAX: (765) 378-4195
TOLL FREE: (800) 428-0461
WWW.BMTR.COM

TENNESSEE CLAIMS OFFICE
14611 W COMMERCE RD
DALEVILLE, IN 47334-9702
TEL: (765) 378-0261
FAX: (765) 378-4195
TOLL FREE: (800) 428-0461
WWW.BMTR.COM

TEXAS CLAIMS OFFICE
14611 W COMMERCE RD
DALEVILLE, IN 47334-9702
TEL: (765) 378-0261
FAX: (765) 378-4195
TOLL FREE: (800) 428-0461
WWW.BMTR.COM

UTAH CLAIMS OFFICE
14611 W COMMERCE RD
DALEVILLE, IN 47334-9702
TEL: (765) 378-0261
FAX: (765) 378-4195
TOLL FREE: (800) 428-0461
WWW.BMTR.COM

VERMONT CLAIMS OFFICE
14611 W COMMERCE RD
DALEVILLE, IN 47334-9702
TEL: (765) 378-0261
FAX: (765) 378-4195
TOLL FREE: (800) 428-0461
WWW.BMTR.COM

VIRGINIA CLAIMS OFFICE
14611 W COMMERCE RD
DALEVILLE, IN 47334-9702
TEL: (765) 378-0261
FAX: (765) 378-4195
TOLL FREE: (800) 428-0461
WWW.BMTR.COM

Insurance Directory

WASHINGTON CLAIMS OFFICE
14611 W COMMERCE RD
DALEVILLE, IN 47334-9702
TEL: (765) 378-0261
FAX: (765) 378-4195
TOLL FREE: (800) 428-0461
WWW.BMTR.COM

WEST VIRGINIA CLAIMS OFFICE
14611 W COMMERCE RD
DALEVILLE, IN 47334-9702
TEL: (765) 378-0261
FAX: (765) 378-4195
TOLL FREE: (800) 428-0461
WWW.BMTR.COM

WISCONSIN CLAIMS OFFICE
14611 W COMMERCE RD
DALEVILLE, IN 47334-9702
TEL: (765) 378-0261
FAX: (765) 378-4195
TOLL FREE: (800) 428-0461
WWW.BMTR.COM

WYOMING CLAIMS OFFICE
14611 W COMMERCE RD
DALEVILLE, IN 47334-9702
TEL: (765) 378-0261
FAX: (765) 378-4195
TOLL FREE: (800) 428-0461
WWW.BMTR.COM

BURLINGTON NORTHERN & SANTA FE RAILWAY CO

TEXAS CLAIMS OFFICE
4200 DEEN RD
FT WORTH, TX 76106
TEL: (817) 740-7345
FAX: (817) 740-7350

BURNHAM SERVICE CORP

GEORGIA CLAIMS OFFICE
1630 PHOENIX BLVD
PO BOX 100541
ATLANTA, GA 30384-0541
TEL: (706) 563-1120

BUSINESS ADMINISTRATORS & CONSULTANTS, INC

OHIO CLAIMS OFFICE
6331 E LIVINGSTON AVE
PO BOX 107
REYNOLDSBURG, OH 43068-0107
TEL: (614) 863-8780
FAX: (614) 863-9137
TOLL FREE: (800) 521-2654

BUSINESS COUNCIL OF NEW YORK

NEW YORK CLAIMS OFFICE
12 CORPORATE WOODS BLVD
ALBANY, NY 12211
TEL: (518) 465-1571
FAX: (518) 432-7033
TOLL FREE: (800) 692-5483
WWW.BCYS.ORG

BUSINESS PLANNERS, INC

295 MADISON AVE, STE 1801
NEW YORK, NY 10017
TEL: (212) 867-6614
FAX: (212) 867-5927

BUSINESSMEN'S ASSURANCE CO OF AMERICA

MISSOURI CLAIMS OFFICE
PO BOX 419458
KANSAS CITY, MO 64141-6458
TEL: (816) 753-8000
FAX: (816) 751-5837
TOLL FREE: (800) 262-5433
WWW.BMA.COM

BUSINESSMEN'S INSURANCE CO

FLORIDA CLAIMS OFFICE
HANSWARD MANAGEMENT SERVICES CO
1320 S DIXIE HWY, STE 350
CORAL GABLES, FL 33146
TEL: (305) 443-2898
FAX: (305) 447-8842

BUSTER BROWN APPAREL, INC

TENNESSEE CLAIMS OFFICE
2001 WHEELER AVE
PO BOX 5008
CHATTANOOGA, TN 37406-3853
TEL: (423) 629-2531
FAX: (423) 493-2463

C & A

PENNSYLVANIA CLAIMS OFFICE
PO BOX 16010
READING, PA 19612-6010
TEL: (610) 320-4000
FAX: (610) 320-4766
TOLL FREE: (800) 345-7542

C.F.S. HEALTH GROUP

MARYLAND CLAIMS OFFICE
BLUE CROSS & BLUE SHIELD OF MARYLAND SUBSIDIARY
10455 MILL RUN CIR
PO BOX 819
OWINGS MILLS, MD 21117-0819
TEL: (410) 654-9394
FAX: (410) 998-5177
TOLL FREE: (800) 553-3745

C. L. FRATES INSURANCE CO

NATIONAL CLAIMS OFFICE
BANK INSURE
5005 N LINCOLN BLVD
PO BOX 26104
OKLAHOMA CITY, OK 73126-0104
TEL: (405) 290-5600
TOLL FREE: (800) 682-1630
WWW.BANKINSURE.COM

C & O EMPLOYEES' HOSPITAL ASSOCIATION

ILLINOIS CLAIMS OFFICE
543 CHURCH ST
CLIFTON FORGE, VA 24422-1199
TEL: (540) 862-5728
FAX: (540) 862-3552

INDIANA CLAIMS OFFICE
543 CHURCH ST
CLIFTON FORGE, VA 24422-1199
TEL: (540) 862-5728
FAX: (540) 862-3552

KENTUCKY CLAIMS OFFICE
543 CHURCH ST
CLIFTON FORGE, VA 24422-1199
TEL: (540) 862-5728
FAX: (540) 862-3552

OHIO CLAIMS OFFICE
543 CHURCH ST
CLIFTON FORGE, VA 24422-1199
TEL: (540) 862-5728
FAX: (540) 862-3552

VIRGINIA CLAIMS OFFICE
543 CHURCH ST
CLIFTON FORGE, VA 24422-1199
TEL: (540) 862-5728
FAX: (540) 862-3552

WEST VIRGINIA CLAIMS OFFICE
543 CHURCH ST
CLIFTON FORGE, VA 24422-1199
TEL: (540) 862-5728
FAX: (540) 862-3552

C. R. ENGLAND, INC

UTAH CLAIMS OFFICE
4701 W 2100 S
PO BOX 27728
SALT LAKE CITY, UT 84127-0728
TEL: (801) 972-2712
FAX: (801) 977-5765

CABELL HUNTINGTON HOSPITAL INC

WEST VIRGINIA CLAIMS OFFICE
1340 HAL GREER BLVD
HUNTINGTON, WV 25701-0195
TEL: (304) 526-2063
FAX: (304) 526-2008
WWW.CABELL HUNTINGTON.ORG

CABOT SAFETY CORP

NATIONAL CLAIMS OFFICE
AEARO CO
90 MECHANIC ST
SOUTHBRIDGE, MA 01550-2555
TEL: (508) 764-5705
FAX: (508) 764-5648
WWW.AEARO.COM

CADBURY BEVERAGES, INC

CONNECTICUT CLAIMS OFFICE
MOTTS NORTH AMERICA
6 HIGH RIDGE PARK
PO BOX 3800
STAMFORD, CT 06905-0800
TEL: (203) 329-0911
FAX: (203) 968-7653
WWW.MOTTS.COM

CADENCE GROUP LIFE HEALTH & DISABILITY

CALIFORNIA CLAIMS OFFICE
2655 SEELY AVE- BLDG 5
SAN JOSE, CA 95134
TEL: (408) 943-1234
FAX: (408) 943-0513
WWW.CADENCE.COM

CAHABA GBA - GEORGIA MEDICARE OPERATIONS

GEORGIA CLAIMS OFFICE
BLUE CROSS & BLUE SHIELD OF ALABAMA
12052 MIDDLEGROUND RD, STE A
PO BOX 3076
SAVANNAH, GA 31402
TEL: (912) 927-0934
FAX: (912) 927-6946
WWW.GAMEDICARE.COM

CAL FARM INSURANCE CO

CALIFORNIA CLAIMS OFFICE
ATTN: HEALTH CLAIMS PROCESSING
1601 EXPOSITION BLVD
SACRAMENTO, CA 95815-5103
TEL: (916) 924-4000
FAX: (916) 646-4168
IN-STATE: (800) 888-8250
WWW.CALFARM.COM

PO BOX 13200
SACRAMENTO, CA 95813-3200
TEL: (916) 924-0266
FAX: (916) 646-3942
TOLL FREE: (800) 444-6844
WWW.CALFARM.COM

PO BOX 11407
SANTA ANA, CA 92711-1407
TEL: (949) 222-0818
FAX: (949) 252-0873
TOLL FREE: (800) 666-8989
WWW.CALFARM.COM

3455 W SHAW AVE, STE 108
FRESNO, CA 93711
TEL: (559) 277-8021
FAX: (559) 228-0991
IN-STATE: (800) 472-0400

NATIONAL CLAIMS OFFICE
3481 CENTRAL PKY, STE 100
CINCINNATI, OH 45223
TEL: (513) 221-1140
FAX: (513) 872-7509

CALCO, INC

ALASKA CLAIMS OFFICE
445 E 5TH AVE
PO BOX 101422
ANCHORAGE, AK 99510-1422
TEL: (907) 276-8177
FAX: (907) 278-7438

CALENDS GROUP

FLORIDA CLAIMS OFFICE
5972 STELLHORN RD
FT WAYNE, IN 46815-7113
TEL: (219) 485-0273
FAX: (219) 485-5297
TOLL FREE: (800) 274-0225

ILLINOIS CLAIMS OFFICE
5972 STELLHORN RD
FT WAYNE, IN 46815-7113
TEL: (219) 485-0273
FAX: (219) 485-5297
TOLL FREE: (800) 274-0225

INDIANA CLAIMS OFFICE
5972 STELLHORN RD
FT WAYNE, IN 46815-7113
TEL: (219) 485-0273
FAX: (219) 485-5297
TOLL FREE: (800) 274-0225
E-MAIL: CALENDS1@AOL.COM

KENTUCKY CLAIMS OFFICE
5972 STELLHORN RD
FT WAYNE, IN 46815-7113
TEL: (219) 485-0273
FAX: (219) 485-5297
TOLL FREE: (800) 274-0225

MICHIGAN CLAIMS OFFICE
5972 STELLHORN RD
FT WAYNE, IN 46815-7113
TEL: (219) 485-0273
FAX: (219) 485-5297
TOLL FREE: (800) 274-0225

OHIO CLAIMS OFFICE
5972 STELLHORN RD
FT WAYNE, IN 46815-7113
TEL: (219) 485-0273
FAX: (219) 485-5297
TOLL FREE: (800) 274-0225

PENNSYLVANIA CLAIMS OFFICE
5972 STELLHORN RD
FT WAYNE, IN 46815-7113
TEL: (219) 485-0273
FAX: (219) 485-5297
TOLL FREE: (800) 274-0225

TENNESSEE CLAIMS OFFICE
5972 STELLHORN RD
FT WAYNE, IN 46815-7113
TEL: (219) 485-0273
FAX: (219) 485-5297
TOLL FREE: (800) 274-0225

CALIBER GROUP INSURANCE

OHIO CLAIMS OFFICE
AETNA HEALTH CARE
PO BOX 5569
AKRON, OH 44334-0569
TEL: (330) 665-4622
FAX: (330) 665-8559
TOLL FREE: (800) 344-1412

CALIFORNIA ASSOCIATION OF EMPLOYERS

CALIFORNIA CLAIMS OFFICE
1485 RESPONSE RD, STE 107
SACRAMENTO, CA 95815
TEL: (916) 921-1312
FAX: (916) 921-6010
TOLL FREE: (800) 399-5331
E-MAIL: INFO@EMPLOYERS.ORG

CALIFORNIA BENEFITS DENTAL PLAN

4911 WARNER AVE, STE 203
HUNTINGTON BEACH, CA 92649-4473
TEL: (714) 540-4255
FAX: (714) 540-4754
TOLL FREE: (800) 350-3999

CALIFORNIA CASUALTY INSURANCE CO

ARIZONA CLAIMS OFFICE
2510 W DUNLAP AVE #220
PO BOX 42630
PHOENIX, AZ 85080
FAX: (800) 803-1398
TOLL FREE: (800) 841-4736
WWW.CALCAS.COM

CALIFORNIA CLAIMS OFFICE
PO BOX 39700
COLORADO SPRINGS, CO 80949
TEL: (719) 532-8000
FAX: (800) 840-9295
TOLL FREE: (800) 800-9410
WWW.CALCAS.COM

COLORADO CLAIMS OFFICE
PO BOX 39700
COLORADO SPRINGS, CO 80949
TEL: (719) 532-8000
FAX: (800) 840-9295
TOLL FREE: (800) 800-9410
WWW.CALCAS.COM

KANSAS CLAIMS OFFICE
7000 SQUIBB RD, STE 205
PO BOX 9100
MISSION, KS 66202-1700
TEL: (913) 671-3310
FAX: (913) 677-1686
TOLL FREE: (800) 346-6850

KENTUCKY CLAIMS OFFICE
7000 SQUIBB RD, STE 205
PO BOX 9100
MISSION, KS 66202-1700
TEL: (913) 671-3310
FAX: (913) 677-1686
TOLL FREE: (800) 346-6850

MARYLAND CLAIMS OFFICE
7000 SQUIBB RD, STE 205
PO BOX 9100
MISSION, KS 66202-1700
TEL: (913) 671-3310
FAX: (913) 677-1686
TOLL FREE: (800) 346-6850

NEVADA CLAIMS OFFICE
4045 S SPENCER ST, STE A51
PO BOX 60185
LAS VEGAS, NV 89160-0185
TOLL FREE: (800) 223-9229
WWW.CALCAS.COM

4045 S SPENCER ST, STE A51
PO BOX 60185
LAS VEGAS, NV 85080
TOLL FREE: (800) 346-6850

7000 SQUIBB RD, STE 205
PO BOX 9100
MISSION, KS 66202-1700
TEL: (913) 671-3310
FAX: (913) 677-1686
TOLL FREE: (800) 346-6850

NEW MEXICO CLAIMS OFFICE
1460 TRINITY DR, STE 4
PO BOX 418
LOS ALAMOS, NM 87544-0418
TEL: (505) 662-4224
FAX: (505) 662-6984
IN-STATE: (800) 841-1231

2510 W DUNLAP AVE #220
PO BOX 42630
PHOENIX, AZ 85080
FAX: (800) 803-1398
TOLL FREE: (800) 841-4736
WWW.CALCAS.COM

CALIFORNIA CASUALTY MANAGEMENT CO

IDAHO CLAIMS OFFICE
2510 W DUNLAP AVE #220
PO BOX 42630
PHOENIX, AZ 85080
FAX: (800) 803-1398
TOLL FREE: (800) 841-4736
WWW.CALCAS.COM

NEVADA CLAIMS OFFICE
2510 W DUNLAP AVE #220
PO BOX 42630
PHOENIX, AZ 85080
FAX: (800) 803-1398
TOLL FREE: (800) 841-4736
WWW.CALCAS.COM

OREGON CLAIMS OFFICE
2510 W DUNLAP AVE #220
PO BOX 42630
PHOENIX, AZ 85080
FAX: (800) 803-1398
TOLL FREE: (800) 841-4736
WWW.CALCAS.COM

UTAH CLAIMS OFFICE
2510 W DUNLAP AVE #220
PO BOX 42630
PHOENIX, AZ 85080
FAX: (800) 803-1398
TOLL FREE: (800) 841-4736
WWW.CALCAS.COM

WYOMING CLAIMS OFFICE
2510 W DUNLAP AVE #220
PO BOX 42630
PHOENIX, AZ 85080
FAX: (800) 803-1398
TOLL FREE: (800) 841-4736
WWW.CALCAS.COM

CALIFORNIA CEDAR PRODUCTS CO

CALIFORNIA CLAIMS OFFICE
DELTA BENEFITS (HEALTH INSURANCE)
400 FRESNO AVE
PO BOX 528
STOCKTON, CA 95201-3028
TEL: (209) 944-5800
FAX: (209) 944-9072
WWW.CALCEDAR.COM

CALIFORNIA COMPENSATION INSURANCE CO

SUPERIOR NATIONAL
21700 E COPLEY DR, STE 300
PO BOX 4909
DIAMOND BAR, CA 91765
TEL: (909) 860-0083
FAX: (909) 396-9795
TOLL FREE: (800) 477-3179
WWW.SUPERIOR.COM

SUPERIOR NATIONAL
1300 E SHAW, STE 164
PO BOX 9060
CALABASAS, CA 91372
TEL: (559) 440-0222
FAX: (559) 221-6530
TOLL FREE: (800) 955-3179
WWW.SUPERIOR.COM

SUPERIOR NATIONAL
30 RAGSDALE DR, STE 101
PO BOX 1431
MONTEREY, CA 93940
TEL: (831) 656-8900
FAX: (831) 657-2155
TOLL FREE: (800) 391-3179
WWW.SUPERIOR.COM

SUPERIOR NATIONAL
PO BOX 800
NOVATO, CA 94948-0800
TEL: (415) 883-2503
FAX: (415) 382-9373
TOLL FREE: (800) 388-3179
WWW.SUPERIOR.COM

SUPERIOR NATIONAL
681 S PARKER ST- BLDG B, STE 200
PO BOX 11027
ORANGE, CA 92856
TEL: (714) 480-8300
FAX: (714) 571-5915
TOLL FREE: (800) 379-3179
WWW.SUPERIOR.COM

SUPERIOR NATIONAL
PO BOX 1240
RANCHO CORDOVA, CA 95741
TOLL FREE: (800) 688-3179
WWW.SUPERIOR.COM

SUPERIOR NATIONAL
3636 NOBEL DR, STE 300
PO BOX 85208
SAN DIEGO, CA 92186-5208
TEL: (619) 642-0065
FAX: (619) 642-5751
TOLL FREE: (800) 677-3179
WWW.SUPERIOR.COM

SUPERIOR NATIONAL
1731 TECHNOLOGY DR, STE 150
PO BOX 447
SAN JOSE, CA 95110
TEL: (408) 437-5425
FAX: (408) 437-1833
TOLL FREE: (800) 766-3179
WWW.SUPERIOR.COM

SUPERIOR NATIONAL
PO BOX 4425
WOODLAND HILLS, CA 91365-4425
TEL: (818) 888-2102
FAX: (818) 347-3298
TOLL FREE: (800) 866-3179
WWW.SUPERIOR.COM

C

CALIFORNIA IRONWORKERS WELFARE PLAN
131 N EL MOLINO AVE, STE 330
PASADENA, CA 91101-1878
TEL: (626) 792-7337
FAX: (626) 792-7667
TOLL FREE: (800) 527-4613

CALIFORNIA MOTOR CAR DEALERS ASSOCIATION
420 CULVER BLVD
PLAYA DEL REY, CA 90293-7706
TEL: (310) 306-6232
FAX: (310) 822-6733
TOLL FREE: (800) 445-8290
IN-STATE: (800) 262-6232
WWW.CMCDA.COM

CALMAR, INC
333 S TURNBULL CYN RD
PO BOX 1203
INDUSTRY, CA 91745-1203
TEL: (626) 330-3161
FAX: (626) 937-2755
WWW.CALMAR.COM

CAM ADMINISTRATIVE SERVICES, INC
MICHIGAN CLAIMS OFFICE
25800 NORTHWESTERN HWY, STE 700
PO BOX 5131
SOUTHFIELD, MI 48086-5131
TEL: (248) 827-1050
FAX: (248) 827-2112
TOLL FREE: (800) 732-8906

CAMBRIDGE BENEFIT SERVICES
2600 HORIZON DR SE
PO BOX 1687
GRAND RAPIDS, MI 49501
TEL: (616) 954-3300
FAX: (616) 942-7610
TOLL FREE: (800) 766-9780

CAMELOT MUSIC INC
OHIO CLAIMS OFFICE
WELFARE BENEFITS
8000 FREEDOM AVE NW
PO BOX 2169
NORTH CANTON, OH 44720-0169
TEL: (330) 494-2283
FAX: (330) 494-0394
WWW.CAMELOTMUSIC.COM

CAMERON MUTUAL INSURANCE CO
ARKANSAS CLAIMS OFFICE
214 MCWELWAIN
CAMERON, MO 65804
TEL: (816) 632-6511
FAX: (816) 632-1022

MISSOURI CLAIMS OFFICE
1330 N KINGS HWY
PO BOX 777
CAPE GIRARDEAU, MO 63702-0777
TEL: (573) 334-7981
FAX: (573) 334-6363

PO BOX 5007
FRAMPTON, MO 65801-5007
TEL: (417) 881-1176
FAX: (417) 881-2590
TOLL FREE: (800) 776-1176

CAMPBELL SOUP CO
NEW JERSEY CLAIMS OFFICE
1 CAMPBELL PL
CAMDEN, NJ 08103-1799
TEL: (609) 342-4800
FAX: (609) 342-3878
WWW.CAMPBELLSOUP.COM

TEXAS CLAIMS OFFICE
500 NW LOOP 286
PO BOX 9016
PARIS, TX 75461-9016
TEL: (903) 784-3341
FAX: (903) 784-0986
WWW.CAMPBELLSOUP.COM

CANADA LIFE ASSURANCE CO
ALBERTA CLAIMS OFFICE
GROUP LIFE & HEALTH
330 UNIVERSITY AVE
TORONTO, ON M5G-1R8
TEL: (416) 597-1456
FAX: (416) 597-8266
TOLL FREE: (800) 387-4492
E-MAIL: INFO@CANADALIFE.COM
WWW.CANADALIFE.COM

BRITISH COLUMBIA CLAIMS OFFICE
GROUP LIFE & HEALTH
330 UNIVERSITY AVE
TORONTO, ON M5G-1R8
TEL: (416) 597-1456
FAX: (416) 597-8266
TOLL FREE: (800) 387-4492
E-MAIL: INFO@CANADALIFE.COM
WWW.CANADALIFE.COM

GEORGIA CLAIMS OFFICE
GROUP DEPT
6201 POWERS FERRY RD
PO BOX 105087
ATLANTA, GA 30348
TEL: (770) 953-1959
FAX: (800) 333-4150
TOLL FREE: (800) 333-2542

MANITOBA CLAIMS OFFICE
GROUP LIFE & HEALTH
330 UNIVERSITY AVE
TORONTO, ON M5G-1R8
TEL: (416) 597-1456
FAX: (416) 597-8266
TOLL FREE: (800) 387-4492
E-MAIL: INFO@CANADALIFE.COM
WWW.CANADALIFE.COM

NEW BRUNSWICK CLAIMS OFFICE
GROUP LIFE & HEALTH
330 UNIVERSITY AVE
TORONTO, ON M5G-1R8
TEL: (416) 597-1456
FAX: (416) 597-8266
TOLL FREE: (800) 387-4492
E-MAIL: INFO@CANADALIFE.COM
WWW.CANADALIFE.COM

NEWFOUNDLAND CLAIMS OFFICE
GROUP LIFE & HEALTH
330 UNIVERSITY AVE
TORONTO, ON M5G-1R8
TEL: (416) 597-1456
FAX: (416) 597-8266
TOLL FREE: (800) 387-4492
E-MAIL: INFO@CANADALIFE.COM
WWW.CANADALIFE.COM

NOVA SCOTIA CLAIMS OFFICE
GROUP LIFE & HEALTH
330 UNIVERSITY AVE
TORONTO, ON M5G-1R8
TEL: (416) 597-1456
FAX: (416) 597-8266
TOLL FREE: (800) 387-4492
E-MAIL: INFO@CANADALIFE.COM
WWW.CANADALIFE.COM

ONTARIO CLAIMS OFFICE
GROUP LIFE & HEALTH
330 UNIVERSITY AVE
TORONTO, ON M5G-1R8
TEL: (416) 597-1456
FAX: (416) 597-8266
TOLL FREE: (800) 387-4492
E-MAIL: INFO@CANADALIFE.COM
WWW.CANADALIFE.COM

PRINCE EDWARD ISLAND CLAIMS OFFICE
GROUP LIFE & HEALTH
330 UNIVERSITY AVE
TORONTO, ON M5G-1R8
TEL: (416) 597-1456
FAX: (416) 597-8266
TOLL FREE: (800) 387-4492
E-MAIL: INFO@CANADALIFE.COM
WWW.CANADALIFE.COM

QUEBEC CLAIMS OFFICE
GROUP LIFE & HEALTH
330 UNIVERSITY AVE
TORONTO, ON M5G-1R8
TEL: (416) 597-1456
FAX: (416) 597-8266
TOLL FREE: (800) 387-4492
E-MAIL: INFO@CANADALIFE.COM
WWW.CANADALIFE.COM

Casualty/Liability Dental Disability 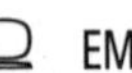 EMC  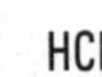 HCPCS 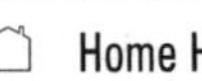 Home Health 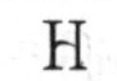 H HMO Medical

SASKATCHEWAN CLAIMS OFFICE
GROUP LIFE & HEALTH
330 UNIVERSITY AVE
TORONTO, ON M5G-1R8
TEL: (416) 597-1456
FAX: (416) 597-8266
TOLL FREE: (800) 387-4492
E-MAIL: INFO@CANADALIFE.COM
WWW.CANADALIFE.COM

℞ ✂ 🦷 6d ♿ 💻

CANAL INSURANCE CO

SOUTH CAROLINA CLAIMS OFFICE
400 E STONE AVE
PO BOX 7
GREENVILLE, SC 29602
TEL: (864) 242-5365
FAX: (864) 271-7667
TOLL FREE: (800) 868-7538

🔨

CANON COCHRAN MANAGEMENT SERVICES, INC

ILLINOIS CLAIMS OFFICE
2 E MAIN TOWN CTR BLDG
PO BOX 1430
DANVILLE, IL 61834-1430
TEL: (217) 446-1089
FAX: (217) 443-0927
TOLL FREE: (800) 634-3506
E-MAIL: CCMSI@CCMSI.COM
WWW.CCMSI.COM

✂ 🦷 6d

CAPITAL ASSURANCE CO

FLORIDA CLAIMS OFFICE
SKANDEE SOUTHEAST COMPANIES
55 ALHAMBRA PLZ
PO BOX 149063
CORAL GABLES, FL 33114-9063
TEL: (305) 461-7400
FAX: (305) 461-4303
TOLL FREE: (800) 999-5198

🔨

CAPITAL BLUE CROSS

PENNSYLVANIA CLAIMS OFFICE
2500 ELMERTON AVE
HARRISBURG, PA 17110
TEL: (717) 541-7000
FAX: (717) 541-6072
TOLL FREE: (800) 958-5558
WWW.CAPBLUECROSS.COM

☂ ⌂ ℞ ⛑ 3 H 💻 ⓜ

CAPITAL BLUE CROSS & PENNSYLVANIA BLUE SHIELD

2500 ELMERTON AVE
HARRISBURG, PA 17110
TEL: (717) 541-7000
FAX: (717) 541-6072
TOLL FREE: (800) 958-5558
WWW.CAPBLUECROSS.COM

☂ ⌂ ℞ ✂ 🦷 6d ♿ 🔨 ♜

CAPITAL CITY INSURANCE CO, INC

SOUTH CAROLINA CLAIMS OFFICE
3850 FERNANDINA RD
PO BOX 21627
COLUMBIA, SC 29221
TEL: (803) 781-7118
FAX: (803) 781-1714

☂ ℞ ⛑ ✂ 🦷 ♿ 3 H 🔨 💻 ☆

CAPITAL DISTRICT PHYSICIANS' HEALTH PLAN, INC

NEW YORK CLAIMS OFFICE
17 COLUMBIA CIR
ALBANY, NY 12203-5190
TEL: (518) 862-3700
FAX: (518) 452-0003
TOLL FREE: (800) 777-CARE
E-MAIL: INFO@CDPHP.COM
WWW.CDPHP.COM

☂ ℞ ✂ 🦷 6d H ♜

CAPITAL HEALTH PLAN

FLORIDA CLAIMS OFFICE
2140 CENTERVILLE PL
PO BOX 15349
TALLAHASSEE, FL 32317-5349
TEL: (850) 383-3377
FAX: (850) 383-3441

H ♜

CAPITAL SECURITY INSURANCE CO

GEORGIA CLAIMS OFFICE
MONUMENTAL LIFE INSURANCE CO
JASPER STA- UNIT 4
PO BOX 999
RIDGELAND, SC 29936
TEL: (843) 717-2748
FAX: (843) 717-2649
TOLL FREE: (800) 933-4643

✂ ♿

SOUTH CAROLINA CLAIMS OFFICE
MONUMENTAL LIFE INSURANCE CO
JASPER STA- UNIT 4
PO BOX 999
RIDGELAND, SC 29936
TEL: (843) 717-2748
FAX: (843) 717-2649
TOLL FREE: (800) 933-4643

✂ ♿

CAPITOL CASUALTY INSURANCE

NEBRASKA CLAIMS OFFICE
130-132 S 13TH, STE 200
PO BOX 83246
LINCOLN, NE 68501-3246
TEL: (402) 475-9900
FAX: (402) 475-8005
TOLL FREE: (800) 488-4671

⛑ 🔨

CAPITOL INDEMNITY CORP

WISCONSIN CLAIMS OFFICE
4610 UNIVERSITY AVE
PO BOX 5900
MADISON, WI 53705-0900
TEL: (608) 231-4450
FAX: (608) 231-3995

⛑ 🔨

CARDAY ASSOCIATES, INC

MARYLAND CLAIMS OFFICE
4600 POWDER MILL RD
DENTSVILLE, MD 20705
TEL: (301) 937-9300
FAX: (301) 902-0437

✂ 🦷 6d ♿ 3

CARDINAL DISTRIBUTION INCORPORATED EMPLOYEE

OHIO CLAIMS OFFICE
CARDINAL HEALTH
5555 GLENDON CT
DUBLIN, OH 43016
TEL: (614) 717-5000
FAX: (614) 717-6000
TOLL FREE: (800) 234-8701

☂

CARE AMERICA HEALTH PLANS

CALIFORNIA CLAIMS OFFICE
CARE AMERICA/ BLUE SHIELD
6300 CANOGA AVE
PO BOX 946
WOODLAND HILLS, CA 91365
TEL: (818) 228-5050
FAX: (818) 228-5103
TOLL FREE: (800) 827-2273
WWW.CAREAMERICA.COM

☂ ⌂ ℞ ⛑ ♿ 3 H 🔨 💻 ☆
♜ 

CARE CHOICES HEALTH PLANS

IOWA CLAIMS OFFICE
PREFERRED CHOICE
522 4TH ST- TERRE CENTRE, STE 250
SIOUX CITY, IA 51101-1748
TEL: (712) 252-2344
FAX: (712) 294-7018
TOLL FREE: (800) 535-6252

⌂ ✂ H ♜

CARE MANAGEMENT 2000, INC

NEW JERSEY CLAIMS OFFICE
258 PARK ST
UPPER MONTCLAIR, NJ 07043
TEL: (973) 655-0120
FAX: (973) 655-0402
E-MAIL: CM2000INC@AOL.COM

☂ ⌂

CAREFIRST BLUE CROSS & BLUE SHIELD

MARYLAND CLAIMS OFFICE
10455 MILL RUN CIR
PO BOX 820
OWINGS MILLS, MD 21117-0820
TEL: (410) 654-8670
FAX: (410) 998-5809
TOLL FREE: (800) 445-6036
WWW.CAREFIRST.COM

☂ ⌂ ℞ ⛑ ✂ 🦷 6d 3 H 🔨
☆ ⓜ

CAREMARK MEDICAL & DENTAL PLAN

NATIONAL CLAIMS OFFICE
MED PARTNERS, INC
2211 SANDERS RD
NORTHBROOK, IL 60062-6126
TEL: (847) 559-4700
FAX: (847) 559-3905

℞ ✂ 🦷 ♿ 🔨 💻 ♜

C

CARETON HEALTH CARE
PO BOX 22987
KNOXVILLE, TN 37933
FAX: (423) 778-4620
TOLL FREE: (800) 976-7747

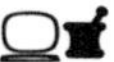

CARILION HEALTH PLANS
VIRGINIA CLAIMS OFFICE
110 W CAMPBELL AVE
PO BOX 1531
ROANOKE, VA 24007
TEL: (540) 343-6101
FAX: (540) 343-0748
WWW.CARILION.COM

CARLSON COMPANIES, INC
MINNESOTA CLAIMS OFFICE
ADMINISTRATION DEPT
PO BOX 59159
MINNEAPOLIS, MN 55459
TEL: (612) 540-5000

CARLTEN HEALTHCARE
TENNESSEE CLAIMS OFFICE
1021 W OAKLAND AVE, STE 300
JOHNSON CITY, TN 37604
TEL: (423) 952-3180
FAX: (423) 952-3188

H

CARNEGIE-MELLON UNIVERSITY
PENNSYLVANIA CLAIMS OFFICE
WHITFIELD HALL
143 N CRAIG ST
PITTSBURGH, PA 15213
TEL: (412) 268-4747
FAX: (412) 268-1524
WWW.CMU.EDU/BA/HR/

CAROLINA BENEFIT ADMINISTRATORS OF SOUTH CAROLINA
SOUTH CAROLINA CLAIMS OFFICE
291 S PINE ST
PO BOX 3257
SPARTANBURG, SC 29304
TEL: (864) 573-6937
FAX: (864) 582-2265
TOLL FREE: (800) 476-2295

CAROLINA CASUALTY INSURANCE CO, INC
FLORIDA CLAIMS OFFICE
8381 DIX ELLIS TRL, STE 400
PO BOX 2575
JACKSONVILLE, FL 32203
TEL: (904) 363-0900
FAX: (904) 363-8097
TOLL FREE: (800) 874-8053
WWW.CAROLINACAS.COM

CAROLINA CONTINENTAL INSURANCE CO
SOUTH CAROLINA CLAIMS OFFICE
2801 DEVINE ST
PO BOX 1807
COLUMBIA, SC 29202
TEL: (803) 256-6265
FAX: (803) 779-4406
TOLL FREE: (800) 433-3036

CAROLINA MEDICORP INCORPORATED CHOICEPLAN
NORTH CAROLINA CLAIMS OFFICE
3333 SILAS CREEK PKY
WINSTON-SALEM, NC 27103-3013
TEL: (336) 718-5000
FAX: (336) 718-9856

CARPENTERS COMBINED FUNDS
PENNSYLVANIA CLAIMS OFFICE
495 MANSFIELD AVE- 1ST FL
PITTSBURGH, PA 15205-4376
TEL: (412) 922-5330
FAX: (412) 922-3420
IN-STATE: (800) 242-2539

CARPENTERS HEALTH & WELFARE TRUST OF SOUTHERN CALIFORNIA
ARIZONA CLAIMS OFFICE
520 S VIRGIL AVE
PO BOX 76827
LOS ANGELES, CA 90076
TEL: (213) 386-8590
FAX: (213) 739-9329
TOLL FREE: (800) 252-9255

H

CALIFORNIA CLAIMS OFFICE
520 S VIRGIL AVE
PO BOX 76827
LOS ANGELES, CA 90076
TEL: (213) 386-8590
FAX: (213) 739-9329
TOLL FREE: (800) 252-9255

H

NEVADA CLAIMS OFFICE
520 S VIRGIL AVE
PO BOX 76827
LOS ANGELES, CA 90076
TEL: (213) 386-8590
FAX: (213) 739-9329
TOLL FREE: (800) 252-9255

H

CASUALTY INSURANCE CO
ILLINOIS CLAIMS OFFICE
FREMONT COMPENSATION INSURANCE
321 N CLARK ST, STE 600
PO BOX 109060
CHICAGO, IL 60610-4789
TEL: (312) 321-1680
FAX: (312) 321-5600
TOLL FREE: (800) 799-4877
WWW.FREMONTCOMP.COM

CASUALTY RECIPROCAL EXCHANGE
MISSOURI CLAIMS OFFICE
DODSON GROUP
9201 STATE LINE RD
PO BOX 419497
KANSAS CITY, MO 64141-6497
TEL: (816) 361-3400
FAX: (800) 825-5035
TOLL FREE: (800) 825-3760
WWW.DODSONGROUP.COM

CATHOLIC KNIGHTS OF AMERICA
3525 HAMPTON AVE
SAINT LOUIS, MO 63139-1917
TEL: (314) 351-1029
FAX: (314) 351-9937

CATO CORP EMPLOYEE
NORTH CAROLINA CLAIMS OFFICE
8100 DENMARK RD
PO BOX 34216
CHARLOTTE, NC 28234
TEL: (704) 554-8510
FAX: (704) 551-7547

CAVALIER FORD
VIRGINIA CLAIMS OFFICE
1515 S MILITARY HWY
CHESAPEAKE, VA 23320-2607
TEL: (757) 424-1111
FAX: (757) 420-7750
WWW.CAVFORD.COM

CELINA MUTUAL INSURANCE CO
OHIO CLAIMS OFFICE
1 INSURANCE SQ
CELINA, OH 45822-1690
TEL: (419) 586-5181
FAX: (419) 586-8343
IN-STATE: (800) 552-5181

CELTIC LIFE INSURANCE CO
ILLINOIS CLAIMS OFFICE
CELTIC INDIVIDUAL HEALTH
200 S WACKER DR, STE 900
PO BOX 06410
CHICAGO, IL 60606-5802
TEL: (312) 332-5401
TOLL FREE: (800) 477-7870
WWW.CELTIC_NET.COM

Casualty/Liability Dental Disability EMC HCPCS Home Health H HMO 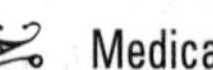 Medical

CEMARA ADMINISTRATORS INC

KANSAS CLAIMS OFFICE
3450 N ROCK RD, STE 605
PO BOX 8902
WICHITA, KS 67208-0902
TEL: (316) 631-3939
FAX: (316) 631-3788
TOLL FREE: (800) 285-1551

CEMETERY WORKERS WELFARE FUND

NEW YORK CLAIMS OFFICE
2409 38TH AVE
LONG ISLAND CITY, NY 11101
TEL: (718) 729-7400
FAX: (718) 729-0253

CENTRAL BENEFITS MUTUAL INSURANCE CO

OHIO CLAIMS OFFICE
255 E MAIN ST
PO BOX 182042
COLUMBUS, OH 43218
TEL: (614) 464-5711
FAX: (614) 464-8444
TOLL FREE: (800) 333-5711
WWW.CENTRALBENEFITS.COM

CENTRAL DATA SERVICES, INC

PENNSYLVANIA CLAIMS OFFICE
503 MARTINDALE ST, 5TH FL
PITTSBURGH, PA 15212
TEL: (412) 321-6172
FAX: (412) 237-1444

CENTRAL ILLINOIS CARPENTERS

ILLINOIS CLAIMS OFFICE
2400 N MAIN ST, STE 100
EAST PEORIA, IL 61611-1735
TEL: (309) 699-7200
FAX: (309) 699-7032

CENTRAL INSURANCE CO

OHIO CLAIMS OFFICE
ALL AMERICA INSURANCE CO
800 S WASHINGTON ST
PO BOX 351
VAN WERT, OH 45891
TEL: (419) 238-1010
WWW.CENTRAL-INSURANCE.COM

CENTRAL INSURANCE SERVICES

TEXAS CLAIMS OFFICE
2185 N GLENVILLE DR
PO BOX 833879
RICHARDSON, TX 75083-3879
TEL: (972) 699-2770
FAX: (972) 699-2788

CENTRAL MAINE POWER

MAINE CLAIMS OFFICE
83 EDISON DR
AUGUSTA, ME 04336
TEL: (207) 623-3521
FAX: (207) 626-9888
WWW.CMPCO.COM

CENTRAL MINNESOTA GROUP HEALTH PLAN

MINNESOTA CLAIMS OFFICE
HEALTH PARTNERS
314 10TH AVE S
WAITE PARK, MN 56387
TEL: (320) 259-7356
FAX: (612) 203-2414
TOLL FREE: (800) 284-3142

CENTRAL MUTUAL INSURANCE CO

MASSACHUSETTS CLAIMS OFFICE
404 WYMAN ST, STE 360
PO BOX 9124
WALTHAM, MA 02454
TEL: (781) 890-1752
FAX: (781) 890-3525
TOLL FREE: (800) 359-2233
WWW.CENTRAL-INSURANCE.COM

OHIO CLAIMS OFFICE
800 S WASHINGTON ST
PO BOX 351
VAN WERT, OH 45891
TEL: (419) 238-1010
FAX: (800) 736-7026
TOLL FREE: (800) 736-7000
WWW.CENTRAL-INSURANCE.COM

CENTRAL NATIONAL INSURANCE CO OF OMAHA

NEBRASKA CLAIMS OFFICE
11128 JOHN GALT BLVD #200
OMAHA, NE 68137
TEL: (402) 970-8600
FAX: (402) 970-8642

CENTRAL PENNSYLVANIA TEAMSTERS HEALTH & WELFARE FUND

NATIONAL CLAIMS OFFICE
1055 SPRING ST
PO BOX 15224
READING, PA 19612-5224
TEL: (610) 320-5500
FAX: (610) 320-9209
TOLL FREE: (800) 331-0420
IN-STATE: (800) 422-8330

CENTRAL RESERVE LIFE INSURANCE CO OF NORTH AMERICA

OHIO CLAIMS OFFICE
17800 ROYALTON RD
STRONGSVILLE, OH 44136-5197
TEL: (440) 572-2400
FAX: (440) 572-8386
TOLL FREE: (800) 321-3997
E-MAIL: CLAIMS@CENTRALRESERVE.COM
WWW.CENTRALRESERVE.COM

CENTRAL STATES HEALTH & LIFE INSURANCE CO OF OMAHA

NATIONAL CLAIMS OFFICE
PO BOX 34952
OMAHA, NE 68134-9832
TEL: (402) 397-1111
FAX: (402) 399-3497
TOLL FREE: (800) 541-2363

CENTRAL UNITED LIFE INSURANCE CO

2727 ALLEN PKY- WORTHAM TWR- 6TH FL
PO BOX 2728
HOUSTON, TX 77252-2728
TEL: (713) 529-0045
FAX: (713) 529-5863
TOLL FREE: (800) 669-9030

CENTRAL VALLEY SCHOOL TRUST

CALIFORNIA CLAIMS OFFICE
3459 W SHAW AVE
FRESNO, CA 93711
TEL: (559) 276-0766
FAX: (559) 276-0856
TOLL FREE: (800) 288-9870
WWW.CVTRUST.ORG

CENTRIS GROUP, INC

650 TOWN CTR DR, STE 1600
PO BOX 2010
COSTA MESA, CA 92626-2010
TEL: (714) 549-1600
FAX: (714) 436-9494
TOLL FREE: (800) 872-3634

CENTURION FINANCIAL, INC

OHIO CLAIMS OFFICE
OHIO MUTUAL GROUP
1725 HOPLEY AVE
PO BOX 111
BUCYRUS, OH 44820-3569
TEL: (419) 562-3011
FAX: (419) 562-0995
IN-STATE: (800) 589-9750

CENTURION LIFE INSURANCE CO

IOWA CLAIMS OFFICE
206 8TH ST
DES MOINES, IA 50309-3805
TEL: (515) 557-7307
FAX: (515) 557-7158
TOLL FREE: (800) 903-7306

C

CENTURY FURNITURE

NORTH CAROLINA CLAIMS OFFICE
401 11TH ST NW
PO BOX 608
HICKORY, NC 28603
TEL: (828) 328-1851
FAX: (828) 328-2176
WWW.CENTURYFURNITURE.COM

CENTURY LIFE INSURANCE

OKLAHOMA CLAIMS OFFICE
100 NW 63RD, STE 300
OKLAHOMA CITY, OK 73116
TEL: (405) 879-0099
FAX: (405) 840-8237
TOLL FREE: (800) 659-1751

CENTURY PLANNERS, LLC

ILLINOIS CLAIMS OFFICE
13537 BARRETT PKY DR, STE 305
BALLWIN, MO 63021
TEL: (314) 822-9992
FAX: (314) 822-9177
TOLL FREE: (800) 776-2452
E-MAIL: CPLLTD@ANET-STL.COM
WWW.CENTURYPLANNERS.COM

MISSOURI CLAIMS OFFICE
13537 BARRETT PKY DR, STE 305
BALLWIN, MO 63021
TEL: (314) 822-9992
FAX: (314) 822-9177
TOLL FREE: (800) 776-2452
E-MAIL: CPLLTD@ANET-STL.COM
WWW.CENTURYPLANNERS.COM

CERTIFIED LIFE INSURANCE CO

NATIONAL CLAIMS OFFICE
BANKERS' LIFE & CASUALTY
222 MERCHANDISE MART PLZ
PO BOX 66933
CHICAGO, IL 60666-0933
TEL: (312) 396-6000
FAX: (312) 396-5951
TOLL FREE: (800) 621-3724

CGU

ALABAMA CLAIMS OFFICE
3555 KOGER BLVD, STE 200
DULUTH, GA 30096
TEL: (678) 380-8734
FAX: (678) 380-7595
TOLL FREE: (800) 762-5573
WWW.CUUSA.COM

GEORGIA CLAIMS OFFICE
3555 KOGER BLVD, STE 200
DULUTH, GA 30096
TEL: (678) 380-8734
FAX: (678) 380-7595
TOLL FREE: (800) 762-5573
IN-STATE: (800) 222-6003
WWW.CUUSA.COM

ILLINOIS CLAIMS OFFICE
HAWKEYE SECURITY
PO BOX 6004
CHESTERFIELD, MO 63006
TEL: (636) 728-1090
TOLL FREE: (800) 558-1396

INDIANA CLAIMS OFFICE
300 N MERIDIAN, STE 1250
PO BOX 40680
INDIANAPOLIS, IN 46240
TEL: (317) 632-1451
FAX: (317) 686-5662
TOLL FREE: (800) 686-1451
WWW.CUUSA.COM

PO BOX 5109
MISHAWAKA, IN 46546
TEL: (219) 273-2773
IN-STATE: (800) 241-1493

KENTUCKY CLAIMS OFFICE
300 N MERIDIAN, STE 1250
PO BOX 40680
INDIANAPOLIS, IN 46240
TEL: (317) 632-1451
FAX: (317) 686-5662
TOLL FREE: (800) 686-1451
WWW.CUUSA.COM

MAINE CLAIMS OFFICE
COMMERCIAL UNION-YORK INSURANCE COMPANY
304 HANCOCK ST, STE 3A
PO BOX 1719
BANGOR, ME 04402-1719
TEL: (207) 990-1111
FAX: (207) 947-3667
IN-STATE: (800) 622-9100
WWW.CUUSA.COM

COMMERCIAL UNION
PO BOX 527
PORTLAND, ME 04112-0527
TEL: (207) 774-1431
FAX: (207) 871-0393

PO BOX 1719
BANGOR, ME 04402-1719
TEL: (207) 990-1111
FAX: (207) 947-3667
TOLL FREE: (800) 622-9100

MASSACHUSETTS CLAIMS OFFICE
PO BOX 1719
BANGOR, ME 04402-1719
TEL: (207) 990-1111
FAX: (207) 947-3667
TOLL FREE: (800) 622-9100

1 BEACON ST
BOSTON, MA 02108
TEL: (617) 725-6000
FAX: (617) 725-6702

MISSOURI CLAIMS OFFICE
HAWKEYE SECURITY
PO BOX 6004
CHESTERFIELD, MO 63006
TEL: (636) 728-1090
TOLL FREE: (800) 558-1396

NATIONAL CLAIMS OFFICE
1 BEACON ST
BOSTON, MA 02108
TEL: (617) 725-6059

2455 CORPORATE WEST DR
PO BOX 5202
LISLE, IL 60532
TEL: (630) 505-4100
FAX: (630) 505-1780
TOLL FREE: (800) 323-2298
WWW.CGU.COM

1 BEACON ST
PO BOX 9003
BOSTON, MA 02205-9003
TEL: (508) 549-8820
FAX: (617) 725-6262
WWW.CGU.COM

100 CORPORATE CTR DR
CAMP HILL, PA 17011
TEL: (717) 766-1700
FAX: (717) 795-2611
WWW.CGU.COM

801 N BRAND BLVD- 8TH FL
PO BOX 29037
GLENDALE, CA 91209-9037
TEL: (818) 247-5001
FAX: (818) 637-5818
TOLL FREE: (800) 464-2457
WWW.CGU-INSURANCE.COM

504 S SERVICE RD E
PO DRAWER 1300
RUSTON, LA 71273-1300
TEL: (318) 255-2622
FAX: (318) 254-4522
TOLL FREE: (800) 551-5100

178 MAIN ST
PO BOX 339
WATERVILLE, ME 04901
TEL: (207) 877-7269
FAX: (207) 877-3067
IN-STATE: (800) 322-0489

175 DWIGHT RD
LONGMEADOW, MA 01106-1761
TEL: (978) 532-6880
WWW.CGU.COM

8 ESSEX CTR DR
PO BOX 6029
PEABODY, MA 01961-6029
TEL: (978) 532-6880
FAX: (978) 977-9015
IN-STATE: (800) 332-3995

100 CORPORATE PKY, STE 200
PO BOX 5135
BUFFALO, NY 14240-5135
TEL: (716) 862-5500
FAX: (716) 833-4698
TOLL FREE: (800) 828-7212
IN-STATE: (800) 462-7267

NEW YORK CLAIMS OFFICE
201 N SERVICE
MELVILLE, NY 11747
TEL: (516) 423-4400
TOLL FREE: (800) 950-7080
IN-STATE: (800) 888-0995

OKLAHOMA CLAIMS OFFICE
PO BOX 3269
TULSA, OK 74102
TEL: (918) 459-8141
IN-STATE: (800) 522-9271

VIRGINIA CLAIMS OFFICE
2108 W LABURNUM AVE, STE 210
PO BOX 85126
RICHMOND, VA 23285-5126
TEL: (804) 278-9946
FAX: (804) 213-4302
TOLL FREE: (800) 423-8153
IN-STATE: (800) 260-5200

CGU HAWKEYE UNITED SECURITY INSURANCE CO

ARIZONA CLAIMS OFFICE
10303 E DRY CREEK RD, STE 300
PO BOX 5150
DENVER, CO 80217-9580
TEL: (303) 768-8674
FAX: (720) 875-2648
TOLL FREE: (800) 654-0190

COLORADO CLAIMS OFFICE
10303 E DRY CREEK RD, STE 300
PO BOX 5150
DENVER, CO 80217-9580
TEL: (303) 768-8674
FAX: (720) 875-2648
TOLL FREE: (800) 654-0190

IDAHO CLAIMS OFFICE
10303 E DRY CREEK RD, STE 300
PO BOX 5150
DENVER, CO 80217-9580
TEL: (303) 768-8674
FAX: (720) 875-2648
TOLL FREE: (800) 654-0190

IOWA CLAIMS OFFICE
4200 UNIVERSITY AVE
PO BOX 1848
WEST DES MOINES, IA 50306
TEL: (515) 222-4000
FAX: (515) 222-4251
TOLL FREE: (800) 747-7833
WWW.CGU-HAWKEYE.COM

MONTANA CLAIMS OFFICE
10303 E DRY CREEK RD, STE 300
PO BOX 5150
DENVER, CO 80217-9580
TEL: (303) 768-8674
FAX: (720) 875-2648
TOLL FREE: (800) 654-0190

NEVADA CLAIMS OFFICE
10303 E DRY CREEK RD, STE 300
PO BOX 5150
DENVER, CO 80217-9580
TEL: (303) 768-8674
FAX: (720) 875-2648
TOLL FREE: (800) 654-0190

UTAH CLAIMS OFFICE
10303 E DRY CREEK RD, STE 300
PO BOX 5150
DENVER, CO 80217-9580
TEL: (303) 768-8674
FAX: (720) 875-2648
TOLL FREE: (800) 654-0190

CGU INSURANCE

CALIFORNIA CLAIMS OFFICE
GENERAL ACCIDENT INSURANCE
1340 TREAT BLVD, STE 400
PO BOX 8098
WALNUT CREEK, CA 94596
TEL: (510) 938-1141
FAX: (925) 942-6198
TOLL FREE: (800) 766-5421
IN-STATE: (800) 537-8855

NATIONAL CLAIMS OFFICE
1 BEACON ST
BOSTON, MA 02108
TEL: (617) 725-6000
FAX: (215) 625-1251

CGU INSURANCE CO

OHIO CLAIMS OFFICE
10560 ASHVIEW PL, STE 155
CINCINNATI, OH 45242-3738
TEL: (513) 554-6600
FAX: (513) 554-6695
TOLL FREE: (800) 582-0497
IN-STATE: (800) 582-0497

17800 JEFFERSON PARK W, STE 107
MIDDLEBURG HEIGHTS, OH 44130-3467
TEL: (440) 243-4023
FAX: (440) 243-0421
IN-STATE: (800) 362-9944

CGU INSURANCE / GENERAL ACCIDENT

OKLAHOMA CLAIMS OFFICE
8282 S MEMORIAL
PO BOX 3269
TULSA, OK 74102
TEL: (918) 459-8141
FAX: (918) 461-0793
TOLL FREE: (800) 234-8141

CGU INTERNS CO

NATIONAL CLAIMS OFFICE
5910 N CENTRAL EXPRESS WY, STE 500
DALLAS, TX 75206
TEL: (214) 739-3919
FAX: (214) 346-7717
IN-STATE: (800) 443-2533

CHAMPUS

ALABAMA CLAIMS OFFICE
PALMETTO GOVERNMENT BENEFIT ADMINISTRATORS, REGIONS 3 & 4
PO BOX 202000
FLORENCE, SC 29502-2000
TEL: (843) 665-7822
TOLL FREE: (800) 403-3950
WWW.HUMANAMILITARY.COM

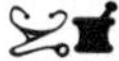

ALASKA CLAIMS OFFICE
PALMETTO GOVERNMENT BENEFIT ADMINISTRATORS REGION 7 & 8
PO BOX 870020
SURFSIDE BEACH, CA 29587-8720
TEL: (843) 650-6100
TOLL FREE: (800) 225-4816
WWW.TRICARE.OSD.MIL

ARIZONA CLAIMS OFFICE
PALMETTO GOVERNMENT BENEFIT ADMINISTRATORS REGION 7 & 8
PO BOX 870020
SURFSIDE BEACH, CA 29587-8720
TEL: (843) 650-6100
TOLL FREE: (800) 225-4816
WWW.TRICARE.OSD.MIL

ARKANSAS CLAIMS OFFICE
FOUNDATION HEALTH FEDERAL SERVICES
1313 W BROADWAY
PO BOX 8999
MADISON, WI 53707-8999
TEL: (608) 221-4711
FAX: (608) 223-3611
TOLL FREE: (800) 406-2832
WWW.FHFS.COM

COLORADO CLAIMS OFFICE
PALMETTO GOVERNMENT BENEFIT ADMINISTRATORS REGION 7 & 8
PO BOX 870020
SURFSIDE BEACH, CA 29587-8720
TEL: (843) 650-6100
TOLL FREE: (800) 225-4816
WWW.TRICARE.OSD.MIL

CONNECTICUT CLAIMS OFFICE
TRICARE - REGION 1 CLAIMS
PO BOX 7011
CAMDEN, SC 29020-7011
TOLL FREE: (800) 578-1294
WWW.OCHAMPUS.MIL

DELAWARE CLAIMS OFFICE
TRICARE - REGION 1 CLAIMS
PO BOX 7011
CAMDEN, SC 29020-7011
TOLL FREE: (800) 578-1294
WWW.OCHAMPUS.MIL

DISTRICT OF COLUMBIA CLAIMS OFFICE
TRICARE - REGION 1 CLAIMS
PO BOX 7011
CAMDEN, SC 29020-7011
TOLL FREE: (800) 578-1294
WWW.OCHAMPUS.MIL

FLORIDA CLAIMS OFFICE
PALMETTO GOVERNMENT BENEFIT
ADMINISTRATORS, REGIONS 3 & 4
PO BOX 202000
FLORENCE, SC 29502-2000
TEL: (843) 665-7822
TOLL FREE: (800) 403-3950
WWW.HUMANAMILITARY.COM

FOUNDATION HEALTH FEDERAL SERVICES
1313 W BROADWAY
PO BOX 8999
MADISON, WI 53707-8999
TEL: (608) 221-4711
FAX: (608) 223-3611
TOLL FREE: (800) 406-2832
WWW.FHFS.COM

GEORGIA CLAIMS OFFICE
PALMETTO GOVERNMENT BENEFIT
ADMINISTRATORS, REGIONS 3 & 4
PO BOX 202000
FLORENCE, SC 29502-2000
TEL: (843) 665-7822
TOLL FREE: (800) 403-3950
WWW.HUMANAMILITARY.COM

FOUNDATION HEALTH FEDERAL SERVICES
1313 W BROADWAY
PO BOX 8999
MADISON, WI 53707-8999
TEL: (608) 221-4711
FAX: (608) 223-3611
TOLL FREE: (800) 406-2832
WWW.FHFS.COM

GUAM CLAIMS OFFICE
WPS TRICARE SERVICES OVERSEAS
1717 W BROADWAY
PO BOX 7985
MADISON, WI 53707-7985
TEL: (608) 259-4848
WWW.WPSIC.COM/TRICARE

IDAHO CLAIMS OFFICE
PALMETTO GOVERNMENT BENEFIT
ADMINISTRATORS, REGIONS 3 & 4
PO BOX 100598
FLORENCE, SC 29501-0598
TEL: (843) 665-7822
TOLL FREE: (800) 403-3950
WWW.HUMANAMILITARY.COM

ILLINOIS CLAIMS OFFICE
TRICARE - REGIONS 2 & 5 CLAIMS
PO BOX 7021
CAMDEN, SC 29020-7021
TOLL FREE: (800) 613-7124
WWW.ANTHEM-INC.COM

INDIANA CLAIMS OFFICE
TRICARE - REGIONS 2 & 5 CLAIMS
PO BOX 7021
CAMDEN, SC 29020-7021
TOLL FREE: (800) 613-7124
WWW.ANTHEM-INC.COM

IOWA CLAIMS OFFICE
PALMETTO GOVERNMENT BENEFIT
ADMINISTRATORS, REGIONS 3 & 4
PO BOX 100598
FLORENCE, SC 29501-0598
TEL: (843) 665-7822
TOLL FREE: (800) 403-3950
WWW.HUMANAMILITARY.COM

KANSAS CLAIMS OFFICE
FOUNDATION HEALTH FEDERAL SERVICES
1313 W BROADWAY
PO BOX 8999
MADISON, WI 53707-8999
TEL: (608) 221-4711
FAX: (608) 223-3611
TOLL FREE: (800) 406-2832
WWW.FHFS.COM

KENTUCKY CLAIMS OFFICE
PALMETTO GOVERNMENT BENEFIT
ADMINISTRATORS, REGIONS 3 & 4
PO BOX 100598
FLORENCE, SC 29501-0598
TEL: (843) 665-7822
TOLL FREE: (800) 403-3950
WWW.HUMANAMILITARY.COM

LOUISIANA CLAIMS OFFICE
FOUNDATION HEALTH FEDERAL SERVICES
1313 W BROADWAY
PO BOX 8999
MADISON, WI 53707-8999
TEL: (608) 221-4711
FAX: (608) 223-3611
TOLL FREE: (800) 406-2832
WWW.FHFS.COM

MAINE CLAIMS OFFICE
TRICARE - REGION 1 CLAIMS
PO BOX 7011
CAMDEN, SC 29020-7011
TOLL FREE: (800) 578-1294
WWW.OCHAMPUS.MIL

MARYLAND CLAIMS OFFICE
TRICARE - REGION 1 CLAIMS
PO BOX 7011
CAMDEN, SC 29020-7011
TOLL FREE: (800) 578-1294
WWW.OCHAMPUS.MIL

MASSACHUSETTS CLAIMS OFFICE
TRICARE - REGION 1 CLAIMS
PO BOX 7011
CAMDEN, SC 29020-7011
TOLL FREE: (800) 578-1294
WWW.OCHAMPUS.MIL

MICHIGAN CLAIMS OFFICE
TRICARE - REGIONS 2 & 5 CLAIMS
PO BOX 7021
CAMDEN, SC 29020-7021
TOLL FREE: (800) 578-1294
WWW.ANTHEM-INC.COM

MINNESOTA CLAIMS OFFICE
PALMETTO GOVERNMENT BENEFIT
ADMINISTRATORS, REGIONS 3 & 4
PO BOX 100598
FLORENCE, SC 29501-0598
TEL: (843) 665-7822
TOLL FREE: (800) 403-3950
WWW.HUMANAMILITARY.COM

MISSISSIPPI CLAIMS OFFICE
PALMETTO GOVERNMENT BENEFIT
ADMINISTRATORS, REGIONS 3 & 4
PO BOX 202000
FLORENCE, SC 29502-2000
TEL: (843) 665-7822
TOLL FREE: (800) 403-3950
WWW.HUMANAMILITARY.COM

FOUNDATION HEALTH FEDERAL SERVICES
1313 W BROADWAY
PO BOX 8999
MADISON, WI 53707-8999
TEL: (608) 221-4711
FAX: (608) 223-3611
TOLL FREE: (800) 406-2832
WWW.FHFS.COM

MISSOURI CLAIMS OFFICE
FOUNDATION HEALTH FEDERAL SERVICES
1313 W BROADWAY
PO BOX 8999
MADISON, WI 53707-8999
TEL: (608) 221-4711
FAX: (608) 223-3611
TOLL FREE: (800) 406-2832
WWW.FHFS.COM

MONTANA CLAIMS OFFICE
PALMETTO GOVERNMENT BENEFIT
ADMINISTRATORS REGION 7 & 8
PO BOX 870020
SURFSIDE BEACH, CA 29587-8720
TEL: (843) 650-6100
TOLL FREE: (800) 225-4816
WWW.TRICARE.OSD.MIL

NEBRASKA CLAIMS OFFICE
PALMETTO GOVERNMENT BENEFIT
ADMINISTRATORS REGION 7 & 8
PO BOX 870020
SURFSIDE BEACH, CA 29587-8720
TEL: (843) 650-6100
TOLL FREE: (800) 225-4816
WWW.TRICARE.OSD.MIL

C

NEVADA CLAIMS OFFICE
PALMETTO GOVERNMENT BENEFIT
ADMINISTRATORS REGION 7 & 8
PO BOX 870020
SURFSIDE BEACH, CA 29587-8720
TEL: (843) 650-6100
TOLL FREE: (800) 225-4816
WWW.TRICARE.OSD.MIL

NEW HAMPSHIRE CLAIMS OFFICE
TRICARE - REGION 1 CLAIMS
PO BOX 7011
CAMDEN, SC 29020-7011
TOLL FREE: (800) 578-1294
WWW.OCHAMPUS.MIL

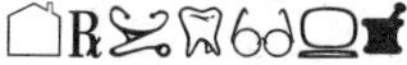

NEW JERSEY CLAIMS OFFICE
TRICARE - REGION 1 CLAIMS
PO BOX 7011
CAMDEN, SC 29020-7011
TOLL FREE: (800) 578-1294
WWW.OCHAMPUS.MIL

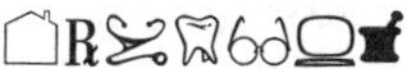

NEW MEXICO CLAIMS OFFICE
PALMETTO GOVERNMENT BENEFIT
ADMINISTRATORS REGION 7 & 8
PO BOX 870020
SURFSIDE BEACH, CA 29587-8720
TEL: (843) 650-6100
TOLL FREE: (800) 225-4816
WWW.TRICARE.OSD.MIL

NEW YORK CLAIMS OFFICE
TRICARE - REGION 1 CLAIMS
PO BOX 7011
CAMDEN, SC 29020-7011
TOLL FREE: (800) 578-1294
WWW.OCHAMPUS.MIL

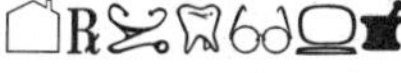

NORTH CAROLINA CLAIMS OFFICE
TRICARE - REGIONS 2 & 5 CLAIMS
PO BOX 7021
CAMDEN, SC 29020-7021
TOLL FREE: (800) 613-7124
WWW.ANTHEM-INC.COM

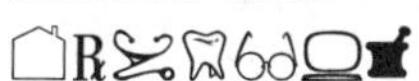

NORTH DAKOTA CLAIMS OFFICE
PALMETTO GOVERNMENT BENEFIT
ADMINISTRATORS REGION 7 & 8
PO BOX 870020
SURFSIDE BEACH, CA 29587-8720
TEL: (843) 650-6100
TOLL FREE: (800) 225-4816
WWW.TRICARE.OSD.MIL

OHIO CLAIMS OFFICE
TRICARE - REGION 1 CLAIMS
PO BOX 7021
CAMDEN, SC 29020-7021
TOLL FREE: (800) 613-7124
WWW.ANTHEM-INC.COM

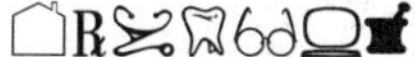

OKLAHOMA CLAIMS OFFICE
FOUNDATION HEALTH FEDERAL SERVICES
1313 W BROADWAY
PO BOX 8999
MADISON, WI 53707-8999
TEL: (608) 221-4711
FAX: (608) 223-3611
TOLL FREE: (800) 406-2832
WWW.FHFS.COM

OREGON CLAIMS OFFICE
PALMETTO GOVERNMENT BENEFIT
ADMINISTRATORS REGION 7 & 8
PO BOX 870020
SURFSIDE BEACH, CA 29587-8720
TEL: (843) 650-6100
TOLL FREE: (800) 225-4816
WWW.TRICARE.OSD.MIL

PENNSYLVANIA CLAIMS OFFICE
TRICARE - REGION 1 CLAIMS
PO BOX 7011
CAMDEN, SC 29020-7011
TOLL FREE: (800) 578-1294
WWW.OCHAMPUS.MIL

PUERTO RICO CLAIMS OFFICE
WPS TRICARE SERVICES OVERSEAS
1717 W BROADWAY
PO BOX 7985
MADISON, WI 53707-7985
TEL: (608) 259-4848
WWW.WPSIC.COM/TRICARE

RHODE ISLAND CLAIMS OFFICE
TRICARE - REGION 1 CLAIMS
PO BOX 7011
CAMDEN, SC 29020-7011
TOLL FREE: (800) 578-1294
WWW.OCHAMPUS.MIL

SOUTH CAROLINA CLAIMS OFFICE
PALMETTO GOVERNMENT BENEFIT
ADMINISTRATORS, REGIONS 3 & 4
PO BOX 202000
FLORENCE, SC 29502-2000
TEL: (843) 665-7822
TOLL FREE: (800) 403-3950
WWW.HUMANAMILITARY.COM

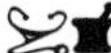

SOUTH DAKOTA CLAIMS OFFICE
PALMETTO GOVERNMENT BENEFIT
ADMINISTRATORS REGION 7 & 8
PO BOX 870020
SURFSIDE BEACH, CA 29587-8720
TEL: (843) 650-6100
TOLL FREE: (800) 225-4816
WWW.TRICARE.OSD.MIL

TENNESSEE CLAIMS OFFICE
PALMETTO GOVERNMENT BENEFIT
ADMINISTRATORS, REGIONS 3 & 4
PO BOX 202000
FLORENCE, SC 29502-2000
TEL: (843) 665-7822
TOLL FREE: (800) 403-3950
WWW.HUMANAMILITARY.COM

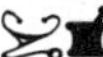

FOUNDATION HEALTH FEDERAL SERVICES
1313 W BROADWAY
PO BOX 8999
MADISON, WI 53707-8999
TEL: (608) 221-4711
FAX: (608) 223-3611
TOLL FREE: (800) 406-2832
WWW.FHFS.COM

TEXAS CLAIMS OFFICE
FOUNDATION HEALTH FEDERAL SERVICES
1313 W BROADWAY
PO BOX 8999
MADISON, WI 53707-8999
TEL: (608) 221-4711
FAX: (608) 223-3611
TOLL FREE: (800) 406-2832
WWW.FHFS.COM

UTAH CLAIMS OFFICE
PALMETTO GOVERNMENT BENEFIT
ADMINISTRATORS REGION 7 & 8
PO BOX 870020
SURFSIDE BEACH, CA 29587-8720
TEL: (843) 650-6100
TOLL FREE: (800) 225-4816
WWW.TRICARE.OSD.MIL

VERMONT CLAIMS OFFICE
TRICARE - REGION 1 CLAIMS
PO BOX 7011
CAMDEN, SC 29020-7011
TOLL FREE: (800) 578-1294
WWW.OCHAMPUS.MIL

VIRGIN ISLANDS CLAIMS OFFICE
WPS TRICARE SERVICES OVERSEAS
1717 W BROADWAY
PO BOX 7985
MADISON, WI 53707-7985
TEL: (608) 259-4848
WWW.WPSIC.COM/TRICARE

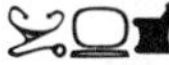

VIRGINIA CLAIMS OFFICE
TRICARE - REGIONS 2 & 5 CLAIMS
PO BOX 7021
CAMDEN, SC 29020-7021
TOLL FREE: (800) 613-7124
WWW.ANTHEM-INC.COM

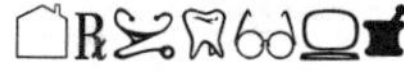

TRICARE - REGION 1 CLAIMS
PO BOX 7011
CAMDEN, SC 29020-7011
TOLL FREE: (800) 578-1294
WWW.OCHAMPUS.MIL

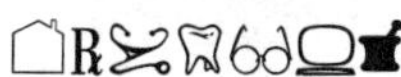

WASHINGTON CLAIMS OFFICE
PALMETTO GOVERNMENT BENEFIT
ADMINISTRATORS REGION 7 & 8
PO BOX 870020
SURFSIDE BEACH, CA 29587-8720
TEL: (843) 650-6100
TOLL FREE: (800) 225-4816
WWW.TRICARE.OSD.MIL

WEST VIRGINIA CLAIMS OFFICE
TRICARE - REGIONS 2 & 5 CLAIMS
PO BOX 7021
CAMDEN, SC 29020-7021
TOLL FREE: (800) 613-7124
WWW.ANTHEM-INC.COM

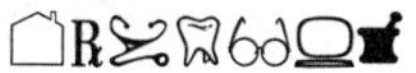

C

TRICARE - REGION 1 CLAIMS
PO BOX 7011
CAMDEN, SC 29020-7011
TOLL FREE: (800) 578-1294
WWW.OCHAMPUS.MIL

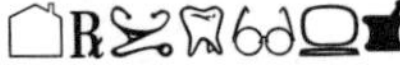

WISCONSIN CLAIMS OFFICE
TRICARE - REGIONS 2 & 5 CLAIMS
PO BOX 7021
CAMDEN, SC 29020-7021
TOLL FREE: (800) 613-7124
WWW.ANTHEM-INC.COM

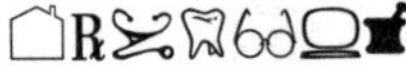

WYOMING CLAIMS OFFICE
PALMETTO GOVERNMENT BENEFIT ADMINISTRATORS REGION 7 & 8
PO BOX 870020
SURFSIDE BEACH, CA 29587-8720
TEL: (843) 650-6100
TOLL FREE: (800) 225-4816
WWW.TRICARE.OSD.MIL

CHARTER BENEFIT ADMINISTRATORS

TENNESSEE CLAIMS OFFICE
133 HOLIDAY CT, STE 210
PO BOX 681329
FRANKLIN, TN 37067
TEL: (615) 794-0001
FAX: (615) 794-0004
WWW.CHARTERBENEFITS.COM

CHER BUMPS & ASSOCIATES

OKLAHOMA CLAIMS OFFICE
6100 N ROBINSON, STE 204
PO BOX 548805
OKLAHOMA CITY, OK 73154-8805
TEL: (405) 840-6022
FAX: (405) 858-7361
TOLL FREE: (888) 840-8924

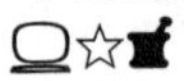

CHEROKEE NATIONAL LIFE INSURANCE CO

GEORGIA CLAIMS OFFICE
2960 RIVERSIDE DR
PO BOX 6097
MACON, GA 31213-1399
TEL: (912) 477-0400
FAX: (912) 471-0178
TOLL FREE: (800) 849-4265

CHESTER COUNTY MUTUAL INSURANCE CO

PENNSYLVANIA CLAIMS OFFICE
RIDGEWOOD CORP CTR 410 BOOT RD
PO BOX 1019
DOWNINGTON, PA 19335-0919
TEL: (610) 873-4000
FAX: (610) 873-4856

CHESTERFIELD RESOURCES, INC

OHIO CLAIMS OFFICE
PO BOX 1884
AKRON, OH 44309-1884
TEL: (330) 896-2232 / 896-4337
FAX: (330) 896-6186

CHEVRON WORKERS' COMPENSATION GROUP

CALIFORNIA CLAIMS OFFICE
575 MARKET
PO BOX 7300
SAN FRANCISCO, CA 94120-7300
TEL: (415) 894-3100
FAX: (415) 894-9887

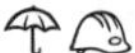

CHICAGO AREA IB OF T LOCAL 703

ILLINOIS CLAIMS OFFICE
300 S ASHLAND AVE, RM 502
PO BOX 66930
CHICAGO, IL 60666
TEL: (312) 738-1350
FAX: (312) 693-7907

CHICAGO DISTRICT COUNCIL OF CARPENTERS

12 E ERIE ST
CHICAGO, IL 60611
TEL: (312) 787-9455
FAX: (312) 951-1515
TOLL FREE: (800) 972-6489

CHICAGO MUTUAL INSURANCE CO

300 S WACKER DR, STE 1250
CHICAGO, IL 60606
TEL: (312) 347-1200
FAX: (312) 347-1205
TOLL FREE: (800) 736-5745
IN-STATE: (888) 262-8864

CHILDREN'S HOSPITAL MEDICAL CENTER OF AKRON

OHIO CLAIMS OFFICE
1 PERKINS SQ
AKRON, OH 44308-1813
TEL: (330) 379-8330
FAX: (330) 258-3176
IN-STATE: (800) 262-0333

CHILDREN'S HOSPITAL OF ORANGE COUNTY

CALIFORNIA CLAIMS OFFICE
455 S MAIN ST
PO BOX 21333
PASADENA, CA 91185-3333
TEL: (714) 532-8440
FAX: (714) 532-8833
WWW.CHOC.ORG

CHOICECARE HEALTH PLANS, INC

OHIO CLAIMS OFFICE
CHOICECARE HUMANA
655 EDEN PARK DR, STE 400
PO BOX 3188
CINCINNATI, OH 45201
TEL: (513) 784-5200
FAX: (513) 784-5310
TOLL FREE: (800) 543-7158
WWW.CHOICECARE.COM

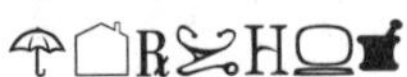

CHRISTIAN FAMILY FINANCIAL CONCEPTS, INC

WISCONSIN CLAIMS OFFICE
INSURANCE MARKETING
4630 N 109TH ST
PO BOX 18625
MILWAUKEE, WI 53218
TEL: (414) 466-4321
FAX: (414) 466-4326

CHRISTIAN FIDELITY LIFE INSURANCE CO

TEXAS CLAIMS OFFICE
2001 BATES DR
WAXAHACHIE, TX 75167-4812
TEL: (972) 937-4420

CHUBB CORPORATION

NATIONAL CLAIMS OFFICE
WORLD HEADQUARTERS
15 MOUNTAIN VIEW RD
PO BOX 1615
WARREN, NJ 07059
TEL: (908) 903-2000
FAX: (908) 903-2027
TOLL FREE: (800) 252-4670
WWW.CHUBB.COM

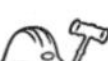

CHUBB GROUP OF INSURANCE COMPANIES

ALABAMA CLAIMS OFFICE
CHUBB & SON
1000 URVAN CENTER DR, STE 205
BIRMINGHAM, AL 35242
TEL: (205) 968-5400
FAX: (205) 968-5471
TOLL FREE: (800) 252-4670
WWW.CHUBB.COM

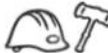

4500 WESTOWN PKY, STE 201, REGENCY 5 WEST
WEST DES MOINES, IA 50266-1066
TEL: (515) 224-2150
FAX: (515) 224-2159
TOLL FREE: (800) 248-7229
WWW.CHUBB.COM

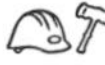

ALBERTA CLAIMS OFFICE
CHUBB & SON
6200 COURTNEY CAMPBELL CSWY, STE 700
PO BOX 31527
TAMPA, FL 33607-1489
TEL: (813) 281-7400
FAX: (813) 281-1007
TOLL FREE: (800) 252-4670
IN-STATE: (800) 226-2482
WWW.CHUBB.COM

Casualty/Liability · Dental · Disability · EMC · HCPCS · Home Health · HMO · Medical

CHUBB & SON
5020 RICHARD LN, STE 201
PO BOX 2063
MECHANICSBURG, PA 17055-0740
TEL: (717) 791-6000
FAX: (717) 791-6040
TOLL FREE: (800) 252-4670
IN-STATE: (800) 909-0900
WWW.CHUBB.COM

CHUBB & SON
1 LIBERTY PL- 1650 MARKET ST
PHILADELPHIA, PA 19103-7301
TEL: (215) 569-9660
FAX: (215) 981-8183
TOLL FREE: (800) 252-4670
IN-STATE: (800) 523-4738
WWW.CHUBB.COM

AMERICAN SAMOA CLAIMS OFFICE
CHUBB & SON
1 LIBERTY PL- 1650 MARKET ST
PHILADELPHIA, PA 19103-7301
TEL: (215) 569-9660
FAX: (215) 981-8183
TOLL FREE: (800) 252-4670
IN-STATE: (800) 523-4738
WWW.CHUBB.COM

ARIZONA CLAIMS OFFICE
CHUBB & SON
2929 N CENTRAL AVE, STE 1600
PHOENIX, AZ 85012-2722
TEL: (602) 248-4500
FAX: (602) 248-4545
TOLL FREE: (800) 252-4670
WWW.CHUBB.COM

4500 WESTOWN PKY, STE 201, REGENCY 5 WEST
WEST DES MOINES, IA 50266-1066
TEL: (515) 224-2150
FAX: (515) 224-2159
TOLL FREE: (800) 248-7229
WWW.CHUBB.COM

BRITISH COLUMBIA CLAIMS OFFICE
CHUBB & SON
5020 RICHARD LN, STE 201
PO BOX 2063
MECHANICSBURG, PA 17055-0740
TEL: (717) 791-6000
FAX: (717) 791-6040
TOLL FREE: (800) 252-4670
IN-STATE: (800) 909-0900
WWW.CHUBB.COM

CHUBB & SON
1 LIBERTY PL- 1650 MARKET ST
PHILADELPHIA, PA 19103-7301
TEL: (215) 569-9660
FAX: (215) 981-8183
TOLL FREE: (800) 252-4670
IN-STATE: (800) 523-4738
WWW.CHUBB.COM

CHUBB & SON
251 N ILLINOIS ST, STE 1100- CAPITAL CTR
INDIANAPOLIS, IN 46204-1927
TEL: (317) 321-6000
FAX: (317) 321-6061
TOLL FREE: (800) 252-4670
WWW.CHUBB.COM

CALIFORNIA CLAIMS OFFICE
CHUBB & SON
801 S FIGUEROA ST- 21ST FL
PO BOX 30850
LOS ANGELES, CA 90030-0850
TEL: (213) 612-0880
FAX: (213) 612-5728
TOLL FREE: (800) 252-4670
IN-STATE: (800) 262-4459
WWW.CHUBB.COM

CHUBB & SON
100 BAY VIEW CIR, STE 6000
PO BOX 2620
NEWPORT BEACH, CA 92658-2620
TEL: (949) 823-4900
FAX: (949) 823-4909
TOLL FREE: (800) 252-4670
WWW.CHUBB.COM

CHUBB & SON
5050 HOPYARD RD, STE 400
PLEASANTON, CA 94588-3321
TEL: (925) 598-6000
FAX: (925) 598-6146
TOLL FREE: (800) 252-4670
WWW.CHUBB.COM

CHUBB & SON
101 W BROADWAY, STE 1340
SAN DIEGO, CA 92101-3505
TEL: (619) 525-8000
FAX: (619) 525-8070
TOLL FREE: (800) 252-4670
WWW.CHUBB.COM

CHUBB & SON
2 EMBARCADERO CTR, STE 1500
SAN FRANCISCO, CA 94111
TEL: (415) 989-3000
FAX: (415) 397-9575
TOLL FREE: (800) 252-4670
WWW.CHUBB.COM

CHUBB & SON
5050 HOPYARD, STE 400
PLEASANTON, CA 94588
TEL: (925) 598-6000
TOLL FREE: (800) 252-4670
WWW.CHUBB.COM

4500 WESTOWN PKY, STE 201, REGENCY 5 WEST
WEST DES MOINES, IA 50266-1066
TEL: (515) 224-2150
FAX: (515) 224-2159
TOLL FREE: (800) 248-7229
WWW.CHUBB.COM

COLORADO CLAIMS OFFICE
CHUBB & SON
6400 S FIDDLERS GRN CIR, STE 1600
PO BOX 6520
ENGLEWOOD, CO 80155-6520
TEL: (303) 770-8700
FAX: (303) 721-6705
TOLL FREE: (800) 252-4670
WWW.CHUBB.COM

4500 WESTOWN PKY, STE 201, REGENCY 5 WEST
WEST DES MOINES, IA 50266-1066
TEL: (515) 224-2150
FAX: (515) 224-2159
TOLL FREE: (800) 248-7229
WWW.CHUBB.COM

CONNECTICUT CLAIMS OFFICE
CHUBB & SON
555 LONG WHARF DR
PO BOX 1903
NEW HAVEN, CT 06511-5941
TEL: (203) 782-4000
FAX: (203) 782-4126
TOLL FREE: (800) 252-4670
WWW.CHUBB.COM

4500 WESTOWN PKY, STE 201, REGENCY 5 WEST
WEST DES MOINES, IA 50266-1066
TEL: (515) 224-2150
FAX: (515) 224-2159
TOLL FREE: (800) 248-7229
WWW.CHUBB.COM

DISTRICT OF COLUMBIA CLAIMS OFFICE
CHUBB & SON
1801 K ST NW, STE 700 K
WASHINGTON, DC 20006
TEL: (202) 822-3200
FAX: (202) 822-3269
TOLL FREE: (800) 252-4670
WWW.CHUBB.COM

4500 WESTOWN PKY, STE 201, REGENCY 5 WEST
WEST DES MOINES, IA 50266-1066
TEL: (515) 224-2150
FAX: (515) 224-2159
TOLL FREE: (800) 248-7229
WWW.CHUBB.COM

FLORIDA CLAIMS OFFICE
REPUBLIC SECURITY BLDG
1301 CONGRESS AVE, STE 110
BOYNTON BEACH, FL 33426
TEL: (561) 734-2280
FAX: (800) 300-2538
TOLL FREE: (800) 252-4670
WWW.CHUBB.COM

C

4500 WESTOWN PKY, STE 201, REGENCY 5 WEST
WEST DES MOINES, IA 50266-1066
TEL: (515) 224-2150
FAX: (515) 224-2159
TOLL FREE: (800) 248-7229
WWW.CHUBB.COM

GEORGIA CLAIMS OFFICE
4500 WESTOWN PKY, STE 201, REGENCY 5 WEST
WEST DES MOINES, IA 50266-1066
TEL: (515) 224-2150
FAX: (515) 224-2159
TOLL FREE: (800) 248-7229
WWW.CHUBB.COM

GUAM CLAIMS OFFICE
CHUBB & SON
1 LIBERTY PL- 1650 MARKET ST
PHILADELPHIA, PA 19103-7301
TEL: (215) 569-9660
FAX: (215) 981-8183
TOLL FREE: (800) 252-4670
IN-STATE: (800) 523-4738
WWW.CHUBB.COM

ILLINOIS CLAIMS OFFICE
500 PARK BLVD, STE 600
ITASCA, IL 60143-2625
TEL: (630) 875-6000
FAX: (630) 875-6060
TOLL FREE: (800) 252-4670
WWW.CHUBB.COM

4500 WESTOWN PKY, STE 201, REGENCY 5 WEST
WEST DES MOINES, IA 50266-1066
TEL: (515) 224-2150
FAX: (515) 224-2159
TOLL FREE: (800) 248-7229
WWW.CHUBB.COM

INDIANA CLAIMS OFFICE
4500 WESTOWN PKY, STE 201, REGENCY 5 WEST
WEST DES MOINES, IA 50266-1066
TEL: (515) 224-2150
FAX: (515) 224-2159
TOLL FREE: (800) 248-7229
WWW.CHUBB.COM

IOWA CLAIMS OFFICE
4500 WESTOWN PKY, STE 201, REGENCY 5 WEST
WEST DES MOINES, IA 50266-1066
TEL: (515) 224-2150
FAX: (515) 224-2159
TOLL FREE: (800) 248-7229
WWW.CHUBB.COM

MANITOBA CLAIMS OFFICE
CHUBB & SON
1 LIBERTY PL- 1650 MARKET ST
PHILADELPHIA, PA 19103-7301
TEL: (215) 569-9660
FAX: (215) 981-8183
TOLL FREE: (800) 252-4670
IN-STATE: (800) 523-4738
WWW.CHUBB.COM

CHUBB & SON
251 N ILLINOIS ST, STE 1100- CAPITAL CTR
INDIANAPOLIS, IN 46204-1927
TEL: (317) 321-6000
FAX: (317) 321-6061
TOLL FREE: (800) 252-4670
WWW.CHUBB.COM

MARYLAND CLAIMS OFFICE
ST PAUL PLZ- 25TH FL
200 SAINT PAUL PL, STE 2500
BALTIMORE, MD 21202-2038
TEL: (410) 659-6500
FAX: (410) 659-6591
TOLL FREE: (800) 252-4670
WWW.CHUBB.COM

4500 WESTOWN PKY, STE 201, REGENCY 5 WEST
WEST DES MOINES, IA 50266-1066
TEL: (515) 224-2150
FAX: (515) 224-2159
TOLL FREE: (800) 248-7229
WWW.CHUBB.COM

MASSACHUSETTS CLAIMS OFFICE
4500 WESTOWN PKY, STE 201, REGENCY 5 WEST
WEST DES MOINES, IA 50266-1066
TEL: (515) 224-2150
FAX: (515) 224-2159
TOLL FREE: (800) 248-7229
WWW.CHUBB.COM

MEXICO CLAIMS OFFICE
CHUBB & SON
5020 RICHARD LN, STE 201
PO BOX 2063
MECHANICSBURG, PA 17055-0740
TEL: (717) 791-6000
FAX: (717) 791-6040
TOLL FREE: (800) 252-4670
IN-STATE: (800) 909-0900
WWW.CHUBB.COM

CHUBB & SON
1 LIBERTY PL- 1650 MARKET ST
PHILADELPHIA, PA 19103-7301
TEL: (215) 569-9660
FAX: (215) 981-8183
TOLL FREE: (800) 252-4670
IN-STATE: (800) 523-4738
WWW.CHUBB.COM

FEDERAL INSURANCE COMPANY
3445 PIEDMONT RD NE, STE 900
ATLANTA, GA 30326-1276
TEL: (404) 266-4000
FAX: (404) 264-6840
TOLL FREE: (800) 252-4670
WWW.CHUBB.COM

CHUBB & SON
251 N ILLINOIS ST, STE 1100- CAPITAL CTR
INDIANAPOLIS, IN 46204-1927
TEL: (317) 321-6000
FAX: (317) 321-6061
TOLL FREE: (800) 252-4670
WWW.CHUBB.COM

MICHIGAN CLAIMS OFFICE
4500 WESTOWN PKY, STE 201, REGENCY 5 WEST
WEST DES MOINES, IA 50266-1066
TEL: (515) 224-2150
FAX: (515) 224-2159
TOLL FREE: (800) 248-7229
WWW.CHUBB.COM

MINNESOTA CLAIMS OFFICE
4500 WESTOWN PKY, STE 201, REGENCY 5 WEST
WEST DES MOINES, IA 50266-1066
TEL: (515) 224-2150
FAX: (515) 224-2159
TOLL FREE: (800) 248-7229
WWW.CHUBB.COM

MISSOURI CLAIMS OFFICE
4500 WESTOWN PKY, STE 201, REGENCY 5 WEST
WEST DES MOINES, IA 50266-1066
TEL: (515) 224-2150
FAX: (515) 224-2159
TOLL FREE: (800) 248-7229
WWW.CHUBB.COM

NATIONAL CLAIMS OFFICE
NORTHERN ZONE ADMINISTRATIVE OFFICE
SEARS TWR- 233 S WACKER DR, STE 4700
CHICAGO, IL 60606-6303
TEL: (312) 454-4200
FAX: (312) 454-4401
TOLL FREE: (800) 252-4670
WWW.CHUBB.COM

NORTH AMERICAN UNDERWRITING SERVICES (NAUS)
25 INDEPENDENCE BLVD
PO BOX 1615
WARREN, NJ 07059
TEL: (908) 903-7056
FAX: (908) 903-7040
TOLL FREE: (800) 252-4670
WWW.CHUBB.COM

CHUBB & SON
6200 COURTNEY CAMPBELL CSWY, STE 700
PO BOX 31527
TAMPA, FL 33607-1489
TEL: (813) 281-7400
FAX: (813) 281-1007
TOLL FREE: (800) 252-4670
IN-STATE: (800) 226-2482
WWW.CHUBB.COM

FEDERAL INSURANCE COMPANY
3445 PIEDMONT RD NE, STE 900
ATLANTA, GA 30326-1276
TEL: (404) 266-4000
FAX: (404) 264-6840
TOLL FREE: (800) 252-4670
WWW.CHUBB.COM

CHUBB & SON
251 N ILLINOIS ST, STE 1100- CAPITAL CTR
INDIANAPOLIS, IN 46204-1927
TEL: (317) 321-6000
FAX: (317) 321-6061
TOLL FREE: (800) 252-4670
WWW.CHUBB.COM

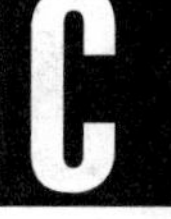

2400 PROVIDIAN CTR
400 W MARKET ST, STE 2400
LOUISVILLE, KY 40202-3368
TEL: (502) 568-8500
FAX: (502) 568-8502
TOLL FREE: (800) 248-7229
WWW.CHUBB.COM

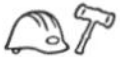

CHUBB & SON
1 FINANCIAL CTR
BOSTON, MA 02111-2697
TEL: (617) 439-4440
FAX: (800) 300-2538
TOLL FREE: (800) 252-4670
WWW.CHUBB.COM

5750 NEW KING ST, STE 200
PO BOX 7078
TROY, MI 48098-2696
TEL: (313) 641-7900
TOLL FREE: (800) 252-4670
WWW.CHUBB.COM

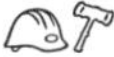

CHUBB & SON
1000 PILLSBURY CTR- 200 S 6TH ST, STE 1000
MINNEAPOLIS, MN 55402-1470
TEL: (612) 373-7300
FAX: (612) 373-7436
TOLL FREE: (800) 252-4670
IN-STATE: (800) 525-0614
WWW.CHUBB.COM

CHUBB & SON
7733 FORSYTH, STE 1300
CLAYTON, MO 63105
TEL: (314) 889-4400
FAX: (314) 862-5687
TOLL FREE: (800) 252-4670
WWW.CHUBB.COM

10 PETTICOAT LN- 3RD FL
PO BOX 13167
KANSAS CITY, MO 64199-3167
TEL: (816) 292-4500
FAX: (816) 292-4600
TOLL FREE: (800) 252-4670
IN-STATE: (800) 821-7851
WWW.CHUBB.COM

700 RTE 202-206 N
PO BOX 6980
BRIDGEWATER, NJ 08807-0975
TEL: (908) 253-8000
FAX: (908) 704-0140
TOLL FREE: (800) 699-9916
WWW.CHUBB.COM

600 INDEPENDENCE PKY
PO BOX 4700
CHESAPEAKE, VA 23327-4700
FAX: (800) 300-2538
TOLL FREE: (800) 252-4670
IN-STATE: (800) 535-0498
WWW.CHUBB.COM

111 WINNER'S CIR
PO BOX 15039
ALBANY, NY 12212-5039
TEL: (518) 437-8000
FAX: (518) 437-8010
TOLL FREE: (800) 252-4670
WWW.CHUBB.COM

OLYMPIC TWRS- 300 PEARL ST, STE 900
BUFFALO, NY 14202-2501
TEL: (716) 855-0831
FAX: (716) 855-1006
TOLL FREE: (800) 252-4670
WWW.CHUBB.COM

CHUBB & SON
55 WATER ST
NEW YORK, NY 10041
TEL: (212) 612-4000
TOLL FREE: (800) 252-4670
IN-STATE: (800) 884-4669
WWW.CHUBB.COM

1221 AVE OF THE AMERICAS- 25TH FL
PO BOX 15039
NEW YORK, NY 10020-1001
TEL: (212) 403-2800
TOLL FREE: (800) 252-4670
WWW.CHUBB.COM

CHUBB & SON
333 EARLE OVINGTON BLVD
UNIONDALE, NY 11553-3644
TEL: (516) 745-8200
FAX: (516) 745-8498
TOLL FREE: (800) 252-4670
WWW.CHUBB.COM

CHUBB & SON
2200 1ST UNION CTR- 301 S COLLEGE ST
CHARLOTTE, NC 28202-6027
TEL: (704) 372-1230
FAX: (704) 342-2750
TOLL FREE: (800) 252-4670
WWW.CHUBB.COM

312 WALNUT ST- 18TH FL
CINCINNATI, OH 45202-4035
TEL: (513) 721-0601
FAX: (513) 721-0095
TOLL FREE: (800) 252-4670
WWW.CHUBB.COM

CHUBB & SON
BANK ONE CTR- 600 SUPERIOR AVE E- 11TH FL
CLEVELAND, OH 44114-2609
TEL: (216) 687-1700
FAX: (216) 987-8601
TOLL FREE: (800) 252-4670
IN-STATE: (800) 362-2052
WWW.CHUBB.COM

PIONEER TWR- 888 SW 5TH AVE, STE 400
PO BOX 2018
PORTLAND, OR 97204-2018
TEL: (503) 221-4240
FAX: (503) 294-5425
TOLL FREE: (800) 252-4670
IN-STATE: (800) 362-4822
WWW.CHUBB.COM

CHUBB & SON
2 WARREN PL- 6120 S YALE, STE 450
TULSA, OK 74136-4222
TEL: (918) 493-5600
FAX: (918) 493-5697
TOLL FREE: (800) 252-4670
WWW.CHUBB.COM

CHUBB & SON
5020 RICHARD LN, STE 201
PO BOX 2063
MECHANICSBURG, PA 17055-0740
TEL: (717) 791-6000
FAX: (717) 791-6040
TOLL FREE: (800) 252-4670
IN-STATE: (800) 909-0900
WWW.CHUBB.COM

CHUBB & SON
1 LIBERTY PL- 1650 MARKET ST
PHILADELPHIA, PA 19103-7301
TEL: (215) 569-9660
FAX: (215) 981-8183
TOLL FREE: (800) 252-4670
IN-STATE: (800) 523-4738
WWW.CHUBB.COM

CHUBB & SON
5TH AVE PL- 120 5TH AVE
PITTSBURGH, PA 15222-3008
TEL: (412) 391-6585
FAX: (412) 456-8979
TOLL FREE: (800) 252-4670
IN-STATE: (800) 248-5254
WWW.CHUBB.COM

AMER CTR I- 3100 W END AVE, STE 900
NASHVILLE, TN 37203-1386
TEL: (615) 298-6000
FAX: (615) 298-6005
TOLL FREE: (800) 252-4670
WWW.CHUBB.COM

CHUBB & SON
2000 W LOOP S, STE 1800
HOUSTON, TX 77027-3511
TEL: (713) 297-4600
FAX: (713) 297-4750
TOLL FREE: (800) 252-4670
WWW.CHUBB.COM

CHUBB & SON
NATIONS BANK PLZ- 300 CONVENT ST, STE 2300
SAN ANTONIO, TX 78205
TEL: (210) 223-6600
FAX: (210) 978-8703
TOLL FREE: (800) 252-4670
WWW.CHUBB.COM

CHUBB & SON
323 LAW & COMMERCE BLDG
BLUEFIELD, WV 24701-3032
TEL: (304) 327-6138
TOLL FREE: (800) 252-4670
WWW.CHUBB.COM

C

4101 COX RD, STE 301
PO BOX 5336
GLEN ALLEN, VA 23058-5336
TEL: (804) 935-6300
FAX: (804) 935-6333
TOLL FREE: (800) 252-4670
WWW.CHUBB.COM

CHUBB & SON
2 PLZ E- 330 E KILBOURNE AVE, STE 1450
PO BOX 3146
MILWAUKEE, WI 53202-3146
TEL: (414) 271-2955
FAX: (414) 271-8617
TOLL FREE: (800) 252-4670
IN-STATE: (800) 362-4822
WWW.CHUBB.COM

600 INDEPENDENCE PKY
PO BOX 4700
CHESAPEAKE, VA 23327-4700
TEL: (757) 222-4822
FAX: (800) 300-2538
TOLL FREE: (800) 252-4670
IN-STATE: (800) 535-0498
WWW.CHUBB.COM

NEW BRUNSWICK CLAIMS OFFICE
CHUBB & SON
1 LIBERTY PL- 1650 MARKET ST
PHILADELPHIA, PA 19103-7301
TEL: (215) 569-9660
FAX: (215) 981-8183
TOLL FREE: (800) 252-4670
IN-STATE: (800) 523-4738
WWW.CHUBB.COM

FEDERAL INSURANCE COMPANY
3445 PIEDMONT RD NE, STE 900
ATLANTA, GA 30326-1276
TEL: (404) 266-4000
FAX: (404) 264-6840
TOLL FREE: (800) 252-4670
WWW.CHUBB.COM

CHUBB & SON
251 N ILLINOIS ST, STE 1100- CAPITAL CTR
INDIANAPOLIS, IN 46204-1927
TEL: (317) 321-6000
FAX: (317) 321-6061
TOLL FREE: (800) 252-4670
WWW.CHUBB.COM

NEW JERSEY CLAIMS OFFICE
1 INDEPENDENCE WAY
PRINCETON, NJ 08543-5242
TEL: (609) 734-6400
FAX: (609) 734-6493
TOLL FREE: (800) 252-4670
WWW.CHUBB.COM

4500 WESTOWN PKY, STE 201, REGENCY 5 WEST
WEST DES MOINES, IA 50266-1066
TEL: (515) 224-2150
FAX: (515) 224-2159
TOLL FREE: (800) 248-7229
WWW.CHUBB.COM

NEW YORK CLAIMS OFFICE
EASTERN ZONE ADMINISTRATIVE OFFICE
3 GANNETT DR
WHITE PLAINS, NY 10604-3410
TEL: (914) 642-8600
FAX: (914) 642-8700
TOLL FREE: (800) 252-4670
WWW.CHUBB.COM

CHUBB & SON
700 CLINTON SQUARE
ROCHESTER, NY 14604-1717
TEL: (716) 238-8000
FAX: (716) 232-6497
TOLL FREE: (800) 252-4670
WWW.CHUBB.COM

4500 WESTOWN PKY, STE 201, REGENCY 5 WEST
WEST DES MOINES, IA 50266-1066
TEL: (515) 224-2150
FAX: (515) 224-2159
TOLL FREE: (800) 248-7229
WWW.CHUBB.COM

NEWFOUNDLAND CLAIMS OFFICE
FEDERAL INSURANCE COMPANY
3445 PIEDMONT RD NE, STE 900
ATLANTA, GA 30326-1276
TEL: (404) 266-4000
FAX: (404) 264-6840
TOLL FREE: (800) 252-4670
WWW.CHUBB.COM

CHUBB & SON
251 N ILLINOIS ST, STE 1100- CAPITAL CTR
INDIANAPOLIS, IN 46204-1927
TEL: (317) 321-6000
FAX: (317) 321-6061
TOLL FREE: (800) 252-4670
WWW.CHUBB.COM

NORTH CAROLINA CLAIMS OFFICE
4500 WESTOWN PKY, STE 201, REGENCY 5 WEST
WEST DES MOINES, IA 50266-1066
TEL: (515) 224-2150
FAX: (515) 224-2159
TOLL FREE: (800) 248-7229
WWW.CHUBB.COM

NOVA SCOTIA CLAIMS OFFICE
CHUBB & SON
1 LIBERTY PL- 1650 MARKET ST
PHILADELPHIA, PA 19103-7301
TEL: (215) 569-9660
FAX: (215) 981-8183
TOLL FREE: (800) 252-4670
IN-STATE: (800) 523-4738
WWW.CHUBB.COM

CHUBB & SON
251 N ILLINOIS ST, STE 1100- CAPITAL CTR
INDIANAPOLIS, IN 46204-1927
TEL: (317) 321-6000
FAX: (317) 321-6061
TOLL FREE: (800) 252-4670
WWW.CHUBB.COM

OHIO CLAIMS OFFICE
4500 WESTOWN PKY, STE 201, REGENCY 5 WEST
WEST DES MOINES, IA 50266-1066
TEL: (515) 224-2150
FAX: (515) 224-2159
TOLL FREE: (800) 248-7229
WWW.CHUBB.COM

OKLAHOMA CLAIMS OFFICE
4500 WESTOWN PKY, STE 201, REGENCY 5 WEST
WEST DES MOINES, IA 50266-1066
TEL: (515) 224-2150
FAX: (515) 224-2159
TOLL FREE: (800) 248-7229
WWW.CHUBB.COM

ONTARIO CLAIMS OFFICE
CHUBB & SON
6200 COURTNEY CAMPBELL CSWY, STE 700
PO BOX 31527
TAMPA, FL 33607-1489
TEL: (813) 281-7400
FAX: (813) 281-1007
TOLL FREE: (800) 252-4670
IN-STATE: (800) 226-2482
WWW.CHUBB.COM

CHUBB & SON
5020 RICHARD LN, STE 201
PO BOX 2063
MECHANICSBURG, PA 17055-0740
TEL: (717) 791-6000
FAX: (717) 791-6040
TOLL FREE: (800) 252-4670
IN-STATE: (800) 909-0900
WWW.CHUBB.COM

CHUBB & SON
1 LIBERTY PL- 1650 MARKET ST
PHILADELPHIA, PA 19103-7301
TEL: (215) 569-9660
FAX: (215) 981-8183
TOLL FREE: (800) 252-4670
IN-STATE: (800) 523-4738
WWW.CHUBB.COM

CHUBB & SON
251 N ILLINOIS ST, STE 1100- CAPITAL CTR
INDIANAPOLIS, IN 46204-1927
TEL: (317) 321-6000
FAX: (317) 321-6061
TOLL FREE: (800) 252-4670
WWW.CHUBB.COM

4500 WESTOWN PKY, STE 201, REGENCY 5 WEST
WEST DES MOINES, IA 50266-1066
TEL: (515) 224-2150
FAX: (515) 224-2159
TOLL FREE: (800) 248-7229
WWW.CHUBB.COM

OREGON CLAIMS OFFICE
4500 WESTOWN PKY, STE 201, REGENCY 5
WEST
WEST DES MOINES, IA 50266-1066
TEL: (515) 224-2150
FAX: (515) 224-2159
TOLL FREE: (800) 248-7229
WWW.CHUBB.COM

PENNSYLVANIA CLAIMS OFFICE
4500 WESTOWN PKY, STE 201, REGENCY 5
WEST
WEST DES MOINES, IA 50266-1066
TEL: (515) 224-2150
FAX: (515) 224-2159
TOLL FREE: (800) 248-7229
WWW.CHUBB.COM

PRINCE EDWARD ISLAND CLAIMS OFFICE
CHUBB & SON
251 N ILLINOIS ST, STE 1100- CAPITAL CTR
INDIANAPOLIS, IN 46204-1927
TEL: (317) 321-6000
FAX: (317) 321-6061
TOLL FREE: (800) 252-4670
WWW.CHUBB.COM

PUERTO RICO CLAIMS OFFICE
CHUBB & SON
5020 RICHARD LN, STE 201
PO BOX 2063
MECHANICSBURG, PA 17055-0740
TEL: (717) 791-6000
FAX: (717) 791-6040
TOLL FREE: (800) 252-4670
IN-STATE: (800) 909-0900
WWW.CHUBB.COM

CHUBB & SON
1 LIBERTY PL- 1650 MARKET ST
PHILADELPHIA, PA 19103-7301
TEL: (215) 569-9660
FAX: (215) 981-8183
TOLL FREE: (800) 252-4670
IN-STATE: (800) 523-4738
WWW.CHUBB.COM

QUEBEC CLAIMS OFFICE
CHUBB & SON
6200 COURTNEY CAMPBELL CSWY, STE 700
PO BOX 31527
TAMPA, FL 33607-1489
TEL: (813) 281-7400
FAX: (813) 281-1007
TOLL FREE: (800) 252-4670
IN-STATE: (800) 226-2482
WWW.CHUBB.COM

CHUBB & SON
5020 RICHARD LN, STE 201
PO BOX 2063
MECHANICSBURG, PA 17055-0740
TEL: (717) 791-6000
FAX: (717) 791-6040
TOLL FREE: (800) 252-4670
IN-STATE: (800) 909-0900
WWW.CHUBB.COM

CHUBB & SON
1 LIBERTY PL- 1650 MARKET ST
PHILADELPHIA, PA 19103-7301
TEL: (215) 569-9660
FAX: (215) 981-8183
TOLL FREE: (800) 252-4670
IN-STATE: (800) 523-4738
WWW.CHUBB.COM

CHUBB & SON
251 N ILLINOIS ST, STE 1100- CAPITAL CTR
INDIANAPOLIS, IN 46204-1927
TEL: (317) 321-6000
FAX: (317) 321-6061
TOLL FREE: (800) 252-4670
WWW.CHUBB.COM

4500 WESTOWN PKY, STE 201, REGENCY 5
WEST
WEST DES MOINES, IA 50266-1066
TEL: (515) 224-2150
FAX: (515) 224-2159
TOLL FREE: (800) 248-7229
WWW.CHUBB.COM

SASKATCHEWAN CLAIMS OFFICE
CHUBB & SON
251 N ILLINOIS ST, STE 1100- CAPITAL CTR
INDIANAPOLIS, IN 46204-1927
TEL: (317) 321-6000
FAX: (317) 321-6061
TOLL FREE: (800) 252-4670
WWW.CHUBB.COM

TENNESSEE CLAIMS OFFICE
4500 WESTOWN PKY, STE 201, REGENCY 5
WEST
WEST DES MOINES, IA 50266-1066
TEL: (515) 224-2150
FAX: (515) 224-2159
TOLL FREE: (800) 248-7229
WWW.CHUBB.COM

TEXAS CLAIMS OFFICE
SOUTHERN ZONE ADMINISTRATIVE OFFICE
1445 ROSS AVE, STE 4200
DALLAS, TX 75202-2785
TEL: (214) 754-0777
FAX: (214) 754-8129
TOLL FREE: (800) 252-4670
IN-STATE: (800) 873-0777
WWW.CHUBB.COM

4500 WESTOWN PKY, STE 201, REGENCY 5
WEST
WEST DES MOINES, IA 50266-1066
TEL: (515) 224-2150
FAX: (515) 224-2159
TOLL FREE: (800) 248-7229
WWW.CHUBB.COM

UTAH CLAIMS OFFICE
4500 WESTOWN PKY, STE 201, REGENCY 5
WEST
WEST DES MOINES, IA 50266-1066
TEL: (515) 224-2150
FAX: (515) 224-2159
TOLL FREE: (800) 248-7229
WWW.CHUBB.COM

VIRGINIA CLAIMS OFFICE
4500 WESTOWN PKY, STE 201, REGENCY 5
WEST
WEST DES MOINES, IA 50266-1066
TEL: (515) 224-2150
FAX: (515) 224-2159
TOLL FREE: (800) 248-7229
WWW.CHUBB.COM

WASHINGTON CLAIMS OFFICE
CHUBB & SON
601 UNION ST, STE 3800
SEATTLE, WA 98101-2337
TEL: (206) 624-2100
FAX: (206) 224-4878
TOLL FREE: (800) 252-4670
WWW.CHUBB.COM

4500 WESTOWN PKY, STE 201, REGENCY 5
WEST
WEST DES MOINES, IA 50266-1066
TEL: (515) 224-2150
FAX: (515) 224-2159
TOLL FREE: (800) 248-7229
WWW.CHUBB.COM

WEST VIRGINIA CLAIMS OFFICE
4500 WESTOWN PKY, STE 201, REGENCY 5
WEST
WEST DES MOINES, IA 50266-1066
TEL: (515) 224-2150
FAX: (515) 224-2159
TOLL FREE: (800) 248-7229
WWW.CHUBB.COM

WISCONSIN CLAIMS OFFICE
4500 WESTOWN PKY, STE 201, REGENCY 5
WEST
WEST DES MOINES, IA 50266-1066
TEL: (515) 224-2150
FAX: (515) 224-2159
TOLL FREE: (800) 248-7229
WWW.CHUBB.COM

CHURCH MUTUAL INSURANCE CO

NATIONAL CLAIMS OFFICE
3000 SCHUSTER LN
PO BOX 342
MERRILL, WI 54452-3098
TEL: (715) 536-5577
FAX: (715) 539-4651
TOLL FREE: (800) 542-3465
WWW.CHURCHHILL-MUTUAL.COM

CHURCHILL ADMINISTRATIVE PLANS, INC

NEW JERSEY CLAIMS OFFICE
270 SYLVAN AVE
ENGLEWOOD CLIFFS, NJ 07632
TEL: (201) 871-8400

C

CIGNA CORP

CALIFORNIA CLAIMS OFFICE
CIGNA HEALTHCARE'S FRESNO SERVICE CTR
1630 E SHAW AVE, STE 106
PO BOX 24005
FRESNO, CA 93779
TEL: (209) 222-2500
TOLL FREE: (800) 841-4143
WWW.CIGNAHEALTHCARE.COM

CONNECTICUT CLAIMS OFFICE
CIGNA HEALTHCARE OF THE NORTHEAST
32 VALLEY ST
PO BOX 8015
BRISTOL, CT 06010
TEL: (860) 583-3874
FAX: (860) 585-6476
TOLL FREE: (800) 345-9458

CIGNA P & C- NEW ENGLAND WORKERS' COMP CTR
PO BOX 5001
HARTFORD, CT 06102-5001
FAX: (860) 769-4807
TOLL FREE: (800) 824-6076

DELAWARE CLAIMS OFFICE
CIGNA WORLDWIDE INSURANCE CO- WORKERS' COMP DIVISION
1 BEAVER VALLEY RD
PO BOX 15050
WILMINGTON, DE 19850-5527
TEL: (302) 479-6000
WWW.CIGNA.COM

FLORIDA CLAIMS OFFICE
CIGNA HEALTHCARE OF SOUTH FLORIDA
2220 PARK LAKE DR, STE 100
PO BOX 49400
ATLANTA, GA 30359
TEL: (770) 723-7894
FAX: (770) 723-7890
TOLL FREE: (800) 942-2471
IN-STATE: (800) 526-7431

GEORGIA CLAIMS OFFICE
CIGNA HEALTHCARE OF SOUTH FLORIDA
2220 PARK LAKE DR, STE 100
PO BOX 49400
ATLANTA, GA 30359
TEL: (770) 723-7894
FAX: (770) 723-7890
TOLL FREE: (800) 942-2471
IN-STATE: (800) 526-7431

MASSACHUSETTS CLAIMS OFFICE
CIGNA P & C- NEW ENGLAND WORKERS' COMP CTR
PO BOX 5001
HARTFORD, CT 06102-5001
TEL: (860) 769-4544
FAX: (860) 769-4807
TOLL FREE: (800) 824-6076

NATIONAL CLAIMS OFFICE
1601 CHESTNUT ST- TWO LIBERTY PL
PHILADELPHIA, PA 19192-1550
TEL: (215) 761-1000

CIGNA HEALTHCARE OF ARIZONA, INC
600 E TAYLOR
PO BOX 9321
SHERMAN, TX 75091-9321
TEL: (903) 892-8167
FAX: (903) 892-6271
TOLL FREE: (800) 525-5803
IN-STATE: (800) 238-8801
WWW.CIGNA.COM

CIGNA HEALTHCARE OF ARIZONA, TUCSON
600 E TAYLOR
PO BOX 9328
SHERMAN, TX 75091-9328
TEL: (903) 892-8167
FAX: (903) 892-6271
TOLL FREE: (800) 525-5803
IN-STATE: (800) 238-8801
WWW.CIGNA.COM

RISK TRANSFER- CASUALTY/LIABILITY CLAIMS
7TH FLOOR
PO BOX 152035
IRVING, TX 75015
FAX: (972) 869-8669
TOLL FREE: (800) 250-1643
WWW.CIGNA.COM

WESTERN CLAIMS CENTER
10860 GOLD CTR DR, STE 455
PO BOX 13088
RANCHO CORDOVA, CA 95670
TEL: (916) 636-3700
FAX: (916) 636-3984
TOLL FREE: (800) 824-6643
IN-STATE: (800) 421-2471
WWW.CIGNA.COM

9740 APPALOOSA DR
PO BOX 85490
SAN DIEGO, CA 92121
TEL: (619) 693-4600
FAX: (619) 693-4881
TOLL FREE: (800) 822-2994
WWW.CIGNA.COM

CIGNA HEALTHCARE CONNECTICUT GENERAL SERVICE CENTER
4025 W MINERAL KING
PO BOX 5038
VISALIA, CA 93278-5038
TEL: (209) 738-2000
FAX: (209) 738-2050
TOLL FREE: (800) 272-2471
WWW.CIGNA.COM

4582 S ULSTER, STE 700
PO BOX 2941
DENVER, CO 80237
TEL: (303) 721-3000
FAX: (303) 721-3222
TOLL FREE: (800) 742-4135
WWW.CIGNA.COM

CIGNA HEALTHCARE OF COLORADO
600 E TAYLOR
PO BOX 9025
SHERMAN, TX 75091-9025
TEL: (903) 892-8167
FAX: (903) 892-6271
TOLL FREE: (800) 525-5803
IN-STATE: (800) 238-8801
WWW.CIGNA.COM

CIGNA HEALTHCARE HOME OFC- BLOOMFIELD OFC COMPLEX
900 COTTAGE GROVE RD- WILDE BLDG
HARTFORD, CT 06152
TEL: (860) 726-6000
WWW.CIGNA.COM

CIGNA HEALTHCARE OF GEORGIA
100 PEACHTREE ST NW, STE 700
ATLANTA, GA 30303
TEL: (404) 681-7000
TOLL FREE: (800) 526-5481
WWW.CIGNA.COM

MEDICARE
2 VANTAGE WY
PO BOX 22599
NASHVILLE, TN 37202
TEL: (615) 244-5650
FAX: (615) 782-4651
IN-STATE: (800) 627-2782
WWW.CIGNA.COM

CONNECTICUT GENERAL (UNITED AIRLINE EMPLOYEE DEPT)
21 HERITAGE DR
BOURBONNAIS, IL 60914
TEL: (815) 939-4566
FAX: (815) 935-3499
TOLL FREE: (800) 654-8777
WWW.CIGNA.COM

CIGNA HEALTHCARE
13300 HICKMAN RD
CLIVE, IA 50325
TEL: (515) 223-9600
FAX: (515) 226-8662
WWW.CIGNA.COM

CIGNA HEALTHCARE OF KANSAS
600 E TAYLOR
PO BOX 9303
SHERMAN, TX 75091-9303
TEL: (903) 892-8167
FAX: (903) 892-6271
TOLL FREE: (800) 525-5803
IN-STATE: (800) 238-8801
WWW.CIGNA.COM

CIGNA HEALTHCARE OF LOUISIANA, BATON ROUGE
600 E TAYLOR
PO BOX 9022
SHERMAN, TX 75091-9022
TEL: (903) 892-8167
FAX: (903) 892-6271
TOLL FREE: (800) 525-5803
IN-STATE: (800) 238-8801
WWW.CIGNA.COM

Insurance Directory

CIGNA HEALTHCARE OF LOUISIANA, SHREVEPORT
600 E TAYLOR
PO BOX 9305
SHERMAN, TX 75091-9305
TEL: (903) 892-8167
FAX: (903) 892-6271
TOLL FREE: (800) 525-5803
IN-STATE: (800) 238-8801
WWW.CIGNA.COM

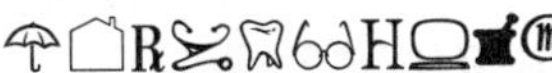

CIGNA HEALTHCARE OF MID-ATLANTIC
9700 PATUXENT WOOD DR
COLUMBIA, MD 21046
TEL: (410) 720-5800
FAX: (410) 720-5860
TOLL FREE: (800) 542-2471
WWW.CIGNA.COM

CIGNA MEDICAL HEALTH PLAN
24750 LAHSER DR
PO BOX 5013
SOUTHFIELD, MI 48086
TEL: (248) 353-9800
FAX: (248) 353-0431
WWW.CIGNA.COM

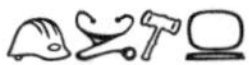

CIGNA DENTAL HEALTH PLAN
26913 NORTHWESTERN HWY, STE 300
PO BOX 183
SOUTHFIELD, MI 48037
TEL: (810) 354-8330
FAX: (810) 948-6240
TOLL FREE: (800) 523-4626
WWW.CIGNA.COM

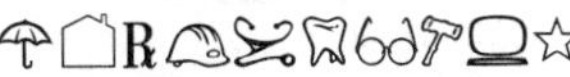

CIGNA HEALTHCARE
PO BOX 64143
SAINT PAUL, MN 55164-0143
TEL: (651) 454-7500
FAX: (612) 455-8751
TOLL FREE: (800) 292-9902
WWW.CIGNA.COM

CIGNA HEALTHCARE OF MISSISSIPPI
600 E TAYLOR
PO BOX 9338
SHERMAN, TX 75091-9338
TEL: (903) 892-8167
FAX: (903) 892-6271
TOLL FREE: (800) 525-5803
IN-STATE: (800) 238-8801
WWW.CIGNA.COM

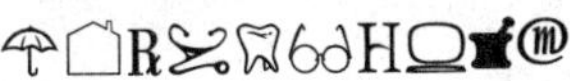

CIGNA HEALTHCARE
PO BOX 3310 STA DR
ALBUQUERQUE, NM 87190-3310
TOLL FREE: (800) 237-6039
WWW.CIGNA.COM

CIGNA HEALTHCARE
32 VALLEY ST
BRISTOL, CT 06010
TEL: (860) 583-3874
TOLL FREE: (800) 462-7482
IN-STATE: (800) 722-0445
WWW.CIGNA.COM

CIGNA HEALTHCARE
263 RT 17K
NEWBURGH, NY 12550-8310
TEL: (914) 564-3400
FAX: (914) 564-4997
TOLL FREE: (800) 431-4949
WWW.CIGNA.COM

CIGNA HEALTHCARE
255 EAST AVE
ROCHESTER, NY 14604
TEL: (716) 258-1744
FAX: (716) 258-1780
TOLL FREE: (800) 532-9288
WWW.CIGNA.COM

CIGNA HEALTHCARE OF NORTH CAROLINA
4421 STUART ANDREWS BLVD, STE 500
PO BOX 30575
CHARLOTTE, NC 28217
TEL: (704) 561-8600
FAX: (704) 561-8691
TOLL FREE: (800) 235-5707
WWW.CIGNA.COM

CIGNA HEALTHCARE
4198 COX RD- 2ND FL
PO BOX 6839
GLEN ALLEN, VA 23060
TEL: (804) 346-3600
FAX: (804) 346-3605
TOLL FREE: (800) 445-8113

CIGNA HEALTHCARE OF OHIO
1000 POLARIS PKY
PO BOX 182331
COLUMBUS, OH 43240
TEL: (614) 785-1310
FAX: (614) 786-7777
WWW.CIGNA.COM

CIGNA HEALTHCARE
1 S HOLARIS PKY
PO BOX 16672
COLUMBUS, OH 43240
TEL: (614) 785-1310
FAX: (614) 786-7777
WWW.CIGNA.COM

CIGNA HEALTHCARE OF OKLAHOMA
600 E TAYLOR
PO BOX 9336
SHERMAN, TX 75091-9336
TEL: (903) 892-8167
FAX: (903) 892-6271
TOLL FREE: (800) 525-5803
IN-STATE: (800) 238-8801
WWW.CIGNA.COM

CIGNA HEALTHCARE OF OREGON / WASHINGTON
1630 E SHAW AVE, STE 106
PO BOX 24022
FRESNO, CA 93779-4022
TEL: (209) 222-2500
TOLL FREE: (800) 245-2471
IN-STATE: (800) 428-8891
WWW.CIGNA.COM/HEALTHCARE

CIGNA HEALTHCARE
PO BOX 2300
PITTSBURGH, PA 15230
TEL: (412) 562-2960
TOLL FREE: (800) 338-7691
WWW.CIGNA.COM

CIGNA LIFE INSURANCE COMPANIES- CANADA
250 YOUNGS ST, STE 1400
PO BOX 14
TORONTO, ON M5B-2L7
TEL: (416) 591-1225
FAX: (416) 591-9399
TOLL FREE: (800) 668-7029
WWW.CIGNA.COM

CIGNA HEALTHCARE
4198 COX RD- 2ND FL
PO BOX 6839
RICHMOND, VA 23030
TEL: (804) 346-3600
FAX: (804) 346-3613
TOLL FREE: (800) 445-8113
WWW.CIGNA.COM

CIGNA HEALTHCARE OF MEMPHIS, TENNESSEE
600 E TAYLOR
PO BOX 9337
SHERMAN, TX 75091-9337
TEL: (903) 892-8167
FAX: (903) 892-6271
TOLL FREE: (800) 525-5803
IN-STATE: (800) 238-8801
WWW.CIGNA.COM

CIGNA GROUP INSURANCE
12225 GREENVILLE AVE
STE 655, LB179
PO BOX 9384
DALLAS, TX 75243-9384
TEL: (972) 234-3404
FAX: (972) 907-7194
TOLL FREE: (800) 352-0611
WWW.CIGNA.COM

CIGNA HEALTHCARE OF TEXAS, INC
600 E TAYLOR
PO BOX 2546
SHERMAN, TX 75091-2546
TEL: (903) 892-8167
FAX: (903) 892-6271
TOLL FREE: (800) 525-5803
IN-STATE: (800) 238-8801
WWW.CIGNA.COM

CIGNA HEALTHCARE OF VIRGINIA
4050 INNSLAKE DR, STE 300
PO BOX 31353
RICHMOND, VA 23294
TEL: (804) 273-1100
FAX: (804) 273-1219
TOLL FREE: (800) 533-1708
WWW.CIGNA.COM

CIGNA PROPERTY & CASUALTY
PO BOX 13088
SACRAMENTO, CA 95813-4088
TEL: (916) 636-3700
FAX: (916) 636-3984
TOLL FREE: (800) 824-6643
WWW.CIGNA.COM

CIGNA HEALTH CARE OF CONNECTICUT
900 COTTAGE GROVE RD A-118
HARTFORD, CT 06152
TEL: (860) 725-2000
TOLL FREE: (800) 458-5508
WWW.CIGNA.COM

CIGNA HEALTH PLAN OF KANSAS
7400 W 110TH ST, STE 600
OVERLAND PARK, KS 66210
TEL: (913) 451-3706
TOLL FREE: (800) 832-3211
WWW.CIGNA.COM

CIGNA HEALTHCARE
8182 MARYLAND AVE, STE 900
SAINT LOUIS, MO 63105
TEL: (314) 726-7850
FAX: (314) 726-7764
TOLL FREE: (800) 727-6226
IN-STATE: (800) 541-7526
WWW.CIGNA.COM

CIGNA HEALTHCARE NORTH TAMPA
11707 CLUB DR
TAMPA, FL 33612
TEL: (813) 972-4171
FAX: (813) 971-6038
WWW.CIGNA.COM

CIGNA HEALTHCARE OF TENNESSEE
6555 QUINCE RD, STE 215
MEMPHIS, TN 38119
TOLL FREE: (800) 346-6301
WWW.CIGNA.COM

CIGNA HEALTHPLAN OF LOUISIANA, NEW ORLEANS
3838 N CSWY BLVD #2800-B
METAIRIE, LA 70002
TEL: (504) 832-1994
FAX: (504) 831-7499
TOLL FREE: (800) 654-3106
IN-STATE: (800) 238-8801
WWW.CIGNA.COM

CIGNA WORKERS COMPENSATION
31 READ'S WAY- NEW CASTLE CORP COMMONS
PO BOX 15558
NEW CASTLE, DE 19720
FAX: (302) 479-6242
TOLL FREE: (800) 648-9431
WWW.CIGNA.COM

CIGNA PROPERTY CASUALTY
600 E LAS COLINAS BLVD
IRVING, TX 75039
TEL: (972) 869-8700
FAX: (972) 869-8389
TOLL FREE: (800) 250-1645
WWW.CIGNA.COM

CIGNA WORKERS COMP
8310 N CAPITOL TX HWY, STE 175
AUSTIN, TX 78731
TEL: (512) 383-1500
WWW.CIGNA.COM

CIGNA WORLDWIDE INSURANCE CO- INTERNATIONAL CLAIMS
1 BEAVER VALLEY RD
PO BOX 15050
WILMINGTON, DE 19850-5050
TEL: (302) 479-6000
TOLL FREE: (800) 441-2668
WWW.CIGNA.COM

CIGNA WORLDWIDE INSURANCE CO
1 BEAVER VALLEY RD
PO BOX 15408
WILMINGTON, DE 19850
TEL: (302) 324-1841
TOLL FREE: (800) 441-7150
WWW.CIGNA.COM

7555 GOODWIN RD
PO BOX 188002
CHATTANOOGA, TN 37422-8002
TEL: (423) 490-2100
FAX: (423) 499-3280
WWW.CIGNA.COM

CIGNA HEALTHCARE OF TENNESSEE
ONE CORP CTR DR, STE 500-472-50
PO BOX 9339
SHERMAN, TX 75091
TEL: (903) 892-8167
TOLL FREE: (800) 492-2224
WWW.CIGNA.COM

CIGNA HEALTHCARE OF ILLINOIS INC
1700 HIGGINS, STE 600
DES PLAINES, IL 60018
TEL: (815) 939-4566
FAX: (815) 939-0473
TOLL FREE: (800) 541-7526
WWW.CIGNA.COM

NEW HAMPSHIRE CLAIMS OFFICE
CIGNA P & C- NEW ENGLAND WORKERS' COMP CTR
PO BOX 5001
HARTFORD, CT 06102-5001
FAX: (860) 769-4807
TOLL FREE: (800) 824-6076

NEW YORK CLAIMS OFFICE
CIGNA P & C- NEW ENGLAND WORKERS' COMP CTR
PO BOX 5001
HARTFORD, CT 06102-5001
FAX: (860) 769-4807
TOLL FREE: (800) 824-6076

OKLAHOMA CLAIMS OFFICE
CIGNA HEALTHCARE
5100 N BROOKLINE- 9TH FL
OKLAHOMA CITY, OK 73112
TOLL FREE: (800) 245-2471
IN-STATE: (800) 245-2471

PENNSYLVANIA CLAIMS OFFICE
CIGNA WORKERS COMPENSATION
1 BEAVER VALLEY RD
PO BOX 15050
WILMINGTON, DE 19850
FAX: (302) 479-6242
TOLL FREE: (800) 648-9431
WWW.CIGNA.COM

RHODE ISLAND CLAIMS OFFICE
CIGNA P & C- NEW ENGLAND WORKERS' COMP CTR
PO BOX 5001
HARTFORD, CT 06102-5001
FAX: (860) 769-4807
TOLL FREE: (800) 824-6076

VERMONT CLAIMS OFFICE
CIGNA P & C- NEW ENGLAND WORKERS' COMP CTR
PO BOX 5001
HARTFORD, CT 06102-5001
FAX: (860) 769-4807
TOLL FREE: (800) 824-6076

CINCINNATI EQUITABLE

OHIO CLAIMS OFFICE
525 VINE ST, STE 2100
PO BOX 3428
CINCINNATI, OH 45201-3428
TEL: (513) 621-1826
FAX: (513) 621-4531
IN-STATE: (800) 621-1826

CINCINNATI INSURANCE CO

ALABAMA CLAIMS OFFICE
3150 HOLCOMB BRDIGE RD, STE 350
PO BOX 920338
NORCROSS, GA 30092-0338
TEL: (770) 662-8753
FAX: (770) 417-4635
WWW.CINFIN.COM

GEORGIA CLAIMS OFFICE
3150 HOLCOMB BRDIGE RD, STE 350
PO BOX 920338
NORCROSS, GA 30092-0338
TEL: (770) 662-8753
FAX: (770) 417-4635
WWW.CINFIN.COM

NATIONAL CLAIMS OFFICE
CINCINNATI CASUALTY CO
PO BOX 42536
SAINT PETERSBURG, FL 33742-4536
TEL: (813) 576-1442
FAX: (813) 576-2958
IN-STATE: (800) 677-1442
WWW.CINFIN.COM

SOUTH CAROLINA CLAIMS OFFICE
3150 HOLCOMB BRDIGE RD, STE 350
PO BOX 920338
NORCROSS, GA 30092-0338
TEL: (770) 662-8753
FAX: (770) 417-4635
WWW.CINFIN.COM

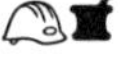

TENNESSEE CLAIMS OFFICE
3150 HOLCOMB BRDIGE RD, STE 350
PO BOX 920338
NORCROSS, GA 30092-0338
TEL: (770) 662-8753
FAX: (770) 417-4635
WWW.CINFIN.COM

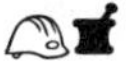

CINCINNATI LIFE INSURANCE CO

NATIONAL CLAIMS OFFICE
6200 S GILMORE
PO BOX 145496
CINCINNATI, OH 45250-5496
TEL: (513) 870-2149
FAX: (513) 870-2969

CITATION INSURANCE CO

CALIFORNIA CLAIMS OFFICE
SEQUOIA INSURANCE CO
2100 W ORANGEWOOD AVE, STE 200
PO BOX 14206
ORANGE, CA 92863-1206
TEL: (714) 456-1900
FAX: (714) 456-1950
TOLL FREE: (800) 648-1112
IN-STATE: (800) 888-5440

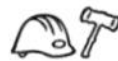

CITGO PETROLEUM CORP

OKLAHOMA CLAIMS OFFICE
BENEFITS OFFICE
PO BOX 3758
TULSA, OK 74102-3758
TEL: (918) 495-4759

CITIZENS INSURANCE CO OF AMERICA

INDIANA CLAIMS OFFICE
3950 PRIORITY WAY S DR, STE 200
PO BOX 80812
INDIANAPOLIS, IN 46240
TEL: (317) 580-9980
FAX: (317) 580-9981
TOLL FREE: (800) 289-2422
WWW.ALLMERICA.COM

MICHIGAN CLAIMS OFFICE
ALLMERICA
2501 14TH AVE S
PO BOX 1028
ESCANABA, MI 49829-1028
FAX: (906) 789-1533
TOLL FREE: (800) 349-0013
WWW.ALLMERICA.COM

ALL AMERICA
814 S OTSEGO
PO BOX 477
GAYLORD, MI 49734
TEL: (517) 732-7583
FAX: (517) 732-2937
TOLL FREE: (800) 444-7583
WWW.ALLMERICA.COM

4100 EMBASSY DR SE
PO BOX 3337
GRAND RAPIDS, MI 49501
TEL: (616) 942-2425
FAX: (616) 940-0769
IN-STATE: (800) 999-9621

OAKLAND CLAIMS COMPLEX
25300 TELEGRAPH RD, STE 375
PO BOX 5122
SOUTHFIELD, MI 48086-5122
TEL: (810) 352-7000
FAX: (810) 352-5052
TOLL FREE: (800) 288-9560
WWW.ALLMERICA.COM

NATIONAL CLAIMS OFFICE
CORPORATE OFFICE
645 W GRAND RIVER
HOWELL, MI 48843
TEL: (517) 546-2160
FAX: (517) 546-1667
TOLL FREE: (800) 388-1300
WWW.ALLMERICA.COM

OHIO CLAIMS OFFICE
ALLMERICA INSURANCE
8101 N HIGH ST, STE 40
PO BOX 342250
COLUMBUS, OH 43235
TEL: (614) 846-6511
FAX: (614) 846-3252
TOLL FREE: (800) 417-7289
WWW.ALLMERICA.COM

CITIZENS SECURITY LIFE INSURANCE CO

ALABAMA CLAIMS OFFICE
12910 SHELBYVILLE RD, STE 300
PO BOX 436149
LOUISVILLE, KY 40253-6149
TEL: (502) 244-2420
FAX: (502) 244-2439
TOLL FREE: (800) 843-7752

ARKANSAS CLAIMS OFFICE
12910 SHELBYVILLE RD, STE 300
PO BOX 436149
LOUISVILLE, KY 40253-6149
TEL: (502) 244-2420
FAX: (502) 244-2439
TOLL FREE: (800) 843-7752

DISTRICT OF COLUMBIA CLAIMS OFFICE
12910 SHELBYVILLE RD, STE 300
PO BOX 436149
LOUISVILLE, KY 40253-6149
TEL: (502) 244-2420
FAX: (502) 244-2439
TOLL FREE: (800) 843-7752

FLORIDA CLAIMS OFFICE
12910 SHELBYVILLE RD, STE 300
PO BOX 436149
LOUISVILLE, KY 40253-6149
TEL: (502) 244-2420
FAX: (502) 244-2439
TOLL FREE: (800) 843-7752

GEORGIA CLAIMS OFFICE
12910 SHELBYVILLE RD, STE 300
PO BOX 436149
LOUISVILLE, KY 40253-6149
TEL: (502) 244-2420
FAX: (502) 244-2439
TOLL FREE: (800) 843-7752

INDIANA CLAIMS OFFICE
12910 SHELBYVILLE RD, STE 300
PO BOX 436149
LOUISVILLE, KY 40253-6149
TEL: (502) 244-2420
FAX: (502) 244-2439
TOLL FREE: (800) 843-7752

KENTUCKY CLAIMS OFFICE
12910 SHELBYVILLE RD, STE 300
PO BOX 436149
LOUISVILLE, KY 40253-6149
TEL: (502) 244-2420
FAX: (502) 244-2439
TOLL FREE: (800) 843-7752

LOUISIANA CLAIMS OFFICE
12910 SHELBYVILLE RD, STE 300
PO BOX 436149
LOUISVILLE, KY 40253-6149
TEL: (502) 244-2420
FAX: (502) 244-2439
TOLL FREE: (800) 843-7752

MARYLAND CLAIMS OFFICE
12910 SHELBYVILLE RD, STE 300
PO BOX 436149
LOUISVILLE, KY 40253-6149
TEL: (502) 244-2420
FAX: (502) 244-2439
TOLL FREE: (800) 843-7752

MISSISSIPPI CLAIMS OFFICE
12910 SHELBYVILLE RD, STE 300
PO BOX 436149
LOUISVILLE, KY 40253-6149
TEL: (502) 244-2420
FAX: (502) 244-2439
TOLL FREE: (800) 843-7752

MISSOURI CLAIMS OFFICE
12910 SHELBYVILLE RD, STE 300
PO BOX 436149
LOUISVILLE, KY 40253-6149
TEL: (502) 244-2420
FAX: (502) 244-2439
TOLL FREE: (800) 843-7752

NEW JERSEY CLAIMS OFFICE
12910 SHELBYVILLE RD, STE 300
PO BOX 436149
LOUISVILLE, KY 40253-6149
TEL: (502) 244-2420
FAX: (502) 244-2439
TOLL FREE: (800) 843-7752

NORTH CAROLINA CLAIMS OFFICE
12910 SHELBYVILLE RD, STE 300
PO BOX 436149
LOUISVILLE, KY 40253-6149
TEL: (502) 244-2420
FAX: (502) 244-2439
TOLL FREE: (800) 843-7752

OHIO CLAIMS OFFICE
12910 SHELBYVILLE RD, STE 300
PO BOX 436149
LOUISVILLE, KY 40253-6149
TEL: (502) 244-2420
FAX: (502) 244-2439
TOLL FREE: (800) 843-7752

PENNSYLVANIA CLAIMS OFFICE
12910 SHELBYVILLE RD, STE 300
PO BOX 436149
LOUISVILLE, KY 40253-6149
TEL: (502) 244-2420
FAX: (502) 244-2439
TOLL FREE: (800) 843-7752

SOUTH CAROLINA CLAIMS OFFICE
12910 SHELBYVILLE RD, STE 300
PO BOX 436149
LOUISVILLE, KY 40253-6149
TEL: (502) 244-2420
FAX: (502) 244-2439
TOLL FREE: (800) 843-7752

CITRUS INSURANCE TRUST

CALIFORNIA CLAIMS OFFICE
25060 AVE STANFORD, STE 200
VALENCIA, CA 91355-3446
TEL: (661) 257-4744
FAX: (661) 295-0430
WWW.APASCO.COM

CITY MARKET FOOD & PHARMACY

COLORADO CLAIMS OFFICE
CORPORATE OFFICES
105 W COLORADO AVE
PO BOX 729
GRAND JUNCTION, CO 81502
TEL: (970) 241-0750
FAX: (970) 242-5209

CITY OF AMARILLO GROUP HEALTH PLAN

TEXAS CLAIMS OFFICE
909 E 7TH
PO BOX 1971
AMARILLO, TX 79105-1971
TEL: (806) 378-4209
FAX: (806) 378-9488

CITY OF EULESS EMPLOYEE BENEFITS PLAN

201 N ECTOR DR
EULESS, TX 76039-3543
TEL: (817) 685-1475
FAX: (817) 685-1819

CITY OF LONG BEACH

CALIFORNIA CLAIMS OFFICE
CITY HALL
333 W OCEAN BLVD- 8TH FL
LONG BEACH, CA 90802-4664
TEL: (562) 570-2245
FAX: (562) 570-2220

CITY OF LOS ANGELES WORKERS COMPENSATION DIVISION

700 E TEMPLE, STE 210
LOS ANGELES, CA 90012-4111
TEL: (213) 847-9405
FAX: (213) 847-9037

3

CITY OF MESA EMPLOYEE BENEFITS

ARIZONA CLAIMS OFFICE
20 E MAIN ST, STE 220
PO BOX 1466
MESA, AZ 85211-1466
TEL: (480) 644-2299
FAX: (480) 644-3013

R

CITY PUBLIC SERVICE GROUP HEALTH PLAN

TEXAS CLAIMS OFFICE
145 NAVARRO
PO BOX 1771
SAN ANTONIO, TX 78296-1771
TEL: (210) 978-2900
FAX: (210) 978-3351

R

CIVIL SERVICE EMPLOYEES INSURANCE CO

ARIZONA CLAIMS OFFICE
CSE INSURANCE GROUP
2720 GATEWAY OAKS DR, STE 300
PO BOX 13506
SACRAMENTO, CA 95853-4506
TEL: (916) 564-5126
FAX: (800) 332-0262
TOLL FREE: (800) 282-6848
WWW.CSE-INSURANCE.COM

CALIFORNIA CLAIMS OFFICE
CSE INSURANCE GROUP
2720 GATEWAY OAKS DR, STE 300
PO BOX 13506
SACRAMENTO, CA 95853-4506
TEL: (916) 564-5126
FAX: (800) 332-0262
TOLL FREE: (800) 282-6848
WWW.CSE-INSURANCE.COM

IDAHO CLAIMS OFFICE
CSE INSURANCE GROUP
2720 GATEWAY OAKS DR, STE 300
PO BOX 13506
SACRAMENTO, CA 95853-4506
TEL: (916) 564-5126
FAX: (800) 332-0262
TOLL FREE: (800) 282-6848
WWW.CSE-INSURANCE.COM

OREGON CLAIMS OFFICE
CSE INSURANCE GROUP
2720 GATEWAY OAKS DR, STE 300
PO BOX 13506
SACRAMENTO, CA 95853-4506
TEL: (916) 564-5126
FAX: (800) 332-0262
TOLL FREE: (800) 282-6848
WWW.CSE-INSURANCE.COM

UTAH CLAIMS OFFICE
CSE INSURANCE GROUP
2720 GATEWAY OAKS DR, STE 300
PO BOX 13506
SACRAMENTO, CA 95853-4506
TEL: (916) 564-5126
FAX: (800) 332-0262
TOLL FREE: (800) 282-6848
WWW.CSE-INSURANCE.COM

WASHINGTON CLAIMS OFFICE
CSE INSURANCE GROUP
2720 GATEWAY OAKS DR, STE 300
PO BOX 13506
SACRAMENTO, CA 95853-4506
TEL: (916) 564-5126
FAX: (800) 332-0262
TOLL FREE: (800) 282-6848
WWW.CSE-INSURANCE.COM

CIVIL SERVICE EMPLOYEES INSURANCE GROUP

ARIZONA CLAIMS OFFICE
99 S LAKE AVE- 4TH FL
PO BOX 7006
PASADENA, CA 91109-7006
TEL: (626) 793-6300
FAX: (800) 223-4131
TOLL FREE: (800) 282-6848
WWW.CSE-INSURANCE.COM

H

CALIFORNIA CLAIMS OFFICE
99 S LAKE AVE- 4TH FL
PO BOX 7006
PASADENA, CA 91109-7006
TEL: (626) 793-6300
FAX: (800) 223-4131
TOLL FREE: (800) 282-6848
WWW.CSE-INSURANCE.COM

H

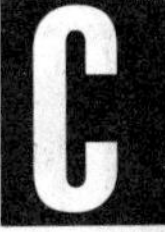

UTAH CLAIMS OFFICE
99 S LAKE AVE- 4TH FL
PO BOX 7006
PASADENA, CA 91109-7006
TEL: (626) 793-6300
FAX: (800) 223-4131
TOLL FREE: (800) 282-6848
WWW.CSE-INSURANCE.COM

CLAIMS ADMINISTRATION CORP

DISTRICT OF COLUMBIA CLAIMS OFFICE
15400 CALHOON DR
ROCKVILLE, MD 20885
TEL: (301) 738-1216
FAX: (301) 517-2126
TOLL FREE: (800) 410-7778

MARYLAND CLAIMS OFFICE
15400 CALHOON DR
ROCKVILLE, MD 20885
TEL: (301) 738-1216
FAX: (301) 517-2126
TOLL FREE: (800) 410-7778

CLAIMS ADMINISTRATION SERVICES, INC

NATIONAL CLAIMS OFFICE
6401 CONGRESS AVE, STE 230
PO BOX 3968
BOCA RATON, FL 33427-3968
TEL: (561) 241-9500
FAX: (561) 241-9709
TOLL FREE: (800) 388-5190
E-MAIL: INFO@CASI.COM

CLAIMSWARE, INC

MANAGEMED
PO BOX 6125
GREENVILLE, SC 29606-6125
TEL: (864) 234-8200
FAX: (864) 234-8202
TOLL FREE: (800) 992-8088

CLARK UNITED PROVIDERS

WASHINGTON CLAIMS OFFICE
SWMD (SOUTHWEST WASHINGTON MEDICAL DIRECTORY)
505 NE 87TH AVE, STE 1147
VANCOUVER, WA 98664
TEL: (360) 896-7093
FAX: (360) 896-7625
TOLL FREE: (800) 315-7862
IN-STATE: (800) 315-7862

CMS CAP MANAGEMENT SYSTEMS

CALIFORNIA CLAIMS OFFICE
12966 EUCLID ST, STE 500
GARDEN GROVE, CA 92840
TEL: (714) 590-5000
FAX: (714) 590-5100
IN-STATE: (800) 611-0111

CNA

NATIONAL CLAIMS OFFICE
CNA PLZ- 333 S WABASH AVE
CHICAGO, IL 60685
TEL: (312) 822-5000
FAX: (312) 822-6419
TOLL FREE: (800) 262-4473
WWW.CNA.COM

1800 E IMPERIAL HWY
PO BOX 2300
BREA, CA 92821
TEL: (714) 255-2200
FAX: (714) 255-2366
TOLL FREE: (800) 262-8714
WWW.CNA.COM

3075 E IMPERIAL HWY
PO BOX 6500
BREA, CA 92822
TEL: (714) 255-2200
FAX: (714) 572-4572
TOLL FREE: (800) 262-8714
WWW.CNA.COM

10333 E DRY CREEK RD, STE 300
PO BOX 17369
ENGLEWOOD, CO 80112
TEL: (303) 858-4100
FAX: (303) 858-4429
TOLL FREE: (800) 262-5303
IN-STATE: (800) 262-5303
WWW.CNA.COM

PO BOX 154
ORLANDO, FL 32802-0154
TEL: (407) 677-2100
FAX: (407) 677-2236
TOLL FREE: (800) 432-9988
WWW.CNA.COM

707 ORLANDO CENTRAL PKY
PO BOX 598210
ORLANDO, FL 32809-3925
TEL: (407) 859-2100
FAX: (407) 858-5377
TOLL FREE: (800) 303-9744
WWW.CNA.COM

200 S WACKER DR
CHICAGO, IL 60606-5894
TEL: (312) 876-5000
TOLL FREE: (800) 955-2303
WWW.CNA.COM

1411 OPUS PL
PO BOX 1562
DOWNERS GROVE, IL 60515
TEL: (630) 719-3000
FAX: (630) 719-3318
TOLL FREE: (800) 262-4554
WWW.CNA.COM

8403 COLESVILLE RD
SILVER SPRING, MD 20910
TEL: (301) 650-5000
FAX: (301) 650-5277
WWW.CNA.COM

1250 HANCOCK ST
PO BOX 9167
QUINCY, MA 02269-9167
TEL: (617) 984-4500
FAX: (617) 984-4545
TOLL FREE: (800) 972-5550
WWW.CNA.COM

400 GALLERIA OFC CTR, STE 300
PO BOX 5159
SOUTHFIELD, MI 48086-5159
TEL: (248) 351-6000
FAX: (248) 351-6100
TOLL FREE: (800) 262-2710
WWW.CNA.COM

NINE ENTIN RD
PARSIPPANY, NJ 07054
TEL: (973) 541-3300
FAX: (973) 515-6767
TOLL FREE: (800) 262-3249
WWW.CNA.COM

175 PINELAWN RD
PO BOX 609
MELVILLE, NY 11747
TEL: (516) 756-7300
FAX: (516) 756-7570
TOLL FREE: (800) 732-9109
WWW.CNA.COM

333 GLEN ST
PO BOX 5000
GLENS FALLS, NY 12801
FAX: (877) 329-5677
TOLL FREE: (800) 262-1145
IN-STATE: (800) 426-3692
WWW.CNA.COM

40 WALTZ ST
NEW YORK, NY 10005
TEL: (212) 440-3000
FAX: (212) 440-7130

ONE TELERGY PKY
PO BOX 4736
SYRACUSE, NY 13221-4736
TEL: (315) 431-6000
FAX: (315) 431-6005
IN-STATE: (800) 262-6344
WWW.CNA.COM

1111 E BROAD ST
PO BOX 182644
COLUMBUS, OH 43218-2644
TEL: (614) 251-5374
FAX: (614) 326-5677
TOLL FREE: (800) 613-7872
WWW.CNA.COM

1111 E BROAD ST
PO BOX 1499
COLUMBUS, OH 43205
TEL: (614) 251-5000
FAX: (614) 251-5000
TOLL FREE: (800) 955-7720
WWW.CNA.COM

2 CHATHAM CTR- 112 WASHINGTON PL
PO BOX 2872
PITTSBURGH, PA 15219
TEL: (412) 562-4100
FAX: (412) 562-4111
TOLL FREE: (800) 262-9759
WWW.CNA.COM

100 CNA DR
PO BOX 305123
NASHVILLE, TN 37214
TEL: (615) 871-1400
FAX: (615) 902-7250
TOLL FREE: (800) 251-5852
WWW.CNA.COM

600 N PEARL ST, STE 1400F
DALLAS, TX 75381
TEL: (214) 220-1300
IN-STATE: (800) 262-1113
WWW.CNA.COM

PO BOX 27537
HOUSTON, TX 77227-7537
TEL: (713) 663-5200
FAX: (713) 663-5398
TOLL FREE: (800) 262-3370
WWW.CNA.COM

6805 CAPITOL OF TX HWY, STE 260
HOUSTON, TX 78731
TEL: (512) 502-6400
FAX: (512) 502-6440
TOLL FREE: (800) 999-0972
WWW.CNA.COM

PO BOX 1236
MILWAUKEE, WI 53201-1236
TEL: (414) 821-4500
FAX: (414) 821-4544
TOLL FREE: (800) 262-4554
WWW.CNA.COM

OREGON CLAIMS OFFICE
CNA — OREGON CLAIMS OFFICE
8625 SW CASCADE BLVD
BEAVERTON, OR 97008
TEL: (503) 526-6800
FAX: (503) 526-6810
TOLL FREE: (800) 881-1350

WASHINGTON CLAIMS OFFICE
CNA — OREGON CLAIMS OFFICE
8625 SW CASCADE BLVD
BEAVERTON, OR 97008
TEL: (503) 526-6800
FAX: (503) 526-6810
TOLL FREE: (800) 881-1350

CO-OP INSURANCE COMPANIES

VERMONT CLAIMS OFFICE
292 COLONIAL DR
PO BOX 5890
MIDDLEBURY, VT 05753
TEL: (802) 388-7917
FAX: (802) 388-0069
IN-STATE: (800) 639-4017

COAST BENEFITS

NEVADA CLAIMS OFFICE
3850 S VALLEY VIEW BLVD
PO BOX 80040
LAS VEGAS, NV 89180-0040
TEL: (702) 889-1155
FAX: (702) 889-1284

COASTCAST CORP

NATIONAL CLAIMS OFFICE
3025 E VICTORIA ST
PO BOX 9076
RANCHO DOMINGUEZ, CA 90224
TEL: (310) 638-0595
FAX: (310) 631-6820

COLLIN COUNTY COURTHOUSE

TEXAS CLAIMS OFFICE
HUMAN RESOURCE OFFICE
210 S MCDONALD ST, STE 612
MCKINNEY, TX 75069-5667
TEL: (972) 548-4604
WWW.CO.COLLIN.TX.US.COM

COLONIAL INSURANCE CO

NATIONAL CLAIMS OFFICE
5525 PARKCENTER CIR
DUBLIN, OH 43017
TEL: (614) 854-8635
TOLL FREE: (800) 854-6845

COLONIAL LIFE & ACCIDENT INSURANCE CO

SOUTH CAROLINA CLAIMS OFFICE
1200 COLONIAL LIFE BLVD
PO BOX 1365
COLUMBIA, SC 29202-1365
TEL: (803) 798-7000
FAX: (800) 880-9325
TOLL FREE: (800) 325-4368

COLORADO FARM BUREAU MUTUAL INSURANCE CO

COLORADO CLAIMS OFFICE
9177 E MINERAL CIR
PO BOX 5647
DENVER, CO 80217
TEL: (303) 749-7500
FAX: (303) 749-7748

COLORADO PREFERRED PHYSICIAN ORGANIZATION

WEST CARE
4891 INDEPENDENCE ST, STE 285
PO BOX 897
WHEAT RIDGE, CO 80034
TEL: (303) 467-3667
FAX: (303) 467-3791

H

COLUMBIA INSURANCE GROUP

ARKANSAS CLAIMS OFFICE
124 IOWA AVE
PO BOX 2180
SALINA, KS 67402-2180
TEL: (913) 825-5531
FAX: (913) 825-0338
TOLL FREE: (800) 998-8902
WWW.COLINSGRP.COM

IOWA CLAIMS OFFICE
124 IOWA AVE
PO BOX 2180
SALINA, KS 67402-2180
TEL: (913) 825-5531
FAX: (913) 825-0338
TOLL FREE: (800) 998-8902
WWW.COLINSGRP.COM

KANSAS CLAIMS OFFICE
124 IOWA AVE
PO BOX 2180
SALINA, KS 67402-2180
TEL: (913) 825-5531
FAX: (913) 825-0338
TOLL FREE: (800) 998-8902
WWW.COLINSGRP.COM

MISSOURI CLAIMS OFFICE
124 IOWA AVE
PO BOX 2180
SALINA, KS 67402-2180
TEL: (913) 825-5531
FAX: (913) 825-0338
TOLL FREE: (800) 998-8902
WWW.COLINSGRP.COM

NEBRASKA CLAIMS OFFICE
124 IOWA AVE
PO BOX 2180
SALINA, KS 67402-2180
TEL: (913) 825-5531
FAX: (913) 825-0338
TOLL FREE: (800) 998-8902
WWW.COLINSGRP.COM

OHIO CLAIMS OFFICE
124 IOWA AVE
PO BOX 2180
SALINA, KS 67402-2180
TEL: (913) 825-5531
FAX: (913) 825-0338
TOLL FREE: (800) 998-8902
WWW.COLINSGRP.COM

OKLAHOMA CLAIMS OFFICE
124 IOWA AVE
PO BOX 2180
SALINA, KS 67402-2180
TEL: (913) 825-5531
FAX: (913) 825-0338
TOLL FREE: (800) 998-8902
WWW.COLINSGRP.COM

COLUMBIA INSURANCE GROUP, INC
NATIONAL CLAIMS OFFICE
2102 WHITE GATE DR
PO BOX 618
COLUMBIA, MO 65205
TEL: (573) 474-6193
FAX: (573) 474-8209
TOLL FREE: (800) 877-3579
WWW.COLINSGRP.COM

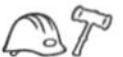

COLUMBIA UNIVERSAL LIFE INSURANCE CO
11211 TAYLOR DRAPER LN
PO BOX 200225
AUSTIN, TX 78720-0225
TEL: (512) 345-3200
FAX: (512) 343-7599
TOLL FREE: (800) 880-1370
WWW.COLUMBIA-UNIVERSAL.COM

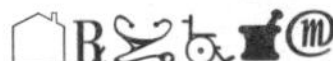

COLUMBUS LIFE INSURANCE CO
OHIO CLAIMS OFFICE
400 E 4TH ST
PO BOX 5737
CINCINNATI, OH 45201-5737
TEL: (513) 361-6700
FAX: (513) 361-6939
TOLL FREE: (800) 677-9595
E-MAIL: CLIENT.SERVICES@COLUMBUSLIFE.COM
WWW.COLUMBUSLIFE.COM

COMAIR INC
NATIONAL CLAIMS OFFICE
2258 TOWER DR
PO BOX 75021
ERLANGER, KY 41018
TEL: (606) 525-2550
FAX: (606) 767-2962

COMBINED BENEFITS ADMINISTRATIONS
CALIFORNIA CLAIMS OFFICE
CBA ADMINISTRATORS
4704 W JENNIFER AVE
FRESNO, CA 93722
TEL: (209) 275-3984
FAX: (209) 271-0419
TOLL FREE: (800) 709-4734

COMBINED INSURANCE
ILLINOIS CLAIMS OFFICE
5050 N BROADWAY ST
CHICAGO, IL 60640-3007
TEL: (773) 275-8000
FAX: (773) 769-8955
TOLL FREE: (800) 225-4500

COMBINED INSURANCE CO OF AMERICA
NATIONAL CLAIMS OFFICE
AON CORP
5050 N BROADWAY
CHICAGO, IL 60640
TEL: (773) 275-8000
FAX: (773) 765-1850
TOLL FREE: (800) 225-4500
WWW.COMBINEDINSURANCE.COM

COMBINED LIFE INSURANCE CO OF NEW YORK
11 BRITISH AMERICAN BLVD
LATHAM, NY 12110
TEL: (518) 220-9333
FAX: (518) 220-2921

COMBINED UNDERWRITERS LIFE INSURANCE CO
TEXAS CLAIMS OFFICE
LIFELINE UNDERWRITERS LIFE INSURANCE CO
307 N GLENWOOD
PO BOX 2503
TYLER, TX 75710-2503
TEL: (903) 597-3761
FAX: (903) 597-3767
TOLL FREE: (800) 872-6339

COMCAR INDUSTRIES, INC
FLORIDA CLAIMS OFFICE
111 HAVENDALE BLVD
PO BOX 67
AUBURNDALE, FL 33823
TEL: (941) 967-1101
FAX: (941) 551-1442
TOLL FREE: (800) 524-1101

COMMERCE INSURANCE CO
MASSACHUSETTS CLAIMS OFFICE
11 GORE RD
WEBSTER, MA 01570-2209
TEL: (508) 943-9000
FAX: (508) 949-5930
IN-STATE: (800) 221-1605
WWW.COMMERCEINSURANCE.COM

COMMERCIAL GENERAL UNION
NATIONAL CLAIMS OFFICE
COMMERCIAL UNION INSURANCE CO
10490 LITTLE PATUXENT PKY, STE 400
COLUMBIA, MD 21044
TEL: (410) 527-0333
IN-STATE: (800) 638-8842

COMMERCIAL TRAVELERS MUTUAL INSURANCE CO
NEW YORK CLAIMS OFFICE
70 GENESSEE ST
UTICA, NY 13502-3503
TEL: (315) 797-5200
FAX: (315) 797-3198
TOLL FREE: (800) 422-6200

COMMERCIAL UNION INSURANCE CO OF AMERICA
NATIONAL CLAIMS OFFICE
108 MYRTLE ST
NORTH QUINCY, MA 02171
TEL: (617) 786-2000
FAX: (617) 786-2386
TOLL FREE: (800) 343-5660
WWW.CGU.COM

COMMONWEALTH HEALTH ALLIANCE
PRIMARY SELECT
1650 STATE FARM BLVD
PO BOX 1323
CHARLOTTESVILLE, VA 22902
TEL: (804) 977-3500
FAX: (804) 979-5626
TOLL FREE: (800) 677-1867

COMMUNITY HEALTH PLAN OF OHIO
OHIO CLAIMS OFFICE
1915 TAMARACK RD
NEWARK, OH 43055-1300
TEL: (740) 348-1400
FAX: (740) 348-1500
TOLL FREE: (800) 806-2756

COMPANION HEALTH CARE CORP
SOUTH CAROLINA CLAIMS OFFICE
200 ARBOR LAKE DR, STE 200
PO BOX 6170
COLUMBIA, SC 29260-6170
TEL: (803) 786-8466
FAX: (803) 714-6443
TOLL FREE: (800) 327-3183
WWW.BCBSSC

COMPANION LIFE INSURANCE CO
NATIONAL CLAIMS OFFICE
BLUE CROSS & BLUE SHIELD OF SOUTH CAROLINA
51 CLEMSON RD, STE C
PO BOX 100102
COLUMBIA, SC 29229-6504
TEL: (803) 735-1251
FAX: (803) 735-0736
TOLL FREE: (800) 753-0404
E-MAIL: C.LIFECOMPANIONGROUP.COM

COMPCARE HEALTH SERVICES INSURANCE CO
401 W MICHIGAN ST
PO BOX 1581
MILWAUKEE, WI 53201-1581
TEL: (414) 226-6744
FAX: (414) 226-6478
TOLL FREE: (800) 492-4049

COMPDENT
ALABAMA CLAIMS OFFICE
PO BOX 4605
CHICAGO, IL 60680
FAX: (312) 829-9767
TOLL FREE: (800) 793-8068
IN-STATE: (800) 837-2341
WWW.COMPDENT.COM

C

ARKANSAS CLAIMS OFFICE
PO BOX 4605
CHICAGO, IL 60680
FAX: (312) 829-9767
TOLL FREE: (800) 793-8068
IN-STATE: (800) 837-2341
WWW.COMPDENT.COM

FLORIDA CLAIMS OFFICE
PO BOX 4605
CHICAGO, IL 60680
FAX: (312) 829-9767
TOLL FREE: (800) 793-8068
IN-STATE: (800) 837-2341
WWW.COMPDENT.COM

GEORGIA CLAIMS OFFICE
PO BOX 4605
CHICAGO, IL 60680
FAX: (312) 829-9767
TOLL FREE: (800) 793-8068
IN-STATE: (800) 837-2341
WWW.COMPDENT.COM

ILLINOIS CLAIMS OFFICE
PO BOX 4605
CHICAGO, IL 60680
FAX: (312) 829-9767
TOLL FREE: (800) 793-8068
IN-STATE: (800) 837-2341
WWW.COMPDENT.COM

INDIANA CLAIMS OFFICE
PO BOX 4605
CHICAGO, IL 60680
FAX: (312) 829-9767
TOLL FREE: (800) 793-8068
IN-STATE: (800) 837-2341
WWW.COMPDENT.COM

KANSAS CLAIMS OFFICE
PO BOX 4605
CHICAGO, IL 60680
FAX: (312) 829-9767
TOLL FREE: (800) 793-8068
IN-STATE: (800) 837-2341
WWW.COMPDENT.COM

KENTUCKY CLAIMS OFFICE
PO BOX 4605
CHICAGO, IL 60680
FAX: (312) 829-9767
TOLL FREE: (800) 793-8068
IN-STATE: (800) 837-2341
WWW.COMPDENT.COM

LOUISIANA CLAIMS OFFICE
PO BOX 4605
CHICAGO, IL 60680
FAX: (312) 829-9767
TOLL FREE: (800) 793-8068
IN-STATE: (800) 837-2341
WWW.COMPDENT.COM

MISSISSIPPI CLAIMS OFFICE
PO BOX 4605
CHICAGO, IL 60680
FAX: (312) 829-9767
TOLL FREE: (800) 793-8068
IN-STATE: (800) 837-2341
WWW.COMPDENT.COM

MISSOURI CLAIMS OFFICE
PO BOX 4605
CHICAGO, IL 60680
FAX: (312) 829-9767
TOLL FREE: (800) 793-8068
IN-STATE: (800) 837-2341
WWW.COMPDENT.COM

NORTH CAROLINA CLAIMS OFFICE
PO BOX 4605
CHICAGO, IL 60680
FAX: (312) 829-9767
TOLL FREE: (800) 793-8068
IN-STATE: (800) 837-2341
WWW.COMPDENT.COM

OHIO CLAIMS OFFICE
PO BOX 4605
CHICAGO, IL 60680
FAX: (312) 829-9767
TOLL FREE: (800) 793-8068
IN-STATE: (800) 837-2341
WWW.COMPDENT.COM

SOUTH CAROLINA CLAIMS OFFICE
PO BOX 4605
CHICAGO, IL 60680
FAX: (312) 829-9767
TOLL FREE: (800) 793-8068
IN-STATE: (800) 837-2341
WWW.COMPDENT.COM

TENNESSEE CLAIMS OFFICE
PO BOX 4605
CHICAGO, IL 60680
FAX: (312) 829-9767
TOLL FREE: (800) 793-8068
IN-STATE: (800) 837-2341
WWW.COMPDENT.COM

TEXAS CLAIMS OFFICE
PO BOX 4605
CHICAGO, IL 60680
FAX: (312) 829-9767
TOLL FREE: (800) 793-8068
IN-STATE: (800) 837-2341
WWW.COMPDENT.COM

WEST VIRGINIA CLAIMS OFFICE
PO BOX 4605
CHICAGO, IL 60680
FAX: (312) 829-9767
TOLL FREE: (800) 793-8068
IN-STATE: (800) 837-2341
WWW.COMPDENT.COM

COMPDENT CORP

ALABAMA CLAIMS OFFICE
100 MANSELL CT E, STE 400
PO BOX 769729
ROSWELL, GA 30076
TEL: (770) 552-7101
FAX: (770) 998-6871
TOLL FREE: (800) 633-1262
WWW.COMPDENT.COM

ARKANSAS CLAIMS OFFICE
100 MANSELL CT E, STE 400
PO BOX 769729
ROSWELL, GA 30076
TEL: (770) 552-7101
FAX: (770) 998-6871
TOLL FREE: (800) 633-1262
WWW.COMPDENT.COM

FLORIDA CLAIMS OFFICE
100 MANSELL CT E, STE 400
PO BOX 769729
ROSWELL, GA 30076
TEL: (770) 552-7101
FAX: (770) 998-6871
TOLL FREE: (800) 633-1262
WWW.COMPDENT.COM

GEORGIA CLAIMS OFFICE
100 MANSELL CT E, STE 400
PO BOX 769729
ROSWELL, GA 30076
TEL: (770) 552-7101
FAX: (770) 998-6871
TOLL FREE: (800) 633-1262
WWW.COMPDENT.COM

ILLINOIS CLAIMS OFFICE
100 MANSELL CT E, STE 400
PO BOX 769729
ROSWELL, GA 30076
TEL: (770) 552-7101
FAX: (770) 998-6871
TOLL FREE: (800) 633-1262
WWW.COMPDENT.COM

INDIANA CLAIMS OFFICE
100 MANSELL CT E, STE 400
PO BOX 769729
ROSWELL, GA 30076
TEL: (770) 552-7101
FAX: (770) 998-6871
TOLL FREE: (800) 633-1262
WWW.COMPDENT.COM

KANSAS CLAIMS OFFICE
100 MANSELL CT E, STE 400
PO BOX 769729
ROSWELL, GA 30076
TEL: (770) 552-7101
FAX: (770) 998-6871
TOLL FREE: (800) 633-1262
WWW.COMPDENT.COM

KENTUCKY CLAIMS OFFICE
100 MANSELL CT E, STE 400
PO BOX 769729
ROSWELL, GA 30076
TEL: (770) 552-7101
FAX: (770) 998-6871
TOLL FREE: (800) 633-1262
WWW.COMPDENT.COM

LOUISIANA CLAIMS OFFICE
100 MANSELL CT E, STE 400
PO BOX 769729
ROSWELL, GA 30076
TEL: (770) 552-7101
FAX: (770) 998-6871
TOLL FREE: (800) 633-1262
WWW.COMPDENT.COM

MISSISSIPPI CLAIMS OFFICE
100 MANSELL CT E, STE 400
PO BOX 769729
ROSWELL, GA 30076
TEL: (770) 552-7101
FAX: (770) 998-6871
TOLL FREE: (800) 633-1262
WWW.COMPDENT.COM

MISSOURI CLAIMS OFFICE
100 MANSELL CT E, STE 400
PO BOX 769729
ROSWELL, GA 30076
TEL: (770) 552-7101
FAX: (770) 998-6871
TOLL FREE: (800) 633-1262
WWW.COMPDENT.COM

NORTH CAROLINA CLAIMS OFFICE
100 MANSELL CT E, STE 400
PO BOX 769729
ROSWELL, GA 30076
TEL: (770) 552-7101
FAX: (770) 998-6871
TOLL FREE: (800) 633-1262
WWW.COMPDENT.COM

OHIO CLAIMS OFFICE
100 MANSELL CT E, STE 400
PO BOX 769729
ROSWELL, GA 30076
TEL: (770) 552-7101
FAX: (770) 998-6871
TOLL FREE: (800) 633-1262
WWW.COMPDENT.COM

SOUTH CAROLINA CLAIMS OFFICE
100 MANSELL CT E, STE 400
PO BOX 769729
ROSWELL, GA 30076
TEL: (770) 552-7101
FAX: (770) 998-6871
TOLL FREE: (800) 633-1262
WWW.COMPDENT.COM

TENNESSEE CLAIMS OFFICE
100 MANSELL CT E, STE 400
PO BOX 769729
ROSWELL, GA 30076
TEL: (770) 552-7101
FAX: (770) 998-6871
TOLL FREE: (800) 633-1262
WWW.COMPDENT.COM

TEXAS CLAIMS OFFICE
100 MANSELL CT E, STE 400
PO BOX 769729
ROSWELL, GA 30076
TEL: (770) 552-7101
FAX: (770) 998-6871
TOLL FREE: (800) 633-1262
WWW.COMPDENT.COM

WEST VIRGINIA CLAIMS OFFICE
100 MANSELL CT E, STE 400
PO BOX 769729
ROSWELL, GA 30076
TEL: (770) 552-7101
FAX: (770) 998-6871
TOLL FREE: (800) 633-1262
WWW.COMPDENT.COM

COMPENSATION PROGRAMS OF OHIO, INC

OHIO CLAIMS OFFICE
1123 N CANFIELD NILES RD
PO BOX 230
AUSTINTOWN, OH 44515
TEL: (330) 652-9821
FAX: (330) 652-0397
TOLL FREE: (800) 733-7709

COMPREHENSIVE BENEFITS ADMINISTRATORS, INC

VERMONT CLAIMS OFFICE
30 AIRPORT RD
PO BOX 2365
SOUTH BURLINGTON, VT 05407-2365
TEL: (802) 864-8321
FAX: (802) 864-8115
TOLL FREE: (800) 525-8788

COMPREHENSIVE CARE SERVICES

MINNESOTA CLAIMS OFFICE
AFFILIATE OF BLUE CROSS & BLUE SHIELD OF MINNESOTA
1200 YANKEE DOODLE RD
PO BOX 64668
EGAN, MN 55122
TEL: (612) 456-5940
FAX: (612) 456-1582
TOLL FREE: (800) 365-2735

COMPREHENSIVE HEALTH SERVICES INC

NATIONAL CLAIMS OFFICE
THE WELLNESS PLAN
2875 W GRAND BLVD
DETROIT, MI 48202
TEL: (313) 875-4200
TOLL FREE: (800) 875-9355

COMPUTER SCIENCE CORP

800 N PEARL ST
PO BOX 4444
ALBANY, NY 12204-0444
TEL: (518) 447-9200
FAX: (518) 447-9240
IN-STATE: (800) 522-5518

CONCENTRA MANAGED CARE, INC

MASSACHUSETTS CLAIMS OFFICE
312 UNION WHARF
BOSTON, MA 02109
TEL: (617) 367-2163
FAX: (617) 367-8519
WWW.CONCENTRAMC.COM

CONCORD GENERAL

MAINE CLAIMS OFFICE
CONCORD GROUP INSURANCE
510 S ST
PO BOX 2048
CONCORD, NH 03302-2048
TEL: (603) 225-1141
FAX: (603) 225-5659
TOLL FREE: (800) 888-6050

MASSACHUSETTS CLAIMS OFFICE
CONCORD GROUP INSURANCE
510 S ST
PO BOX 2048
CONCORD, NH 03302-2048
TEL: (603) 225-1141
FAX: (603) 225-5659
TOLL FREE: (800) 888-6050

NEW HAMPSHIRE CLAIMS OFFICE
CONCORD GROUP INSURANCE
510 S ST
PO BOX 2048
CONCORD, NH 03302-2048
TEL: (603) 225-1141
FAX: (603) 225-5659
TOLL FREE: (800) 888-6050

VERMONT CLAIMS OFFICE
CONCORD GROUP INSURANCE
510 S ST
PO BOX 2048
CONCORD, NH 03302-2048
TEL: (603) 225-1141
FAX: (603) 225-5659
TOLL FREE: (800) 888-6050

CONCORD GROUP INSURANCE

AIRPORT RD
PO BOX 870
MONTPELIER, VT 05601
TEL: (802) 229-0355
FAX: (802) 229-0715
TOLL FREE: (800) 660-3838

CONCORD GROUP INSURANCE CO

MAINE CLAIMS OFFICE
CORPORATE OFFICE
4 BOUTON ST
CONCORD, NH 03301-5023
TEL: (603) 224-4086
FAX: (603) 224-2614
TOLL FREE: (800) 852-3380

MASSACHUSETTS CLAIMS OFFICE
CORPORATE OFFICE
4 BOUTON ST
CONCORD, NH 03301-5023
TEL: (603) 224-4086
FAX: (603) 224-2614
TOLL FREE: (800) 852-3380

NATIONAL CLAIMS OFFICE
308 CENTER ST
PO BOX 300
AUBURN, ME 04212
TEL: (207) 784-7337
FAX: (207) 784-3600
TOLL FREE: (800) 482-7443

NEW HAMPSHIRE CLAIMS OFFICE
CORPORATE OFFICE
4 BOUTON ST
CONCORD, NH 03301-5023
TEL: (603) 224-4086
FAX: (603) 224-2614
TOLL FREE: (800) 852-3380

VERMONT CLAIMS OFFICE
CORPORATE OFFICE
4 BOUTON ST
CONCORD, NH 03301-5023
TEL: (603) 224-4086
FAX: (603) 224-2614
TOLL FREE: (800) 852-3380

CONESTOGA LIFE ASSURANCE CO

NATIONAL CLAIMS OFFICE
360 REED RD, STE 100
BROOMALL, PA 19008
TEL: (610) 543-9090
FAX: (610) 543-4277
TOLL FREE: (800) 468-8009
WWW.CONESTOGALIFEANDHEALTH.COM

CONNECTICARE INC & AFFILIATES

CONNECTICUT CLAIMS OFFICE
30 BATTERSON PARK RD
PO BOX 546
FARMINGTON, CT 06032
TEL: (860) 674-5700
FAX: (860) 674-5728
TOLL FREE: (800) 251-7722
WWW.CONNECTICARE.COM

CONSECO

INDIANA CLAIMS OFFICE
JEFFERSON NATIONAL LIFE INSURANCE
11815 N PENN ST
PO BOX 1951
CARMEL, IN 46032
TEL: (317) 817-3700
FAX: (317) 817-3345
TOLL FREE: (800) 824-2726
WWW.CONSECO.COM

NATIONAL CLAIMS OFFICE
11815 N PENNSYLVANIA ST
CARMEL, IN 46032
TEL: (317) 817-6200
FAX: (317) 817-3604
TOLL FREE: (800) 441-3978
IN-STATE: (800) 888-4918
WWW.CONSECO.COM

CONSECO CO

INDIANA CLAIMS OFFICE
11815 N PENN ST
CARMEL, IN 46032
TEL: (317) 817-3700
FAX: (317) 817-3345
TOLL FREE: (800) 824-2726
WWW.CONSECO.COM

CONSECO DIRECT LIFE INSURANCE CO

PENNSYLVANIA CLAIMS OFFICE
399 MARKET ST
PHILADELPHIA, PA 19181-1250
TEL: (215) 928-8000
TOLL FREE: (800) 523-4000

CONSOLIDATED AMERICAN INSURANCE CO

NATIONAL CLAIMS OFFICE
CEIBELS
1501 LADY ST
PO BOX 1
COLUMBIA, SC 29202
TEL: (803) 748-2000
FAX: (803) 748-8438
TOLL FREE: (800) 525-8835

CONSOLIDATED ASSOCIATION OF RAILROAD EMPLOYEES CARE

4912 MIDWAY DR
PO BOX 6130
TEMPLE, TX 76503
TEL: (254) 773-1330
FAX: (254) 774-8029
TOLL FREE: (800) 334-1330

CONSOLIDATED HEALTH PLANS

MASSACHUSETTS CLAIMS OFFICE
195 STAFFORD ST
SPRINGFIELD, MA 01104-3503
TEL: (413) 733-4540
FAX: (413) 781-2937
TOLL FREE: (800) 633-7867
E-MAIL: CHP@VGERNET.NET

CONSOLIDATED INTERNATIONAL, INC

DELAWARE CLAIMS OFFICE
INTERNATIONAL AMERICAN MANAGEMENT
1415 FOULK RD, STE 205
WILMINGTON, DE 19803
TEL: (302) 479-2100
FAX: (302) 479-2103
TOLL FREE: (800) 533-7628

CONSOLIDATED NATURAL GAS CO

PENNSYLVANIA CLAIMS OFFICE
625 LIBERTY AVE- CNG TWR
PITTSBURGH, PA 15222-3199
TEL: (412) 227-1000
WWW.CNG.COM

CONSOLIDATED RAIL CORPORATION

2001 MARKET ST 18B
PHILADELPHIA, PA 19101-1406
TEL: (215) 209-4415

CONSTRUCTION INDUSTRY LABORERS WELFARE FUND

MISSOURI CLAIMS OFFICE
116 COMMERCE DR
JEFFERSON CITY, MO 65109-1196
TEL: (573) 893-2446
FAX: (573) 893-4369

CONSTRUCTION INDUSTRY WELFARE FUND

ILLINOIS CLAIMS OFFICE
34 E SPRINGFIELD AVE
CHAMPAIGN, IL 61820
TEL: (217) 352-5269
FAX: (217) 352-5297

CONSUMER HEALTH NETWORK

CONNECTICUT CLAIMS OFFICE
371 HOES LN, STE 101
PISCATAWAY, NJ 08854
TEL: (732) 562-0888
FAX: (732) 562-9616
TOLL FREE: (800) 225-4246
E-MAIL: MARKETING@4CHN.COM
WWW.4CHN.COM

NEW JERSEY CLAIMS OFFICE
371 HOES LN, STE 101
PISCATAWAY, NJ 08854
TEL: (732) 562-0888
FAX: (732) 562-9616
TOLL FREE: (800) 225-4246
E-MAIL: MARKETING@4CHN.COM
WWW.4CHN.COM

NEW YORK CLAIMS OFFICE
371 HOES LN, STE 101
PISCATAWAY, NJ 08854
TEL: (732) 562-0888
FAX: (732) 562-9616
TOLL FREE: (800) 225-4246
E-MAIL: MARKETING@4CHN.COM
WWW.4CHN.COM

CONTAINER SUPPLY CO

CALIFORNIA CLAIMS OFFICE
12571 WESTERN
PO BOX 5367
GARDEN GROVE, CA 92841
TEL: (714) 892-8321
FAX: (714) 892-3824

Insurance Directory

CONTECH CONSTRUCTION PRODUCTS INC

NATIONAL CLAIMS OFFICE
1001 GROVE ST
PO BOX 800
MIDDLETOWN, OH 45042
TEL: (513) 425-2199
FAX: (513) 425-2604
WWW.CONTECH-CPI.COM

CONTINENTAL GENERAL INSURANCE CO

MASSACHUSETTS CLAIMS OFFICE
8901 INDIAN HILLS DR
PO BOX 247007
OMAHA, NE 68124-7007
TEL: (402) 397-3200
FAX: (402) 392-7771
TOLL FREE: (800) 545-8905

NEBRASKA CLAIMS OFFICE
8901 INDIAN HILLS DR
PO BOX 247007
OMAHA, NE 68124-7007
TEL: (402) 397-3200
FAX: (402) 392-7771
TOLL FREE: (800) 545-8905
IN-STATE: (800) 397-3200
WWW.CONTINENTALGENERAL.COM

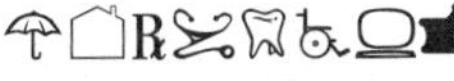

CONTINENTAL LIFE & ACCIDENT

ILLINOIS CLAIMS OFFICE
CONSECO
304 N MAIN ST
PO BOX 1300
ROCKFORD, IL 61105-1300
TEL: (815) 987-5000
FAX: (815) 720-2829
TOLL FREE: (800) 221-3770

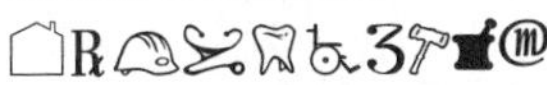

CONTINENTAL LIFE INSURANCE CO

ARIZONA CLAIMS OFFICE
101 CONTINENTAL PL
PO BOX 1188
BRENTWOOD, TN 37024
TEL: (615) 377-1300
FAX: (615) 373-0272
TOLL FREE: (800) 264-4000

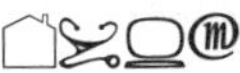

ARKANSAS CLAIMS OFFICE
101 CONTINENTAL PL
PO BOX 1188
BRENTWOOD, TN 37024
TEL: (615) 377-1300
FAX: (615) 373-0272
TOLL FREE: (800) 264-4000

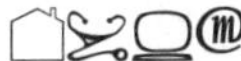

COLORADO CLAIMS OFFICE
101 CONTINENTAL PL
PO BOX 1188
BRENTWOOD, TN 37024
TEL: (615) 377-1300
FAX: (615) 373-0272
TOLL FREE: (800) 264-4000

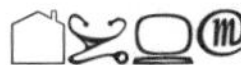

FLORIDA CLAIMS OFFICE
101 CONTINENTAL PL
PO BOX 1188
BRENTWOOD, TN 37024
TEL: (615) 377-1300
FAX: (615) 373-0272
TOLL FREE: (800) 264-4000

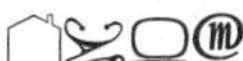

GEORGIA CLAIMS OFFICE
101 CONTINENTAL PL
PO BOX 1188
BRENTWOOD, TN 37024
TEL: (615) 377-1300
FAX: (615) 373-0272
TOLL FREE: (800) 264-4000

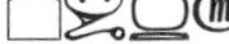

IDAHO CLAIMS OFFICE
101 CONTINENTAL PL
PO BOX 1188
BRENTWOOD, TN 37024
TEL: (615) 377-1300
FAX: (615) 373-0272
TOLL FREE: (800) 264-4000

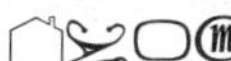

ILLINOIS CLAIMS OFFICE
101 CONTINENTAL PL
PO BOX 1188
BRENTWOOD, TN 37024
TEL: (615) 377-1300
FAX: (615) 373-0272
TOLL FREE: (800) 264-4000

INDIANA CLAIMS OFFICE
101 CONTINENTAL PL
PO BOX 1188
BRENTWOOD, TN 37024
TEL: (615) 377-1300
FAX: (615) 373-0272
TOLL FREE: (800) 264-4000

KENTUCKY CLAIMS OFFICE
101 CONTINENTAL PL
PO BOX 1188
BRENTWOOD, TN 37024
TEL: (615) 377-1300
FAX: (615) 373-0272
TOLL FREE: (800) 264-4000

LOUISIANA CLAIMS OFFICE
101 CONTINENTAL PL
PO BOX 1188
BRENTWOOD, TN 37024
TEL: (615) 377-1300
FAX: (615) 373-0272
TOLL FREE: (800) 264-4000

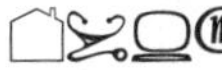

MISSISSIPPI CLAIMS OFFICE
101 CONTINENTAL PL
PO BOX 1188
BRENTWOOD, TN 37024
TEL: (615) 377-1300
FAX: (615) 373-0272
TOLL FREE: (800) 264-4000

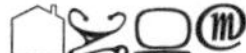

MISSOURI CLAIMS OFFICE
101 CONTINENTAL PL
PO BOX 1188
BRENTWOOD, TN 37024
TEL: (615) 377-1300
FAX: (615) 373-0272
TOLL FREE: (800) 264-4000

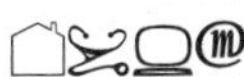

MONTANA CLAIMS OFFICE
101 CONTINENTAL PL
PO BOX 1188
BRENTWOOD, TN 37024
TEL: (615) 377-1300
FAX: (615) 373-0272
TOLL FREE: (800) 264-4000

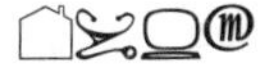

NEBRASKA CLAIMS OFFICE
101 CONTINENTAL PL
PO BOX 1188
BRENTWOOD, TN 37024
TEL: (615) 377-1300
FAX: (615) 373-0272
TOLL FREE: (800) 264-4000

NEW MEXICO CLAIMS OFFICE
101 CONTINENTAL PL
PO BOX 1188
BRENTWOOD, TN 37024
TEL: (615) 377-1300
FAX: (615) 373-0272
TOLL FREE: (800) 264-4000

NORTH CAROLINA CLAIMS OFFICE
101 CONTINENTAL PL
PO BOX 1188
BRENTWOOD, TN 37024
TEL: (615) 377-1300
FAX: (615) 373-0272
TOLL FREE: (800) 264-4000

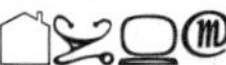

OHIO CLAIMS OFFICE
101 CONTINENTAL PL
PO BOX 1188
BRENTWOOD, TN 37024
TEL: (615) 377-1300
FAX: (615) 373-0272
TOLL FREE: (800) 264-4000

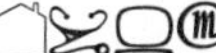

OKLAHOMA CLAIMS OFFICE
101 CONTINENTAL PL
PO BOX 1188
BRENTWOOD, TN 37024
TEL: (615) 377-1300
FAX: (615) 373-0272
TOLL FREE: (800) 264-4000

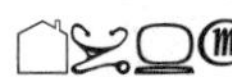

PENNSYLVANIA CLAIMS OFFICE
101 CONTINENTAL PL
PO BOX 1188
BRENTWOOD, TN 37024
TEL: (615) 377-1300
FAX: (615) 373-0272
TOLL FREE: (800) 264-4000

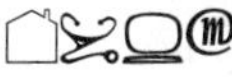

C

SOUTH CAROLINA CLAIMS OFFICE
101 CONTINENTAL PL
PO BOX 1188
BRENTWOOD, TN 37024
TEL: (615) 377-1300
FAX: (615) 373-0272
TOLL FREE: (800) 264-4000

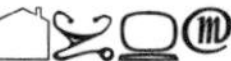

TENNESSEE CLAIMS OFFICE
101 CONTINENTAL PL
PO BOX 1188
BRENTWOOD, TN 37024
TEL: (615) 377-1300
FAX: (615) 373-0272
TOLL FREE: (800) 264-4000

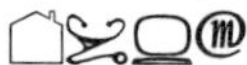

TEXAS CLAIMS OFFICE
101 CONTINENTAL PL
PO BOX 1188
BRENTWOOD, TN 37024
TEL: (615) 377-1300
FAX: (615) 373-0272
TOLL FREE: (800) 264-4000

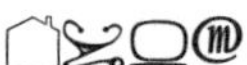

UTAH CLAIMS OFFICE
101 CONTINENTAL PL
PO BOX 1188
BRENTWOOD, TN 37024
TEL: (615) 377-1300
FAX: (615) 373-0272
TOLL FREE: (800) 264-4000

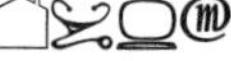

VIRGINIA CLAIMS OFFICE
101 CONTINENTAL PL
PO BOX 1188
BRENTWOOD, TN 37024
TEL: (615) 377-1300
FAX: (615) 373-0272
TOLL FREE: (800) 264-4000

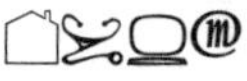

WEST VIRGINIA CLAIMS OFFICE
101 CONTINENTAL PL
PO BOX 1188
BRENTWOOD, TN 37024
TEL: (615) 377-1300
FAX: (615) 373-0272
TOLL FREE: (800) 264-4000

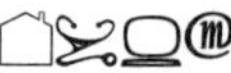

CONTINENTAL WESTERN INSURANCE CO

IOWA CLAIMS OFFICE
1924 ST ANDREWS DR NE
PO BOX 218
CEDAR RAPIDS, IA 52233-0218
TEL: (319) 393-5192
FAX: (319) 393-0243
TOLL FREE: (800) 396-3380

NATIONAL CLAIMS OFFICE
CONTINENTAL WESTERN CASUALTY
11201 DOUGLAS AVE
PO BOX 1594
DES MOINES, IA 50306-1594
TEL: (515) 278-3000
FAX: (515) 278-3382
TOLL FREE: (800) 235-2942
WWW.CONTWESTINS.COM

3641 S WEST PLZ
PO BOX 4566
TOPEKA, KS 66604-0566
TEL: (785) 267-3022
FAX: (785) 267-7669
TOLL FREE: (800) 454-8936

100 N 84TH ST
PO BOX 82558
LINCOLN, NE 68501-2558
TEL: (402) 483-4100
FAX: (402) 483-6415
IN-STATE: (800) 742-7337

CONTRA COSTA HEALTH PLAN

CALIFORNIA CLAIMS OFFICE
595 CENTER AVE, STE 100
MARTINEZ, CA 94553
TEL: (925) 313-6080
FAX: (925) 313-6002

COOK & CO INC

NATIONAL CLAIMS OFFICE
1025 PLAIN ST
PO BOX 1068
MARSHFIELD, MA 02050-0702
TEL: (781) 837-7300
FAX: (781) 837-5668
TOLL FREE: (800) 281-9696
WWW.COOKANDCOMPANY.COM

COOK GROUP HEALTH PLAN TRUST

INDIANA CLAIMS OFFICE
PO BOX 1608
BLOOMINGTON, IN 47402
TEL: (812) 331-1025
FAX: (812) 331-8990

COOPERATIVA DE SEGUROS

PUERTO RICO CLAIMS OFFICE
DE VIDA DE PUERTO RICO
PO BOX 363428
SAN JUAN, PR 00936-3428
TEL: (787) 751-5656
FAX: (787) 756-8548

COOPERATIVE BENEFIT ADMINISTRATORS

NATIONAL CLAIMS OFFICE
PO BOX 6249
LINCOLN, NE 68506-0249
TEL: (402) 483-9200
FAX: (402) 483-9201

COORDINATED HEALTH PARTNERS, INC

RHODE ISLAND CLAIMS OFFICE
15 LA SALLE SQ
PROVIDENCE, RI 02903
TEL: (401) 459-5500
TOLL FREE: (800) 528-4141
WWW.BCBSRI.COM

H

COPPS CORP.

WISCONSIN CLAIMS OFFICE
2828 WAYNE ST
PO BOX 187
STEVENS POINT, WI 54481-4169
TEL: (715) 344-5900
FAX: (715) 344-7378
WWW.COPPS.COM

CORESOURCE

NATIONAL CLAIMS OFFICE
14440 MYERLAKE CIR
CLEARWATER, FL 33760
TEL: (813) 530-5947
FAX: (813) 530-4186
TOLL FREE: (800) 253-2107

NORTH CAROLINA CLAIMS OFFICE
6100 FAIRVIEW RD, STE 1000
CHARLOTTE, NC 28210-3291
TEL: (704) 552-0900
FAX: (704) 552-8635
TOLL FREE: (800) 327-5462
IN-STATE: (800) 821-0345

CORESOURCE, INC

NATIONAL CLAIMS OFFICE
4801 SOUTHWICK DR, STE 400
PO BOX 168
MATTESON, IL 60443
TEL: (708) 747-7400
FAX: (708) 747-2142
TOLL FREE: (800) 848-3012

PO BOX 879
ANDERSON, IN 46015
TEL: (765) 778-8511
FAX: (765) 778-8039
TOLL FREE: (800) 331-1199

4210 SHAWNEE MISSION PKY, STE 302A
SHAWNEE MISSION, KS 66205
TEL: (913) 384-3735
FAX: (913) 384-0326
TOLL FREE: (800) 545-1769

4940 CAMPBELL BLVD, STE 200
BALTIMORE, MD 21236
TEL: (410) 931-5060
FAX: (410) 931-3653
TOLL FREE: (800) 624-7130

3717 NATIONAL DR, STE 217
PO BOX 31547
RALEIGH, NC 27622
TEL: (919) 782-9020
FAX: (919) 782-5939
TOLL FREE: (800) 451-9446

229 HUBER VLG BLVD
PO BOX 6118
WESTERVILLE, OH 43081-6118
TEL: (614) 890-0070
FAX: (614) 794-0736
TOLL FREE: (800) 282-3920

NEW JERSEY CLAIMS OFFICE
940 W VALLEY RD
PO BOX 6994
WAYNE, PA 19087
TEL: (610) 687-5924
FAX: (610) 687-1959
TOLL FREE: (800) 345-1166

PENNSYLVANIA CLAIMS OFFICE
26-28 W KING ST
PO BOX 83301
LANCASTER, PA 17608
TEL: (717) 295-9201
FAX: (717) 295-9368
TOLL FREE: (800) 223-3943
WWW.TRUSTMARKINSURANCE.COM

940 W VALLEY RD
PO BOX 6994
WAYNE, PA 19087
TEL: (610) 687-5924
FAX: (610) 687-1959
TOLL FREE: (800) 345-1166

CORESTAR

ILLINOIS CLAIMS OFFICE
JACKSON CLAIM CENTER
146 INDUSTRIAL PARK
JACKSON, MN 56143-9511
TEL: (507) 847-5740
FAX: (507) 847-2358
TOLL FREE: (800) 274-6965

MINNESOTA CLAIMS OFFICE
JACKSON CLAIM CENTER
146 INDUSTRIAL PARK
JACKSON, MN 56143-9511
TEL: (507) 847-5740
FAX: (507) 847-2358
TOLL FREE: (800) 274-6965

CORNHUSKER CASUALTY CO

NEBRASKA CLAIMS OFFICE
BERKSHIRE HATHAWAY HOMESTATE COMPANIES
9290 W DODGE RD, STE 300
OMAHA, NE 68114-3363
TEL: (402) 393-7255
FAX: (402) 393-7619
TOLL FREE: (800) 488-2930

CORPORATE BENEFIT SERVICE, INC

NORTH CAROLINA CLAIMS OFFICE
145 SCALEY BARK, STE B
PO BOX 12953
CHARLOTTE, NC 28209-2953
TEL: (704) 373-0447
FAX: (704) 342-2777
TOLL FREE: (800) 277-9746

CORPORATE BENEFIT SERVICES OF AMERICA, INC

NATIONAL CLAIMS OFFICE
10159 WAYZATA BLVD
MINNETONKA, MN 55305-1503
TEL: (612) 546-0062
FAX: (612) 541-0193
TOLL FREE: (800) 925-2272
E-MAIL: CUSTOMER.SERVICE@CBSAINC.COM
WWW.CBSAINC.COM

CORPORATE DIVERSIFIED SERVICES

NEBRASKA CLAIMS OFFICE
2401 S 73RD ST, STE 1
PO BOX 2835
OMAHA, NE 68103-2835
TEL: (402) 393-3133
FAX: (402) 398-3773
TOLL FREE: (800) 642-4089

CORPORATE SYSTEMS ADMINISTRATION, INC

TENNESSEE CLAIMS OFFICE
4722 LAKE PARK DR
PO BOX 4985
JOHNSON CITY, TN 37602-4985
TEL: (423) 282-3420
FAX: (423) 282-2999
TOLL FREE: (800) 829-7566
WWW.CSABENEFITS.COM

CORVEL CORP

NATIONAL CLAIMS OFFICE
10260 SW GREENBERG RD, STE 1165
PORTLAND, OR 97223
TEL: (503) 244-2093
FAX: (503) 244-2189
WWW.CORVEL.COM

ADMINISTRATION OFFICES
1300 SW 5TH AVE, STE 2500
PORTLAND, OR 97201
TEL: (503) 222-3144
FAX: (503) 222-0225
WWW.CORVEL.COM

COTTAGE HEALTH SYSTEM

CALIFORNIA CLAIMS OFFICE
CLAIMS PROCESSING CENTER
2400 BATH ST
PO BOX 689
SANTA BARBARA, CA 93102-0689
TEL: (805) 569-8220
FAX: (805) 569-8218

COTTON STATES INSURANCE COMPANIES

GEORGIA CLAIMS OFFICE
244 PERIMETER CENTER PKY
PO BOX 105303
ATLANTA, GA 30348
FAX: (800) 457-1660
TOLL FREE: (800) 457-1658

COUNTRY COMPANIES

NATIONAL CLAIMS OFFICE
411 WILLIAMSBURG AVE
GENEVA, IL 60134
TEL: (630) 232-2595
FAX: (630) 232-7802

COUNTRY MUTUAL & COUNTRY CASUALTY

3440 38TH AVE
MOLINE, IL 61265
TEL: (309) 757-1650
FAX: (309) 757-0063

2449 N DIRKSEN PKY
SPRINGFIELD, IL 62702
TEL: (217) 753-5220
FAX: (217) 753-3922
TOLL FREE: (800) 701-5220

COUNTRY PREFERRED
2150 COUNTRY DR S
PO BOX 2209
SALEM, OR 97308
TEL: (503) 581-1730
FAX: (503) 375-2797
TOLL FREE: (800) 767-3157

COUNTRY PREFERRED
2150 COUNTRY DR S
PO BOX 2209
SALEM, OR 97308-2209
TEL: (503) 581-1730
FAX: (503) 375-2797
TOLL FREE: (800) 767-3157

COUNTRY-WIDE INSURANCE CO

40 WALL ST- 13-15TH FLOORS
NEW YORK, NY 10005
TEL: (212) 344-8700
FAX: (212) 514-7291

COUNTY OF LOS ANGELES

CALIFORNIA CLAIMS OFFICE
1436 GOODRICH BLVD
COMMERCE, CA 90022
TEL: (213) 738-2279

COVENANT ADMINISTRATORS, INC

NATIONAL CLAIMS OFFICE
11330 LAKEFIELD DR, STE 100
PO BOX 740042
ATLANTA, GA 30374
TEL: (770) 242-6100
FAX: (770) 239-3989
TOLL FREE: (800) 374-6101

COVENTRY HEALTHCARE

6705 ROCKLEDGE DR, STE 900
BETHESDA, MD 20817
TEL: (301) 581-0600
TOLL FREE: (800) 843-7421
WWW.CZTY.COM

COX INSURANCE GROUP, INC

COLORADO CLAIMS OFFICE
5170 COMMERCE CIR
PO BOX 17008
INDIANAPOLIS, IN 46237
TEL: (317) 887-0030
FAX: (317) 888-7145

☆

C

INDIANA CLAIMS OFFICE
5170 COMMERCE CIR
PO BOX 17008
INDIANAPOLIS, IN 46237
TEL: (317) 887-0030
FAX: (317) 888-7145

☆

CPIC LIFE

CALIFORNIA CLAIMS OFFICE
PO BOX 3007
LODI, CA 95241-1911
TEL: (209) 367-3415
FAX: (209) 367-3450
TOLL FREE: (800) 642-5599
IN-STATE: (800) 537-0666

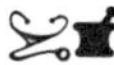

CRAWFORD & CO

ALASKA CLAIMS OFFICE
4341 B ST, STE 301
ANCHORAGE, AK 99503
TEL: (907) 561-5222
FAX: (907) 561-7383
IN-STATE: (888) 549-5222
WWW.CRAWFORDANDCOMPANY.COM

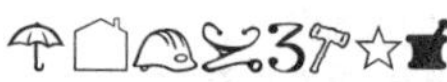

CALIFORNIA CLAIMS OFFICE
6312 VARIEL AVE, STE 218
WOODLAND HILLS, CA 91367
TEL: (818) 593-2900
FAX: (818) 593-2901
TOLL FREE: (800) 241-2541
WWW.CRAWFORDANDCOMPANY.COM

ILLINOIS CLAIMS OFFICE
1900 E GOLF RD, STE 700 & 800
PO BOX 681519
SCHAUMBURG, IL 60168
TEL: (847) 517-4175
FAX: (847) 517-4181
TOLL FREE: (800) 545-2213
WWW.CRAWFORDANDCOMPANY.COM

NATIONAL CLAIMS OFFICE
5620 GLENRIDGE DR NE
PO BOX 5047
ATLANTA, GA 30302
TEL: (404) 256-0830
FAX: (678) 443-3532
TOLL FREE: (800) 241-2541
WWW.CRAWFORDANDCOMPANY.COM

7878 N 16TH ST, STE 230
PHOENIX, AZ 85020
TEL: (602) 943-5444
FAX: (602) 216-9478
TOLL FREE: (800) 242-1252
WWW.CRAWFORDANDCOMPANY.COM

10802 EXECUTIVE CTR DR, STE 208
LITTLE ROCK, AR 72211
TEL: (501) 225-4494
FAX: (501) 224-9536
TOLL FREE: (800) 241-2541
IN-STATE: (800) 431-4494
WWW.CRAWFORDANDCOMPANY.COM

1550 S BASCOM AVE, STE 120
PO BOX 5640
CAMPBELL, CA 95150
TEL: (408) 371-5331
FAX: (408) 371-7504
WWW.CRAWFORDANDCOMPANY.COM

562 MANZANITA AVE, STE 9
PO BOX 349010
CHICO, CA 95834-9010
TEL: (530) 343-8795
FAX: (916) 928-0332
WWW.CRAWFORDANDCOMPANY.COM

400 CORPORATE PT
PO BOX 92091
CULVER CITY, CA 90230
TEL: (310) 642-4400
WWW.CRAWFORDANDCOMPANY.COM

10411 OLD PLACERVILLE RD, STE 200
SACRAMENTO, CA 95827-2508
TEL: (916) 364-7487
FAX: (916) 364-0660
WWW.CRAWFORDANDCOMPANY.COM

3870 MURPHY CANYON RD, STE 100
PO BOX 85305
SAN DIEGO, CA 92186-5305
TEL: (619) 292-6210
FAX: (619) 292-0973
WWW.CRAWFORDANDCOMPANY.COM

711 KAPIOLANI BLVD, STE 900
PO BOX 4218
HONOLULU, OAHU, HI 96812-4218
TEL: (808) 591-2376
FAX: (808) 596-0380
WWW.CRAWFORDANDCOMPANY.COM

FRANKLIN BUS PRK- 146 S COLE RD
BOISE, ID 83709
TEL: (208) 375-5021
FAX: (208) 375-4514
WWW.CRAWFORDANDCOMPANY.COM

625 CENTRAL AVE W, STE 100
PO BOX 3007
GREAT FALLS, MT 59403
TEL: (406) 761-7230
FAX: (406) 454-0454
WWW.CRAWFORDANDCOMPANY.COM

12725 SW 66TH AVE, STE 207
PORTLAND, OR 97223-2548
TEL: (503) 639-2111
FAX: (503) 620-0676
WWW.CRAWFORDANDCOMPANY.COM

CRAWFORD OF CALIFORNIA

CALIFORNIA CLAIMS OFFICE
CRAWFORD & CO
500 AIRPORT BLVD, STE 415
PO BOX 4208
BURLINGAME, CA 94010
TEL: (650) 342-6470
FAX: (650) 342-6492
TOLL FREE: (800) 241-2541

CREDIT INSURANCE SERVICES

NATIONAL CLAIMS OFFICE
101 W FRIENDLY AVE
PO BOX 21848
GREENSBORO, NC 27401
TEL: (336) 805-3455
FAX: (336) 805-2026
TOLL FREE: (800) 879-1703

CRESTAR TECHNOLOGY

MARYLAND CLAIMS OFFICE
1001 SEMMES AVE
PO BOX 27546
RICHMOND, VA 23261
TEL: (804) 319-1200
FAX: (804) 319-1847
TOLL FREE: (800) 205-7816

CRUM & FORSTER INSURANCE

ALABAMA CLAIMS OFFICE
3700 MANSELL RD, STE 500
PO BOX 1454
ATLANTA, GA 30301
TEL: (678) 461-7000
FAX: (678) 461-7062
TOLL FREE: (800) 225-0348
WWW.CFINS.COM

ALASKA CLAIMS OFFICE
6404 INTERNATIONAL PKY, STE 1000
PLANO, TX 75093
TEL: (972) 380-3000
FAX: (972) 380-3176
TOLL FREE: (800) 690-5520
WWW.CSINS.COM

ARIZONA CLAIMS OFFICE
6404 INTERNATIONAL PKY, STE 1000
PLANO, TX 75093
TEL: (972) 380-3000
FAX: (972) 380-3176
TOLL FREE: (800) 690-5520
WWW.CSINS.COM

ARKANSAS CLAIMS OFFICE
6404 INTERNATIONAL PKY, STE 1000
PLANO, TX 75093
TEL: (972) 380-3000
FAX: (972) 380-3176
TOLL FREE: (800) 690-5520
WWW.CSINS.COM

CALIFORNIA CLAIMS OFFICE
6404 INTERNATIONAL PKY, STE 1000
PLANO, TX 75093
TEL: (972) 380-3000
FAX: (972) 380-3176
TOLL FREE: (800) 690-5520
WWW.CSINS.COM

COLORADO CLAIMS OFFICE
6404 INTERNATIONAL PKY, STE 1000
PLANO, TX 75093
TEL: (972) 380-3000
FAX: (972) 380-3176
TOLL FREE: (800) 690-5520
WWW.CSINS.COM

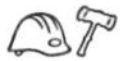

CONNECTICUT CLAIMS OFFICE
665 WINDING BRK DR
PO BOX 8000
GLASTONBURY, CT 06033
TEL: (860) 659-3561
FAX: (860) 659-8070
IN-STATE: (800) 842-8224
WWW.CFINS.COM

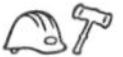

GEORGIA CLAIMS OFFICE
3700 MANSELL RD, STE 500
PO BOX 1454
ATLANTA, GA 30301
TEL: (678) 461-7000
FAX: (678) 461-7062
TOLL FREE: (800) 225-0348
WWW.CFINS.COM

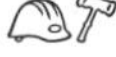

HAWAII CLAIMS OFFICE
6404 INTERNATIONAL PKY, STE 1000
PLANO, TX 75093
TEL: (972) 380-3000
FAX: (972) 380-3176
TOLL FREE: (800) 690-5520
WWW.CSINS.COM

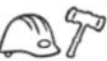

IDAHO CLAIMS OFFICE
6404 INTERNATIONAL PKY, STE 1000
PLANO, TX 75093
TEL: (972) 380-3000
FAX: (972) 380-3176
TOLL FREE: (800) 690-5520
WWW.CSINS.COM

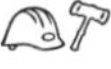

ILLINOIS CLAIMS OFFICE
400 N EXECUTIVE DR
BROOKFIELD, WI 53008-0977
TEL: (414) 784-0044
FAX: (414) 784-6297
TOLL FREE: (800) 242-4566
WWW.CFINS.COM

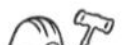

INDIANA CLAIMS OFFICE
INSURANCE / NORTHRIVER INSURANCE
4445 LK FOREST DR, STE 700
PO BOX 429583
CINCINNATI, OH 45242
TEL: (513) 563-3400
FAX: (513) 563-3402
TOLL FREE: (800) 777-2786
WWW.CFINS.COM

IOWA CLAIMS OFFICE
400 N EXECUTIVE DR
BROOKFIELD, WI 53008-0977
TEL: (414) 784-0044
FAX: (414) 784-6297
TOLL FREE: (800) 242-4566
WWW.CFINS.COM

KANSAS CLAIMS OFFICE
10975 GRAND VIEW, STE 300
PO BOX 2942
SHAWNEE MISSION, KS 66201
TEL: (913) 345-2044
FAX: (913) 345-2048
TOLL FREE: (800) 255-0454

6404 INTERNATIONAL PKY, STE 1000
PLANO, TX 75093
TEL: (972) 380-3000
FAX: (972) 380-3176
TOLL FREE: (800) 690-5520
WWW.CSINS.COM

KENTUCKY CLAIMS OFFICE
INSURANCE / NORTHRIVER INSURANCE
4445 LK FOREST DR, STE 700
PO BOX 429583
CINCINNATI, OH 45242
TEL: (513) 563-3400
FAX: (513) 563-3402
TOLL FREE: (800) 777-2786
WWW.CFINS.COM

MEXICO CLAIMS OFFICE
1 UNIVERSITY PL- 8801 J.M. KEYNES DR
PO BOX 560188
CHARLOTTE, NC 28256
TEL: (704) 510-2500
FAX: (704) 549-1059
TOLL FREE: (800) 438-9578
IN-STATE: (800) 528-1386

MICHIGAN CLAIMS OFFICE
300 GALLERIA OFFICENTRE
27710 NORTHWESTERN HWY, STE 200
PO BOX 5118
SOUTHFIELD, MI 48034
TEL: (810) 827-4440
FAX: (810) 827-4737
IN-STATE: (800) 572-7396

400 N EXECUTIVE DR
BROOKFIELD, WI 53008-0977
TEL: (414) 784-0044
FAX: (414) 784-6297
TOLL FREE: (800) 242-4566
WWW.CFINS.COM

MINNESOTA CLAIMS OFFICE
7900 INTERNATIONAL DR, STE 700
BLOOMINGTON, MN 55425
TEL: (612) 858-0400
FAX: (612) 858-0493
IN-STATE: (800) 328-8323
WWW.CFINS.COM

400 N EXECUTIVE DR
BROOKFIELD, WI 53008-0977
TEL: (414) 784-0044
FAX: (414) 784-6297
TOLL FREE: (800) 242-4566
WWW.CFINS.COM

MISSISSIPPI CLAIMS OFFICE
3700 MANSELL RD, STE 500
PO BOX 1454
ATLANTA, GA 30301
TEL: (678) 461-7000
FAX: (678) 461-7062
TOLL FREE: (800) 225-0348
WWW.CFINS.COM

MISSOURI CLAIMS OFFICE
6404 INTERNATIONAL PKY, STE 1000
PLANO, TX 75093
TEL: (972) 380-3000
FAX: (972) 380-3176
TOLL FREE: (800) 690-5520
WWW.CSINS.COM

MONTANA CLAIMS OFFICE
6404 INTERNATIONAL PKY, STE 1000
PLANO, TX 75093
TEL: (972) 380-3000
FAX: (972) 380-3176
TOLL FREE: (800) 690-5520
WWW.CSINS.COM

NATIONAL CLAIMS OFFICE
QUADRANT, STE 500- 5445 DTC PKY
PO BOX 5090
DENVER, CO 80217
TEL: (303) 773-2000
FAX: (303) 846-1970
TOLL FREE: (800) 255-3445
IN-STATE: (800) 255-3445
WWW.CSINS.COM

275 BATTERY ST- 7TH FL
PO BOX 7791
SAN FRANCISCO, CA 94120
TEL: (415) 658-3200
TOLL FREE: (800) 972-4848

601 S LAKE DESTINY RD, STE 300
PO BOX 945075
MAITLAND, FL 32794
TEL: (407) 660-0402
FAX: (407) 660-0280
IN-STATE: (800) 423-3060

CITY FINANCIAL TWR
201 MERCHANT ST, STE 1960
HONOLULU, HI 96813
TEL: (808) 536-3655
FAX: (808) 533-7006
IN-STATE: (800) 232-9492
WWW.CFINS.COM

1111 W 22ND ST
PO BOX 4942
OAK BROOK, IL 60523
TEL: (630) 954-1280
FAX: (630) 954-5250
TOLL FREE: (800) 233-1399
IN-STATE: (800) 558-4219

C

1111 W 22ND ST
PO BOX 4942
OAK BROOK, IL 60523
TEL: (630) 954-1280
FAX: (630) 954-5250
TOLL FREE: (800) 233-1399
IN-STATE: (800) 558-4219

4445 LK FOREST DR, STE 700
PO BOX 429583
CINCINNATI, OH 45242
TEL: (513) 563-3400
FAX: (513) 563-3447
TOLL FREE: (800) 777-2786

89 S ST- LINCOLN PLZ- 5TH FL
BOSTON, MA 02111
TEL: (617) 330-7575
FAX: (617) 345-0415
TOLL FREE: (800) REPORTING
IN-STATE: (800) 258-5815

200 INTERNATIONAL CIR, STE 4500
PO BOX 8042
HUNT VALLEY, MD 21030-1331
FAX: (410) 785-0583
TOLL FREE: (800) 521-0858
WWW.CFINS.COM

89 S ST- LINCOLN PLZ- 5TH FL
BOSTON, MA 02111
TEL: (617) 330-7575
FAX: (617) 345-0415
IN-STATE: (800) 258-5815

275 BATTERY ST- 7TH FL
PO BOX 7791
SAN FRANCISCO, CA 94111
TEL: (415) 658-3200
TOLL FREE: (800) 972-4848

55 S LAKE AVE, STE 700
PO BOX 91596
PASADENA, CA 91109
TEL: (626) 397-4700
FAX: (626) 397-4778
TOLL FREE: (800) 331-5595
WWW.CFINS.COM

275 BATTERY ST- 7TH FL
PO BOX 7791
SAN FRANCISCO, CA 94111
TEL: (415) 658-3200
FAX: (415) 658-3202
TOLL FREE: (800) 972-4848
WWW.CSINS.COM

305 MADISON AVE
MORRISTOWN, NJ 07960
TEL: (973) 490-6600
FAX: (973) 490-6682
TOLL FREE: (800) 690-5520
WWW.CSINS.COM

QUADRANT, STE 500, 5445 DTC PKY
PO BOX 5090
DENVER, CO 80217
TEL: (303) 773-2000
FAX: (303) 846-1970
TOLL FREE: (800) 255-3445

225 GREENFIELD PKY
PO BOX 4865
LIVERPOOL, NY 13088
TEL: (315) 445-2433
IN-STATE: (800) 962-2925
WWW.CFINS.COM

2 WORLD TRADE CTR
NEW YORK, NY 10048
TEL: (212) 390-5100
FAX: (212) 390-5199
TOLL FREE: (800) 442-2124

1 UNIVERSITY PL- 8801 J.M. KEYNES DR
PO BOX 560188
CHARLOTTE, NC 28256
TEL: (704) 510-2500
FAX: (704) 549-1059
TOLL FREE: (800) 438-9578
IN-STATE: (800) 528-1386

R 3 H

UNITED STATES FIRE
7900 INTERNATIONAL DR, STE 700
BLOOMINGTON, MN 55425
TEL: (612) 858-0400
FAX: (612) 858-0493
IN-STATE: (800) 328-8323
WWW.CFINS.COM

3

7900 INTERNATIONAL DR, STE 700
BLOOMINGTON, MN 55425
TEL: (612) 858-0400
FAX: (612) 858-0493
TOLL FREE: (800) 328-8323
WWW.CFINS.COM

3

6404 INTERNATIONAL PKY, STE 1000
PLANO, TX 75093
TEL: (972) 380-3000
FAX: (972) 380-3176
TOLL FREE: (800) 527-5531
WWW.CSINS.COM

ONE LINCOLN PLZ, 89 S ST- 5TH FL
BOSTON, MA 02111
TEL: (617) 330-7575
FAX: (617) 345-0415
TOLL FREE: (800) REPORTING
IN-STATE: (800) 258-5815

PO BOX 7791
SAN FRANCISCO, CA 94111
TEL: (415) 658-3200
FAX: (415) 658-3208
TOLL FREE: (800) 972-4848

1601 5TH AVE, STE 1450
SEATTLE, WA 98101
TEL: (206) 623-6045
FAX: (206) 667-9115
TOLL FREE: (800) 233-6733

US FIRE INSURANCE CO
QUADRANT, STE 500, 5445 DTC PKY
PO BOX 5090
DENVER, CO 80217-5090
TEL: (303) 773-2000
FAX: (303) 846-1970
TOLL FREE: (800) 255-3445
IN-STATE: (800) 874-9798

NEBRASKA CLAIMS OFFICE
6404 INTERNATIONAL PKY, STE 1000
PLANO, TX 75093
TEL: (972) 380-3000
FAX: (972) 380-3176
TOLL FREE: (800) 690-5520
WWW.CSINS.COM

NEVADA CLAIMS OFFICE
6404 INTERNATIONAL PKY, STE 1000
PLANO, TX 75093
TEL: (972) 380-3000
FAX: (972) 380-3176
TOLL FREE: (800) 690-5520
WWW.CSINS.COM

NEW MEXICO CLAIMS OFFICE
6404 INTERNATIONAL PKY, STE 1000
PLANO, TX 75093
TEL: (972) 380-3000
FAX: (972) 380-3176
TOLL FREE: (800) 690-5520
WWW.CSINS.COM

NORTH DAKOTA CLAIMS OFFICE
400 N EXECUTIVE DR
BROOKFIELD, WI 53008-0977
TEL: (414) 784-0044
FAX: (414) 784-6297
TOLL FREE: (800) 242-4566
WWW.CFINS.COM

OHIO CLAIMS OFFICE
U.S. FIRE INSURANCE / NORTHRIVER INSURANCE
4445 LK FOREST DR, STE 700
PO BOX 429583
CINCINNATI, OH 45242
TEL: (513) 563-3400
FAX: (513) 563-3402
TOLL FREE: (800) 777-2786
WWW.CFINS.COM

3

OREGON CLAIMS OFFICE
6404 INTERNATIONAL PKY, STE 1000
PLANO, TX 75093
TEL: (972) 380-3000
FAX: (972) 380-3176
TOLL FREE: (800) 527-5531

6404 INTERNATIONAL PKY, STE 1000
PLANO, TX 75093
TEL: (972) 380-3000
FAX: (972) 380-3176
TOLL FREE: (800) 690-5520
WWW.CSINS.COM

PENNSYLVANIA CLAIMS OFFICE
COMMERCE CT- 4 STA SQ, STE 620
PITTSBURGH, PA 15219-1115
TEL: (412) 392-4000
FAX: (412) 392-0277
IN-STATE: (800) 245-2505

RHODE ISLAND CLAIMS OFFICE
89 S ST- LINCOLN PLZ- 5TH FL
BOSTON, MA 02111
TEL: (617) 330-7575
FAX: (617) 345-0415
IN-STATE: (800) 258-5815

SOUTH DAKOTA CLAIMS OFFICE
400 N EXECUTIVE DR
BROOKFIELD, WI 53008-0977
TEL: (414) 784-0044
FAX: (414) 784-6297
TOLL FREE: (800) 242-4566
WWW.CFINS.COM

UTAH CLAIMS OFFICE
6404 INTERNATIONAL PKY, STE 1000
PLANO, TX 75093
TEL: (972) 380-3000
FAX: (972) 380-3176
TOLL FREE: (800) 690-5520
WWW.CSINS.COM

WASHINGTON CLAIMS OFFICE
6404 INTERNATIONAL PKY, STE 1000
PLANO, TX 75093
TEL: (972) 380-3000
FAX: (972) 380-3176
TOLL FREE: (800) 690-5520
WWW.CSINS.COM

WISCONSIN CLAIMS OFFICE
400 N EXECUTIVE DR
BROOKFIELD, WI 53008-0977
TEL: (414) 784-0044
FAX: (414) 784-6297
TOLL FREE: (800) 242-4566
WWW.CFINS.COM

WYOMING CLAIMS OFFICE
6404 INTERNATIONAL PKY, STE 1000
PLANO, TX 75093
TEL: (972) 380-3000
FAX: (972) 380-3176
TOLL FREE: (800) 690-5520
WWW.CSINS.COM

CSA BENEFIT

NATIONAL CLAIMS OFFICE
BLUE CROSS BLUE SHIELD
4625 S WENDLER DR, STE 211
PO BOX 13466
PHOENIX, AZ 85002
TEL: (602) 431-3502
FAX: (602) 431-3637
TOLL FREE: (800) 382-8383

CTI ADMINISTRATIORS, INC

CTI INC
100 COURT AVE STE 306
DES MOINES, IA 50309-2200
TEL: (515) 244-7322
FAX: (515) 244-8650
TOLL FREE: (800) 245-8813

CULLEN ASSOCIATES, INC

GEORGIA CLAIMS OFFICE
4626 MILLER RD, UNIT C
COLUMBUS, GA 31909
TEL: (706) 563-9200
FAX: (706) 562-0220

CUMBERLAND MUTUAL FIRE INSURANCE CO

NEW JERSEY CLAIMS OFFICE
633 SHILOH PIKE
PO BOX 556
BRIDGETON, NJ 08302-1452
TEL: (609) 451-4050
FAX: (609) 455-8468
TOLL FREE: (800) 232-6992
WWW.CUMBERLAND GROUP.COM

CUNA MUTUAL GROUP

NATIONAL CLAIMS OFFICE
CUMIS INSURANCE
5190 MINERAL POINT RD
PO BOX 391
MADISON, WI 53701-0391
TEL: (608) 238-5851
FAX: (608) 238-0830
TOLL FREE: (800) 356-2644
WWW.CUNAMUTUAL.COM

5910 MINERAL POINT RD
PO BOX 1648
MADISON, WI 53701
TEL: (909) 627-2644
FAX: (608) 238-0830
TOLL FREE: (800) 548-9390
WWW.CUNAMUTUAL.COM

CUNA MUTUAL INSURANCE GROUP

5910 MINERAL PT RD
PO BOX 391
MADISON, WI 53701-0391
TEL: (608) 238-5851
FAX: (608) 238-0830
TOLL FREE: (800) 356-2644
WWW.CUNAMUTUAL.COM

CUNNINGHAM LINDSEY INC

CALIFORNIA CLAIMS OFFICE
3030 SATURN ST, STE 102
PO BOX 9219
BREA, CA 92822
TEL: (714) 993-9801
FAX: (714) 993-6410
WWW.CUNNINGHAMLINDSEY.COM

9370 SKY PARK CT, STE 200
SAN DIEGO, CA 92123
TEL: (619) 569-8877
FAX: (619) 569-9849

TEXAS CLAIMS OFFICE
3910 BROOKSIDE DR
PO BOX 6030
TYLER, TX 75711
TEL: (903) 561-6700
FAX: (903) 581-2536
TOLL FREE: (800) 581-7165
WWW.CUNNINGHAMLINDSEY.COM

CYPRESS INSURANCE CO

CALIFORNIA CLAIMS OFFICE
395 OYSTER PT BLVD, STE 401
PO BOX 1930
SAN FRANCISCO, CA 94083-1930
TEL: (650) 635-0444
FAX: (650) 635-0443
TOLL FREE: (800) 834-3848

NATIONAL CLAIMS OFFICE
465 N HALSTEAD ST
PO BOX 7008
PASADENA, CA 91109
TEL: (626) 351-1180
FAX: (626) 351-1622
TOLL FREE: (800) 834-3848

DAIRYLAND INSURANCE CO

ARIZONA CLAIMS OFFICE
SENTRY CLAIMS CENTER
9060 E VIA LINDA
PO BOX 29460
PHOENIX, AZ 85038-9460
TEL: (602) 860-7800
FAX: (602) 860-7702
TOLL FREE: (800) 833-2244

DAKOTACARE

SOUTH DAKOTA CLAIMS OFFICE
1323 S MINNESOTA AVE
SIOUX FALLS, SD 57105-0624
TEL: (605) 334-4000
FAX: (605) 336-0270
TOLL FREE: (800) 628-3778
IN-STATE: (800) 325-5598
WWW.DAKOTACARE.COM

D

D

DBL SERVICES, INC
NATIONAL CLAIMS OFFICE
515 OLIVE ST, STE 700
PO BOX 66714
SAINT LOUIS, MO 63166-6714
TEL: (314) 241-8665
FAX: (314) 241-3628
TOLL FREE: (800) 844-7979
IN-STATE: (800) 241-8665

DC CHARTERED HEALTH PLAN, INC
DISTRICT OF COLUMBIA CLAIMS OFFICE
820 FIRST ST NE, STE LL100
WASHINGTON, DC 20002
TEL: (202) 408-4710
FAX: (202) 408-4730
TOLL FREE: (800) 799-4710
WWW.CHARTER-HEALTH.COM

DCA HEALTHCARE MANAGEMENT GROUP
NORTH DAKOTA CLAIMS OFFICE
13100 WAYZATA BLVD
MINNETONKA, MN 55305-1840
TEL: (612) 541-7500
FAX: (612) 541-5999
TOLL FREE: (800) 284-4464

DCA INC
NATIONAL CLAIMS OFFICE
3405 ANNAPOLIS LN N, STE 100
PLYMOUTH, MN 55447
TEL: (612) 278-4000
FAX: (612) 278-4601
TOLL FREE: (800) 284-4464

DCI/DIALYSIS CLINIC, INC
TENNESSEE CLAIMS OFFICE
1600 HAYES ST, STE 300
NASHVILLE, TN 37203-3028
TEL: (615) 327-3061
FAX: (615) 327-0527

DEACONESS MEDICAL CENTER
MONTANA CLAIMS OFFICE
PO BOX 37000
BILLINGS, MT 59107-7000
TEL: (406) 657-4000
FAX: (406) 657-3864
TOLL FREE: (800) 225-1246

DEAN HEALTH PLAN HMO
ILLINOIS CLAIMS OFFICE
1277 DEMING WAY
PO BOX 56099
MADISON, WI 53705
TEL: (608) 828-1301
FAX: (608) 836-1210
TOLL FREE: (800) 279-1301
IN-STATE: (800) 356-7344
WWW.DEANCARE.COM

IOWA CLAIMS OFFICE
1277 DEMING WAY
PO BOX 56099
MADISON, WI 53705
TEL: (608) 828-1301
FAX: (608) 836-1210
TOLL FREE: (800) 279-1301
IN-STATE: (800) 356-7344
WWW.DEANCARE.COM

WISCONSIN CLAIMS OFFICE
1277 DEMING WAY
PO BOX 56099
MADISON, WI 53705
TEL: (608) 828-1301
FAX: (608) 836-1210
TOLL FREE: (800) 279-1301
IN-STATE: (800) 356-7344
WWW.DEANCARE.COM

DEEP SOUTH SURPLUS OF TEXAS
ARKANSAS CLAIMS OFFICE
PO BOX 143-0099
IRVING, TX 75014
TEL: (214) 860-0265
FAX: (214) 860-0292
TOLL FREE: (800) 239-6871

GEORGIA CLAIMS OFFICE
PO BOX 143-0099
IRVING, TX 75014
TEL: (214) 860-0265
FAX: (214) 860-0292
TOLL FREE: (800) 239-6871

LOUISIANA CLAIMS OFFICE
PO BOX 143-0099
IRVING, TX 75014
TEL: (214) 860-0265
FAX: (214) 860-0292
TOLL FREE: (800) 239-6871

MISSISSIPPI CLAIMS OFFICE
PO BOX 143-0099
IRVING, TX 75014
TEL: (214) 860-0265
FAX: (214) 860-0292
TOLL FREE: (800) 239-6871

TEXAS CLAIMS OFFICE
PO BOX 143-0099
IRVING, TX 75014
TEL: (214) 860-0265
FAX: (214) 860-0292
TOLL FREE: (800) 239-6871

DEKALB GENETICS CORP
ILLINOIS CLAIMS OFFICE
3100 SYCAMORE RD
DEKALB, IL 60115-9621
TEL: (815) 758-3461
FAX: (815) 895-2846
IN-STATE: (800) 892-6990

DELMARVA HEALTH PLAN, INC
DELAWARE CLAIMS OFFICE
301 BAY ST, STE 401
PO BOX 2410
EASTON, MD 21601
TEL: (410) 822-7223
FAX: (410) 822-8152
TOLL FREE: (800) 334-3427
IN-STATE: (800) 334-3427
WWW.CAREFIRST.COM

MARYLAND CLAIMS OFFICE
301 BAY ST, STE 401
PO BOX 2410
EASTON, MD 21601
TEL: (410) 822-7223
FAX: (410) 822-8152
TOLL FREE: (800) 334-3427
IN-STATE: (800) 334-3427
WWW.CAREFIRST.COM

DELOITTE & TOUCHE
NATIONAL CLAIMS OFFICE
10 WESTPORT RD
PO BOX 820
WILTON, CT 06897
TEL: (203) 761-3000
FAX: (203) 834-2200
WWW.US.DELOIT.COM

DELTA CASUALTY CO
FLORIDA CLAIMS OFFICE
4711 N CLARK ST
CHICAGO, IL 60640-4632
TEL: (773) 878-8500
FAX: (773) 769-0687

ILLINOIS CLAIMS OFFICE
4711 N CLARK ST
CHICAGO, IL 60640-4632
TEL: (773) 878-8500
FAX: (773) 769-0687

DELTA DENTAL INSURANCE CO
ARIZONA CLAIMS OFFICE
DELTA DENTAL OF ARIZONA
15648 N 35TH AVE, STE 111
PO BOX 43000
PHOENIX, AZ 85080-3000
TEL: (602) 938-3131
FAX: (602) 588-3636
TOLL FREE: (800) 352-6132

DISTRICT OF COLUMBIA CLAIMS OFFICE
DELTA DENTAL OF THE DISTRICT OF COLUMBIA
ONE DELTA DR
MECHANICSBURG, PA 17055-6999
TEL: (717) 766-8500
FAX: (717) 766-8711
TOLL FREE: (800) 932-0783

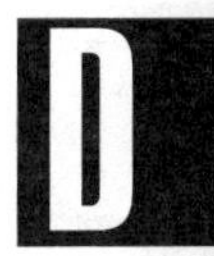

IDAHO CLAIMS OFFICE
DELTA DENTAL OF IDAHO
200 N FOURTH ST, STE 102
PO BOX 2870
BOISE, ID 83701
TEL: (208) 344-4546
FAX: (208) 344-4649
TOLL FREE: (800) 388-3490
IN-STATE: (800) 356-7586

INDIANA CLAIMS OFFICE
DELTA DENTAL OF MICHIGAN
PO BOX 9085
FARMINGTON HILLS, MI 48333-9085
TEL: (517) 347-5200
FAX: (517) 347-5248
TOLL FREE: (800) 462-7283
WWW.DELTADENTALIN.COM

MICHIGAN CLAIMS OFFICE
DELTAL DENTAL OF MICHIGAN
PO BOX 9085
FARMINGTON HILLS, MI 48333-9085
TEL: (517) 347-5200
FAX: (517) 347-5248
TOLL FREE: (800) 462-7283
WWW.DELTADENTALMI.COM

MINNESOTA CLAIMS OFFICE
DELTA DENTAL OF MINNESOTA
7807 CREEKBRIDGE CIR
PO BOX 330
MINNEAPOLIS, MN 55440
TEL: (612) 944-0391
FAX: (612) 944-4182
TOLL FREE: (800) 553-9536

MISSOURI CLAIMS OFFICE
DELTA DENTAL OF MISSOURI
8390 DELMAR BLVD
PO BOX 16921
SAINT LOUIS, MO 63105
TEL: (314) 993-9090
FAX: (314) 993-5120
TOLL FREE: (800) 392-1167
IN-STATE: (800) 392-1167

NATIONAL CLAIMS OFFICE
1000 MANSELL EXCHNG W- BLDG 100, STE 100
PO BOX 1809
ALPHARETTA, GA 30023-1809
TEL: (770) 645-8700
FAX: (770) 518-4757
TOLL FREE: (800) 521-2651

PO BOX 1809
ALPHARETTA, GA 30023-1809
TEL: (770) 645-8700
FAX: (770) 518-4757
TOLL FREE: (800) 521-2651

1000 MANSELL EXCHNG W- BLDG 100, STE 100
PO BOX 1809
ALPHARETTA, GA 30023-1809
TEL: (770) 645-8700
FAX: (770) 518-4757
TOLL FREE: (800) 521-2651
WWW.DELTADENTAL.COM

ONE DELTA DR
MECHANICSBURG, PA 17055-6999
TEL: (717) 766-8500
FAX: (717) 766-8719
TOLL FREE: (800) 932-0783

DELTA DENTAL OF NEW YORK
ONE DELTA DR
MECHANICSBURG, PA 17055-6999
TEL: (717) 766-8500
FAX: (717) 766-8719
TOLL FREE: (800) 932-0783
WWW.DELTADENTAL.COM

DELTA DENTAL OF PENNSYLVANIA
ONE DELTA DR
MECHANICSBURG, PA 17055-6999
TEL: (717) 766-8500
FAX: (717) 766-8719
TOLL FREE: (800) 932-0783
WWW.DELTADENTAL.COM

DELTA DENTAL OF ARKANSAS
100 SHADOW OAKS DR
PO BOX 15965
LITTLE ROCK, AR 72231-5965
TEL: (501) 835-3400
FAX: (501) 835-9520
TOLL FREE: (800) 462-5410

DELTA DENTAL OF PUERTO RICO
AVE DE DIEGO ESQ LOIZA ST, STE 75
PO BOX 9020992
SAN JUAN, PR 00902-0992
TEL: (787) 728-6120
FAX: (787) 268-7952
TOLL FREE: (800) 260-6120

DELTA DENTAL PLAN OF TENNESSEE
240 VENTURE CIR
NASHVILLE, TN 37228
TEL: (615) 255-3175
FAX: (615) 244-8108
TOLL FREE: (800) 223-3104
IN-STATE: (800) 223-3104
WWW.DELTADENTALTN.COM

DELTA DENTAL OF WYOMING
PO BOX 29
CHEYENNE, WY 82003
TEL: (307) 632-3313
FAX: (307) 632-7309
TOLL FREE: (800) 735-3379

SOUTH DAKOTA CLAIMS OFFICE
DELTA DENTAL OF SOUTH DAKOTA
720 N EUCLID
PO BOX 1157
PIERRE, SD 57501
TEL: (605) 224-7345
FAX: (605) 224-0909
TOLL FREE: (800) 627-3961
E-MAIL: DDPSD@DTGNET.COM

DELTA DENTAL OF CALIFORNIA

NATIONAL CLAIMS OFFICE
PO BOX 7736
SAN FRANCISCO, CA 94120
TEL: (415) 972-8300
FAX: (415) 972-8366
TOLL FREE: (888) 335-8227
E-MAIL: CMS@DELTA.ORG
WWW.DELTADENTALCA.ORG

DELTA DENTAL OF KANSAS, INC

KANSAS CLAIMS OFFICE
1010 N MAIN ST
PO BOX 49198
WICHITA, KS 67201-9198
TEL: (316) 264-1099
FAX: (316) 264-5912
TOLL FREE: (800) 733-5823
WWW.DELTADENTALKS.COM

DELTA DENTAL OF RHODE ISLAND

NATIONAL CLAIMS OFFICE
10 CHARLES ST
PO BOX 1517
PROVIDENCE, RI 02901-1517
TEL: (401) 453-0808
TOLL FREE: (800) 598-6684
WWW.DELTADENTALRI.COM

DELTA DENTAL OF WEST VIRGINIA

ONE DELTA DR
MECHANICSBURG, PA 17055-6999
TEL: (717) 766-8500
FAX: (717) 766-8719
TOLL FREE: (800) 932-0783
WWW.DELTADENTAL.COM

DELTA DENTAL PLAN OF ILLINOIS

ILLINOIS CLAIMS OFFICE
DELTA DENTAL OF ILLINOIS
2001 BUTTERFIELD RD, STE 900
PO BOX 9500
DOWNERS GROVE, IL 60515
TEL: (630) 964-2400
FAX: (630) 964-2494
TOLL FREE: (800) 452-1987
IN-STATE: (800) 323-1743
WWW.DELTADENTALIL.COM

DELTA DENTAL PLAN OF KENTUCKY

NATIONAL CLAIMS OFFICE
PO BOX 242810
LOUISVILLE, KY 40224-2810
TEL: (502) 423-1863
FAX: (502) 327-5715
TOLL FREE: (800) 955-2030
WWW.DDPKY.COM

DELTA DENTAL PLAN OF MASSACHUSETTS

PO BOX 9695
BOSTON, MA 02114
TEL: (617) 886-1000
FAX: (617) 886-1199
TOLL FREE: (800) 872-0500
WWW.DELTAMASS.COM

DELTA DENTAL PLAN OF MICHIGAN
OHIO CLAIMS OFFICE
DELTA DENTAL OF MICHIGAN
PO BOX 9085
FARMINGTON HILLS, MI 48333-9085
TEL: (517) 347-5200
FAX: (517) 347-5248
TOLL FREE: (800) 462-7283
WWW.DELTADENTALOH.COM

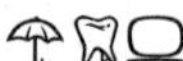

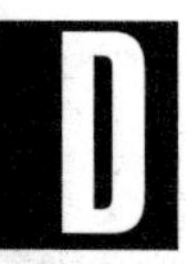

DELTA DENTAL PLAN OF NEBRASKA
NATIONAL CLAIMS OFFICE
8601 W DODGE RD, STE 116
OMAHA, NE 68114
TEL: (402) 397-4878
FAX: (402) 397-6401
TOLL FREE: (800) 553-9536

DELTA DENTAL PLAN OF NEW JERSEY INC
DELTA DENTAL OF NEW JERSEY
1639 RT 10
PO BOX 222
PARSIPPANY, NJ 07054
TEL: (973) 285-4000
FAX: (973) 285-4141
TOLL FREE: (800) 321-0142
WWW.DELTADENTALNJ.COM

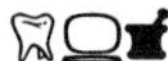

DELTA DENTAL PLAN OF NEW MEXICO
NEW MEXICO CLAIMS OFFICE
2500 LOUISIANA BLVD NE, STE 600
ALBUQUERQUE, NM 87110
TEL: (505) 883-4777
FAX: (505) 883-7444
TOLL FREE: (800) 999-0963

DELTA DENTAL PLAN OF NORTH CAROLINA
NATIONAL CLAIMS OFFICE
333 SIX FORKS RD, STE 180
RALEIGH, NC 27609
TEL: (919) 832-6015
FAX: (919) 832-6061
TOLL FREE: (800) 662-8856

DELTA DENTAL PLAN OF OHIO
2500 CORPORATE EXCHANGE DR
PO BOX 29979
COLUMBUS, OH 43229
TEL: (614) 890-1117
FAX: (614) 890-1274
TOLL FREE: (800) 282-0749
IN-STATE: (800) 537-5527
WWW.DELTADENTALOH.COM

DELTA DENTAL PLAN OF OKLAHOMA
PO BOX 54709
OKLAHOMA CITY, OK 73154
TEL: (405) 682-1992
FAX: (405) 681-1134
TOLL FREE: (800) 522-0188
WWW.DELTADENTALOK.COM

DELTA DENTAL PLAN OF VIRGINIA
4818 STARKEY RD SW
ROANOKE, VA 24014-4010
TEL: (540) 989-8000
FAX: (540) 774-7797
TOLL FREE: (800) 367-3531
IN-STATE: (800) 237-6060

DELTA DENTAL PLAN OF WISCONSIN
WISCONSIN CLAIMS OFFICE
2801 HOOVER RD
PO BOX 828
STEVENS POINT, WI 54481
TEL: (715) 344-6087
FAX: (715) 344-1067
TOLL FREE: (800) 236-3713
E-MAIL: OPERATIONS@DELTADENTALWI.COM
WWW.DELTADENTALWI.COM

DENTAL BENEFIT PROVIDERS
NATIONAL CLAIMS OFFICE
7200 WISCONSIN, STE 800
PO BOX 30640
BETHESDA, MD 20814
TEL: (301) 986-5600
FAX: (301) 986-7965
TOLL FREE: (800) 445-9090

311 CALIFORNIA ST, STE 550
SAN FRANCISCO, CA 94104
TEL: (310) 414-6950
FAX: (415) 391-1161
TOLL FREE: (800) 445-9090

H

DENTAL PLAN OF COLORADO
COLORADO CLAIMS OFFICE
4582 S ULSTER ST PKY, STE 800
PO BOX 173803
DENVER, CO 80217-3803
TEL: (303) 741-9300
FAX: (303) 741-9350
TOLL FREE: (800) 610-0201

DENTALCOMP, INC
PENNSYLVANIA CLAIMS OFFICE
3501 N FRONT ST
HARRISBURG, PA 17110
TEL: (717) 221-1026
FAX: (717) 221-1027
TOLL FREE: (888) 221-1026
WWW.DENTALCOMP.COM

DEPARTMENT OF MEDICAL ASSISTANCE
NATIONAL CLAIMS OFFICE
EDS
PO BOX 105013
TUCKER, GA 30085-5013
TEL: (404) 298-1228
TOLL FREE: (800) 766-4456

DEPARTMENT OF WATER & POWER CITY OF LOS ANGELES
CALIFORNIA CLAIMS OFFICE
111 N HOPE ST
PO BOX 5111
LOS ANGELES, CA 90051
TEL: (213) 367-4211

DESERET MUTUAL
NATIONAL CLAIMS OFFICE
60 E SOUTH TEMPLE
PO BOX 45530
SALT LAKE CITY, UT 84145-0530
TEL: (801) 578-5600
FAX: (801) 578-5903
TOLL FREE: (800) 777-3622
WWW.DMBA.COM

DETROIT & VICINITY TROWEL TRADES
MICHIGAN CLAIMS OFFICE
2075 W BIG BEAVER RD, STE 750
TROY, MI 48084-3446
TEL: (248) 822-0100
FAX: (248) 822-0126

DIAMOND G EMPLOYEE BENEFIT PLAN
NATIONAL CLAIMS OFFICE
102 COILE ST
PO BOX 877
GREENEVILLE, TN 37744-0877
TEL: (423) 639-1163
FAX: (423) 639-7270

DICTAPHONE CORP
3191 BROAD BRIDGE AVE
STRATFORD, CT 06614
TEL: (203) 381-7000
FAX: (203) 386-8566
IN-STATE: (800) 942-6374

H

DILLON COMPANIES INC
KANSAS CLAIMS OFFICE
700 E 30TH ST
PO BOX 1266
HUTCHINSON, KS 67504-1266
TEL: (316) 663-6801
FAX: (800) 663-1915
TOLL FREE: (800) 345-8385

℞

DIRECT RESPONSE INSURANCE ADMINISTRATIVE SERVICES, INC

NATIONAL CLAIMS OFFICE
7930 CENTURY BLVD
PO BOX 96
MINNEAPOLIS, MN 55440
TEL: (612) 556-5600
FAX: (612) 941-1017
TOLL FREE: (800) 438-8218

7930 CENTURY BLVD
PO BOX 96
MINNEAPOLIS, MN 55440
TEL: (612) 556-5600
FAX: (612) 941-1017
TOLL FREE: (800) 328-2791

DISABILITY MANAGEMENT SERVICES, INC

MASSACHUSETTS CLAIMS OFFICE
MASSACHUSETTS CASUALTY INSURANCE CO
711 ATLANTIC AVE
PO BOX 9099
BOSTON, MA 02205-9099
TEL: (617) 728-8000
FAX: (617) 338-4419
TOLL FREE: (800) 462-9897

DISTRICT 6 HEALTH FUND

NATIONAL CLAIMS OFFICE
18 E 31ST ST
NEW YORK, NY 10016-6702
TEL: (212) 696-5545
FAX: (212) 696-5556
TOLL FREE: (800) 331-1070

DIVERSIFIED GROUP ADMINISTRATORS

311 S CENTRAL
PO BOX 330
CANONSBURG, PA 15317-0330
TEL: (724) 746-8700
FAX: (724) 746-8508
TOLL FREE: (800) 221-8490
IN-STATE: (800) 222-2322

DIVERSIFIED GROUP ADMINISTRATORS, INC

TEXAS CLAIMS OFFICE
8625 KING GEORGE, STE 400
PO BOX 35828
DALLAS, TX 75235
TEL: (214) 688-5550
FAX: (214) 688-5551
TOLL FREE: (800) 394-7887
WWW.DGATPA.COM

DIVISION 1181 ATU NEW YORK WELFARE

NATIONAL CLAIMS OFFICE
10149 WOODHAVEN BLVD
OZONE PARK, NY 11416-2300
TEL: (718) 845-5800
FAX: (718) 641-0122

DIVISION OF HEALTH CARE FINANCING

UTAH CLAIMS OFFICE
BUREAU OF MEDICAL OPERATIONS
288 N 1460 W, 3RD FL
PO BOX 143106
SALT LAKE CITY, UT 84114-3106
TEL: (801) 538-6155
FAX: (801) 538-6805
IN-STATE: (800)662-9651
WWW.HLUNIX.EX.STATE.UT.US/MEDICAID

DODSON INSURANCE GROUP

MISSOURI CLAIMS OFFICE
CASUALTY RECIPROCAL EXCHANGE
9801 STATE LINE RD
PO BOX 419497
KANSAS CITY, MO 64141-6497
TEL: (816) 361-3400
FAX: (816) 825-5035
TOLL FREE: (800) 818-6610

NATIONAL CLAIMS OFFICE
98201 STATE LINE RD
PO BOX 419497
KANSAS CITY, MO 64141-6497
TEL: (816) 361-3400
FAX: (800) 825-5035
TOLL FREE: (800) 818-6610
WWW.DODSONGROUP.COM

DOLLAR GENERAL CORP

427 BEACH ST
SCOTTSVILLE, TN 42164
TEL: (502) 237-5444
FAX: (615) 783-2060
TOLL FREE: (800) 489-2419

DONEGAL MUTUAL INSURANCE CO

DELAWARE CLAIMS OFFICE
1195 RIVER RD
PO BOX 302
MARIETTA, PA 17547-0302
TEL: (717) 426-1931
FAX: (717) 426-7013
TOLL FREE: (800) 877-0600
WWW.DONEGAL.COM

GEORGIA CLAIMS OFFICE
1195 RIVER RD
PO BOX 302
MARIETTA, PA 17547-0302
TEL: (717) 426-1931
FAX: (717) 426-7013
TOLL FREE: (800) 877-0600
WWW.DONEGAL.COM

NEW HAMPSHIRE CLAIMS OFFICE
1195 RIVER RD
PO BOX 302
MARIETTA, PA 17547-0302
TEL: (717) 426-1931
FAX: (717) 426-7013
TOLL FREE: (800) 877-0600
WWW.DONEGAL.COM

PENNSYLVANIA CLAIMS OFFICE
1195 RIVER RD
PO BOX 302
MARIETTA, PA 17547-0302
TEL: (717) 426-1931
FAX: (717) 426-7013
TOLL FREE: (800) 877-0600
WWW.DONEGAL.COM

VIRGINIA CLAIMS OFFICE
1195 RIVER RD
PO BOX 302
MARIETTA, PA 17547-0302
TEL: (717) 426-1931
FAX: (717) 426-7013
TOLL FREE: (800) 877-0600
WWW.DONEGAL.COM

DONOVAN BENEFIT SYSTEMS, INC

NATIONAL CLAIMS OFFICE
440 LOUISIANA ST, STE 1600
PO BOX 2326
HOUSTON, TX 77252-2326
TEL: (713) 860-1800
FAX: (713) 223-2615
TOLL FREE: (800) 847-5797

DUNCANSON & HOLT GROUP(S)

100 WALL ST, 5TH FL
NEW YORK, NY 10005
TEL: (212) 487-9670
FAX: (212) 487-9680
WWW.DHGROUP.COM

DUNN-EDWARDS CORP

ARIZONA CLAIMS OFFICE
4885 E 52ND PL
PO BOX 2213
LOS ANGELES, CA 90040-2828
TEL: (323) 771-3330
FAX: (323) 773-8094
TOLL FREE: (800) 537-4098

CALIFORNIA CLAIMS OFFICE
4885 E 52ND PL
PO BOX 2213
LOS ANGELES, CA 90040-2828
TEL: (323) 771-3330
FAX: (323) 773-8094
TOLL FREE: (800) 537-4098

COLORADO CLAIMS OFFICE
4885 E 52ND PL
PO BOX 2213
LOS ANGELES, CA 90040-2828
TEL: (323) 771-3330
FAX: (323) 773-8094
TOLL FREE: (800) 537-4098

NEVADA CLAIMS OFFICE
4885 E 52ND PL
PO BOX 2213
LOS ANGELES, CA 90040-2828
TEL: (323) 771-3330
FAX: (323) 773-8094
TOLL FREE: (800) 537-4098

NEW MEXICO CLAIMS OFFICE
4885 E 52ND PL
PO BOX 2213
LOS ANGELES, CA 90040-2828
TEL: (323) 771-3330
FAX: (323) 773-8094
TOLL FREE: (800) 537-4098

TEXAS CLAIMS OFFICE
4885 E 52ND PL
PO BOX 2213
LOS ANGELES, CA 90040-2828
TEL: (323) 771-3330
FAX: (323) 773-8094
TOLL FREE: (800) 537-4098

E.B.A. & M. CORP

NATIONAL CLAIMS OFFICE
30501 AGOURA RD, STE 102
PO BOX 5079
WESTLAKE VILLAGE, CA 91359-5079
TEL: (805) 497-4581
FAX: (818) 991-2194
TOLL FREE: (800) 776-1545

EAGLE INSURANCE GROUP

ALASKA CLAIMS OFFICE
4025 DELRIDGE WAY SW, STE 300
PO BOX 47088
SEATTLE, WA 98146
TEL: (206) 933-5200
FAX: (206) 938-0194
TOLL FREE: (800) 372-2255

ARKANSAS CLAIMS OFFICE
4025 DELRIDGE WAY SW, STE 300
PO BOX 47088
SEATTLE, WA 98146
TEL: (206) 933-5200
FAX: (206) 938-0194
TOLL FREE: (800) 372-2255

CALIFORNIA CLAIMS OFFICE
4025 DELRIDGE WAY SW, STE 300
PO BOX 47088
SEATTLE, WA 98146
TEL: (206) 933-5200
FAX: (206) 938-0194
TOLL FREE: (800) 372-2255

COLORADO CLAIMS OFFICE
4025 DELRIDGE WAY SW, STE 300
PO BOX 47088
SEATTLE, WA 98146
TEL: (206) 933-5200
FAX: (206) 938-0194
TOLL FREE: (800) 372-2255

CONNECTICUT CLAIMS OFFICE
4025 DELRIDGE WAY SW, STE 300
PO BOX 47088
SEATTLE, WA 98146
TEL: (206) 933-5200
FAX: (206) 938-0194
TOLL FREE: (800) 372-2255

FLORIDA CLAIMS OFFICE
4025 DELRIDGE WAY SW, STE 300
PO BOX 47088
SEATTLE, WA 98146
TEL: (206) 933-5200
FAX: (206) 938-0194
TOLL FREE: (800) 372-2255

GEORGIA CLAIMS OFFICE
4025 DELRIDGE WAY SW, STE 300
PO BOX 47088
SEATTLE, WA 98146
TEL: (206) 933-5200
FAX: (206) 938-0194
TOLL FREE: (800) 372-2255

HAWAII CLAIMS OFFICE
4025 DELRIDGE WAY SW, STE 300
PO BOX 47088
SEATTLE, WA 98146
TEL: (206) 933-5200
FAX: (206) 938-0194
TOLL FREE: (800) 372-2255

LOUISIANA CLAIMS OFFICE
4025 DELRIDGE WAY SW, STE 300
PO BOX 47088
SEATTLE, WA 98146
TEL: (206) 933-5200
FAX: (206) 938-0194
TOLL FREE: (800) 372-2255

WASHINGTON CLAIMS OFFICE
4025 DELRIDGE WAY SW, STE 300
PO BOX 47088
SEATTLE, WA 98146
TEL: (206) 933-5200
FAX: (206) 938-0194
TOLL FREE: (800) 372-2255

EAGLE PACIFIC INSURANCE CO

NATIONAL CLAIMS OFFICE
4300 B ST, STE 403
ANCHORAGE, AK 99503-5929
TEL: (907) 563-6303
FAX: (907) 562-6246
TOLL FREE: (800) 770-6303

EASTERN BENEFIT SYSTEMS OF CENTENNIAL FINANCIAL GROUP

NEW JERSEY CLAIMS OFFICE
200 FREEWAY DR E
EAST ORANGE, NJ 07018
TEL: (973) 676-6100
FAX: (973) 676-6794
TOLL FREE: (800) 524-0227
IN-STATE: (800) 772-3610

EASTERN SHORE TEAMSTERS

NATIONAL CLAIMS OFFICE
1323 N SALISBURY BLVD
SALISBURY, MD 21801-3674
TEL: (410) 742-1031
FAX: (410) 742-1059
TOLL FREE: (800) 532-7849

EAU CLAIRE HEALTH PROTECTION PLAN

3430 OAKWOOD MALL DR
PO BOX 1060
EAU CLAIRE, WI 54702
TEL: (715) 835-6174
FAX: (715) 838-0220
TOLL FREE: (800) 835-6174

EBI CO

10 WATERSIDE
FARMINGTON, CT 06032
TEL: (860) 674-6600
FAX: (860) 678-5190
TOLL FREE: (800) 842-8343
IN-STATE: (800) 842-8343

EBI COMPANIES

PO BOX 4322
WOODLAND HILLS, CA 91365-4322
TEL: (818) 226-6800
FAX: (818) 226-6449
TOLL FREE: (800) 439-9964
IN-STATE: (800) 439-9964
WWW.EBICO.COM

2443 WARRENVILLE RD, STE 115
LISLE, IL 60532
TEL: (630) 505-1565
FAX: (630) 505-1573
TOLL FREE: (800) 832-0237

1400 11TH AVE, STE B
HELENA, MT 59601
TEL: (406) 449-6795
FAX: (406) 442-9960
IN-STATE: (800) 421-1194

5335 SW MEADOWS RD, STE 400
PO BOX 3725
PORTLAND, OR 97208
TEL: (503) 620-3700
FAX: (503) 624-5300
TOLL FREE: (800) 888-5933

602 OFFICE CENTER DR, STE 150
FORT WASHINGTON, PA 19034
TEL: (215) 245-0600
FAX: (215) 274-1260
IN-STATE: (800) 562-6795
WWW.EBICOMPANIES.COM

PENNSYLVANIA CLAIMS OFFICE
FOSTER PLAZA 10
680 ANDERSEN DR
PITTSBURGH, PA 15220-2700
TEL: (412) 922-5900
FAX: (412) 281-2605
TOLL FREE: (800) 472-1512

EDUCATORS HEALTH CARE, INC

IDAHO CLAIMS OFFICE
EDUCATORS MUTUAL INSURANCE
852 E ARROWHEAD LN
MURRAY, UT 84107-5298
TEL: (801) 262-7476
FAX: (801) 269-9734
TOLL FREE: (800) 644-5411

UTAH CLAIMS OFFICE
EDUCATORS MUTUAL INSURANCE
852 E ARROWHEAD LN
MURRAY, UT 84107-5298
TEL: (801) 262-7476
FAX: (801) 269-9734
TOLL FREE: (800) 644-5411

EDUCATORS MUTUAL LIFE INSURANCE CO

MASSACHUSETTS CLAIMS OFFICE
202 N PRINCE ST
PO BOX 83888
LANCASTER, PA 17608-3888
TEL: (717) 397-2751
FAX: (717) 397-1821
TOLL FREE: (800) 233-0307
E-MAIL: CALLCENTER@EMLIFE.COM

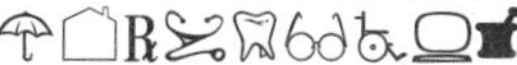

PENNSYLVANIA CLAIMS OFFICE
202 N PRINCE ST
PO BOX 83888
LANCASTER, PA 17608-3888
TEL: (717) 397-2751
FAX: (717) 397-1821
TOLL FREE: (800) 233-0307
E-MAIL: CALLCENTER@EMLIFE.COM

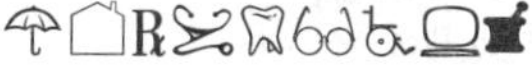

RHODE ISLAND CLAIMS OFFICE
202 N PRINCE ST
PO BOX 83888
LANCASTER, PA 17608-3888
TEL: (717) 397-2751
FAX: (717) 397-1821
TOLL FREE: (800) 233-0307
E-MAIL: CALLCENTER@EMLIFE.COM

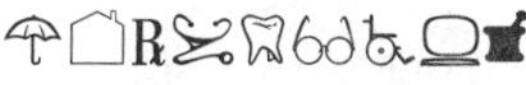

SOUTH CAROLINA CLAIMS OFFICE
202 N PRINCE ST
PO BOX 83888
LANCASTER, PA 17608-3888
TEL: (717) 397-2751
FAX: (717) 397-1821
TOLL FREE: (800) 233-0307
E-MAIL: CALLCENTER@EMLIFE.COM

ELCA BOARD OF PENSIONS

NATIONAL CLAIMS OFFICE
800 MARQUETTE AVE, STE 1050
PO BOX 59093
MINNEAPOLIS, MN 55459-0093
TEL: (612) 333-7651
FAX: (612) 334-5407
IN-STATE: (800) 352-2876
WWW.ELCABOP.ORG

ELECTRIC INSURANCE CO

152 CONANT ST
PO BOX 1036
BEVERLY, MA 01915-1659
TEL: (978) 921-0660
FAX: (978) 524-5361
TOLL FREE: (800) 227-2757

ELECTRONIC DATA SYSTEMS

EDS
PO BOX 15508
SACRAMENTO, CA 95852
TEL: (916) 636-1100
FAX: (916) 636-1056
IN-STATE: (800) 541-5555

ELI LILLY & CO

INDIANA CLAIMS OFFICE
LILLY CORPORATE CTR
INDIANAPOLIS, IN 46285-0001
TEL: (317) 276-2913
FAX: (317) 277-0882
TOLL FREE: (800) 428-4411

EMERALD HEALTH NETWORK, INC

OHIO CLAIMS OFFICE
1100 SUPERIOR AVE- 16TH FL
PO BOX 94808
CLEVELAND, OH 44101-4808
TEL: (216) 479-2030
FAX: (216) 241-4158
TOLL FREE: (800) 683-6830
WWW.EMERALDHEALTH.COM

EMPIRE BLUE CROSS & BLUE SHIELD

NEW YORK CLAIMS OFFICE
11 CORPORATE WOODS BLVD
PO BOX 11800
ALBANY, NY 12211-0800
TEL: (518) 367-4737
FAX: (518) 367-5373
WWW.EMPIREHEALTHCARE.COM

EMPIRE FIRE & MARINE INSURANCE CO

NATIONAL CLAIMS OFFICE
13810 SMB PKY
OMAHA, NE 68154-5202
TEL: (402) 963-5000
FAX: (402) 963-5048
TOLL FREE: (800) 228-9283

EMPIRE INSURANCE GROUP/ ALL CITY INSURANCE CO

NEW YORK CLAIMS OFFICE
35 STREET ADAM ST
BROOKLYN, NY 11201
TEL: (718) 422-4000

EMPIRE MEDICARE SERVICES

PO BOX 4846
SYRACUSE, NY 13221-4846
TEL: (315) 442-4400
FAX: (315) 442-4815
TOLL FREE: (800) 442-8430

EMPLOYEE BENEFIT ASSOCIATION

OHIO CLAIMS OFFICE
2858 W MARKET ST, STE N
PO BOX 5427
AKRON, OH 44333
TEL: (330) 867-9050
FAX: (330) 867-7029
TOLL FREE: (800) 624-2564

EMPLOYEE BENEFIT CLAIMS, INC

NATIONAL CLAIMS OFFICE
820 PARISH ST
PITTSBURGH, PA 15220-3405
TEL: (412) 922-0780
FAX: (412) 922-3071
TOLL FREE: (800) 922-4966

EMPLOYEE BENEFIT INSURANCE

CALIFORNIA CLAIMS OFFICE
E.B.I.
PO BOX 4322
WOODLAND HILLS, CA 91365-4322
TEL: (818) 226-6800
FAX: (818) 226-6449
TOLL FREE: (800) 439-9964
WWW.EBICO.COM

EMPLOYEE BENEFIT MANAGEMENT SERVICES INC

NATIONAL CLAIMS OFFICE
EBMS
PO BOX 21367
BILLINGS, MT 59104-1367
TEL: (406) 245-3575
FAX: (406) 652-5380
TOLL FREE: (800) 777-3575
WWW.EBMSTPA.COM

EMPLOYEE BENEFIT PLAN ADMINISTRATORS

CONNECTICUT CLAIMS OFFICE
CT PIPE TRADES BENEFIT FUNDS ADMINISTRATORS INC
210 MAIN ST
MANCHESTER, CT 06040
TEL: (860) 643-6401
FAX: (860) 643-6818
TOLL FREE: (800) 848-2129

EMPLOYEE BENEFIT SERVICES

NATIONAL CLAIMS OFFICE
1312 N HEARNE AVE, STE 100
PO BOX 70100
SHREVEPORT, LA 71137-0100
TEL: (318) 424-1987
FAX: (318) 424-9702
TOLL FREE: (800) 488-6360

EMPLOYEE BENEFIT SYSTEMS CORP

IOWA CLAIMS OFFICE
1701 MT PLEASANT ST, STE 1
PO BOX 1053
BURLINGTON, IA 52601-2799
TEL: (319) 752-3200
FAX: (319) 754-4480
TOLL FREE: (800) 373-1327
E-MAIL: EBS4BENEFITS@LISCO.NET

EMPLOYEE BENEFIT TRUST

ILLINOIS CLAIMS OFFICE
PO BOX 6279
SPRINGFIELD, IL 62708-6279
TEL: (217) 544-8379
FAX: (217) 544-8385
TOLL FREE: (800) 654-4222

EMPLOYEE SECURITY, INC

MARYLAND CLAIMS OFFICE
5565 STERRETT PL, STE 300
COLUMBIA, MD 21044-2608
TEL: (301) 596-1611
FAX: (410) 997-3796
TOLL FREE: (800) 638-1134

EMPLOYER PLAN SERVICES, INC

NATIONAL CLAIMS OFFICE
2180 N LOOP W, STE 400
HOUSTON, TX 77018
TEL: (713) 932-8917
FAX: (713) 932-1162
TOLL FREE: (800) 447-6588
WWW.ETSIBENEFITSINC.COM

EMPLOYERS INSURANCE CO OF NEVADA

NEVADA CLAIMS OFFICE
STATE INDUSTRIAL INSURANCE SYSTEM
515 E MUSSER
CARSON CITY, NV 89714
TEL: (775) 687-5220
FAX: (775) 687-8959
TOLL FREE: (800) 553-5115
WWW.EMPLOYERSINSCO.COM

1700 W CHARLESTON AVE
PO BOX 26929
LAS VEGAS, NV 89102
TEL: (702) 388-3100
FAX: (702) 388-0083
TOLL FREE: (800) 767-1446
WWW.EMPLOYERSINSCO.COM

EMPLOYERS REINSURANCE CORP

NATIONAL CLAIMS OFFICE
5200 METCALF AVE
PO BOX 2991
OVERLAND PARK, KS 66202-1296
TEL: (913) 676-5200
FAX: (913) 676-5221
TOLL FREE: (800) 255-6931
WWW.ERCGROUP.COM

EMS ADMINISTRATIVE SERVICE CORP

EMS
1115 W LANCASTER AVE
FT WORTH, TX 76102-4509
TEL: (817) 335-2582
FAX: (817) 335-9734

ENTERPRISE LIFE INSURANCE CO

1901 GATEWAY
PO BOX 167667
IRVING, TX 75016
TEL: (972) 751-5544
FAX: (972) 445-8382
TOLL FREE: (800) 527-1984

EPIC LIFE INSURANCE CO, INC

6801 SOUTH TOWNE DR
PO BOX 8924
MADISON, WI 53708-8924
TEL: (608) 223-2100
FAX: (608) 223-2159
TOLL FREE: (800) 236-8809
WWW.WPS.COM

EQUAFAX HEALTH CORP

CENTRA HEALTH CARE
PO BOX 6000
HOUSTON, TX 73534
TEL: (580) 252-9355
FAX: (580) 282-5810
TOLL FREE: (800) 228-4912

EQUITABLE LIFE & CASUALTY INSURANCE CO

ARIZONA CLAIMS OFFICE
3 TRIAD CTR, STE 200- 345 W NORTH TEMPLE
PO BOX 2460
SALT LAKE CITY, UT 84110-2460
TEL: (801) 521-2500
FAX: (801) 579-3790
TOLL FREE: (800) 352-5150
E-MAIL: INFO@EQUILIFE.COM

COLORADO CLAIMS OFFICE
3 TRIAD CTR, STE 200- 345 W NORTH TEMPLE
PO BOX 2460
SALT LAKE CITY, UT 84110-2460
TEL: (801) 521-2500
FAX: (801) 579-3790
TOLL FREE: (800) 352-5150
E-MAIL: INFO@EQUILIFE.COM

IDAHO CLAIMS OFFICE
3 TRIAD CTR, STE 200- 345 W NORTH TEMPLE
PO BOX 2460
SALT LAKE CITY, UT 84110-2460
TEL: (801) 521-2500
FAX: (801) 579-3790
TOLL FREE: (800) 352-5150
E-MAIL: INFO@EQUILIFE.COM

NEW MEXICO CLAIMS OFFICE
3 TRIAD CTR, STE 200- 345 W NORTH TEMPLE
PO BOX 2460
SALT LAKE CITY, UT 84110-2460
TEL: (801) 521-2500
FAX: (801) 579-3790
TOLL FREE: (800) 352-5150
E-MAIL: INFO@EQUILIFE.COM

UTAH CLAIMS OFFICE
3 TRIAD CTR, STE 200- 345 W NORTH TEMPLE
PO BOX 2460
SALT LAKE CITY, UT 84110-2460
TEL: (801) 521-2500
FAX: (801) 579-3790
TOLL FREE: (800) 352-5150
E-MAIL: INFO@EQUILIFE.COM

WYOMING CLAIMS OFFICE
3 TRIAD CTR, STE 200- 345 W NORTH TEMPLE
PO BOX 2460
SALT LAKE CITY, UT 84110-2460
TEL: (801) 521-2500
FAX: (801) 579-3790
TOLL FREE: (800) 352-5150
E-MAIL: INFO@EQUILIFE.COM

EQUITABLE PLAN SERVICES, INC

OKLAHOMA CLAIMS OFFICE
12312 SAINT ANDREWS DR
PO BOX 770466
OKLAHOMA CITY, OK 73177
TEL: (405) 755-2929
FAX: (405) 755-1185
TOLL FREE: (800) 749-2631

EQUITY MUTUAL INSURANCE CO

NATIONAL CLAIMS OFFICE
9201 STATE LINE RD
PO BOX 419497
KANSAS CITY, MO 64141-6497
TEL: (816) 361-3400
FAX: (800) 825-5035
TOLL FREE: (800) 818-6610

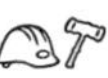

ERIE INSURANCE CO

ILLINOIS CLAIMS OFFICE
PO BOX 9031
CANTON, OH 44711-9031
TEL: (330) 492-4990
FAX: (330) 493-4609
TOLL FREE: (800) 362-6541
IN-STATE: (800) 535-4694

E

INDIANA CLAIMS OFFICE
7223 ENGLE RD, STE 100
PO BOX 9326
FT WAYNE, IN 46899-0326
TEL: (219) 432-5375
FAX: (800) 535-4684
IN-STATE: (800) 892-5655

PO BOX 9031
CANTON, OH 44711-9031
TEL: (330) 492-4990
FAX: (330) 493-4609
TOLL FREE: (800) 362-6541
IN-STATE: (800) 535-4694

PO BOX 4286
BETHLEHEM, PA 18018-0286
TEL: (610) 865-1911
FAX: (610) 974-7355
TOLL FREE: (800) 322-9026

MARYLAND CLAIMS OFFICE
12121 TECH RD
PO BOX 4409
SILVER SPRING, MD 20914-0409
TEL: (301) 622-5200
FAX: (301) 680-7601
TOLL FREE: (800) 492-2709
WWW.ERIE-INSURANCE.COM

R

PO BOX 9031
CANTON, OH 44711-9031
TEL: (330) 492-4990
FAX: (330) 493-4609
TOLL FREE: (800) 362-6541
IN-STATE: (800) 535-4694

NATIONAL CLAIMS OFFICE
COLLEGE PARK PLZ, STE 206
PO BOX 999
JOHNSTOWN, PA 15907
TEL: (814) 266-8936
FAX: (814) 269-0292
TOLL FREE: (800) 241-4209
E-MAIL: ERIE-INSURANCE.COM

301 COMMONWEALTH DR
PO BOX 516
WARRENDALE, PA 15086-0516
TEL: (724) 776-4000
FAX: (724) 772-7700
TOLL FREE: (800) 922-1824

OHIO CLAIMS OFFICE
PO BOX 9031
CANTON, OH 44711-9031
TEL: (330) 492-4990
FAX: (330) 493-4609
TOLL FREE: (800) 362-6541
IN-STATE: (800) 535-4694

PO BOX 4286
BETHLEHEM, PA 18018-0286
TEL: (610) 865-1911
FAX: (610) 974-7355
TOLL FREE: (800) 322-9026

3700 POPPLERS ST
PO BOX 598
PARKERSBURG, WV 26102-0598
TEL: (304) 485-6900
FAX: (304) 420-2099
TOLL FREE: (800) 642-1948

PENNSYLVANIA CLAIMS OFFICE
100 ERIE INSURANCE PL
ERIE, PA 16530-1699
TEL: (814) 451-5000
FAX: (814) 451-5060
TOLL FREE: (800) 458-0811

PO BOX 4286
BETHLEHEM, PA 18018-0286
TEL: (610) 865-1911
FAX: (610) 974-7355
TOLL FREE: (800) 322-9026

1400 N PROVIDENCE RD
MEDIA, PA 19063-2094
TEL: (610) 891-6400
FAX: (610) 892-3697
TOLL FREE: (800) 821-2902

PO BOX 605
MURRYSVILLE, PA 15668
TEL: (724) 325-7700
FAX: (724) 325-7715
TOLL FREE: (800) 553-3367
WWW.ERIE-INSURANCE.COM

PO BOX 9031
CANTON, OH 44711-9031
TEL: (330) 492-4990
FAX: (330) 493-4609
TOLL FREE: (800) 362-6541
IN-STATE: (800) 535-4694

VIRGINIA CLAIMS OFFICE
100 PELHAM DR
PO BOX 1207
WAYNESBORO, VA 22980-0863
TEL: (540) 943-7000
FAX: (540) 942-8781
TOLL FREE: (800) 542-2250

PO BOX 9031
CANTON, OH 44711-9031
TEL: (330) 492-4990
FAX: (330) 493-4609
TOLL FREE: (800) 362-6541
IN-STATE: (800) 535-4694

WEST VIRGINIA CLAIMS OFFICE
3700 POPPLERS ST
PO BOX 598
PARKERSBURG, WV 26102-0598
TEL: (304) 485-6900
FAX: (304) 420-2099
TOLL FREE: (800) 642-1948

PO BOX 9031
CANTON, OH 44711-9031
TEL: (330) 492-4990
FAX: (330) 493-4609
TOLL FREE: (800) 362-6541
IN-STATE: (800) 535-4694

PO BOX 4286
BETHLEHEM, PA 18018-0286
TEL: (610) 865-1911
FAX: (610) 974-7355
TOLL FREE: (800) 322-9026

ERIE INSURANCE GROUP

ILLINOIS CLAIMS OFFICE
250 E 96 ST, STE 201
PO BOX 80129
INDIANAPOLIS, IN 46280-0129
TEL: (317) 848-3420
FAX: (800) 535-4691
TOLL FREE: (800) 624-1620

7100 FOREST AVE, STE 200
PO BOX 28120
RICHMOND, VA 23228-0120
TEL: (804) 662-5400
FAX: (804) 264-4555
TOLL FREE: (800) 322-3743

INDIANA CLAIMS OFFICE
250 E 96 ST, STE 201
PO BOX 80129
INDIANAPOLIS, IN 46280-0129
TEL: (317) 848-3420
FAX: (800) 535-4691
TOLL FREE: (800) 624-1620

2820 ELECTRIC RD, STE 100
PO BOX 20769
ROANOKE, VA 24018-0524
TEL: (540) 989-8950
FAX: (540) 776-1234
TOLL FREE: (800) 533-3743

MARYLAND CLAIMS OFFICE
250 E 96 ST, STE 201
PO BOX 80129
INDIANAPOLIS, IN 46280-0129
TEL: (317) 848-3420
FAX: (800) 535-4691
TOLL FREE: (800) 624-1620

7100 FOREST AVE, STE 200
PO BOX 28120
RICHMOND, VA 23228-0120
TEL: (804) 662-5400
FAX: (804) 264-4555
TOLL FREE: (800) 322-3743

2820 ELECTRIC RD, STE 100
PO BOX 20769
ROANOKE, VA 24018-0524
TEL: (540) 989-8950
FAX: (540) 776-1234
TOLL FREE: (800) 533-3743

MISSOURI CLAIMS OFFICE
7100 FOREST AVE, STE 200
PO BOX 28120
RICHMOND, VA 23228-0120
TEL: (804) 662-5400
FAX: (804) 264-4555
TOLL FREE: (800) 322-3743

NATIONAL CLAIMS OFFICE
18544 BREEZE HILL DR
PO BOX 4158
HAGERSTOWN, MD 21741-4158
TEL: (301) 797-5185
FAX: (301) 714-9218
TOLL FREE: (800) 533-5602

NEW YORK CLAIMS OFFICE
7100 FOREST AVE, STE 200
PO BOX 28120
RICHMOND, VA 23228-0120
TEL: (804) 662-5400
FAX: (804) 264-4555
TOLL FREE: (800) 322-3743

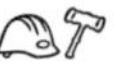

2820 ELECTRIC RD, STE 100
PO BOX 20769
ROANOKE, VA 24018-0524
TEL: (540) 989-8950
FAX: (540) 776-1234
TOLL FREE: (800) 533-3743

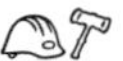

NORTH CAROLINA CLAIMS OFFICE
125 EDINBURGH S
PO BOX 730
CORY, NC 27512-0730
TEL: (919) 460-4473
FAX: (919) 481-0768
TOLL FREE: (800) 533-3982

OHIO CLAIMS OFFICE
250 E 96 ST, STE 201
PO BOX 80129
INDIANAPOLIS, IN 46280-0129
TEL: (317) 848-3420
FAX: (800) 535-4691
TOLL FREE: (800) 624-1620

7100 FOREST AVE, STE 200
PO BOX 28120
RICHMOND, VA 23228-0120
TEL: (804) 662-5400
FAX: (804) 264-4555
TOLL FREE: (800) 322-3743

2820 ELECTRIC RD, STE 100
PO BOX 20769
ROANOKE, VA 24018-0524
TEL: (540) 989-8950
FAX: (540) 776-1234
TOLL FREE: (800) 533-3743

PENNSYLVANIA CLAIMS OFFICE
4901 LOUISE DR
PO BOX 2013
MECHANICSBURG, PA 17055-0710
TEL: (717) 795-8200
FAX: (717) 795-2315
TOLL FREE: (800) 382-1304

250 E 96 ST, STE 201
PO BOX 80129
INDIANAPOLIS, IN 46280-0129
TEL: (317) 848-3420
FAX: (800) 535-4691
TOLL FREE: (800) 624-1620

7100 FOREST AVE, STE 200
PO BOX 28120
RICHMOND, VA 23228-0120
TEL: (804) 662-5400
FAX: (804) 264-4555
TOLL FREE: (800) 322-3743

2820 ELECTRIC RD, STE 100
PO BOX 20769
ROANOKE, VA 24018-0524
TEL: (540) 989-8950
FAX: (540) 776-1234
TOLL FREE: (800) 533-3743

SOUTH CAROLINA CLAIMS OFFICE
7100 FOREST AVE, STE 200
PO BOX 28120
RICHMOND, VA 23228-0120
TEL: (804) 662-5400
FAX: (804) 264-4555
TOLL FREE: (800) 322-3743

TENNESSEE CLAIMS OFFICE
2820 ELECTRIC RD, STE 100
PO BOX 20769
ROANOKE, VA 24018-0524
TEL: (540) 989-8950
FAX: (540) 776-1234
TOLL FREE: (800) 533-3743

VIRGINIA CLAIMS OFFICE
7100 FOREST AVE, STE 200
PO BOX 28120
RICHMOND, VA 23228-0120
TEL: (804) 662-5400
FAX: (804) 264-4555
TOLL FREE: (800) 322-3743

2820 ELECTRIC RD, STE 100
PO BOX 20769
ROANOKE, VA 24018-0524
TEL: (540) 989-8950
FAX: (540) 776-1234
TOLL FREE: (800) 533-3743

250 E 96 ST, STE 201
PO BOX 80129
INDIANAPOLIS, IN 46280-0129
TEL: (317) 848-3420
FAX: (800) 535-4691
TOLL FREE: (800) 624-1620

WEST VIRGINIA CLAIMS OFFICE
250 E 96 ST, STE 201
PO BOX 80129
INDIANAPOLIS, IN 46280-0129
TEL: (317) 848-3420
FAX: (800) 535-4691
TOLL FREE: (800) 624-1620

7100 FOREST AVE, STE 200
PO BOX 28120
RICHMOND, VA 23228-0120
TEL: (804) 662-5400
FAX: (804) 264-4555
TOLL FREE: (800) 322-3743

2820 ELECTRIC RD, STE 100
PO BOX 20769
ROANOKE, VA 24018-0524
TEL: (540) 989-8950
FAX: (540) 776-1234
TOLL FREE: (800) 533-3743

ERIN GROUP ADMINISTRATORS, INC

NATIONAL CLAIMS OFFICE
1871 SANTA BARBARA DR
PO BOX 7777
LANCASTER, PA 17604-7777
TEL: (717) 581-1300
FAX: (717) 581-1318
TOLL FREE: (800) 433-3746

ERISA ADMINISTRATIVE SERVICES, INC

ARIZONA CLAIMS OFFICE
3108 N 24TH ST- BLDG B
PHOENIX, AZ 85016-7313
TEL: (602) 956-3516
FAX: (602) 956-1943
WWW.CSERISA.COM

COLORADO CLAIMS OFFICE
10520 E BETHANY DR- BLDG 7
AURORA, CO 80014
TEL: (303) 745-0147
FAX: (303) 745-7010
WWW.CSERISA.COM

NEW MEXICO CLAIMS OFFICE
1200 SAN PEDRO NE
ALBUQUERQUE, NM 87110
TEL: (505) 262-1821
FAX: (505) 262-1822
WWW.CSERISA.COM

1429 SECOND ST
SANTA FE, NM 87505
TEL: (505) 988-4974
FAX: (505) 988-8943
WWW.CSERISA.COM

TEXAS CLAIMS OFFICE
12325 HYMEADOW DR- BLDG 4
AUSTIN, TX 78750-0001
TEL: (512) 250-9397
FAX: (512) 335-7298
TOLL FREE: (800) 933-7472
WWW.CSERISA.COM

UTAH CLAIMS OFFICE
2156 W 2200 S
SALT LAKE CITY, UT 84119-1326
TEL: (801) 973-1001
FAX: (801) 973-1007
WWW.CSERISA.COM

ESIS CO
CALIFORNIA CLAIMS OFFICE
SIGMA
39300 CIVIC CTR DR, STE 300
PO BOX 5025
FREMONT, CA 94537-5025
TEL: (510) 790-4600
FAX: (510) 790-4631
TOLL FREE: (800) 525-0615

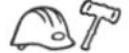

EVEREADY INSURANCE CO
NEW YORK CLAIMS OFFICE
59 MAIDEN LN
NEW YORK, NY 10038-4510
TEL: (212) 412-4700
FAX: (212) 363-1350
TOLL FREE: (800) 826-8285
IN-STATE: (800) 826-8285

EXCESS REINSURANCE UNDERWRITERS AGENCY, INC
NATIONAL CLAIMS OFFICE
307 S EVERGREEN AVE
PO BOX 667
WOODBURY, NJ 08096-7667
TEL: (609) 468-1800
FAX: (609) 468-2655
E-MAIL: ACCESS@WORLDNET.ATT.NET

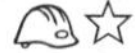

EXCLUSIVE HEALTHCARE, INC
NEBRASKA CLAIMS OFFICE
10250 REGENCY CIR, STE 250
PO BOX 31488
OMAHA, NE 68131-0488
TEL: (402) 351-2700
FAX: (402) 255-1665
TOLL FREE: (800) 617-2871
WWW.MUTUALOFOMAHA.COM

H

EXECUTIVE RESOURCES, INC
ALABAMA CLAIMS OFFICE
ASSOCIATION RESOURCES
3140 CAHABA HTS RD, STE 102
PO BOX 43000
BIRMINGHAM, AL 35243
TEL: (205) 967-1250
FAX: (205) 967-5631

EYE CARE OF WISCONSIN, INC
WISCONSIN CLAIMS OFFICE
8633 N PORT WASHINGTON RD
FOX POINT, WI 53217-2213
TEL: (414) 351-3030
FAX: (414) 351-3603

FALLON COMMUNITY HEALTH PLAN, INC
MASSACHUSETTS CLAIMS OFFICE
10 CHESTNUT ST- ONE CHESTNUT PL
PO BOX 15121
WORCESTER, MA 01615
TEL: (508) 799-2100
FAX: (508) 797-4292
TOLL FREE: (800) 333-2535
WWW.FCHP.ORG

H

FAMILY FINANCIAL LIFE INSURANCE CO
NATIONAL CLAIMS OFFICE
2555 SEVERN AVE
PO BOX 19685
NEW ORLEANS, LA 70179-0685
TEL: (504) 456-0101
FAX: (504) 456-6727
TOLL FREE: (800) 348-1555

FAMILY HEALTH PLAN COOPERATIVE
WISCONSIN CLAIMS OFFICE
11524 W THEO TRECKER WY
PO BOX 44260
MILWAUKEE, WI 53214-7260
TEL: (414) 256-0006
FAX: (414) 302-2298
TOLL FREE: (800) 236-3471
WWW.FAMILYHP.ORG

H

FAMILY HEALTH PLAN OF OHIO
MICHIGAN CLAIMS OFFICE
2200 JEFFERSON AVE- 6TH FL
PO BOX 4708
TOLEDO, OH 43610
TEL: (419) 241-6501
FAX: (419) 241-5441
TOLL FREE: (800) 231-8274
WWW.FAMILYHEALTHPLAN.ORG

OHIO CLAIMS OFFICE
2200 JEFFERSON AVE- 6TH FL
PO BOX 4708
TOLEDO, OH 43610
TEL: (419) 241-6501
FAX: (419) 241-5441
TOLL FREE: (800) 231-8274
WWW.FAMILYHEALTHPLAN.ORG

FARM BUREAU MUTUAL INSURANCE CO
IDAHO CLAIMS OFFICE
529 BROADWAY AVE S
BUHL, ID 83316
TEL: (208) 543-6438
FAX: (208) 543-6439

194 E COMMERCIAL
WEISER, ID 83672-2511
TEL: (208) 549-1414
FAX: (208) 549-1433

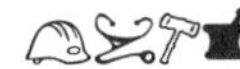

FARM BUREAU MUTUAL INSURANCE CO OF IDAHO
HOME OFFICE
1001 N 7TH ST
PO BOX 4848
POCATELLO, ID 83205-4848
TEL: (208) 232-7914
FAX: (208) 233-9388
E-MAIL: IDFBHA@MICRON.NET
WWW.FBINSURANCE.COM

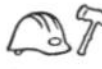

S E MAIN & HWY 93
PO BOX 735
CHALLIS, ID 83226-0735
TEL: (208) 879-2553
FAX: (208) 879-4280

WESTERN FARM BUREAU LIFE INSURANCE CO
444 E 5TH N
PO BOX 1148
BURLEY, ID 83318-1148
TEL: (208) 678-0431
FAX: (208) 678-5368

345 MAIN
PO BOX 428
GRAND VIEW, ID 83624-0428
TEL: (208) 834-2766
FAX: (208) 834-2526

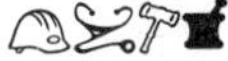

124 W FRANKLIN
PO BOX 210
MERIDIAN, ID 83680-0210
TEL: (208) 888-1821
FAX: (208) 888-3769

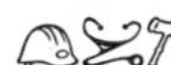

FARM BUREAU INSURANCE SERVICES
1630 BOND AVE
REXBURG, ID 83440
TEL: (208) 356-4439
FAX: (208) 356-4448

WESTERN COMMUNITY INSURANCE CO
170 S 2ND E
PO BOX 506
SODA SPRINGS, ID 83276-0506
TEL: (208) 547-3315
FAX: (208) 547-3316

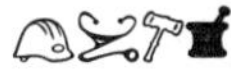

FARM BUREAU TOWN & COUNTRY INSURANCE CO OF MISSOURI
MISSOURI CLAIMS OFFICE
701 S COUNTRY CLUB DR
PO BOX 658
JEFFERSON CITY, MO 65101-0658
TEL: (573) 893-1400
FAX: (573) 893-6822

FARM FAMILY CASUALTY
CONNECTICUT CLAIMS OFFICE
344 RTE 9 W
PO BOX 656
ALBANY, NY 12201-0656
TEL: (518) 431-5000
FAX: (518) 431-5977
TOLL FREE: (800) 948-3276
WWW.FARMFAMILY.COM

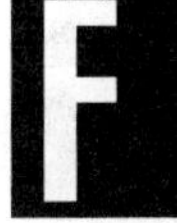

DELAWARE CLAIMS OFFICE
344 RTE 9 W
PO BOX 656
ALBANY, NY 12201-0656
TEL: (518) 431-5000
FAX: (518) 431-5977
TOLL FREE: (800) 948-3276
WWW.FARMFAMILY.COM

MAINE CLAIMS OFFICE
344 RTE 9 W
PO BOX 656
ALBANY, NY 12201-0656
TEL: (518) 431-5000
FAX: (518) 431-5977
TOLL FREE: (800) 948-3276
WWW.FARMFAMILY.COM

MARYLAND CLAIMS OFFICE
344 RTE 9 W
PO BOX 656
ALBANY, NY 12201-0656
TEL: (518) 431-5000
FAX: (518) 431-5977
TOLL FREE: (800) 948-3276
WWW.FARMFAMILY.COM

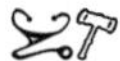

MASSACHUSETTS CLAIMS OFFICE
344 RTE 9 W
PO BOX 656
ALBANY, NY 12201-0656
TEL: (518) 431-5000
FAX: (518) 431-5977
TOLL FREE: (800) 948-3276
WWW.FARMFAMILY.COM

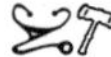

MISSOURI CLAIMS OFFICE
344 RTE 9 W
PO BOX 656
ALBANY, NY 12201-0656
TEL: (518) 431-5000
FAX: (518) 431-5977
TOLL FREE: (800) 948-3276
WWW.FARMFAMILY.COM

NEW YORK CLAIMS OFFICE
344 RTE 9 W
PO BOX 656
ALBANY, NY 12201-0656
TEL: (518) 431-5000
FAX: (518) 431-5977
TOLL FREE: (800) 948-3276
WWW.FARMFAMILY.COM

PENNSYLVANIA CLAIMS OFFICE
344 RTE 9 W
PO BOX 656
ALBANY, NY 12201-0656
TEL: (518) 431-5000
FAX: (518) 431-5977
TOLL FREE: (800) 948-3276
WWW.FARMFAMILY.COM

RHODE ISLAND CLAIMS OFFICE
344 RTE 9 W
PO BOX 656
ALBANY, NY 12201-0656
TEL: (518) 431-5000
FAX: (518) 431-5977
TOLL FREE: (800) 948-3276
WWW.FARMFAMILY.COM

VERMONT CLAIMS OFFICE
344 RTE 9 W
PO BOX 656
ALBANY, NY 12201-0656
TEL: (518) 431-5000
FAX: (518) 431-5977
TOLL FREE: (800) 948-3276
WWW.FARMFAMILY.COM

VIRGINIA CLAIMS OFFICE
344 RTE 9 W
PO BOX 656
ALBANY, NY 12201-0656
TEL: (518) 431-5000
FAX: (518) 431-5977
TOLL FREE: (800) 948-3276
WWW.FARMFAMILY.COM

FARM FAMILY CASUALTY INSURANCE

NEW YORK CLAIMS OFFICE
41 LIBERTY ST, STE 1
BATAVIA, NY 14020
TEL: (716) 343-5010
FAX: (716) 343-8197
TOLL FREE: (800) 544-5010

FARMERS ALLIANCE MUTUAL INSURANCE CO

COLORADO CLAIMS OFFICE
1122 N MAIN
PO BOX 1401
MC PHERSON, KS 67460-1401
TEL: (316) 241-2200
FAX: (316) 241-5482
TOLL FREE: (800) 362-1075
WWW.FAMI.COM

IDAHO CLAIMS OFFICE
1122 N MAIN
PO BOX 1401
MC PHERSON, KS 67460-1401
TEL: (316) 241-2200
FAX: (316) 241-5482
TOLL FREE: (800) 362-1075
WWW.FAMI.COM

KANSAS CLAIMS OFFICE
1122 N MAIN
PO BOX 1401
MC PHERSON, KS 67460-1401
TEL: (316) 241-2200
FAX: (316) 241-5482
TOLL FREE: (800) 362-1075
WWW.FAMI.COM

MINNESOTA CLAIMS OFFICE
1122 N MAIN
PO BOX 1401
MC PHERSON, KS 67460-1401
TEL: (316) 241-2200
FAX: (316) 241-5482
TOLL FREE: (800) 362-1075
WWW.FAMI.COM

MISSOURI CLAIMS OFFICE
1122 N MAIN
PO BOX 1401
MC PHERSON, KS 67460-1401
TEL: (316) 241-2200
FAX: (316) 241-5482
TOLL FREE: (800) 362-1075
WWW.FAMI.COM

MONTANA CLAIMS OFFICE
1122 N MAIN
PO BOX 1401
MC PHERSON, KS 67460-1401
TEL: (316) 241-2200
FAX: (316) 241-5482
TOLL FREE: (800) 362-1075
WWW.FAMI.COM

NEBRASKA CLAIMS OFFICE
1122 N MAIN
PO BOX 1401
MC PHERSON, KS 67460-1401
TEL: (316) 241-2200
FAX: (316) 241-5482
TOLL FREE: (800) 362-1075
WWW.FAMI.COM

NEW MEXICO CLAIMS OFFICE
1122 N MAIN
PO BOX 1401
MC PHERSON, KS 67460-1401
TEL: (316) 241-2200
FAX: (316) 241-5482
TOLL FREE: (800) 362-1075
WWW.FAMI.COM

NORTH DAKOTA CLAIMS OFFICE
1122 N MAIN
PO BOX 1401
MC PHERSON, KS 67460-1401
TEL: (316) 241-2200
FAX: (316) 241-5482
TOLL FREE: (800) 362-1075
WWW.FAMI.COM

OKLAHOMA CLAIMS OFFICE
1122 N MAIN
PO BOX 1401
MC PHERSON, KS 67460-1401
TEL: (316) 241-2200
FAX: (316) 241-5482
TOLL FREE: (800) 362-1075
WWW.FAMI.COM

SOUTH CAROLINA CLAIMS OFFICE
1122 N MAIN
PO BOX 1401
MC PHERSON, KS 67460-1401
TEL: (316) 241-2200
FAX: (316) 241-5482
TOLL FREE: (800) 362-1075
WWW.FAMI.COM

FARMERS AUTO INSURANCE ASSOCIATION

ILLINOIS CLAIMS OFFICE
PEKIN INSURANCE CO
2505 COURT ST
PO BOX 129
PEKIN, IL 61558-0001
TEL: (309) 346-1161
FAX: (309) 346-8265
TOLL FREE: (800) 322-0160
WWW.PEKININSURANCE.COM

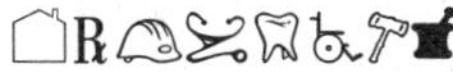

INDIANA CLAIMS OFFICE
PEKIN INSURANCE CO
2505 COURT ST
PO BOX 129
PEKIN, IL 61558-0001
TEL: (309) 346-1161
FAX: (309) 346-8265
TOLL FREE: (800) 322-0160
WWW.PEKININSURANCE.COM

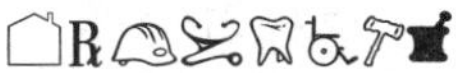

IOWA CLAIMS OFFICE
PEKIN INSURANCE CO
2505 COURT ST
PO BOX 129
PEKIN, IL 61558-0001
TEL: (309) 346-1161
FAX: (309) 346-8265
TOLL FREE: (800) 322-0160
WWW.PEKININSURANCE.COM

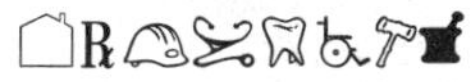

WISCONSIN CLAIMS OFFICE
PEKIN INSURANCE CO
2505 COURT ST
PO BOX 129
PEKIN, IL 61558-0001
TEL: (309) 346-1161
FAX: (309) 346-8265
TOLL FREE: (800) 322-0160
WWW.PEKININSURANCE.COM

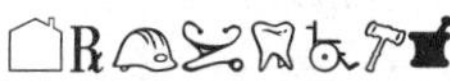

FARMERS CASUALTY INSURANCE CO

IOWA CLAIMS OFFICE
1300 WOODLAND AVE
PO BOX 65150
WEST DES MOINES, IA 50265-0150
TEL: (515) 223-9438
FAX: (515) 223-8065
TOLL FREE: (800) 666-3226

KANSAS CLAIMS OFFICE
1300 WOODLAND AVE
PO BOX 65150
WEST DES MOINES, IA 50265-0150
TEL: (515) 223-9438
FAX: (515) 223-8065
TOLL FREE: (800) 666-3226

FARMERS HOME GROUP

ARIZONA CLAIMS OFFICE
1550 E 78TH ST
PO BOX 9420
MINNEAPOLIS, MN 55440-9420
TEL: (612) 861-4511
FAX: (612) 861-2147

4568 S HIGHLAND DR
PO BOX 17347
SALT LAKE CITY, UT 84117
TEL: (801) 272-6161
FAX: (801) 272-1066
TOLL FREE: (800) 726-3496

CALIFORNIA CLAIMS OFFICE
1550 E 78TH ST
PO BOX 9420
MINNEAPOLIS, MN 55440-9420
TEL: (612) 861-4511
FAX: (612) 861-2147

4568 S HIGHLAND DR
PO BOX 17347
SALT LAKE CITY, UT 84117
TEL: (801) 272-6161
FAX: (801) 272-1066
TOLL FREE: (800) 726-3496

IDAHO CLAIMS OFFICE
1550 E 78TH ST
PO BOX 9420
MINNEAPOLIS, MN 55440-9420
TEL: (612) 861-4511
FAX: (612) 861-2147

4568 S HIGHLAND DR
PO BOX 17347
SALT LAKE CITY, UT 84117
TEL: (801) 272-6161
FAX: (801) 272-1066
TOLL FREE: (800) 726-3496

MINNESOTA CLAIMS OFFICE
1550 E 78TH ST
PO BOX 9420
MINNEAPOLIS, MN 55440-9420
TEL: (612) 861-4511
FAX: (612) 861-2147

4568 S HIGHLAND DR
PO BOX 17347
SALT LAKE CITY, UT 84117
TEL: (801) 272-6161
FAX: (801) 272-1066
TOLL FREE: (800) 726-3496

NATIONAL CLAIMS OFFICE
3021 W MAGNOLIA BLVD
PO BOX 7129
BURBANK, CA 91510
TEL: (818) 843-5550
FAX: (818) 843-2760
TOLL FREE: (800) 660-0605

NEVADA CLAIMS OFFICE
4568 S HIGHLAND DR
PO BOX 17347
SALT LAKE CITY, UT 84117
TEL: (801) 272-6161
FAX: (801) 272-1066
TOLL FREE: (800) 726-3496

NORTH CAROLINA CLAIMS OFFICE
4568 S HIGHLAND DR
PO BOX 17347
SALT LAKE CITY, UT 84117
TEL: (801) 272-6161
FAX: (801) 272-1066
TOLL FREE: (800) 726-3496

NORTH DAKOTA CLAIMS OFFICE
1550 E 78TH ST
PO BOX 9420
MINNEAPOLIS, MN 55440-9420
TEL: (612) 861-4511
FAX: (612) 861-2147

OREGON CLAIMS OFFICE
4568 S HIGHLAND DR
PO BOX 17347
SALT LAKE CITY, UT 84117
TEL: (801) 272-6161
FAX: (801) 272-1066
TOLL FREE: (800) 726-3496

SOUTH DAKOTA CLAIMS OFFICE
1550 E 78TH ST
PO BOX 9420
MINNEAPOLIS, MN 55440-9420
TEL: (612) 861-4511
FAX: (612) 861-2147

UTAH CLAIMS OFFICE
4568 S HIGHLAND DR
PO BOX 17347
SALT LAKE CITY, UT 84117
TEL: (801) 272-6161
FAX: (801) 272-1066
TOLL FREE: (800) 726-3496

1550 E 78TH ST
PO BOX 9420
MINNEAPOLIS, MN 55440-9420
TEL: (612) 861-4511
FAX: (612) 861-2147

WASHINGTON CLAIMS OFFICE
4568 S HIGHLAND DR
PO BOX 17347
SALT LAKE CITY, UT 84117
TEL: (801) 272-6161
FAX: (801) 272-1066
TOLL FREE: (800) 726-3496

WYOMING CLAIMS OFFICE
4568 S HIGHLAND DR
PO BOX 17347
SALT LAKE CITY, UT 84117
TEL: (801) 272-6161
FAX: (801) 272-1066
TOLL FREE: (800) 726-3496

FARMERS INSURANCE EXCHANGE

NATIONAL CLAIMS OFFICE
PO BOX 9075
VAN NUYS, CA 91409
TEL: (805) 583-7400
FAX: (805) 526-4573

F

FARMERS INSURANCE GROUP

ARIZONA CLAIMS OFFICE
SALT LAKE CITY SOUTH BRANCH CLAIMS
9135 S REDWOOD RD
PO BOX 95530
SOUTH JORDAN, UT 84095
TEL: (801) 566-0054
FAX: (801) 352-0310

CALIFORNIA CLAIMS OFFICE
PO BOX 10149
VAN NUYS, CA 91410-0149
TEL: (805) 583-7567
FAX: (805) 583-7467
WWW.FARMERSINSURANCE.COM

SALT LAKE CITY SOUTH BRANCH CLAIMS
9135 S REDWOOD RD
PO BOX 95530
SOUTH JORDAN, UT 84095
TEL: (801) 566-0054
FAX: (801) 352-0310

COLORADO CLAIMS OFFICE
SALT LAKE CITY SOUTH BRANCH CLAIMS
9135 S REDWOOD RD
PO BOX 95530
SOUTH JORDAN, UT 84095
TEL: (801) 566-0054
FAX: (801) 352-0310

IDAHO CLAIMS OFFICE
SALT LAKE CITY SOUTH BRANCH CLAIMS
9135 S REDWOOD RD
PO BOX 95530
SOUTH JORDAN, UT 84095
TEL: (801) 566-0054
FAX: (801) 352-0310

NATIONAL CLAIMS OFFICE
PO BOX 3887
MERCED, CA 95344-3887
TEL: (209) 383-5333
FAX: (209) 383-5955

SALT LAKE CITY NORTH BRANCH CLAIMS
1485 E 3900 S
PO BOX 17357
SALT LAKE CITY, UT 84117-0357
TEL: (801) 272-8081
FAX: (801) 278-7949

4680 WILSHIRE BLVD
PO BOX 2478
LOS ANGELES, CA 90051-0478
TEL: (323) 932-3200

NEVADA CLAIMS OFFICE
SALT LAKE CITY SOUTH BRANCH CLAIMS
9135 S REDWOOD RD
PO BOX 95530
SOUTH JORDAN, UT 84095
TEL: (801) 566-0054
FAX: (801) 352-0310

UTAH CLAIMS OFFICE
PO BOX 9756
OGDEN, UT 84409
TEL: (801) 394-5706
FAX: (801) 393-8567

1180 S 800 E
PO BOX 970 430
OREM, UT 84097
TEL: (801) 224-0166
FAX: (801) 224-1639
IN-STATE: (800) 258-0203

SALT LAKE CITY SOUTH BRANCH CLAIMS
9135 S REDWOOD RD
PO BOX 95530
SOUTH JORDAN, UT 84095
TEL: (801) 566-0054
FAX: (801) 352-0310

WASHINGTON CLAIMS OFFICE
SALT LAKE CITY SOUTH BRANCH CLAIMS
9135 S REDWOOD RD
PO BOX 95530
SOUTH JORDAN, UT 84095
TEL: (801) 566-0054
FAX: (801) 352-0310

WYOMING CLAIMS OFFICE
SALT LAKE CITY SOUTH BRANCH CLAIMS
9135 S REDWOOD RD
PO BOX 95530
SOUTH JORDAN, UT 84095
TEL: (801) 566-0054
FAX: (801) 352-0310

FARMINGTON MEDICAL ASSOCIATES

NATIONAL CLAIMS OFFICE
260 OCOHITIOTE RD
FRAMINGHAM, MA 01701
TEL: (508) 879-0077
TOLL FREE: (800) 458-4929

H

FARMLAND INSURANCE CO

PO BOX 2660
BLOOMINGTON, IL 61702-2660
TEL: (309) 662-0491
FAX: (309) 663-0242
IN-STATE: (800) 322-9351

PO BOX 2650
HUTCHINSON, KS 67504-2650
TEL: (316) 663-6011
FAX: (316) 663-9459
TOLL FREE: (800) 499-6011

PO BOX 3125
MANKATO, MN 56002-3125
TEL: (507) 387-3161
FAX: (507) 387-1499
TOLL FREE: (800) 301-0298

TEXAS CLAIMS OFFICE
PO BOX 15445
AMARILLO, TX 79105-5445
TEL: (806) 358-8795
FAX: (806) 358-3727

FARMLAND MUTUAL

IOWA CLAIMS OFFICE
1620 S 70TH
PO BOX 6065
LINCOLN, NE 68506-0065
TEL: (402) 489-8292
FAX: (402) 489-8255
TOLL FREE: (800) 536-7594

NEBRASKA CLAIMS OFFICE
1620 S 70TH
PO BOX 6065
LINCOLN, NE 68506-0065
TEL: (402) 489-8292
FAX: (402) 489-8255
TOLL FREE: (800) 536-7594

WYOMING CLAIMS OFFICE
1620 S 70TH
PO BOX 6065
LINCOLN, NE 68506-0065
TEL: (402) 489-8292
FAX: (402) 489-8255
TOLL FREE: (800) 536-7594

FARMLAND MUTUAL/ NATIONWIDE AGRA BUSINESS

NATIONAL CLAIMS OFFICE
1963 BELL AVE
DES MOINES, IA 50315-1000
TEL: (515) 245-8800
FAX: (515) 245-4005
TOLL FREE: (800) 247-2484

FBD CONSULTING, INC

KANSAS CLAIMS OFFICE
5101 COLLEGE BLVD, STE 100
LEAWOOD, KS 66211
TEL: (913) 319-8800
FAX: (913) 319-8902
TOLL FREE: (800) 969-4015
WWW.FBDCONSULT.COM

FEDERAL EXPRESS CORP

NATIONAL CLAIMS OFFICE
4009 AIRWAYS BLVD
PO BOX 727
MEMPHIS, TN 38194-9326
TEL: (901) 397-4800
FAX: (901) 397-4136
TOLL FREE: (800) 525-4478

FEDERATED AMERICAN INSURANCE CO

WASHINGTON CLAIMS OFFICE
15805 NE 24TH ST
PO BOX 90701
BELLEVUE, WA 98009-0701
TEL: (206) 364-6010
FAX: (206) 365-6116
TOLL FREE: (800) 562-6565

F

FEDERATED GUARANTY LIFE INSURANCE COMPANIES

ALABAMA CLAIMS OFFICE
ALPHA MUTUAL INSURANCE COMPANIES
2108 E S BLVD
PO BOX 11000
MONTGOMERY, AL 36191-0001
TEL: (334) 288-3900
FAX: (334) 288-0905
IN-STATE: (800) 392-5705

GEORGIA CLAIMS OFFICE
ALPHA MUTUAL INSURANCE COMPANIES
2108 E S BLVD
PO BOX 11000
MONTGOMERY, AL 36191-0001
TEL: (334) 288-3900
FAX: (334) 228-0905
IN-STATE: (800) 392-5705

MISSISSIPPI CLAIMS OFFICE
ALPHA MUTUAL INSURANCE COMPANIES
2108 E S BLVD
PO BOX 11000
MONTGOMERY, AL 36191-0001
TEL: (334) 288-3900
FAX: (334) 228-0905
IN-STATE: (800) 392-5705

FEDERATED MUTUAL INSURANCE CO

ALABAMA CLAIMS OFFICE
2701 N ROCKY PT DR, STE 1200
PO BOX 31716
TAMPA, FL 33631-3716
TEL: (813) 287-0155
FAX: (813) 287-0785
IN-STATE: (800) 237-8292
WWW.FEDERATEDINS.COM

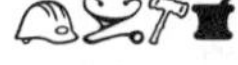

ARIZONA CLAIMS OFFICE
2400 W DUNLAP AVE, STE 250
PO BOX 35910
PHOENIX, AZ 85021
TEL: (602) 944-5566
FAX: (602) 943-6020

CALIFORNIA CLAIMS OFFICE
11050 OLSON DR, STE 100
PO BOX 3150
RANCHO CORDOVA, CA 95741
TEL: (916) 631-0345
FAX: (916) 631-0275
TOLL FREE: (800) 423-1842

FLORIDA CLAIMS OFFICE
2701 N ROCKY PT DR, STE 1200
PO BOX 31716
TAMPA, FL 33631-3716
TEL: (813) 287-0155
FAX: (813) 287-0785
IN-STATE: (800) 237-8292
WWW.FEDERATEDINS.COM

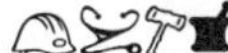

GEORGIA CLAIMS OFFICE
2701 N ROCKY PT DR, STE 1200
PO BOX 31716
TAMPA, FL 33631-3716
TEL: (813) 287-0155
FAX: (813) 287-0785
IN-STATE: (800) 237-8292
WWW.FEDERATEDINS.COM

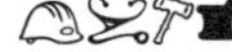

IOWA CLAIMS OFFICE
5000 W TOWN T PARKWAY, STE 240
PO BOX 65509
WEST DES MOINES, IA 50265
TEL: (515) 225-6661
FAX: (515) 225-3768
TOLL FREE: (800) 247-4004

MISSISSIPPI CLAIMS OFFICE
2701 N ROCKY PT DR, STE 1200
PO BOX 31716
TAMPA, FL 33631-3716
TEL: (813) 287-0155
FAX: (813) 287-0785
IN-STATE: (800) 237-8292
WWW.FEDERATEDINS.COM

NATIONAL CLAIMS OFFICE
PO BOX 28477
ATLANTA, GA 30358-0477
TEL: (404) 257-1511
FAX: (800) 416-0027
TOLL FREE: (800) 241-4945

8060 KNUE RD
PO BOX 50487
INDIANAPOLIS, IN 46250-0487
TEL: (317) 849-7550
FAX: (317) 845-8841
TOLL FREE: (800) 428-4143

8060 KNUE RD, STE 200
PO BOX 50487
INDIANAPOLIS, IN 46250-0487
FAX: (810) 643-7981
TOLL FREE: (800) 541-3612

78700 FRANCE
PO BOX 390850
EDINA, MN 55439-0850
TEL: (612) 831-4300
FAX: (612) 820-2387
TOLL FREE: (800) 328-9291

PO BOX 328
OWATONNA, MN 55060
TEL: (507) 455-5200
TOLL FREE: (800) 533-0472

10895 LOWELL
PO BOX 419444
KANSAS CITY, MO 64141
TEL: (913) 451-1962
FAX: (913) 451-1875
TOLL FREE: (800) 445-0109

PO BOX 50487
INDIANAPOLIS, IN 46250-0487
TEL: (317) 849-7550
FAX: (317) 845-8841
TOLL FREE: (800) 428-4143

PO BOX 305129
NASHVILLE, TN 37214
TEL: (615) 391-4139
FAX: (615) 391-4618
TOLL FREE: (800) 338-5568

PO BOX 328
OWATONNA, MN 55060
TEL: (507) 455-5200
FAX: (507) 455-5452
TOLL FREE: (800) 533-0472
WWW.FEDERATEDINSURANCE.COM

NEVADA CLAIMS OFFICE
11050 OLSON DR, STE 100
PO BOX 3150
RANCHO CORDOVA, CA 95741
TEL: (916) 631-0345
FAX: (916) 631-0275
TOLL FREE: (800) 423-1842

NORTH CAROLINA CLAIMS OFFICE
2701 N ROCKY PT DR, STE 1200
PO BOX 31716
TAMPA, FL 33631-3716
TEL: (813) 287-0155
FAX: (813) 287-0785
IN-STATE: (800) 237-8292
WWW.FEDERATEDINS.COM

SOUTH CAROLINA CLAIMS OFFICE
2701 N ROCKY PT DR, STE 1200
PO BOX 31716
TAMPA, FL 33631-3716
TEL: (813) 287-0155
FAX: (813) 287-0785
IN-STATE: (800) 237-8292
WWW.FEDERATEDINS.COM

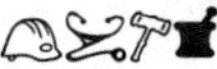

TENNESSEE CLAIMS OFFICE
2701 N ROCKY PT DR, STE 1200
PO BOX 31716
TAMPA, FL 33631-3716
TEL: (813) 287-0155
FAX: (813) 287-0785
IN-STATE: (800) 237-8292
WWW.FEDERATEDINS.COM

TEXAS CLAIMS OFFICE
860 AIRPORT FWY W, STE 500
PO BOX 1548
HURST, TX 76053-1548
TEL: (817) 581-7111
FAX: (817) 581-2970
TOLL FREE: (800) 633-6040

VIRGINIA CLAIMS OFFICE
2701 N ROCKY PT DR, STE 1200
PO BOX 31716
TAMPA, FL 33631-3716
TEL: (813) 287-0155
FAX: (813) 287-0785
IN-STATE: (800) 237-8292
WWW.FEDERATEDINS.COM

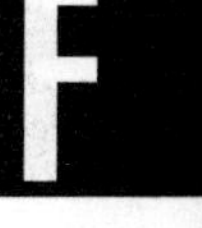

FEWELL & ASSOCIATES AMERICAN INVESTORS

ARKANSAS CLAIMS OFFICE
PO BOX 8212
LITTLE ROCK, AR 72221-8212
TEL: (501) 227-6660
FAX: (501) 227-4430
TOLL FREE: (800) 467-0028

FIC INSURANCE

NATIONAL CLAIMS OFFICE
FINANCIAL INDUSTRY CORP INSURANCE
701 BRAZOS ST, STE 1400
PO BOX 149138
AUSTIN, TX 78714-9138
TEL: (512) 404-5000
FAX: (512) 404-5210
TOLL FREE: (800) 925-6000
IN-STATE: (800) 925-6000
WWW.FICGROUP.COM

F

FIDELIO INSURANCE CO

MARYLAND CLAIMS OFFICE
2826 MT CARMEL AVE
GLENSIDE, PA 19038-2245
TEL: (215) 885-2443
FAX: (215) 576-5849
IN-STATE: (800) 262-4949

NEW JERSEY CLAIMS OFFICE
2826 MT CARMEL AVE
GLENSIDE, PA 19038-2245
TEL: (215) 885-2443
FAX: (215) 576-5849
IN-STATE: (800) 262-4949

NEW YORK CLAIMS OFFICE
2826 MT CARMEL AVE
GLENSIDE, PA 19038-2245
TEL: (215) 885-2443
FAX: (215) 576-5849
IN-STATE: (800) 262-4949

PENNSYLVANIA CLAIMS OFFICE
2826 MT CARMEL AVE
GLENSIDE, PA 19038-2245
TEL: (215) 885-2443
FAX: (215) 576-5849
IN-STATE: (800) 262-4949

FIDELITY & DEPOSIT CO OF MARYLAND

NATIONAL CLAIMS OFFICE
210 N CHARLES ST
PO BOX 1227
BALTIMORE, MD 21203-4098
TEL: (410) 539-0800
FAX: (800) 626-2508
TOLL FREE: (800) 626-2508

FIDELITY SECURITY LIFE INSURANCE CO

PO BOX 418131
KANSAS CITY, MO 64141-9131
TEL: (816) 756-1060
FAX: (816) 968-0560
TOLL FREE: (800) 821-7303

FINANCIAL BENEFIT, INC

IOWA CLAIMS OFFICE
PO BOX 13163
KANSAS CITY, MO 64199-3163
TEL: (816) 842-2081
FAX: (816) 842-2081

KANSAS CLAIMS OFFICE
PO BOX 13163
KANSAS CITY, MO 64199-3163
TEL: (816) 842-2081
FAX: (816) 842-2081

MISSOURI CLAIMS OFFICE
PO BOX 13163
KANSAS CITY, MO 64199-3163
TEL: (816) 842-2081
FAX: (816) 842-2081

NEBRASKA CLAIMS OFFICE
PO BOX 13163
KANSAS CITY, MO 64199-3163
TEL: (816) 842-2081
FAX: (816) 842-2081

FINANCIAL INDEMNITY CO

ARIZONA CLAIMS OFFICE
21650 OXNARD ST, STE 1800
PO BOX 10360
WOODLAND HILLS, CA 91410-0360
TEL: (818) 313-8500
FAX: (818) 340-3587
TOLL FREE: (800) 777-4342

CALIFORNIA CLAIMS OFFICE
21650 OXNARD ST, STE 1800
PO BOX 10360
WOODLAND HILLS, CA 91410-0360
TEL: (818) 313-8500
FAX: (818) 340-3587
TOLL FREE: (800) 777-4342

COLORADO CLAIMS OFFICE
21650 OXNARD ST, STE 1800
PO BOX 10360
WOODLAND HILLS, CA 91410-0360
TEL: (818) 313-8500
FAX: (818) 340-3587
TOLL FREE: (800) 777-4342

IDAHO CLAIMS OFFICE
21650 OXNARD ST, STE 1800
PO BOX 10360
WOODLAND HILLS, CA 91410-0360
TEL: (818) 313-8500
FAX: (818) 340-3587
TOLL FREE: (800) 777-4342

KANSAS CLAIMS OFFICE
21650 OXNARD ST, STE 1800
PO BOX 10360
WOODLAND HILLS, CA 91410-0360
TEL: (818) 313-8500
FAX: (818) 340-3587
TOLL FREE: (800) 777-4342

LOUISIANA CLAIMS OFFICE
21650 OXNARD ST, STE 1800
PO BOX 10360
WOODLAND HILLS, CA 91410-0360
TEL: (818) 313-8500
FAX: (818) 340-3587
TOLL FREE: (800) 777-4342

NEVADA CLAIMS OFFICE
21650 OXNARD ST, STE 1800
PO BOX 10360
WOODLAND HILLS, CA 91410-0360
TEL: (818) 313-8500
FAX: (818) 340-3587
TOLL FREE: (800) 777-4342

OKLAHOMA CLAIMS OFFICE
21650 OXNARD ST, STE 1800
PO BOX 10360
WOODLAND HILLS, CA 91410-0360
TEL: (818) 313-8500
FAX: (818) 340-3587
TOLL FREE: (800) 777-4342

SOUTH DAKOTA CLAIMS OFFICE
21650 OXNARD ST, STE 1800
PO BOX 10360
WOODLAND HILLS, CA 91410-0360
TEL: (818) 313-8500
FAX: (818) 340-3587
TOLL FREE: (800) 777-4342

UTAH CLAIMS OFFICE
21650 OXNARD ST, STE 1800
PO BOX 10360
WOODLAND HILLS, CA 91410-0360
TEL: (818) 313-8500
FAX: (818) 340-3587
TOLL FREE: (800) 777-4342

WASHINGTON CLAIMS OFFICE
21650 OXNARD ST, STE 1800
PO BOX 10360
WOODLAND HILLS, CA 91410-0360
TEL: (818) 313-8500
FAX: (818) 340-3587
TOLL FREE: (800) 777-4342

WYOMING CLAIMS OFFICE
21650 OXNARD ST, STE 1800
PO BOX 10360
WOODLAND HILLS, CA 91410-0360
TEL: (818) 313-8500
FAX: (818) 340-3587
TOLL FREE: (800) 777-4342

FINANCIAL INSURANCE CENTER

NATIONAL CLAIMS OFFICE
UNION FIDELITY OFC PRK
TREVOSE, PA 19049-6511
TEL: (215) 953-3000
FAX: (215) 953-4494
TOLL FREE: (800) 626-6557

FIRE & CASUALTY INSURANCE CO OF CONNECTICUT

9 FARM SPGS RD
PO BOX 4310
FARMINGTON, CT 06032
TEL: (860) 674-6600
FAX: (860) 674-6797
TOLL FREE: (800) 243-7060
WWW.ORIONCAPITAL.COM

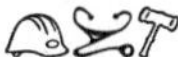

FIREMAN'S FUND INSURANCE CO

ALASKA CLAIMS OFFICE
2995 PROSPECT PARK DR
RANCHO CORDOVA, CA 95670
TEL: (916) 852-4500
FAX: (916) 852-4536
TOLL FREE: (800) 852-7212

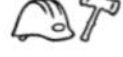

ARIZONA CLAIMS OFFICE
2995 PROSPECT PARK DR
RANCHO CORDOVA, CA 95670
TEL: (916) 852-4500
FAX: (916) 852-4536
TOLL FREE: (800) 852-7212

CALIFORNIA CLAIMS OFFICE
SPEARE TWR, 11TH FL
PO BOX 193136
SAN FRANCISCO, CA 94119
TEL: (415) 777-9900
FAX: (415) 541-4560
TOLL FREE: (800) 227-1700
IN-STATE: (800) 553-8205
WWW.THE-FUND.COM

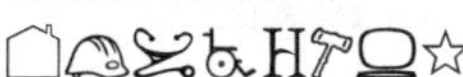

NWRCCC
PO BOX 808036
PETALUMA, CA 94975-8036
TEL: (415) 899-4700
FAX: (415) 899-4087
TOLL FREE: (800) 825-8607
WWW.THE'FUND.COM

2995 PROSPECT PARK DR
RANCHO CORDOVA, CA 95670
TEL: (916) 852-4500
FAX: (916) 852-4536
TOLL FREE: (800) 852-7212

6300 CANOGA AVE
PO BOX 9304
VAN NUYS, CA 91409-9304
TEL: (818) 703-8110
FAX: (818) 715-7311
TOLL FREE: (800) 543-3979

195 SCOTT SWAMP RD
PO BOX 4049
FARMINGTON, CT 06034-4049
TEL: (860) 677-3500
FAX: (800) 448-9733
TOLL FREE: (800) 446-1677

COLORADO CLAIMS OFFICE
2995 PROSPECT PARK DR
RANCHO CORDOVA, CA 95670
TEL: (916) 852-4500
FAX: (916) 852-4536
TOLL FREE: (800) 852-7212

CONNECTICUT CLAIMS OFFICE
195 SCOTT SWAMP RD
PO BOX 4049
FARMINGTON, CT 06034-4049
TEL: (860) 677-3500
FAX: (800) 448-9733
TOLL FREE: (800) 446-1677

PO BOX 26705
GREENSBORO, NC 27407-6705
TEL: (336) 855-9113
FAX: (336) 856-6078
TOLL FREE: (800) 222-3701
WWW.FFUND.COM

DELAWARE CLAIMS OFFICE
PO BOX 26705
GREENSBORO, NC 27407-6705
TEL: (336) 855-9113
FAX: (336) 856-6078
TOLL FREE: (800) 222-3701
WWW.FFUND.COM

FLORIDA CLAIMS OFFICE
5310 CYPRESS CENTER DR
PO BOX 18025
TAMPA, FL 33679-8025
TEL: (813) 287-3000
FAX: (813) 287-3288
IN-STATE: (800) 282-2711

PO BOX 26705
GREENSBORO, NC 27407-6705
TEL: (336) 855-9113
FAX: (336) 856-6078
TOLL FREE: (800) 222-3701
WWW.FFUND.COM

GEORGIA CLAIMS OFFICE
PO BOX 26705
GREENSBORO, NC 27407-6705
TEL: (336) 855-9113
FAX: (336) 856-6078
TOLL FREE: (800) 222-3701
WWW.FFUND.COM

HAWAII CLAIMS OFFICE
1001 BISHOP ST- PAUAHI TWR, STE 1900
PO BOX 2079
HONOLULU, HI 96805-2079
TEL: (808) 523-6500
FAX: (808) 523-6586
IN-STATE: (800) 272-3391

ILLINOIS CLAIMS OFFICE
PO BOX 26705
GREENSBORO, NC 27407-6705
TEL: (336) 855-9113
FAX: (336) 856-6078
TOLL FREE: (800) 222-3701
WWW.FFUND.COM

INDIANA CLAIMS OFFICE
PO BOX 26705
GREENSBORO, NC 27407-6705
TEL: (336) 855-9113
FAX: (336) 856-6078
TOLL FREE: (800) 222-3701
WWW.FFUND.COM

IOWA CLAIMS OFFICE
PO BOX 26705
GREENSBORO, NC 27407-6705
TEL: (336) 855-9113
FAX: (336) 856-6078
TOLL FREE: (800) 222-3701
WWW.FFUND.COM

MAINE CLAIMS OFFICE
PO BOX 26705
GREENSBORO, NC 27407-6705
TEL: (336) 855-9113
FAX: (336) 856-6078
TOLL FREE: (800) 222-3701
WWW.FFUND.COM

MARYLAND CLAIMS OFFICE
9690 DEERECO RD
TIMONIUM, MD 21093
TEL: (410) 560-4600
FAX: (410) 560-4653
IN-STATE: (800) 492-4758

PO BOX 26705
GREENSBORO, NC 27407-6705
TEL: (336) 855-9113
FAX: (336) 856-6078
TOLL FREE: (800) 222-3701
WWW.FFUND.COM

727 CRAIG RD
PO BOX 419083
SAINT LOUIS, MO 63141-9083
TEL: (314) 569-7800
FAX: (800) 343-0589
TOLL FREE: (800) 222-8062

1100 WALNUT, STE 3000
PO BOX 13206
KANSAS CITY, MO 64199-3206
TEL: (816) 556-9200
FAX: (816) 556-9357
TOLL FREE: (800) 552-8028
IN-STATE: (800) 892-7678

195 SCOTT SWAMP RD
PO BOX 4049
FARMINGTON, CT 06034-4049
TEL: (860) 677-3500
FAX: (800) 448-9733
TOLL FREE: (800) 446-1677

F

MASSACHUSETTS CLAIMS OFFICE
JOHN HANCOCK TOWER
BOSTON, MA 02117
TEL: (617) 236-5200
FAX: (617) 375-3760
TOLL FREE: (800) 647-7011

PO BOX 26705
GREENSBORO, NC 27407-6705
TEL: (336) 855-9113
FAX: (336) 856-6078
TOLL FREE: (800) 222-3701
WWW.FFUND.COM

MISSOURI CLAIMS OFFICE
1100 WALNUT, STE 3000
PO BOX 13206
KANSAS CITY, MO 64199-3206
TEL: (816) 556-9200
FAX: (816) 556-9357
TOLL FREE: (800) 552-8028
IN-STATE: (800) 892-7678

727 CRAIG RD
PO BOX 419083
SAINT LOUIS, MO 63141-9083
TEL: (314) 569-7800
FAX: (800) 343-0589
TOLL FREE: (800) 222-8062

9690 DEERECO RD
TIMONIUM, MD 21093
TEL: (410) 560-4600
FAX: (410) 560-4653
IN-STATE: (800) 492-4758

NATIONAL CLAIMS OFFICE
AMERICAN INSURANCE CO
777 SAN MARIN DR
NOVATO, CA 94998-0002
TEL: (415) 899-2000
FAX: (415) 899-3600
TOLL FREE: (800) 227-1700
WWW.THE-FUND.COM

3400 RIVERSIDE DR, STE 300
PO BOX 7780
BURBANK, CA 91510
TEL: (818) 972-8000
FAX: (818) 972-8533
TOLL FREE: (800) 221-5490

777 SAN MARIN DR
NOVATO, CA 94998
TEL: (415) 899-2000
FAX: (415) 899-3600

SOUTHERN STATES REGIONAL WC CENTER
11605 HAYNES BRIDGE RD
PO BOX 740174
ATLANTA, GA 30374
TEL: (678) 393-4067
FAX: (678) 393-4100
TOLL FREE: (800) 282-6351

PO BOX 8217
LITTLE ROCK, AR 72221-8217
TEL: (501) 228-1000
FAX: (501) 228-1003
TOLL FREE: (800) 367-8421
IN-STATE: (800) 482-9346

PO BOX 50550
ONTARIO, CA 91761-1055
TEL: (909) 605-9696
FAX: (909) 975-6080
TOLL FREE: (800) 544-5343

PO BOX 193136
SAN FRANCISCO, CA 94119-3136
TEL: (415) 777-9900
FAX: (415) 541-4242
TOLL FREE: (800) 553-8205
WWW.THE-FUND.COM

17542 E 17TH ST
PO BOX 1975
SANTA ANA, CA 92702-1975
TEL: (714) 669-0911
FAX: (714) 669-7581
IN-STATE: (800) 422-2036

7887 E BELLVIEW
ENGLEWOOD, CO 80111
TEL: (303) 224-5000
FAX: (303) 224-5173

233 S WACKER DR, STE 2000
CHICAGO, IL 60606-6308
TEL: (312) 441-5400
FAX: (312) 441-6260
TOLL FREE: (800) 544-9358
WWW.THE-FUND.COM

PO BOX 9431
MINNETONKA, MN 55440-9431
TEL: (612) 546-8421
FAX: (612) 541-8223
TOLL FREE: (800) 742-0510

538 BROAD HOLLOW RD
MELVILLE, NY 11747
TOLL FREE: (800) 582-1998

7887 E BELLEVIEW AVE, STE 300
ENGLEWOOD, CO 80111
TEL: (303) 224-5000
FAX: (800) 622-7630
TOLL FREE: (800) 432-5158

101 SW MAINE, STE 710
PO BOX 3825
PORTLAND, OR 97208
TEL: (503) 226-3761
FAX: (503) 778-2309

PO BOX 650594
DALLAS, TX 75265-0594
TEL: (214) 220-4000
FAX: (214) 220-4153
TOLL FREE: (800) 442-7090

NEVADA CLAIMS OFFICE
2995 PROSPECT PARK DR
RANCHO CORDOVA, CA 95670
TEL: (916) 852-4500
FAX: (916) 852-4536
TOLL FREE: (800) 852-7212

NEW HAMPSHIRE CLAIMS OFFICE
PO BOX 26705
GREENSBORO, NC 27407-6705
TEL: (336) 855-9113
FAX: (336) 856-6078
TOLL FREE: (800) 222-3701
WWW.FFUND.COM

NEW JERSEY CLAIMS OFFICE
PO BOX 26705
GREENSBORO, NC 27407-6705
TEL: (336) 855-9113
FAX: (336) 856-6078
TOLL FREE: (800) 222-3701
WWW.FFUND.COM

NEW MEXICO CLAIMS OFFICE
2995 PROSPECT PARK DR
RANCHO CORDOVA, CA 95670
TEL: (916) 852-4500
FAX: (916) 852-4536
TOLL FREE: (800) 852-7212

NEW YORK CLAIMS OFFICE
PO BOX 26705
GREENSBORO, NC 27407-6705
TEL: (336) 855-9113
FAX: (336) 856-6078
TOLL FREE: (800) 222-3701
WWW.FFUND.COM

NORTH CAROLINA CLAIMS OFFICE
PO BOX 26705
GREENSBORO, NC 27407-6705
TEL: (336) 855-9113
FAX: (336) 856-6078
TOLL FREE: (800) 222-3701
WWW.FFUND.COM

195 SCOTT SWAMP RD
PO BOX 4049
FARMINGTON, CT 06034-4049
TEL: (860) 677-3500
FAX: (800) 448-9733
TOLL FREE: (800) 446-1677

OHIO CLAIMS OFFICE
PO BOX 26705
GREENSBORO, NC 27407-6705
TEL: (336) 855-9113
FAX: (336) 856-6078
TOLL FREE: (800) 222-3701
WWW.FFUND.COM

OREGON CLAIMS OFFICE
2995 PROSPECT PARK DR
RANCHO CORDOVA, CA 95670
TEL: (916) 852-4500
FAX: (916) 852-4536
TOLL FREE: (800) 852-7212

PENNSYLVANIA CLAIMS OFFICE
PO BOX 26705
GREENSBORO, NC 27407-6705
TEL: (336) 855-9113
FAX: (336) 856-6078
TOLL FREE: (800) 222-3701
WWW.FFUND.COM

RHODE ISLAND CLAIMS OFFICE
PO BOX 26705
GREENSBORO, NC 27407-6705
TEL: (336) 855-9113
FAX: (336) 856-6078
TOLL FREE: (800) 222-3701
WWW.FFUND.COM

SOUTH CAROLINA CLAIMS OFFICE
PO BOX 26705
GREENSBORO, NC 27407-6705
TEL: (336) 855-9113
FAX: (336) 856-6078
TOLL FREE: (800) 222-3701
WWW.FFUND.COM

VERMONT CLAIMS OFFICE
PO BOX 26705
GREENSBORO, NC 27407-6705
TEL: (336) 855-9113
FAX: (336) 856-6078
TOLL FREE: (800) 222-3701
WWW.FFUND.COM

VIRGINIA CLAIMS OFFICE
PO BOX 26705
GREENSBORO, NC 27407-6705
TEL: (336) 855-9113
FAX: (336) 856-6078
TOLL FREE: (800) 222-3701
WWW.FFUND.COM

WASHINGTON CLAIMS OFFICE
2995 PROSPECT PARK DR
RANCHO CORDOVA, CA 95670
TEL: (916) 852-4500
FAX: (916) 852-4536
TOLL FREE: (800) 852-7212

2101 4TH AVE, STE 1100
SEATTLE, WA 98121-2317
TEL: (206) 728-7530
FAX: (206) 728-5236
TOLL FREE: (800) 441-3888

PO BOX 26705
GREENSBORO, NC 27407-6705
TEL: (336) 855-9113
FAX: (336) 856-6078
TOLL FREE: (800) 222-3701
WWW.FFUND.COM

WEST VIRGINIA CLAIMS OFFICE
PO BOX 26705
GREENSBORO, NC 27407-6705
TEL: (336) 855-9113
FAX: (336) 856-6078
TOLL FREE: (800) 222-3701
WWW.FFUND.COM

FIREMAN'S INSURANCE CO OF WASHINGTON, DC

DELAWARE CLAIMS OFFICE
7315 WISCONSIN AVE, STE 300 W
BETHESDA, MD 20814
TEL: (301) 941-0100
FAX: (301) 652-9809
TOLL FREE: (800) 333-4190

DISTRICT OF COLUMBIA CLAIMS OFFICE
7315 WISCONSIN AVE, STE 300 W
BETHESDA, MD 20814
TEL: (301) 941-0100
FAX: (301) 652-9809
TOLL FREE: (800) 333-4190

MARYLAND CLAIMS OFFICE
7315 WISCONSIN AVE, STE 300 W
BETHESDA, MD 20814
TEL: (301) 941-0100
FAX: (301) 652-9809
TOLL FREE: (800) 333-4190

NORTH DAKOTA CLAIMS OFFICE
7315 WISCONSIN AVE, STE 300 W
BETHESDA, MD 20814
TEL: (301) 941-0100
FAX: (301) 652-9809
TOLL FREE: (800) 333-4190

PENNSYLVANIA CLAIMS OFFICE
7315 WISCONSIN AVE, STE 300 W
BETHESDA, MD 20814
TEL: (301) 941-0100
FAX: (301) 652-9809
TOLL FREE: (800) 333-4190

VIRGINIA CLAIMS OFFICE
7315 WISCONSIN AVE, STE 300 W
BETHESDA, MD 20814
TEL: (301) 941-0100
FAX: (301) 652-9809
TOLL FREE: (800) 333-4190

FIRST AMERICAN ADMINISTRATORS

IOWA CLAIMS OFFICE
512 MAIN ST, STE 200
PO BOX 8150
RAPID CITY, SD 57709-8150
TEL: (605) 343-2509
FAX: (605) 343-8887

MINNESOTA CLAIMS OFFICE
512 MAIN ST, STE 200
PO BOX 8150
RAPID CITY, SD 57709-8150
TEL: (605) 343-2509
FAX: (605) 343-8887

MONTANA CLAIMS OFFICE
512 MAIN ST, STE 200
PO BOX 8150
RAPID CITY, SD 57709-8150
TEL: (605) 343-2509
FAX: (605) 343-8887

NEBRASKA CLAIMS OFFICE
512 MAIN ST, STE 200
PO BOX 8150
RAPID CITY, SD 57709-8150
TEL: (605) 343-2509
FAX: (605) 343-8887

SOUTH DAKOTA CLAIMS OFFICE
512 MAIN ST, STE 200
PO BOX 8150
RAPID CITY, SD 57709-8150
TEL: (605) 343-2509
FAX: (605) 343-8887

WYOMING CLAIMS OFFICE
512 MAIN ST, STE 200
PO BOX 8150
RAPID CITY, SD 57709-8150
TEL: (605) 343-2509
FAX: (605) 343-8887

FIRST AMERICAN INSURANCE CO

NATIONAL CLAIMS OFFICE
3100 BROADWAY, STE 1300
KANSAS CITY, MO 64111
TEL: (816) 531-7668
FAX: (816) 531-0189
TOLL FREE: (800) 821-5546
WWW.FAIC.COM

FIRST ASSURANCE LIFE INSURANCE CO

LOUISIANA CLAIMS OFFICE
9016 BLUE BONNET BLVD
PO DRAWER 83480
BATON ROUGE, LA 70884-3480
TEL: (504) 769-9923
IN-STATE: (800) 272-8000
WWW.THELDSGROUP.COM

FIRST CARE

TEXAS CLAIMS OFFICE
3310 DANVERS
AMARILLO, TX 79106-3504
TEL: (806) 356-5151
FAX: (806) 356-5178
TOLL FREE: (800) 365-1051

FIRST EXCESS & REINSURANCE CORP

KANSAS CLAIMS OFFICE
6329 GLENWOOD, STE 300
PO BOX 29164
OVERLAND PARK, KS 66201-9164
TEL: (913) 676-5520
FAX: (913) 676-5222
WWW.GEREINSURANCE.COM

FIRST HEALTH

ALASKA CLAIMS OFFICE
4411 BUSINESS PARK BLVD, STE 16
ANCHORAGE, AK 99503
TEL: (907) 561-5650
FAX: (907) 563-1082

NATIONAL CLAIMS OFFICE
3540 WILSHIRE BLVD
PO BOX 54170
LOS ANGELES, CA 90010-2307
TEL: (213) 383-1100
FAX: (213) 738-0386
TOLL FREE: (800) 421-9064
IN-STATE: (800) 872-4474

F

PO BOX GG
BOISE, ID 83707
TEL: (800) 962-7809
TOLL FREE: (800) 554-4954

PO BOX GG
BOISE, ID 83707
TOLL FREE: (800) 527-0772

333 ROUSER RD
CORAOPOLIS, PA 15108
TEL: (412) 269-1178
FAX: (412) 269-0645

FORMERLY ALTA HEALTH CARE STRATEGIES
2650 S DECKER LAKE DR
SALT LAKE CITY, UT 84119
TEL: (801) 954-6550
FAX: (801) 954-6662
TOLL FREE: (800) 572-2089

2650 DECKER LN
PO BOX 30110
WEST VALLEY CITY, UT 84130
TEL: (801) 973-7300
FAX: (801) 974-6716
TOLL FREE: (800) 572-2089

11301 W LAKE PARK DR.
PO BOX 26199
MILWAUKEE, WI 53224-6199
TEL: (414) 577-2140
FAX: (414) 577-1999
TOLL FREE: (800) 558-9056

FIRST INSURANCE CO OF HAWAII

HAWAII CLAIMS OFFICE
1100 WARD AVE
PO BOX 2866
HONOLULU, HI 96803-2866
TEL: (808) 527-7777
FAX: (808) 527-7511
IN-STATE: (800) 272-5202
WWW.FICOH.COM

FIRST INTEGRATED HEALTH

CALIFORNIA CLAIMS OFFICE
19191 S VERMONT, STE 700
PO BOX 5279
TORRANCE, CA 90510-5279
TEL: (310) 532-8887
FAX: (310) 532-2824
TOLL FREE: (800) 433-3554
WWW.FIH.COM

FIRST LIFE INSURANCE CO

OKLAHOMA CLAIMS OFFICE
501 W I-44 SERVICE RD, STE 400
PO BOX 548801
OKLAHOMA CITY, OK 73154-8801
TEL: (405) 848-0179
FAX: (405) 841-8758
TOLL FREE: (800) 725-7887

FIRST OPTION HEALTH PLAN

NATIONAL CLAIMS OFFICE
3501 ST HWY 66
NEPTUNE, NJ 07754
TEL: (732) 918-6700
FAX: (732) 918-6991
TOLL FREE: (800) 977-3288

FIRST PRIORITY HEALTH

70 N MAIN ST
WILKES-BARRE, PA 18711
TEL: (570) 829-6011
FAX: (570) 819-8181
TOLL FREE: (800) 829-8599
IN-STATE: (800) 822-8753

PENNSYLVANIA CLAIMS OFFICE
PO BOX 3500
WILKES-BARRE, PA 18773-3500
FAX: (717) 831-2240
TOLL FREE: (800) 822-8753

H

FIRST RELIANCE STANDARD LIFE INSURANCE CO

NEW YORK CLAIMS OFFICE
11 W 42ND ST
NEW YORK, NY 10036
TEL: (212) 303-8400
TOLL FREE: (800) 882-8700
WWW.RSL.COM

FIRST SECURITY INSURANCE, INC

UTAH CLAIMS OFFICE
405 S MAIN, 8TH FL
PO BOX 957
SALT LAKE CITY, UT 84110-0957
TEL: (801) 246-1900
FAX: (801) 531-1452
TOLL FREE: (800) 385-3194
IN-STATE: (800) 356-5909

FIRST UNITED AMERICAN LIFE INSURANCE CO

NEW YORK CLAIMS OFFICE
1020 7TH N ST
PO BOX 3125
SYRACUSE, NY 13220-3125
TEL: (315) 451-2544
FAX: (315) 451-7679

FIRST UNUM LIFE INSURANCE CO

CHRISTIANIA BLDG
120 WHITE PLNS RD, STE 300
TARRYTOWN, NY 10591
TEL: (914) 524-4000
FAX: (800) 356-5815
TOLL FREE: (800) 321-0745

FIRST VIRGINIA LIFE INSURANCE CO

MARYLAND CLAIMS OFFICE
6402 ARLINGTON BLVD, STE 1120
FALLS CHURCH, VA 22042-2300
TEL: (703) 241-4401
FAX: (703) 533-6429
TOLL FREE: (800) 382-3365

TENNESSEE CLAIMS OFFICE
6402 ARLINGTON BLVD, STE 1120
FALLS CHURCH, VA 22042-2300
TEL: (703) 241-4401
FAX: (703) 533-6429
TOLL FREE: (800) 382-3365

VIRGINIA CLAIMS OFFICE
6402 ARLINGTON BLVD, STE 1120
FALLS CHURCH, VA 22042-2300
TEL: (703) 241-4401
FAX: (703) 533-6429
TOLL FREE: (800) 382-3365

FLEX CORP

TEXAS CLAIMS OFFICE
HAND & ASSOC
5700 NW CENTRAL DR, STE 300
HOUSTON, TX 77092-2092
TEL: (713) 460-4850
FAX: (713) 460-0361
IN-STATE: (800) 856-3539

FLORIDA EMPLOYERS INSURANCE SERVICE CORP

FLORIDA CLAIMS OFFICE
2601 CATTLEMEN RD
PO BOX 25248
SARASOTA, FL 34277
TEL: (941) 955-2811
FAX: (941) 951-3602
TOLL FREE: (800) 226-7148

FLORIDA FARM BUREAU MUTUAL INSURANCE CO

NATIONAL CLAIMS OFFICE
5700 SW 34TH ST
PO BOX 147030
GAINESVILLE, FL 32614-7030
TEL: (352) 378-8100
FAX: (352) 374-1579
TOLL FREE: (800) 330-3327

F

FLORIDA FIRST HEALTH PLAN

FLORIDA CLAIMS OFFICE
3425 LK ALFRED RD
PO BOX 9126
WINTER HAVEN, FL 33883-9126
TEL: (941) 293-0785
FAX: (941) 297-9095
TOLL FREE: (800) 226-3155
IN-STATE: (800) 226-3155

FLORIDA HEALTH CARE PLAN, INC

1340 RIDGEWOOD AVE
HOLLY HILL, FL 32117
TEL: (904) 676-7100
FAX: (904) 676-7148
TOLL FREE: (800) 352-9824

H

FLORISTS MUTUAL INSURANCE CO

ILLINOIS CLAIMS OFFICE
500 SAINT LOUIS ST
EDWARDSVILLE, IL 62025
TEL: (618) 656-4240
FAX: (618) 656-7581
TOLL FREE: (800) 851-7740
WWW.PLANTNET.COM

FOLKSAMERICA GROUP

NEW YORK CLAIMS OFFICE
ONE LIBERTY PLZ
NEW YORK, NY 10006
TEL: (212) 312-2500
FAX: (212) 385-2279

FORD LIFE INSURANCE CO

MICHIGAN CLAIMS OFFICE
THE AMERICAN RD
DEARBORN, MI 48121
TEL: (313) 322-3000
FAX: (313) 323-9479
TOLL FREE: (800) 765-5433
IN-STATE: (800) 392-3673

FOREIGN SERVICE BENEFIT PLAN

NATIONAL CLAIMS OFFICE
AMERICAN FOREIGN SERVICE PROTECTIVE ASSOCIATION
1716 N ST NW
WASHINGTON, DC 20036-2907
TEL: (202) 833-4910
FAX: (202) 833-4918
E-MAIL: AFSPA@AFSPA.ORG
WWW.AFSPA.ORG

FOREMOST CORP OF AMERICA

MICHIGAN CLAIMS OFFICE
5600 BEECHTREE LN
PO BOX 2739
GRAND RAPIDS, MI 49501-2450
TEL: (616) 942-3000
FAX: (616) 956-3567
TOLL FREE: (800) 527-3907
WWW.FOREMOST.COM

FORREST T. JONES & CO, INC

MISSOURI CLAIMS OFFICE
FIDELITY SECURITY LIFE INSURANCE
3130 BROADWAY ST
PO BOX 418131
KANSAS CITY, MO 64141-9131
TEL: (816) 756-1060
FAX: (816) 968-0568
TOLL FREE: (800) 821-7303

FORTIS BENEFITS INSURANCE CO

ALABAMA CLAIMS OFFICE
FORTIS BENEFIT
PO BOX 3195
MILWAUKEE, WI 53201-3195
TEL: (972) 238-7400
FAX: (972) 238-1019
TOLL FREE: (800) 444-6254
WWW.FORTIS.COM

ARIZONA CLAIMS OFFICE
FORTIS BENEFIT
PO BOX 3195
MILWAUKEE, WI 53201-3195
TEL: (972) 238-7400
FAX: (972) 238-1019
TOLL FREE: (800) 444-6254
WWW.FORTIS.COM

ARKANSAS CLAIMS OFFICE
FORTIS BENEFIT
PO BOX 3195
MILWAUKEE, WI 53201-3195
TEL: (972) 238-7400
FAX: (972) 238-1019
TOLL FREE: (800) 444-6254
WWW.FORTIS.COM

CALIFORNIA CLAIMS OFFICE
FORTIS BENEFIT
PO BOX 3195
MILWAUKEE, WI 53201-3195
TEL: (972) 238-7400
FAX: (972) 238-1019
TOLL FREE: (800) 444-6254
WWW.FORTIS.COM

COLORADO CLAIMS OFFICE
FORTIS BENEFIT
PO BOX 3195
MILWAUKEE, WI 53201-3195
TEL: (972) 238-7400
FAX: (972) 238-1019
TOLL FREE: (800) 444-6254
WWW.FORTIS.COM

CONNECTICUT CLAIMS OFFICE
FORTIS BENEFIT
PO BOX 3195
MILWAUKEE, WI 53201-3195
TEL: (972) 238-7400
FAX: (972) 238-1019
TOLL FREE: (800) 444-6254
WWW.FORTIS.COM

DELAWARE CLAIMS OFFICE
FORTIS BENEFIT
PO BOX 3195
MILWAUKEE, WI 53201-3195
TEL: (972) 238-7400
FAX: (972) 238-1019
TOLL FREE: (800) 444-6254
WWW.FORTIS.COM

DISTRICT OF COLUMBIA CLAIMS OFFICE
FORTIS BENEFIT
PO BOX 3195
MILWAUKEE, WI 53201-3195
TEL: (972) 238-7400
FAX: (972) 238-1019
TOLL FREE: (800) 444-6254
WWW.FORTIS.COM

FLORIDA CLAIMS OFFICE
FORTIS BENEFIT
PO BOX 3195
MILWAUKEE, WI 53201-3195
TEL: (972) 238-7400
FAX: (972) 238-1019
TOLL FREE: (800) 444-6254
WWW.FORTIS.COM

GEORGIA CLAIMS OFFICE
FORTIS BENEFIT
1950 SPECTRUM CIR, STE B100
MARIETTA, GA 30067-6052
FAX: (770) 916-0905
TOLL FREE: (800) 955-1586

FORTIS BENEFIT
PO BOX 3195
MILWAUKEE, WI 53201-3195
TEL: (972) 238-7400
FAX: (972) 238-1019
TOLL FREE: (800) 444-6254
WWW.FORTIS.COM

IDAHO CLAIMS OFFICE
FORTIS BENEFIT
PO BOX 3195
MILWAUKEE, WI 53201-3195
TEL: (972) 238-7400
FAX: (972) 238-1019
TOLL FREE: (800) 444-6254
WWW.FORTIS.COM

ILLINOIS CLAIMS OFFICE
FORTIS BENEFIT
PO BOX 3195
MILWAUKEE, WI 53201-3195
TEL: (972) 238-7400
FAX: (972) 238-1019
TOLL FREE: (800) 444-6254
WWW.FORTIS.COM

INDIANA CLAIMS OFFICE
FORTIS BENEFIT
PO BOX 3195
MILWAUKEE, WI 53201-3195
TEL: (972) 238-7400
FAX: (972) 238-1019
TOLL FREE: (800) 444-6254
WWW.FORTIS.COM

IOWA CLAIMS OFFICE
FORTIS BENEFIT
PO BOX 2940
CLINTON, IA 52733
TEL: (612) 920-8055
FAX: (612) 920-4577
TOLL FREE: (800) 325-8385
WWW.FORTIS.COM

FIRST FORTIS LIFE INSURANCE
PO BOX 2941
CLINTON, IA 52733
TEL: (612) 920-8055
FAX: (612) 920-4577
TOLL FREE: (800) 325-8385
WWW.FORTIS.COM

FORTIS BENEFIT
PO BOX 3195
MILWAUKEE, WI 53201-3195
TEL: (972) 238-7400
FAX: (972) 238-1019
TOLL FREE: (800) 444-6254
WWW.FORTIS.COM

KANSAS CLAIMS OFFICE
FORTIS BENEFIT
PO BOX 3195
MILWAUKEE, WI 53201-3195
TEL: (972) 238-7400
FAX: (972) 238-1019
TOLL FREE: (800) 444-6254
WWW.FORTIS.COM

KENTUCKY CLAIMS OFFICE
FORTIS BENEFIT
PO BOX 3195
MILWAUKEE, WI 53201-3195
TEL: (972) 238-7400
FAX: (972) 238-1019
TOLL FREE: (800) 444-6254
WWW.FORTIS.COM

LOUISIANA CLAIMS OFFICE
FORTIS BENEFIT
PO BOX 3195
MILWAUKEE, WI 53201-3195
TEL: (972) 238-7400
FAX: (972) 238-1019
TOLL FREE: (800) 444-6254
WWW.FORTIS.COM

MAINE CLAIMS OFFICE
FORTIS BENEFIT
PO BOX 3195
MILWAUKEE, WI 53201-3195
TEL: (972) 238-7400
FAX: (972) 238-1019
TOLL FREE: (800) 444-6254
WWW.FORTIS.COM

MARYLAND CLAIMS OFFICE
FORTIS BENEFIT
PO BOX 3195
MILWAUKEE, WI 53201-3195
TEL: (972) 238-7400
FAX: (972) 238-1019
TOLL FREE: (800) 444-6254
WWW.FORTIS.COM

MASSACHUSETTS CLAIMS OFFICE
FORTIS BENEFIT
PO BOX 2940
CLINTON, IA 52733
TEL: (612) 920-8055
FAX: (612) 920-4577
TOLL FREE: (800) 325-8385
WWW.FORTIS.COM

FIRST FORTIS LIFE INSURANCE
PO BOX 2941
CLINTON, IA 52733
TEL: (612) 920-8055
FAX: (612) 920-4577
TOLL FREE: (800) 325-8385
WWW.FORTIS.COM

FORTIS BENEFIT
PO BOX 3195
MILWAUKEE, WI 53201-3195
TEL: (972) 238-7400
FAX: (972) 238-1019
TOLL FREE: (800) 444-6254
WWW.FORTIS.COM

MICHIGAN CLAIMS OFFICE
FORTIS BENEFIT
PO BOX 3195
MILWAUKEE, WI 53201-3195
TEL: (972) 238-7400
FAX: (972) 238-1019
TOLL FREE: (800) 444-6254
WWW.FORTIS.COM

MINNESOTA CLAIMS OFFICE
FORTIS BENEFIT
PO BOX 2940
CLINTON, IA 52733
TEL: (612) 920-8055
FAX: (612) 920-4577
TOLL FREE: (800) 325-8385
WWW.FORTIS.COM

FIRST FORTIS LIFE INSURANCE
PO BOX 2941
CLINTON, IA 52733
TEL: (612) 920-8055
FAX: (612) 920-4577
TOLL FREE: (800) 325-8385
WWW.FORTIS.COM

FORTIS BENEFIT
PO BOX 3195
MILWAUKEE, WI 53201-3195
TEL: (972) 238-7400
FAX: (972) 238-1019
TOLL FREE: (800) 444-6254
WWW.FORTIS.COM

MISSISSIPPI CLAIMS OFFICE
FORTIS BENEFIT
PO BOX 3195
MILWAUKEE, WI 53201-3195
TEL: (972) 238-7400
FAX: (972) 238-1019
TOLL FREE: (800) 444-6254
WWW.FORTIS.COM

MISSOURI CLAIMS OFFICE
FORTIS BENEFIT
PO BOX 3195
MILWAUKEE, WI 53201-3195
TEL: (972) 238-7400
FAX: (972) 238-1019
TOLL FREE: (800) 444-6254
WWW.FORTIS.COM

MONTANA CLAIMS OFFICE
FORTIS BENEFIT
PO BOX 3195
MILWAUKEE, WI 53201-3195
TEL: (972) 238-7400
FAX: (972) 238-1019
TOLL FREE: (800) 444-6254
WWW.FORTIS.COM

NEBRASKA CLAIMS OFFICE
FORTIS BENEFIT
PO BOX 3195
MILWAUKEE, WI 53201-3195
TEL: (972) 238-7400
FAX: (972) 238-1019
TOLL FREE: (800) 444-6254
WWW.FORTIS.COM

NEVADA CLAIMS OFFICE
FORTIS BENEFIT
PO BOX 3195
MILWAUKEE, WI 53201-3195
TEL: (972) 238-7400
FAX: (972) 238-1019
TOLL FREE: (800) 444-6254
WWW.FORTIS.COM

NEW HAMPSHIRE CLAIMS OFFICE
FORTIS BENEFIT
PO BOX 3195
MILWAUKEE, WI 53201-3195
TEL: (972) 238-7400
FAX: (972) 238-1019
TOLL FREE: (800) 444-6254
WWW.FORTIS.COM

NEW JERSEY CLAIMS OFFICE
FORTIS BENEFIT
PO BOX 3195
MILWAUKEE, WI 53201-3195
TEL: (972) 238-7400
FAX: (972) 238-1019
TOLL FREE: (800) 444-6254
WWW.FORTIS.COM

NEW MEXICO CLAIMS OFFICE
FORTIS BENEFIT
PO BOX 3195
MILWAUKEE, WI 53201-3195
TEL: (972) 238-7400
FAX: (972) 238-1019
TOLL FREE: (800) 444-6254
WWW.FORTIS.COM

NORTH CAROLINA CLAIMS OFFICE
FORTIS BENEFIT
PO BOX 3195
MILWAUKEE, WI 53201-3195
TEL: (972) 238-7400
FAX: (972) 238-1019
TOLL FREE: (800) 444-6254
WWW.FORTIS.COM

NORTH DAKOTA CLAIMS OFFICE
FORTIS BENEFIT
PO BOX 3195
MILWAUKEE, WI 53201-3195
TEL: (972) 238-7400
FAX: (972) 238-1019
TOLL FREE: (800) 444-6254
WWW.FORTIS.COM

OHIO CLAIMS OFFICE
FORTIS BENEFIT
PO BOX 3195
MILWAUKEE, WI 53201-3195
TEL: (972) 238-7400
FAX: (972) 238-1019
TOLL FREE: (800) 444-6254
WWW.FORTIS.COM

OKLAHOMA CLAIMS OFFICE
FORTIS BENEFIT
PO BOX 3195
MILWAUKEE, WI 53201-3195
TEL: (972) 238-7400
FAX: (972) 238-1019
TOLL FREE: (800) 444-6254
WWW.FORTIS.COM

OREGON CLAIMS OFFICE
FORTIS BENEFIT
PO BOX 3195
MILWAUKEE, WI 53201-3195
TEL: (972) 238-7400
FAX: (972) 238-1019
TOLL FREE: (800) 444-6254
WWW.FORTIS.COM

PENNSYLVANIA CLAIMS OFFICE
FORTIS BENEFIT
PO BOX 3195
MILWAUKEE, WI 53201-3195
TEL: (972) 238-7400
FAX: (972) 238-1019
TOLL FREE: (800) 444-6254
WWW.FORTIS.COM

RHODE ISLAND CLAIMS OFFICE
FORTIS BENEFIT
PO BOX 3195
MILWAUKEE, WI 53201-3195
TEL: (972) 238-7400
FAX: (972) 238-1019
TOLL FREE: (800) 444-6254
WWW.FORTIS.COM

SOUTH CAROLINA CLAIMS OFFICE
FORTIS BENEFIT
PO BOX 3195
MILWAUKEE, WI 53201-3195
TEL: (972) 238-7400
FAX: (972) 238-1019
TOLL FREE: (800) 444-6254
WWW.FORTIS.COM

SOUTH DAKOTA CLAIMS OFFICE
FORTIS BENEFIT
PO BOX 3195
MILWAUKEE, WI 53201-3195
TEL: (972) 238-7400
FAX: (972) 238-1019
TOLL FREE: (800) 444-6254
WWW.FORTIS.COM

TENNESSEE CLAIMS OFFICE
FORTIS BENEFIT
PO BOX 3195
MILWAUKEE, WI 53201-3195
TEL: (972) 238-7400
FAX: (972) 238-1019
TOLL FREE: (800) 444-6254
WWW.FORTIS.COM

TEXAS CLAIMS OFFICE
FORTIS BENEFIT
PO BOX 3195
MILWAUKEE, WI 53201-3195
TEL: (972) 238-7400
FAX: (972) 238-1019
TOLL FREE: (800) 444-6254
WWW.FORTIS.COM

UTAH CLAIMS OFFICE
FORTIS BENEFIT
PO BOX 3195
MILWAUKEE, WI 53201-3195
TEL: (972) 238-7400
FAX: (972) 238-1019
TOLL FREE: (800) 444-6254
WWW.FORTIS.COM

VERMONT CLAIMS OFFICE
FORTIS BENEFIT
PO BOX 3195
MILWAUKEE, WI 53201-3195
TEL: (972) 238-7400
FAX: (972) 238-1019
TOLL FREE: (800) 444-6254
WWW.FORTIS.COM

VIRGINIA CLAIMS OFFICE
FORTIS BENEFIT
PO BOX 3195
MILWAUKEE, WI 53201-3195
TEL: (972) 238-7400
FAX: (972) 238-1019
TOLL FREE: (800) 444-6254
WWW.FORTIS.COM

WASHINGTON CLAIMS OFFICE
FORTIS BENEFIT
PO BOX 3195
MILWAUKEE, WI 53201-3195
TEL: (972) 238-7400
FAX: (972) 238-1019
TOLL FREE: (800) 444-6254
WWW.FORTIS.COM

WEST VIRGINIA CLAIMS OFFICE
FORTIS BENEFIT
PO BOX 3195
MILWAUKEE, WI 53201-3195
TEL: (972) 238-7400
FAX: (972) 238-1019
TOLL FREE: (800) 444-6254
WWW.FORTIS.COM

WISCONSIN CLAIMS OFFICE
FORTIS BENEFIT
PO BOX 2940
CLINTON, IA 52733
TEL: (612) 920-8055
FAX: (612) 920-4577
TOLL FREE: (800) 325-8385
WWW.FORTIS.COM

FIRST FORTIS LIFE INSURANCE
PO BOX 2941
CLINTON, IA 52733
TEL: (612) 920-8055
FAX: (612) 920-4577
TOLL FREE: (800) 325-8385
WWW.FORTIS.COM

FORTIS BENEFIT
PO BOX 3195
MILWAUKEE, WI 53201-3195
TEL: (972) 238-7400
FAX: (972) 238-1019
TOLL FREE: (800) 444-6254
WWW.FORTIS.COM

WYOMING CLAIMS OFFICE
FORTIS BENEFIT
PO BOX 3195
MILWAUKEE, WI 53201-3195
TEL: (972) 238-7400
FAX: (972) 238-1019
TOLL FREE: (800) 444-6254
WWW.FORTIS.COM

FORTIS HEALTH

MASSACHUSETTS CLAIMS OFFICE
501 W MICHIGAN
PO BOX 624
MILWAUKEE, WI 53201-0624
TEL: (414) 271-3011
FAX: (414) 224-0472
TOLL FREE: (800) 800-8463
WWW.FORTIS.COM

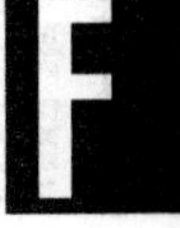

MINNESOTA CLAIMS OFFICE
501 W MICHIGAN
PO BOX 624
MILWAUKEE, WI 53201-0624
TEL: (414) 271-3011
FAX: (414) 224-0472
TOLL FREE: (800) 800-8463
WWW.FORTIS.COM

WISCONSIN CLAIMS OFFICE
501 W MICHIGAN
PO BOX 624
MILWAUKEE, WI 53201-0624
TEL: (414) 271-3011
FAX: (414) 224-0472
TOLL FREE: (800) 800-8463
WWW.FORTIS.COM

FORTUNE INSURANCE CO

FLORIDA CLAIMS OFFICE
MOBILE AMERICA INSURANCE GROUP
10475 FORTUNE PARKWAY, STE 110
PO BOX 24814
JACKSONVILLE, FL 32241-4814
TEL: (352) 363-6339

FOUNDATION HEALTH

CALIFORNIA CLAIMS OFFICE
AMERIMED
3400 DATA DR
RANCHO CORDOVA, CA 95670
TEL: (916) 631-5000
FAX: (916) 631-5152
TOLL FREE: (800) 634-7148
WWW.FHS.COM

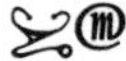

FOX-EVERETT, INC

MISSISSIPPI CLAIMS OFFICE
3780 I-55 N FRONTAGE RD, STE 200
PO BOX 23096
JACKSON, MS 39225-3095
TEL: (601) 981-6000
FAX: (601) 718-5399

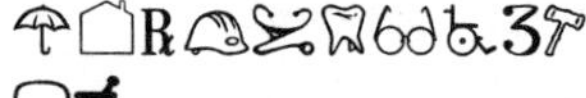
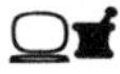

F

FRANK M. VACCARO & ASSOCIATES, INC

PENNSYLVANIA CLAIMS OFFICE
1 NESHAMINY INTERPLEX, STE 303
TREVOSE, PA 19053
TEL: (215) 638-3682
FAX: (215) 638-1294
TOLL FREE: (800) 883-3682

FRANKENMUTH MUTUAL INSURANCE CO

MICHIGAN CLAIMS OFFICE
1 MUTUAL AVE
FRANKENMUTH, MI 48787-0040
TEL: (517) 652-6121
FAX: (517) 652-6231
TOLL FREE: (800) 234-4433

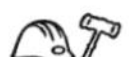

FRANKLIN MUTUAL INSURANCE CO

NEW JERSEY CLAIMS OFFICE
FMI
5 BROAD ST
PO BOX 400
BRANCHVILLE, NJ 07826-0400
TEL: (973) 948-3120
FAX: (973) 948-7190
TOLL FREE: (800) 842-0551

FRED MEYER

OREGON CLAIMS OFFICE
3800 S E 22ND ST AVE
PO BOX 42121
PORTLAND, OR 97242
TEL: (503) 232-8844
FAX: (503) 797-5579
TOLL FREE: (800) 858-9202

FREE STATE HEALTH PLAN

MARYLAND CLAIMS OFFICE
100 S CHARLES ST- TWR II
BALTIMORE, MD 21201
TEL: (410) 544-6500
FAX: (410) 544-8628
TOLL FREE: (800) 445-6036

H

VIRGINIA CLAIMS OFFICE
CARE FIRST, BLUE CROSS & BLUE SHIELD
100 S CHARLES ST- TWR II
BALTIMORE, MD 21201
TEL: (410) 528-7000
FAX: (410) 528-7014
TOLL FREE: (800) 367-3387
WWW.CAREFIRST.COM

H

WASHINGTON CLAIMS OFFICE
CARE FIRST, BLUE CROSS & BLUE SHIELD
100 S CHARLES ST- TWR II
BALTIMORE, MD 21201
TEL: (410) 528-7000
FAX: (410) 528-7014
TOLL FREE: (800) 367-3387
WWW.CAREFIRST.COM

H

FREMONT

ARIZONA CLAIMS OFFICE
2141 E HYLAND, STE 200
PO BOX 44037
PHOENIX, AZ 85064
TEL: (602) 852-5300
FAX: (602) 852-5360
TOLL FREE: (800) 677-3259

FREMONT COMP

IDAHO CLAIMS OFFICE
1471 SHORELINE DR #200
BOISE, ID 83702
TEL: (208) 336-4210
FAX: (208) 344-3071
TOLL FREE: (800) 635-5164
IN-STATE: (800) 632-5109

MONTANA CLAIMS OFFICE
1471 SHORELINE DR #200
BOISE, ID 83702
TEL: (208) 336-4210
FAX: (208) 344-3071
TOLL FREE: (800) 635-5164
IN-STATE: (800) 632-5109

UTAH CLAIMS OFFICE
1471 SHORELINE DR #200
BOISE, ID 83702
TEL: (208) 336-4210
FAX: (208) 344-3071
TOLL FREE: (800) 635-5164
IN-STATE: (800) 632-5109

FREMONT COMPENSATION

HAWAII CLAIMS OFFICE
201 MERCHANT ST, STE 1800
HONOLULU, HI 96813-2982
TEL: (808) 521-1477
FAX: (808) 521-5982
IN-STATE: (800) 232-9492

FREMONT COMPENSATION INSURANCE CO

ALASKA CLAIMS OFFICE
INDUSTRIAL INDEMNITY
4341 B ST, STE 400
ANCHORAGE, AK 99503-5923
TEL: (907) 762-6400
FAX: (907) 561-6523

ARIZONA CLAIMS OFFICE
2390 E CAMELBACK
PO BOX 44090
PHOENIX, AZ 85064
TEL: (602) 553-4100
FAX: (602) 553-4177
TOLL FREE: (800) 274-5111
IN-STATE: (800) 274-5111

ARKANSAS CLAIMS OFFICE
520 MARYVILLE CENTER DR, STE 400
PO BOX 419069
SAINT LOUIS, MO 63141
TEL: (314) 542-4600
FAX: (314) 542-4627
TOLL FREE: (800) 336-3661
WWW.FREMONTCOMP.COM

CALIFORNIA CLAIMS OFFICE
500 N BRAND BLVD
PO BOX 29069
GLENDALE, CA 91209-9069
TEL: (818) 502-5200
FAX: (818) 502-5246
IN-STATE: (800) 540-3502

3255 CAMINO DEL RIO S
PO BOX 85615
SAN DIEGO, CA 92168
TEL: (619) 563-0288
FAX: (619) 521-2745
IN-STATE: (800) 540-3502

255 CALIFORNIA ST
PO BOX 7928
SAN FRANCISCO, CA 94120-7928
TEL: (415) 362-3333
FAX: (415) 627-5448
TOLL FREE: (800) 794-0568
IN-STATE: (800) 652-1637
WWW.FREMONT.COM

INDUSTRIAL INDEMNITY CO
255 CALIFORNIA ST
PO BOX 7468
SAN FRANCISCO, CA 94111
TEL: (415) 627-5000
FAX: (415) 296-3099
IN-STATE: (800) 464-0556
WWW.INSWEB.COM

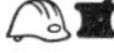

3530 WILSHIRE BLVD, STE 500
PO BOX 512252
LOS ANGELES, CA 90010-0252
TEL: (213) 739-4200
FAX: (213) 739-8519

PO BOX 15709
SACRAMENTO, CA 95852-1709
TEL: (916) 394-4000
FAX: (916) 614-6790
TOLL FREE: (800) 365-3787

3255 CAMINO DEL RIO S
PO BOX 85365
SAN DIEGO, CA 92108-5365
TEL: (619) 521-2700
FAX: (619) 521-3603
IN-STATE: (800) 995-4460

IDAHO CLAIMS OFFICE
2390 E CAMELBACK
PO BOX 44090
PHOENIX, AZ 85064
TEL: (602) 553-4100
FAX: (602) 553-4177
TOLL FREE: (800) 274-5111
IN-STATE: (800) 274-5111

IOWA CLAIMS OFFICE
520 MARYVILLE CENTER DR, STE 400
PO BOX 419069
SAINT LOUIS, MO 63141
TEL: (314) 542-4600
FAX: (314) 542-4627
TOLL FREE: (800) 336-3661
WWW.FREMONTCOMP.COM

KANSAS CLAIMS OFFICE
520 MARYVILLE CENTER DR, STE 400
PO BOX 419069
SAINT LOUIS, MO 63141
TEL: (314) 542-4600
FAX: (314) 542-4627
TOLL FREE: (800) 336-3661
WWW.FREMONTCOMP.COM

KENTUCKY CLAIMS OFFICE
520 MARYVILLE CENTER DR, STE 400
PO BOX 419069
SAINT LOUIS, MO 63141
TEL: (314) 542-4600
FAX: (314) 542-4627
TOLL FREE: (800) 336-3661
WWW.FREMONTCOMP.COM

MICHIGAN CLAIMS OFFICE
520 MARYVILLE CENTER DR, STE 400
PO BOX 419069
SAINT LOUIS, MO 63141
TEL: (314) 542-4600
FAX: (314) 542-4627
TOLL FREE: (800) 336-3661
WWW.FREMONTCOMP.COM

MINNESOTA CLAIMS OFFICE
520 MARYVILLE CENTER DR, STE 400
PO BOX 419069
SAINT LOUIS, MO 63141
TEL: (314) 542-4600
FAX: (314) 542-4627
TOLL FREE: (800) 336-3661
WWW.FREMONTCOMP.COM

MISSOURI CLAIMS OFFICE
520 MARYVILLE CENTER DR, STE 400
PO BOX 419069
SAINT LOUIS, MO 63141
TEL: (314) 542-4600
FAX: (314) 542-4627
TOLL FREE: (800) 336-3661
WWW.FREMONTCOMP.COM

NEW MEXICO CLAIMS OFFICE
2390 E CAMELBACK
PO BOX 44090
PHOENIX, AZ 85064
TEL: (602) 553-4100
FAX: (602) 553-4177
TOLL FREE: (800) 274-5111
IN-STATE: (800) 274-5111

NORTH DAKOTA CLAIMS OFFICE
520 MARYVILLE CENTER DR, STE 400
PO BOX 419069
SAINT LOUIS, MO 63141
TEL: (314) 542-4600
FAX: (314) 542-4627
TOLL FREE: (800) 336-3661
WWW.FREMONTCOMP.COM

OKLAHOMA CLAIMS OFFICE
520 MARYVILLE CENTER DR, STE 400
PO BOX 419069
SAINT LOUIS, MO 63141
TEL: (314) 542-4600
FAX: (314) 542-4627
TOLL FREE: (800) 336-3661
WWW.FREMONTCOMP.COM

OREGON CLAIMS OFFICE
101 SW MAIN ST, STE 600
PORTLAND, OR 97204
TEL: (503) 795-3600
FAX: (503) 795-3605
TOLL FREE: (800) 782-0681

SOUTH DAKOTA CLAIMS OFFICE
520 MARYVILLE CENTER DR, STE 400
PO BOX 419069
SAINT LOUIS, MO 63141
TEL: (314) 542-4600
FAX: (314) 542-4627
TOLL FREE: (800) 336-3661
WWW.FREMONTCOMP.COM

TENNESSEE CLAIMS OFFICE
520 MARYVILLE CENTER DR, STE 400
PO BOX 419069
SAINT LOUIS, MO 63141
TEL: (314) 542-4600
FAX: (314) 542-4627
TOLL FREE: (800) 336-3661
WWW.FREMONTCOMP.COM

UTAH CLAIMS OFFICE
2390 E CAMELBACK
PO BOX 44090
PHOENIX, AZ 85064
TEL: (602) 553-4100
FAX: (602) 553-4177
TOLL FREE: (800) 274-5111
IN-STATE: (800) 274-5111

WASHINGTON CLAIMS OFFICE
1601 FIFTH AVE, STE 1300
SEATTLE, WA 98101
TEL: (206) 667-3800
FAX: (206) 667-3998
TOLL FREE: (800) 288-9636

WISCONSIN CLAIMS OFFICE
520 MARYVILLE CENTER DR, STE 400
PO BOX 419069
SAINT LOUIS, MO 63141
TEL: (314) 542-4600
FAX: (314) 542-4627
TOLL FREE: (800) 336-3661
WWW.FREMONTCOMP.COM

FREMONT INDEMNITY

CALIFORNIA CLAIMS OFFICE
1888 CENTURY PK E, STE 800
LOS ANGELES, CA 90067
TEL: (310) 712-5858
FAX: (310) 712-5893
TOLL FREE: (800) 362-7001

FREMONT MUTUAL INSURANCE CO

MICHIGAN CLAIMS OFFICE
933 E MAIN ST
FREMONT, MI 49412-9751
TEL: (616) 924-0300
FAX: (616) 924-0880
WWW.FMIC.COM

FRINGE BENEFIT COORDINATORS

FLORIDA CLAIMS OFFICE
1239 NW 10TH AVE
GAINESVILLE, FL 32601-4154
TEL: (352) 372-2028
FAX: (352) 372-9805
IN-STATE: (800) 654-1452

FRINGE BENEFITS FUND

MICHIGAN CLAIMS OFFICE
LABORERS METROPOLITAN DETROIT HEALTH CARE FUND
241 E SAGINAW, STE 601
EAST LANSING, MI 48823-2791
TEL: (517) 351-3400
FAX: (517) 351-6442
IN-STATE: (800) 228-0048

FRONT RANGE MEDICAL GROUP

COLORADO CLAIMS OFFICE
9351 GRANT ST, STE 360
THORNTON, CO 80229
TEL: (303) 452-4224
FAX: (303) 452-4136

FRONTIER INSURANCE GROUP

NEW YORK CLAIMS OFFICE
195 LK LOUISE MARIE RD
ROCK HILL, NY 12775-8000
TEL: (914) 796-2100
FAX: (914) 791-5053
TOLL FREE: (800) 836-2100
WWW.FTR.COM

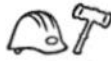

GAB ROBINS NORTH AMERICA

CALIFORNIA CLAIMS OFFICE
3230 E IMPERIAL HWY, STE 312
BREA, CA 92821-6746
TEL: (714) 528-5300
FAX: (714) 577-5872

2542 S BASCOM AVE, STE 215
CAMPBELL, CA 95008
TEL: (408) 371-9510
FAX: (408) 371-0432
WWW.GABROBINS.COM

G

PO BOX 269037
SACRAMENTO, CA 95827-9037
TEL: (916) 853-6600
FAX: (916) 853-3203

3350 SHELBY ST, STE 300
ONTARIO, CA 91764
TEL: (909) 980-0498
FAX: (909) 980-0458

IDAHO CLAIMS OFFICE
9110 W BARNES
BOISE, ID 83709
TEL: (208) 322-2822
FAX: (208) 375-3078
WWW.GABROBINS.COM

ROBINS NORTH AMERICA, INC
445 W 17TH ST
PO BOX 50797
IDAHO FALLS, ID 83402
TEL: (208) 529-4477
FAX: (208) 529-4482
WWW.GABROBINS.COM

MONTANA CLAIMS OFFICE
1941 HARRISON AVE, STE E
BUTTE, MT 59701
TEL: (406) 723-3247
FAX: (406) 782-6456
WWW.GABROBINS.COM

NATIONAL CLAIMS OFFICE
1661 E CAMEL BACK, STE 260
PO BOX 32419
PHOENIX, AZ 85064-2419
TEL: (602) 248-4130
FAX: (602) 248-4139
WWW.GABROBINS.COM

3700 S WESTPORT AVE
SIOUX FALLS, SD 57106
TEL: (605) 362-8991
FAX: (605) 362-8879

NEW JERSEY CLAIMS OFFICE
9 CAMPUS DR
PO BOX 316
PARSIPPANY, NJ 07054-0316
TEL: (201) 993-3400
FAX: (201) 993-3432
TOLL FREE: (800) 422-4436
E-MAIL: ANSWERS@GABROBINS.COM
WWW.GABROBINSNA.COM

TENNESSEE CLAIMS OFFICE
965 RDG LK BLVD, STE 208
MEMPHIS, TN 38120-0416
TEL: (901) 761-7830
FAX: (901) 767-6403
WWW.GABROBINS.COM

TEXAS CLAIMS OFFICE
1341 W MOCKINGBIRD LN, STE 900 W
DALLAS, TX 75247-6907
TEL: (214) 631-4455
FAX: (214) 631-4261
WWW.GABROBINS.COM

701 SAN JACINTO
CONROE, TX 77301-2539
TEL: (409) 833-7541
FAX: (713) 270-3800
WWW.GABROBINS.COM

WYOMING CLAIMS OFFICE
400 2ND ST, STE A
PO BOX 1373
ROCK SPRINGS, WY 82902-1373
TEL: (307) 382-2660
FAX: (307) 382-8147
WWW.GABROBINS.COM

GAINSCO, INC

NATIONAL CLAIMS OFFICE
GENERAL AGENTS INS CO OF AMERICA/MGA INS CO/GAINSCO COUNTY MUTUAL
500 COMMERCE
PO BOX 2933
FT WORTH, TX 76113-2933
TEL: (817) 336-2500
FAX: (800) 690-9650
TOLL FREE: (800) 438-4246
E-MAIL: CLAIMS@GAINSCO.COM
WWW.GAINSCO.COM

GALILEO INTERNATIONAL

ILLINOIS CLAIMS OFFICE
9700 W HIGGINS RD, STE 400
ROSEMONT, IL 60018-4708
TEL: (847) 518-4000
FAX: (847) 518-4085
WWW.GALILEO.COM

GALLAGHER-BASSETT SERVICES, INC

PO BOX 5227
LISLE, IL 60532
TEL: (630) 773-3800
FAX: (630) 493-3800
IN-STATE: (800) 323-1726

GALLATIN MEDICAL CLINICS

CALIFORNIA CLAIMS OFFICE
10720 PARAMOUNT BLVD
PO BOX 868
DOWNEY, CA 90241-3306
TEL: (562) 923-6511
FAX: (562) 861-6884

GALLO UNION HEALTH PLAN

DELTA HEALTH SYSTEMS
1234 W OAK
PO BOX 669
STOCKTON, CA 95201
TEL: (209) 948-8483
FAX: (209) 475-4926
TOLL FREE: (800) 422-6099

GAN NORTH AMERICA INSURANCE CO

NEW YORK CLAIMS OFFICE
120 WALL ST- 14TH FL
NEW YORK, NY 10005
TEL: (212) 943-8070
FAX: (212) 709-1840
TOLL FREE: (800) 944-5567

GARDNER FAMILY HEALTH NETWORK, INC

CALIFORNIA CLAIMS OFFICE
ALVISO HEALTH CENTER
1621 GOLD ST
PO BOX 1240
ALVISO, CA 95002-1240
TEL: (408) 262-7944
FAX: (408) 935-3988

GARDNER & WHITE

INDIANA CLAIMS OFFICE
8902 N MERIDIAN ST, STE 202
PO BOX 40619
INDIANAPOLIS, IN 46260-5307
TEL: (317) 581-1580
FAX: (317) 587-0780
TOLL FREE: (800) 347-5737

GATES MCDONALD

OHIO CLAIMS OFFICE
NATIONWIDE MUTUAL INSURANCE CO
3455 MILL RUN DR
HILLIARD, OH 43026-9079
TEL: (614) 777-3000
FAX: (614) 777-3352
TOLL FREE: (800) 336-4733

GE CAPITOL INSURANCE

NATIONAL CLAIMS OFFICE
30851 W AGORA RD
PO DRAWER 3199
WESTLAKE VILLAGE, CA 91359
TEL: (818) 889-2520
FAX: (800) 463-0183
TOLL FREE: (800) 999-3643
IN-STATE: (800) 421-7135

GEICO INSURANCE

ALASKA CLAIMS OFFICE
GEICO WEST
14111 DANIELSON ST
PO BOX 509090
SAN DIEGO, CA 92150-9090
TOLL FREE: (800) 341-8000
IN-STATE: (800) 654-5896

Insurance Directory

ARIZONA CLAIMS OFFICE
GEICO WEST
14111 DANIELSON ST
PO BOX 509090
SAN DIEGO, CA 92150-9090
TOLL FREE: (800) 341-8000
IN-STATE: (800) 654-5896

CALIFORNIA CLAIMS OFFICE
GEICO WEST
14111 DANIELSON ST
PO BOX 509090
SAN DIEGO, CA 92150-9090
TOLL FREE: (800) 341-8000
IN-STATE: (800) 654-5896

HAWAII CLAIMS OFFICE
GEICO WEST
14111 DANIELSON ST
PO BOX 509090
SAN DIEGO, CA 92150-9090
TOLL FREE: (800) 341-8000
IN-STATE: (800) 654-5896

IDAHO CLAIMS OFFICE
GEICO WEST
14111 DANIELSON ST
PO BOX 509090
SAN DIEGO, CA 92150-9090
TOLL FREE: (800) 341-8000
IN-STATE: (800) 654-5896

MONTANA CLAIMS OFFICE
GEICO WEST
14111 DANIELSON ST
PO BOX 509090
SAN DIEGO, CA 92150-9090
TOLL FREE: (800) 341-8000
IN-STATE: (800) 654-5896

NEVADA CLAIMS OFFICE
GEICO WEST
14111 DANIELSON ST
PO BOX 509090
SAN DIEGO, CA 92150-9090
TOLL FREE: (800) 341-8000
IN-STATE: (800) 654-5896

OREGON CLAIMS OFFICE
GEICO WEST
14111 DANIELSON ST
PO BOX 509090
SAN DIEGO, CA 92150-9090
TOLL FREE: (800) 341-8000
IN-STATE: (800) 654-5896

UTAH CLAIMS OFFICE
GEICO WEST
14111 DANIELSON ST
PO BOX 509090
SAN DIEGO, CA 92150-9090
TOLL FREE: (800) 341-8000
IN-STATE: (800) 654-5896

WASHINGTON CLAIMS OFFICE
GEICO WEST
14111 DANIELSON ST
PO BOX 509090
SAN DIEGO, CA 92150-9090
TOLL FREE: (800) 341-8000
IN-STATE: (800) 654-5896

GEM INSURANCE CO

ARIZONA CLAIMS OFFICE
525 E 100 S
PO BOX 115
PUEBLO, CO 81002-0115
FAX: (888) 359-5304
TOLL FREE: (800) 888-7164

NEVADA CLAIMS OFFICE
525 E 100 S
PO BOX 115
PUEBLO, CO 81002-0115
FAX: (888) 359-5304
TOLL FREE: (800) 888-7164

NEW MEXICO CLAIMS OFFICE
525 E 100 S
PO BOX 115
PUEBLO, CO 81002-0115
FAX: (888) 359-5304
TOLL FREE: (800) 888-7164

TEXAS CLAIMS OFFICE
525 E 100 S
PO BOX 115
PUEBLO, CO 81002-0115
FAX: (888) 359-5304
TOLL FREE: (800) 888-7164

UTAH CLAIMS OFFICE
525 E 100 S
PO BOX 115
PUEBLO, CO 81002-0115
FAX: (888) 359-5304
TOLL FREE: (800) 888-7164

GENENTECH INC GROUP

CALIFORNIA CLAIMS OFFICE
460 PT SAN BRUNO BLVD
SAN FRANCISCO, CA 94080-4918
TEL: (650) 225-1000
FAX: (650) 225-6000
TOLL FREE: (800) 626-3553
WWW.GENE.COM

GENERAL AMERICAN LIFE INSURANCE CO

NATIONAL CLAIMS OFFICE
719 TEACO RD
PO BOX 882
KENNETT, MO 63857-3749
TEL: (314) 843-8700
FAX: (314) 525-5740
TOLL FREE: (800) 633-8989

521 COLEMAN CT DR
PO BOX 5126
ROCKFORD, IL 61108
TEL: (815) 227-4800
FAX: (815) 395-4888
TOLL FREE: (800) 854-7309
WWW.GENM.COM

OHIO CLAIMS OFFICE
5455 RINGS RD, STE 550
DUBLIN, OH 43016
TEL: (614) 717-2557
FAX: (614) 717-2588
TOLL FREE: (800) 445-7119

TEXAS CLAIMS OFFICE
275 W CAMPBELL RD, STE 401
RICHARDSON, TX 75080
TEL: (972) 238-5000
IN-STATE: (800) 541-3234

GENERAL INSURANCE EXCHANGE AGENCY, INC

OHIO CLAIMS OFFICE
4301 DARROW RD
PO BOX 1849
STOW, OH 44224-0849
TEL: (330) 688-4322
FAX: (330) 688-4904
TOLL FREE: (800) 968-7222
WWW.CHANDLER-GROUP.COM

GENERAL REINSURANCE CORP

NATIONAL CLAIMS OFFICE
695 E MAIN
STAMFORD, CT 06904
TEL: (212) 341-8000
FAX: (203) 328-6432
TOLL FREE: (800) 431-9994

GENISUS HEALTH VENTURES, INC

PENNSYLVANIA CLAIMS OFFICE
101 E STATE ST
KENNETT SQUARE, PA 19348
TEL: (610) 444-6350
FAX: (610) 925-4353
TOLL FREE: (800) 628-4928

GEORGE N. PEGULA AGENCY

CATHLOC AGENCY
430 PENN AVE
PO BOX 3658
SCRANTON, PA 18503
TEL: (570) 343-4745
FAX: (570) 961-5779
TOLL FREE: (800) 233-4697

GEORGE WASHINGTON UNIVERSITY HEALTH PLAN

DISTRICT OF COLUMBIA CLAIMS OFFICE
4550 MONTGOMERY AVE, STE 800
BETHESDA NORTH, MD 20814
TEL: (301) 941-2000
TOLL FREE: (800) 333-4947

MARYLAND CLAIMS OFFICE
4550 MONTGOMERY AVE, STE 800
BETHESDA NORTH, MD 20814
TEL: (301) 941-2000
TOLL FREE: (800) 333-4947

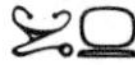

VIRGINIA CLAIMS OFFICE
4550 MONTGOMERY AVE, STE 800
BETHESDA NORTH, MD 20814
TEL: (301) 941-2000
TOLL FREE: (800) 333-4947

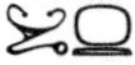

GEORGIA BANKERS ASSOCIATION INSURANCE

GEORGIA CLAIMS OFFICE
50 HURT PLZ, STE 1050
ATLANTA, GA 30303-2916
TEL: (404) 522-1501
FAX: (404) 522-9848
WWW.GABANKERS.COM

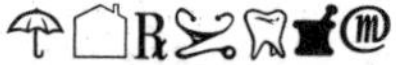

GEORGIA FARM BUREAU MUTUAL INSURANCE CO

1620 BASH RD
PO BOX 7008
MACON, GA 31209-7008
TEL: (912) 474-8411
FAX: (912) 474-8492
TOLL FREE: (800) 342-1192

GERBER LIFE INSURANCE CO

FLORIDA CLAIMS OFFICE
204 W MAIN ST
FREMONT, MI 49412
TEL: (616) 928-2000
FAX: (616) 928-2322
TOLL FREE: (800) 628-0560

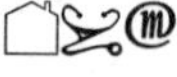

MICHIGAN CLAIMS OFFICE
204 W MAIN ST
FREMONT, MI 49412
TEL: (616) 928-2000
FAX: (616) 928-2322
TOLL FREE: (800) 628-0560

PO BOX 2088
GRAND RAPIDS, MI 49501-2088
TEL: (616) 928-2000
TOLL FREE: (800) 628-0011

NATIONAL CLAIMS OFFICE
66 CHURCH ST
WHITE PLAINS, NY 10601-1901
TEL: (914) 761-4404
FAX: (914) 761-4772
TOLL FREE: (800) 253-3074

NEW YORK CLAIMS OFFICE
204 W MAIN ST
FREMONT, MI 49412
TEL: (616) 928-2000
FAX: (616) 928-2322
TOLL FREE: (800) 628-0560

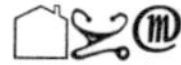

GERLING AMERICA INSURANCE CO

ALABAMA CLAIMS OFFICE
717 5TH AVE
NEW YORK, NY 10022
TEL: (212) 752-8900
FAX: (212) 888-3720
WWW.GERLING.COM

ALASKA CLAIMS OFFICE
717 5TH AVE
NEW YORK, NY 10022
TEL: (212) 752-8900
FAX: (212) 888-3720
WWW.GERLING.COM

ARIZONA CLAIMS OFFICE
717 5TH AVE
NEW YORK, NY 10022
TEL: (212) 752-8900
FAX: (212) 888-3720
WWW.GERLING.COM

ARKANSAS CLAIMS OFFICE
717 5TH AVE
NEW YORK, NY 10022
TEL: (212) 752-8900
FAX: (212) 888-3720
WWW.GERLING.COM

CALIFORNIA CLAIMS OFFICE
717 5TH AVE
NEW YORK, NY 10022
TEL: (212) 752-8900
FAX: (212) 888-3720
WWW.GERLING.COM

COLORADO CLAIMS OFFICE
717 5TH AVE
NEW YORK, NY 10022
TEL: (212) 752-8900
FAX: (212) 888-3720
WWW.GERLING.COM

CONNECTICUT CLAIMS OFFICE
717 5TH AVE
NEW YORK, NY 10022
TEL: (212) 752-8900
FAX: (212) 888-3720
WWW.GERLING.COM

DELAWARE CLAIMS OFFICE
717 5TH AVE
NEW YORK, NY 10022
TEL: (212) 752-8900
FAX: (212) 888-3720
WWW.GERLING.COM

DISTRICT OF COLUMBIA CLAIMS OFFICE
717 5TH AVE
NEW YORK, NY 10022
TEL: (212) 752-8900
FAX: (212) 888-3720
WWW.GERLING.COM

FLORIDA CLAIMS OFFICE
717 5TH AVE
NEW YORK, NY 10022
TEL: (212) 752-8900
FAX: (212) 888-3720
WWW.GERLING.COM

GEORGIA CLAIMS OFFICE
717 5TH AVE
NEW YORK, NY 10022
TEL: (212) 752-8900
FAX: (212) 888-3720
WWW.GERLING.COM

HAWAII CLAIMS OFFICE
717 5TH AVE
NEW YORK, NY 10022
TEL: (212) 752-8900
FAX: (212) 888-3720
WWW.GERLING.COM

IDAHO CLAIMS OFFICE
717 5TH AVE
NEW YORK, NY 10022
TEL: (212) 752-8900
FAX: (212) 888-3720
WWW.GERLING.COM

ILLINOIS CLAIMS OFFICE
717 5TH AVE
NEW YORK, NY 10022
TEL: (212) 752-8900
FAX: (212) 888-3720
WWW.GERLING.COM

INDIANA CLAIMS OFFICE
717 5TH AVE
NEW YORK, NY 10022
TEL: (212) 752-8900
FAX: (212) 888-3720
WWW.GERLING.COM

IOWA CLAIMS OFFICE
717 5TH AVE
NEW YORK, NY 10022
TEL: (212) 752-8900
FAX: (212) 888-3720
WWW.GERLING.COM

KANSAS CLAIMS OFFICE
717 5TH AVE
NEW YORK, NY 10022
TEL: (212) 752-8900
FAX: (212) 888-3720
WWW.GERLING.COM

KENTUCKY CLAIMS OFFICE
717 5TH AVE
NEW YORK, NY 10022
TEL: (212) 752-8900
FAX: (212) 888-3720
WWW.GERLING.COM

LOUISIANA CLAIMS OFFICE
717 5TH AVE
NEW YORK, NY 10022
TEL: (212) 752-8900
FAX: (212) 888-3720
WWW.GERLING.COM

MAINE CLAIMS OFFICE
717 5TH AVE
NEW YORK, NY 10022
TEL: (212) 752-8900
FAX: (212) 888-3720
WWW.GERLING.COM
3 ☂ ☆

MARYLAND CLAIMS OFFICE
717 5TH AVE
NEW YORK, NY 10022
TEL: (212) 752-8900
FAX: (212) 888-3720
WWW.GERLING.COM
3 ☂ ☆

MASSACHUSETTS CLAIMS OFFICE
717 5TH AVE
NEW YORK, NY 10022
TEL: (212) 752-8900
FAX: (212) 888-3720
WWW.GERLING.COM
3 ☂ ☆

MICHIGAN CLAIMS OFFICE
717 5TH AVE
NEW YORK, NY 10022
TEL: (212) 752-8900
FAX: (212) 888-3720
WWW.GERLING.COM
3 ☂ ☆

MINNESOTA CLAIMS OFFICE
717 5TH AVE
NEW YORK, NY 10022
TEL: (212) 752-8900
FAX: (212) 888-3720
WWW.GERLING.COM
3 ☂ ☆

MISSISSIPPI CLAIMS OFFICE
717 5TH AVE
NEW YORK, NY 10022
TEL: (212) 752-8900
FAX: (212) 888-3720
WWW.GERLING.COM
3 ☂ ☆

MISSOURI CLAIMS OFFICE
717 5TH AVE
NEW YORK, NY 10022
TEL: (212) 752-8900
FAX: (212) 888-3720
WWW.GERLING.COM
3 ☂ ☆

MONTANA CLAIMS OFFICE
717 5TH AVE
NEW YORK, NY 10022
TEL: (212) 752-8900
FAX: (212) 888-3720
WWW.GERLING.COM
3 ☂ ☆

NEBRASKA CLAIMS OFFICE
717 5TH AVE
NEW YORK, NY 10022
TEL: (212) 752-8900
FAX: (212) 888-3720
WWW.GERLING.COM
3 ☂ ☆

NEVADA CLAIMS OFFICE
717 5TH AVE
NEW YORK, NY 10022
TEL: (212) 752-8900
FAX: (212) 888-3720
WWW.GERLING.COM
3 ☂ ☆

NEW HAMPSHIRE CLAIMS OFFICE
717 5TH AVE
NEW YORK, NY 10022
TEL: (212) 752-8900
FAX: (212) 888-3720
WWW.GERLING.COM
3 ☂ ☆

NEW MEXICO CLAIMS OFFICE
717 5TH AVE
NEW YORK, NY 10022
TEL: (212) 752-8900
FAX: (212) 888-3720
WWW.GERLING.COM
3 ☂ ☆

NEW YORK CLAIMS OFFICE
717 5TH AVE
NEW YORK, NY 10022
TEL: (212) 752-8900
FAX: (212) 888-3720
WWW.GERLING.COM
3 ☂ ☆

NORTH CAROLINA CLAIMS OFFICE
717 5TH AVE
NEW YORK, NY 10022
TEL: (212) 752-8900
FAX: (212) 888-3720
WWW.GERLING.COM
3 ☂ ☆

NORTH DAKOTA CLAIMS OFFICE
717 5TH AVE
NEW YORK, NY 10022
TEL: (212) 752-8900
FAX: (212) 888-3720
WWW.GERLING.COM
3 ☂ ☆

OHIO CLAIMS OFFICE
717 5TH AVE
NEW YORK, NY 10022
TEL: (212) 752-8900
FAX: (212) 888-3720
WWW.GERLING.COM
3 ☂ ☆

OKLAHOMA CLAIMS OFFICE
717 5TH AVE
NEW YORK, NY 10022
TEL: (212) 752-8900
FAX: (212) 888-3720
WWW.GERLING.COM
3 ☂ ☆

OREGON CLAIMS OFFICE
717 5TH AVE
NEW YORK, NY 10022
TEL: (212) 752-8900
FAX: (212) 888-3720
WWW.GERLING.COM
3 ☂ ☆

PENNSYLVANIA CLAIMS OFFICE
717 5TH AVE
NEW YORK, NY 10022
TEL: (212) 752-8900
FAX: (212) 888-3720
WWW.GERLING.COM
3 ☂ ☆

RHODE ISLAND CLAIMS OFFICE
717 5TH AVE
NEW YORK, NY 10022
TEL: (212) 752-8900
FAX: (212) 888-3720
WWW.GERLING.COM
3 ☂ ☆

SOUTH CAROLINA CLAIMS OFFICE
717 5TH AVE
NEW YORK, NY 10022
TEL: (212) 752-8900
FAX: (212) 888-3720
WWW.GERLING.COM
3 ☂ ☆

SOUTH DAKOTA CLAIMS OFFICE
717 5TH AVE
NEW YORK, NY 10022
TEL: (212) 752-8900
FAX: (212) 888-3720
WWW.GERLING.COM
3 ☂ ☆

TENNESSEE CLAIMS OFFICE
717 5TH AVE
NEW YORK, NY 10022
TEL: (212) 752-8900
FAX: (212) 888-3720
WWW.GERLING.COM
3 ☂ ☆

TEXAS CLAIMS OFFICE
717 5TH AVE
NEW YORK, NY 10022
TEL: (212) 752-8900
FAX: (212) 888-3720
WWW.GERLING.COM
3 ☂ ☆

UTAH CLAIMS OFFICE
717 5TH AVE
NEW YORK, NY 10022
TEL: (212) 752-8900
FAX: (212) 888-3720
WWW.GERLING.COM
3 ☂ ☆

VERMONT CLAIMS OFFICE
717 5TH AVE
NEW YORK, NY 10022
TEL: (212) 752-8900
FAX: (212) 888-3720
WWW.GERLING.COM
3 ☂ ☆

VIRGINIA CLAIMS OFFICE
717 5TH AVE
NEW YORK, NY 10022
TEL: (212) 752-8900
FAX: (212) 888-3720
WWW.GERLING.COM
3 ☂ ☆

WASHINGTON CLAIMS OFFICE
717 5TH AVE
NEW YORK, NY 10022
TEL: (212) 752-8900
FAX: (212) 888-3720
WWW.GERLING.COM
3 ☂ ☆

G

WEST VIRGINIA CLAIMS OFFICE
717 5TH AVE
NEW YORK, NY 10022
TEL: (212) 752-8900
FAX: (212) 888-3720
WWW.GERLING.COM

WISCONSIN CLAIMS OFFICE
717 5TH AVE
NEW YORK, NY 10022
TEL: (212) 752-8900
FAX: (212) 888-3720
WWW.GERLING.COM

WYOMING CLAIMS OFFICE
717 5TH AVE
NEW YORK, NY 10022
TEL: (212) 752-8900
FAX: (212) 888-3720
WWW.GERLING.COM

GERLING CANADA

ONTARIO CLAIMS OFFICE
480 UNIVERSITY AVE, STE 1700
TORONTO, ON M5G-1V6
TEL: (416) 598-4651
FAX: (416) 598-5478

GERLING GLOBAL LIFE REINSURANCE CO

CALIFORNIA CLAIMS OFFICE
480 UNIVERSITY AVE
TORONTO, ON M5G-1V6
TEL: (416) 598-4677
FAX: (416) 598-3901
TOLL FREE: (800) 263-1747

QUEBEC CLAIMS OFFICE
480 UNIVERSITY AVE
TORONTO, ON M5G-1V6
TEL: (416) 598-4677
FAX: (416) 598-3901
TOLL FREE: (800) 263-1747

GERLING GLOBAL REINSURANCE CORP

NATIONAL CLAIMS OFFICE
110 WILLIAM ST- 7TH FL
NEW YORK, NY 10038-3991
TEL: (212) 225-1000
FAX: (212) 346-0953
TOLL FREE: (800) 255-5530

GILBERT-MAGILL CO

MISSOURI CLAIMS OFFICE
920 MAIN ST, STE 1800
PO BOX 410249
KANSAS CITY, MO 64141-0249
TEL: (816) 474-3535
FAX: (816) 842-5795
TOLL FREE: (800) 522-2460

GILLETTE CO

NATIONAL CLAIMS OFFICE
ONE GILLETTE WY
BOSTON, MA 02127
TEL: (617) 421-7000

GILSBAR, INC

LOUISIANA CLAIMS OFFICE
2100 COVINGTON CTR
PO BOX 998
COVINGTON, LA 70434-0998
TEL: (504) 892-3520
FAX: (504) 898-1666
TOLL FREE: (800) 445-7227
E-MAIL: GILSBAR@GILSBAR.COM
WWW.GILSBAR.COM

GLOBE LIFE & ACCIDENT INSURANCE CO

NATIONAL CLAIMS OFFICE
GLOBE LIFE CENTER
204 N ROBINSON
PO BOX 268844
OKLAHOMA CITY, OK 73126-8844
TEL: (405) 270-1400
TOLL FREE: (800) 654-5433

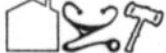

GMP EMPLOYERS RETIREE TRUST

FLORIDA CLAIMS OFFICE
5245 BIG PINE WY SE
FT MYERS, FL 33907-5998
TEL: (941) 936-6242
FAX: (941) 936-3438

GOLDEN RULE LIFE INSURANCE CO

ILLINOIS CLAIMS OFFICE
712 11TH ST
LAWRENCEVILLE, IL 62439-2395
TEL: (618) 943-8000
FAX: (618) 943-8031

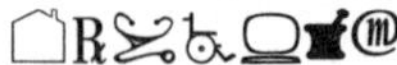

NATIONAL CLAIMS OFFICE
7440 WOODLAND DR
INDIANAPOLIS, IN 46278-1719
TEL: (317) 297-4123
FAX: (317) 298-4410
IN-STATE: (800) 265-7791
WWW.GOLDENRULE.COM

GOLDEN STATE MUTUAL LIFE INSURANCE CO

1999 W ADAMS BLVD
PO BOX 512332
LOS ANGELES, CA 90051-0332
TEL: (323) 731-1131
TOLL FREE: (800) 225-5476
WWW.GSMLIFE.COM

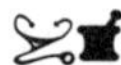

GOOD SAMARITAN WOUND CENTER

1020 E OGDEN AVE, STE 106
NAPERVILLE, IL 60563
TEL: (630) 428-9600
FAX: (630) 428-9215
TOLL FREE: (800) 435-4011
WWW.CURITIVE.COM

GOODVILLE MUTUAL CASUALTY CO

PENNSYLVANIA CLAIMS OFFICE
625 W MAIN
PO BOX 489
NEW HOLLAND, PA 17557-0489
TEL: (717) 354-4921
FAX: (717) 354-5158

GOULD MEDICAL FOUNDATION

CALIFORNIA CLAIMS OFFICE
PO BOX 254708
SACRAMENTO, CA 95865
TEL: (209) 524-2221
FAX: (209) 524-4562
IN-STATE: (800) 564-6853

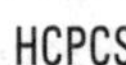

GOVERNMENT EMPLOYEES HOSPITAL ASSOCIATION

NATIONAL CLAIMS OFFICE
17306 E 24 HWY
PO BOX 4665
INDEPENDENCE, MO 64051-4665
TEL: (816) 257-3500
TOLL FREE: (800) 821-6136
WWW.GEHA.COM

GRAIN DEALER MUTUAL INSURANCE CO

COLORADO CLAIMS OFFICE
11906 ARBOR ST
OMAHA, NE 68144-2938
TEL: (402) 334-9100
FAX: (402) 334-3180
TOLL FREE: (800) 228-9780

INDIANA CLAIMS OFFICE
1752 N MERIDIAN ST
PO BOX 1747
INDIANAPOLIS, IN 46206-1747
TEL: (317) 923-2453
FAX: (800) 300-5446
TOLL FREE: (800) 428-7081
WWW.GRAINDEALERS.COM

IOWA CLAIMS OFFICE
11906 ARBOR ST
OMAHA, NE 68144-2938
TEL: (402) 334-9100
FAX: (402) 334-3180
TOLL FREE: (800) 228-9780

KANSAS CLAIMS OFFICE
11906 ARBOR ST
OMAHA, NE 68144-2938
TEL: (402) 334-9100
FAX: (402) 334-3180
TOLL FREE: (800) 228-9780

MISSOURI CLAIMS OFFICE
11906 ARBOR ST
OMAHA, NE 68144-2938
TEL: (402) 334-9100
FAX: (402) 334-3180
TOLL FREE: (800) 228-9780

NEBRASKA CLAIMS OFFICE
11906 ARBOR ST
OMAHA, NE 68144-2938
TEL: (402) 334-9100
FAX: (402) 334-3180
TOLL FREE: (800) 228-9780

WASHINGTON CLAIMS OFFICE
11906 ARBOR ST
OMAHA, NE 68144-2938
TEL: (402) 334-9100
FAX: (402) 334-3180
TOLL FREE: (800) 228-9780

GRAND PACIFIC LIFE INSURANCE CO, LTD

HAWAII CLAIMS OFFICE
1164 BISHOP ST, STE 500
PO BOX 420
HONOLULU, HI 96809-0420
TEL: (808) 548-3363
FAX: (808) 548-5122
TOLL FREE: (800) 326-4754
WWW.GPLI.COM

GRAND VALLEY CORP

MICHIGAN CLAIMS OFFICE
829 FOREST HILLS AVE SE
GRAND RAPIDS, MI 49546-2325
TEL: (616) 949-2410
FAX: (616) 949-4978

GRANGE INSURANCE ASSOCIATION

CALIFORNIA CLAIMS OFFICE
ROCKY MOUNTAIN FIRE & CASUALTY CO
200 CEDAR ST
PO BOX C-21089
SEATTLE, WA 98111-3809
TEL: (206) 448-4911
FAX: (206) 448-9023
TOLL FREE: (800) 247-2643

2260 S XANADU WAY, STE 225
AURORA, CO 80014
TEL: (303) 369-8100
FAX: (303) 369-2030
TOLL FREE: (800)247-7758

COLORADO CLAIMS OFFICE
2260 S XANADU WAY, STE 225
AURORA, CO 80014
TEL: (303) 369-8100
FAX: (303) 369-2030
TOLL FREE: (800)247-7758

ROCKY MOUNTAIN FIRE & CASUALTY CO
200 CEDAR ST
PO BOX C-21089
SEATTLE, WA 98111-3809
TEL: (206) 448-4911
FAX: (206) 448-9023
TOLL FREE: (800) 247-2643

GEORGIA CLAIMS OFFICE
6415 MUTUAL DR
PO BOX 12010
FT WAYNE, IN 46862-2010
TEL: (219) 483-1636
FAX: (219) 484-6475
IN-STATE: (800) 589-5590

IDAHO CLAIMS OFFICE
ROCKY MOUNTAIN FIRE & CASUALTY CO
200 CEDAR ST
PO BOX C-21089
SEATTLE, WA 98111-3809
TEL: (206) 448-4911
FAX: (206) 448-9023
TOLL FREE: (800) 247-2643

ILLINOIS CLAIMS OFFICE
6415 MUTUAL DR
PO BOX 12010
FT WAYNE, IN 46862-2010
TEL: (219) 483-1636
FAX: (219) 484-6475
IN-STATE: (800) 589-5590

INDIANA CLAIMS OFFICE
6415 MUTUAL DR
PO BOX 12010
FT WAYNE, IN 46862-2010
TEL: (219) 483-1636
FAX: (219) 484-6475
IN-STATE: (800) 589-5590

KENTUCKY CLAIMS OFFICE
2425 REGENCY RD
PO BOX 8035
LEXINGTON, KY 40533-8035
TEL: (606) 278-5481
FAX: (800) 837-0802
TOLL FREE: (800) 837-0801

MONTANA CLAIMS OFFICE
ROCKY MOUNTAIN FIRE & CASUALTY CO
200 CEDAR ST
PO BOX C-21089
SEATTLE, WA 98111-3809
TEL: (206) 448-4911
FAX: (206) 448-9023
TOLL FREE: (800) 247-2643

OHIO CLAIMS OFFICE
6415 MUTUAL DR
PO BOX 12010
FT WAYNE, IN 46862-2010
TEL: (219) 483-1636
FAX: (219) 484-6475
IN-STATE: (800) 589-5590

OREGON CLAIMS OFFICE
2501 SE COLUMBIA WAY, STE 160
PO BOX 1117
VANCOUVER, WA 98666
TEL: (360) 696-0235
FAX: (360) 696-3095
TOLL FREE: (800) 368-8881
IN-STATE: (800) 368-8881

ROCKY MOUNTAIN FIRE & CASUALTY CO
200 CEDAR ST
PO BOX C-21089
SEATTLE, WA 98111-3809
TEL: (206) 448-4911
FAX: (206) 448-9023
TOLL FREE: (800) 247-2643

TENNESSEE CLAIMS OFFICE
6415 MUTUAL DR
PO BOX 12010
FT WAYNE, IN 46862-2010
TEL: (219) 483-1636
FAX: (219) 484-6475
IN-STATE: (800) 589-5590

WASHINGTON CLAIMS OFFICE
ROCKY MOUNTAIN FIRE & CASUALTY CO
200 CEDAR ST
PO BOX C-21089
SEATTLE, WA 98111-3809
TEL: (206) 448-4911
FAX: (206) 448-9023
TOLL FREE: (800) 247-2643

ROCKY MOUNTAIN FIRE & CASUALTY CO
13112 NE 20TH ST- BLDG C-2, STE 1
BELLEVUE, WA 98005-9888
TEL: (425) 869-4949
FAX: (425) 869-9653
TOLL FREE: (800) 826-3197

2501 SE COLUMBIA WAY, STE 160
PO BOX 1117
VANCOUVER, WA 98666
TEL: (360) 696-0235
FAX: (360) 696-3095
TOLL FREE: (800) 368-8881
IN-STATE: (800) 368-8881

2260 S XANADU WAY, STE 225
AURORA, CO 80014
TEL: (303) 369-8100
FAX: (303) 369-2030
TOLL FREE: (800)247-7758

WYOMING CLAIMS OFFICE
ROCKY MOUNTAIN FIRE & CASUALTY CO
200 CEDAR ST
PO BOX C-21089
SEATTLE, WA 98111-3809
TEL: (206) 448-4911
FAX: (206) 448-9023
TOLL FREE: (800) 247-2643

2260 S XANADU WAY, STE 225
AURORA, CO 80014
TEL: (303) 369-8100
FAX: (303) 369-2030
TOLL FREE: (800)247-7758

GRANGE MUTUAL CASUALTY CO

GEORGIA CLAIMS OFFICE
2060 WATSON BLVD
PO BOX 8049
WARNER ROBINS, GA 31095-8049
TEL: (912) 922-4494
FAX: (912) 923-3085
TOLL FREE: (800) 342-3785

OHIO CLAIMS OFFICE
650 S FRONT ST
PO BOX 1218
COLUMBUS, OH 43216
TEL: (614) 445-2900
FAX: (614) 445-8363
TOLL FREE: (800) 422-0550
WWW.GRANGEINSURANCE.COM

GRANGE MUTUAL INSURANCE CO

NEW HAMPSHIRE CLAIMS OFFICE
17 WAKEFIELD ST
PO BOX 1150
ROCHESTER, NH 03866-1150
TEL: (603) 332-6933
FAX: (603) 332-1586
IN-STATE: (800) 244-7358

GRAY INSURANCE CO

LOUISIANA CLAIMS OFFICE
3601 N I-10 SERVICE RD W
PO BOX 6202
METAIRIE, LA 70009-6202
TEL: (504) 888-7790
FAX: (504) 887-5658
WWW.GRAYINSCO.COM

GRE INDIANA INSURANCE GROUP

WISCONSIN CLAIMS OFFICE
N 14 W 24200 TWR PL
PO BOX 936
PEWAUKEE, WI 53072-0936
TEL: (414) 547-3636
FAX: (414) 524-6578
TOLL FREE: (800) 846-2331

GRE INSURANCE GROUP

ILLINOIS CLAIMS OFFICE
300 W WASHINGTON, STE 501
CHICAGO, IL 60606
TEL: (312) 470-0233
FAX: (312) 470-0290
TOLL FREE: (800) 677-8565

NATIONAL CLAIMS OFFICE
ALBANY INSURANCE CO
61 BROADWAY- 32ND FL
NEW YORK, NY 10006
TEL: (212) 208-4100
FAX: (212) 514-6928
WWW.GRE-INSURANCE.COM

LIBERTY MUTUAL
1504 SANTA ROSA RD, STE 100
PO BOX K-187
RICHMOND, VA 23288
TEL: (804) 288-7947
FAX: (804) 288-4617
TOLL FREE: (800) 677-4595

NEW JERSEY CLAIMS OFFICE
600 COLLEGE RD E
PRINCETON, NJ 08540
TEL: (609) 275-2600
TOLL FREE: (800) 955-5513

6281 TRI-RIDGE BLVD
LOVELAND, OH 45140
TEL: (513) 576-3200
FAX: (800) 436-9611
TOLL FREE: (800) 436-9600
IN-STATE: (800) 436-9600

OHIO CLAIMS OFFICE
6281 TRI-RIDGE BLVD
LOVELAND, OH 45140
TEL: (513) 576-3200
FAX: (800) 436-9611
TOLL FREE: (800) 436-9600
IN-STATE: (800) 436-9600

600 COLLEGE RD E
PRINCETON, NJ 08540
TEL: (609) 275-2600
TOLL FREE: (800) 955-5513

GREAT AMERICAN INSURANCE COMPANIES

CONNECTICUT CLAIMS OFFICE
11353 REED HARTMAN HWY
PO BOX 405015
CINCINNATI, OH 45240-5015
TEL: (513) 530-8700
FAX: (513) 530-8455
TOLL FREE: (800) 545-4269
IN-STATE: (800) 572-7440
WWW.OCAS.COM

FLORIDA CLAIMS OFFICE
2701 MAITLAND CTR PKY, STE 125
MAITLAND, FL 32751
TEL: (407) 667-0022
FAX: (407) 667-8931
TOLL FREE: (800) 241-4353

OHIO CASUALTY
3105 GLENWOOD AVE
PO BOX 29557
RALEIGH, NC 27626
TEL: (919) 783-1400
FAX: (919) 571-7458
TOLL FREE: (800) 654-2138

GEORGIA CLAIMS OFFICE
OHIO CASUALTY
3105 GLENWOOD AVE
PO BOX 29557
RALEIGH, NC 27626
TEL: (919) 783-1400
FAX: (919) 571-7458
TOLL FREE: (800) 654-2138

LOUISIANA CLAIMS OFFICE
OHIO CASUALTY
3105 GLENWOOD AVE
PO BOX 29557
RALEIGH, NC 27626
TEL: (919) 783-1400
FAX: (919) 571-7458
TOLL FREE: (800) 654-2138

MARYLAND CLAIMS OFFICE
10480 LITTLE PATUXENT PKY, STE 350
PO BOX 1146
COLUMBIA, MD 21044-0146
TEL: (410) 740-9525
FAX: (410) 740-9736
TOLL FREE: (800) 492-9331

OHIO CASUALTY
10480 LITTLE PATUXENT, STE 350
PO BOX 1146
COLUMBIA, MD 21044-0146
TEL: (410) 740-9525
FAX: (410) 740-9736
TOLL FREE: (800) 492-9331

MINNESOTA CLAIMS OFFICE
11353 REED HARTMAN HWY
PO BOX 405015
CINCINNATI, OH 45240-5015
TEL: (513) 530-8700
FAX: (513) 530-8455
TOLL FREE: (800) 545-4269
IN-STATE: (800) 572-7440
WWW.OCAS.COM

MISSISSIPPI CLAIMS OFFICE
OHIO CASUALTY
3105 GLENWOOD AVE
PO BOX 29557
RALEIGH, NC 27626
TEL: (919) 783-1400
FAX: (919) 571-7458
TOLL FREE: (800) 654-2138

NATIONAL CLAIMS OFFICE
OHIO CASUALTY
750 E SIPY DR S, STE 300
PO BOX 14180
ORANGE, CA 92863-1580
TEL: (714) 740-2400
FAX: (714) 740-3150
TOLL FREE: (800) 637-9975

NEW JERSEY CLAIMS OFFICE
OHIO CASUALTY
500 LANIDEX CTR
PO BOX 318
PARSIPPANY, NJ 07054-0318
TEL: (973) 887-4800
FAX: (973) 952-9737
IN-STATE: (800) 222-0305

NEW YORK CLAIMS OFFICE
OHIO CASUALTY
251 SALINA MEADOWS PKY
PO BOX 4931
SYRACUSE, NY 13221-4931
TEL: (315) 451-2130
FAX: (315) 451-5971
TOLL FREE: (800) 393-1144
IN-STATE: (800) 962-5479

NORTH CAROLINA CLAIMS OFFICE
OHIO CASUALTY
3105 GLENWOOD AVE
PO BOX 29557
RALEIGH, NC 27626
TEL: (919) 783-1400
FAX: (919) 571-7458
TOLL FREE: (800) 654-2138

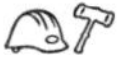

OHIO CLAIMS OFFICE
OHIO CASUALTY
580 WALNUT ST
CINCINNATI, OH 45202
TEL: (513) 369-5000
FAX: (513) 369-5693

11353 REED HARTMAN HWY
PO BOX 405015
CINCINNATI, OH 45240-5015
TEL: (513) 530-8700
FAX: (513) 530-8455
TOLL FREE: (800) 545-4269
IN-STATE: (800) 572-7440
WWW.OCAS.COM

OHIO CASUALTY
11353 REED HARTMAN HWY
PO BOX 429563
CINCINNATI, OH 45242-9563
TEL: (513) 530-8700
FAX: (513) 530-8455
TOLL FREE: (800) 348-4269

OKLAHOMA CLAIMS OFFICE
OHIO CASUALTY
3105 GLENWOOD AVE
PO BOX 29557
RALEIGH, NC 27626
TEL: (919) 783-1400
FAX: (919) 571-7458
TOLL FREE: (800) 654-2138

PENNSYLVANIA CLAIMS OFFICE
OHIO CASUALTY
10480 LITTLE PATUXENT, STE 350
PO BOX 1146
COLUMBIA, MD 21044-0146
TEL: (410) 740-9525
FAX: (410) 740-9736
TOLL FREE: (800) 492-9331

SOUTH CAROLINA CLAIMS OFFICE
OHIO CASUALTY
3105 GLENWOOD AVE
PO BOX 29557
RALEIGH, NC 27626
TEL: (919) 783-1400
FAX: (919) 571-7458
TOLL FREE: (800) 654-2138

TENNESSEE CLAIMS OFFICE
OHIO CASUALTY
3105 GLENWOOD AVE
PO BOX 29557
RALEIGH, NC 27626
TEL: (919) 783-1400
FAX: (919) 571-7458
TOLL FREE: (800) 654-2138

UTAH CLAIMS OFFICE
OHIO CASUALTY
11353 REED HARTMAN HWY
PO BOX 429563
CINCINNATI, OH 45242-9563
TEL: (513) 530-8700
FAX: (513) 530-8455
TOLL FREE: (800) 348-4269

WASHINGTON CLAIMS OFFICE
OHIO CASUALTY
11353 REED HARTMAN HWY
PO BOX 429563
CINCINNATI, OH 45242-9563
TEL: (513) 530-8700
FAX: (513) 530-8455
TOLL FREE: (800) 348-4269

GREAT ATLANTIC LIFE INSURANCE CO

FLORIDA CLAIMS OFFICE
2090 PALM BEACH LKS BLVD, STE 200
WEST PALM BEACH, FL 33409-6596
TEL: (561) 683-0202
FAX: (561) 689-3829

SOUTH CAROLINA CLAIMS OFFICE
2090 PALM BEACH LKS BLVD, STE 200
WEST PALM BEACH, FL 33409-6596
TEL: (561) 683-0202
FAX: (561) 689-3829

TENNESSEE CLAIMS OFFICE
2090 PALM BEACH LKS BLVD, STE 200
WEST PALM BEACH, FL 33409-6596
TEL: (561) 683-0202
FAX: (561) 689-3829

GREAT NORTHERN INSURANCE CO

NATIONAL CLAIMS OFFICE
CHUBB GROUP INSURANCE
200 S 6TH ST, STE 1000
MINNEAPOLIS, MN 55402-1470
TEL: (612) 373-7300
FAX: (612) 373-7318
TOLL FREE: (800) 525-0614
WWW.CHUBB.COM

GREAT REPUBLIC LIFE INSURANCE CO

ALASKA CLAIMS OFFICE
1900 W HARRISON
SEATTLE, WA 98119-1650
TEL: (206) 285-1422
FAX: (206) 282-5865
TOLL FREE: (800) 388-7330
E-MAIL: GRLIC@AOL.COM

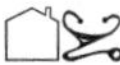

ARIZONA CLAIMS OFFICE
1900 W HARRISON
SEATTLE, WA 98119-1650
TEL: (206) 285-1422
FAX: (206) 282-5865
TOLL FREE: (800) 388-7330
E-MAIL: GRLIC@AOL.COM

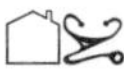

IDAHO CLAIMS OFFICE
1900 W HARRISON
SEATTLE, WA 98119-1650
TEL: (206) 285-1422
FAX: (206) 282-5865
TOLL FREE: (800) 388-7330
E-MAIL: GRLIC@AOL.COM

NEVADA CLAIMS OFFICE
1900 W HARRISON
SEATTLE, WA 98119-1650
TEL: (206) 285-1422
FAX: (206) 282-5865
TOLL FREE: (800) 388-7330
E-MAIL: GRLIC@AOL.COM

OREGON CLAIMS OFFICE
1900 W HARRISON
SEATTLE, WA 98119-1650
TEL: (206) 285-1422
FAX: (206) 282-5865
TOLL FREE: (800) 388-7330
E-MAIL: GRLIC@AOL.COM

UTAH CLAIMS OFFICE
1900 W NICKERSON
SEATTLE, WA 98119-1650
TEL: (206) 285-1422
FAX: (206) 282-5865
TOLL FREE: (800) 388-7330
E-MAIL: GRLIC@AOL.COM

WASHINGTON CLAIMS OFFICE
1900 W HARRISON
SEATTLE, WA 98119-1650
TEL: (206) 285-1422
FAX: (206) 282-5865
TOLL FREE: (800) 388-7330
E-MAIL: GRLIC@AOL.COM

GREAT SOUTHERN LIFE INSURANCE CO

TEXAS CLAIMS OFFICE
PO BOX 13487
KANSAS CITY, MO 64199-3487
TEL: (214) 954-8100
FAX: (214) 954-8491
TOLL FREE: (800) 231-0801

GREAT WEST CASUALTY CO

NATIONAL CLAIMS OFFICE
1100 W 29TH ST
PO BOX 277
SOUTH SIOUX CITY, NE 68876-0277
TEL: (402) 494-2411
FAX: (402) 494-7450
TOLL FREE: (800) 228-8602
WWW.GWCCNET.COM

GREAT WEST LIFE

DISTRICT OF COLUMBIA CLAIMS OFFICE
5350 SPECTRUM DR
PO BOX 920
FREDERICK, MD 21705
TEL: (800) 685-4030
FAX: (301) 846-4179
TOLL FREE: (800) 685-4030

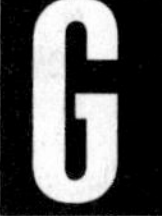

MARYLAND CLAIMS OFFICE
5350 SPECTRUM DR
PO BOX 920
FREDERICK, MD 21705
TEL: (800) 685-4030
FAX: (301) 846-4179
TOLL FREE: (800) 685-4030

NATIONAL CLAIMS OFFICE
1740 TECHNOLOGY DR, STE 300
PO BOX 1120
SAN JOSE, CA 95108
FAX: (408) 453-7963
TOLL FREE: (800) 685-1050
WWW.1HEALTHPLAN.COM

1511 N WEST SHORE BLVD, STE 850
PO BOX 31251
TAMPA, FL 33631-3251
FAX: (813) 281-0019
TOLL FREE: (800) 333-5251
WWW.1HEALTHPLAN.COM

2 MERIDIAN PLZ- 10401 N MERIDIAN ST, STE 330
PO BOX 80817
INDIANAPOLIS, IN 46280-0817
FAX: (317) 575-1102
TOLL FREE: (800) 685-4040
WWW.GWLA.COM

14 E FIRST ST- 4TH FL
PO BOX 5011
FORT SCOTT, KS 66701
FAX: (316) 223-5986
TOLL FREE: (800) 685-3040
WWW.GWLA.COM

90 WOODBRIDGE CTR DR, STE 700
PO BOX 4015
ISELIN, NJ 08830
TEL: (800) 685-4020
FAX: (732) 602-0657
TOLL FREE: (800) 685-2070
WWW.GWLA.COM

ONE HEALTH PLAN
PO BOX 7000
CORAOPOLIS, PA 15108
TEL: (412) 269-3700
FAX: (412) 269-3234
TOLL FREE: (800) 333-8583
WWW.GWL.COM

NEW ENGLAND
10000 N CENTRAL EXPY, STE 800
DALLAS, TX 75231
FAX: (214) 987-0827
TOLL FREE: (800) 685-3020
WWW.GWL.COM

1802 DEL RANGE BLVD, STE 200
CHEYENNE, WY 82001
TOLL FREE: (800) 288-9575

OHIO CLAIMS OFFICE
25145 COUNTRY CLUB BLVD
PO BOX 8020
NORTH OLMSTED, OH 44070-8020
FAX: (440) 777-1474
TOLL FREE: (800) 678-5764

VIRGINIA CLAIMS OFFICE
5350 SPECTRUM DR
PO BOX 920
FREDERICK, MD 21705
TEL: (800) 685-4030
FAX: (301) 846-4179
TOLL FREE: (800) 685-4030

GREAT-WEST LIFE & ANNUITY

NATIONAL CLAIMS OFFICE
PO BOX 950
DENVER, CO 80201
FAX: (303) 790-1998
TOLL FREE: (800) 685-2020
WWW.GWLA.COM

OREGON CLAIMS OFFICE
1800 S W 1ST AVE, STE 410
PO BOX 429
PORTLAND, OR 97207-0429
FAX: (503) 224-2202
TOLL FREE: (800) 685-1020

PENNSYLVANIA CLAIMS OFFICE
200 GILBRALTER RD, STE 350
PO BOX 1000
HORSHAM, PA 19044-1000
TEL: (215) 956-9410
FAX: (215) 674-9517
TOLL FREE: (800) 685-4010

GREAT-WEST LIFE ASSURANCE CO

CALIFORNIA CLAIMS OFFICE
455 MARKET ST, STE 2000
SAN FRANCISCO, CA 94105-2403
TEL: (415) 777-4646
FAX: (415) 957-9842
TOLL FREE: (800) 685-1040

GEORGIA CLAIMS OFFICE
PO BOX 88260
ATLANTA, GA 30356-8260
TOLL FREE: (800) 685-3030
WWW.1HEALTHPLAN.COM

NATIONAL CLAIMS OFFICE
CORPORATE HEADQUARTERS
8515 E ORCHARD RD
PO BOX 1700
DENVER, CO 80201
TEL: (303) 689-3000
FAX: (303) 689-3198
TOLL FREE: (800) 537-2033

500 N CENTRAL AVE- 3RD FL
PO BOX 10188
GLENDALE, CA 91209-3188
TEL: (818) 247-7053
FAX: (818) 247-2360
TOLL FREE: (800) 423-3002
WWW.ONEHEALTH.COM

6250 RIVER RD
PO BOX 5004
ROSEMONT, IL 60018
FAX: (847) 986-9200
TOLL FREE: (800) 284-6143

200 RENAISSANCE CTR, STE 1700
DETROIT, MI 48243-1209
FAX: (313) 259-6870
TOLL FREE: (800) 685-2030

900 2ND AVE S, STE 650
MINNEAPOLIS, MN 55402-3341
FAX: (612) 673-9738
TOLL FREE: (800) 685-2010
WWW.GWLA.COM

1377 DUBLIN RD
PO BOX 963
COLUMBUS, OH 43216
TEL: (614) 486-2908
FAX: (614) 486-3402
TOLL FREE: (800) 685-2040
WWW.ONEHEALTHPLAN.COM

10000 N CENTRAL EXPY, STE 800
DALLAS, TX 75231
TOLL FREE: (800) 685-3020
IN-STATE: (800) 442-3042

CORPORATE OFFICE FOR CANADA
60 OSBOURNE ST N
PO BOX 6000
WINNIPEG, MB R3C-3A5
TEL: (204) 942-3589
FAX: (204) 946-8960
TOLL FREE: (800) 665-0551
IN-STATE: (800) 957-9777

WASHINGTON CLAIMS OFFICE
SEATTLE BPO
3005 112TH AVE NE, STE 210
PO BOX 97313
BELLEVUE, WA 98009-9313
TEL: (425) 822-4173
FAX: (425) 827-3072
TOLL FREE: (800) 685-1010
WWW.GWLA.COM

GREATER GEORGIA LIFE INSURANCE CO

GEORGIA CLAIMS OFFICE
BLUE CROSS BLUE SHIELD OF GEORGIA
3 RAVINIA DR, STE 1700
PO BOX 4445
ATLANTA, GA 30302-4445
TEL: (706) 571-0230
FAX: (706) 571-4486
TOLL FREE: (800) 851-8544
WWW.BCBSGA.COM

GREATER MARSHFIELD HEALTH PLAN

WISCONSIN CLAIMS OFFICE
100 N OAK AVE
MARSHFIELD, WI 54449
TEL: (715) 387-5621

GREATER NEW YORK MUTUAL INSURANCE CO

CONNECTICUT CLAIMS OFFICE
95 GLASTONBURY BLVD- 2ND FL
GLASTONBURY, CT 06033
TEL: (860) 652-7090
FAX: (860) 652-7095
IN-STATE: (800) 842-8354

200 MADISON AVE
NEW YORK, NY 10016-6023
TEL: (212) 683-9700
FAX: (212) 779-1499
IN-STATE: (800) 522-5504

MASSACHUSETTS CLAIMS OFFICE
95 GLASTONBURY BLVD- 2ND FL
GLASTONBURY, CT 06033
TEL: (860) 652-7090
FAX: (860) 652-7095
IN-STATE: (800) 842-8354

NEW JERSEY CLAIMS OFFICE
200 MADISON AVE
NEW YORK, NY 10016-6023
TEL: (212) 683-9700
FAX: (212) 779-1499
IN-STATE: (800) 522-5504

95 GLASTONBURY BLVD- 2ND FL
GLASTONBURY, CT 06033
TEL: (860) 652-7090
FAX: (860) 652-7095
IN-STATE: (800) 842-8354

NEW YORK CLAIMS OFFICE
200 MADISON AVE
NEW YORK, NY 10016-6023
TEL: (212) 683-9700
FAX: (212) 779-1499
IN-STATE: (800) 522-5504

95 GLASTONBURY BLVD- 2ND FL
GLASTONBURY, CT 06033
TEL: (860) 652-7090
FAX: (860) 652-7095
IN-STATE: (800) 842-8354

GREENBAY HEALTH PROTECTION PLAN

NATIONAL CLAIMS OFFICE
NATIONWIDE INSURANCE
2000 WESTWOOD DR
PO BOX 8012
WAUSAU, WI 54401-7802
TEL: (715) 847-7111
FAX: (715) 847-7699
TOLL FREE: (800) 826-9781

GROCER'S INSURANCE GROUP

6605 SE LAKE RD
PO BOX 22146
PORTLAND, OR 97269
TEL: (503) 833-1600
FAX: (503) 833-1699
TOLL FREE: (800) 777-3602
WWW.GROCINS.COM

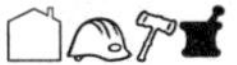

GROUP ADMINISTRATION AGENCY, INC

ILLINOIS CLAIMS OFFICE
20 N WACKER DR, STE 2700
CHICAGO, IL 60606-3167
TEL: (312) 372-0973
FAX: (312) 372-8226
TOLL FREE: (800) 621-1666

GROUP ADMINISTRATIVE CONCEPTS

NATIONAL CLAIMS OFFICE
1207 N TIMES, STE 1
PO BOX 24420
TAMPA, FL 33623-4420
TEL: (813) 877-6021
FAX: (813) 877-6312
TOLL FREE: (800) 275-2147

GROUP BENEFIT ADMINISTRATORS

IDAHO CLAIMS OFFICE
621 S 3200 W
PO BOX 30749
SALT LAKE CITY, UT 84130-0749
TEL: (801) 972-1177
FAX: (801) 972-3364
TOLL FREE: (800) 657-5377

MONTANA CLAIMS OFFICE
621 S 3200 W
PO BOX 30749
SALT LAKE CITY, UT 84130-0749
TEL: (801) 972-1177
FAX: (801) 972-3364
TOLL FREE: (800) 657-5377

UTAH CLAIMS OFFICE
621 S 3200 W
PO BOX 30749
SALT LAKE CITY, UT 84130-0749
TEL: (801) 972-1177
FAX: (801) 972-3364
TOLL FREE: (800) 657-5377

WYOMING CLAIMS OFFICE
621 S 3200 W
PO BOX 30749
SALT LAKE CITY, UT 84130-0749
TEL: (801) 972-1177
FAX: (801) 972-3364
TOLL FREE: (800) 657-5377

GROUP BENEFIT SERVICES, INC

NATIONAL CLAIMS OFFICE
6 N PARK, STE 310
HUNT VALLEY, MD 21030
TEL: (410) 832-1300
FAX: (410) 832-1315
TOLL FREE: (800) 638-6085
WWW.G-B-S.COM

GROUP BENEFITS UNLIMITED

ILLINOIS CLAIMS OFFICE
1000 PLAZA DR, STE 300
CHAMBERG, IL 60173
TEL: (847) 330-6000
FAX: (847) 330-9400
TOLL FREE: (800) 772-0666

GROUP DEKKO INTERNATIONAL, INC

INDIANA CLAIMS OFFICE
6928 N 400 E
PO BOX 2000
KENDALLVILLE, IN 46755
TEL: (219) 347-0700
FAX: (219) 347-9537
TOLL FREE: (800) 829-9449

IOWA CLAIMS OFFICE
6928 N 400 E
PO BOX 2000
KENDALLVILLE, IN 46755
TEL: (219) 347-0700
FAX: (219) 347-9537
TOLL FREE: (800) 829-9449

WISCONSIN CLAIMS OFFICE
6928 N 400 E
PO BOX 2000
KENDALLVILLE, IN 46755
TEL: (219) 347-0700
FAX: (219) 347-9537
TOLL FREE: (800) 829-9449

GROUP DIVERSIFIED SERVICES, INC

NEW YORK CLAIMS OFFICE
33 E MERRICK RD
VALLEY STREAM, NY 11580-5814
TEL: (516) 872-0200

GROUP HEALTH COOPERATIVE OF EAU CLAIRE

WISCONSIN CLAIMS OFFICE
2503 N HILLCREST PKY
PO BOX 3217
EAU CLAIRE, WI 54702-3217
TEL: (715) 836-8552
FAX: (715) 836-7683

H

GROUP HEALTH COOPERATIVE OF PUGET SOUND

CALIFORNIA CLAIMS OFFICE
521 WALL ST
PO BOX 3485
SEATTLE, WA 98124-1585
FAX: (206) 901-4612
TOLL FREE: (888) 901-4636
WWW.GHC.ORG

WASHINGTON CLAIMS OFFICE
521 WALL ST
PO BOX 3485
SEATTLE, WA 98124-1585
FAX: (206) 901-4612
TOLL FREE: (888) 901-4636
WWW.GHC.ORG

GROUP HEALTH COOPERATIVE OF SOUTH CENTRAL WISCONSIN

WISCONSIN CLAIMS OFFICE
PO BOX 44971
MADISON, WI 53744-4971
TEL: (608) 251-4156
FAX: (608) 257-3842

GROUP HEALTH & LIFE INSURANCE

INDIANA CLAIMS OFFICE
PO BOX 1601
FT WAYNE, IN 46802
TEL: (219) 461-4000
FAX: (219) 461-4737

GROUP HEALTH MANAGERS

MICHIGAN CLAIMS OFFICE
26205 FIVE-MILE RD
REDFORD, MI 48239-3154
TEL: (313) 535-7100
FAX: (313) 535-8472
TOLL FREE: (800) 992-2508

GROUP HEALTH NORTHWEST

IDAHO CLAIMS OFFICE
GROUP HEALTH CO
2010 N LAKEWOOD DR
COEUR D'ALENE, ID 83814-2635
TEL: (208) 664-5174
FAX: (208) 664-9315
WWW.GHNW.COM

NATIONAL CLAIMS OFFICE
CORP CTR- 5615 W SUNSET HWY
PO BOX 204
SPOKANE, WA 99210
TEL: (509) 838-9100
FAX: (509) 838-3292
TOLL FREE: (800) 497-2210
IN-STATE: (800) 377-8853
WWW.GHNW.ORG

WASHINGTON CLAIMS OFFICE
5615 W SUNSET HIGH
PO BOX 204
SPOKANE, WA 99210-0204
TEL: (509) 838-9100
FAX: (509) 458-0368
TOLL FREE: (800) 767-4670
IN-STATE: (800) 838-9100
WWW.GHNW.ORG

GROUP HEALTH CO
2010 N LAKEWOOD DR
COEUR D'ALENE, ID 83814-2635
TEL: (208) 664-5174
FAX: (208) 664-9315
WWW.GHNW.COM

GROUP HEALTH PLAN OF ST. LOUIS

ILLINOIS CLAIMS OFFICE
111 CORPERATE OFFICE DR, STE 400
EARTH CITY, MO 63145
TEL: (314) 453-1700
FAX: (314) 506-1958
TOLL FREE: (800) 743-3901
WWW.GHP.COM

GROUP HEALTH PLAN OF ST LOUIS

MISSOURI CLAIMS OFFICE
111 CORPERATE OFFICE DR, STE 400
EARTH CITY, MO 63145
TEL: (314) 453-1700
FAX: (314) 506-1555
TOLL FREE: (800) 743-3901
WWW.GHP.COM

GROUP INSURANCE PLAN CHATTANOOGA

FLORIDA CLAIMS OFFICE
1500 N DALE MABRY HWY E 6
PO BOX 31601
TAMPA, FL 33631-3601
TEL: (813) 871-4664
FAX: (813) 871-4601

GROUP INSURANCE PLAN FOR EMPLOYEES

TENNESSEE CLAIMS OFFICE
100 PLUMLEY DR
PO BOX 758
PARIS, TN 38242
TEL: (901) 642-5582
FAX: (901) 642-6872

GROUP INSURANCE SERVICE CENTER

MASSACHUSETTS CLAIMS OFFICE
1020 PLAIN ST
PO BOX 9120
MARSHFIELD, MA 02050-9120
TEL: (781) 837-6171
FAX: (781) 837-5738
TOLL FREE: (800) 242-4472
IN-STATE: (800) 242-3834

GROUP MAJOR MEDICAL EXPENSE

MISSOURI CLAIMS OFFICE
PO BOX 6614
SAINT LOUIS, MO 63166-6149
TEL: (314) 554-6490

GROUP & PENSION ADMINISTRATORS

TEXAS CLAIMS OFFICE
300 MUNICIPAL DR
PO BOX 830827
RICHARDSON, TX 75080
TEL: (972) 238-7900
FAX: (972) 669-8155
TOLL FREE: (800) 827-7223

GROUP SERVICES & ADMINISTRATION, INC

KANSAS CLAIMS OFFICE
3113 CLASSEN BLVD
OKLAHOMA CITY, OK 73118-3818
TEL: (405) 528-4400
FAX: (405) 528-5558
TOLL FREE: (800) 475-4445

MISSOURI CLAIMS OFFICE
3113 CLASSEN BLVD
OKLAHOMA CITY, OK 73118-3818
TEL: (405) 528-4400
FAX: (405) 528-5558
TOLL FREE: (800) 475-4445

OKLAHOMA CLAIMS OFFICE
3113 CLASSEN BLVD
OKLAHOMA CITY, OK 73118-3818
TEL: (405) 528-4400
FAX: (405) 528-5558
TOLL FREE: (800) 475-4445

TEXAS CLAIMS OFFICE
3113 CLASSEN BLVD
OKLAHOMA CITY, OK 73118-3818
TEL: (405) 528-4400
FAX: (405) 528-5558
TOLL FREE: (800) 475-4445

GROUP SERVICES, INC

IOWA CLAIMS OFFICE
3066 VICTORIA DR
BETTENDORF, IA 52722-2793
TEL: (319) 332-5552
FAX: (319) 332-7826
TOLL FREE: (800) 925-8846

GUAM MEMORIAL HEALTH PLAN

GUAM CLAIMS OFFICE
142 W SEATON BLVD
AGANA, GU 96910-5136
TEL: (671) 646-4647

H

GUARANTEE LIFE

NATIONAL CLAIMS OFFICE
8801 INDIAN HILLS DR
PO BOX 2640
OMAHA, NE 681103-2640
TEL: (402) 361-7300
FAX: (402) 361-2893
TOLL FREE: (800) 423-2765

GUARANTEE RESERVE LIFE INSURANCE CO

ILLINOIS CLAIMS OFFICE
530 RIVER OAKS W
CALUMET CITY, IL 60409
TEL: (708) 868-4232
FAX: (708) 891-8886
TOLL FREE: (800) 323-8764

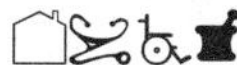

GUARANTEE TRUST LIFE INSURANCE CO

1275 MILWAUKEE AVE
PO BOX 1144
GLENVIEW, IL 60025
TEL: (847) 699-0600
FAX: (847) 699-1048
TOLL FREE: (800) 338-7452
WWW.GTLIC.COM

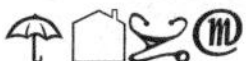

GUARDIAN LIFE INSURANCE CO OF AMERICA

NATIONAL CLAIMS OFFICE
7 HANOVER SQ
NEW YORK, NY 10004
TEL: (212) 598-8400
FAX: (212) 598-8344
TOLL FREE: (800) 441-6455
WWW.THEGUARDIAN.COM

THE GUARDIAN
700 LONGWATER DR
PO BOX 9128
NORWELL, MA 02061-9128
TEL: (781) 871-4890
FAX: (781) 982-8641
TOLL FREE: (800) 524-4542
WWW.THEGUARDIAN.COM

THE GUARDIAN SHORT TERM DISABILITY
3900 BURGESS PL
PO BOX 26160
BETHLEHEM, PA 18002-6160
TEL: (610) 861-0733
FAX: (610) 807-8270
TOLL FREE: (800) 268-2525
WWW.THEGUARDIAN.COM

THE GUARDIAN
777 E MAGNESIUM
PO BOX 2467
SPOKANE, WA 99210
TEL: (509) 468-6000
FAX: (509) 468-6420
TOLL FREE: (800) 695-4542
WWW.THEGUARDIAN.COM

GUICARPENTER

NEW YORK CLAIMS OFFICE
2 WORLD TRADE CENTER
NEW YORK, NY 10048
TEL: (212) 323-1000
FAX: (212) 313-4600
TOLL FREE: (800) 645-3020

GUIDANT INSURANCE GROUP

ILLINOIS CLAIMS OFFICE
3125 SANDY TRL
PO BOX 531460
INDIANAPOLIS, IN 46253-1460
TEL: (317) 293-2008
FAX: (317) 293-2084
TOLL FREE: (800) 678-2143

INDIANA CLAIMS OFFICE
3125 SANDY TRL
PO BOX 531460
INDIANAPOLIS, IN 46253-1460
TEL: (317) 293-2008
FAX: (317) 293-2084
TOLL FREE: (800) 678-2143

MICHIGAN CLAIMS OFFICE
3125 SANDY TRL
PO BOX 531460
INDIANAPOLIS, IN 46253-1460
TEL: (317) 293-2008
FAX: (317) 293-2084
TOLL FREE: (800) 678-2143

OHIO CLAIMS OFFICE
3125 SANDY TRL
PO BOX 531460
INDIANAPOLIS, IN 46253-1460
TEL: (317) 293-2008
FAX: (317) 293-2084
TOLL FREE: (800) 678-2143

GUIDEONE INSURANCE

ALABAMA CLAIMS OFFICE
PO BOX 360810
BIRMINGHAM, AL 35236
TEL: (205) 823-4511
TOLL FREE: (800) 826-7644
IN-STATE: (800) 247-4176

2100 RIVER CHASE CTR- BLDG 100, STE 100
BIRMINGHAM, AL 35244
TEL: (205) 987-0440
FAX: (205) 987-5282

36 CAROL VILLA DR
PO BOX 211088
MONTGOMERY, AL 36121-1088
TEL: (334) 272-0957

ARIZONA CLAIMS OFFICE
3220 S FAIR LN, STE 19A
TEMPE, AZ 85282
TEL: (602) 431-9420
TOLL FREE: (800) 647-7456

PO BOX 2588
GUASTI, CA 94743-2588
TEL: (909) 944-1744
FAX: (909) 944-1071

ARKANSAS CLAIMS OFFICE
2305 W PARK PL, STE A
PO BOX P
STONE MOUNTAIN, GA 30087
TEL: (770) 469-6006
FAX: (770) 879-2773
TOLL FREE: (800) 659-1232

1204 S HARVARD
PO BOX 4756
TULSA, OK 74159-3328
TEL: (918) 582-7700
FAX: (918) 582-3053
TOLL FREE: (800) 777-0404

CALIFORNIA CLAIMS OFFICE
2351 SUNSET BLVD, STE 170-305
ROCKLIN, CA 95765
TEL: (916) 624-3288
FAX: (916) 624-3278
TOLL FREE: (800) 647-9324

PO BOX 2588
GUASTI, CA 94743-2588
TEL: (909) 944-1744
FAX: (909) 944-1071

COLORADO CLAIMS OFFICE
320 N ACADEMY BLVD, STE 303
COLORADO SPRINGS, CO 80909
TEL: (719) 550-9686
FAX: (719) 550-9693
TOLL FREE: (800) 652-2062

PO BOX 4227
ENGLEWOOD, CO 80155
TEL: (303) 220-8460
TOLL FREE: (800) 652-2062

DELAWARE CLAIMS OFFICE
2305 W PARK PL, STE A
PO BOX P
STONE MOUNTAIN, GA 30087
TEL: (770) 469-6006
FAX: (770) 879-2773
TOLL FREE: (800) 659-1232

DISTRICT OF COLUMBIA CLAIMS OFFICE
2305 W PARK PL, STE A
PO BOX P
STONE MOUNTAIN, GA 30087
TEL: (770) 469-6006
FAX: (770) 879-2773
TOLL FREE: (800) 659-1232

FLORIDA CLAIMS OFFICE
PO BOX 271488
TAMPA, FL 33688-1488
TEL: (813) 933-8699
FAX: (813) 933-8821

G

GEORGIA CLAIMS OFFICE
512 OAK ST NW
PO BOX 4279
EASTMAN, GA 31023-4279
TEL: (912) 374-2085
FAX: (912) 374-7094

359 C COMMERCIAL DR
SAVANNAH, GA 31406
TEL: (912) 352-0641
FAX: (912) 354-7073

2305 W PARK PL, STE A
PO BOX P
STONE MOUNTAIN, GA 30087
TEL: (770) 469-6006
FAX: (770) 879-2773
TOLL FREE: (800) 659-1232

IDAHO CLAIMS OFFICE
8201 SOUTHPARK LN, STE 150
LITTLETON, CO 80120
TEL: (303) 795-2432
FAX: (303) 347-1091
TOLL FREE: (800) 652-2062

IOWA CLAIMS OFFICE
GUIDANT SPECIALTY MUTUAL
1111 ASHWORTH RD
WEST DES MOINES, IA 50265-3538
TEL: (515) 225-5000
FAX: (515) 267-5311
TOLL FREE: (800) 247-4180

KENTUCKY CLAIMS OFFICE
3830 TAYLORSVILLE RD, STE 4
PO BOX 206489
LOUISVILLE, KY 40252
TEL: (502) 459-9300
FAX: (502) 451-0538
TOLL FREE: (800) 777-5783

LOUISIANA CLAIMS OFFICE
PO BOX 360810
BIRMINGHAM, AL 35236
TEL: (205) 823-4511
TOLL FREE: (800) 826-7644
IN-STATE: (800) 247-4176

320 WESTWAY PL, STE 521
PO BOX 180009
ARLINGTON, TX 76096
TEL: (817) 465-1441
FAX: (817) 465-2925
TOLL FREE: (800) 441-1554

MARYLAND CLAIMS OFFICE
2305 W PARK PL, STE A
PO BOX P
STONE MOUNTAIN, GA 30087
TEL: (770) 469-6006
FAX: (770) 879-2773
TOLL FREE: (800) 659-1232

MINNESOTA CLAIMS OFFICE
14101 W SOUTHCROSS DR, STE 400
PO BOX 1039
BURNSVILLE, MN 55337
TEL: (612) 895-5194
FAX: (612) 890-1729
TOLL FREE: (800) 778-7814
WWW.GUIDEONE.COM

MISSISSIPPI CLAIMS OFFICE
2100 RIVER CHASE CTR- BLDG 100, STE 100
BIRMINGHAM, AL 35244
TEL: (205) 987-0440
FAX: (205) 987-5282

PO BOX 360810
BIRMINGHAM, AL 35236
TEL: (205) 823-4511
TOLL FREE: (800) 826-7644
IN-STATE: (800) 247-4176

MONTANA CLAIMS OFFICE
15407 1ST AVE S
SEATTLE, WA 98148
TEL: (206) 433-8040
TOLL FREE: (800) 647-9324

3825 ATHERTON RD, STE 500
ROCKLIN, CA 95765
TEL: (916) 624-3288
FAX: (916) 624-3378
TOLL FREE: (800) 647-9324

NEBRASKA CLAIMS OFFICE
11110 FORT ST, STE 102
PO BOX 34070
OMAHA, NE 68134-0070
TEL: (402) 493-4186
FAX: (402) 493-4752
TOLL FREE: (800) 376-6423

NEVADA CLAIMS OFFICE
2351 SUNSET BLVD, STE 170-305
ROCKLIN, CA 95765
TEL: (916) 624-3288
FAX: (916) 624-3278
TOLL FREE: (800) 647-9324

3220 S FAIR LN, STE 19A
TEMPE, AZ 85282
TEL: (602) 431-9420
TOLL FREE: (800) 647-7456

PO BOX 2588
GUASTI, CA 94743-2588
TEL: (909) 944-1744
FAX: (909) 944-1071

NEW MEXICO CLAIMS OFFICE
3220 S FAIR LN, STE 19A
TEMPE, AZ 85282
TEL: (602) 431-9420
TOLL FREE: (800) 647-7456

PO BOX 2588
GUASTI, CA 94743-2588
TEL: (909) 944-1744
FAX: (909) 944-1071

NORTH CAROLINA CLAIMS OFFICE
2305 W PARK PL, STE A
PO BOX P
STONE MOUNTAIN, GA 30087
TEL: (770) 469-6006
FAX: (770) 879-2773
TOLL FREE: (800) 659-1232

NORTH DAKOTA CLAIMS OFFICE
14101 W SOUTHCROSS DR, STE 400
PO BOX 1039
BURNSVILLE, MN 55337
TEL: (612) 895-5194
FAX: (612) 890-1729
TOLL FREE: (800) 778-7814
WWW.GUIDEONE.COM

OHIO CLAIMS OFFICE
1231 LYONS RD- BLDG F
DAYTON, OH 45458
TEL: (937) 434-4815
FAX: (937) 434-1735
IN-STATE: (800) 826-9013

OKLAHOMA CLAIMS OFFICE
1204 S HARVARD
PO BOX 4756
TULSA, OK 74159-3328
TEL: (918) 582-7700
FAX: (918) 582-3053
TOLL FREE: (800) 777-0404

OREGON CLAIMS OFFICE
2351 SUNSET BLVD, STE 170-305
ROCKLIN, CA 95765
TEL: (916) 624-3288
FAX: (916) 624-3278
TOLL FREE: (800) 647-9324

PENNSYLVANIA CLAIMS OFFICE
5425 JONESTOWN RD, STE 101
PO BOX 126157
HARRISBURG, PA 17112-6157
TEL: (717) 657-1215
FAX: (717) 657-1343
TOLL FREE: (800) 778-7816

SOUTH DAKOTA CLAIMS OFFICE
14101 W SOUTHCROSS DR, STE 400
PO BOX 1039
BURNSVILLE, MN 55337
TEL: (612) 895-5194
FAX: (612) 890-1729
TOLL FREE: (800) 778-7814
WWW.GUIDEONE.COM

TENNESSEE CLAIMS OFFICE
2305 W PARK PL, STE A
PO BOX P
STONE MOUNTAIN, GA 30087
TEL: (770) 469-6006
FAX: (770) 879-2773
TOLL FREE: (800) 659-1232

3830 TAYLORSVILLE RD, STE 4
PO BOX 206489
LOUISVILLE, KY 40252
TEL: (502) 459-9300
FAX: (502) 451-0538
TOLL FREE: (800) 777-5783

TEXAS CLAIMS OFFICE
320 WESTWAY PL, STE 521
PO BOX 180009
ARLINGTON, TX 76096
TEL: (817) 465-1441
FAX: (817) 465-2925
TOLL FREE: (800) 441-1554

11999 KATY FWY, STE 270
PO BOX 79520
HOUSTON, TX 77279-9520
TEL: (281) 496-0399
FAX: (281) 496-5349
TOLL FREE: (800) 826-7670

4415 71ST ST, STE 11
PO BOX 64897
LUBBOCK, TX 79464
TEL: (806) 795-9389
FAX: (806) 792-1752

UTAH CLAIMS OFFICE
835 E 4800 S, STE 220
SALT LAKE CITY, UT 84107
TEL: (801) 263-3933
FAX: (801) 263-8652

PO BOX 2588
GUASTI, CA 94743-2588
TEL: (909) 944-1744
FAX: (909) 944-1071

VIRGINIA CLAIMS OFFICE
2305 W PARK PL, STE A
PO BOX P
STONE MOUNTAIN, GA 30087
TEL: (770) 469-6006
FAX: (770) 879-2773
TOLL FREE: (800) 659-1232

WEST VIRGINIA CLAIMS OFFICE
2305 W PARK PL, STE A
PO BOX P
STONE MOUNTAIN, GA 30087
TEL: (770) 469-6006
FAX: (770) 879-2773
TOLL FREE: (800) 659-1232

3830 TAYLORSVILLE RD, STE 4
PO BOX 206489
LOUISVILLE, KY 40252
TEL: (502) 459-9300
FAX: (502) 451-0538
TOLL FREE: (800) 777-5783

GULF GUARANTY EMPLOYEE BENEFIT SERVICES, INC

MISSISSIPPI CLAIMS OFFICE
4785 I-55 N, STE 106
PO BOX 14977
JACKSON, MS 39236-4977
TEL: (601) 981-9505
FAX: (601) 981-6805
TOLL FREE: (800) 890-7337

GULF INSURANCE CO

GEORGIA CLAIMS OFFICE
64 PERIMETER CTR E, STE 900
PO BOX 5059
ATLANTA, GA 30302-5059
TEL: (678) 443-3600
FAX: (678) 443-3331

NATIONAL CLAIMS OFFICE
PO BOX 446
DALLAS, TX 75221
TEL: (972) 650-2800
FAX: (972) 650-3636
TOLL FREE: (800) 994-3890

GULF SOUTH HEALTH PLANS, INC

LOUISIANA CLAIMS OFFICE
5615 CORPORATE BLVD, STE 3
PO BOX 14449
BATON ROUGE, LA 70898-4449
TEL: (225) 237-1700
FAX: (225) 237-1792
TOLL FREE: (800) 634-8595
WWW.GENERALHEALTH.ORG

GULFCO LIFE INSURANCE CO

660 N MAIN
PO BOX 157
MARKSVILLE, LA 71351-0157
TEL: (318) 253-7564
FAX: (318) 253-4903

H.E.R.E.I.U. WELFARE FUNDS

NATIONAL CLAIMS OFFICE
HOTEL EMPLOYEES & RESTAURANT EMPLOYEES INT'L UNION
711 N COMMONS DR
PO BOX 6020
AURORA, IL 60598
TEL: (630) 236-5100
FAX: (630) 236-4394

HALLMARK INSURANCE ADMINISTRATORS, INC

ILLINOIS CLAIMS OFFICE
BLUE CROSS & BLUE SHIELD OF ILLINOIS
75 EXECUTIVE DR, STE 300
PO BOX 2036
AURORA, IL 60507-2036
TEL: (630) 978-7878
FAX: (630) 978-8460
TOLL FREE: (800) 538-8833
WWW.BCBSIL.COM

HANOVER INSURANCE CO

ALABAMA CLAIMS OFFICE
ALLMERICA FINANCIAL
1455 LINCOLN PKY
PO BOX 105319
ATLANTA, GA 30348
TEL: (770) 353-6200
FAX: (770) 353-6169
TOLL FREE: (800) 343-4801
IN-STATE: (800) 523-2873
WWW.ALLMERICA.COM

ARKANSAS CLAIMS OFFICE
ALL AMERICAN FINANCIAL
10816 EXECUTIVE CTR DR
PO BOX 24868
LITTLE ROCK, AR 72221
TEL: (501) 223-8249
FAX: (501) 223-8766
TOLL FREE: (800) 332-5513
IN-STATE: (800) 332-5513
WWW.ALLAMERICA.COM

CALIFORNIA CLAIMS OFFICE
ALL AMERICAN FINANCIAL
2200 PROFESSIONAL, STE 200
PO BOX 15380
ROSEVILLE, CA 95661
TEL: (916) 773-8077
FAX: (916) 773-8853
TOLL FREE: (800) 688-8077
IN-STATE: (800) 955-8850
WWW.ALLAMERICA.COM

CONNECTICUT CLAIMS OFFICE
ALLMERICA FINANCIAL
538 PRESTON AVE
PO BOX 1002
MERIDEN, CT 06450-7521
TEL: (203) 639-0778
FAX: (203) 639-1004
TOLL FREE: (800) 922-3272
WWW.ALLAMERICA.COM

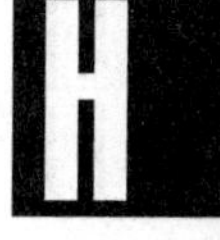

FLORIDA CLAIMS OFFICE
ALL AMERICAN FINANCIAL
3740 ST JOHNS BLUFF RD, STE 9
JACKSONVILLE, FL 32224
TEL: (904) 641-3410
FAX: (904) 641-3696
IN-STATE: (800) 888-4954
WWW.ALLAMERICA.COM

GEORGIA CLAIMS OFFICE
ALLMERICA FINANCIAL
1455 LINCOLN PKY
PO BOX 105319
ATLANTA, GA 30348
TEL: (770) 353-6200
FAX: (770) 353-6169
TOLL FREE: (800) 343-4801
WWW.ALLMERICA.COM

ILLINOIS CLAIMS OFFICE
ALL AMERICAN FINANCIAL
333 W PIERCE RD
PO BOX 478
ITASCA, IL 60143-3116
TEL: (630) 773-2882
FAX: (630) 773-8766
TOLL FREE: (800) 288-8963
WWW.ALLAMERICA.COM

KANSAS CLAIMS OFFICE
ALL AMERICAN FINANCIAL
PO BOX 29117
SHAWNEE MISSION, KS 66201-1417
TEL: (913) 752-8505
FAX: (913) 752-8585
IN-STATE: (800) 288-5128
WWW.ALLAMERICA.COM

LOUISIANA CLAIMS OFFICE
ALL AMERICAN FINANCIAL
2400 VETERANS BLVD, STE 400
PO BOX 1758
KENNER, LA 70063-1758
TEL: (504) 464-6012
FAX: (504) 469-7563
TOLL FREE: (800) 477-7661
IN-STATE: (800) 477-7661
WWW.ALLAMERICA.COM

MAINE CLAIMS OFFICE
ALL AMERICAN FINANCIAL
27 PEARL ST
PO BOX 9801
PORTLAND, ME 04104-5004
TEL: (207) 771-5000
FAX: (207) 771-5008
TOLL FREE: (800) 492-0532
IN-STATE: (800) 492-0532
WWW.ALLAMERICA.COM

MASSACHUSETTS CLAIMS OFFICE
ALL AMERICAN FINANCIAL
100 CENTURY DR
PO BOX 2449
WORCESTER, MA 01605-0081
TEL: (413) 538-9211
IN-STATE: (800) 435-2022
WWW.ALLAMERICA.COM

ALL AMERICAN FINANCIAL
100 CENTURY DR
PO BOX 15145
WORCESTER, MA 01615-0081
TEL: (603) 472-9990
FAX: (800) 399-4734
IN-STATE: (800) 421-9990
WWW.ALLAMERICA.COM

MISSOURI CLAIMS OFFICE
ALL AMERICAN FINANCIAL
10816 EXECUTIVE CTR DR
PO BOX 24868
LITTLE ROCK, AR 72221
TEL: (501) 223-8249
FAX: (501) 223-8766
TOLL FREE: (800) 332-5513
IN-STATE: (800) 332-5513
WWW.ALLAMERICA.COM

NATIONAL CLAIMS OFFICE
ALL AMERICAN FINANCIAL
440 LINCOLN ST
PO BOX 01653
WORCESTER, MA 01605
TEL: (508) 853-7200
FAX: (508) 856-9092
TOLL FREE: (800) 922-8427
WWW.ALLAMERICA.COM

ALL AMERICAN FINANCIAL
PO BOX 21258
TULSA, OK 74121-1258
TEL: (918) 488-8700
FAX: (918) 497-2288
IN-STATE: (800) 256-9038
WWW.ALLAMERICA.COM

NEW HAMPSHIRE CLAIMS OFFICE
ALL AMERICAN FINANCIAL
100 CENTURY DR
PO BOX 15145
WORCESTER, MA 01615-0081
TEL: (603) 472-9990
FAX: (800) 399-4734
IN-STATE: (800) 421-9990
WWW.ALLAMERICA.COM

NEW JERSEY CLAIMS OFFICE
ALL AMERICAN FINANCIAL
860 CENTENNIAL AVE
PO BOX 1090
PISCATAWAY, NJ 08855-1383
TEL: (732) 457-0577
FAX: (732) 980-9650
IN-STATE: (800) 257-5720
WWW.ALLAMERICA.COM

ALLMERICAN FINANCIAL
1 HUNTINGTON QUAD, STE 2S04
MELVILLE, NY 11747
TEL: (516) 756-1650
FAX: (516) 756-1699
TOLL FREE: (800) 233-6622
WWW.ALLMERICA.COM

NEW YORK CLAIMS OFFICE
ALLMERICAN FINANCIAL
1 HUNTINGTON QUAD, STE 2S04
MELVILLE, NY 11747
TEL: (516) 756-1650
FAX: (516) 756-1699
TOLL FREE: (800) 233-6622
WWW.ALLMERICA.COM

ALL AMERICAN FINANCIAL
103 COMMERCE BLVD
PO BOX 4898
SYRACUSE, NY 13221-4898
TEL: (315) 451-3970
FAX: (800) 955-7668
TOLL FREE: (800) 888-4925
WWW.ALLAMERICA.COM

NORTH CAROLINA CLAIMS OFFICE
ALL AMERICAN FINANCIAL
7130 GLEN FOREST DR, STE 400
PO BOX 85612
RICHMOND, VA 23285-5612
TEL: (804) 288-3113
FAX: (804) 288-6946
TOLL FREE: (800) 552-3960
IN-STATE: (800) 552-3960
WWW.ALLAMERICA.COM

OKLAHOMA CLAIMS OFFICE
ALL AMERICAN FINANCIAL
10816 EXECUTIVE CTR DR
PO BOX 24868
LITTLE ROCK, AR 72221
TEL: (501) 223-8249
FAX: (501) 223-8766
TOLL FREE: (800) 332-5513
IN-STATE: (800) 332-5513
WWW.ALLAMERICA.COM

PENNSYLVANIA CLAIMS OFFICE
ALL AMERICAN FINANCIAL
860 CENTENNIAL AVE
PO BOX 1090
PISCATAWAY, NJ 08855-1383
TEL: (732) 457-0577
FAX: (732) 980-9650
IN-STATE: (800) 257-5720
WWW.ALLAMERICA.COM

SOUTH CAROLINA CLAIMS OFFICE
ALL AMERICAN FINANCIAL
7130 GLEN FOREST DR, STE 400
PO BOX 85612
RICHMOND, VA 23285-5612
TEL: (804) 288-3113
FAX: (804) 288-6946
TOLL FREE: (800) 552-3960
IN-STATE: (800) 552-3960
WWW.ALLAMERICA.COM

TEXAS CLAIMS OFFICE
ALL AMERICAN FINANCIAL
2400 VETERANS BLVD, STE 400
PO BOX 1758
KENNER, LA 70063-1758
TEL: (504) 464-6012
FAX: (504) 469-7563
TOLL FREE: (800) 477-7661
IN-STATE: (800) 477-7661
WWW.ALLAMERICA.COM

VIRGINIA CLAIMS OFFICE
ALL AMERICAN FINANCIAL
7130 GLEN FOREST DR, STE 400
PO BOX 85612
RICHMOND, VA 23285-5612
TEL: (804) 288-3113
FAX: (804) 288-6946
TOLL FREE: (800) 552-3960
IN-STATE: (800) 552-3960
WWW.ALLAMERICA.COM

HARBISON-FISCHER

TEXAS CLAIMS OFFICE
PO BOX 2477
FT WORTH, TX 76113
TEL: (817) 297-2211
FAX: (817) 297-9679

HARCO NATIONAL INSURANCE CO

ALABAMA CLAIMS OFFICE
2850 W GOLF RD
PO BOX 68309
SCHAUMBURG, IL 60168-0309
TEL: (847) 734-4100
FAX: (847) 734-4210
TOLL FREE: (800) 822-4429

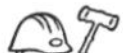

ALASKA CLAIMS OFFICE
2850 W GOLF RD
PO BOX 68309
SCHAUMBURG, IL 60168-0309
TEL: (847) 734-4100
FAX: (847) 734-4210
TOLL FREE: (800) 822-4429

ARIZONA CLAIMS OFFICE
2850 W GOLF RD
PO BOX 68309
SCHAUMBURG, IL 60168-0309
TEL: (847) 734-4100
FAX: (847) 734-4210
TOLL FREE: (800) 822-4429

ARKANSAS CLAIMS OFFICE
2850 W GOLF RD
PO BOX 68309
SCHAUMBURG, IL 60168-0309
TEL: (847) 734-4100
FAX: (847) 734-4210
TOLL FREE: (800) 822-4429

CALIFORNIA CLAIMS OFFICE
2850 W GOLF RD
PO BOX 68309
SCHAUMBURG, IL 60168-0309
TEL: (847) 734-4100
FAX: (847) 734-4210
TOLL FREE: (800) 822-4429

COLORADO CLAIMS OFFICE
2850 W GOLF RD
PO BOX 68309
SCHAUMBURG, IL 60168-0309
TEL: (847) 734-4100
FAX: (847) 734-4210
TOLL FREE: (800) 822-4429

CONNECTICUT CLAIMS OFFICE
2850 W GOLF RD
PO BOX 68309
SCHAUMBURG, IL 60168-0309
TEL: (847) 734-4100
FAX: (847) 734-4210
TOLL FREE: (800) 822-4429

DELAWARE CLAIMS OFFICE
2850 W GOLF RD
PO BOX 68309
SCHAUMBURG, IL 60168-0309
TEL: (847) 734-4100
FAX: (847) 734-4210
TOLL FREE: (800) 822-4429

DISTRICT OF COLUMBIA CLAIMS OFFICE
2850 W GOLF RD
PO BOX 68309
SCHAUMBURG, IL 60168-0309
TEL: (847) 734-4100
FAX: (847) 734-4210
TOLL FREE: (800) 822-4429

FLORIDA CLAIMS OFFICE
2850 W GOLF RD
PO BOX 68309
SCHAUMBURG, IL 60168-0309
TEL: (847) 734-4100
FAX: (847) 734-4210
TOLL FREE: (800) 822-4429

GEORGIA CLAIMS OFFICE
2850 W GOLF RD
PO BOX 68309
SCHAUMBURG, IL 60168-0309
TEL: (847) 734-4100
FAX: (847) 734-4210
TOLL FREE: (800) 822-4429

IDAHO CLAIMS OFFICE
2850 W GOLF RD
PO BOX 68309
SCHAUMBURG, IL 60168-0309
TEL: (847) 734-4100
FAX: (847) 734-4210
TOLL FREE: (800) 822-4429

ILLINOIS CLAIMS OFFICE
2850 W GOLF RD
PO BOX 68309
SCHAUMBURG, IL 60168-0309
TEL: (847) 734-4100
FAX: (847) 734-4210
TOLL FREE: (800) 822-4429

INDIANA CLAIMS OFFICE
2850 W GOLF RD
PO BOX 68309
SCHAUMBURG, IL 60168-0309
TEL: (847) 734-4100
FAX: (847) 734-4210
TOLL FREE: (800) 822-4429

IOWA CLAIMS OFFICE
2850 W GOLF RD
PO BOX 68309
SCHAUMBURG, IL 60168-0309
TEL: (847) 734-4100
FAX: (847) 734-4210
TOLL FREE: (800) 822-4429

KANSAS CLAIMS OFFICE
2850 W GOLF RD
PO BOX 68309
SCHAUMBURG, IL 60168-0309
TEL: (847) 734-4100
FAX: (847) 734-4210
TOLL FREE: (800) 822-4429

KENTUCKY CLAIMS OFFICE
2850 W GOLF RD
PO BOX 68309
SCHAUMBURG, IL 60168-0309
TEL: (847) 734-4100
FAX: (847) 734-4210
TOLL FREE: (800) 822-4429

LOUISIANA CLAIMS OFFICE
2850 W GOLF RD
PO BOX 68309
SCHAUMBURG, IL 60168-0309
TEL: (847) 734-4100
FAX: (847) 734-4210
TOLL FREE: (800) 822-4429

MAINE CLAIMS OFFICE
2850 W GOLF RD
PO BOX 68309
SCHAUMBURG, IL 60168-0309
TEL: (847) 734-4100
FAX: (847) 734-4210
TOLL FREE: (800) 822-4429

MASSACHUSETTS CLAIMS OFFICE
2850 W GOLF RD
PO BOX 68309
SCHAUMBURG, IL 60168-0309
TEL: (847) 734-4100
FAX: (847) 734-4210
TOLL FREE: (800) 822-4429

MICHIGAN CLAIMS OFFICE
2850 W GOLF RD
PO BOX 68309
SCHAUMBURG, IL 60168-0309
TEL: (847) 734-4100
FAX: (847) 734-4210
TOLL FREE: (800) 822-4429

MINNESOTA CLAIMS OFFICE
2850 W GOLF RD
PO BOX 68309
SCHAUMBURG, IL 60168-0309
TEL: (847) 734-4100
FAX: (847) 734-4210
TOLL FREE: (800) 822-4429

MISSISSIPPI CLAIMS OFFICE
2850 W GOLF RD
PO BOX 68309
SCHAUMBURG, IL 60168-0309
TEL: (847) 734-4100
FAX: (847) 734-4210
TOLL FREE: (800) 822-4429

H

MISSOURI CLAIMS OFFICE
2850 W GOLF RD
PO BOX 68309
SCHAUMBURG, IL 60168-0309
TEL: (847) 734-4100
FAX: (847) 734-4210
TOLL FREE: (800) 822-4429

MONTANA CLAIMS OFFICE
2850 W GOLF RD
PO BOX 68309
SCHAUMBURG, IL 60168-0309
TEL: (847) 734-4100
FAX: (847) 734-4210
TOLL FREE: (800) 822-4429

NEBRASKA CLAIMS OFFICE
2850 W GOLF RD
PO BOX 68309
SCHAUMBURG, IL 60168-0309
TEL: (847) 734-4100
FAX: (847) 734-4210
TOLL FREE: (800) 822-4429

NEVADA CLAIMS OFFICE
2850 W GOLF RD
PO BOX 68309
SCHAUMBURG, IL 60168-0309
TEL: (847) 734-4100
FAX: (847) 734-4210
TOLL FREE: (800) 822-4429

NEW HAMPSHIRE CLAIMS OFFICE
2850 W GOLF RD
PO BOX 68309
SCHAUMBURG, IL 60168-0309
TEL: (847) 734-4100
FAX: (847) 734-4210
TOLL FREE: (800) 822-4429

NEW JERSEY CLAIMS OFFICE
2850 W GOLF RD
PO BOX 68309
SCHAUMBURG, IL 60168-0309
TEL: (847) 734-4100
FAX: (847) 734-4210
TOLL FREE: (800) 822-4429

NEW MEXICO CLAIMS OFFICE
2850 W GOLF RD
PO BOX 68309
SCHAUMBURG, IL 60168-0309
TEL: (847) 734-4100
FAX: (847) 734-4210
TOLL FREE: (800) 822-4429

NEW YORK CLAIMS OFFICE
2850 W GOLF RD
PO BOX 68309
SCHAUMBURG, IL 60168-0309
TEL: (847) 734-4100
FAX: (847) 734-4210
TOLL FREE: (800) 822-4429

NORTH CAROLINA CLAIMS OFFICE
2850 W GOLF RD
PO BOX 68309
SCHAUMBURG, IL 60168-0309
TEL: (847) 734-4100
FAX: (847) 734-4210
TOLL FREE: (800) 822-4429

NORTH DAKOTA CLAIMS OFFICE
2850 W GOLF RD
PO BOX 68309
SCHAUMBURG, IL 60168-0309
TEL: (847) 734-4100
FAX: (847) 734-4210
TOLL FREE: (800) 822-4429

OHIO CLAIMS OFFICE
2850 W GOLF RD
PO BOX 68309
SCHAUMBURG, IL 60168-0309
TEL: (847) 734-4100
FAX: (847) 734-4210
TOLL FREE: (800) 822-4429

OKLAHOMA CLAIMS OFFICE
2850 W GOLF RD
PO BOX 68309
SCHAUMBURG, IL 60168-0309
TEL: (847) 734-4100
FAX: (847) 734-4210
TOLL FREE: (800) 822-4429

OREGON CLAIMS OFFICE
2850 W GOLF RD
PO BOX 68309
SCHAUMBURG, IL 60168-0309
TEL: (847) 734-4100
FAX: (847) 734-4210
TOLL FREE: (800) 822-4429

PENNSYLVANIA CLAIMS OFFICE
2850 W GOLF RD
PO BOX 68309
SCHAUMBURG, IL 60168-0309
TEL: (847) 734-4100
FAX: (847) 734-4210
TOLL FREE: (800) 822-4429

SOUTH CAROLINA CLAIMS OFFICE
2850 W GOLF RD
PO BOX 68309
SCHAUMBURG, IL 60168-0309
TEL: (847) 734-4100
FAX: (847) 734-4210
TOLL FREE: (800) 822-4429

SOUTH DAKOTA CLAIMS OFFICE
2850 W GOLF RD
PO BOX 68309
SCHAUMBURG, IL 60168-0309
TEL: (847) 734-4100
FAX: (847) 734-4210
TOLL FREE: (800) 822-4429

TENNESSEE CLAIMS OFFICE
2850 W GOLF RD
PO BOX 68309
SCHAUMBURG, IL 60168-0309
TEL: (847) 734-4100
FAX: (847) 734-4210
TOLL FREE: (800) 822-4429

TEXAS CLAIMS OFFICE
2850 W GOLF RD
PO BOX 68309
SCHAUMBURG, IL 60168-0309
TEL: (847) 734-4100
FAX: (847) 734-4210
TOLL FREE: (800) 822-4429

UTAH CLAIMS OFFICE
2850 W GOLF RD
PO BOX 68309
SCHAUMBURG, IL 60168-0309
TEL: (847) 734-4100
FAX: (847) 734-4210
TOLL FREE: (800) 822-4429

VERMONT CLAIMS OFFICE
2850 W GOLF RD
PO BOX 68309
SCHAUMBURG, IL 60168-0309
TEL: (847) 734-4100
FAX: (847) 734-4210
TOLL FREE: (800) 822-4429

VIRGINIA CLAIMS OFFICE
2850 W GOLF RD
PO BOX 68309
SCHAUMBURG, IL 60168-0309
TEL: (847) 734-4100
FAX: (847) 734-4210
TOLL FREE: (800) 822-4429

WASHINGTON CLAIMS OFFICE
2850 W GOLF RD
PO BOX 68309
SCHAUMBURG, IL 60168-0309
TEL: (847) 734-4100
FAX: (847) 734-4210
TOLL FREE: (800) 822-4429

WEST VIRGINIA CLAIMS OFFICE
2850 W GOLF RD
PO BOX 68309
SCHAUMBURG, IL 60168-0309
TEL: (847) 734-4100
FAX: (847) 734-4210
TOLL FREE: (800) 822-4429

WISCONSIN CLAIMS OFFICE
2850 W GOLF RD
PO BOX 68309
SCHAUMBURG, IL 60168-0309
TEL: (847) 734-4100
FAX: (847) 734-4210
TOLL FREE: (800) 822-4429

WYOMING CLAIMS OFFICE
2850 W GOLF RD
PO BOX 68309
SCHAUMBURG, IL 60168-0309
TEL: (847) 734-4100
FAX: (847) 734-4210
TOLL FREE: (800) 822-4429

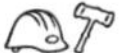

HARFORD MUTUAL INSURANCE CO

MARYLAND CLAIMS OFFICE
200 N MAIN ST
BEL AIR, MD 21014
TEL: (410) 838-4000
FAX: (410) 838-8675
TOLL FREE: (800) 638-3669

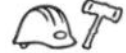

HARLEYSVILLE INSURANCE CO

10010 JCT DR, STE 200
PO BOX 2000
ANNAPOLIS JUNCTION, MD 20701
TEL: (301) 604-6644
FAX: (301) 776-9708
TOLL FREE: (800) 544-0800

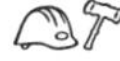

5250 LOGANS FERRY RD
PO BOX 119
PITTSBURGH, PA 15230-0119
TEL: (724) 327-8889
FAX: (724) 327-6859
TOLL FREE: (800) 233-8222
WWW.HARLEYSVILLEGROUP.COM

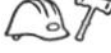

NATIONAL CLAIMS OFFICE
308 HARPER DR
PO BOX 1016
MOORESTOWN, NJ 08057
TEL: (609) 642-9779
FAX: (609) 642-9416
TOLL FREE: (800) 322-5521

NEW JERSEY CLAIMS OFFICE
308 HARPER DR
PO BOX 1016
MOORESTOWN, NJ 08057
TEL: (856) 642-9779
FAX: (856) 642-9416
TOLL FREE: (800) 322-2251
WWW.HARLEYSVILLEGROUP.COM

5250 LOGANS FERRY RD
PO BOX 119
PITTSBURGH, PA 15230-0119
TEL: (724) 327-8889
FAX: (724) 327-6859
TOLL FREE: (800) 233-8222
WWW.HARLEYSVILLEGROUP.COM

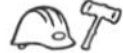

NEW YORK CLAIMS OFFICE
5250 LOGANS FERRY RD
PO BOX 119
PITTSBURGH, PA 15230-0119
TEL: (724) 327-8889
FAX: (724) 327-6859
TOLL FREE: (800) 233-8222
WWW.HARLEYSVILLEGROUP.COM

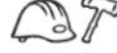

NORTH CAROLINA CLAIMS OFFICE
5700 EXECUTIVE CTR DR, STE 110
PO BOX 25518
CHARLOTTE, NC 28229-5518
TEL: (704) 563-3000
FAX: (704) 537-0227
TOLL FREE: (800) 468-8439

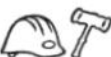

3511 W MARKET ST, STE 200
PO BOX 22300
GREENSBORO, NC 27420
TEL: (336) 852-4800
FAX: (336) 852-3940
TOLL FREE: (800) 822-1726

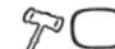

5250 LOGANS FERRY RD
PO BOX 119
PITTSBURGH, PA 15230-0119
TEL: (724) 327-8889
FAX: (724) 327-6859
TOLL FREE: (800) 233-8222
WWW.HARLEYSVILLEGROUP.COM

PENNSYLVANIA CLAIMS OFFICE
355 MAPLE AVE
HARLEYSVILLE, PA 19438-2297
TEL: (215) 256-3300
FAX: (215) 256-3435
TOLL FREE: (800) 523-6344

1300 VIRGINIA DR, STE 310
FT WASHINGTON, PA 19034-3221
TEL: (215) 628-9300
FAX: (215) 628-4096
TOLL FREE: (800) 455-7881

2700 COMMERCE DR
PO BOX 6237
HARRISBURG, PA 17112-6237
TEL: (717) 657-8100
FAX: (717) 657-2877
TOLL FREE: (800) 222-3459

5250 LOGANS FERRY RD
PO BOX 119
PITTSBURGH, PA 15230-0119
TEL: (724) 327-8889
FAX: (724) 327-6859
TOLL FREE: (800) 233-8222
WWW.HARLEYSVILLEGROUP.COM

VIRGINIA CLAIMS OFFICE
6800 PARAGON PL, STE 626
RICHMOND, VA 23230-1643
TEL: (540) 563-9780
FAX: (540) 563-9769
TOLL FREE: (800) 368-3440
IN-STATE: (800) 552-3808

5250 LOGANS FERRY RD
PO BOX 119
PITTSBURGH, PA 15230-0119
TEL: (724) 327-8889
FAX: (724) 327-6859
TOLL FREE: (800) 233-8222
WWW.HARLEYSVILLEGROUP.COM

HARRINGTON BENEFIT SERVICES

OHIO CLAIMS OFFICE
HEALTHPLAN SERVICES, INC
130 W 2ND ST, STE 400
PO BOX 1391
DAYTON, OH 45401-1391
TEL: (937) 226-8610
FAX: (937) 226-8628
TOLL FREE: (800) 222-2733
IN-STATE: (800) 523-9398

HEALTHPLAN SERVICES, INC
3041 MORSE XING
PO BOX 16789
COLUMBUS, OH 43216-6789
TEL: (614) 470-7000
FAX: (614) 470-7171
TOLL FREE: (800) 848-4623
IN-STATE: (800) 848-2664

HARRIS METHODIST HEALTH PLAN

TEXAS CLAIMS OFFICE
611 RYAN PLZ DR, STE 900
PO BOX 90100
ARLINGTON, TX 76011
TEL: (817) 878-5800
FAX: (817) 462-7235
TOLL FREE: (800) 633-8598
WWW.HMHP.COM

HARTFORD FINANCIAL GROUP INC

NATIONAL CLAIMS OFFICE
HARTFORD PLZ
HARTFORD, CT 06115-2013
TEL: (860) 547-5000
FAX: (860) 547-8800
TOLL FREE: (800) 243-5860
WWW.ATTHEHARTFORD.COM

HARTFORD INSURANCE CO

ALABAMA CLAIMS OFFICE
WORKER'S COMP CLAIMS
101 S HALL LN
PO BOX 940669
MAITLAND, FL 32751
TEL: (407) 875-5000
FAX: (407) 875-8188
TOLL FREE: (800) 824-1732

ARIZONA CLAIMS OFFICE
9630 N 25 AVE, STE 300
PO BOX 39700
PHOENIX, AZ 85069-9700
TEL: (602) 943-9612
FAX: (602) 944-8448
TOLL FREE: (800) 343-8985
IN-STATE: (800) 343-9612

CALIFORNIA CLAIMS OFFICE
555 POITE DR
PO BOX 1170
BREA, CA 92821
TEL: (714) 671-2811
FAX: (714) 256-1287
TOLL FREE: (800) 228-1320
WWW.ATTHEHARTFORD.COM

COLORADO CLAIMS OFFICE
PO BOX 5188
DENVER, CO 80217-5188
TEL: (303) 645-8500
FAX: (303) 768-0689
TOLL FREE: (800) 537-5809

CONNECTICUT CLAIMS OFFICE
55 FARMINGTON
PO BOX 2923
HARTFORD, CT 06104
TEL: (860) 520-1600
FAX: (860) 520-2288
TOLL FREE: (800) 243-6185
WWW.ATTHEHARTFORD.COM

FLORIDA CLAIMS OFFICE
WORKER'S COMP CLAIMS
101 S HALL LN
PO BOX 940669
MAITLAND, FL 32751
TEL: (407) 875-5000
FAX: (407) 875-8188
TOLL FREE: (800) 824-1732

2502 ROCKY PT DR, STE 400
PO BOX 30773
TAMPA, FL 33630-3773
TEL: (813) 286-8243
FAX: (813) 286-8997
TOLL FREE: (800) 243-5860

GEORGIA CLAIMS OFFICE
ALL AMERICA FINANCIAL
50 GLENLAKE PKY
PO BOX 88140
ATLANTA, GA 30328
TEL: (770) 730-3331
FAX: (770) 804-1563
TOLL FREE: (800) 282-5855

HAWAII CLAIMS OFFICE
1001 BISHOP ST, STE 1700
PO BOX 1140
HONOLULU, HI 96807
TEL: (808) 546-5750
FAX: (808) 538-0214
WWW.ATTHEHARTFORD.COM

ILLINOIS CLAIMS OFFICE
12647 OLIVE BLVD
PO BOX 790043
SAINT LOUIS, MO 63179-0043
TEL: (314) 275-8100
FAX: (314) 275-2695
TOLL FREE: (800) 444-7857
WWW.THEHARTFORD.COM

INDIANA CLAIMS OFFICE
8910 PURDUE RD
PO BOX 68930
INDIANAPOLIS, IN 46268-0930
TEL: (317) 876-7076
FAX: (317) 872-7805
TOLL FREE: (800) 962-6170

IOWA CLAIMS OFFICE
ALL AMERICA FINANCIAL
1125 S 103RD ST, STE 200
PO BOX 3993
OMAHA, NE 68124
TEL: (402) 399-8833
FAX: (402) 399-2049
TOLL FREE: (800) 642-8950
WWW.ATTHEHARTFORD.COM

KANSAS CLAIMS OFFICE
7300 W 110 ST
PO BOX 2927
OVERLAND PARK, KS 66201
TEL: (913) 451-2324
FAX: (913) 469-6834
TOLL FREE: (800) 255-6440
WWW.THEHARTFORD.COM

LOUISIANA CLAIMS OFFICE
WORKER'S COMP CLAIMS
101 S HALL LN
PO BOX 940669
MAITLAND, FL 32751
TEL: (407) 875-5000
FAX: (407) 875-8188
TOLL FREE: (800) 824-1732

MAINE CLAIMS OFFICE
24 NEW ENGLAND EXECUTIVE PRK
PO BOX 3004
BURLINGTON, MA 01803
TEL: (781) 313-8699
FAX: (781) 270-9805
TOLL FREE: (800) 775-5457

MASSACHUSETTS CLAIMS OFFICE
24 NEW ENGLAND EXECUTIVE PRK
PO BOX 3004
BURLINGTON, MA 01803
TEL: (781) 313-8699
FAX: (781) 270-9805
TOLL FREE: (800) 775-5457

MISSISSIPPI CLAIMS OFFICE
WORKER'S COMP CLAIMS
101 S HALL LN
PO BOX 940669
MAITLAND, FL 32751
TEL: (407) 875-5000
FAX: (407) 875-8188
TOLL FREE: (800) 824-1732

MISSOURI CLAIMS OFFICE
12647 OLIVE BLVD
PO BOX 790043
SAINT LOUIS, MO 63179-0043
TEL: (314) 275-8100
FAX: (314) 275-2695
TOLL FREE: (800) 444-7857
WWW.THEHARTFORD.COM

7300 W 110 ST
PO BOX 2927
OVERLAND PARK, KS 66201
TEL: (913) 451-2324
FAX: (913) 469-6834
TOLL FREE: (800) 255-6440
WWW.THEHARTFORD.COM

MONTANA CLAIMS OFFICE
PO BOX 6310
GREAT FALLS, MT 59406
TEL: (406) 454-3274
FAX: (406) 454-0504
TOLL FREE: (800) 394-1822

NATIONAL CLAIMS OFFICE
3520 NW 58TH ST
OKLAHOMA CITY, OK 73112
FAX: (405) 947-4167
TOLL FREE: (800) 444-6562

2 ARMSTRONG RD
PO BOX 1000
SHELTON, CT 06484-1000
TEL: (203) 925-0010
FAX: (203) 925-0313
TOLL FREE: (800) 766-9119

215 SHUMAN BLVD
PO BOX 3118
NAPERVILLE, IL 60566
TEL: (630) 369-2100
FAX: (630) 369-2178
TOLL FREE: (800) 843-7006

2 PARK EXEC DR
PO BOX 5340
MANCHESTER, NH 03108
TEL: (603) 623-8045
FAX: (603) 622-9976
TOLL FREE: (800) 258-6213
IN-STATE: (800) 562-8225
WWW.ATTHEHARTFORD.COM

RED BANK CLAIMS CENTER
230 HALF MILE RD
PO BOX 7002
RED BANK, NJ 07701-7002
TEL: (732) 747-5445
FAX: (732) 219-0767
TOLL FREE: (800) 498-6569

ROCKAWAY 80 CORPORATE CTR
100 ENTERPRISE DR
PO BOX 2000
ROCKAWAY, NJ 07866
TEL: (973) 361-3700
FAX: (973) 361-2742
TOLL FREE: (800) 626-7740
IN-STATE: (800) 252-7824

1 PARK PL- 300 S STATE
PO BOX 4771
SYRACUSE, NY 13201
TEL: (315) 474-6531
TOLL FREE: (800) 962-8867

5832 FARM POND LN
PO BOX 25268
CHARLOTTE, NC 28229-5268
TEL: (704) 535-2851
FAX: (704) 531-9222
TOLL FREE: (800) 879-9144
WWW.ATTHEHARTFORD.COM

ALL AMERICA FINANCIAL
6480 ROCKSIDE WDS BLVD S, STE 200
PO BOX 318041
INDEPENDENCE, OH 44131-2222
TEL: (216) 447-1000
FAX: (216) 328-9020
TOLL FREE: (800) 777-3086
WWW.ATTHEHARTFORD.COM

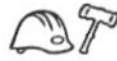

150 S WARNER RD- 3RD FL
PO BOX 61560
KING OF PRUSSIA, PA 19406
TEL: (610) 254-0591
FAX: (610) 341-0291
TOLL FREE: (800) 610-4456
IN-STATE: (800) 732-0011

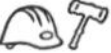

SPECIALTY RISK SERVICES
828 ROYAL PKY, STE 200
PO BOX 305104
NASHVILLE, TN 37230
TEL: (615) 883-4324
FAX: (615) 874-0636
TOLL FREE: (800) 327-3636

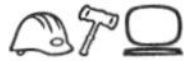

5285 SHAWNEE RD, STE 300
PO BOX 13168
ALEXANDRIA, VA 22312-0970
TEL: (703) 914-2400
FAX: (703) 354-0917
TOLL FREE: (800) 933-4551

720 OLIVE WAY, STE 300
PO BOX 1875
SEATTLE, WA 98111-1875
TEL: (206) 583-0053
FAX: (206) 583-0574
TOLL FREE: (800) 552-7667

NEBRASKA CLAIMS OFFICE
ALL AMERICA FINANCIAL
1125 S 103RD ST, STE 200
PO BOX 3993
OMAHA, NE 68124
TEL: (402) 399-8833
FAX: (402) 399-2049
TOLL FREE: (800) 642-8950
WWW.ATTHEHARTFORD.COM

NEW HAMPSHIRE CLAIMS OFFICE
24 NEW ENGLAND EXECUTIVE PRK
PO BOX 3004
BURLINGTON, MA 01803
TEL: (781) 313-8699
FAX: (781) 270-9805
TOLL FREE: (800) 775-5457

NORTH DAKOTA CLAIMS OFFICE
ALL AMERICA FINANCIAL
1125 S 103RD ST, STE 200
PO BOX 3993
OMAHA, NE 68124
TEL: (402) 399-8833
FAX: (402) 399-2049
TOLL FREE: (800) 642-8950
WWW.ATTHEHARTFORD.COM

OKLAHOMA CLAIMS OFFICE
ONE CORP PLZ- 3520 NW 58TH ST
OKLAHOMA CITY, OK 73112
TEL: (405) 947-0511
FAX: (405) 947-0928
TOLL FREE: (800) 444-6562

OREGON CLAIMS OFFICE
ALL AMERICA FINANCIAL
7678 S W MOHAWK ST
PO BOX 1188
TUALATIN, OR 97062
TEL: (503) 691-0758
FAX: (503) 691-0693
TOLL FREE: (800) 647-1627
IN-STATE: (800) 452-0380
WWW.ATTHEHARTFORD.COM

RHODE ISLAND CLAIMS OFFICE
55 FARMINGTON
PO BOX 2923
HARTFORD, CT 06104
TEL: (860) 520-1600
FAX: (860) 520-2288
TOLL FREE: (800) 243-6185
WWW.ATTHEHARTFORD.COM

SOUTH CAROLINA CLAIMS OFFICE
ALL AMERICA FINANCIAL
1125 S 103RD ST, STE 200
PO BOX 3993
OMAHA, NE 68124
TEL: (402) 399-8833
FAX: (402) 399-2049
TOLL FREE: (800) 642-8950
WWW.ATTHEHARTFORD.COM

TEXAS CLAIMS OFFICE
17855 DALLAS PKY, STE 490
PO BOX 1630
DALLAS, TX 75221
TEL: (972) 807-4600
FAX: (972) 807-4499
TOLL FREE: (800) 443-3783

17855 DALLAS PKY
PO BOX 802517
DALLAS, TX 75380
TEL: (972) 807-4400
FAX: (972) 991-1228
TOLL FREE: (800) 677-1412
WWW.THDHARTFORD.COM

450 GEARS RD, STE 500
PO BOX 4626
HOUSTON, TX 77210-4626
TEL: (281) 874-9600
FAX: (281) 877-3980
TOLL FREE: (800) 392-7805

VERMONT CLAIMS OFFICE
24 NEW ENGLAND EXECUTIVE PARK
PO BOX 3004
BURLINGTON, MA 01803
TEL: (781) 313-8699
FAX: (781) 270-9805
TOLL FREE: (800) 775-5457

VIRGINIA CLAIMS OFFICE
4480 COX RD, STE 200
GLEN ALLEN, VA 23060
TEL: (804) 747-7011
FAX: (804) 747-6338
TOLL FREE: (800) 333-7216

WISCONSIN CLAIMS OFFICE
125 S 84 ST, STE 400
PO BOX 14248
MILWAUKEE, WI 53214
TEL: (414) 475-5885
FAX: (414) 475-1205
TOLL FREE: (800) 825-3825

HARTFORD INSURANCE GROUP

NEW YORK CLAIMS OFFICE
20 CORPORATE WOODS BLVD
PO BOX 1690
ALBANY, NY 12201-1690
TEL: (518) 431-0500
FAX: (518) 447-9106
TOLL FREE: (800) 342-3235

HARTFORD LIFE

MINNESOTA CLAIMS OFFICE
505 N HWY 169
PO BOX 59179
MINNEAPOLIS, MN 55459
TEL: (612) 545-2100
FAX: (612) 591-9493
TOLL FREE: (800) 541-6757
WWW.THEHARTFORD.COM

HARVARD INDUSTRIES

NATIONAL CLAIMS OFFICE
3 WERNER WAY, STE 210
LEBANON, NJ 08833
TEL: (908) 437-4100
FAX: (908) 236-0071
WWW.HARVARDIND.COM

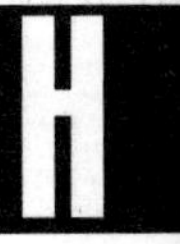

HARVARD PILGRIM HEALTH CARE

MASSACHUSETTS CLAIMS OFFICE
ONE HOPPIN ST
PROVIDENCE, RI 02903
TEL: (401) 331-3000
FAX: (401) 331-0496
TOLL FREE: (800) 444-1210
WWW.HARVARDPILGRIM.ORG

NEW HAMPSHIRE CLAIMS OFFICE
ONE HOPPIN ST
PROVIDENCE, RI 02903
TEL: (401) 331-3000
FAX: (401) 331-0496
TOLL FREE: (800) 444-1210
WWW.HARVARDPILGRIM.ORG

RHODE ISLAND CLAIMS OFFICE
ONE HOPPIN ST
PROVIDENCE, RI 02903
TEL: (401) 331-3000
FAX: (401) 331-0496
TOLL FREE: (800) 444-1210
WWW.HARVARDPILGRIM.ORG

HARVARD PILGRIM HEALTH CARE, INC

MASSACHUSETTS CLAIMS OFFICE
HARVARD COMMUNITY HEALTH PLAN
20 OVERLAND ST
BOSTON, MA 02215
TEL: (617) 421-6300
FAX: (617) 421-6315
TOLL FREE: (800) 338-4247

HARVARD UNIVERSITY GROUP HEALTH PLAN

UNIVERSITY HEALTH SERVICES
75 MT AUBURN ST
CAMBRIDGE, MA 02138-4901
TEL: (617) 495-2008
FAX: (617) 496-6125
WWW.UHF.HARVARD.EDU

HAWAII MEDICAL SERVICE ASSOCIATION

HAWAII CLAIMS OFFICE
BLUE CROSS & BLUE SHIELD OF HAWAII
818 KEEAUMOKU ST
PO BOX 860
HONOLULU, HI 96808
TEL: (808) 948-6111
FAX: (808) 948-6555
TOLL FREE: (800) 776-4672
WWW.HMSA.COM

HAWORTH, INC

MICHIGAN CLAIMS OFFICE
1 HAWORTH CTR 2-31G
HOLLAND, MI 49423
TEL: (616) 393-3000
FAX: (616) 393-1551
WWW.HAWORTH.COM

HEALTH ADMINISTRATION SERVICES

TEXAS CLAIMS OFFICE
HAS
100 GLENBOROUGH DR, STE 450
HOUSTON, TX 77067-3610
TEL: (281) 873-8682
FAX: (281) 872-5351
TOLL FREE: (800) 749-2714

HEALTH ADVANTAGE

ARKANSAS CLAIMS OFFICE
HMO ARKANSAS
26 CORPORATE HILL DR
PO BOX 8069
LITTLE ROCK, AR 72203
TEL: (501) 221-3733
FAX: (501) 221-7103
TOLL FREE: (800) 243-1329
IN-STATE: (800) 225-1891

HEALTH AGENCIES OF THE WEST, INC

CALIFORNIA CLAIMS OFFICE
500 N STATE COLLEGE BLVD, STE 1450
ORANGE, CA 92868-1664
TEL: (714) 634-7550
FAX: (714) 634-7555
TOLL FREE: (800) 556-0800
E-MAIL: HAWADMIN@AOL.COM

HEALTH ALLIANCE MEDICAL PLANS

NATIONAL CLAIMS OFFICE
102 MAIN ST
URBANA, IL 61801
TEL: (217) 337-8100
FAX: (217) 337-8008
TOLL FREE: (800) 851-3379
WWW.HEALTHALLIANCE.ORG

HEALTH ALLIANCE OF THE SOUTH

GEORGIA CLAIMS OFFICE
SOUTH GEORGIA PARTNERS
808 GORDON AVE
PO BOX 1939
THOMASVILLE, GA 31799-1993
TEL: (912) 226-4122
FAX: (912) 226-1408
TOLL FREE: (800) 341-6216

HEALTH ALLIANCE PLAN OF MICHIGAN

MICHIGAN CLAIMS OFFICE
HAP
2850 W GRAND BLVD
DETROIT, MI 48202-2692
TEL: (313) 872-8100
FAX: (313) 874-7496
TOLL FREE: (800) 422-4641
IN-STATE: (800) 367-3292
WWW.HAPCORP.ORG

HEALTH AMERICA

PENNSYLVANIA CLAIMS OFFICE
2575 INTERSTATE DR
HARRISBURG, PA 17110
TEL: (412) 553-7300
FAX: (412) 553-7384
TOLL FREE: (800) 735-2202
WWW.HEALTHAMERICA.CVTY.COM

HEALTH BENEFIT, INC

PO BOX 1040
WILLOW GROVE, PA 19090
TEL: (215) 957-1700
FAX: (215) 957-1717

HEALTH BENEFIT TRUST FUND LOCAL 94

NEW YORK CLAIMS OFFICE
331-337 W 44TH ST
NEW YORK, NY 10036-5454
TEL: (212) 541-9880
FAX: (212) 245-7886
WWW.LOCAL94.COM

HEALTH BENEFITS FUND

INDIANA CLAIMS OFFICE
1233 SHELBY ST
INDIANAPOLIS, IN 46203
TEL: (317) 639-3573
FAX: (317) 639-3548
TOLL FREE: (800) 859-6862
IN-STATE: (800) 859-6862
WWW.INSTABN.COM

HEALTH CARE ADMINISTRATORS

OKLAHOMA CLAIMS OFFICE
HEALTH CARE SOLUTIONS
2401 CHANDLER RD, STE 300
PO BOX 1309
MUSKOGEE, OK 74402
TEL: (918) 687-1261
FAX: (918) 682-7984
TOLL FREE: (800) 749-1422

HEALTH CARE ADMINISTRATORS, INC

INDIANA CLAIMS OFFICE
ARNET HEALTH PLANS
415 N 26TH ST, STE 101
PO BOX 6108
LAFAYETTE, IN 47903-6108
TEL: (765) 474-5455
FAX: (765) 448-7799
TOLL FREE: (888) 448-7447

HEALTH CARE BENEFITS, INC

TEXAS CLAIMS OFFICE
1001 E CAMPBELL RD
PO BOX 833889
RICHARDSON, TX 75083-3889
TEL: (972) 669-4660
FAX: (972) 669-8663

HEALTH CARE PARTNERS HEALTH PLAN

821 E SE LOOP 323, STE 200
PO BOX 130217
TYLER, TX 75713
TEL: (903) 581-2600
FAX: (903) 509-5726
TOLL FREE: (800) 477-2287

HEALTH CARE PLAN

NEW YORK CLAIMS OFFICE
28 CHURCH ST- RM 100
BUFFALO, NY 14202-3998
TEL: (716) 847-1480
FAX: (716) 857-6220
TOLL FREE: (800) 427-8490
WWW.UNIVERAHEALTHCARE.ORG

H

HEALTH CARE SERVICE CORP

ILLINOIS CLAIMS OFFICE
BLUE CROSS & BLUE SHIELD
300 E RANDOLPH ST
PO BOX 1364
CHICAGO, IL 60690
TEL: (312) 938-6000

H

MICHIGAN CLAIMS OFFICE
BLUE CROSS & BLUE SHIELD
300 E RANDOLPH ST
PO BOX 1364
CHICAGO, IL 60690
TEL: (312) 938-6000

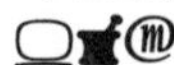

TEXAS CLAIMS OFFICE
BLUE CROSS & BLUE SHIELD
300 E RANDOLPH ST
PO BOX 1364
CHICAGO, IL 60690
TEL: (312) 938-6000

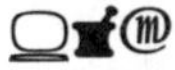

HEALTH CLAIM SERVICES, INC

FLORIDA CLAIMS OFFICE
1211 S MILITARY TRL
PO BOX 9615
DEERFIELD BEACH, FL 33442-9615
TEL: (954) 480-2744
FAX: (954) 480-9661
TOLL FREE: (800) 222-3560

HEALTH CLAIMS ADMINISTRATION, INC

NATIONAL CLAIMS OFFICE
20 E CASS ST
JOLIET, IL 60432-1015
TEL: (815) 740-4251
FAX: (815) 740-4262
TOLL FREE: (800) 435-0155

HEALTH ECONOMICS GROUP, INC

NEW YORK CLAIMS OFFICE
625 PANORAMA TRL- BLDG 3
ROCHESTER, NY 14625
TEL: (716) 385-3390
FAX: (716) 385-4787
TOLL FREE: (800) 666-6690

HEALTH FIRST

OHIO CLAIMS OFFICE
278 BARKS RD W
PO BOX 1820
MARION, OH 43301-1820
TEL: (740) 387-6355
FAX: (740) 383-3840
TOLL FREE: (800) 858-1472
E-MAIL: HFIRSTDP@ACC-NET.COM

HEALTH FIRST, INC

TEXAS CLAIMS OFFICE
HEALTH PLAN
821 E SE LOOP 323, II AMERICAN CTR, STE 200
PO BOX 130217
TYLER, TX 75713
TEL: (903) 581-2600
FAX: (903) 509-5726
TOLL FREE: (800) 477-2287
IN-STATE: (800) 477-2287

HEALTH FUTURE, INC

OREGON CLAIMS OFFICE
825 E MAIN ST, STE D
MEDFORD, OR 97504-7156
TEL: (503) 772-3062
IN-STATE: (800) 452-2558
WWW.HEALTHFUTURELLC.COM

HEALTH GUARD

PENNSYLVANIA CLAIMS OFFICE
280 GRANITE RUN DR, STE 105
LANCASTER, PA 17601-6810
TEL: (717) 560-9049
FAX: (717) 560-9413
TOLL FREE: (800) 269-4606
WWW.HGUARD.COM

HEALTH GUARD SERVICES, INC

NATIONAL CLAIMS OFFICE
322 N COMMERCIAL
PO BOX 5348
BELLINGHAM, WA 98227
TEL: (360) 647-3849
FAX: (360) 392-9100
TOLL FREE: (800) 688-0010

HEALTH INSURANCE PLAN OF GREATER NEW YORK

FLORIDA CLAIMS OFFICE
7 W 34TH ST
NEW YORK, NY 10001-8100
TEL: (212) 630-5000
FAX: (212) 630-5062
TOLL FREE: (800) 447-8255
WWW.HIPUSA.COM

NEW YORK CLAIMS OFFICE
7 W 34TH ST
NEW YORK, NY 10001-8100
TEL: (212) 630-5000
FAX: (212) 630-5062
TOLL FREE: (800) 447-8255
WWW.HIPUSA.COM

HEALTH MANAGEMENT ASSOCIATES

NATIONAL CLAIMS OFFICE
1600 W BROADWAY RD, STE 385
TEMPE, AZ 85282
TEL: (480) 921-8944
FAX: (480) 894-5230
TOLL FREE: (800) 331-9562
E-MAIL: HMA@VERDINET.COM

HEALTH NET

CALIFORNIA CLAIMS OFFICE
FOUNDATION HEALTH SYSTEMS
21600 OXIDE ST
PO BOX 9103
WOODLAND HILLS, CA 91367-9103
TEL: (818) 676-6775
FAX: (818) 676-8755
TOLL FREE: (800) 522-0088
WWW.HEALTHNET.COM

KANSAS CLAIMS OFFICE
2300 MAIN ST, STE 700
KANSAS CITY, MO 64108
TEL: (816) 221-8400
FAX: (816) 221-7709
TOLL FREE: (800) 468-1442
WWW.HEALTH NET_KC.COM

MISSOURI CLAIMS OFFICE
2300 MAIN ST, STE 700
KANSAS CITY, MO 64108
TEL: (816) 221-8400
FAX: (816) 221-7709
TOLL FREE: (800) 468-1442
WWW.HEALTH NET_KC.COM

HEALTH NET HMO, INC

TENNESSEE CLAIMS OFFICE
44 VANTAGE WAY, STE 300
PO BOX 20000
NASHVILLE, TN 37202
TEL: (615) 291-7022
FAX: (615) 401-4647
TOLL FREE: (800) 881-9466
IN-STATE: (800) 314-3258

HEALTH NETWORK AMERICA, INC

NATIONAL CLAIMS OFFICE
187 MONMOUTH PKY
WEST LONG BRANCH, NJ 07764
TEL: (732) 222-2229
FAX: (732) 222-4584
TOLL FREE: (800) 332-7772
WWW.HEALTHNETWORKAMERICA.COM

HEALTH NEW ENGLAND

MASSACHUSETTS CLAIMS OFFICE
ONE MONARCH PL
SPRINGFIELD, MA 01144-1006
TEL: (413) 787-4000
FAX: (413) 731-7498
TOLL FREE: (800) 842-4464

HEALTH OPTIONS, INC

FLORIDA CLAIMS OFFICE
CENTRAL FLORIDA HEALTH OPTIONS
3191 MAGUIRE BLVD, STE 125
ORLANDO, FL 32803-3723
TEL: (407) 894-7200
FAX: (407) 894-2305
IN-STATE: (800) 545-6565

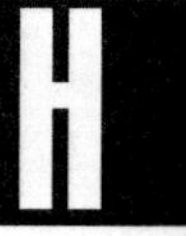

HEALTH OPTIONS OF SOUTH FLORIDA

8400 NW 33 ST, STE 100
PO BOX 025314
MIAMI, FL 33122
TEL: (305) 591-9955
TOLL FREE: (800) 283-8268

H

HEALTH PARTNERS

ALABAMA CLAIMS OFFICE
851 S BELTLINE HWY, STE 610
MOBILE, AL 36606
TEL: (334) 470-8500
FAX: (334) 470-8551
IN-STATE: (800) 735-2439

H

MINNESOTA CLAIMS OFFICE
8100 34TH AVE S
PO BOX 1309
BLOOMINGTON, MN 55440-1309
TEL: (612) 883-5000
FAX: (612) 883-6100
TOLL FREE: (800) 444-4558
WWW.HEALTHPARTNERS.COM

PO BOX 1309
MINNEAPOLIS, MN 55440-1309
TEL: (612) 883-6000
FAX: (612) 883-6100
TOLL FREE: (800) 828-1159
WWW.HEALTHPARTNER.COM

PENNSYLVANIA CLAIMS OFFICE
841 CHESTNUT ST, STE 900
PHILADELPHIA, PA 19107
TEL: (215) 849-9606
FAX: (215) 849-7097
TOLL FREE: (888) 991-9023

HEALTH PLAN

OHIO CLAIMS OFFICE
52160 NATIONAL RD E
ST. CLAIRSVILLE, OH 43950-9306
TEL: (740) 695-7605
FAX: (740) 695-8103
TOLL FREE: (800) 624-6961
WWW.HEALTHPLAN.ORG

WEST VIRGINIA CLAIMS OFFICE
52160 NATIONAL RD E
ST. CLAIRSVILLE, OH 43950-9306
TEL: (740) 695-7605
FAX: (740) 695-8103
TOLL FREE: (800) 624-6961
WWW.HEALTHPLAN.ORG

HEALTH PLAN ADMINISTRATORS, INC

CONNECTICUT CLAIMS OFFICE
30 SHELTER ROCK RD
PO BOX 3986
DANBURY, CT 06810
TEL: (203) 794-1703
FAX: (203) 748-7528

NATIONAL CLAIMS OFFICE
3703 N MAIN ST
PO BOX 2638
ROCKFORD, IL 61132
TEL: (815) 633-5800
FAX: (815) 633-0277
TOLL FREE: (800) 397-5800

NEW YORK CLAIMS OFFICE
30 SHELTER ROCK RD
PO BOX 3986
DANBURY, CT 06810
TEL: (203) 794-1703
FAX: (203) 748-7528

HEALTH PLAN OF NEVADA, INC

NEVADA CLAIMS OFFICE
SIERRA HEALTH SERVICES
2724 TENAYA
PO BOX 15645
LAS VEGAS, NV 89114-5645
TEL: (702) 242-7444
FAX: (702) 242-9038

HEALTH PLAN OF THE REDWOODS

CALIFORNIA CLAIMS OFFICE
3033 CLEVELAND AVE
SANTA ROSA, CA 95403-2126
TEL: (707) 544-2273
FAX: (707) 525-4261
IN-STATE: (800) 248-2070
WWW.HPR.ORG

HEALTH PLAN SERVICES

CALIFORNIA CLAIMS OFFICE
3501 FRONTAGE RD
PO BOX 30098
TAMPA, FL 33630-3098
TEL: (813) 289-1000
FAX: (813) 289-7937
TOLL FREE: (800) 237-7767
E-MAIL: HEALTHCARE.COM
WWW.HPS.COM

FLORIDA CLAIMS OFFICE
CORPORATE OFFICE
3501 FRONTAGE RD
PO BOX 30098
TAMPA, FL 33630-3098
TEL: (813) 289-1000
FAX: (813) 289-7937
TOLL FREE: (800) 237-7767
E-MAIL: HEALTHCARE.COM
WWW.HPS.COM

3501 E FRONTAGE RD
PO BOX 30098
TAMPA, FL 33630-3098
TEL: (813) 289-1000
FAX: (813) 289-7937
TOLL FREE: (800) 237-7767
WWW.HEALTHPLAN.COM

NATIONAL CLAIMS OFFICE
PO BOX 1069
NASHUA, NH 03061-1069
FAX: (603) 598-8701
TOLL FREE: (800) 832-0311

OHIO CLAIMS OFFICE
3501 FRONTAGE RD
PO BOX 30098
TAMPA, FL 33630-3098
TEL: (813) 289-1000
FAX: (813) 289-7937
TOLL FREE: (800) 237-7767
E-MAIL: HEALTHCARE.COM
WWW.HPS.COM

OKLAHOMA CLAIMS OFFICE
3501 FRONTAGE RD
PO BOX 30098
TAMPA, FL 33630-3098
TEL: (813) 289-1000
FAX: (813) 289-7937
TOLL FREE: (800) 237-7767
E-MAIL: HEALTHCARE.COM
WWW.HPS.COM

TEXAS CLAIMS OFFICE
3501 FRONTAGE RD
PO BOX 30098
TAMPA, FL 33630-3098
TEL: (813) 289-1000
FAX: (813) 289-7937
TOLL FREE: (800) 237-7767
E-MAIL: HEALTHCARE.COM
WWW.HPS.COM

HEALTH PLAN SOUTHEAST

FLORIDA CLAIMS OFFICE
3520 THOMASVILLE RD, STE 200
PO BOX 13700
TALLAHASSEE, FL 32317-3700
TEL: (850) 668-3000
FAX: (850) 668-3133
TOLL FREE: (800) 833-2169
WWW.HPSE.COM

HEALTH PLUS OF MICHIGAN

MICHIGAN CLAIMS OFFICE
2050 S LINDEN RD
PO BOX 1700
FLINT, MI 48501-1700
TEL: (810) 230-2000
FAX: (810) 230-2090
TOLL FREE: (800) 332-9161
WWW.HEALTHPLUS.COM

HEALTH RISK MANAGEMENT

5250 LOVERS LN
PO BOX 4022
KALAMAZOO, MI 49002-1564
TEL: (616) 381-7995
FAX: (616) 382-1525
TOLL FREE: (800) 253-0966
IN-STATE: (800) 632-5674

NATIONAL CLAIMS OFFICE
10900 HAMPSHIRE AVE S
PO BOX 226
MINNEAPOLIS, MN 55440-0226
TEL: (612) 829-3500
FAX: (612) 829-3622
TOLL FREE: (800) 642-4456

HEALTH SERVICES BENEFITS ADMINISTRATION
CALIFORNIA CLAIMS OFFICE
HEALTH SERVICES FOUNDATION
160 AIRWAY BLVD
LIVERMORE, CA 94550
TEL: (925) 449-7070
FAX: (925) 443-2035
IN-STATE: (800) 528-4357

HEALTH SERVICES MEDICAL CORP
NEW YORK CLAIMS OFFICE
UNIVERA
8278 WILLETT PKY
BALDWINSVILLE, NY 13027
TEL: (315) 638-2133
FAX: (315) 638-0985
TOLL FREE: (800) 388-3264
WWW.PHPHMO.COM

HEALTH SOURCE NORTH CAROLINA
NORTH CAROLINA CLAIMS OFFICE
701 CORPORATE CTR DR
PO BOX 28087
RALEIGH, NC 27607
TEL: (919) 854-7000
FAX: (919) 854-7114
TOLL FREE: (800) 849-9300

HEALTH SOUTH OF ERIE
NATIONAL CLAIMS OFFICE
143 E 2ND ST
ERIE, PA 16507-1403
TEL: (814) 878-1235
FAX: (814) 878-1239
TOLL FREE: (800) 234-4574

HEALTH SPECIAL RISK, INC
MINNESOTA CLAIMS OFFICE
4001 N JOSEY LN
CARROLLTON, TX 75007
TEL: (972) 482-6474
FAX: (972) 492-4946
TOLL FREE: (800) 328-1114
E-MAIL: HSRTEXAS@COMPETEK.NET

NATIONAL CLAIMS OFFICE
4001 N JOSEY LN
CARROLLTON, TX 75007
TEL: (972) 492-6474
FAX: (972) 492-4946
TOLL FREE: (800) 328-1114
E-MAIL: HSRTEXAS@AIRMAIL.NET
WWW.HEALTHSPECIALRISK.COM

HEALTH & WELFARE FUND LOCAL 716
INDIANA CLAIMS OFFICE
849 S MERIDIAN
INDIANAPOLIS, IN 46225
TEL: (317) 266-0314
FAX: (317) 266-0611

HEALTH & WELFARE FUND OF THE EXCAV LOCAL 731
ILLINOIS CLAIMS OFFICE
PO BOX 1407
LAGRANGE PARK, IL 60526
TEL: (708) 352-0202
FAX: (708) 352-0310

HEALTHCARE AMERICA PLANS, INC
KANSAS CLAIMS OFFICE
453 S WEBB RD, STE 200
PO BOX 780467
WICHITA, KS 67278-0467
TEL: (316) 687-1600
FAX: (316) 616-2076
TOLL FREE: (800) 475-4274

HEALTHCARE CENTER AT CHRISTIANA
DELAWARE CLAIMS OFFICE
CHRISTIANA CARE HEALTH SERVICES
200 HYGEIA DR
PO BOX 15965
NEWARK, DE 19850-5965
TEL: (302) 623-0100
FAX: (302) 623-0117

HEALTHCARE MANAGEMENT ALTERNATIVES, INC
PENNSYLVANIA CLAIMS OFFICE
100 PENN SQUARE EAST STE 900
PO BOX 41566
PHILADELPHIA, PA 19107
TEL: (215) 832-4500
FAX: (215) 832-4583
TOLL FREE: (800) 345-3627

HEALTHCARE PARTNERS MEDICAL GROUP, INC
CALIFORNIA CLAIMS OFFICE
PO BOX 6099
TORRANCE, CA 90504
TEL: (310) 965-1100
FAX: (310) 352-6219

HEALTHFIRST, INC
SOUTH CAROLINA CLAIMS OFFICE
PO BOX 17709
GREENVILLE, SC 29606
TEL: (864) 289-3000
FAX: (864) 289-3053
TOLL FREE: (800) 832-7713
WWW.HEALTHFIRST.COM

HEALTHNOW
NEW YORK CLAIMS OFFICE
HMO OF BLUE CROSS OF WESTERN NEW YORK, INC
1901 MAIN ST
PO BOX 159
BUFFALO, NY 14240-1199
TEL: (716) 887-6900
FAX: (716) 887-7912
TOLL FREE: (800) 950-0052
WWW.HEALTHNOWNY.COM

HEALTHPLAN MANAGEMENT, INC
NATIONAL CLAIMS OFFICE
101 N WAUKEGAN RD, STE 700
LAKE BLUFF, IL 60044
TEL: (847) 234-8870
FAX: (847) 234-9244
TOLL FREE: (800) 562-2506

HEALTHPLEX, INC
NEW JERSEY CLAIMS OFFICE
DENTCARE
60 CHARLES LINDBERGH BLVD
UNIONDALE, NY 11553
TEL: (516) 542-2200
FAX: (516) 794-3186
TOLL FREE: (800) 468-0608
E-MAIL: HEALTHPLEX@AOL.COM
WWW.HEALTHPLEX.COM

NEW YORK CLAIMS OFFICE
DENTCARE
60 CHARLES LINDBERGH BLVD
UNIONDALE, NY 11553
TEL: (516) 542-2200
FAX: (516) 794-3186
TOLL FREE: (800) 468-0608
E-MAIL: HEALTHPLEX@AOL.COM
WWW.HEALTHPLEX.COM

HEALTHPOINT, INC
INDIANA CLAIMS OFFICE
HEALTHPOINT LLC
8900 KEYSTONE XING, STE 480
INDIANAPOLIS, IN 46240
TEL: (317) 574-8181

HEALTHRIGHT, INC
CONNECTICUT CLAIMS OFFICE
134 STATE ST
MERIDEN, CT 06450
TEL: (203) 630-3356
FAX: (203) 630-0108
TOLL FREE: (800) 474-1444

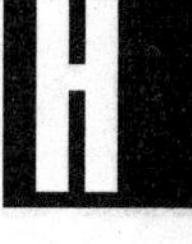

HEALTHSOURCE
MAINE CLAIMS OFFICE
HEALTHSOURCE OF MAINE
2 STONEWWOD DR
PO BOX 447
FREEPORT, ME 04032-0447
TEL: (207) 865-5000
FAX: (207) 865-5632
IN-STATE: (800) 642-5551

MASSACHUSETTS CLAIMS OFFICE
HEALTHSOURCE OF NEW HAMPSHIRE
2 COLLEGE PARK DR
HOOKSETT, NH 03106
TEL: (603) 225-5077
FAX: (603) 268-7981
TOLL FREE: (800) 531-3121
IN-STATE: (800) 531-3121
WWW.CIGNA.COM

NEW HAMPSHIRE CLAIMS OFFICE
HEALTHSOURCE OF NEW HAMPSHIRE
2 COLLEGE PARK DR
HOOKSETT, NH 03106
TEL: (603) 225-5077
FAX: (603) 268-7981
TOLL FREE: (800) 531-3121
IN-STATE: (800) 531-3121
WWW.CIGNA.COM

NEW YORK CLAIMS OFFICE
5794 WIDEWATERS PKY- 2ND FL
PO BOX 1498
SYRACUSE, NY 13201-1498
TEL: (315) 449-1100
FAX: (315) 449-2200
TOLL FREE: (800) 999-0874
WWW.SIGNA.COM

HELLER ASSOCIATES

NATIONAL CLAIMS OFFICE
2755 BRISTOL ST, STE 250
COSTA MESA, CA 92626-5956
TEL: (714) 549-7052
FAX: (714) 549-4816
IN-STATE: (800) 552-2929
E-MAIL: CLAIMS@HELLERTPA.COM
WWW.HELLERTPA.COM

2235 FLAMINGO RD #406
LAS VEGAS, NV 89119
TEL: (714) 549-7052
FAX: (714) 549-4816
E-MAIL: CLAIMS@HELLERTPA.COM
WWW.HELLERTPA.COM

8228 MAYFIELD RD, STE 5-B
CHESTERLAND, OH 44026
TEL: (714) 549-7052
FAX: (714) 549-4816
E-MAIL: CLAIMS@HELLERTPA.COM
WWW.HELLERTPA.COM

HELMSMAN MANAGEMENT SERVICES

CALIFORNIA CLAIMS OFFICE
LIBERTY MUTUAL
101 N BRAND BLVD, STE 1400
PO BOX 29073
GLENDALE, CA 91203
TEL: (818) 240-1234
FAX: (818) 598-0596
TOLL FREE: (800) 281-1120
WWW.LIBERTYMUTUAL.COM

HENRY FORD HEALTH SYSTEM

MICHIGAN CLAIMS OFFICE
2799 W GRAND BLVD
DETROIT, MI 48202-2608
TEL: (313) 876-2600
FAX: (313) 916-3000
IN-STATE: (800) 999-4340

OHIO CLAIMS OFFICE
2799 W GRAND BLVD
DETROIT, MI 48202-2608
TEL: (313) 876-2600
FAX: (313) 916-3000
IN-STATE: (800) 999-4340

HEP ADMINISTRATORS, INC

ILLINOIS CLAIMS OFFICE
100 S MAIN ST, STE 400
OCONOMOWOC, WI 53066
TEL: (414) 567-9695
FAX: (414) 567-1814
TOLL FREE: (800) 437-4940

WISCONSIN CLAIMS OFFICE
100 S MAIN ST, STE 400
OCONOMOWOC, WI 53066
TEL: (414) 567-9695
FAX: (414) 567-1814
TOLL FREE: (800) 437-4940

HERBERT L. JAMISON & CO LLC

NEW JERSEY CLAIMS OFFICE
N. JAMISON SPECIAL RISK, INC
100 EXECUTIVE DR, STE 200
WEST ORANGE, NJ 07052-3362
TEL: (973) 731-0806
FAX: (973) 731-3035
TOLL FREE: (800) 526-4766
WWW.JAMISONGROUP.COM

HERITAGE INSURANCE MANAGERS, INC

TEXAS CLAIMS OFFICE
PO BOX 659570
SAN ANTONIO, TX 78265-9570
TEL: (210) 829-7467
FAX: (210) 822-4113
TOLL FREE: (800) 456-7480
E-MAIL: SALES@HERITAGE-INS.COM
WWW.HERITAGE-INS.COM

HERITAGE MUTUAL INSURANCE CO

ILLINOIS CLAIMS OFFICE
2800 S TAYLOR DR
PO BOX 58
SHEBOYGAN, WI 53082-0058
TEL: (920) 458-9131
FAX: (920) 458-1618
TOLL FREE: (800) 242-7611
IN-STATE: (800) 242-3620
WWW.HERITAGEINSURANCE.COM

IOWA CLAIMS OFFICE
2800 S TAYLOR DR
PO BOX 58
SHEBOYGAN, WI 53082-0058
TEL: (920) 458-9131
FAX: (920) 458-1618
TOLL FREE: (800) 242-7611
IN-STATE: (800) 242-3620
WWW.HERITAGEINSURANCE.COM

KENTUCKY CLAIMS OFFICE
2800 S TAYLOR DR
PO BOX 58
SHEBOYGAN, WI 53082-0058
TEL: (920) 458-9131
FAX: (920) 458-1618
TOLL FREE: (800) 242-7611
IN-STATE: (800) 242-3620
WWW.HERITAGEINSURANCE.COM

MICHIGAN CLAIMS OFFICE
2800 S TAYLOR DR
PO BOX 58
SHEBOYGAN, WI 53082-0058
TEL: (920) 458-9131
FAX: (920) 458-1618
TOLL FREE: (800) 242-7611
IN-STATE: (800) 242-3620
WWW.HERITAGEINSURANCE.COM

MINNESOTA CLAIMS OFFICE
2800 S TAYLOR DR
PO BOX 58
SHEBOYGAN, WI 53082-0058
TEL: (920) 458-9131
FAX: (920) 458-1618
TOLL FREE: (800) 242-7611
IN-STATE: (800) 242-3620
WWW.HERITAGEINSURANCE.COM

NEBRASKA CLAIMS OFFICE
2800 S TAYLOR DR
PO BOX 58
SHEBOYGAN, WI 53082-0058
TEL: (920) 458-9131
FAX: (920) 458-1618
TOLL FREE: (800) 242-7611
IN-STATE: (800) 242-3620
WWW.HERITAGEINSURANCE.COM

NORTH DAKOTA CLAIMS OFFICE
2800 S TAYLOR DR
PO BOX 58
SHEBOYGAN, WI 53082-0058
TEL: (920) 458-9131
FAX: (920) 458-1618
TOLL FREE: (800) 242-7611
IN-STATE: (800) 242-3620
WWW.HERITAGEINSURANCE.COM

SOUTH DAKOTA CLAIMS OFFICE
2800 S TAYLOR DR
PO BOX 58
SHEBOYGAN, WI 53082-0058
TEL: (920) 458-9131
FAX: (920) 458-1618
TOLL FREE: (800) 242-7611
IN-STATE: (800) 242-3620
WWW.HERITAGEINSURANCE.COM

WISCONSIN CLAIMS OFFICE
2800 S TAYLOR DR
PO BOX 58
SHEBOYGAN, WI 53082-0058
TEL: (920) 458-9131
FAX: (920) 458-1618
TOLL FREE: (800) 242-7611
IN-STATE: (800) 242-3620
WWW.HERITAGEINSURANCE.COM

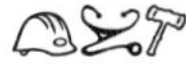

HERRINGTON BENEFIT SERVICES

NATIONAL CLAIMS OFFICE
55 E JACKSON BLVD
CHICAGO, IL 60604-4103
TEL: (312) 346-1451
FAX: (312) 663-9902
IN-STATE: (800) 828-8563

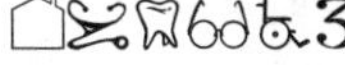

HIGHLANDS INSURANCE

CONNECTICUT CLAIMS OFFICE
1000 LENOX DR
PO BOX 6426
LAWRENCEVILLE, NJ 08648-0426
TEL: (609) 896-1921
FAX: (609) 219-1773
TOLL FREE: (800) 252-4655
IN-STATE: (800) 431-3800

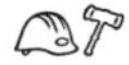

FLORIDA CLAIMS OFFICE
4011 W CHASE BLVD
RALEIGH, NC 27607
TOLL FREE: (800) 735-1168

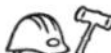

NEW JERSEY CLAIMS OFFICE
1000 LENOX DR
PO BOX 6426
LAWRENCEVILLE, NJ 08648-0426
TEL: (609) 896-1921
FAX: (609) 219-1773
TOLL FREE: (800) 252-4655
IN-STATE: (800) 431-3800

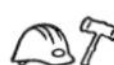

NEW YORK CLAIMS OFFICE
1000 LENOX DR
PO BOX 6426
LAWRENCEVILLE, NJ 08648-0426
TEL: (609) 896-1921
FAX: (609) 219-1773
TOLL FREE: (800) 252-4655
IN-STATE: (800) 431-3800

PENNSYLVANIA CLAIMS OFFICE
1000 LENOX DR
PO BOX 6426
LAWRENCEVILLE, NJ 08648-0426
TEL: (609) 896-1921
FAX: (609) 219-1773
TOLL FREE: (800) 252-4655
IN-STATE: (800) 431-3800

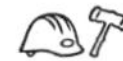

HIGHLANDS INSURANCE GROUP

ARKANSAS CLAIMS OFFICE
15661 RED HILL AVE, STE 100
PO BOX 2058
TUSTIN, CA 92781-2058
TEL: (714) 259-5700
FAX: (714) 258-8311
IN-STATE: (800) 477-6644

CALIFORNIA CLAIMS OFFICE
15661 RED HILL AVE, STE 100
PO BOX 2058
TUSTIN, CA 92781-2058
TEL: (714) 259-5700
FAX: (714) 258-8311
IN-STATE: (800) 477-6644

COLORADO CLAIMS OFFICE
15661 RED HILL AVE, STE 100
PO BOX 2058
TUSTIN, CA 92781-2058
TEL: (714) 259-5700
FAX: (714) 258-8311
IN-STATE: (800) 477-6644

IDAHO CLAIMS OFFICE
15661 RED HILL AVE, STE 100
PO BOX 2058
TUSTIN, CA 92781-2058
TEL: (714) 259-5700
FAX: (714) 258-8311
IN-STATE: (800) 477-6644

ILLINOIS CLAIMS OFFICE
18650 W CORPORATE DR
PO BOX 504
MILWAUKEE, WI 53201-0504
TEL: (414) 792-3000
FAX: (414) 792-3271
TOLL FREE: (800) 873-6644
WWW.HIGHLANDSINSURANCE.COM

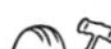

INDIANA CLAIMS OFFICE
4011 WESTCHASE BLVD- 3RD FL
PO BOX 27257
RALEIGH, NC 27611
TEL: (919) 836-2000
FAX: (919) 836-2040
TOLL FREE: (800) 849-2000

18650 W CORPORATE DR
PO BOX 504
MILWAUKEE, WI 53201-0504
TEL: (414) 792-3000
FAX: (414) 792-3271
TOLL FREE: (800) 873-6644
WWW.HIGHLANDSINSURANCE.COM

IOWA CLAIMS OFFICE
15661 RED HILL AVE, STE 100
PO BOX 2058
TUSTIN, CA 92781-2058
TEL: (714) 259-5700
FAX: (714) 258-8311
IN-STATE: (800) 477-6644

KANSAS CLAIMS OFFICE
15661 RED HILL AVE, STE 100
PO BOX 2058
TUSTIN, CA 92781-2058
TEL: (714) 259-5700
FAX: (714) 258-8311
IN-STATE: (800) 477-6644

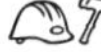

MINNESOTA CLAIMS OFFICE
18650 W CORPORATE DR
PO BOX 504
MILWAUKEE, WI 53201-0504
TEL: (414) 792-3000
FAX: (414) 792-3271
TOLL FREE: (800) 873-6644
WWW.HIGHLANDSINSURANCE.COM

MISSOURI CLAIMS OFFICE
15661 RED HILL AVE, STE 100
PO BOX 2058
TUSTIN, CA 92781-2058
TEL: (714) 259-5700
FAX: (714) 258-8311
IN-STATE: (800) 477-6644

MONTANA CLAIMS OFFICE
15661 RED HILL AVE, STE 100
PO BOX 2058
TUSTIN, CA 92781-2058
TEL: (714) 259-5700
FAX: (714) 258-8311
IN-STATE: (800) 477-6644

NEBRASKA CLAIMS OFFICE
15661 RED HILL AVE, STE 100
PO BOX 2058
TUSTIN, CA 92781-2058
TEL: (714) 259-5700
FAX: (714) 258-8311
IN-STATE: (800) 477-6644

NEVADA CLAIMS OFFICE
15661 RED HILL AVE, STE 100
PO BOX 2058
TUSTIN, CA 92781-2058
TEL: (714) 259-5700
FAX: (714) 258-8311
IN-STATE: (800) 477-6644

NORTH CAROLINA CLAIMS OFFICE
4011 WESTCHASE BLVD- 3RD FL
PO BOX 27257
RALEIGH, NC 27611
TEL: (919) 836-2000
FAX: (919) 836-2040
TOLL FREE: (800) 849-2000

SOUTH DAKOTA CLAIMS OFFICE
15661 RED HILL AVE, STE 100
PO BOX 2058
TUSTIN, CA 92781-2058
TEL: (714) 259-5700
FAX: (714) 258-8311
IN-STATE: (800) 477-6644

WISCONSIN CLAIMS OFFICE
18650 W CORPORATE DR
PO BOX 504
MILWAUKEE, WI 53201-0504
TEL: (414) 792-3000
FAX: (414) 792-3271
TOLL FREE: (800) 873-6644
WWW.HIGHLANDSINSURANCE.COM

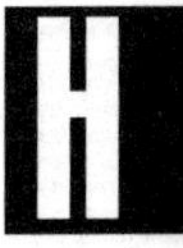

HIGHLANDS NORTHWESTERN NATIONAL INSURANCE CO

IOWA CLAIMS OFFICE
6955 VISTA DR
PO BOX 9108
DES MOINES, IA 50306
TEL: (515) 224-6480
FAX: (800) 285-5677
TOLL FREE: (800) 289-6644
IN-STATE: (800) 289-6644

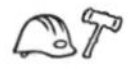

KANSAS CLAIMS OFFICE
6955 VISTA DR
PO BOX 9108
DES MOINES, IA 50306
TEL: (515) 224-6480
FAX: (800) 285-5677
TOLL FREE: (800) 289-6644
IN-STATE: (800) 289-6644

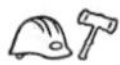

MISSOURI CLAIMS OFFICE
6955 VISTA DR
PO BOX 9108
DES MOINES, IA 50306
TEL: (515) 224-6480
FAX: (800) 285-5677
TOLL FREE: (800) 289-6644
IN-STATE: (800) 289-6644

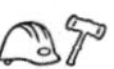

NEBRASKA CLAIMS OFFICE
6955 VISTA DR
PO BOX 9108
DES MOINES, IA 50306
TEL: (515) 224-6480
FAX: (800) 285-5677
TOLL FREE: (800) 289-6644
IN-STATE: (800) 289-6644

SOUTH DAKOTA CLAIMS OFFICE
6955 VISTA DR
PO BOX 9108
DES MOINES, IA 50306
TEL: (515) 224-6480
FAX: (800) 285-5677
TOLL FREE: (800) 289-6644
IN-STATE: (800) 289-6644

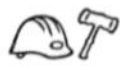

HINGHAM MUTUAL FIRE INSURANCE CO

CONNECTICUT CLAIMS OFFICE
230 BEAL ST
HINGHAM, MA 02043
TEL: (781) 749-0841
FAX: (781) 749-4477
IN-STATE: (800) 341-8200

MASSACHUSETTS CLAIMS OFFICE
230 BEAL ST
HINGHAM, MA 02043
TEL: (781) 749-0841
FAX: (781) 749-4477
IN-STATE: (800) 341-8200

230 BEAL ST
HINGHAM, MA 02043
TEL: (781) 749-0841
FAX: (781) 749-4477
TOLL FREE: (800) 341-8200

NEW HAMPSHIRE CLAIMS OFFICE
230 BEAL ST
HINGHAM, MA 02043
TEL: (781) 749-0841
FAX: (781) 749-4477
TOLL FREE: (800) 341-8200

RHODE ISLAND CLAIMS OFFICE
230 BEAL ST
HINGHAM, MA 02043
TEL: (781) 749-0841
FAX: (781) 749-4477
TOLL FREE: (800) 341-8200

VERMONT CLAIMS OFFICE
230 BEAL ST
HINGHAM, MA 02043
TEL: (781) 749-0841
FAX: (781) 749-4477
IN-STATE: (800) 341-8200

HIP HEALTH PLAN OF FLORIDA, INC

FLORIDA CLAIMS OFFICE
300 S PARK RD
HOLLYWOOD, FL 33021
TEL: (954) 961-0005
FAX: (954) 986-6209
TOLL FREE: (800) 447-5116

NEW YORK CLAIMS OFFICE
300 S PARK RD
HOLLYWOOD, FL 33021
TEL: (954) 961-0005
FAX: (954) 986-6209
TOLL FREE: (800) 447-5116

HMA, INC

ARIZONA CLAIMS OFFICE
DBA HEALTH MANAGEMENT ASSOCIATES, INC
PO BOX 2069
COTTONWOOD, AZ 86326
TEL: (602) 921-8944
FAX: (602) 894-5230
TOLL FREE: (800) 448-3585

COLORADO CLAIMS OFFICE
DBA HEALTH MANAGEMENT ASSOCIATES, INC
PO BOX 2069
COTTONWOOD, AZ 86326
TEL: (602) 921-8944
FAX: (602) 894-5230
TOLL FREE: (800) 448-3585

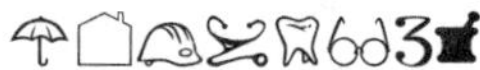

NEVADA CLAIMS OFFICE
DBA HEALTH MANAGEMENT ASSOCIATES, INC
PO BOX 2069
COTTONWOOD, AZ 86326
TEL: (602) 921-8944
FAX: (602) 894-5230
TOLL FREE: (800) 448-3585

HMO BLUE OF EL PASO

TEXAS CLAIMS OFFICE
BLUE CROSS & BLUE SHIELD OF TEXAS
4150 PINNACLE ST, STE 203
EL PASO, TX 79902-1035
TEL: (915) 496-6600
FAX: (915) 496-6697
TOLL FREE: (800) 831-0576

HMO COLORADO, INC

COLORADO CLAIMS OFFICE
BLUE CROSS BLUE SHIELD OF COLORADO
700 BROADWAY
DENVER, CO 80273
TEL: (303) 831-0801
FAX: (303) 861-9018
TOLL FREE: (800) 544-3879
IN-STATE: (800) 533-5643
WWW.BCBSCO.COM

HMO ILLINOIS

ILLINOIS CLAIMS OFFICE
HEALTH CARE SERVICE CORPORATION
300 E RANDOLPH
PO BOX LA3694
CHICAGO, IL 60690
TEL: (312) 653-6000
FAX: (800) 260-6840
TOLL FREE: (800) 892-2803
WWW.BCBSIL.COM

HMO MONTANA

MONTANA CLAIMS OFFICE
PLAN OF BLUE CROSS AND BLUE SHIELD OF MT
404 FULLER AVE
PO BOX 5004
GREAT FALLS, MT 59403
TEL: (406) 447-8600
TOLL FREE: (800) 447-7828
WWW.BCBSMT.COM

HMO NEBRASKA

IOWA CLAIMS OFFICE
2401 S 73RD ST, STE 2
PO BOX 241739
OMAHA, NE 68124-5739
TEL: (402) 392-2800
FAX: (402) 392-2761
TOLL FREE: (800) 843-2373

NEBRASKA CLAIMS OFFICE
2401 S 73RD ST, STE 2
PO BOX 241739
OMAHA, NE 68124-5739
TEL: (402) 392-2800
FAX: (402) 392-2761
TOLL FREE: (800) 843-2373

HMO NEW MEXICO, INC

COLORADO CLAIMS OFFICE
12800 INDIAN SCHOOL NE
PO BOX 11968
ALBUQUERQUE, NM 87112
TEL: (505) 291-6945
TOLL FREE: (800) 423-1630
IN-STATE: (800) 423-1630

NEVADA CLAIMS OFFICE
12800 INDIAN SCHOOL NE
PO BOX 11968
ALBUQUERQUE, NM 87112
TEL: (505) 291-6945
TOLL FREE: (800) 423-1630
IN-STATE: (800) 423-1630

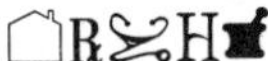

NEW MEXICO CLAIMS OFFICE
12800 INDIAN SCHOOL NE
PO BOX 11968
ALBUQUERQUE, NM 87112
TEL: (505) 291-6945
TOLL FREE: (800) 423-1630
IN-STATE: (800) 423-1630

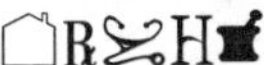

HMO REGENCE CARE

WASHINGTON CLAIMS OFFICE
1800 9TH AVE
PO BOX 91005
SEATTLE, WA 98111-9105
TEL: (206) 340-6600
FAX: (206) 389-6719
TOLL FREE: (800) 222-6129

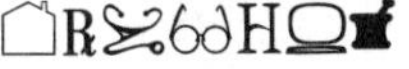

HMO TEXAS HEALTH CHOICE

TEXAS CLAIMS OFFICE
11011 RICHMOND AVE, STE 900
HOUSTON, TX 77043
TEL: (713) 952-6868
FAX: (713) 974-1650

H

HOLY CROSS RESOURCES, INC

INDIANA CLAIMS OFFICE
ST MARY'S LOURDES HALL
3575 MOREAU CT
SOUTH BEND, IN 46628-4320
TEL: (219) 283-4600
FAX: (219) 283-4709
TOLL FREE: (800) 348-2616
WWW.HCRI.ORG

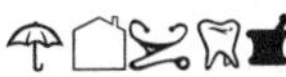

HOLYOKE MUTUAL INSURANCE CO

MASSACHUSETTS CLAIMS OFFICE
HOLYOKE SQ
PO BOX 2006
SALEM, MA 01970-6506
TEL: (978) 744-6123
FAX: (978) 744-5677
TOLL FREE: (800) 225-2533
E-MAIL: INFO@HOLYOKEMUTUAL.COM
WWW.HOLYOKEMUTUAL.COM

HOMETOWN HEALTH NETWORK

OHIO CLAIMS OFFICE
100 LILLIAN GISH BLVD, STE 301
MASSILLON, OH 44647
TEL: (330) 837-6880
FAX: (330) 837-6869
IN-STATE: (800) 426-9013
WWW.HOMETOWNHEALTHNET.COM

HOMETOWN HEALTH PLAN

NEVADA CLAIMS OFFICE
400 S WELLS AVE
RENO, NV 89502-1823
TEL: (775) 325-3000
FAX: (775) 982-3160
TOLL FREE: (800) 336-0123
IN-STATE: (800) 336-0123
WWW.WASHOEHEALTH.COM

HORACE MANN COMPANIES

NATIONAL CLAIMS OFFICE
1 HORACE MANN PLZ
SPRINGFIELD, IL 62715
TEL: (217) 789-2500
FAX: (217) 788-5161
TOLL FREE: (800) 999-1030
WWW.HORACEMANN.COM

HOSPITAL BENEFITS, INC

CALIFORNIA CLAIMS OFFICE
217 N WESTMONTE DR, STE 3033
PO BOX 162148
ALTAMONTE SPG, FL 32716
TEL: (407) 862-0311
FAX: (407) 862-0201
TOLL FREE: (800) 883-0311

FLORIDA CLAIMS OFFICE
217 N WESTMONTE DR, STE 3033
PO BOX 162148
ALTAMONTE SPG, FL 32716
TEL: (407) 862-0311
FAX: (407) 862-0201
TOLL FREE: (800) 883-0311

GEORGIA CLAIMS OFFICE
217 N WESTMONTE DR, STE 3033
PO BOX 162148
ALTAMONTE SPG, FL 32716
TEL: (407) 862-0311
FAX: (407) 862-0201
TOLL FREE: (800) 883-0311

MINNESOTA CLAIMS OFFICE
217 N WESTMONTE DR, STE 3033
PO BOX 162148
ALTAMONTE SPG, FL 32716
TEL: (407) 862-0311
FAX: (407) 862-0201
TOLL FREE: (800) 883-0311

TEXAS CLAIMS OFFICE
217 N WESTMONTE DR, STE 3033
PO BOX 162148
ALTAMONTE SPG, FL 32716
TEL: (407) 862-0311
FAX: (407) 862-0201
TOLL FREE: (800) 883-0311

WISCONSIN CLAIMS OFFICE
217 N WESTMONTE DR, STE 3033
PO BOX 162148
ALTAMONTE SPG, FL 32716
TEL: (407) 862-0311
FAX: (407) 862-0201
TOLL FREE: (800) 883-0311

HSB INDUSTRIAL RISK INSURERS

NATIONAL CLAIMS OFFICE
85 WOODLAND ST
PO BOX 5010
HARTFORD, CT 06102-5010
TEL: (860) 520-7300
FAX: (860) 549-5780
TOLL FREE: (800) 243-8308

HUMAN RESOURCE BENEFIT ADMINISTRATION

16 INVERNESS PL E- BLDG A
ENGLEWOOD, CO 80112
TEL: (303) 792-3311
FAX: (303) 790-0599
TOLL FREE: (800) 742-4722

HUMANA

WISCONSIN CLAIMS OFFICE
PO BOX 12359
MILWAUKEE, WI 53212-0359
TEL: (414) 223-3300
FAX: (414) 223-7777
TOLL FREE: (800) 289-0260
WWW.HUMANA.COM

HUMANA/ EMPLOYERS HEALTH INSURANCE CO

ALABAMA CLAIMS OFFICE
4626 FREY ST
PO BOX 5620
MADISON, WI 53705-0620
FAX: (608) 231-6522
IN-STATE: (800) 833-6910

ARKANSAS CLAIMS OFFICE
4626 FREY ST
PO BOX 5620
MADISON, WI 53705-0620
FAX: (608) 231-6522
IN-STATE: (800) 833-6910

FLORIDA CLAIMS OFFICE
4626 FREY ST
PO BOX 5620
MADISON, WI 53705-0620
FAX: (608) 231-6522
IN-STATE: (800) 833-6910

GEORGIA CLAIMS OFFICE
4626 FREY ST
PO BOX 5620
MADISON, WI 53705-0620
FAX: (608) 231-6522
IN-STATE: (800) 833-6910

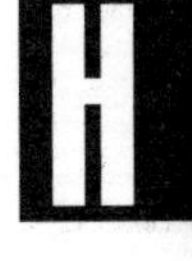

KANSAS CLAIMS OFFICE
4626 FREY ST
PO BOX 5620
MADISON, WI 53705-0620
FAX: (608) 231-6522
IN-STATE: (800) 833-6910

KENTUCKY CLAIMS OFFICE
4626 FREY ST
PO BOX 5620
MADISON, WI 53705-0620
FAX: (608) 231-6522
IN-STATE: (800) 833-6910

LOUISIANA CLAIMS OFFICE
4626 FREY ST
PO BOX 5620
MADISON, WI 53705-0620
FAX: (608) 231-6522
IN-STATE: (800) 833-6910

MISSISSIPPI CLAIMS OFFICE
4626 FREY ST
PO BOX 5620
MADISON, WI 53705-0620
FAX: (608) 231-6522
IN-STATE: (800) 833-6910

MISSOURI CLAIMS OFFICE
4626 FREY ST
PO BOX 5620
MADISON, WI 53705-0620
FAX: (608) 231-6522
IN-STATE: (800) 833-6910

NATIONAL CLAIMS OFFICE
1100 EMPLOYERS BLVD
GREEN BAY, WI 54344
TEL: (920) 336-1100
FAX: (920) 337-7660
TOLL FREE: (800) 558-4444
IN-STATE: (800) 822-6275

NORTH CAROLINA CLAIMS OFFICE
4626 FREY ST
PO BOX 5620
MADISON, WI 53705-0620
FAX: (608) 231-6522
IN-STATE: (800) 833-6910

SOUTH DAKOTA CLAIMS OFFICE
4626 FREY ST
PO BOX 5620
MADISON, WI 53705-0620
FAX: (608) 231-6522
IN-STATE: (800) 833-6910

TENNESSEE CLAIMS OFFICE
4626 FREY ST
PO BOX 5620
MADISON, WI 53705-0620
FAX: (608) 231-6522
IN-STATE: (800) 833-6910

WEST VIRGINIA CLAIMS OFFICE
4626 FREY ST
PO BOX 5620
MADISON, WI 53705-0620
FAX: (608) 231-6522
IN-STATE: (800) 833-6910

WISCONSIN CLAIMS OFFICE
4626 FREY ST
PO BOX 5620
MADISON, WI 53705-0620
FAX: (608) 231-6522
IN-STATE: (800) 833-6910

HUMANA HEALTH CARE PLAN, INC

KENTUCKY CLAIMS OFFICE
500 W MAIN
LOUISVILLE, KY 40202
TEL: (502) 580-5251
FAX: (502) 580-3127
TOLL FREE: (800) 448-6262
WWW.HUMANA.COM

TEXAS CLAIMS OFFICE
HUMANA, INC
8119 DATAPOINT
PO BOX 400040
SAN ANTONIO, TX 78229
TEL: (210) 615-3000
FAX: (210) 615-3165
TOLL FREE: (800) 638-2639
IN-STATE: (800) 448-6262
WWW.HUMANA.COM

HUMANA HEALTH CARE PLAN, INC / CHOICE CARE

OHIO CLAIMS OFFICE
655 EDEN PARK DR, STE 400
CINCINNATI, OH 45202
TEL: (513) 784-5200
TOLL FREE: (800) 521-3508
WWW.HUMANA.COM

HUMANA, INC

ALABAMA CLAIMS OFFICE
500 W MAIN ST
LOUISVILLE, KY 40202-1438
TEL: (502) 580-1000
FAX: (502) 580-3127
TOLL FREE: (800) 448-6262
IN-STATE: (800) 486-2620
WWW.HUMANA.COM

ARIZONA CLAIMS OFFICE
500 W MAIN ST
LOUISVILLE, KY 40202-1438
TEL: (502) 580-1000
FAX: (502) 580-3127
TOLL FREE: (800) 448-6262
IN-STATE: (800) 486-2620
WWW.HUMANA.COM

CALIFORNIA CLAIMS OFFICE
500 W MAIN ST
LOUISVILLE, KY 40202-1438
TEL: (502) 580-1000
FAX: (502) 580-3127
TOLL FREE: (800) 448-6262
IN-STATE: (800) 486-2620
WWW.HUMANA.COM

COLORADO CLAIMS OFFICE
500 W MAIN ST
LOUISVILLE, KY 40202-1438
TEL: (502) 580-1000
FAX: (502) 580-3127
TOLL FREE: (800) 448-6262
IN-STATE: (800) 486-2620
WWW.HUMANA.COM

DISTRICT OF COLUMBIA CLAIMS OFFICE
500 W MAIN ST
LOUISVILLE, KY 40202-1438
TEL: (502) 580-1000
FAX: (502) 580-3127
TOLL FREE: (800) 448-6262
IN-STATE: (800) 486-2620
WWW.HUMANA.COM

FLORIDA CLAIMS OFFICE
500 W MAIN ST
LOUISVILLE, KY 40202-1438
TEL: (502) 580-1000
FAX: (502) 580-3127
TOLL FREE: (800) 448-6262
IN-STATE: (800) 486-2620
WWW.HUMANA.COM

GEORGIA CLAIMS OFFICE
500 W MAIN ST
LOUISVILLE, KY 40202-1438
TEL: (502) 580-1000
FAX: (502) 580-3127
TOLL FREE: (800) 448-6262
IN-STATE: (800) 486-2620
WWW.HUMANA.COM

ILLINOIS CLAIMS OFFICE
500 W MAIN ST
LOUISVILLE, KY 40202-1438
TEL: (502) 580-1000
FAX: (502) 580-3127
TOLL FREE: (800) 448-6262
IN-STATE: (800) 486-2620
WWW.HUMANA.COM

INDIANA CLAIMS OFFICE
500 W MAIN ST
LOUISVILLE, KY 40202-1438
TEL: (502) 580-1000
FAX: (502) 580-3127
TOLL FREE: (800) 448-6262
IN-STATE: (800) 486-2620
WWW.HUMANA.COM

KANSAS CLAIMS OFFICE
500 W MAIN ST
LOUISVILLE, KY 40202-1438
TEL: (502) 580-1000
FAX: (502) 580-3127
TOLL FREE: (800) 448-6262
IN-STATE: (800) 486-2620
WWW.HUMANA.COM

KENTUCKY CLAIMS OFFICE
500 W MAIN ST
LOUISVILLE, KY 40202-1438
TEL: (502) 580-1000
FAX: (502) 580-3127
TOLL FREE: (800) 448-6262
IN-STATE: (800) 486-2620
WWW.HUMANA.COM

101 PROSPEROUS PL, STE 300
LEXINGTON, KY 40509-1845
TEL: (606) 263-1400
FAX: (606) 263-1488
TOLL FREE: (800) 426-2600
IN-STATE: (800) 221-8390
WWW.HUMANA.COM

MARYLAND CLAIMS OFFICE
500 W MAIN ST
LOUISVILLE, KY 40202-1438
TEL: (502) 580-1000
FAX: (502) 580-3127
TOLL FREE: (800) 448-6262
IN-STATE: (800) 486-2620
WWW.HUMANA.COM

MICHIGAN CLAIMS OFFICE
500 W MAIN ST
LOUISVILLE, KY 40202-1438
TEL: (502) 580-1000
FAX: (502) 580-3127
TOLL FREE: (800) 448-6262
IN-STATE: (800) 486-2620
WWW.HUMANA.COM

MINNESOTA CLAIMS OFFICE
500 W MAIN ST
LOUISVILLE, KY 40202-1438
TEL: (502) 580-1000
FAX: (502) 580-3127
TOLL FREE: (800) 448-6262
IN-STATE: (800) 486-2620
WWW.HUMANA.COM

MISSOURI CLAIMS OFFICE
10450 HOLMES RD, STE 200
KANSAS CITY, MO 64131
TEL: (816) 941-8900
FAX: (816) 942-6782
WWW.HUMANA.COM

NEBRASKA CLAIMS OFFICE
500 W MAIN ST
LOUISVILLE, KY 40202-1438
TEL: (502) 580-1000
FAX: (502) 580-3127
TOLL FREE: (800) 448-6262
IN-STATE: (800) 486-2620
WWW.HUMANA.COM

NORTH CAROLINA CLAIMS OFFICE
500 W MAIN ST
LOUISVILLE, KY 40202-1438
TEL: (502) 580-1000
FAX: (502) 580-3127
TOLL FREE: (800) 448-6262
IN-STATE: (800) 486-2620
WWW.HUMANA.COM

OHIO CLAIMS OFFICE
500 W MAIN ST
LOUISVILLE, KY 40202-1438
TEL: (502) 580-1000
FAX: (502) 580-3127
TOLL FREE: (800) 448-6262
IN-STATE: (800) 486-2620
WWW.HUMANA.COM

TENNESSEE CLAIMS OFFICE
500 W MAIN ST
LOUISVILLE, KY 40202-1438
TEL: (502) 580-1000
FAX: (502) 580-3127
TOLL FREE: (800) 448-6262
IN-STATE: (800) 486-2620
WWW.HUMANA.COM

TEXAS CLAIMS OFFICE
500 W MAIN ST
LOUISVILLE, KY 40202-1438
TEL: (502) 580-1000
FAX: (502) 580-3127
TOLL FREE: (800) 448-6262
IN-STATE: (800) 486-2620
WWW.HUMANA.COM

VIRGINIA CLAIMS OFFICE
500 W MAIN ST
LOUISVILLE, KY 40202-1438
TEL: (502) 580-1000
FAX: (502) 580-3127
TOLL FREE: (800) 448-6262
IN-STATE: (800) 486-2620
WWW.HUMANA.COM

WISCONSIN CLAIMS OFFICE
500 W MAIN ST
LOUISVILLE, KY 40202-1438
TEL: (502) 580-1000
FAX: (502) 580-3127
TOLL FREE: (800) 448-6262
IN-STATE: (800) 486-2620
WWW.HUMANA.COM

HUMANA P.C.A.

TEXAS CLAIMS OFFICE
PO BOX 9420
AUSTIN, TX 78766-9420
TEL: (512) 338-6100
TOLL FREE: (800) 234-7912

HUMANA/ WISCONSIN HEALTH ORGANIZATION

WISCONSIN CLAIMS OFFICE
111 W PLEASANT ST
MILWAUKEE, WI 53212
TEL: (414) 223-3300
TOLL FREE: (800) 289-0906
IN-STATE: (800) 777-0184

IBA HEALTH & LIFE ASSURANCE CO

INDIANA CLAIMS OFFICE
PHYSICIANS HEALTH PLAN OF SW MICHIGAN
106 FARMERS ALLEY, STE 300
PO BOX 51100
KALAMAZOO, MI 49005
TEL: (616) 341-8000
FAX: (616) 341-6832
TOLL FREE: (800) 722-3644
WWW.IBAHEALTH.COM

MICHIGAN CLAIMS OFFICE
PHYSICIANS HEALTH PLAN OF SW MICHIGAN
106 FARMERS ALLEY, STE 300
PO BOX 51100
KALAMAZOO, MI 49005
TEL: (616) 341-8000
FAX: (616) 341-6832
TOLL FREE: (800) 722-3644
WWW.IBAHEALTH.COM

IDAHO FARM BUREAU MUTUAL INSURANCE CO

IDAHO CLAIMS OFFICE
57 W WASHINGTON ST
PO BOX 266
ABERDEEN, ID 83210-0266
TEL: (208) 397-4111
FAX: (208) 397-4112

435 LINCOLN
PO BOX 239
AMERICAN FALLS, ID 83211-0239
TEL: (208) 226-5066
FAX: (208) 226-7929

225 W GRAND
PO BOX 824
ARCO, ID 83213-0824
TEL: (208) 527-3431
FAX: (208) 527-3432

WESTERN COMMUNITY INSURANCE CO
124 N OAK
PO BOX 668
BLACKFOOT, ID 83221-0668
TEL: (208) 785-2410
FAX: (208) 785-2422

8620 W EMERALD, STE 100
BOISE, ID 83704
TEL: (208) 375-3411
FAX: (208) 375-2180

6426 KOOTENAI ST
PO BOX 1387
BONNERS FERRY, ID 83805-1387
TEL: (208) 267-5502
FAX: (208) 267-5503

4122 CLEVELAND BLVD
PO BOX 849
CALDWELL, ID 83606-0849
TEL: (208) 459-1604
FAX: (208) 459-1664

6912 N GOVERNMENT WY
DALTON GARDENS, ID 83815-8747
TEL: (208) 772-6662
FAX: (208) 772-2553

29 N MAIN
PO BOX 67
DRIGGS, ID 83422-0067
TEL: (208) 354-2775
FAX: (208) 354-8114

906 S WASHINGTON
PO BOX 156
EMMETT, ID 83617-0156
TEL: (208) 365-5382
FAX: (208) 365-2465

131 3RD AVE E
GOODING, ID 83330-1101
TEL: (208) 934-8405
FAX: (208) 934-8406

711 N MAIN
PO BOX 609
HAILEY, ID 83333-0609
TEL: (208) 788-3529
FAX: (208) 788-3619

118 W IDAHO
PO BOX 1197
HOMEDALE, ID 83620-1197
TEL: (208) 337-4041
FAX: (208) 337-4042

BONNEVILLE COUNTY FARM BUREAU
956 LINCOLN
PO BOX 2948
IDAHO FALLS, ID 83403-2948
TEL: (208) 522-2652
FAX: (208) 522-2675

200 E AVE A
PO BOX C
JEROME, ID 83338-0326
TEL: (208) 324-4378
FAX: (208) 324-4393

602 E MAIN ST
PO BOX 284
KENDRICK, ID 83537-0134
TEL: (208) 289-3462
FAX: (208) 289-3463

2007 14TH AVE
LEWISTON, ID 83501-3019
TEL: (208) 743-5533
FAX: (208) 743-5535

34 N MAIN
MALAD, ID 83252-1247
TEL: (208) 766-2259
FAX: (208) 766-4211

470 WASHINGTON ST
MONTPELIER, ID 83254-1545
TEL: (208) 847-0851
FAX: (208) 847-0856

530 S ASBURY STE 3
PO BOX 8901
MOSCOW, ID 83843-1401
TEL: (208) 882-1531
FAX: (208) 882-9149

140 E 2ND N
PO BOX 673
MOUNTAIN HOME, ID 83647-0673
TEL: (208) 587-8484
FAX: (208) 587-8121

1501 26TH ST, STE C
OROFINO, ID 83544
TEL: (208) 476-4722
FAX: (208) 476-7348

235 N MAIN
PAYETTE, ID 83661-2852
TEL: (208) 642-4414
FAX: (208) 642-4415

200 W ALAMEDA
PO BOX 4848
POCATELLO, ID 83205
TEL: (208) 233-9442
FAX: (208) 233-4167

33 S 1ST E
PO BOX 311
PRESTON, ID 83263-0311
TEL: (208) 852-2364
FAX: (208) 852-2365

102 W FREMONT
PO BOX 306
RIGBY, ID 83442-0306
TEL: (208) 745-7776
FAX: (208) 745-7786

112 CENTER ST
PO BOX 1924
SALMON, ID 83467-1924
TEL: (208) 756-3335
FAX: (208) 756-3357

WESTERN COMMUNITY INSURANCE CO
920 KOOTENAI CUTOFF RD
SANDPOINT, ID 83864
TEL: (208) 263-3161
FAX: (208) 263-1348

325 E MAIN
PO BOX 528
SAINT ANTHONY, ID 83445-0528
TEL: (208) 624-3171
FAX: (208) 624-3173

414 MAIN AVE
SAINT MARIES, ID 83861-2059
TEL: (208) 245-5568
FAX: (208) 245-5569

2732 KIMBERLY RD
PO BOX 1788
TWIN FALLS, ID 83303-1788
TEL: (208) 733-7212
FAX: (208) 733-6586

435 LINCOLN
PO BOX 239
AMERICAN FALLS, ID 83211-0239
TEL: (208) 226-5066
FAX: (208) 226-7929

530 S ASBURY
PO BOX 8901
MOSCOW, ID 83843-1401
TEL: (208) 882-1531
FAX: (208) 882-9149

225 W GRAND
PO BOX 824
ARCO, ID 83213-0824
TEL: (208) 527-3431
FAX: (208) 527-3432

IDAHO STATE INSURANCE FUND

1215 W STATE ST
PO BOX 83720
BOISE, ID 83720-0044
TEL: (208) 334-2370
FAX: (208) 334-3253
TOLL FREE: (800) 334-2370
WWW.STATE.ID.US/ISIF

IDEALIFE INSURANCE CO

CONNECTICUT CLAIMS OFFICE
AMERICAN ADMINISTRATIVE INSURANCE GROUP
PO BOX 9100
CLEARWATER, FL 33758
TEL: (813) 791-1369
FAX: (813) 725-4190
TOLL FREE: (800) 554-8744

IDS LIFE INSURANCE CO OF NEW YORK

NEW YORK CLAIMS OFFICE
20 MADISON AVE, EXT 122203
PO BOX 5144
ALBANY, NY 12205-5144
TEL: (518) 869-8613
FAX: (518) 869-8753
TOLL FREE: (800) 797-9000

IFG CO

NATIONAL CLAIMS OFFICE
238 INTERNATIONAL RD
BURLINGTON, NC 27215
TEL: (336) 586-2800
FAX: (336) 586-2808

IHC HEALTH PLANS

IDAHO CLAIMS OFFICE
INTERMOUNTAIN HEALTH CARE
4646 W LAKE PARK BLVD
SALT LAKE CITY, UT 84120-8212
TEL: (801) 442-5000
FAX: (801) 442-5003
TOLL FREE: (800) 538-5038
IN-STATE: (800) 442-5038
E-MAIL: WEBMASTER@IHC.COM
WWW.IHC.COM

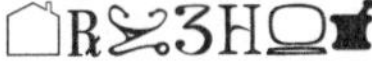

UTAH CLAIMS OFFICE
INTERMOUNTAIN HEALTH CARE
4646 W LAKE PARK BLVD
SALT LAKE CITY, UT 84120-8212
TEL: (801) 442-5000
FAX: (801) 442-5003
TOLL FREE: (800) 538-5038
IN-STATE: (800) 442-5038
E-MAIL: WEBMASTER@IHC.COM
WWW.IHC.COM

INTERMOUNTAIN HEALTH CARE
4646 W LAKE PARK BLVD
PO BOX 30192
SALT LAKE CITY, UT 84130-0192
TEL: (801) 442-5000
FAX: (801) 442-5752
TOLL FREE: (800) 442-5038
IN-STATE: (800) 442-5038

WYOMING CLAIMS OFFICE
INTERMOUNTAIN HEALTH CARE
4646 W LAKE PARK BLVD
SALT LAKE CITY, UT 84120-8212
TEL: (801) 442-5000
FAX: (801) 442-5003
TOLL FREE: (800) 538-5038
IN-STATE: (800) 442-5038
E-MAIL: WEBMASTER@IHC.COM
WWW.IHC.COM

ILLINOIS EMCASCO INSURANCE CO

ILLINOIS CLAIMS OFFICE
815 COMMERCE DR
OAK BROOK, IL 60523
TEL: (630) 573-4900
FAX: (630) 573-4947
TOLL FREE: (800) 942-7448

ILLINOIS EMPLOYEE BENEFITS CORP

28 N 1ST ST
PO BOX 470
GENEVA, IL 60134-0470
TEL: (630) 232-7166
FAX: (630) 232-7172
TOLL FREE: (800) 448-5825

IOWA CLAIMS OFFICE
28 N 1ST ST
PO BOX 470
GENEVA, IL 60134-0470
TEL: (630) 232-7166
FAX: (630) 232-7172
TOLL FREE: (800) 448-5825

ILLINOIS MASONIC COMMUNITY HEALTH PLAN

ILLINOIS CLAIMS OFFICE
836 W WELLINGTON
CHICAGO, IL 60657-5147
TEL: (773) 296-7167
FAX: (773) 296-5598

ILLINOIS MUTUAL LIFE INSURANCE CO

300 SW ADAMS ST
PEORIA, IL 61634-0002
TEL: (309) 674-8255
FAX: (309) 674-8137
TOLL FREE: (800) 437-7355

IMI CORNELIUS

MINNESOTA CLAIMS OFFICE
1 CORNELIUS PL
ANOKA, MN 55303-1592
TEL: (612) 421-6120
FAX: (612) 422-7762
TOLL FREE: (800) 238-3600

IMT INSURANCE CO

IOWA CLAIMS OFFICE
4445 CORPORATE DR
PO BOX 9208
WEST DES MOINES, IA 50306-9208
TEL: (515) 327-2777
FAX: (515) 327-2892
TOLL FREE: (800) 274-3531

1108 PIERCE ST
PO BOX 723
SIOUX CITY, IA 51102-0723
TEL: (712) 255-5336
FAX: (712) 255-4935
TOLL FREE: (800) 365-5519

SOUTH DAKOTA CLAIMS OFFICE
3900 W TECHNOLOGY CIRCLE, STE 3
PO BOX 88137
SIOUX FALLS, SD 57109-1001
TEL: (605) 362-1670
FAX: (605) 362-1669
TOLL FREE: (800) 288-8289

INDEPENDENCE BLUE CROSS

PENNSYLVANIA CLAIMS OFFICE
1901 MARKET ST
PHILADELPHIA, PA 19103-1480
TEL: (215) 241-2400
FAX: (215) 241-4272
TOLL FREE: (800) 626-8144
WWW.IBX.COM

INDEPENDENT HEALTH

NEW YORK CLAIMS OFFICE
511 FARBER LAKES DR
BUFFALO, NY 14221
TEL: (716) 631-3001
FAX: (716) 635-3785
TOLL FREE: (800) 247-1466
WWW.INDEPENDENTHEALTH.COM

INDIANA INSURANCE CO

ILLINOIS CLAIMS OFFICE
103 S COUNTRY FAIR DR
PO BOX 6568
CHAMPAIGN, IL 61826-6568
TEL: (217) 352-7931
FAX: (217) 352-0923
TOLL FREE: (800) 654-2107

INDIANA CLAIMS OFFICE
350 E 96TH ST
PO BOX 1967
INDIANAPOLIS, IN 46206-1967
TEL: (317) 581-6400
FAX: (317) 581-6700
TOLL FREE: (800) 428-2100

4424 VOGEL RD
PO BOX 5629
EVANSVILLE, IN 47716-5629
TEL: (812) 473-3086
FAX: (812) 473-1091
TOLL FREE: (800) 854-4583

LIBERTY MUTUAL
515 PARKPLACE CIR
PO BOX 6429
SOUTH BEND, IN 46660-6429
TEL: (219) 271-0005
FAX: (219) 277-7018
TOLL FREE: (800) 533-4601

KENTUCKY CLAIMS OFFICE
LIBERTY MUTUAL
950 BRECKENRIDGE LN
PO BOX 6707
LOUISVILLE, KY 40206-0707
TEL: (502) 899-2600
FAX: (502) 899-2601
TOLL FREE: (800) 237-3629
IN-STATE: (800) 237-3629

MICHIGAN CLAIMS OFFICE
906 CENTENILLE, STE 250
PO BOX 80080
LANSING, MI 48908-0080
TEL: (517) 323-9606
FAX: (517) 323-7770
TOLL FREE: (800) 345-0575

OHIO CLAIMS OFFICE
LIBERTY MUTUAL
4700 LAKHURST CT
PO BOX 8005
DUBLIN, OH 43016-2005
TEL: (614) 799-4000
FAX: (614) 799-4004
TOLL FREE: (800) 762-4807

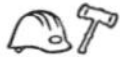

INDIANA INSURANCE COMPANY

INDIANA CLAIMS OFFICE
350 E 96TH ST
PO BOX 1967
INDIANAPOLIS, IN 46206-1967
TEL: (317) 581-6400
FAX: (317) 581-6700
TOLL FREE: (800) 428-2100

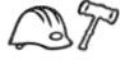

INDIANAPOLIS LIFE

NATIONAL CLAIMS OFFICE
2960 N MERIDIAN ST
PO BOX 1230
INDIANAPOLIS, IN 46206
TEL: (317) 927-6500
FAX: (317) 927-3393
TOLL FREE: (800) 428-7031
E-MAIL: CORPCOMMSG.INDIANAPOLISLIFE.COM
WWW.INDIANAPOLISLIFE.COM

INDIVIDUAL ASSURANCE CO LIFE, HEALTH & ACCIDENT

ARKANSAS CLAIMS OFFICE
1600 OAK ST
KANSAS CITY, MO 64108-1427
TEL: (816) 842-8842
FAX: (816) 218-1390
TOLL FREE: (800) 821-5434

COLORADO CLAIMS OFFICE
1600 OAK ST
KANSAS CITY, MO 64108-1427
TEL: (816) 842-8842
FAX: (816) 218-1390
TOLL FREE: (800) 821-5434

ILLINOIS CLAIMS OFFICE
1600 OAK ST
KANSAS CITY, MO 64108-1427
TEL: (816) 842-8842
FAX: (816) 218-1390
TOLL FREE: (800) 821-5434

IOWA CLAIMS OFFICE
1600 OAK ST
KANSAS CITY, MO 64108-1427
TEL: (816) 842-8842
FAX: (816) 218-1390
TOLL FREE: (800) 821-5434

KANSAS CLAIMS OFFICE
1600 OAK ST
KANSAS CITY, MO 64108-1427
TEL: (816) 842-8842
FAX: (816) 218-1390
TOLL FREE: (800) 821-5434

MISSOURI CLAIMS OFFICE
1600 OAK ST
KANSAS CITY, MO 64108-1427
TEL: (816) 842-8842
FAX: (816) 218-1390
TOLL FREE: (800) 821-5434

NEBRASKA CLAIMS OFFICE
1600 OAK ST
KANSAS CITY, MO 64108-1427
TEL: (816) 842-8842
FAX: (816) 218-1390
TOLL FREE: (800) 821-5434

OHIO CLAIMS OFFICE
1600 OAK ST
KANSAS CITY, MO 64108-1427
TEL: (816) 842-8842
FAX: (816) 218-1390
TOLL FREE: (800) 821-5434

OKLAHOMA CLAIMS OFFICE
1600 OAK ST
KANSAS CITY, MO 64108-1427
TEL: (816) 842-8842
FAX: (816) 218-1390
TOLL FREE: (800) 821-5434

INFINITY GROUP

ALABAMA CLAIMS OFFICE
2204 LAKESHORE DR, STE 125
PO BOX 830695
BIRMINGHAM, AL 35201
TEL: (205) 870-4000
TOLL FREE: (800) 782-2020
WWW.INFINITY-INSURANCE.COM

INSPIRE INSURANCE SOLUTIONS

TEXAS CLAIMS OFFICE
MILLERS INSURANCE GROUP
300 BURNETT
PO BOX 2269
FT. WORTH, TX 76113-2269
TEL: (817) 332-7761
FAX: (800) 872-1029
TOLL FREE: (800) 972-3822

INSURANCE BROKERAGE SERVICES

WISCONSIN CLAIMS OFFICE
3992 N RICHMOND
PO BOX 2579
APPLETON, WI 54913-2579
TEL: (920) 730-8000
FAX: (920) 730-8951
TOLL FREE: (800) 472-1722

INSURANCE CO OF GREATER NEW YORK

NEW YORK CLAIMS OFFICE
GREATER NEW YORK INSURANCE
200 MADISON AVE
NEW YORK, NY 10016-6023
TEL: (212) 683-9700
FAX: (212) 685-0826
IN-STATE: (800) 522-5504

INSURANCE CO OF THE WEST

CALIFORNIA CLAIMS OFFICE
ICW GROUP
11455 EL CAMINO REAL
PO BOX 85563
SAN DIEGO, CA 92186-5563
TEL: (619) 350-2400
FAX: (619) 350-2543
TOLL FREE: (800) 877-1111

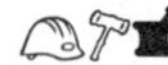

INSURANCE CONSULTANTS, INC

NEBRASKA CLAIMS OFFICE
200 BLACKSTONE CTR
OMAHA, NE 68131
TEL: (402) 345-5000
FAX: (402) 231-4300
TOLL FREE: (800) 662-8855
IN-STATE: (800) 662-8855

INSURANCE CORP OF HANNOVER

CALIFORNIA CLAIMS OFFICE
3435 WILSHIRE BLVD, STE 700
LOS ANGELES, CA 90010
TEL: (213) 380-8822
FAX: (213) 386-2062

INSURANCE MANAGEMENT ADMINISTRATORS OF LOUISIANA

LOUISIANA CLAIMS OFFICE
1325 BARKSDALE BLVD, STE 300
PO BOX 71120
BOSSIER, LA 71171
TEL: (318) 868-0600
FAX: (318) 747-5074

INSURANCE MANAGEMENT ASSOCIATES, INC

KANSAS CLAIMS OFFICE
250 N WATER ST, STE 600
PO BOX 2992
WICHITA, KS 67201
TEL: (316) 267-9221
FAX: (316) 266-6385
TOLL FREE: (800) 288-6732
WWW.IMACORP.COM

INSURANCE & PERSONNEL SERVICES

NEBRASKA CLAIMS OFFICE
2121 N WEBB RD
PO BOX 2160
GRAND ISLAND, NE 68802-2160
TEL: (308) 384-8700
FAX: (308) 384-8423

INSURANCE & RISK MANAGEMENT

NATIONAL CLAIMS OFFICE
INSURANCE CLAIM SERVICE / EMPLOYEE HEALTH
3811 ILLINOIS RD
PO BOX 1705
FT WAYNE, IN 46801-2362
TEL: (219) 436-1616
FAX: (219) 432-4083
TOLL FREE: (800) 395-8601
WWW.INSURANCERISKMGMT.COM

INSURERS ADMINISTRATIVE CORP

ARIZONA CLAIMS OFFICE
2101 W PEORIA AVE, STE 100
PO BOX 39119
PHOENIX, AZ 85029-9119
TEL: (602) 870-1400
FAX: (602) 395-0496
TOLL FREE: (800) 843-3106

INSUREX BENEFITS ADMINISTRATORS

TENNESSEE CLAIMS OFFICE
1835 UNION AVE, STE 400
PO BOX 41779
MEMPHIS, TN 38174-1779
TEL: (901) 725-6435
FAX: (901) 725-6437

INTEGON

MISSOURI CLAIMS OFFICE
18 CORPORATE WOODS BLVD, STE 103
PO BOX 22086
ALBANY, NY 12211
TEL: (518) 447-1879
FAX: (518) 447-1891
TOLL FREE: (800) 322-3682

NEW YORK CLAIMS OFFICE
18 CORPORATE WOODS BLVD, STE 103
PO BOX 22086
ALBANY, NY 12211
TEL: (518) 447-1879
FAX: (518) 447-1891
TOLL FREE: (800) 322-3682

NORTH CAROLINA CLAIMS OFFICE
3060 S CHURCH ST
PO BOX 2510
BURLINGTON, NC 27216
TEL: (336) 538-4000
FAX: (336) 538-4185
TOLL FREE: (800) 323-6848
WWW.INTEGON.COM

PENNSYLVANIA CLAIMS OFFICE
18 CORPORATE WOODS BLVD, STE 103
PO BOX 22086
ALBANY, NY 12211
TEL: (518) 447-1879
FAX: (518) 447-1891
TOLL FREE: (800) 322-3682

INTEGON CORP

NORTH CAROLINA CLAIMS OFFICE
P & C CLAIMS
500 W 5TH ST
PO BOX 3199
WINSTON-SALEM, NC 27102-3199
TEL: (336) 770-2000
FAX: (336) 770-2122
TOLL FREE: (800) 642-0506
WWW.INTEGON.COM

INTEGRATED HEALTH SERVICES

NEW MEXICO CLAIMS OFFICE
SOUTHWEST EMPLOYEE BENEFITS
235 ELM ST NE
PO BOX 30278
ALBUQUERQUE, NM 87190
TEL: (505) 222-8260

INTEGRITY MUTUAL INSURANCE CO

IOWA CLAIMS OFFICE
2121 E CAPITOL DR
PO BOX 539
APPLETON, WI 54912-0539
TEL: (920) 734-4511
FAX: (920) 730-5712
TOLL FREE: (800) 452-3421
WWW.INTEGRITY.INSURANCE.COM

MINNESOTA CLAIMS OFFICE
2121 E CAPITOL DR
PO BOX 539
APPLETON, WI 54912-0539
TEL: (920) 734-4511
FAX: (920) 730-5712
TOLL FREE: (800) 452-3421
WWW.INTEGRITY.INSURANCE.COM

WISCONSIN CLAIMS OFFICE
2121 E CAPITOL DR
PO BOX 539
APPLETON, WI 54912-0539
TEL: (920) 734-4511
FAX: (920) 730-5712
TOLL FREE: (800) 452-3421
WWW.INTEGRITY.INSURANCE.COM

INTER VALLEY HEALTH PLAN

CALIFORNIA CLAIMS OFFICE
300 S PARK AVE
PO BOX 6002
POMONA, CA 91769-6002
TEL: (909) 623-6333
FAX: (909) 622-2907
TOLL FREE: (800) 251-8191
WWW.IVHP.COM

INTER-AMERICAS INSURANCE CORP

KANSAS CLAIMS OFFICE
AMERICAN UNDERWRITERS INSURANCE CO
1035 S 183 RD
PO BOX 9510
WICHITA, KS 67277
TEL: (316) 794-2200
FAX: (316) 794-8470

INTERACTIVE MEDICAL SYSTEMS, INC

NORTH CAROLINA CLAIMS OFFICE
4505 FALLS OF NEUSE, STE 550
PO BOX 19108
RALEIGH, NC 27619
TEL: (919) 877-9933
FAX: (919) 846-8887

SOUTH CAROLINA CLAIMS OFFICE
4505 FALLS OF NEUSE, STE 550
PO BOX 19108
RALEIGH, NC 27619
TEL: (919) 877-9933
FAX: (919) 846-8887

INTERCARE BENEFIT SYSTEMS, INC

COLORADO CLAIMS OFFICE
INTERCARE HEALTH PLAN
5500 GREENWOOD PLZ BLVD
PO BOX 3559
ENGLEWOOD, CO 80111-3559
TEL: (303) 770-5710
FAX: (303) 770-2743
TOLL FREE: (800) 426-7453

INTERCONTINENTAL CORP

INDIANA CLAIMS OFFICE
135 N PENNSYLVANIA ST, STE 770
INDIANAPOLIS, IN 46204
TEL: (317) 238-5700
FAX: (317) 637-6634
TOLL FREE: (800) 962-6831
WWW.INTERCONTINENTALCORP.COM

INTERGROUP OF ARIZONA

ARIZONA CLAIMS OFFICE
930 N FINANCE CTR DR
TUCSON, AZ 85710
TEL: (520) 751-6111
FAX: (520) 290-5176
TOLL FREE: (800) 289-2818

INTERGROUP OF UTAH, INC

UTAH CLAIMS OFFICE
127 S 500 E
SALT LAKE CITY, UT 84102
TEL: (801) 532-7665

INTERMOUNTAIN ADMINISTRATORS, INC

MONTANA CLAIMS OFFICE
2806 GARFIELD
PO BOX 3018
MISSOULA, MT 59806
TEL: (406) 721-2222
FAX: (406) 721-2252
TOLL FREE: (800) 877-1122
WWW.IAI-TPA.COM

MINNESOTA CLAIMS OFFICE
5400 UNIVERSITY AVE
WEST DES MOINES, IA 50266
TEL: (515) 225-5400
FAX: (515) 226-6074

SOUTH DAKOTA CLAIMS OFFICE
5400 UNIVERSITY AVE
WEST DES MOINES, IA 50266
TEL: (515) 225-5400
FAX: (515) 226-6074

UTAH CLAIMS OFFICE
5400 UNIVERSITY AVE
WEST DES MOINES, IA 50266
TEL: (515) 225-5400
FAX: (515) 226-6074

WEST VIRGINIA CLAIMS OFFICE
5400 UNIVERSITY AVE
WEST DES MOINES, IA 50266
TEL: (515) 225-5400
FAX: (515) 226-6074

INTERNATIONAL BENEFIT SERVICES CORP

NATIONAL CLAIMS OFFICE
USI ADMINISTRATORS
4150 INTERNATIONAL PLZ, STE 900
PO BOX 1326
FT WORTH, TX 76101-1326
TEL: (817) 737-1700
FAX: (817) 737-1786
TOLL FREE: (800) 759-0101
E-MAIL: IBSTX@AOL.COM
WWW.IBSUSI.COM

INTERSTATE BANKERS LIFE INSURANCE CO

ILLINOIS CLAIMS OFFICE
8501 W HIGGINS RD, STE 710
CHICAGO, IL 60631-2801
TEL: (773) 693-3930
FAX: (773) 693-3278

INVESTORS HERITAGE LIFE INSURANCE CO

KENTUCKY CLAIMS OFFICE
200 CAPITAL AVE
PO BOX 717
FRANKFORT, KY 40602
TEL: (502) 223-2361
FAX: (502) 227-7205
TOLL FREE: (800) 422-2011
IN-STATE: (800) 372-2997

IOWA FARM BUREAU

IOWA CLAIMS OFFICE
5400 UNIVERSITY AVE
WEST DES MOINES, IA 50266
TEL: (515) 225-5400
FAX: (515) 226-6074

IOWA MUTUAL INSURANCE GROUP

ILLINOIS CLAIMS OFFICE
509 9TH ST
PO BOX 60
DE WITT, IA 52742-0060
TEL: (319) 659-3231
FAX: (800) 365-3407
TOLL FREE: (800) 456-5259

IOWA CLAIMS OFFICE
509 9TH ST
PO BOX 60
DE WITT, IA 52742-0060
TEL: (319) 659-3231
FAX: (800) 365-3407
TOLL FREE: (800) 456-5259

NEBRASKA CLAIMS OFFICE
509 9TH ST
PO BOX 60
DE WITT, IA 52742-0060
TEL: (319) 659-3231
FAX: (800) 365-3407
TOLL FREE: (800) 456-5259

SOUTH DAKOTA CLAIMS OFFICE
509 9TH ST
PO BOX 60
DE WITT, IA 52742-0060
TEL: (319) 659-3231
FAX: (800) 365-3407
TOLL FREE: (800) 456-5259

ISLAND INSURANCE CO, LTD

HAWAII CLAIMS OFFICE
1165 BETHEL ST
PO BOX 1520
HONOLULU, HI 96806-1520
TEL: (808) 545-7740
FAX: (808) 539-9738

IU MEDICAL GROUP PRIMARY CARE

INDIANA CLAIMS OFFICE
MEMBER SERVICES
3901 W 86TH ST, STE 230
PO BOX 78310
INDIANAPOLIS, IN 46278-8310
TEL: (317) 872-2202
FAX: (317) 871-8833
TOLL FREE: (800) 927-7927
WWW.IHUC.COM

J. C. PENNEY INSURANCE

NATIONAL CLAIMS OFFICE
J. C. PENNEY DIRECT MARKETING SERVICES
2700 W PLANO PKY
PO BOX 869090
PLANO, TX 75086
TEL: (972) 881-6000
FAX: (972) 881-6782
TOLL FREE: (800) 692-5246
WWW.JCPENNEYINSURANCEGROUP.COM

J & H, MARSH & MCLENNAN

NEW YORK CLAIMS OFFICE
1166 AVENUE OF THE AMERICAS
NEW YORK, NY 10036
TEL: (212) 574-7000
FAX: (212) 574-7676
WWW.MARSHMAC.COM

J.P. FARLEY CORP

NATIONAL CLAIMS OFFICE
22021 BROOKPARK RD, STE 100
PO BOX 268000
CLEVELAND, OH 44126-8000
TEL: (440) 734-6800
FAX: (440) 734-1668
TOLL FREE: (800) 634-0173
E-MAIL: BENEFITS@JPFARLEY.COM
WWW.JPFARLEY.COM

JARDINE GROUP SERVICES

300 S WACKER DR, STE 700
CHICAGO, IL 60606
TEL: (312) 922-9350
FAX: (312) 922-2849
TOLL FREE: (800) 222-9958

JARDINE GROUP SERVICES CORP

13 CORNELL RD
LATHAM, NY 12110
TEL: (518) 782-3000
FAX: (518) 782-3157
TOLL FREE: (800) 366-5273
WWW.JGSC.COM

JC TAYLOR INSURANCE CO

PENNSYLVANIA CLAIMS OFFICE
320 S 69TH ST
PO BOX 88
UPPER DARBY, PA 19082
TEL: (610) 853-1300
FAX: (610) 853-3823
TOLL FREE: (800) 345-8290

JEFFERSON LIFE INSURANCE CO

TEXAS CLAIMS OFFICE
9304 FOREST LN N, STE 256
PO BOX 749008
DALLAS, TX 75374-9008
TEL: (214) 340-8995
FAX: (214) 340-6114
TOLL FREE: (800) 343-5542

JEFFERSON PILOT FINANCIAL

NATIONAL CLAIMS OFFICE
CHUBB LIFE
1 GRANITE PL
PO BOX 2052
CONCORD, NH 03301-3253
TEL: (603) 226-5000
TOLL FREE: (800) 258-3648
WWW.CHUBB.COM

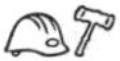

JEFFERSON-PILOT LIFE INSURANCE CO

NORTH CAROLINA CLAIMS OFFICE
JEFFERSON-PILOT FINANCIAL
100 N GREEN ST
PO BOX 21008
GREENSBORO, NC 27420-1008
TEL: (336) 691-3000
FAX: (336) 691-4500
TOLL FREE: (800) 458-1419
IN-STATE: (800) 792-2268

JENKINS & ATHENS INSURANCE SERVICES

CALIFORNIA CLAIMS OFFICE
2552 STANWELL DR
PO BOX 696
CONCORD, CA 94522-0696
TEL: (925) 798-2780
TOLL FREE: (800) 234-6363
E-MAIL: INFO@JENKINS-ATHENS.COM
WWW.JENKINS-ATHENS.COM

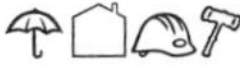

JENSEN ADMINISTRATIVE SERVICES

ARIZONA CLAIMS OFFICE
4885 S 9TH E, STE 202
SALT LAKE CITY, UT 84117-5725
TEL: (801) 266-3256
FAX: (801) 266-4383
TOLL FREE: (800) 345-3248

IDAHO CLAIMS OFFICE
4885 S 9TH E, STE 202
SALT LAKE CITY, UT 84117-5725
TEL: (801) 266-3256
FAX: (801) 266-4383
TOLL FREE: (800) 345-3248

NEVADA CLAIMS OFFICE
4885 S 9TH E, STE 202
SALT LAKE CITY, UT 84117-5725
TEL: (801) 266-3256
FAX: (801) 266-4383
TOLL FREE: (800) 345-3248

UTAH CLAIMS OFFICE
4885 S 9TH E, STE 202
SALT LAKE CITY, UT 84117-5725
TEL: (801) 266-3256
FAX: (801) 266-4383
TOLL FREE: (800) 345-3248

JEWELERS MUTUAL INSURANCE CO

WISCONSIN CLAIMS OFFICE
24 JEWELERS PARK DR
PO BOX 468
NEENAH, WI 54957-0468
TEL: (920) 725-4326
FAX: (920) 725-9401
TOLL FREE: (800) 558-6411
WWW.JEWELERSMUTUAL.COM

JFP BENEFIT MANAGEMENT

MICHIGAN CLAIMS OFFICE
100 S JACKSON ST, STE 200
PO BOX 189
JACKSON, MI 49201
TEL: (517) 784-0535
FAX: (517) 784-0821
IN-STATE: (800) 589-7660
E-MAIL: DPELHAM@IBM.NET

JM FAMILY ENTERPRISES

FLORIDA CLAIMS OFFICE
8019 BAYBERRY RD
JACKSONVILLE, FL 32256-7411
TEL: (904) 443-6650
FAX: (904) 443-6670
TOLL FREE: (800) 736-3936

JMH HEALTH PLAN

1801 NW 9TH AVE, STE 700
MIAMI, FL 33136
TEL: (305) 575-3700
FAX: (305) 545-5212
TOLL FREE: (800) 721-2993

JOHN ALDEN LIFE INSURANCE CO

ARIZONA CLAIMS OFFICE
1005 MAIN ST
PO BOX 1599
BOISE, ID 83702
TEL: (208) 368-7770
FAX: (208) 336-1050
TOLL FREE: (800) 328-4316

COLORADO CLAIMS OFFICE
1005 MAIN ST
PO BOX 1599
BOISE, ID 83702
TEL: (208) 368-7770
FAX: (208) 336-1050
TOLL FREE: (800) 328-4316

CONNECTICUT CLAIMS OFFICE
1005 MAIN ST
PO BOX 1599
BOISE, ID 83701
TEL: (208) 368-7770
FAX: (208) 336-1050
TOLL FREE: (800) 328-4316

FLORIDA CLAIMS OFFICE
7300 CORPORATE CTR DR
PO BOX 020270
MIAMI, FL 33152-0270
TEL: (305) 715-2000
TOLL FREE: (800) 327-7771

IDAHO CLAIMS OFFICE
1005 MAIN ST
PO BOX 1599
BOISE, ID 83702
TEL: (208) 368-7770
FAX: (208) 336-1050
TOLL FREE: (800) 328-4316

ILLINOIS CLAIMS OFFICE
1005 MAIN ST
PO BOX 1599
BOISE, ID 55416-1521
TEL: (208) 368-7770
FAX: (208) 336-1050
TOLL FREE: (800) 328-4316

INDIANA CLAIMS OFFICE
1005 MAIN ST
PO BOX 1599
BOISE, ID 55416-1521
TEL: (208) 368-7770
FAX: (208) 336-1050
TOLL FREE: (800) 328-4316

IOWA CLAIMS OFFICE
1005 MAIN ST
PO BOX 1599
BOISE, ID 55416-1521
TEL: (208) 368-7770
FAX: (208) 336-1050
TOLL FREE: (800) 328-4316

KANSAS CLAIMS OFFICE
1005 MAIN ST
PO BOX 1599
BOISE, ID 55416-1521
TEL: (208) 368-7770
FAX: (208) 336-1050
TOLL FREE: (800) 328-4316

MAINE CLAIMS OFFICE
1005 MAIN ST
PO BOX 1599
BOISE, ID 55416-1521
TEL: (208) 368-7770
FAX: (208) 336-1050
TOLL FREE: (800) 328-4316

J

MASSACHUSETTS CLAIMS OFFICE
1005 MAIN ST
PO BOX 1599
BOISE, ID 55416-1521
TEL: (208) 368-7770
FAX: (208) 336-1050
TOLL FREE: (800) 328-4316

MICHIGAN CLAIMS OFFICE
1005 MAIN ST
PO BOX 1599
BOISE, ID 55416-1521
TEL: (208) 368-7770
FAX: (208) 336-1050
TOLL FREE: (800) 328-4316

MINNESOTA CLAIMS OFFICE
1005 MAIN ST
PO BOX 1599
BOISE, ID 55416-1521
TEL: (208) 368-7770
FAX: (208) 336-1050
TOLL FREE: (800) 328-4316

MISSOURI CLAIMS OFFICE
1005 MAIN ST
PO BOX 1599
BOISE, ID 55416-1521
TEL: (208) 368-7770
FAX: (208) 336-1050
TOLL FREE: (800) 328-4316

MONTANA CLAIMS OFFICE
1005 MAIN ST
PO BOX 1599
BOISE, ID 83702
TEL: (208) 368-7770
FAX: (208) 336-1050
TOLL FREE: (800) 328-4316

NEBRASKA CLAIMS OFFICE
1005 MAIN ST
PO BOX 1599
BOISE, ID 55416-1521
TEL: (208) 368-7770
FAX: (208) 336-1050
TOLL FREE: (800) 328-4316

NEVADA CLAIMS OFFICE
1005 MAIN ST
PO BOX 1599
BOISE, ID 83702
TEL: (208) 368-7770
FAX: (208) 336-1050
TOLL FREE: (800) 328-4316

NEW HAMPSHIRE CLAIMS OFFICE
1005 MAIN ST
PO BOX 1599
BOISE, ID 55416-1521
TEL: (208) 368-7770
FAX: (208) 336-1050
TOLL FREE: (800) 328-4316

NEW MEXICO CLAIMS OFFICE
1005 MAIN ST
PO BOX 1599
BOISE, ID 83702
TEL: (208) 368-7770
FAX: (208) 336-1050
TOLL FREE: (800) 328-4316

NORTH DAKOTA CLAIMS OFFICE
1005 MAIN ST
PO BOX 1599
BOISE, ID 55416-1521
TEL: (208) 368-7770
FAX: (208) 336-1050
TOLL FREE: (800) 328-4316

OREGON CLAIMS OFFICE
FORTIS HEALTH
1005 MAIN ST
PO BOX 1599
BOISE, ID 83702
TEL: (208) 368-7770
FAX: (208) 336-1050
TOLL FREE: (800) 328-4316

RHODE ISLAND CLAIMS OFFICE
FORTIS HEALTH
1005 MAIN ST
PO BOX 1599
BOISE, ID 55416-1521
TOLL FREE: (800) 328-4316

SOUTH DAKOTA CLAIMS OFFICE
FORTIS HEALTH
1005 MAIN ST
PO BOX 1599
BOISE, ID 55416-1521
TOLL FREE: (800) 328-4316

UTAH CLAIMS OFFICE
FORTIS HEALTH
1005 MAIN ST
PO BOX 1599
BOISE, ID 83702
TEL: (208) 368-7770
FAX: (208) 336-1050
TOLL FREE: (800) 328-4316

VERMONT CLAIMS OFFICE
FORTIS HEALTH
1005 MAIN ST
PO BOX 1599
BOISE, ID 55416-1521
TOLL FREE: (800) 328-4316

WASHINGTON CLAIMS OFFICE
FORTIS HEALTH
1005 MAIN ST
PO BOX 1599
BOISE, ID 83702
TEL: (208) 368-7770
FAX: (208) 336-1050
TOLL FREE: (800) 328-4316

WISCONSIN CLAIMS OFFICE
FORTIS HEALTH
1005 MAIN ST
PO BOX 1599
BOISE, ID 55416-1521
TOLL FREE: (800) 328-4316

WYOMING CLAIMS OFFICE
FORTIS HEALTH
1005 MAIN ST
PO BOX 1599
BOISE, ID 83702
TEL: (208) 368-7770
FAX: (208) 336-1050
TOLL FREE: (800) 328-4316

JOHN DEERE HEALTHCARE

ILLINOIS CLAIMS OFFICE
HERITAGE NATIONAL HEALTH PLAN
1300 RIVER DR, STE 200
MOLINE, IL 61265
TEL: (309) 765-1200
FAX: (309) 748-1146
TOLL FREE: (800) 797-1496

IOWA CLAIMS OFFICE
3740 UTICA RDG RD, STE A
BETTENDORF, IA 52722-1624
TEL: (319) 344-4500
FAX: (319) 359-1665
TOLL FREE: (800) 747-1446

HERITAGE NATIONAL HEALTH PLAN
3022 AIRPORT BLVD
PO BOX 9000
WATERLOO, IA 50704
TEL: (319) 292-4330
FAX: (319) 291-7838
TOLL FREE: (800) 798-7378

TENNESSEE CLAIMS OFFICE
HERITAGE NATIONAL HEALTH PLAN
2578 E STONE DR, STE A
KINGSPORT, TN 37660
TEL: (423) 378-5122
FAX: (423) 378-4752
TOLL FREE: (800) 229-6602

H

JOHN DEERE INSURANCE CO

ILLINOIS CLAIMS OFFICE
3400 80TH ST
MOLINE, IL 61265-5886
TEL: (309) 765-4100
FAX: (309) 765-8660
TOLL FREE: (800) 635-3377

JOHN DEERE TRANSPORTATION

WISCONSIN CLAIMS OFFICE
20300 WATERTOWER, STE 100
PO BOX 2051
BROOKFIELD, WI 53045
TEL: (414) 717-0602
FAX: (414) 717-0575
TOLL FREE: (800) 558-9257

JOHN DEERE TRANSPORTATION INSURANCE

FLORIDA CLAIMS OFFICE
9440 PHILLIPS HWY, STE 7
PO BOX 24847
JACKSONVILLE, FL 32241-4847
TEL: (904) 262-3441
FAX: (904) 262-4169
TOLL FREE: (800) 255-5814
IN-STATE: (800) 255-5814

JOHN MUIR MEDICAL CENTER

CALIFORNIA CLAIMS OFFICE
1601 YGNACIO VLY RD
WALNUT CREEK, CA 94598-3122
TEL: (925) 939-3000

JOHN P. PEARL & ASSOCIATES

ILLINOIS CLAIMS OFFICE
1200 E GLEN AVE
PEORIA HEIGHTS, IL 61614-5348
TEL: (309) 693-1900
FAX: (309) 688-5444
TOLL FREE: (800) 447-4982
IN-STATE: (800) 322-2488
WWW.PEARLINS.COM

3

JOHNS HOPKINS MEDICAL SERVICES CORPORATION

MARYLAND CLAIMS OFFICE
3100 WYMAN PK DR
BALTIMORE, MD 21211
TEL: (410) 338-3624
FAX: (410) 338-3214

R H

JOINT WELFARE FUND, LOCAL 164 IBEW

NEW JERSEY CLAIMS OFFICE
65 W CENTURY RD
PARAMUS, NJ 07652
TEL: (201) 225-1641
FAX: (201) 225-0628

R H

K & K INSURANCE GROUP

INDIANA CLAIMS OFFICE
1712 MAGNAVOX WAY
PO BOX 2338
FT WAYNE, IN 46804-1538
TEL: (219) 459-5000
FAX: (219) 459-5910
TOLL FREE: (800) 237-2917
WWW.K&KINSURANCE.COM

KAISER FOUNDATION HEALTH PLAN

MASSACHUSETTS CLAIMS OFFICE
DENTAL DEPT
31 HALL DR
AMHERST, MA 01002
TEL: (413) 256-4370
FAX: (413) 256-4419

KAISER FOUNDATION HEALTH PLAN OF CALIFORNIA

NATIONAL CLAIMS OFFICE
425 MARKET ST, STE 925
SAN FRANCISCO, CA 94105
TEL: (415) 512-6000
FAX: (415) 512-6030
IN-STATE: (800) 464-4000
WWW.KAIPERM.ORG

H

KAISER / GROUP HEALTH

WASHINGTON CLAIMS OFFICE
521 WALL ST
SEATTLE, WA 98121
TEL: (206) 448-5600
FAX: (206) 901-4612
TOLL FREE: (800) 901-4636
WWW.GHC.ORG

H

KAISER PERMANENTE

CALIFORNIA CLAIMS OFFICE
393 E WALNUT ST- 3RD FL
PO BOX 7102
PASADENA, CA 91109-9880
FAX: (626) 683-2030
TOLL FREE: (888) 634-1300
WWW.KAISERPERMANENTE.ORG

H

3495 PIEDMONT RD NE- BLDG 9
ATLANTA, GA 30305
TEL: (404) 233-0555
FAX: (404) 364-4791
TOLL FREE: (800) 611-1811
WWW.KAISERPERMANENTE.ORG

H

COLORADO CLAIMS OFFICE
3495 PIEDMONT RD NE- BLDG 9
ATLANTA, GA 30305
TEL: (404) 233-0555
FAX: (404) 364-4791
TOLL FREE: (800) 611-1811
WWW.KAISERPERMANENTE.ORG

H

CONNECTICUT CLAIMS OFFICE
PO BOX 15109
ALBANY, NY 12212
TEL: (518) 783-1864
FAX: (518) 782-0845
TOLL FREE: (800) 638-0668
WWW.KAISERPERMANENTE.ORG

H

DISTRICT OF COLUMBIA CLAIMS OFFICE
2101 E JEFFERSON ST
ROCKVILLE, MD 20849
TEL: (301) 816-2424
FAX: (301) 816-7461
TOLL FREE: (800) 368-5784
IN-STATE: (800) 777-7902
WWW.KAISERPERMANENTE.ORG

H

GEORGIA CLAIMS OFFICE
3495 PIEDMONT RD NE- BLDG 9
ATLANTA, GA 30305
TEL: (404) 233-0555
FAX: (404) 364-4791
TOLL FREE: (800) 611-1811
WWW.KAISERPERMANENTE.ORG

H

HAWAII CLAIMS OFFICE
711 KAPIOLANI BLVD
PO BOX 31000
HONOLULU, HI 96849-5086
TEL: (808) 597-5340
FAX: (808) 597-5300
TOLL FREE: (800) 596-5955
IN-STATE: (800) 596-5955
WWW.KAISERPERMANENTE.ORG

H

3495 PIEDMONT RD NE- BLDG 9
ATLANTA, GA 30305
TEL: (404) 233-0555
FAX: (404) 364-4791
TOLL FREE: (800) 611-1811
WWW.KAISERPERMANENTE.ORG

H

KANSAS CLAIMS OFFICE
10561 BARKLEY, STE 200
OVERLAND PARK, KS 66212-1883
TEL: (913) 967-4600
FAX: (913) 642-0209
WWW.KAISERPERMANENTE.ORG

H

3495 PIEDMONT RD NE- BLDG 9
ATLANTA, GA 30305
TEL: (404) 233-0555
FAX: (404) 364-4791
TOLL FREE: (800) 611-1811
WWW.KAISERPERMANENTE.ORG

H

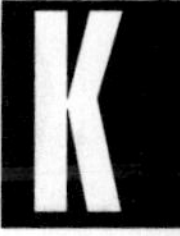

MARYLAND CLAIMS OFFICE
2101 E JEFFERSON ST
PO BOX 6233
ROCKVILLE, MD 20849-6233
TEL: (301) 816-2424
FAX: (301) 816-7461
TOLL FREE: (800) 368-5784
IN-STATE: (800) 777-7902
WWW.KAISERPERMANENTE.ORG

MASSACHUSETTS CLAIMS OFFICE
PO BOX 15109
ALBANY, NY 12212
TEL: (518) 783-1864
FAX: (518) 782-0845
TOLL FREE: (800) 638-0668
WWW.KAISERPERMANENTE.ORG

COMMUNITY HEALTH PLAN
ONE CHP PLZ
LATHAM, NY 12110
TEL: (518) 783-1864
TOLL FREE: (800) 638-0668
WWW.KAISERPERMANENTE.ORG

MISSISSIPPI CLAIMS OFFICE
3495 PIEDMONT RD NE- BLDG 9
ATLANTA, GA 30305
TEL: (404) 233-0555
FAX: (404) 364-4791
TOLL FREE: (800) 611-1811
WWW.KAISERPERMANENTE.ORG

MISSOURI CLAIMS OFFICE
10561 BARKLEY, STE 200
OVERLAND PARK, KS 66212-1883
TEL: (913) 967-4600
FAX: (913) 642-0209
WWW.KAISERPERMANENTE.ORG

NATIONAL CLAIMS OFFICE
KAISER FOUNDATION HEALTH PLAN OF MASSACHUSETTS, INC
76 BATTERSON PARK RD
PO BOX 4011
FARMINGTON, CT 06034-4011
TEL: (860) 678-6000
FAX: (860) 678-6170
TOLL FREE: (800) 344-5682
WWW.KAISERPERMANENTE.ORG

PO BOX 40669
RALEIGH, NC 27629
TEL: (919) 981-6000
FAX: (919) 981-6052
TOLL FREE: (800) 221-5347
WWW.KAISERPERMANENTE.ORG

4909 ST HWY 28, STE 10
COOPERSTOWN, NY 13326-1301
TEL: (607) 547-9244
FAX: (607) 547-9435
TOLL FREE: (800) 562-5750
WWW.KAISERPERMANENTE.ORG

NEW YORK CLAIMS OFFICE
PO BOX 15109
ALBANY, NY 12212
TEL: (518) 783-1864
FAX: (518) 782-0845
TOLL FREE: (800) 638-0668
WWW.KAISERPERMANENTE.ORG

COMMUNITY HEALTH PLAN
ONE CHP PLZ
LATHAM, NY 12110
TEL: (518) 783-1864
TOLL FREE: (800) 638-0668
WWW.KAISERPERMANENTE.ORG

210 WESTCHESTER AVE
WHITE PLAINS, NY 10604-2914
TEL: (914) 682-0700
FAX: (914) 682-6403
TOLL FREE: (800) 305-1992
WWW.KAISERPERMANENTE.ORG

NORTH CAROLINA CLAIMS OFFICE
3495 PIEDMONT RD NE- BLDG 9
ATLANTA, GA 30305
TEL: (404) 233-0555
FAX: (404) 364-4791
TOLL FREE: (800) 611-1811
WWW.KAISERPERMANENTE.ORG

COMMUNITY HEALTH PLAN
ONE CHP PLZ
LATHAM, NY 12110
TEL: (518) 783-1864
TOLL FREE: (800) 638-0668
WWW.KAISERPERMANENTE.ORG

OHIO CLAIMS OFFICE
N PT TWR- 1001 LAKESIDE AVE, STE 1200
CLEVELAND, OH 44114-1153
TEL: (216) 621-5600
FAX: (216) 621-7354
WWW.KAISERPERMANENTE.ORG

3495 PIEDMONT RD NE- BLDG 9
ATLANTA, GA 30305
TEL: (404) 233-0555
FAX: (404) 364-4791
TOLL FREE: (800) 611-1811
WWW.KAISERPERMANENTE.ORG

OREGON CLAIMS OFFICE
500 NE MULTNOMAH, STE 100
PORTLAND, OR 97232-2099
TEL: (503) 813-2800
FAX: (503) 813-2710
TOLL FREE: (800) 813-2000
WWW.KAISERPERMANENTE.ORG

3495 PIEDMONT RD NE- BLDG 9
ATLANTA, GA 30305
TEL: (404) 233-0555
FAX: (404) 364-4791
TOLL FREE: (800) 611-1811
WWW.KAISERPERMANENTE.ORG

TEXAS CLAIMS OFFICE
3495 PIEDMONT RD NE- BLDG 9
ATLANTA, GA 30305
TEL: (404) 233-0555
FAX: (404) 364-4791
TOLL FREE: (800) 611-1811
WWW.KAISERPERMANENTE.ORG

VERMONT CLAIMS OFFICE
PO BOX 15109
ALBANY, NY 12212
TEL: (518) 783-1864
FAX: (518) 782-0845
TOLL FREE: (800) 638-0668
WWW.KAISERPERMANENTE.ORG

VIRGINIA CLAIMS OFFICE
2101 E JEFFERSON ST
ROCKVILLE, MD 20852
TEL: (301) 468-6000
TOLL FREE: (800) 368-5784
IN-STATE: (800) 777-7902
WWW.KAISERPERMANENTE.ORG

KAISER PERMANENTE NE DIVISION

NEW YORK CLAIMS OFFICE
ATTN: DOC PREPARATION DEPT
1 CHP PLAZA
PO BOX 15109
LATHAM, NY 12110
TEL: (518) 783-1864
FAX: (518) 785-1109
TOLL FREE: (800) 638-0668
IN-STATE: (800) 597-3872
WWW.KAISERPERMANENTE.ORG

KANAWHA HEALTHCARE SOLUTIONS, INC

SOUTH CAROLINA CLAIMS OFFICE
545 N PLEASANTBURG DR, STE 202
PO BOX 5150
GREENVILLE, SC 29606
TEL: (864) 235-6474
FAX: (864) 240-3170
TOLL FREE: (800) 476-5150
IN-STATE: (800) 476-5150

KANAWHA INSURANCE CO

210 S WHITE ST
PO BOX 610
LANCASTER, SC 29721-0610
TEL: (803) 283-5556
FAX: (803) 283-5313
TOLL FREE: (800) 635-4252
IN-STATE: (800) 635-4252

KANSAS CITY LIFE INSURANCE CO

MISSOURI CLAIMS OFFICE
3520 BROADWAY
PO BOX 419139
KANSAS CITY, MO 64141-6139
TEL: (816) 753-7299
FAX: (816) 931-4006
TOLL FREE: (800) 874-5254

KANSAS FARM BUREAU & AFFILIATED SERVICES

KANSAS CLAIMS OFFICE
2627 KFB PLZ
MANHATTAN, KS 66503-8154
TEL: (785) 587-6000
FAX: (785) 587-6883
WWW.KFBF.COM

KEENAN & ASSOCIATES

CALIFORNIA CLAIMS OFFICE
2355 CRENSHAW BLVD
PO BOX 11431
TORRANCE, CA 90510-1431
TEL: (310) 212-3344
FAX: (310) 212-3381
IN-STATE: (800) 653-3626
WWW.KEENANASSOC.COM

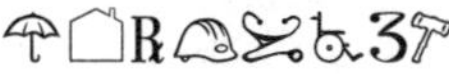

2105 S BASCOM AVE, STE 310
CAMPBELL, CA 95008-3271
TEL: (408) 377-3338
FAX: (408) 371-1796
TOLL FREE: (800) 334-6554
WWW.KEENANASSOCIATES.COM

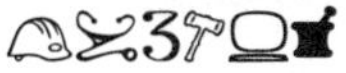

8441 N MELBROOK AVE, STE 104
FRESNO, CA 93720
TEL: (559) 436-6644
FAX: (559) 436-6656
TOLL FREE: (800) 232-5639
WWW.KEENANASSOCIATES.COM

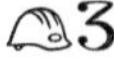

3610 CENTRAL, STE 400
RIVERSIDE, CA 92506-2405
TEL: (909) 788-0330
FAX: (909) 788-8013
TOLL FREE: (800) 654-8347

KEMPER INSURANCE

152 N 3RD ST, STE 710
SAN JOSE, CA 95112
TEL: (408) 297-3002
FAX: (408) 297-3242
TOLL FREE: (800) 552-5344

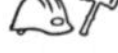

COLORADO CLAIMS OFFICE
10375 E HARVARD, STE 500
PO BOX 5347
DENVER, CO 80217-5347
TEL: (303) 696-1441
FAX: (303) 752-5425
TOLL FREE: (800) 321-9515

FLORIDA CLAIMS OFFICE
EASTERN REGION
CRAGG BLDG- 3452 LAKE LYNDA DR, STE 400
PO BOX 675050
ORLANDO, FL 32867-5050
TEL: (407) 249-4335
FAX: (407) 249-4340
TOLL FREE: (800) 258-0034
WWW.KEMPERINSURANCE.COM

ILLINOIS CLAIMS OFFICE
ONE KEMPER DR
LONG GROVE, IL 60049-0001
TEL: (847) 320-2000
FAX: (847) 320-2494
TOLL FREE: (800) 833-0355
WWW.KEMPERINSURANCE.COM

INDIANA CLAIMS OFFICE
WESTERN REGION
E DR, STE 151- 2780 WATERFRONT PKY
PO BOX 24339
INDIANAPOLIS, IN 46224-0339
TEL: (317) 298-0113
FAX: (317) 297-0310
TOLL FREE: (800) 352-7475

KANSAS CLAIMS OFFICE
1861 N ROCK RD, STE 202
PO BOX 20380
WICHITA, KS 67208-9998
TEL: (316) 681-2001
FAX: (316) 681-2629

MISSISSIPPI CLAIMS OFFICE
EASTERN REGION
WDLNDS OFC PRK- 775 WDLNDS PKY, STE 102
RIDGELAND, MS 39157-5212
TEL: (601) 978-3328
FAX: (601) 978-3466
TOLL FREE: (800) 232-8679
WWW.KEMPERINSURANCE.COM

NORTH CAROLINA CLAIMS OFFICE
EASTERN REGION
SOMERSET BUS CTR- 4505 FALLS OF NEUSE
PO BOX 19308
RALEIGH, NC 27619-9308
TEL: (919) 873-1990
FAX: (919) 873-1895
TOLL FREE: (800) 336-1799
WWW.KEMPERINSURANCE.COM

PENNSYLVANIA CLAIMS OFFICE
HILLSIDE CORPORATE CTR
5001 LOUISE DR, STE 102
MECHANICSBURG, PA 17055-6913
TEL: (717) 691-7460
FAX: (717) 691-7474
TOLL FREE: (800) 437-3357
WWW.KEMPERINSURANCE.COM

KEMPER INSURANCE COMPANIES

ALABAMA CLAIMS OFFICE
SATELLITE OFFICE
1600 SW 80TH TERRACE
PO BOX 189124
PLANTATION, FL 33318-9083
TEL: (954) 452-4000
FAX: (954) 452-4121
TOLL FREE: (800) 800-7885
WWW.KEMPERINSURANCE.COM

EASTERN REGION
1100 CIR 75 PKY, STE 400
ATLANTA, GA 30339-3076
TEL: (770) 984-1990
FAX: (770) 984-2344
TOLL FREE: (800) 452-0753

ALASKA CLAIMS OFFICE
300 ELLIOTT AVE W, STE 500
PO BOX 2377
SEATTLE, WA 98111-2377
TEL: (206) 281-3300
FAX: (206) 298-2040
TOLL FREE: (800) 562-2114
WWW.KEMPERINSURANCE.COM

ARIZONA CLAIMS OFFICE
WESTERN REGION
2400 W DUNLAP AVE, STE 225
PO BOX 37829
PHOENIX, AZ 85069
TEL: (602) 678-5250
FAX: (602) 861-1951
TOLL FREE: (800) 338-5848

CALIFORNIA CLAIMS OFFICE
WESTERN REGION
17800 CASTLETON ST, STE 300
INDUSTRY, CA 91748-1707
TEL: (626) 369-7700
FAX: (626) 369-7714
TOLL FREE: (800) 732-7475
WWW.KEMPERINSURANCE.COM

WESTERN REGION
2 CORP CTR- 1390 WILLOW PASS RD, STE 500
PO BOX 4133
CONCORD, CA 94524_4133
TEL: (925) 677-3400
FAX: (925) 677-3401
TOLL FREE: (800) 874-8523

SATELLITE OFFICE
KOLL CTR ORANGE- 500 N ST CLG BLVD, STE 530
ORANGE, CA 92868-1619
TEL: (714) 939-1210
FAX: (714) 939-6504
WWW.KEMPERINSURANCE.COM

WESTERN REGION
2920 KILGORE RD
PO BOX 15810
SACRAMENTO, CA 95852-0810
TEL: (916) 851-7500
FAX: (916) 851-7730
TOLL FREE: (800) 225-0185

SATELLITE OFFICE
16835 W BERNARDO DR, STE 103
SAN DIEGO, CA 92127
FAX: (619) 673-1439
TOLL FREE: (800) 225-0185
WWW.KEMPERINSURANCE.COM

WESTERN REGION
LINCOLN TOWN CTR- 2677 N MAIN ST, STE 300
PO BOX 25229
SANTA ANA, CA 92799-5229
TEL: (714) 480-3300
FAX: (714) 480-3301
TOLL FREE: (800) 874-2573

WESTERN REGION
17800 CASTLETON ST
PO BOX 925
LA PUENTE, CA 91747-0925
TEL: (626) 369-7786
FAX: (626) 369-8864
TOLL FREE: (800) 732-7475
WWW.KEMPERINSURANCE.COM

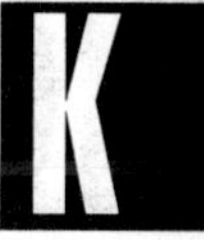

CONNECTICUT CLAIMS OFFICE
EASTERN REGION
10 COLUMBUS BLVD- 4TH FL
PO BOX 2958
HARTFORD, CT 06104-2958
TEL: (860) 527-6438
FAX: (860) 527-9716
TOLL FREE: (800) 348-4869
WWW.KEMPERINSURANCE.COM

FLORIDA CLAIMS OFFICE
BALBONI BLDG- 5601 MARINER ST, STE 400
PO BOX 22437
TAMPA, FL 33622-2437
TEL: (813) 286-2621
FAX: (813) 207-2401
TOLL FREE: (800) 258-1811

GEORGIA CLAIMS OFFICE
EASTERN REGION
6200 CORNERS PKY, STE 500
NORCROSS, GA 30092-3343
TEL: (678) 969-7337
FAX: (678) 969-7363
TOLL FREE: (800) 450-0692
WWW.KEMPERINSURANCE.COM

EASTERN REGION
1100 CIR 75 PKY, STE 400
ATLANTA, GA 30339-3076
TEL: (770) 984-1990
FAX: (770) 984-2344
TOLL FREE: (800) 452-0753

IDAHO CLAIMS OFFICE
300 ELLIOTT AVE W, STE 500
PO BOX 2377
SEATTLE, WA 98111-2377
TEL: (206) 281-3300
FAX: (206) 298-2040
TOLL FREE: (800) 562-2114
WWW.KEMPERINSURANCE.COM

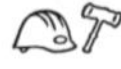

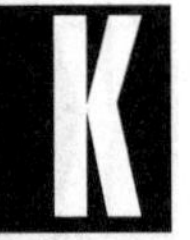

ILLINOIS CLAIMS OFFICE
AMERICAN MANUFACTURERS MUTUAL INSURANCE CO
1 KEMPER DR
LONG GROVE, IL 60049-0001
TEL: (847) 320-2000
FAX: (847) 320-2494
TOLL FREE: (800) 833-0355
WWW.KEMPERINSURANCE.COM

CORPORATE OFFICE
1 KEMPER DR
LONG GROVE, IL 60049-0001
TEL: (847) 320-2000
FAX: (847) 320-4027
TOLL FREE: (800) 833-0355
WWW.KEMPERINSURANCE.COM

WESTERN REGION
1000 TWR LN, STE 325
BENSENVILLE, IL 60101
TEL: (630) 860-3750
FAX: (630) 860-2126
WWW.KEMPERINSURANCE.COM

LUMBERMANS MUTUAL CASUALTY
CLAYTON EXEC CTR- 7980 CLAYTON RD, STE 200
PO BOX 66851
SAINT LOUIS, MO 63166-6851
TEL: (314) 951-4000
FAX: (314) 781-1382
TOLL FREE: (800) 232-3804
WWW.KEMPERINSURANCE.COM

IOWA CLAIMS OFFICE
5101 UTICA RIDGE RD
PO BOX 520
DAVENPORT, IA 52805-0520
TEL: (319) 359-8200
FAX: (319) 355-0189
TOLL FREE: (800) 452-2207
WWW.KEMPERINSURANCE.COM

KANSAS CLAIMS OFFICE
WESTERN REGION
CORPORATE WDS- 9900 W 109 ST
PO BOX 10900
OVERLAND PARK, KS 66225-0900
TEL: (913) 469-7700
FAX: (913) 491-6358
TOLL FREE: (800) 553-1053

LOUISIANA CLAIMS OFFICE
3233 S SHERWOOD FOREST BLVD, STE 112
BATON ROUGE, LA 70816-3233
TEL: (225) 291-4817
WWW.KEMPERINSURANCE.COM

WESTERN REGION
3 LKWY CTR- 3838 N CSWY BLVD, STE 2050
PO BOX 8390
METAIRIE, LA 70011-8390
TEL: (504) 837-5962
FAX: (504) 833-0402
TOLL FREE: (800) 323-1159
WWW.KEMPERINSURANCE.COM

MARYLAND CLAIMS OFFICE
210 W PENNSYLVANIA AVE, STE 350
TOWSON, MD 21204
TEL: (410) 821-4800
FAX: (410) 821-4817
TOLL FREE: (800) 672-4048
WWW.KEMPERINSURANCE.COM

MASSACHUSETTS CLAIMS OFFICE
EASTERN REGION
1 NEW ENGLAND EXEC PRK
PO BOX 979
BURLINGTON, MA 01803-5979
TEL: (781) 229-7900
FAX: (781) 272-4677
TOLL FREE: (800) 258-9546
WWW.KEMPERINSURANCE.COM

MICHIGAN CLAIMS OFFICE
SATELLITE OFFICE
3033 ORCHARD VISTA DR SE, STE 312
PO BOX 171
GRAND RAPIDS, MI 49501-0171
TEL: (616) 949-7080
FAX: (616) 942-5530
TOLL FREE: (800) 832-4553
WWW.KEMPERINSURANCE.COM

WESTERN REGION
17187 N LAUREL PRK DR, STE 330
PO BOX 537902
LIVONIA, MI 48153-7902
TEL: (734) 953-9550
FAX: (734) 953-9034
TOLL FREE: (800) 311-2323
WWW.KEMPERINSURANCE.COM

MINNESOTA CLAIMS OFFICE
WESTERN REGION
8400 NORMANDALE LK BLVD, STE 1700
PO BOX 59053
MINNEAPOLIS, MN 55459-0053
TEL: (612) 820-6100
FAX: (612) 820-6102
TOLL FREE: (800) 345-7270
WWW.KEMPERINSURANCE.COM

MISSISSIPPI CLAIMS OFFICE
EASTERN REGION
1100 CIR 75 PKY, STE 400
ATLANTA, GA 30339-3076
TEL: (770) 984-1990
FAX: (770) 984-2344
TOLL FREE: (800) 452-0753

MISSOURI CLAIMS OFFICE
LUMBERMANS MUTUAL CASUALTY
CLAYTON EXEC CTR- 7980 CLAYTON RD, STE 200
PO BOX 66851
SAINT LOUIS, MO 63166-6851
TEL: (314) 951-4000
FAX: (314) 781-1382
TOLL FREE: (800) 232-3804
WWW.KEMPERINSURANCE.COM

WESTERN REGION
CORPORATE WDS- 9900 W 109 ST
PO BOX 10900
OVERLAND PARK, KS 66225-0900
TEL: (913) 469-7700
FAX: (913) 491-6358
TOLL FREE: (800) 553-1053

MONTANA CLAIMS OFFICE
300 ELLIOTT AVE W, STE 500
PO BOX 2377
SEATTLE, WA 98111-2377
TEL: (206) 281-3300
FAX: (206) 298-2040
TOLL FREE: (800) 562-2114
WWW.KEMPERINSURANCE.COM

NATIONAL CLAIMS OFFICE
EASTERN REGION
81 WELBY RD
PO BOX 51148
NEW BEDFORD, MA 02745-1148
TEL: (800) 258-9546
TOLL FREE: (800) 521-2003
WWW.KEMPERINSURANCE.COM

NEVADA CLAIMS OFFICE
SATELLITE OFFICE
AIRPORT PLZ- 1755 E PLUMB LN, STE 126
RENO, NV 89502-3600
TEL: (702) 348-1400
FAX: (702) 348-0708

NEW JERSEY CLAIMS OFFICE
EASTERN REGION
25 DEFOREST AVE
SUMMIT, NJ 07901-2154
TEL: (908) 522-4000
FAX: (908) 522-4458
TOLL FREE: (800) 700-7572
WWW.KEMPERINSURANCE.COM

NEW MEXICO CLAIMS OFFICE
SATELLITE OFFICE
METRO CTR- 1720 LOUISIANA BLVD NE, STE 206
PO BOX 8768
ALBUQUERQUE, NM 87198-8768
TEL: (505) 255-7788
FAX: (505) 255-6699

NEW YORK CLAIMS OFFICE
EASTERN REGION
BLDG VII- 5784 WIDEWATERS PKY
PO BOX 4780
SYRACUSE, NY 13221
TEL: (315) 449-5685
FAX: (315) 449-8939
TOLL FREE: (800) 357-8999
WWW.KEMPERINSURANCE.COM

EASTERN REGION
300 WESTAGE BUSINESS CTR, STE 320
PO BOX 444
FISHKILL, NY 12524-0444
TEL: (914) 896-0611
FAX: (914) 896-0625
TOLL FREE: (888) 234-0340
WWW.KEMPERINSURANCE.COM

EASTERN REGION
BLDG II- 898 VETERANS MEM HWY- 4TH FL
PO BOX 5000
SMITHTOWN, NY 11787-0880
TEL: (516) 234-2230
FAX: (516) 234-3080
TOLL FREE: (888) 234-0329
WWW.KEMPERINSURANCE.COM

NORTH CAROLINA CLAIMS OFFICE
EASTERN REGION
5 LKPT PLZ- 2709 WATER RDG PKY- 3RD FL
CHARLOTTE, NC 28217-4539
TEL: (704) 329-2500
FAX: (704) 329-2515
TOLL FREE: (800) 532-6500
WWW.KEMPERINSURANCE.COM

OHIO CLAIMS OFFICE
EASTERN REGION
CRYSTAL PT CTR- 202 MONTROSE W AVE, STE 100
PO BOX 4491
AKRON, OH 44321-0491
TEL: (330) 668-9100
FAX: (330) 666-1250
TOLL FREE: (800) 258-5344
WWW.KEMPERINSURANCE.COM

EASTERN REGION
COMM CORP CTR- 445 HUTCHINSON AVE, STE 550
PO BOX 231
WORTHINGTON, OH 43085-0231
TEL: (614) 436-8990
FAX: (614) 431-0877
TOLL FREE: (800) 272-2616
WWW.KEMPERINSURANCE.COM

OKLAHOMA CLAIMS OFFICE
WESTERN REGION
CORPORATE WDS- 9900 W 109 ST
PO BOX 10900
OVERLAND PARK, KS 66225-0900
TEL: (913) 469-7700
FAX: (913) 491-6358
TOLL FREE: (800) 553-1053

ONTARIO CLAIMS OFFICE
EASTERN REGION
320 FRONT ST W- BLDG C, 6TH FL
TORONTO, ON M5V3B6
TEL: (416) 593-6626
FAX: (416) 351-2550
TOLL FREE: (800) 387-2934
WWW.KEMPERINSURANCE.COM

OREGON CLAIMS OFFICE
PACIFIC CORPORATE CENTER
6650 SW REDWOOD LN- BLDG 16, STE 333
PO BOX 2109
LAKE OSWEGO, OR 97035-0035
TEL: (503) 684-8484
FAX: (503) 620-7503
WWW.KEMPERINSURANCE.COM

PENNSYLVANIA CLAIMS OFFICE
EASTERN REGION
1717 ARCH ST
PHILADELPHIA, PA 19103
TEL: (215) 564-3701
FAX: (215) 564-3783
TOLL FREE: (800) 258-2636
WWW.KEMPERINSURANCE.COM

1 CHATHAM CTR, STE 325
PITTSBURGH, PA 15219-3492
TEL: (412) 434-8800
FAX: (412) 281-1982
TOLL FREE: (800) 242-1535
WWW.KEMPER INSURANCE.COM

SOUTH CAROLINA CLAIMS OFFICE
EASTERN REGION
LAURENS BLDG- 750 EXECUTIVE CTR DR, STE 205
PO BOX 5266
GREENVILLE, SC 29606-5266
TEL: (864) 288-1225
FAX: (864) 297-4040
TOLL FREE: (800) 922-9915
E-MAIL: KEMPERINSURANCE.COM

TENNESSEE CLAIMS OFFICE
WESTERN REGION
HIGHLAND RDG III- 545 MARRIOTT DR, STE 700
PO BOX 292769
NASHVILLE, TN 37229-2769
TEL: (615) 872-2500
FAX: (615) 872-2507
TOLL FREE: (800) 647-2039
WWW.KEMPERINSURANCE.COM

TEXAS CLAIMS OFFICE
LAKESIDE SQUARE, 12377 MARIT DR, STE 1400
PO BOX 749003
DALLAS, TX 75374-9003
TEL: (972) 364-5400
FAX: (972) 364-5550
TOLL FREE: (800) 252-1455
WWW.KEMPERINSURANCE.COM

WESTERN REGION
2 NORTHPOINT DR, STE 800
HOUSTON, TX 77060-3237
TEL: (281) 447-8679
FAX: (281) 447-4129
TOLL FREE: (800) 352-9994
WWW.KEMPERINSURANCE.COM

SATELLITE OFFICE
4241 WOODROCK DR, STE 101B
PO BOX 28070
SAN ANTONIO, TX 78228-0070
TEL: (210) 733-1833
FAX: (210) 733-0324
TOLL FREE: (800) 323-6658

VIRGINIA CLAIMS OFFICE
1 MONUMENT PL- 12150 E MONUMENT DR, STE 200
PO BOX 3646
FAIRFAX, VA 22038-4053
TEL: (703) 385-3667
FAX: (703) 293-6690
TOLL FREE: (800) 622-8637
WWW.KEMPERINSURANCE.COM

4805 LK BRK DR
PO BOX 5550
GLEN ALLEN, VA 23058-5550
TEL: (804) 418-6800
FAX: (804) 418-6704
TOLL FREE: (800) 619-1777
WWW.KEMPERINSURANCE.COM

WASHINGTON CLAIMS OFFICE
300 ELLIOTT AVE W, STE 500
PO BOX 2377
SEATTLE, WA 98111-2377
TEL: (206) 281-3300
FAX: (206) 298-2040
TOLL FREE: (800) 562-2114
WWW.KEMPERINSURANCE.COM

WISCONSIN CLAIMS OFFICE
BROOKFIELD LAKES OFFICE PARK
175 N PATRICK BLVD, STE 100
PO BOX 770
BROOKFIELD, WI 53008-0770
TEL: (414) 792-9880
FAX: (414) 792-9818
TOLL FREE: (800) 242-8808
WWW.KEMPERINSURANCE.COM

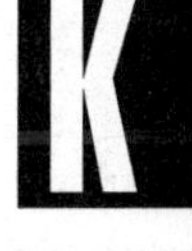

EASTERN REGION
175 N PATRICK BLVD, STE 100
PO BOX 770
BROOKFIELD, WI 53008-0770
TEL: (414) 792-9880
FAX: (414) 792-9818
TOLL FREE: (800) 242-8808
WWW.KEMPERINSURANCE.COM

KEMPTON GROUP

OKLAHOMA CLAIMS OFFICE
PO BOX 54889
OKLAHOMA CITY, OK 73154-1889
TEL: (405) 521-1711
FAX: (405) 521-9804
TOLL FREE: (800) 521-1711
WWW.KEMPTONGROUP.COM

KENTUCKY FARM BUREAU MUTUAL INSURANCE CO

KENTUCKY CLAIMS OFFICE
9201 BUNSEN PKY
PO BOX 20700
LOUISVILLE, KY 40250-0700
TEL: (502) 495-5000
FAX: (502) 495-5177
WWW.KYFB.COM

1382 CAMPBELL LN
PO BOX 51545
BOWLING GREEN, KY 42102-5845
TEL: (502) 782-1300
FAX: (502) 782-1397
TOLL FREE: (800) 538-8656

2909 RING RD
PO BOX 958
ELIZABETHTOWN, KY 42702-0958
TEL: (270) 765-4400
FAX: (270) 765-7756
TOLL FREE: (800) 782-3811

957 WEAVER RD
PO BOX 337
FLORENCE, KY 41022-0337
TEL: (606) 525-6170
FAX: (606) 525-6574
TOLL FREE: (800) 538-8653

1810 E 9TH ST
PO BOX 954
HOPKINSVILLE, KY 42241-0954
TEL: (502) 886-8123
FAX: (502) 885-4190
TOLL FREE: (800) 538-8657

211 PANBOWL LK DR
PO BOX 1210
JACKSON, KY 41339-5210
TEL: (606) 666-2476
FAX: (606) 666-4565
TOLL FREE: (800) 538-8647

3271 RUCKRIEGEL PKY
PO BOX 99595
JEFFERSONTOWN, KY 40269-0595
TEL: (502) 266-6100
FAX: (502) 266-6104
WWW.KYFBINS.COM

2401 MERCHANT ST
PO BOX 12408
LEXINGTON, KY 40583-2408
TEL: (606) 254-8074
FAX: (606) 254-7216
TOLL FREE: (800) 782-3810

1601 SANITA RD
PO BOX 35009
LOUISVILLE, KY 40232-5009
TEL: (502) 456-1664
FAX: (502) 456-1688
TOLL FREE: (800) 782-3812

400 N 7TH ST
PO BOX 363
MAYFIELD, KY 42066-0363
TEL: (502) 247-4787
FAX: (502) 247-7654
TOLL FREE: (800) 538-8654

506 SUNSET DR
PO BOX 890
MOREHEAD, KY 40351
TEL: (606) 784-7536
FAX: (606) 784-8769
TOLL FREE: (800) 538-8649

3036 PARRISH AVE
PO BOX 21369
OWENSBORO, KY 42304-1369
TEL: (502) 684-2165
FAX: (502) 684-4019
TOLL FREE: (800) 538-8655

1215 W HWY 80
PO BOX 860
SOMERSET, KY 42502-0860
TEL: (606) 679-4327
FAX: (606) 679-3453
TOLL FREE: (800) 538-8650

KEYSTONE HEALTH PLAN CENTRAL

PENNSYLVANIA CLAIMS OFFICE
300 CORPORATE CTR DR
PO BOX 898812
CAMP HILL, PA 17089-8812
TEL: (717) 763-3458
FAX: (717) 975-6895
TOLL FREE: (800) 622-2843
WWW.KHPC.COM

H

KEYSTONE HEALTH PLAN EAST, INC

1901 MARKET ST
PHILADELPHIA, PA 19103
TEL: (215) 241-2001
FAX: (215) 241-2040
TOLL FREE: (800) 227-3114

H

KEYSTONE INSURANCE CO

2040 MARKET ST
PHILADELPHIA, PA 19103-5161
TEL: (215) 864-5000
FAX: (215) 864-5438

KEYSTONE MERCY HEALTH PLAN

CLAIMS PROCESSING CTR
200 STEVENS DR
LESTER, PA 19113-1570
TEL: (215) 937-7300
FAX: (215) 937-5300
IN-STATE: (800) 521-6007

KIRKE-VAN ORSDEL

MISSOURI CLAIMS OFFICE
1 METROPOLITAN SQ, STE 800
PO BOX 9007
SAINT LOUIS, MO 63101
TEL: (314) 982-8400
FAX: (314) 621-0181

KITSAP PHYSICIANS SERVICE

WASHINGTON CLAIMS OFFICE
400 WARREN AVE
PO BOX 339
BREMERTON, WA 98337
TEL: (360) 377-5576
FAX: (360) 415-6514
TOLL FREE: (800) 552-7114

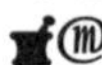

KLAIS & CO

OHIO CLAIMS OFFICE
1867 W MARKET ST
AKRON, OH 44313
TEL: (330) 867-8443
FAX: (330) 867-0827
TOLL FREE: (800) 331-1096

KOHLER CO

WISCONSIN CLAIMS OFFICE
444 HIGHLAND DR
KOHLER, WI 53044-1544
TEL: (920) 457-4441
FAX: (920) 457-0669
TOLL FREE: (800) 456-1675

L.I.U. OF NORTH AMERICA LOCAL 415

NEW JERSEY CLAIMS OFFICE
45 E WASHINGTON AVE
PLEASANTVILLE, NJ 08232-2749
TEL: (609) 646-4138
FAX: (609) 646-1419
E-MAIL: BENEFIT415@AOL.COM

L.P.C.W.I.F.

MICHIGAN CLAIMS OFFICE
5750 15-MILE RD, STE 12
STERLING HEIGHTS, MI 48310
TEL: (810) 954-3540
FAX: (810) 954-3668

LABORERS HEALTH & WELFARE FUNDS

CALIFORNIA CLAIMS OFFICE
4401 SANTA ANITA AVE
PO BOX 8024
EL MONTE, CA 91734-2324
TEL: (626) 442-4500
FAX: (626) 448-7111
TOLL FREE: (800) 887-5679

LABORERS LOCAL 190 WELFARE FUND

NEW YORK CLAIMS OFFICE
668 WEMPLE RD
PO BOX 339
GLENMONT, NY 12077-0339
TEL: (518) 465-1376
FAX: (518) 465-1379

LAFAYETTE LIFE INSURANCE CO

INDIANA CLAIMS OFFICE
1905 TEAL RD
PO BOX 7007
LAFAYETTE, IN 47903-7007
TEL: (765) 477-7411
FAX: (765) 477-3349
TOLL FREE: (800) 443-8793

LAMAR LIFE

ALABAMA CLAIMS OFFICE
PO BOX 66978
CHICAGO, IL 60666-0978
FAX: (312) 396-7911
TOLL FREE: (800) 258-5542

ARKANSAS CLAIMS OFFICE
PO BOX 66978
CHICAGO, IL 60666-0978
FAX: (312) 396-7911
TOLL FREE: (800) 258-5542

CALIFORNIA CLAIMS OFFICE
PO BOX 66978
CHICAGO, IL 60666-0978
FAX: (312) 396-7911
TOLL FREE: (800) 258-5542

FLORIDA CLAIMS OFFICE
PO BOX 66978
CHICAGO, IL 60666-0978
FAX: (312) 396-7911
TOLL FREE: (800) 258-5542

GEORGIA CLAIMS OFFICE
PO BOX 66978
CHICAGO, IL 60666-0978
FAX: (312) 396-7911
TOLL FREE: (800) 258-5542

ILLINOIS CLAIMS OFFICE
PO BOX 66978
CHICAGO, IL 60666-0978
FAX: (312) 396-7911
TOLL FREE: (800) 258-5542

IOWA CLAIMS OFFICE
PO BOX 66978
CHICAGO, IL 60666-0978
FAX: (312) 396-7911
TOLL FREE: (800) 258-5542

KENTUCKY CLAIMS OFFICE
PO BOX 66978
CHICAGO, IL 60666-0978
FAX: (312) 396-7911
TOLL FREE: (800) 258-5542

LOUISIANA CLAIMS OFFICE
PO BOX 66978
CHICAGO, IL 60666-0978
FAX: (312) 396-7911
TOLL FREE: (800) 258-5542

MISSISSIPPI CLAIMS OFFICE
PO BOX 66978
CHICAGO, IL 60666-0978
FAX: (312) 396-7911
TOLL FREE: (800) 258-5542

OKLAHOMA CLAIMS OFFICE
PO BOX 66978
CHICAGO, IL 60666-0978
FAX: (312) 396-7911
TOLL FREE: (800) 258-5542

TENNESSEE CLAIMS OFFICE
PO BOX 66978
CHICAGO, IL 60666-0978
FAX: (312) 396-7911
TOLL FREE: (800) 258-5542

TEXAS CLAIMS OFFICE
PO BOX 66978
CHICAGO, IL 60666-0978
FAX: (312) 396-7911
TOLL FREE: (800) 258-5542

LAMAR LIFE INSURANCE

ILLINOIS CLAIMS OFFICE
CONSECO
222 MERCHANDISE MART PLZ
PO BOX 66978
CHICAGO, IL 60666-0978
TEL: (312) 396-7500
FAX: (312) 396-7911
TOLL FREE: (800) 258-5542

MISSISSIPPI CLAIMS OFFICE
222 MERCHANDISE MART PLZ
PO BOX 66978
CHICAGO, IL 60666
FAX: (312) 396-7910
TOLL FREE: (800) 258-5542
IN-STATE: (800) 521-5542

LANCER CLAIM SERVICE CORP

CALIFORNIA CLAIMS OFFICE
333 CITY BLVD W
PO BOX 7048
ORANGE, CA 92863
TEL: (714) 939-0700
FAX: (714) 978-8023
TOLL FREE: (800) 821-0540
IN-STATE: (800) 645-5324

LANCER CORP

TEXAS CLAIMS OFFICE
6655 LANCER BLVD
SAN ANTONIO, TX 78219
TEL: (210) 310-7000
FAX: (210) 310-7183
TOLL FREE: (800) 729-1500

LANDMARK HEALTH CARE

CALIFORNIA CLAIMS OFFICE
1750 HOWE AVE, STE 300
SACRAMENTO, CA 95825
TEL: (916) 646-3477
FAX: (916) 929-8350
TOLL FREE: (800) 638-4557
WWW.LANDMARKHEALTHCARE.COM

LASALLE CLINIC

WISCONSIN CLAIMS OFFICE
1165 APPLETON RD
PO BOX 8005
MENASHA, WI 54952-8005
TEL: (920) 727-4200
FAX: (920) 727-7637
TOLL FREE: (800) 236-1338

LAWRENCE E. SMITH & ASSOCIATES, INC

MISSOURI CLAIMS OFFICE
1819 CLARKSON RD, STE 300
PO BOX 411216
SAINT LOUIS, MO 63141-1216
TEL: (636) 532-1660
FAX: (636) 532-1737
TOLL FREE: (800) 325-1350

LEMARS MUTUAL INSURANCE CO OF IOWA

IOWA CLAIMS OFFICE
1 PARK LN
PO BOX 1608
LE MARS, IA 51031-1608
TEL: (712) 546-7847
FAX: (712) 546-9648
TOLL FREE: (800) 545-6480
IN-STATE: (800) 352-4945

LEWER AGENCY, INC

NATIONAL CLAIMS OFFICE
4534 WORNALL RD
KANSAS CITY, MO 64111-3211
TEL: (816) 753-4390
FAX: (816) 561-6840
TOLL FREE: (800) 821-7715
WWW.LEWER.COM

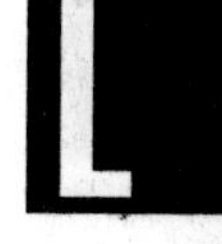

LEXINGTON INSURANCE CO

MASSACHUSETTS CLAIMS OFFICE
200 STATE ST
BOSTON, MA 02109-2694
TEL: (617) 330-1100
FAX: (617) 439-9793
TOLL FREE: (800) 355-4891

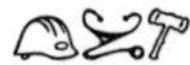

LIBERTY LIFE INSURANCE CO

INDIANA CLAIMS OFFICE
420 HURSTBOURNE LN, STE 203
PO BOX 24348
LOUISVILLE, KY 40224
TEL: (502) 327-9591
FAX: (502) 327-8891
TOLL FREE: (800) 230-8474

KENTUCKY CLAIMS OFFICE
1510 NEW TOWN PIKE, STE A
PO BOX 11668
LEXINGTON, KY 40577
TEL: (606) 255-7959
FAX: (606) 253-3124
TOLL FREE: (800) 230-8480

3716 CAMBERLAIN FALLS HWY
CORBIN, KY 40702
TEL: (606) 528-5808

420 HURSTBOURNE LN, STE 203
PO BOX 24348
LOUISVILLE, KY 40224
TEL: (502) 327-9591
FAX: (502) 327-8891
TOLL FREE: (800) 230-8474

LOUISIANA CLAIMS OFFICE
MAGNOLIA LIFE INSURANCE
2000 WADE HAMPTON BLVD
BOX 789
GREENVILLE, SC 29602
TEL: (864) 609-4770
FAX: (864) 609-4172

SOUTH CAROLINA CLAIMS OFFICE
2000 WADE HAMPTON BLVD
PO BOX 789
GREENVILLE, SC 29602
TEL: (864) 609-8111
FAX: (864) 609-8084
WWW.LIBERTY.COM

LIBERTY MUTUAL

NATIONAL CLAIMS OFFICE
30200 TELEGRAPH RD
PO BOX 33430
DETROIT, MI 48232-5430
TEL: (248) 901-6002
FAX: (248) 901-1742
TOLL FREE: (800) 431-7464
IN-STATE: (800) 572-7390

LIBERTY MUTUAL GROUP

NEW HAMPSHIRE CLAIMS OFFICE
10 CORPORATE DR, STE 100
BEDFORD, NH 03110-5954
TEL: (603) 472-7100
FAX: (603) 472-6910
TOLL FREE: (800) 562-3936
WWW.LIBERTYMUTUAL.COM

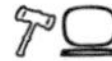

NEW YORK CLAIMS OFFICE
80 GRASSLANDS RD
PO BOX 1207
ELMSFORD, NY 10523-0907
TEL: (914) 347-5200
FAX: (914) 347-6776
TOLL FREE: (800) 245-1700
IN-STATE: (800) 422-0820
WWW.LIBERTYMUTUAL.COM

LIBERTY MUTUAL INSURANCE

ALABAMA CLAIMS OFFICE
1200 CORPORATE DR, STE 100
PO BOX 530605
BIRMINGHAM, AL 35253
TEL: (205) 995-9883
FAX: (205) 995-9458
TOLL FREE: (800) 292-6226
WWW.LIBERTYMUTUAL.COM

ARIZONA CLAIMS OFFICE
2510 W DUNLAP AVE, STE 300
PO BOX 35920
PHOENIX, AZ 85021
TEL: (602) 997-4700
FAX: (602) 997-4755
TOLL FREE: (800) 541-7698
WWW.LIBERTYMUTUAL.COM

ARKANSAS CLAIMS OFFICE
10800 FINANCIAL CTR PKY, STE 300
LITTLE ROCK, AR 72211-3568
TEL: (501) 224-4300
FAX: (501) 224-6915
TOLL FREE: (800) 482-5786
IN-STATE: (800) 482-5786
WWW.LIBERTYMUTUAL.COM

CALIFORNIA CLAIMS OFFICE
1333 E SHAW AVE
FRESNO, CA 93710
TEL: (559) 224-6110
FAX: (559) 224-9352
TOLL FREE: (800) 331-1133
WWW.LIBERTYMUTUAL.COM

3633 E INLAND EMPIRE BLVD- 5TH FL
PO BOX 51486
ONTARIO, CA 91761-0086
TEL: (909) 948-9774
FAX: (909) 987-2515
TOLL FREE: (800) 791-8213
WWW.LIBERTYMUTUAL.COM

HELSMAN MANAGEMENT SERVICE
333 CITY BLVD W, STE 300
PO BOX 11020
ORANGE, CA 92868-1026
TEL: (714) 937-1400
FAX: (714) 634-1791
TOLL FREE: (800) 303-0100

HELMSMAN SERVICES
333 CITY BLVD W, STE 300
PO BOX 11025
ORANGE, CA 92868-1026
TEL: (714) 937-1400
FAX: (714) 634-1791
TOLL FREE: (800) 303-0100

6130 STONERIDGE MALL RD, BLDG 3
PO BOX 9118
PLEASANTON, CA 94566-9118
TEL: (925) 734-9200
FAX: (925) 734-0916
TOLL FREE: (800) 303-0100
IN-STATE: (800) 343-1534
WWW.LIBERTYMUTUAL.COM

1750 HOWE AVE, STE 450
PO BOX 989000
SACRAMENTO, CA 95813-8003
TEL: (916) 564-1792
FAX: (916) 564-2059
TOLL FREE: (800) 821-0967

CONNECTICUT CLAIMS OFFICE
101 BARNES RD
PO BOX 5009
WALLINGFORD, CT 06492
TEL: (203) 294-1505
FAX: (203) 294-0674
TOLL FREE: (800) 458-3749
WWW.LIBERTYMUTUAL.COM

20 WESTERN BLVD
PO BOX 7500
GLASTONBURY, CT 06033-6508
TEL: (860) 659-4111
FAX: (860) 659-9563
TOLL FREE: (800) 245-5558
WWW.LIBERTYMUTUAL.COM

DELAWARE CLAIMS OFFICE
1 MIDDLETON DR
WILMINGTON, DE 19808
TEL: (302) 234-1800
FAX: (302) 234-2267
TOLL FREE: (800) 292-7829
WWW.LIBERTYMUTUAL.COM

FLORIDA CLAIMS OFFICE
6363 NW 6TH WAY, STE 250
PO BOX 407013
FT LAUDERDALE, FL 33340
FAX: (954) 491-4819
TOLL FREE: (800) 275-4103
WWW.LIBERTYMUTUAL.COM

3350 BUSCHWOOD PK DR
PO BOX 31204
TAMPA, FL 33631
TEL: (813) 932-2220
FAX: (813) 932-9874
TOLL FREE: (800) 282-6218
WWW.LIBERTYMUTUAL.COM

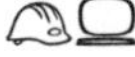

GEORGIA CLAIMS OFFICE
1750 BEAVER RUIN RD
PO BOX 2967
NORCROSS, GA 30091
TEL: (770) 564-0400
FAX: (770) 923-1450
TOLL FREE: (800) 852-8662
IN-STATE: (800) 852-6662
WWW.LIBERTYMUTUAL.COM

2875 BROWNS BRG RD
GAINESVILLE, GA 30504
TEL: (770) 536-8761
FAX: (770) 532-4598
TOLL FREE: (800) 241-9911
IN-STATE: (800) 241-1121
WWW.LIBERTYMUTUAL.COM

HAWAII CLAIMS OFFICE
1601 KAPIOLANI BLVD, STE 1020
PO BOX 30608
HONOLULU, HI 96820
TEL: (808) 979-2020
FAX: (808) 979-2167
TOLL FREE: (800) 352-5957
WWW.LIBERTYMUTUAL.COM

ILLINOIS CLAIMS OFFICE
4505 N ROCKWOOD RD
PO BOX 9340
PEORIA, IL 61612-9340
TEL: (309) 685-7625
FAX: (309) 685-3108
TOLL FREE: (800) 772-1962
IN-STATE: (800) 772-1962
WWW.LIBERTYMUTUAL.COM

7115 WINDSOR LAKE PKY
PO BOX 5013
ROCKFORD, IL 61125-0013
TEL: (815) 282-2600
FAX: (815) 282-6268
TOLL FREE: (800) 862-5757
WWW.LIBERTYMUTUAL.COM

24651 CENTER RDG RD, STE 400
CLEVELAND, OH 44145
TEL: (440) 835-5300
FAX: (440) 871-7865
TOLL FREE: (800) 582-2503
WWW.LIBERTYMUTUAL.COM

INDIANA CLAIMS OFFICE
111 CONGRESSIONAL BLVD, STE 200
PO BOX 7170
CARMEL, IN 46207
TEL: (317) 582-1700
FAX: (317) 582-1758
TOLL FREE: (800) 752-5832
WWW.LIBERTYMUTUAL.COM

24651 CENTER RDG RD, STE 400
CLEVELAND, OH 44145
TEL: (440) 835-5300
FAX: (440) 871-7865
TOLL FREE: (800) 582-2503
WWW.LIBERTYMUTUAL.COM

IOWA CLAIMS OFFICE
2829 W TOWN PARKWAY
PO BOX 10335
DES MOINES, IA 50306-0335
TEL: (515) 225-0843
FAX: (515) 225-8613
TOLL FREE: (800) 342-7011
WWW.LIBERTYMUTUAL.COM

KANSAS CLAIMS OFFICE
10561 BARKLEY ST, STE 400
PO BOX 12805
OVERLAND PARK, KS 66212-1883
TEL: (913) 648-5900
FAX: (913) 648-1856
TOLL FREE: (800) 255-0254
WWW.LIBERTYMUTUAL.COM

KENTUCKY CLAIMS OFFICE
9900 CORPORATE CAMPUS DR, STE 2000
PO BOX 37430
LOUISVILLE, KY 40233
TEL: (502) 425-8450
FAX: (502) 426-2332
TOLL FREE: (800) 292-2073
IN-STATE: (800) 430-2482
WWW.LIBERTYMUTUAL.COM

LOUISIANA CLAIMS OFFICE
COMMERCIAL MARKET CLAIMS
3850 N CSWY BLVD, STE 600
PO BOX 8510
METAIRIE, LA 70011-8510
TEL: (504) 837-7000
FAX: (504) 833-1132
IN-STATE: (800) 520-8844

MARYLAND CLAIMS OFFICE
6101 EXECUTIVE BLVD, STE 100
ROCKVILLE, MD 20852-3947
TEL: (301) 881-9300
FAX: (301) 231-5784
TOLL FREE: (800) 526-3454
IN-STATE: (800) 526-6525
WWW.LIBERTYMUTUAL.COM

MASSACHUSETTS CLAIMS OFFICE
50 DERBY ST
PO BOX 0212
HINGHAM, MA 02018-0212
TEL: (781) 740-1920
FAX: (781) 740-1369
TOLL FREE: (800) 446-4426
WWW.LIBERTYMUTUAL.COM

222 ROSEWOOD DR, 2ND FL
PO BOX 6079
DANZERS, MA 01923-9827
TEL: (978) 774-0300
FAX: (978) 750-6713
TOLL FREE: (800) 566-0323
WWW.LIBERTYMUTUAL.COM

200 LOWDER BRK DR, STE 2100
WESTWOOD, MA 02090-9212
TEL: (781) 326-7100
FAX: (781) 326-2923
TOLL FREE: (800) 762-5026
WWW.LIBERTYMUTUAL.COM

MICHIGAN CLAIMS OFFICE
2450 44TH ST SE
KENTWOOD, MI 49512
TEL: (616) 455-1700
FAX: (616) 455-2623
TOLL FREE: (800) 470-3811
IN-STATE: (800) 632-9567
WWW.LIBERTYMUTUAL.COM

24651 CENTER RDG RD, STE 400
CLEVELAND, OH 44145
TEL: (440) 835-5300
FAX: (440) 871-7865
TOLL FREE: (800) 582-2503
WWW.LIBERTYMUTUAL.COM

MINNESOTA CLAIMS OFFICE
1660 S HWY 100, STE 400
MINNEAPOLIS, MN 55416
TEL: (612) 546-7550
FAX: (612) 593-9334
TOLL FREE: (800) 328-0705
WWW.LIBERTYMUTUAL.COM

MISSISSIPPI CLAIMS OFFICE
795 WOODLANDS PKY, STE 210
PO BOX 12575
RIDGELAND, MS 39157
TEL: (601) 977-0814
FAX: (601) 957-1097
TOLL FREE: (800) 872-4232
WWW.LIBERTYMUTUAL.COM

MISSOURI CLAIMS OFFICE
12250 WEBBER HILL RD
SAINT LOUIS, MO 63127-1599
TEL: (314) 843-0600
FAX: (314) 843-1240
IN-STATE: (800) 392-9223
WWW.LIBERTYMUTUAL.COM

NEBRASKA CLAIMS OFFICE
9290 W DODGE RD, STE 405
OMAHA, NE 68104
TEL: (402) 393-4041
FAX: (402) 392-2321
TOLL FREE: (800) 462-0015
WWW.LIBERTYMUTUAL.COM

NEW JERSEY CLAIMS OFFICE
701 RT 73 S, STE 201
PO BOX 993
MARLTON, NJ 08053-0993
TEL: (609) 596-2234
FAX: (609) 596-4280
TOLL FREE: (800) 486-6152
WWW.LIBERTYMUTUAL.COM

PARK EIGHTY PLZ E
SADDLE BROOK, NJ 07663
TEL: (201) 845-4300
FAX: (201) 845-6746
TOLL FREE: (800) 746-7430
WWW.LIBERTYMUTUAL.COM

100 FRANKLIN SQ DR
PO BOX 6804
SOMERSET, NJ 08873
TEL: (732) 563-6800
FAX: (732) 805-9647
TOLL FREE: (800) 746-7428
WWW.LIBERTYMUTUAL.COM

NEW YORK CLAIMS OFFICE
3 LEAR JET LN
PO BOX 15041
ALBANY, NY 12212-5041
TEL: (518) 782-2541
FAX: (518) 782-2556
TOLL FREE: (800) 252-5730
WWW.LIBERTYMUTUAL.COM

2950 EXPRESS DR S, STE 100
PO BOX 490
ISLANDIA, NY 11722
TEL: (516) 232-3500
FAX: (516) 232-6946
TOLL FREE: (800) 445-0446
IN-STATE: (800) 445-0446
WWW.LIBERTYMUTUAL.COM

5015 CAMPUS WOOD DR
PO BOX 4836
SYRACUSE, NY 13221-4836
TEL: (315) 433-1144
FAX: (315) 433-9850
TOLL FREE: (800) 962-5157
IN-STATE: (800) 962-5157
WWW.LIBERTYMUTUAL.COM

325 ESSJAY RD
PO BOX 9030
WILLIAMSVILLE, NY 14231-9030
TEL: (716) 631-9140
FAX: (716) 631-9173
TOLL FREE: (800) 457-9140

NORTH CAROLINA CLAIMS OFFICE
8514 MCALPINE PARK DR, STE 200
PO BOX 25333
CHARLOTTE, NC 28229-5333
TEL: (704) 362-2208
FAX: (704) 365-4379
TOLL FREE: (800) 532-7706
WWW.LIBERTYMUTUAL.COM

OHIO CLAIMS OFFICE
TOWERS OF KINWOOD
8044 MONTGOMERY RD, STE 650
CINCINNATI, OH 45236
TEL: (513) 984-0550
FAX: (513) 984-9369
IN-STATE: (800) 441-9185
WWW.LIBERTYMUTUAL.COM

24651 CENTER RDG RD, STE 400
CLEVELAND, OH 44145
TEL: (440) 835-5300
FAX: (440) 871-7865
TOLL FREE: (800) 582-2503
WWW.LIBERTYMUTUAL.COM

OKLAHOMA CLAIMS OFFICE
3503 NW 63RD ST, STE 500
OKLAHOMA CITY, OK 73116-2203
TEL: (405) 848-8921
FAX: (405) 843-3435
TOLL FREE: (800) 522-9243
WWW.LIBERTYMUTUAL.COM

PENNSYLVANIA CLAIMS OFFICE
15 KINGS GRANT DR
PO BOX 3632
BALA CYNWYD, PA 19004-1715
TEL: (215) 839-6600
FAX: (610) 660-9051
TOLL FREE: (800) 300-4472
IN-STATE: (800) 300-4472
WWW.LIBERTYMUTUAL.COM

15 KINGS GRANT DR
PO BOX 3632
BALA CYNWYD, PA 19004-1715
TEL: (215) 839-6600
FAX: (610) 660-9051
TOLL FREE: (800) 300-4472
IN-STATE: (800) 300-4472
WWW.LIBERTYMUTUAL.COM

18 SENTRY PARKWEST, STE 200
PO BOX 3051
BLUE BELL, PA 19422
TEL: (215) 641-0400
FAX: (215) 641-4819
TOLL FREE: (800) 345-6222
IN-STATE: (800) 362-5698
WWW.LIBERTYMUTUAL.COM

625 CHERRINGTON PKY
CORAOPOLIS, PA 15108-4300
TEL: (412) 269-1900
FAX: (412) 269-8930
TOLL FREE: (800) 227-2859
WWW.LIBERTYMUTUAL.COM

2501 WILMINGTON RD
NEW CASTLE, PA 16105
TEL: (724) 658-3771
FAX: (724) 652-7224
TOLL FREE: (800) 245-1284
IN-STATE: (800) 245-1700
WWW.LIBERTYMUTUAL.COM

QUEBEC CLAIMS OFFICE
3333 PL CAVENDISH, STE 105
SAINT LAURENT, PQ H4M-2X6
TEL: (514) 335-6660
FAX: (514) 335-6060
TOLL FREE: (800) 731-6660
WWW.LIBERTYMUTUAL.COM

RHODE ISLAND CLAIMS OFFICE
245 WATERMAN ST
PO BOX 9761
PROVIDENCE, RI 02940
TEL: (401) 351-2200
FAX: (401) 351-1729
TOLL FREE: (800) 225-2390
IN-STATE: (800) 422-4718
WWW.LIBERTYMUTUAL.COM

SOUTH CAROLINA CLAIMS OFFICE
100 CENTER POINT CIR, STE 220
PO BOX 2521
COLUMBIA, SC 29202-2521
TEL: (803) 731-0830
FAX: (803) 772-6876
TOLL FREE: (800) 922-3305
WWW.LIBERTYMUTUAL.COM

TENNESSEE CLAIMS OFFICE
5301 VIRGINIA WAY STE 200
PO BOX 300
BRENTWOOD, TN 37024-0300
TEL: (615) 373-9555
FAX: (615) 371-9538
TOLL FREE: (800) 523-6906

2100 STEIN RD
PO BOX 182263
CHATTANOOGA, TN 37411
TEL: (423) 894-2620
FAX: (423) 490-8575
TOLL FREE: (800) 238-3428
WWW.LIBERTYMUTUAL.COM

TEXAS CLAIMS OFFICE
13201 NW FWY, STE 400
PO BOX 40914
HOUSTON, TX 77240
TEL: (713) 460-4650
FAX: (713) 895-8419
TOLL FREE: (800) 533-3170
IN-STATE: (800) 533-3170

2120 WALNUT HILL LN, STE 220
PO BOX 168368
IRVING, TX 75016-8368
TEL: (972) 550-7899
FAX: (972) 714-0850
TOLL FREE: (800) 313-8844
WWW.LIBERTYMUTUAL.COM

UTAH CLAIMS OFFICE
2735 E PARLEY'S WAY, STE 203
PO BOX 45440
SALT LAKE CITY, UT 84102
TEL: (801) 463-7368
FAX: (801) 463-6076
TOLL FREE: (800) 634-4201
WWW.LIBERTYMUTUAL.COM

VERMONT CLAIMS OFFICE
1795 WILLISTON RD
PO BOX 9280
SOUTH BURLINGTON, VT 05407-9280
TEL: (802) 864-0281
FAX: (802) 863-6207
TOLL FREE: (800) 332-0274
WWW.LIBERTYMUTUAL.COM

VIRGINIA CLAIMS OFFICE
4101 COX RD, STE 200
PO BOX 85198
RICHMOND, VA 23261
TEL: (804) 270-6222
FAX: (804) 747-7301
TOLL FREE: (800) 468-6634
WWW.LIBERTYMUTUAL.COM

WASHINGTON CLAIMS OFFICE
14711 NE 29TH PL, STE 101
PO BOX 7149
BELLEVUE, WA 98008
TEL: (425) 861-4441
FAX: (425) 861-5632
TOLL FREE: (800) 542-0814
WWW.LIBERTYMUTUAL.COM

WEST VIRGINIA CLAIMS OFFICE
24651 CENTER RDG RD, STE 400
CLEVELAND, OH 44145
TEL: (440) 835-5300
FAX: (440) 871-7865
TOLL FREE: (800) 582-2503
WWW.LIBERTYMUTUAL.COM

WISCONSIN CLAIMS OFFICE
15700 W BLUEMOUND RD
PO BOX 0915
BROOKFIELD, WI 53008-0915
TEL: (414) 782-9500
FAX: (414) 782-5682
TOLL FREE: (800) 242-5838
WWW.LIBERTYMUTUAL.COM

LIBERTY NORTHWEST

OREGON CLAIMS OFFICE
ONE LIBERTY CENTRE
PO BOX 5255
PORTLAND, OR 97208
TEL: (503) 239-5800
FAX: (503) 239-4108
TOLL FREE: (800) 275-5600
WWW.LIBERTYNORTHWEST.COM

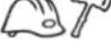

LIFE & HEALTH INSURANCE CO OF AMERICA

NATIONAL CLAIMS OFFICE
2200 WALNUT ST
PHILADELPHIA, PA 19103
TEL: (215) 567-1246
FAX: (215) 567-6444
TOLL FREE: (800) 458-7493
WWW.LIFE-HEALTHAMERICA.COM

LIFE INSURANCE CO OF ALABAMA

ALABAMA CLAIMS OFFICE
310 BROAD ST
PO BOX 349
GADSDEN, AL 35902-0349
TEL: (256) 543-2022
TOLL FREE: (800) 226-2371

LIFE INSURANCE CO OF GEORGIA

ADMINISTRATIVE OFFICES
4850 STREET RD
PO BOX 3013
LANGHORNE, PA 19047-9113
TOLL FREE: (800) 877-7756

LIFE INSURANCE CO OF MISSISSIPPI

MISSISSIPPI CLAIMS OFFICE
715 S PEAR ORCHARD RD, STE 400
PO BOX 6005
RIDGELAND, MS 39158-6005
TEL: (601) 978-6732
FAX: (601) 978-6722
TOLL FREE: (800) 748-8774

LIFE INSURANCE CO OF NORTH AMERICA

NATIONAL CLAIMS OFFICE
CIGNA
255 EAST AVE
ROCHESTER, NY 14604
TEL: (716) 258-1744
FAX: (716) 258-1780
TOLL FREE: (800) 532-9288

LIFE INVESTOR INSURANCE CO OF AMERICA

ARKANSAS CLAIMS OFFICE
1020 W 4TH ST
PO BOX 8063
LITTLE ROCK, AR 72203-8063
TEL: (501) 376-0426
FAX: (501) 371-3196
TOLL FREE: (800) 251-7254

LIFE INVESTORS

IOWA CLAIMS OFFICE
4333 EDGEWOOD RD NE
CEDAR RAPIDS, IA 52499-0001
TEL: (319) 398-8511
TOLL FREE: (800) 347-7082

LIFE INVESTORS INSURANCE CO OF AMERICA

BANKERS UNITED LIFE ASSURANCE CO
815 TRAILWOOD, STE 205
PO BOX 982012
NORTH RICHLAND HILLS, TX 76182-8012
FAX: (817) 285-3030
TOLL FREE: (800) 347-7082

TEXAS CLAIMS OFFICE
BANKERS UNITED LIFE ASSURANCE CO
815 TRAILWOOD, STE 205
PO BOX 982012
NORTH RICHLAND HILLS, TX 76182-8012
FAX: (817) 285-3030
TOLL FREE: (800) 347-7082

LIFE OF AMERICA INSURANCE CO

LIFE OF AMERICA & REPUBLIC AMERICAN
8200 BROOKRIVER DR, STE 600N
DALLAS, TX 75247-3831
TEL: (214) 631-6310
FAX: (214) 638-6431
TOLL FREE: (800) 876-8776

LIFE OF THE SOUTH SERVICE CO

NATIONAL CLAIMS OFFICE
100 W BAY ST, STE 200
PO BOX 44130
JACKSONVILLE, FL 32231-4130
TEL: (904) 350-9600
FAX: (904) 359-2041
TOLL FREE: (800) 888-2738
WWW.LIFE-SOUTH.COM

LIFE REINSURANCE CO

TEXAS CLAIMS OFFICE
800 NW LOOP 410, STE 600 N
PO BOX 792070
SAN ANTONIO, TX 78209-2070
TEL: (210) 357-1000
FAX: (210) 357-1020
TOLL FREE: (800) 229-1024
IN-STATE: (800) 229-1024

LIFEGUARD, INC

CALIFORNIA CLAIMS OFFICE
2840 JUNCTION AVE
SAN JOSE, CA 95134
TEL: (408) 943-9400
FAX: (408) 383-4309
TOLL FREE: (800) 995-0380
WWW.LIFEGUARD.COM

LIFEWISE A PREMERA HEALTH PLAN, INC

OREGON CLAIMS OFFICE
1133 NW WALL ST
PO BOX 7709
BEND, OR 97708-7709
TEL: (541) 388-3307
FAX: (541) 318-2309
TOLL FREE: (800) 777-1502
WWW.PREMERA.COM/LIFEWISE

LINCOLN MUTUAL LIFE & CASUALTY INSURANCE CO

NORTH DAKOTA CLAIMS OFFICE
203 N 10TH ST
PO BOX 1918
FARGO, ND 58107-1918
TEL: (701) 282-1807
FAX: (701) 282-1840
TOLL FREE: (800) 325-6915
IN-STATE: (800) 947-4084
WWW.LML.COM

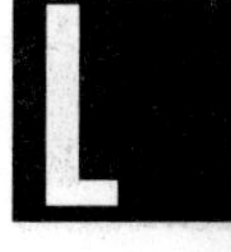

LOCAL 1245 HEALTH FUND
NEW JERSEY CLAIMS OFFICE
170 CHANGE BRG RD- UNIT C6
PO BOX 426
MONTVILLE, NJ 07045-9113
TEL: (973) 882-2900
FAX: (973) 882-1408

LOCAL 138 WELFARE FUND
NEW YORK CLAIMS OFFICE
PO BOX 206
FARMINGDALE, NY 11735-0206
TEL: (516) 694-2140
FAX: (516) 694-7831

LOCAL 318 HEALTH & WELFARE
129-09 26TH AVE
FLUSHING, NY 11354-1931
TEL: (718) 961-3400
FAX: (718) 461-8059

LOCAL 338 HEALTH & WELFARE FUND
97-45 QUEENS BLVD
REGO PARK, NY 11374-2101
TEL: (718) 997-7400
FAX: (718) 997-0821

LOCAL 342 INSURANCE TRUST
501 WILLIAM FLOYD PKY
SHIRLEY, NY 11967-3417
TEL: (516) 395-0600
FAX: (516) 395-1943

LOCAL 365 UAW WELFARE FUND
30-07 39TH AVE
LONG ISLAND CITY, NY 11101
TEL: (718) 392-3600
FAX: (718) 361-9381

LOCAL 802 MUSICIANS HEALTH BENEFIT
322 W 48TH ST
NEW YORK, NY 10036-1308
TEL: (212) 245-4802
FAX: (212) 245-6255

LOCAL UNION 164 IBEW JOINT WELFARE
NEW JERSEY CLAIMS OFFICE
65 W CENTURY RD
PARAMUS, NJ 07652
TEL: (201) 225-1641

LOCAL UNION NO 682 HEALTH & WELFARE
MISSOURI CLAIMS OFFICE
5730 ELIZABETH AVE
SAINT LOUIS, MO 63110-2802
TEL: (314) 647-8350

LOCALS 302 & 612 INTERNATIONAL
WASHINGTON CLAIMS OFFICE
WELFARE & PENSION ADMIN SERV
2815 SECOND AVE #300
PO BOX 34684
SEATTLE, WA 98124-1203
TEL: (206) 441-7574
FAX: (206) 441-9110
TOLL FREE: (800) 331-6158
IN-STATE: (800)732-1121
WWW.WPAS-INC.COM

LOMA LINDA UNIVERSITY ADVENTIST HEALTH SCIENCES CENTER
CALIFORNIA CLAIMS OFFICE
11161 ANDERSON ST, STE 200
PO BOX 1770
LOMA LINDA, CA 92354-0570
TEL: (909) 824-4386
FAX: (909) 824-4775

LONDON LIFE REINSURANCE
PENNSYLVANIA CLAIMS OFFICE
1787 CENTURY PKY W, STE 420
PO BOX 1120
BLUE BELL, PA 19422
TEL: (215) 542-7200
FAX: (215) 542-1295
TOLL FREE: (800) 220-1110
WWW.LONDONLIFE.COM

LONE STAR LIFE INSURANCE CO
TEXAS CLAIMS OFFICE
16980 DALLAS PKY
PO BOX 709009
DALLAS, TX 75370-9009
TEL: (972) 447-6614
FAX: (972) 447-6410
TOLL FREE: (800) 743-0122
E-MAIL: LSLCLMS2@DFW.NET

LOOMIS CO
NATIONAL CLAIMS OFFICE
850 PARK RD N
PO BOX 7011
WYOMISSING, PA 19610
TEL: (610) 374-4040
FAX: (610) 374-6986
TOLL FREE: (800) 782-0392
E-MAIL: LOOMIS@LOOMISCO.COM
WWW.LOOMISCO.COM

LOS ANGELES COUNTY FIRE FIGHTERS LOCAL 1014
CALIFORNIA CLAIMS OFFICE
10824 SAINT JAMES AVE
SOUTH GATE, CA 90280-7199
TEL: (310) 898-3732
FAX: (310) 631-8139
IN-STATE: (800) 660-1014

LOUISIANA FARM BUREAU MUTUAL INSURANCE CO
LOUISIANA CLAIMS OFFICE
9516 AIRLINE HWY
PO BOX 95005
BATON ROUGE, LA 70895-9005
TEL: (225) 922-6200
FAX: (225) 922-6429

LOVE BOX CO
KANSAS CLAIMS OFFICE
C/O WILLIS CORROON CORP OF KS
300 W DOUGLAS, 8TH FL
PO BOX 2697
WICHITA, KS 67202
TEL: (316) 264-5311
FAX: (316) 832-3539
TOLL FREE: (800) 937-5229
WWW.LOVEBOX.COM

LOVELACE HEALTH PLAN, INC
NEW MEXICO CLAIMS OFFICE
4101 INDIAN SCHOOL RD 5200
PO BOX 27107
ALBUQUERQUE, NM 87108
TEL: (505) 262-7363
FAX: (505) 262-3806
TOLL FREE: (800) 808-7363
WWW.LOVELACE.COM

LOYAL AMERICAN LIFE INSURANCE CO
ALABAMA CLAIMS OFFICE
2800 DAUEHIN ST
PO BOX 6959
MOBILE, AL 36660
TEL: (334) 470-6562
FAX: (334) 470-6424
TOLL FREE: (800) 752-7818
IN-STATE: (800) 624-6660

NATIONAL CLAIMS OFFICE
2800 DAUEHIN ST
PO BOX 6959
MOBILE, AL 36660-0959
TEL: (334) 470-6439
FAX: (334) 470-6424
TOLL FREE: (800) 752-7818
IN-STATE: (800) 624-6660

LUFKIN INDUSTRIES, INC
TEXAS CLAIMS OFFICE
423 JEFFERSON ST
PO BOX 849
LUFKIN, TX 75902-0849
TEL: (409) 637-5347
FAX: (409) 637-5475
WWW.LUFKIN.COM

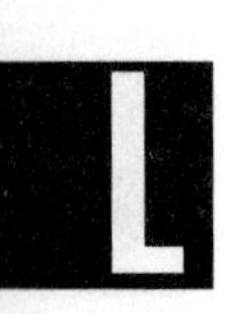

LUKAS INSURANCE CO
MASSACHUSETTS CLAIMS OFFICE
155 MAPLE ST, STE 406
SPRINGFIELD, MA 01105-1828
TEL: (413) 736-4534
FAX: (413) 737-4772
TOLL FREE: (800) 446-3495

LUMBER INSURANCE COMPANIES
ONE SPEEN ST
PO BOX 9165
FRAMINGHAM, MA 01701
TEL: (508) 872-8111
FAX: (508) 872-7968
TOLL FREE: (800) 557-1117
WWW.LUMBERINS.COM

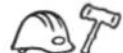

LUMBERMEN'S MUTUAL CASUALTY CO
ILLINOIS CLAIMS OFFICE
KEMPER INSURANCE
ONE KEMPER DR
LONG GROVE, IL 60049-0001
TEL: (847) 320-2000
FAX: (847) 320-2494
TOLL FREE: (800) 833-0355
WWW.KEMPERINSURANCE.COM

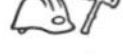

LUTHERAN BROTHERHOOD INSURANCE CO
MINNESOTA CLAIMS OFFICE
625 4TH AVE S
MINNEAPOLIS, MN 55415-1624
TEL: (612) 340-7000
FAX: (612) 340-8682
TOLL FREE: (800) 990-6290
WWW.LUTHBRO.COM

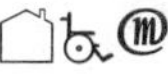

LYNDON INSURANCE CO
MISSOURI CLAIMS OFFICE
520 MARYVILLE CENTER DR, STE 500
SAINT LOUIS, MO 63141
TEL: (314) 275-5200
FAX: (314) 275-5230
TOLL FREE: (800) 288-6060

M.S.I. INSURANCE
MINNESOTA CLAIMS OFFICE
2 PINE TREE DR
PO BOX 64035
SAINT PAUL, MN 55164-0035
TEL: (651) 631-7000
FAX: (651) 631-7460
TOLL FREE: (800) 345-2436
WWW.MSI-INSURANCE.COM

M-CARE ADMINISTRATION
MICHIGAN CLAIMS OFFICE
2301 COMMONWEALTH BLVD
PO BOX 130799
ANN ARBOR, MI 48113-0799
TEL: (734) 747-8700
TOLL FREE: (800) 527-5549

M-PLAN
INDIANA CLAIMS OFFICE
8802 N MERIDIAN ST, STE 100
INDIANAPOLIS, IN 46260-5318
TEL: (317) 571-5300
FAX: (317) 705-3119
TOLL FREE: (800) 878-8802

MACHIGONNE BENEFIT ADMINISTRATORS
MAINE CLAIMS OFFICE
110 FREE ST
PO BOX 3859
PORTLAND, ME 04104-3859
TEL: (207) 822-5855
FAX: (207) 822-5888
TOLL FREE: (800) 245-3529
IN-STATE: (800) 585-6150

MADISON NATIONAL LIFE INSURANCE CO, INC
WISCONSIN CLAIMS OFFICE
6120 UNIVERSITY AVE
PO BOX 5008
MADISON, WI 53705
TEL: (608) 238-2691
FAX: (608) 238-7028
TOLL FREE: (800) 356-9601
E-MAIL: MNLMADISN#@AOL.COM

MAGINNIS & ASSOCIATES, INC
ILLINOIS CLAIMS OFFICE
332 S MICHIGAN AVE
CHICAGO, IL 60604-4301
TEL: (312) 427-1441
FAX: (312) 427-7847
TOLL FREE: (800) 621-3008
WWW.MAGINNIS.COM

MAIL HANDLERS BENEFIT PLAN
FLORIDA CLAIMS OFFICE
PO BOX 45118
JACKSONVILLE, FL 32232-5118
FAX: (602) 668-2554
TOLL FREE: (800) 410-7778
WWW.MHBP.COM

MARYLAND CLAIMS OFFICE
PO BOX 45118
JACKSONVILLE, FL 32232-5118
FAX: (602) 668-2554
TOLL FREE: (800) 410-7778
WWW.MHBP.COM

MAINE BONDING & CASUALTY CO
CONNECTICUT CLAIMS OFFICE
ZURICH GROUP
500 ENTERPRISE DR
PO BOX 150410
HARTFORD, CT 06102
TEL: (860) 257-6700
FAX: (860) 257-6582
TOLL FREE: (800) 257-6500

MAJESTIC UNDERWRITERS, INC
MICHIGAN CLAIMS OFFICE
550 STEPHENSON HWY, STE 407
TROY, MI 48083
TEL: (248) 583-4488
FAX: (248) 583-0904
TOLL FREE: (800) 428-8460

MAKSIN MANAGEMENT CORP
NEW JERSEY CLAIMS OFFICE
KEVON OFFFICE BLDG, STE 160
2500 MCCLELLAN AVE
PENNSAUKEN, NJ 08109-4613
TEL: (609) 486-7400
FAX: (609) 486-7228
TOLL FREE: (800) 257-6250
E-MAIL: MAKSIN@MAKSIN.COM
WWW.MAKSIN.COM

MANAGED BENEFIT ADMINISTRATORS
NATIONAL CLAIMS OFFICE
2868 PROSPECT PARK DR, STE 600
PO BOX 873
RANCHO CORDOVA, CA 95812-0873
TEL: (916) 631-1225
FAX: (916) 636-9705
TOLL FREE: (800) 888-1801

MANAGED BENEFIT ADMINISTRATORS, INC
OKLAHOMA CLAIMS OFFICE
4606 S GARNETT, STE 400
TULSA, OK 74146
TEL: (918) 660-2222
FAX: (918) 660-2266
TOLL FREE: (800) 654-6437

MANAGED CARE CONSULTANTS, INC (MCC)
NEVADA CLAIMS OFFICE
4160 S PECOS RD
PO BOX 12449
LAS VEGAS, NV 89121-5025
TEL: (702) 792-2994
FAX: (702) 433-5465
TOLL FREE: (800) 748-6842

MANAGED HEALTH FUNDING, INC
CALIFORNIA CLAIMS OFFICE
PO BOX 4221
WOODLAND HILLS, CA 91365-4221
TEL: (818) 227-6446
FAX: (818) 227-6466
TOLL FREE: (800) 828-8360

M

OREGON CLAIMS OFFICE
PO BOX 4221
WOODLAND HILLS, CA 91365-4221
TEL: (818) 227-6446
FAX: (818) 227-6466
TOLL FREE: (800) 828-8360

WASHINGTON CLAIMS OFFICE
PO BOX 4221
WOODLAND HILLS, CA 91365-4221
TEL: (818) 227-6446
FAX: (818) 227-6466
TOLL FREE: (800) 828-8360

MANAGED HEALTH, INC
NEW YORK CLAIMS OFFICE
25 BROADWAY, STE 900
NEW YORK, NY 10004
FAX: (212) 801-1799
TOLL FREE: (888) 260-1010

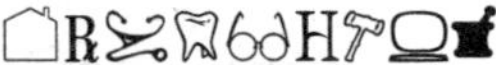

MANAGED HEALTH SERVICES INSURANCE CORP
WISCONSIN CLAIMS OFFICE
2040 W WISCONSIN, STE 452
PO BOX 2973
MILWAUKEE, WI 53201
TEL: (414) 345-4600
FAX: (414) 345-4624
TOLL FREE: (800) 547-1647

H

MANAGED HEALTHCARE CONCEPTS, INC
GEORGIA CLAIMS OFFICE
1100 SPRING ST, STE 610
PO BOX 77436
ATLANTA, GA 30357
TEL: (404) 873-4485
FAX: (404) 873-2590
TOLL FREE: (800) 736-9059

MANAGED HEALTHCARE, INC
TEXAS CLAIMS OFFICE
50 BRIAR HOLLOW, STE 500
HOUSTON, TX 77027-9406
TEL: (713) 961-4671
FAX: (713) 961-5257
TOLL FREE: (800) 635-4735

MANPOWER, INC
WISCONSIN CLAIMS OFFICE
5301 N IRONWOOD RD
PO BOX 2053
MILWAUKEE, WI 53201-2053
TEL: (414) 961-1000
FAX: (414) 906-7847

MANULIFE FINANCIAL
ONTARIO CLAIMS OFFICE
200 BLOOR ST E
TORONTO, ON M4W-1E5
TEL: (416) 926-0100
FAX: (416) 926-5454
TOLL FREE: (800) 387-2747
WWW.MANULIFE.COM

MARRIOTT INTERNATIONAL, INC
DISTRICT OF COLUMBIA CLAIMS OFFICE
1 MARRIOTT DR
WASHINGTON, DC 20058-0001
TEL: (301) 380-9000
FAX: (301) 380-3787
TOLL FREE: (800) 638-8108
WWW.MARRIOTT.COM

MARTIN'S POINT HEALTH CARE
MAINE CLAIMS OFFICE
331 VERANDA ST
PO BOX 9746
PORTLAND, ME 04104-5040
TEL: (207) 774-5801
FAX: (207) 828-2446
TOLL FREE: (800) 322-0280
WWW.MARTINSPOINT.COM

H

NEW HAMPSHIRE CLAIMS OFFICE
331 VERANDA ST
PO BOX 9746
PORTLAND, ME 04104-5040
TEL: (207) 774-5801
FAX: (207) 828-2446
TOLL FREE: (800) 322-0280
WWW.MARTINSPOINT.COM

H

MASS BENEFITS CONSULTANTS
VIRGINIA CLAIMS OFFICE
7212 POPLAR ST
PO BOX 828
ANNANDALE, VA 22003-0828
TEL: (703) 256-7800
TOLL FREE: (800) 221-3083

MASSACHUSETTS MUTUAL LIFE INSURANCE CO
MASSACHUSETTS CLAIMS OFFICE
UNICARE LIFE AND HEALTH
1350 MAIN ST
PO BOX 51130
SPRINGFIELD, MA 01151-5130
TOLL FREE: (800) 288-8630

MINNESOTA CLAIMS OFFICE
333 S 7TH ST, STE 2200
MINNEAPOLIS, MN 55402
TEL: (612) 333-1413
FAX: (612) 333-9041
TOLL FREE: (800) 272-2216
WWW.MASSINSURANCE.COM

MASSMUTUAL LIFE INSURANCE
CONNECTICUT CLAIMS OFFICE
1295 STATE ST
SPRINGFIELD, MA 01111
TEL: (413) 788-8411
FAX: (413) 744-2842
TOLL FREE: (800) 272-2216
WWW.MASSMUTUAL.COM

MASSACHUSETTS CLAIMS OFFICE
1295 STATE ST
SPRINGFIELD, MA 01111
TEL: (413) 788-8411
FAX: (413) 744-2842
TOLL FREE: (800) 272-2216
WWW.MASSMUTUAL.COM

MAURY, DONNELLY & PARR, INC
MARYLAND CLAIMS OFFICE
24 COMMERCE & WATERS ST
BALTIMORE, MD 21202
TEL: (410) 685-4625
FAX: (410) 685-3071
TOLL FREE: (800) 638-9202

MAXICARE HEALTH INSURANCE CO OF WISCONSIN
NATIONAL CLAIMS OFFICE
733 N VAN BUREN, STE 620
MILWAUKEE, WI 53202
TEL: (414) 345-4646
TOLL FREE: (800) 375-6244
WWW.MAXICARE.COM

H

MAXICARE HEALTH PLANS
PO BOX 861059
LOS ANGELES, CA 90086-1059
TEL: (213) 742-0900
FAX: (213) 365-3498
WWW.MAXICARE.COM

H

MAXICARE INDIANA
INDIANA CLAIMS OFFICE
9480 PRIORITY WAY W DR
INDIANAPOLIS, IN 46240-3899
TEL: (317) 844-5775
FAX: (317) 574-0713
IN-STATE: (800) 441-3355
WWW.MAXICARE.COM

H

MAXICARE LOUISIANA, INC
LOUISIANA CLAIMS OFFICE
1515 POYDRAS, STE 1130
NEW ORLEANS, LA 70112
TEL: (504) 523-7080
FAX: (504) 571-5974
IN-STATE: (800) 933-6294

H

MAXICARE OF NORTH CAROLINA, INC
NORTH CAROLINA CLAIMS OFFICE
5550-77 CENTER DR, STE 380
PO BOX 241228
CHARLOTTE, NC 28217
TEL: (704) 525-0880
FAX: (704) 529-0382
TOLL FREE: (800) 822-0012
IN-STATE: (800) 822-0012
WWW.MAXICARE.COM

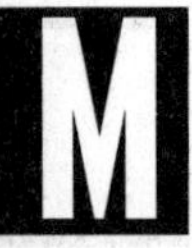

SOUTH CAROLINA CLAIMS OFFICE
5550-77 CENTER DR, STE 380
PO BOX 241228
CHARLOTTE, NC 28217
TEL: (704) 525-0880
FAX: (704) 529-0382
TOLL FREE: (800) 822-0012
IN-STATE: (800) 822-0012
WWW.MAXICARE.COM

MAYO HEALTH PLAN

MINNESOTA CLAIMS OFFICE
MAYO MANAGEMENT SERVICES, INC
21 1ST ST SW, STE 401
ROCHESTER, MN 55902
TEL: (507) 284-8274
FAX: (507) 284-0528
TOLL FREE: (800) 635-6671

MCC BEHAVIORAL CARE

CALIFORNIA CLAIMS OFFICE
801 N BRAND BLVD, STE 1150
GLENDALE, CA 91203
TEL: (818) 551-2200
FAX: (818) 551-2722
TOLL FREE: (800) 554-6931
IN-STATE: (800) 234-3596
WWW.MCC/CARE.COM

H

MCCREARY CORPORATION

FLORIDA CLAIMS OFFICE
700 CENTRAL PKY
STUART, FL 34994-3985
TEL: (561) 287-7650
FAX: (561) 287-1387
TOLL FREE: (800) 431-2221

MD INDIVIDUAL PRACTICE ASSOCIATION

MARYLAND CLAIMS OFFICE
MAMSI
4 TAFT CT
ROCKVILLE, MD 20850-5310
TEL: (301) 762-8205
TOLL FREE: (800) 544-2853
WWW.MAMSI.COM

H

MEAD CORP

OHIO CLAIMS OFFICE
WORLD HEADQUARTERS
COURTHOUSE PLZ NE
DAYTON, OH 45463
TEL: (937) 222-6323
TOLL FREE: (800) 345-6323
WWW.MEAD.COM

MEADOWBROOK INSURANCE GROUP

MICHIGAN CLAIMS OFFICE
26600 TELEGRAPH RD, STE 300
PO BOX 5086
SOUTHFIELD, MI 48086-5086
TEL: (248) 204-8563
FAX: (248) 358-3251
TOLL FREE: (800) 482-2726
IN-STATE: (800) 482-0626

MED-PAY, INC

MISSOURI CLAIMS OFFICE
1650 E BATTLEFIELD, STE 300
PO BOX 10909
SPRINGFIELD, MO 65808
TEL: (417) 886-6886
FAX: (417) 886-2276
TOLL FREE: (800) 777-9087

MEDEX ASSISTANCE CORP

MARYLAND CLAIMS OFFICE
9515 DEERECO RD- 4TH FL
PO BOX 5375
TIMONIUM, MD 21093-5375
TEL: (410) 453-6300
FAX: (410) 453-6331
TOLL FREE: (800) 537-2029
E-MAIL: MEDEXASST@AOL.COM
WWW.MEDEXASSIST.COM

MEDICA

MINNESOTA CLAIMS OFFICE
4614 MIKE COLALILLO DR
DULUTH, MN 55807
TEL: (218) 624-6500
FAX: (218) 624-6761

MEDICAID FISCAL AGENTS

ALABAMA CLAIMS OFFICE
1460 ANN ST
MONTGOMERY, AL 36107
TEL: (334) 834-3330
FAX: (334) 834-5301
IN-STATE: (800) 688-7989

ARIZONA CLAIMS OFFICE
AHCCCS ADMINISTRATION
701 E JEFFERSON
PO BOX 25520
PHOENIX, AZ 85002-9949
TEL: (602) 417-4000
FAX: (602) 253-5472
TOLL FREE: (800) 523-0231
WWW.AHCCCS.STATE.AZ.US

ARKANSAS CLAIMS OFFICE
EDS FEDERAL CORP
PO BOX 8036
LITTLE ROCK, AR 72203-2501
TEL: (501) 374-6608
FAX: (501) 374-0549
IN-STATE: (800) 457-4454
WWW.MEDICAID.STATE.AR.US.COM

COLORADO CLAIMS OFFICE
HEALTHCARE FINANCE & POLICY
700 BROADWAY
PO BOX 173300
DENVER, CO 80217-3300
TEL: (303) 831-0504
TOLL FREE: (800) 443-5747
IN-STATE: (800) 443-5747

CONNECTICUT CLAIMS OFFICE
EDS FEDERAL CORP
PO BOX 2941
HARTFORD, CT 06104-2941
TEL: (860) 832-9259
IN-STATE: (800) 842-8440

DELAWARE CLAIMS OFFICE
EDS
MANOR BRANCH
PO BOX 908
NEW CASTLE, DE 19720
TEL: (302) 454-7154
FAX: (302) 454-7603
IN-STATE: (800) 999-3371

DISTRICT OF COLUMBIA CLAIMS OFFICE
FIRST HEALTH SERVICES
4300 COX RD
PO BOX 3900
GLEN ALLEN, VA 23060
TEL: (804) 965-7400
FAX: (804) 965-7416
TOLL FREE: (800) 884-2822
WWW.FHSC.COM

GEORGIA CLAIMS OFFICE
EDS
736 PARK N BLVD
CLARKSTON, GA 30021
TEL: (404) 297-3700
FAX: (404) 298-1031
TOLL FREE: (800) 766-4456

IDAHO CLAIMS OFFICE
IDAHO STATE MEDICAID
PO BOX 23
BOISE, ID 83707
TEL: (208) 383-4310
FAX: (208) 395-2030
TOLL FREE: (800) 685-3757
IN-STATE: (800) 685-3757

ILLINOIS CLAIMS OFFICE
DEPARTMENT OF PUBLIC AID
201 S GRAND AVE E- PRESCOTT BLOOM BLDG
PO BOX 19105
SPRINGFIELD, IL 62794-9105
TEL: (217) 782-5567
FAX: (217) 524-7194

KANSAS CLAIMS OFFICE
EDS FEDERAL CORP
PO BOX 3571
TOPEKA, KS 66601
TOLL FREE: (800) 933-6593

KENTUCKY CLAIMS OFFICE
DEPT FOR MEDICAID SERVICES
275 E MAIN ST
FRANKFORT, KY 40621-0001
TEL: (502) 564-4321

LOUISIANA CLAIMS OFFICE
UNISYS CORP
8591 UNITED PLZ BLVD
PO BOX 91024
BATON ROUGE, LA 70821-9024
TEL: (504) 237-3200
TOLL FREE: (800) 473-2783

MAINE CLAIMS OFFICE
MEDICAL ASSISTANCE CLAIMS PROCESSING M500
BUREAU OF MED SVCS- 249 WESTERN AVE
AUGUSTA, ME 04333-0001
TEL: (207) 287-3081
IN-STATE: (800) 321-5557

MARYLAND CLAIMS OFFICE
201 W PRESTON ST, RM L9
PO BOX 1935
BALTIMORE, MD 21203
TEL: (410) 767-5503
FAX: (410) 333-7118
TOLL FREE: (800) 445-1159

MASSACHUSETTS CLAIMS OFFICE
UNISYS CORP
5 MIDDLESEX AVE
PO BOX 9101
SOMMERVILLE, MA 02145-9101
TEL: (617) 625-0120
FAX: (617) 576-4087
TOLL FREE: (800) 325-5231

MINNESOTA CLAIMS OFFICE
DEPT OF HUMAN SERVICES
444 LAFAYETTE
PO BOX 3849
SAINT PAUL, MN 55155-3849
TEL: (612) 296-3598
FAX: (612) 282-6744
TOLL FREE: (800) 366-5411

MISSISSIPPI CLAIMS OFFICE
EDS FEDERAL CORP
111 E CAPITOL ST, STE 400
PO BOX 23077
JACKSON, MS 39225-3077
TEL: (601) 960-2800
FAX: (601) 960-2807
TOLL FREE: (800) 884-3222

MISSOURI CLAIMS OFFICE
MISSOURI MEDICAID
PO BOX 5600
JEFFERSON CITY, MO 65102
TEL: (573) 751-2896
TOLL FREE: (800) 392-0938

MONTANA CLAIMS OFFICE
CONSULTEC, INC
PO BOX 8000
HELENA, MT 59604-8000
TEL: (406) 442-1837
FAX: (406) 442-4402
IN-STATE: (800) 624-3958
E-MAIL: CONSULTEC-IIX.COM/

NEBRASKA CLAIMS OFFICE
NEBRASKA DEPT OF HEALTH & HUMAN SVCS
PO BOX 95026
LINCOLN, NE 68509-5026
TEL: (402) 471-9147
FAX: (402) 471-9092
TOLL FREE: (800) 430-3244

NEVADA CLAIMS OFFICE
BLUE CROSS & BLUE SHIELD OF NEVADA
PO BOX 12127
RENO, NV 89510-2127
TEL: (775) 829-4020
FAX: (775) 448-8101
TOLL FREE: (800) 727-4020

NEW HAMPSHIRE CLAIMS OFFICE
EDS FEDERAL CORP
7 EAGLE SQ
PO BOX 2001
CONCORD, NH 03302-2001
TEL: (603) 224-1747
FAX: (603) 225-7964
IN-STATE: (800) 423-8303

NEW JERSEY CLAIMS OFFICE
UNISYS CORP
3705 QUAKERBRIDGE RD, STE 101
TRENTON, NJ 08619-1209
TEL: (609) 584-0200
FAX: (609) 584-8270
TOLL FREE: (800) 776-6334

NEW MEXICO CLAIMS OFFICE
CONSULTEC, I NC
1720 RANDOLPH RD, STE A
PO BOX 25700
ALBUQUERQUE, NM 87125
TEL: (505) 246-9988
FAX: (505) 246-8485
IN-STATE: (800) 282-4477

NORTH CAROLINA CLAIMS OFFICE
EDS FEDERAL CORP OF NORTH CAROLINA
4905 WATEREDGE DR
RALEIGH, NC 27606
TEL: (919) 851-8888
FAX: (919) 851-4014
TOLL FREE: (800) 688-6696

NORTH DAKOTA CLAIMS OFFICE
DEPT OF HUMAN SERVICES, MEDICAL SERVICES
600 E BLVD AVE
BISMARCK, ND 58505-0261
TEL: (701) 328-2321
FAX: (701) 328-1544
TOLL FREE: (800) 755-2604

OHIO CLAIMS OFFICE
DEPT OF HUMAN SERVICES
PO BOX 1461
COLUMBUS, OH 43266-0161
TEL: (614) 728-3288
FAX: (614) 728-3264

OKLAHOMA CLAIMS OFFICE
UNISYS CORP
201 NW 63RD, STE 100
OKLAHOMA CITY, OK 73116
TEL: (405) 841-3400
FAX: (405) 841-3510

PENNSYLVANIA CLAIMS OFFICE
DEPT OF PUBLIC WELFARE
PO BOX 2675
HARRISBURG, PA 17105-2675
TEL: (717) 787-1870
FAX: (717) 787-4639
TOLL FREE: (800) 537-8862

RHODE ISLAND CLAIMS OFFICE
STATE OF RHODE ISLAND MEDICAL SERVICES
600 NEW LONDON AVE
CRANSTON, RI 02920-3037
TEL: (401) 464-3575

SOUTH CAROLINA CLAIMS OFFICE
DHHS- PREVENTIVE CARE
PO BOX 8206
COLUMBIA, SC 29202-8206
TEL: (803) 253-6126
FAX: (803) 253-7512

SOUTH DAKOTA CLAIMS OFFICE
DEPT OF SOCIAL SERVICES- OFFICE OF MEDICAL SERVICES
700 GOVERNORS DR- KNIEP BLDG
PIERRE, SD 57501-2291
TEL: (605) 945-5006
FAX: (605) 773-5246
IN-STATE: (800) 452-7691

TENNESSEE CLAIMS OFFICE
EDS FEDERAL CORP
729 CHURCH ST
NASHVILLE, TN 42743
TEL: (615) 255-8313
FAX: (615) 254-7728
IN-STATE: (800) 821-8186

TEXAS CLAIMS OFFICE
TEXAS DEPT OF HUMAN SERVICES
NATIONAL HERITAGE INSURANCE CO
PO BOX 200555
AUSTIN, TX 78720-0555
TEL: (512) 343-4900
FAX: (512) 343-4951
TOLL FREE: (800) 873-6768

UTAH CLAIMS OFFICE
UTAH STATE DEPT MEDICAID PROCESSING
PO BOX 143106
SALT LAKE CITY, UT 84114-3106
TEL: (801) 538-6451
FAX: (801) 538-6952
TOLL FREE: (800) 662-9651
IN-STATE: (800) 662-9651

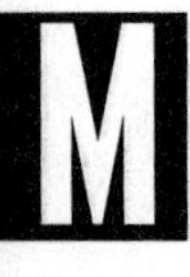

VERMONT CLAIMS OFFICE
EDS FEDERAL CORP
PO BOX 888
WILLISTON, VT 05495-0888
TEL: (802) 878-7871
FAX: (802) 878-3440
IN-STATE: (800) 925-1706

VIRGINIA CLAIMS OFFICE
FIRST HEALTH SERVICES CORP
4300 COX RD
PO BOX 3900
GLEN ALLEN, VA 23060
TEL: (804) 965-7400
FAX: (804) 965-7416
TOLL FREE: (800) 884-2822
IN-STATE: (800) 884-2822
WWW.FHSC.COM

WASHINGTON CLAIMS OFFICE
DEPT OF SOCIAL & HEALTH SERVICES
5000 CAPITAL BLVD
PO BOX 45080
DUMWATER, WA 98501
TEL: (360) 753-1777
FAX: (360) 586-6787
TOLL FREE: (800) 562-3022
IN-STATE: (800) 321-6787

WEST VIRGINIA CLAIMS OFFICE
DEPT OF HEALTH & HUMAN RESOURCES
CAPITOL COMPLEX- BLDG 6
CHARLESTON, WV 25305
TEL: (304) 926-1700
FAX: (304) 926-1776
IN-STATE: (800) 433-3019
WWW.STATE.WV.US

WISCONSIN CLAIMS OFFICE
EDS FEDERAL CORP
6406 BRIDGE RD
MADISON, WI 53784-1846
TEL: (608) 221-4746

MEDICAL ASSOCIATES HEALTH PLANS, INC

ILLINOIS CLAIMS OFFICE
700 LOCUST, STE 230
PO BOX 5002
DUBUQUE, IA 52004-5002
TEL: (319) 556-8070
FAX: (319) 556-5134
TOLL FREE: (800) 747-8900

IOWA CLAIMS OFFICE
700 LOCUST, STE 230
PO BOX 5002
DUBUQUE, IA 52004-5002
TEL: (319) 556-8070
FAX: (319) 556-5134
TOLL FREE: (800) 747-8900

WISCONSIN CLAIMS OFFICE
700 LOCUST, STE 230
PO BOX 5002
DUBUQUE, IA 52004-5002
TEL: (319) 556-8070
FAX: (319) 556-5134
TOLL FREE: (800) 747-8900

MEDICAL CENTER OF OCEAN COUNTY

NEW JERSEY CLAIMS OFFICE
2121 EDGEWATER PL
POINT PLEASANT, NJ 08742-2212
TEL: (732) 892-1100
FAX: (732) 295-6006
WWW.MERIDIANHEALTH.COM

MEDICAL LIFE INSURANCE CO

OHIO CLAIMS OFFICE
1220 HURON RD
CLEVELAND, OH 44115
TEL: (216) 687-6800
FAX: (216) 522-8702
TOLL FREE: (800) 544-9000
WWW.MED-LIFE.COM

MEDICAL MUTUAL OF OHIO

PO BOX 6018
CLEVELAND, OH 44101-1355
TEL: (216) 522-8622
FAX: (216) 694-2910
TOLL FREE: (800) 233-2058

HMO HOME HEALTH OHIO
SUB-REGION OFFICE
2060 READING RD, STE 300
CINCINNATI, OH 45202-1455
TEL: (513) 684-8100
TOLL FREE: (800) 272-1660

MEDICAL NETWORK OF COLORADO SPRINGS

COLORADO CLAIMS OFFICE
555 E PIKES PK AVE
PO BOX 828
COLORADO SPRINGS, CO 80901
TEL: (719) 365-5025
FAX: (719) 365-5004
TOLL FREE: (800) 207-1018

MEDICAL RISK MANAGERS

CONNECTICUT CLAIMS OFFICE
1170 ELLINGTON RD
WINDSOR, CT 06074-4316
TEL: (860) 289-8434
FAX: (860) 289-5937

MEDICARE PART A

WYOMING CLAIMS OFFICE
PO BOX 908
CHEYENNE, WY 82003
TEL: (307) 432-2860
FAX: (307) 632-1654
IN-STATE: (800) 442-2376

MEDICARE — PART A HORIZON BLUE CROSS BLUE SHIELD OF NEW JERSEY

NEW JERSEY CLAIMS OFFICE
33 WASHINGTON ST
PO BOX 1236
NEWARK, NJ 07101-1236
TEL: (973) 456-2112
FAX: (973) 456-2086

MEDICARE — PART A INTERMEDIARIES

ALABAMA CLAIMS OFFICE
BLUE CROSS & BLUE SHIELD OF ALABAMA
450 RIVERCHASE PKY EAST
PO BOX 830139
BIRMINGHAM, AL 35298
TEL: (205) 988-2100
FAX: (205) 981-4841
TOLL FREE: (800) 292-8855

ARIZONA CLAIMS OFFICE
BLUE CROSS & BLUE SHIELD OF ARIZONA, INC
2444 W LAS PAMARITAS DR
PO BOX 13466
PHOENIX, AZ 85002-3466
TEL: (602) 864-4100
FAX: (602) 864-4653
WWW.BCBSAZ.COM

ARKANSAS CLAIMS OFFICE
ARKANSAS BLUE CROSS & BLUE SHIELD
601 GAINES ST
PO BOX 2181
LITTLE ROCK, AR 72203-2181
TEL: (501) 378-2000
FAX: (501) 378-2576
TOLL FREE: (800) 813-8868

CALIFORNIA CLAIMS OFFICE
BLUE CROSS OF CALIFORNIA (WELLPOINT HEALTH NETWORKS)
21555 OXNARD ST
PO BOX 70000
VAN NUYS, CA 91470
TEL: (818) 703-2345
FAX: (818) 703-2848
TOLL FREE: (800) 234-0111
WWW.BLUECROSSCA.COM

CONNECTICUT CLAIMS OFFICE
BLUE CROSS & BLUE SHIELD OF CONNECTICUT, INC
370 BASSETT RD
PO BOX 533
HAVEN, CT 06473-0533
TEL: (203) 239-4911
FAX: (203) 630-4628
IN-STATE: (800) 922-4670
WWW.ANTHEMINC.COM

M

BLUE CROSS & BLUE SHIELD OF CONNECTICUT, INC
370 BASSETT RD
PO BOX 1010
NORTH HAVEN, CT 06473-1010
TEL: (203) 239-4911
FAX: (203) 630-4628
IN-STATE: (800) 922-4670
WWW.ANTHEMINC.COM

DELAWARE CLAIMS OFFICE
MEDICAL SERVICES ASSOCIATION OF PENNSYLVANIA
1800 CENTER ST
PO BOX 890089
CAMP HILL, PA 17089-0089
TEL: (717) 763-3151
FAX: (717) 763-3544

DISTRICT OF COLUMBIA CLAIMS OFFICE
MEDICAL SERVICES ASSOCIATION OF PENNSYLVANIA
1800 CENTER ST
PO BOX 890089
CAMP HILL, PA 17089-0089
TEL: (717) 763-3151
FAX: (717) 763-3544

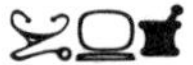

GEORGIA CLAIMS OFFICE
BLUE CROSS & BLUE SHIELD OF GEORGIA, INC
2357 WARM SPGS RD
PO BOX 9048
COLUMBUS, GA 31908-9048
TEL: (706) 571-5371
FAX: (706) 571-5431

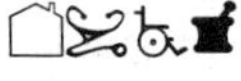

INDIANA CLAIMS OFFICE
ADMINISTER FEDERAL, INC
8115 KNUE RD
INDIANAPOLIS, IN 46250-2804
TEL: (317) 841-4400
FAX: (317) 841-4691
TOLL FREE: (800) 999-7608

IOWA CLAIMS OFFICE
WELLMARK BLUE CROSS & BLUE SHIELD OF IOWA
636 GRAND AVE
STATION 120
DES MOINES, IA 50309
TEL: (515) 245-4834
FAX: (515) 245-3984
WWW.WELLMEDICARE.COM

KANSAS CLAIMS OFFICE
SEE BLUE CROSS & BLUE SHEILD OF KANSAS
133 S TOPEKA
TOPEKA, KS 66601-1712
TEL: (785) 291-7000
FAX: (785) 291-6924

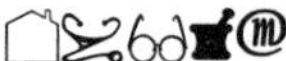

KENTUCKY CLAIMS OFFICE
ADMINASTAR FEDERAL - KENTUCKY
9901 LINN STATION RD
PO BOX 23711
LOUISVILLE, KY 40223-0711
TEL: (502) 425-7776
FAX: (502) 329-8559

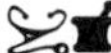

LOUISIANA CLAIMS OFFICE
SOCIAL SECURITY
346 HOLMER RD
MENDON, LA 71055
TEL: (318) 377-7387
TOLL FREE: (800) 772-1213

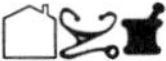

MAINE CLAIMS OFFICE
ASSOC HOSP SVC OF MAINE- DBA BLUE CROSS & BLUE SHIELD OF MAINE
2 GANNETT DR
SOUTH PORTLAND, ME 04106-6911
TEL: (207) 822-8484
FAX: (207) 822-7926
TOLL FREE: (888) 896-4997
E-MAIL: MEDICARE@BCBSME.COM
WWW.AHSMEDICARE.COM

MASSACHUSETTS CLAIMS OFFICE
ASSOC HOSP SVC OF MAINE- DBA BLUE CROSS & BLUE SHIELD OF MAINE
2 GANNETT DR
SOUTH PORTLAND, ME 04106-6911
TEL: (207) 822-8484
FAX: (207) 822-7926
TOLL FREE: (888) 896-4997
E-MAIL: MEDICARE@BCBSME.COM
WWW.AHSMEDICARE.COM

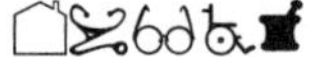

MINNESOTA CLAIMS OFFICE
BLUE CROSS & BLUE SHIELD OF MINNESOTA
PO BOX 64357
SAINT PAUL, MN 55164-0357
TEL: (651) 662-8000
FAX: (651) 662-2745
TOLL FREE: (800) 382-2000

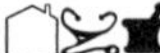

METRAHEALTH INSURANCE CO
450 COLOUMBUS BLVD - 5GB
PO BOX 150450
HARTFORD, CT 06115-0450
TEL: (860) 702-6668
FAX: (860) 702-6587

NORIDIAN MUTUAL INSURANCE CO
4305 13TH AVE SW
FARGO, ND 58103-3309
TEL: (701) 277-2655
FAX: (701) 277-2196

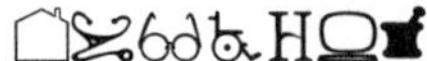

MISSISSIPPI CLAIMS OFFICE
BLUE CROSS & BLUE SHIELD OF MISSISSIPPI, INC
1064 FLINT DR
PO BOX 23035
JACKSON, MS
TEL: (601) 936-0105
FAX: (601) 932-9233

METRAHEALTH INSURANCE CO
450 COLOUMBUS BLVD - 5GB
PO BOX 150450
HARTFORD, CT 06115-0450
TEL: (860) 702-6669
FAX: (860) 702-6587

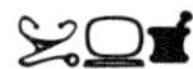

MISSOURI CLAIMS OFFICE
SEE BLUE CROSS & BLUE SHEILD OF KANSAS
133 S TOPEKA
TOPEKA, KS 66601-1712
TEL: (785) 291-7000
FAX: (785) 291-6924

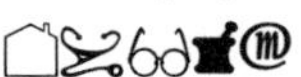

MONTANA CLAIMS OFFICE
BLUE CROSS & BLUE SHIELD OF MONTANA, INC
340 N LAST CHANCE GULCH
PO BOX 4309
HELENA, MT 59604
TEL: (406) 791-4000
FAX: (406) 791-4119
TOLL FREE: (800) 447-7828
WWW.BCBSMT.COM

NATIONAL CLAIMS OFFICE
FIRST COAST SERVICE OPTIONS, INC / BLUE CROSS & BLUE SHIELD OF FLORIDA, INC
532 RIVERSIDE AVENUE- 17TH & 18TH FLS
PO BOX 2711
JACKSONVILLE, FL 32231-0021
TEL: (904) 355-8899
FAX: (904) 791-8296
IN-STATE: (800) 333-7586

NEBRASKA CLAIMS OFFICE
BLUE CROSS & BLUE SHIELD OF NEBRASKA ALSO PROCESSED AT BLUE CROSS AND BLUE SHEILD OF KANSAS
7261 MERCY RD
PO BOX 24563
OMAHA, NE 68124-0563
TEL: (402) 390-1850
FAX: (402) 398-3640

NEW HAMPSHIRE CLAIMS OFFICE
NH- VT HEALTH SERVICE- DBA BLUE CROSS & BLUE SHIELD OF NEW HAMPSHIRE
3000 GOFF FALLS RD
MANCHESTER, NH 03111-0001
TEL: (603) 695-7204
FAX: (603) 695-7741

NEW HAMPSHIRE-VERMONT HEALTH SERVICES- DBA BCBS OF NEW HAMPSHIRE
3000 GOFFS FALLS RD
MANCHESTER, NH 03111-0001
TEL: (603) 695-7204
FAX: (603) 695-7741

NEW YORK CLAIMS OFFICE
BLUE CROSS & BLUE SHIELD OF WESTERN NEW YORK
1901 MAIN ST
PO BOX 80
BUFFALO, NY 14208
TEL: (716) 887-6900
FAX: (716) 887-8981
TOLL FREE: (800) 252-6550
IN-STATE: (800) 695-2583

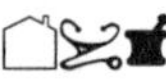

EMPIRE BLUE CROSS AND BLUE SHIELD MEDICARE SERVICES
ONE WORLD TRADE CENTER
PO BOX 1407
NEW YORK, NY 10048
TEL: (212) 476-1000
TOLL FREE: (800) 442-8430

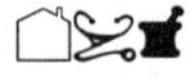

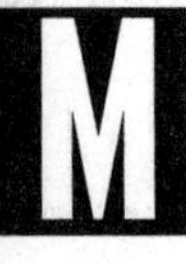

NORTH DAKOTA CLAIMS OFFICE
NORIDIAN MUTUAL INSURANCE CO
4305 13TH AVE SW
FARGO, ND 58103-3309
TEL: (701) 277-2655
FAX: (701) 277-2196

BLUE CROSS BLUE SHIELD OF NORTH DAKOTA
4510 13TH AVE SW
PO BOX 6706
FARGO, ND 58108-6706
TEL: (701) 277-1100
FAX: (701) 282-1002
TOLL FREE: (800) 874-2656
WWW.NORIDIAN.COM

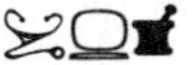

OHIO CLAIMS OFFICE
ANTHEM- DBA COMMUNITY MUTUAL BLUE CROSS & BLUE SHIELD
4361 ERWIN SIMPSON RD
MASON, OH 45050
TEL: (513) 872-8100
FAX: (513) 852-4562

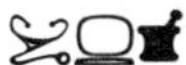

OKLAHOMA CLAIMS OFFICE
GROUP HEALTH SVC OF OK, INC- DBA BLUE CROSS & BLUE SHIELD OF OK
1215 S BOULDER AVE
PO BOX 3404
TULSA, OK 74101
TEL: (918) 560-2090
FAX: (918) 560-3506

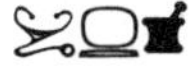

OREGON CLAIMS OFFICE
1600 SW 4TH AVE
PO BOX 8110
PORTLAND, OR 97207
TEL: (503) 721-7007
FAX: (503) 228-3304

PENNSYLVANIA CLAIMS OFFICE
MEDICAL SERVICES ASSOCIATION OF PENNSYLVANIA
1800 CENTER ST
PO BOX 890089
CAMP HILL, PA 17089-0089
TEL: (717) 763-3151
FAX: (717) 763-3544

PUERTO RICO CLAIMS OFFICE
TRIPLE-S INC
1441 ROOSEVELT AVE
PO BOX 71391
SAN JUAN, PR 00936-1391
TEL: (787) 749-4080
FAX: (787) 749-4092

RHODE ISLAND CLAIMS OFFICE
BLUE CROSS & BLUE SHIELD OF RHODE ISLAND
444 WESTMINSTER ST
PROVIDENCE, RI 02903
TEL: (401) 455-0177
FAX: (401) 459-1709
TOLL FREE: (800) 662-5170

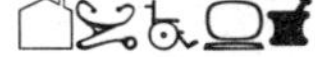

TENNESSEE CLAIMS OFFICE
730 CHESTNUT ST
CHATTANOOGA, TN 37402-1790
TEL: (423) 755-5950

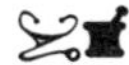

UTAH CLAIMS OFFICE
REGENCE BLUE CROSS & BLUE SHIELD OF UTAH
2890 E COTTONWOOD PKY
PO BOX 30269
SALT LAKE CITY, UT 84130
TEL: (801) 333-2420
FAX: (801) 333-6510

VERMONT CLAIMS OFFICE
NEW HAMPSHIRE-VERMONT HEALTH SERVICES- DBA BCBS OF NH
3000 GOFFS FALLS RD
MANCHESTER, NH 03111-0001
TEL: (603) 695-7204
FAX: (603) 695-7741

NH- VT HEALTH SERVICE- DBA BLUE CROSS & BLUE SHIELD OF NH
3000 GOFF FALLS RD
MANCHESTER, NH 03111-0001
TEL: (603) 695-7204
FAX: (603) 695-7741

WASHINGTON CLAIMS OFFICE
730 CHESTNUT ST
CHATTANOOGA, TN 37402-1790
TEL: (423) 755-5950

WEST VIRGINIA CLAIMS OFFICE
NATIONAL MUTUAL INSURANCE COMPANY
PO BOX 57
COLUMBUS, OH 43216-0057
TEL: (614) 249-7111
FAX: (614) 249-4467
IN-STATE: (800) 848-0106
WWW.NATIONWIDE-MEDICARE.COM

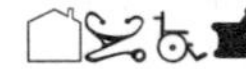

MEDICARE — PART B CARRIERS

ALABAMA CLAIMS OFFICE
BLUE CROSS & BLUE SHEILD OF ALABAMA
PO BOX 830140
BIRMINGHAM, AL 35283-0140
TEL: (205) 981-4842
FAX: (205) 981-4965
TOLL FREE: (800) 292-8855
WWW.BCBSAL.ORG

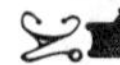

ALASKA CLAIMS OFFICE
BLUE CROSS & BLUE SHIELD OF NORTH DAKOTA
4510 13TH AVE SW
FARGO, ND 58121-0001
TEL: (701) 277-1100
FAX: (701) 282-1002
TOLL FREE: (800) 874-2656
WWW.NORIDIAN.COM

ARIZONA CLAIMS OFFICE
BLUE CROSS & BLUE SHIELD OF NORTH DAKOTA
4510 13TH AVE SW
FARGO, ND 58121-0001
TEL: (701) 277-1100
FAX: (701) 282-1002
TOLL FREE: (800) 874-2656
WWW.NORIDIAN.COM

BLUE CROSS & BLUE SHIELD OF NORTH DAKOTA
4305 16TH AVE S
PO BOX 6704
FARGO, ND 58108-6704
TOLL FREE: (800) 444-4606
IN-STATE: (800) 332-6681

ARKANSAS CLAIMS OFFICE
ARKANSAS BLUE CROSS & BLUE SHIELD
601 GAINES ST
PO BOX 2181
LITTLE ROCK, AR 72203
TEL: (501) 378-2320
FAX: (501) 378-2591
TOLL FREE: (800) 813-8868

ARKANSAS BLUE CROSS & BLUE SHIELD
601 GAINES ST
PO BOX 2181
LITTLE ROCK, AR 72203
TEL: (501) 378-3025
FAX: (501) 378-2804
WWW.ARKMEDICARE.COM

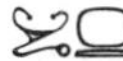

CALIFORNIA CLAIMS OFFICE
TRANSAMERICA OCCIDENTAL LIFE INSURANCE
1149 SOUTH BROADWAY
PO BOX 54905
LOS ANGELES, CA 90054-0905
TEL: (213) 748-2311
FAX: (213) 741-6803
WWW.MEDICARE.TRANSAMERICA.COM

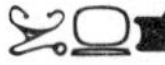

STATE OF CALIFORNIA NATIONAL HERITAGE INSURANCE CO - NORTHERN CALIFORNIA CLAIMS OFFICE
450 W EAST AVE
CHICO, CA 95926
TEL: (530) 896-7025
FAX: (530) 896-7182

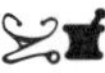

COLORADO CLAIMS OFFICE
BLUE CROSS & BLUE SHEILD OF NORTH DAKOTA
4510 13TH AVE SW
FARGO, ND 58121-0001
TEL: (701) 277-1100
FAX: (701) 282-1002
TOLL FREE: (800) 874-2656
WWW.NORIDIAN.COM

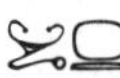

BLUE CROSS & BLUE SHIELD OF NORTH DAKOTA
4305 16TH AVE S
PO BOX 6028
FARGO, ND 58108-6028
TOLL FREE: (800) 444-4606
IN-STATE: (800) 332-6681

M

DISTRICT OF COLUMBIA CLAIMS OFFICE
PENNSYLVANIA BLUE SHIELD
1800 CENTER ST
PO BOX 890101
CAMP HILL, PA 17089-0101
TEL: (717) 731-2333

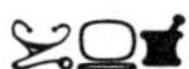

FLORIDA CLAIMS OFFICE
BLUE CROSS & BLUE SHIELD OF FLORIDA
532 RIVERSIDE AVE
PO BOX 2525
JACKSONVILLE, FL 32231-0019
TEL: (904) 634-4994
FAX: (904) 791-8378
IN-STATE: (800) 333-7586

HAWAII CLAIMS OFFICE
BLUE CROSS & BLUE SHIELD OF HAWAII
818 KEEAUMOKU ST
PO BOX 860
HONOLULU, HI 96808
TEL: (808) 948-6247
FAX: (808) 948-6555

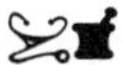

INDIANA CLAIMS OFFICE
ADMINISTAR FEDERAL, INC
8115 KNUE RD
INDIANAPOLIS, IN 46250-2804
TEL: (317) 841-4400
FAX: (317) 841-4691
TOLL FREE: (800) 999-7608

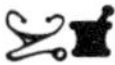

IOWA CLAIMS OFFICE
WELLMARK, INC
636 GRAND AVE, STATION 28
DES MOINES, IA 50309
TEL: (515) 245-4618
FAX: (515) 245-3984
WWW.WELLMEDICARE.COM

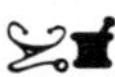

KANSAS CLAIMS OFFICE
BLUE CROSS & BLUE SHIELD OF KANSAS
1133 TOPEKA AVE
PO BOX 239
TOPEKA, KS 66601
TEL: (816) 756-1601
FAX: (913) 291-8532

BLUE CROSS & BLUE SHIELD OF KANSAS
1133 SW TOPEKA BLVD
PO BOX 239
TOPEKA, KS 66629
TEL: (785) 291-4003
FAX: (785) 291-8532

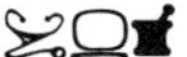

KENTUCKY CLAIMS OFFICE
ADMINISTAR FEDERAL INC
8115 KNUE RD
PO BOX 37630
INDIANAPOLIS, IN 46250-2804
TEL: (317) 841-4400
FAX: (317) 841-4691
TOLL FREE: (800) 999-7608

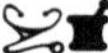

MISSOURI CLAIMS OFFICE
BLUE CROSS & BLUE SHIELD OF KANSAS
1133 SW TOPEKA BLVD
PO BOX 239
TOPEKA, KS 66629
TEL: (816) 756-1601
FAX: (785) 291-8532

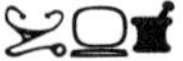

MONTANA CLAIMS OFFICE
BLUE CROSS BLUE SHIELD OF MONTANA
340 N LAST CHANCE GULCH
PO BOX 4310
HELENA, MT 59601
TEL: (406) 791-4000
FAX: (406) 442-9968
IN-STATE: (800) 332-6146
WWW.MEDICARE.BCBSMT.COM

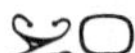

BLUE CROSS BLUE SHIELD OF MONTANA
340 N LAST CHANCE GULCH
PO BOX 4310
HELENA, MT 59601
TEL: (406) 791-4000
FAX: (406) 442-9968
IN-STATE: (800) 332-6146
WWW.MEDICARE.BSBSMT.COM

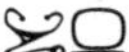

NATIONAL CLAIMS OFFICE
538 PRESTEN AVE
PO BOX 9000
MERIDEN, CT 06454-9000
TEL: (203) 238-4346
FAX: (203) 639-3018
IN-STATE: (800) 982-6819

NEBRASKA CLAIMS OFFICE
BLUE CROSS & BLUE SHIELD OF KANSAS, INC
1133 TOPEKA AVE
PO BOX 239
TOPEKA, KS 66601
TEL: (785) 291-4155
FAX: (785) 291-8532

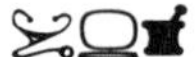

NEVADA CLAIMS OFFICE
BLUE CROSS & BLUE SHIELD OF NORTH DAKOTA
4510 13TH AVE SW
FARGO, ND 58121-0001
TEL: (701) 277-1100
FAX: (701) 282-1002
TOLL FREE: (800) 874-2656
WWW.NORIDIAN.COM

NEW YORK CLAIMS OFFICE
BLUE CROSS & BLUE SHIELD OF WESTERN NEW YORK, INC
1901 MAIN ST
PO BOX 80
BUFFALO, NY 14240-0080
TEL: (716) 887-6900
TOLL FREE: (800) 950-0051

EMPIRE BLUE CROSS & BLUE SHIELD
622 3RD AVE
NEW YORK , NY 10017
TEL: (212) 476-1000
TOLL FREE: (800) 442-8430

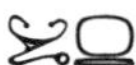

NORTH DAKOTA CLAIMS OFFICE
BLUE CROSS & BLUE SHIELD OF TEXAS
4305 16TH AVE S
PO BOX 6701
FARGO, ND 58103-3373
TOLL FREE: (800) 444-4606
IN-STATE: (800) 332-6681

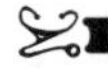

BLUE CROSS & BLUE SHIELD OF NORTH DAKOTA
4510 13TH AVE SW
FARGO, ND 58121-0001
TEL: (701) 277-1100
FAX: (701) 282-1002
TOLL FREE: (800) 874-2656
IN-STATE: (800) 332-6681
WWW.NORIDIAN.COM

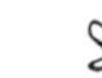

OHIO CLAIMS OFFICE
WEST VA- NATIONWIDE
PO BOX 16788 OR 57
COLUMBUS, OH 43216-0057
TEL: (614) 249-7111
FAX: (616) 249-4467
IN-STATE: (800) 282-0530
WWW.NATIONWIDE-MEDICARE.COM

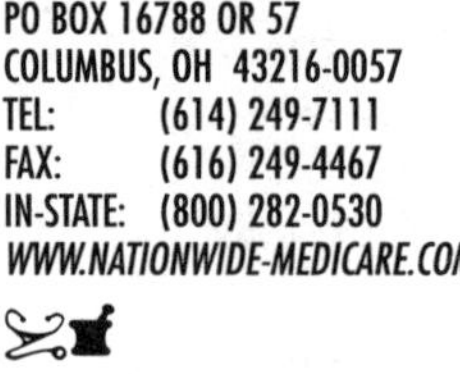

OKLAHOMA CLAIMS OFFICE
SEE ARKANSAS
701 NW 63RD
OKLAHOMA CITY, OK 73116
TEL: (405) 843-9379

OREGON CLAIMS OFFICE
BLUE CROSS & BLUE SHIELD OF NORTH DAKOTA
4510 13TH AVE SW
FARGO, ND 58121-0001
TEL: (701) 277-1100
FAX: (701) 282-1002
TOLL FREE: (800) 874-2656
IN-STATE: (800) 247-2267
WWW.NORIDIAN.COM

BLUE CROSS & BLUE SHIELD OF TEXAS
4305 16TH AVE S
PO BOX 6702
FARGO, ND 58108-6702
TOLL FREE: (800) 444-4606
IN-STATE: (800) 332-6681

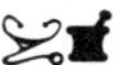

PUERTO RICO CLAIMS OFFICE
TRIPLE-S INC
BOX 71391
SAN JUAN, PR 00936
TEL: (787) 749-4080
FAX: (787) 749-4092

RHODE ISLAND CLAIMS OFFICE
BLUE CROSS & BLUE SHIELD OF RHODE ISLAND
444 WESTMINSTER ST
PROVIDENCE, RI 02903
TEL: (401) 272-3131

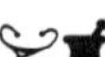

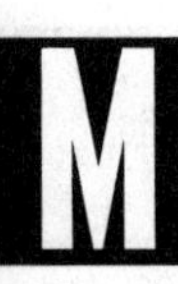

SOUTH CAROLINA CLAIMS OFFICE
BLUE CROSS & BLUE SHIELD OF SOUTH CAROLINA
300 ARBOR LK DR, STE 1300
COLUMBIA, SC 29223
TEL: (803) 788-5568
FAX: (803) 691-2188

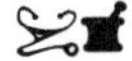

SOUTH DAKOTA CLAIMS OFFICE
BLUE CROSS & BLUE SHIELD OF NORTH DAKOTA
4305 16TH AVE S
PO BOX 6707
FARGO, ND 58108-6707
TOLL FREE: (800) 444-4606
IN-STATE: (800) 332-6681

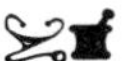

TENNESSEE CLAIMS OFFICE
CONNECTICUT GENERAL LIFE INSURANCE CO (CGLIC)
TWO VANTAGE WAY
PO BOX 1465
NASHVILLE, TN 37228
TEL: (615) 782-4576
FAX: (615) 782-4662
TOLL FREE: (800) 342-8900
WWW.CIGNAMEDICARE.COM

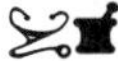

UTAH CLAIMS OFFICE
BLUE CROSS & BLUE SHIELD OF UTAH
2890 COTTONWOOD PKY
PO BOX 30269
SALT LAKE CITY, UT 84130-0269
TEL: (801) 333-2440
FAX: (801) 333-6505
IN-STATE: (800) 426-3477

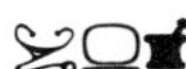

WASHINGTON CLAIMS OFFICE
BLUE CROSS & BLUE SHIELD OF NORTH DAKOTA
4510 13TH AVE SW
FARGO, ND 58121-0001
TEL: (701) 277-1100
FAX: (701) 282-1002
TOLL FREE: (800) 874-2656
WWW.NORIDIAN.COM

BLUE CROSS & BLUE SHIELD OF NORTH DAKOTA
4305 16TH AVE S
PO BOX 6700
FARGO, ND 58108-6700
TOLL FREE: (800) 444-4606
IN-STATE: (800) 332-6681

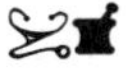

WEST VIRGINIA CLAIMS OFFICE
NATIONAL MUTUAL INSURANCE CO
PO BOX 57
COLUMBUS, OH 43216-0057
TEL: (614) 249-7111
FAX: (614) 249-4467
IN-STATE: (800) 848-0106
WWW.NATIONWIDE-MEDICARE.COM

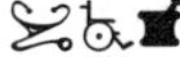

WISCONSIN CLAIMS OFFICE
WISCONSIN PHYSICIANS' SERVICE INSURANCE CORP
PO BOX 1787
MADISON, WI 53701-1787
TEL: (608) 221-3218
IN-STATE: (800) 944-0051
WWW.WPSIC.COM/MEDICARE/INDEX

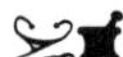

WYOMING CLAIMS OFFICE
BLUE CROSS & BLUE SHIELD OF NORTH DAKOTA
4510 13TH AVE SW
PO BOX 628
FARGO, ND 58121-0001
TEL: (701) 277-1100
FAX: (701) 282-1002
TOLL FREE: (800) 874-2656
WWW.NORIDIAN.COM

BLUE CROSS & BLUE SHIELD OF NORTH DAKOTA
4305 16TH AVE S
PO BOX 6708
FARGO, ND 58108-6708
TOLL FREE: (800) 444-4606
IN-STATE: (800) 332-6681

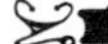

MEDICO LIFE INSURANCE CO

ALABAMA CLAIMS OFFICE
MUTUAL PROTECTIVE
1515 S 75TH ST
PO BOX 3477
OMAHA, NE 68103
TEL: (402) 391-6900
FAX: (402) 391-6489
TOLL FREE: (800) 228-6080

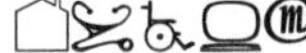

ALASKA CLAIMS OFFICE
MUTUAL PROTECTIVE
1515 S 75TH ST
PO BOX 3477
OMAHA, NE 68103
TEL: (402) 391-6900
FAX: (402) 391-6489
TOLL FREE: (800) 228-6080

ARIZONA CLAIMS OFFICE
MUTUAL PROTECTIVE
1515 S 75TH ST
PO BOX 3477
OMAHA, NE 68103
TEL: (402) 391-6900
FAX: (402) 391-6489
TOLL FREE: (800) 228-6080

ARKANSAS CLAIMS OFFICE
MUTUAL PROTECTIVE
1515 S 75TH ST
PO BOX 3477
OMAHA, NE 68103
TEL: (402) 391-6900
FAX: (402) 391-6489
TOLL FREE: (800) 228-6080

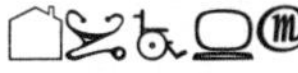

CALIFORNIA CLAIMS OFFICE
MUTUAL PROTECTIVE
1515 S 75TH ST
PO BOX 3477
OMAHA, NE 68103
TEL: (402) 391-6900
FAX: (402) 391-6489
TOLL FREE: (800) 228-6080

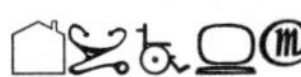

COLORADO CLAIMS OFFICE
MUTUAL PROTECTIVE
1515 S 75TH ST
PO BOX 3477
OMAHA, NE 68103
TEL: (402) 391-6900
FAX: (402) 391-6489
TOLL FREE: (800) 228-6080

DELAWARE CLAIMS OFFICE
MUTUAL PROTECTIVE
1515 S 75TH ST
PO BOX 3477
OMAHA, NE 68103
TEL: (402) 391-6900
FAX: (402) 391-6489
TOLL FREE: (800) 228-6080

DISTRICT OF COLUMBIA CLAIMS OFFICE
MUTUAL PROTECTIVE
1515 S 75TH ST
PO BOX 3477
OMAHA, NE 68103
TEL: (402) 391-6900
FAX: (402) 391-6489
TOLL FREE: (800) 228-6080

FLORIDA CLAIMS OFFICE
MUTUAL PROTECTIVE
1515 S 75TH ST
PO BOX 3477
OMAHA, NE 68103
TEL: (402) 391-6900
FAX: (402) 391-6489
TOLL FREE: (800) 228-6080

GEORGIA CLAIMS OFFICE
MUTUAL PROTECTIVE
1515 S 75TH ST
PO BOX 3477
OMAHA, NE 68103
TEL: (402) 391-6900
FAX: (402) 391-6489
TOLL FREE: (800) 228-6080

HAWAII CLAIMS OFFICE
MUTUAL PROTECTIVE
1515 S 75TH ST
PO BOX 3477
OMAHA, NE 68103
TEL: (402) 391-6900
FAX: (402) 391-6489
TOLL FREE: (800) 228-6080

IDAHO CLAIMS OFFICE
MUTUAL PROTECTIVE
1515 S 75TH ST
PO BOX 3477
OMAHA, NE 68103
TEL: (402) 391-6900
FAX: (402) 391-6489
TOLL FREE: (800) 228-6080

ILLINOIS CLAIMS OFFICE
MUTUAL PROTECTIVE
1515 S 75TH ST
PO BOX 3477
OMAHA, NE 68103
TEL: (402) 391-6900
FAX: (402) 391-6489
TOLL FREE: (800) 228-6080

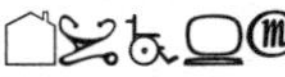

INDIANA CLAIMS OFFICE
MUTUAL PROTECTIVE
1515 S 75TH ST
PO BOX 3477
OMAHA, NE 68103
TEL: (402) 391-6900
FAX: (402) 391-6489
TOLL FREE: (800) 228-6080

IOWA CLAIMS OFFICE
MUTUAL PROTECTIVE
1515 S 75TH ST
PO BOX 3477
OMAHA, NE 68103
TEL: (402) 391-6900
FAX: (402) 391-6489
TOLL FREE: (800) 228-6080

KANSAS CLAIMS OFFICE
MUTUAL PROTECTIVE
1515 S 75TH ST
PO BOX 3477
OMAHA, NE 68103
TEL: (402) 391-6900
FAX: (402) 391-6489
TOLL FREE: (800) 228-6080

KENTUCKY CLAIMS OFFICE
MUTUAL PROTECTIVE
1515 S 75TH ST
PO BOX 3477
OMAHA, NE 68103
TEL: (402) 391-6900
FAX: (402) 391-6489
TOLL FREE: (800) 228-6080

LOUISIANA CLAIMS OFFICE
MUTUAL PROTECTIVE
1515 S 75TH ST
PO BOX 3477
OMAHA, NE 68103
TEL: (402) 391-6900
FAX: (402) 391-6489
TOLL FREE: (800) 228-6080

MARYLAND CLAIMS OFFICE
MUTUAL PROTECTIVE
1515 S 75TH ST
PO BOX 3477
OMAHA, NE 68103
TEL: (402) 391-6900
FAX: (402) 391-6489
TOLL FREE: (800) 228-6080

MASSACHUSETTS CLAIMS OFFICE
MUTUAL PROTECTIVE
1515 S 75TH ST
PO BOX 3477
OMAHA, NE 68103
TEL: (402) 391-6900
FAX: (402) 391-6489
TOLL FREE: (800) 228-6080

MICHIGAN CLAIMS OFFICE
MUTUAL PROTECTIVE
1515 S 75TH ST
PO BOX 3477
OMAHA, NE 68103
TEL: (402) 391-6900
FAX: (402) 391-6489
TOLL FREE: (800) 228-6080

MINNESOTA CLAIMS OFFICE
MUTUAL PROTECTIVE
1515 S 75TH ST
PO BOX 3477
OMAHA, NE 68103
TEL: (402) 391-6900
FAX: (402) 391-6489
TOLL FREE: (800) 228-6080

MISSISSIPPI CLAIMS OFFICE
MUTUAL PROTECTIVE
1515 S 75TH ST
PO BOX 3477
OMAHA, NE 68103
TEL: (402) 391-6900
FAX: (402) 391-6489
TOLL FREE: (800) 228-6080

MISSOURI CLAIMS OFFICE
MUTUAL PROTECTIVE
1515 S 75TH ST
PO BOX 3477
OMAHA, NE 68103
TEL: (402) 391-6900
FAX: (402) 391-6489
TOLL FREE: (800) 228-6080

MONTANA CLAIMS OFFICE
MUTUAL PROTECTIVE
1515 S 75TH ST
PO BOX 3477
OMAHA, NE 68103
TEL: (402) 391-6900
FAX: (402) 391-6489
TOLL FREE: (800) 228-6080

NEBRASKA CLAIMS OFFICE
MUTUAL PROTECTIVE
1515 S 75TH ST
PO BOX 3477
OMAHA, NE 68103
TEL: (402) 391-6900
FAX: (402) 391-6489
TOLL FREE: (800) 228-6080

NEVADA CLAIMS OFFICE
MUTUAL PROTECTIVE
1515 S 75TH ST
PO BOX 3477
OMAHA, NE 68103
TEL: (402) 391-6900
FAX: (402) 391-6489
TOLL FREE: (800) 228-6080

NEW MEXICO CLAIMS OFFICE
MUTUAL PROTECTIVE
1515 S 75TH ST
PO BOX 3477
OMAHA, NE 68103
TEL: (402) 391-6900
FAX: (402) 391-6489
TOLL FREE: (800) 228-6080

NORTH CAROLINA CLAIMS OFFICE
MUTUAL PROTECTIVE
1515 S 75TH ST
PO BOX 3477
OMAHA, NE 68103
TEL: (402) 391-6900
FAX: (402) 391-6489
TOLL FREE: (800) 228-6080

NORTH DAKOTA CLAIMS OFFICE
MUTUAL PROTECTIVE
1515 S 75TH ST
PO BOX 3477
OMAHA, NE 68103
TEL: (402) 391-6900
FAX: (402) 391-6489
TOLL FREE: (800) 228-6080

OHIO CLAIMS OFFICE
MUTUAL PROTECTIVE
1515 S 75TH ST
PO BOX 3477
OMAHA, NE 68103
TEL: (402) 391-6900
FAX: (402) 391-6489
TOLL FREE: (800) 228-6080

OKLAHOMA CLAIMS OFFICE
MUTUAL PROTECTIVE
1515 S 75TH ST
PO BOX 3477
OMAHA, NE 68103
TEL: (402) 391-6900
FAX: (402) 391-6489
TOLL FREE: (800) 228-6080

OREGON CLAIMS OFFICE
MUTUAL PROTECTIVE
1515 S 75TH ST
PO BOX 3477
OMAHA, NE 68103
TEL: (402) 391-6900
FAX: (402) 391-6489
TOLL FREE: (800) 228-6080

PENNSYLVANIA CLAIMS OFFICE
MUTUAL PROTECTIVE
1515 S 75TH ST
PO BOX 3477
OMAHA, NE 68103
TEL: (402) 391-6900
FAX: (402) 391-6489
TOLL FREE: (800) 228-6080

SOUTH CAROLINA CLAIMS OFFICE
MUTUAL PROTECTIVE
1515 S 75TH ST
PO BOX 3477
OMAHA, NE 68103
TEL: (402) 391-6900
FAX: (402) 391-6489
TOLL FREE: (800) 228-6080

SOUTH DAKOTA CLAIMS OFFICE
MUTUAL PROTECTIVE
1515 S 75TH ST
PO BOX 3477
OMAHA, NE 68103
TEL: (402) 391-6900
FAX: (402) 391-6489
TOLL FREE: (800) 228-6080

TENNESSEE CLAIMS OFFICE
MUTUAL PROTECTIVE
1515 S 75TH ST
PO BOX 3477
OMAHA, NE 68103
TEL: (402) 391-6900
FAX: (402) 391-6489
TOLL FREE: (800) 228-6080

TEXAS CLAIMS OFFICE
MUTUAL PROTECTIVE
1515 S 75TH ST
PO BOX 3477
OMAHA, NE 68103
TEL: (402) 391-6900
FAX: (402) 391-6489
TOLL FREE: (800) 228-6080

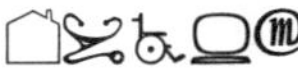

VERMONT CLAIMS OFFICE
MUTUAL PROTECTIVE
1515 S 75TH ST
PO BOX 3477
OMAHA, NE 68103
TEL: (402) 391-6900
FAX: (402) 391-6489
TOLL FREE: (800) 228-6080

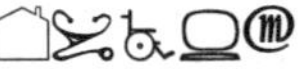

VIRGINIA CLAIMS OFFICE
MUTUAL PROTECTIVE
1515 S 75TH ST
PO BOX 3477
OMAHA, NE 68103
TEL: (402) 391-6900
FAX: (402) 391-6489
TOLL FREE: (800) 228-6080

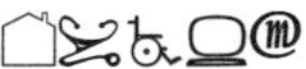

WASHINGTON CLAIMS OFFICE
MUTUAL PROTECTIVE
1515 S 75TH ST
PO BOX 3477
OMAHA, NE 68103
TEL: (402) 391-6900
FAX: (402) 391-6489
TOLL FREE: (800) 228-6080

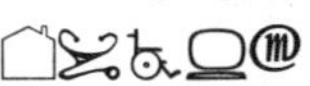

WEST VIRGINIA CLAIMS OFFICE
MUTUAL PROTECTIVE
1515 S 75TH ST
PO BOX 3477
OMAHA, NE 68103
TEL: (402) 391-6900
FAX: (402) 391-6489
TOLL FREE: (800) 228-6080

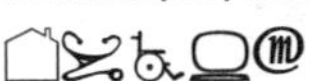

WISCONSIN CLAIMS OFFICE
MUTUAL PROTECTIVE
1515 S 75TH ST
PO BOX 3477
OMAHA, NE 68103
TEL: (402) 391-6900
FAX: (402) 391-6489
TOLL FREE: (800) 228-6080

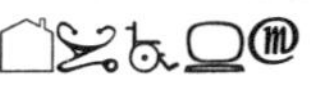

WYOMING CLAIMS OFFICE
MUTUAL PROTECTIVE
1515 S 75TH ST
PO BOX 3477
OMAHA, NE 68103
TEL: (402) 391-6900
FAX: (402) 391-6489
TOLL FREE: (800) 228-6080

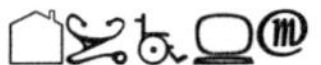

MEDPLAN, INC

NATIONAL CLAIMS OFFICE
UNITED HEALTH CARE
10450 HOLMES RD, STE 100
KANSAS CITY, MO 64131
TEL: (816) 941-8003
FAX: (816) 941-3910
TOLL FREE: (800) 852-4584
IN-STATE: (800) 292-5584

MEGA LIFE & HEALTH INSURANCE

TEXAS CLAIMS OFFICE
PO BOX 809096
DALLAS, TX 75380-9096
TEL: (972) 392-6700
FAX: (972) 851-9032
TOLL FREE: (800) 733-8880

MEIJER, INC

ILLINOIS CLAIMS OFFICE
FRED MEIJER BLDG
2929 WALKER AVE NW BLDG 985
GRAND RAPIDS, MI 49544
TEL: (616) 453-6711
FAX: (616) 365-5755
TOLL FREE: (800) 346-8281

KENTUCKY CLAIMS OFFICE
FRED MEIJER BLDG
2929 WALKER AVE NW BLDG 985
GRAND RAPIDS, MI 49544
TEL: (616) 453-6711
FAX: (616) 365-5755
TOLL FREE: (800) 346-8281

MICHIGAN CLAIMS OFFICE
FRED MEIJER BLDG
2929 WALKER AVE NW BLDG 985
GRAND RAPIDS, MI 49544
TEL: (616) 453-6711
FAX: (616) 365-5755
TOLL FREE: (800) 346-8281

OHIO CLAIMS OFFICE
FRED MEIJER BLDG
2929 WALKER AVE NW BLDG 985
GRAND RAPIDS, MI 49544
TEL: (616) 453-6711
FAX: (616) 365-5755
TOLL FREE: (800) 346-8281

MEMBER SERVICE LIFE INSURANCE CO

OKLAHOMA CLAIMS OFFICE
1400 S BOSTON- 7TH FL
PO BOX 3663
TULSA, OK 74101-3663
TEL: (918) 560-3200
FAX: (918) 560-3223

MEMORIAL SISTERS OF CHARITY HEALTH NETWORK INC

TEXAS CLAIMS OFFICE
MSCH HEALTH NETWORK
9494 SOUTHWEST FWY, STE 300
HOUSTON, TX 77074-1419
TEL: (713) 430-1400
FAX: (713) 778-2375
TOLL FREE: (800) 776-2885
WWW.MSCH.COM

MEMPHIS HOSPITAL SERVICES

TENNESSEE CLAIMS OFFICE
BLUE CROSS & BLUE SHIELD OF TENNESSEE
85 N DANNY THOMAS BLVD
PO BOX 98
MEMPHIS , TN 38101
TEL: (901) 544-2111
FAX: (901) 544-2527
TOLL FREE: (800) 422-2722

MENNONITE MUTUAL AID ASSOCIATION

INDIANA CLAIMS OFFICE
1110 N MAIN ST
PO BOX 483
GOSHEN, IN 46526-0483
TEL: (219) 533-9511
FAX: (219) 533-5264
TOLL FREE: (800) 348-7468

MERCHANTS' & BUSINESSMEN'S MUTUAL INSURANCE CO

PENNSYLVANIA CLAIMS OFFICE
2201 N FRONT ST
PO BOX 1633
HARRISBURG, PA 17105-1633
TEL: (717) 238-8211
FAX: (717) 238-5984
IN-STATE: (800) 323-4863

MERCHANTS INSURANCE GROUP

CONNECTICUT CLAIMS OFFICE
32 CONSTITUTION DR
PO BOX 4981
MANCHESTER, NH 03108
TEL: (603) 472-8881
FAX: (603) 472-8653
TOLL FREE: (800) 258-3574
IN-STATE: (800) 562-1130

MAINE CLAIMS OFFICE
32 CONSTITUTION DR
PO BOX 4981
MANCHESTER, NH 03108
TEL: (603) 472-8881
FAX: (603) 472-8653
TOLL FREE: (800) 258-3574
IN-STATE: (800) 562-1130

MASSACHUSETTS CLAIMS OFFICE
32 CONSTITUTION DR
PO BOX 4981
MANCHESTER, NH 03108
TEL: (603) 472-8881
FAX: (603) 472-8653
TOLL FREE: (800) 258-3574
IN-STATE: (800) 562-1130

NEW HAMPSHIRE CLAIMS OFFICE
32 CONSTITUTION DR
PO BOX 4981
MANCHESTER, NH 03108
TEL: (603) 472-8881
FAX: (603) 472-8653
TOLL FREE: (800) 258-3574
IN-STATE: (800) 562-1130

250 MAIN ST
PO BOX 903
BUFFALO, NY 14240

TEL: (716) 849-3333
FAX: (716) 849-3105
TOLL FREE: (800) 462-1077
IN-STATE: (800) 849-3030

NEW JERSEY CLAIMS OFFICE
309 FELLOWSHIP RD
PO BOX 868
MOORESTOWN, NJ 08057
TEL: (609) 235-8890
FAX: (609) 273-8342

250 MAIN ST
PO BOX 903
BUFFALO, NY 14240

TEL: (716) 849-3333
FAX: (716) 849-3105
TOLL FREE: (800) 462-1077
IN-STATE: (800) 849-3030

NEW YORK CLAIMS OFFICE
250 MAIN ST
PO BOX 903
BUFFALO, NY 14240

TEL: (716) 849-3333
FAX: (716) 849-3105
TOLL FREE: (800) 462-1077
IN-STATE: (800) 849-3030

RHODE ISLAND CLAIMS OFFICE
32 CONSTITUTION DR
PO BOX 4981
MANCHESTER, NH 03108
TEL: (603) 472-8881
FAX: (603) 472-8653
TOLL FREE: (800) 258-3574
IN-STATE: (800) 562-1130

VERMONT CLAIMS OFFICE
32 CONSTITUTION DR
PO BOX 4981
MANCHESTER, NH 03108
TEL: (603) 472-8881
FAX: (603) 472-8653
TOLL FREE: (800) 258-3574
IN-STATE: (800) 562-1130

MERCURY CASUALTY CO

CALIFORNIA CLAIMS OFFICE
CORPORATE OFFICE
4484 WILSHIRE BLVD
PO BOX 54600
LOS ANGELES, CA 90054-0600
TEL: (213) 937-1060
IN-STATE: (800) 431-6654
WWW.MERCURYINSURANCE.COM

555 WEST IMPERIAL HWY
PO BOX 1150
BREA, CA 92622-1150
TEL: (714) 671-6600
FAX: (714) 671-7464
TOLL FREE: (800) 824-6194
IN-STATE: (800) 431-6654

CLAIMS OFC
8825 AERO DR, STE 320
PO BOX 82167
SAN DIEGO, CA 92138-2167
TEL: (619) 569-8500
FAX: (619) 694-4197
WWW.MERCURYINSURANCE.COM

2105 HAMILTON AVE, STE 300
PO BOX 49008
SAN JOSE, CA 95161-9008
TEL: (408) 879-9600
FAX: (408) 879-5575
IN-STATE: (800) 942-5400

FLORIDA CLAIMS OFFICE
4484 WILSHIRE BLVD
PO BOX 54600
LOS ANGELES, CA 90054-0600
TEL: (213) 937-1060
IN-STATE: (800) 431-6654
WWW.MERCURYINSURANCE.COM

GEORGIA CLAIMS OFFICE
4484 WILSHIRE BLVD
PO BOX 54600
LOS ANGELES, CA 90054-0600
TEL: (213) 937-1060
IN-STATE: (800) 431-6654
WWW.MERCURYINSURANCE.COM

ILLINOIS CLAIMS OFFICE
4484 WILSHIRE BLVD
PO BOX 54600
LOS ANGELES, CA 90054-0600
TEL: (213) 937-1060
IN-STATE: (800) 431-6654
WWW.MERCURYINSURANCE.COM

OKLAHOMA CLAIMS OFFICE
4484 WILSHIRE BLVD
PO BOX 54600
LOS ANGELES, CA 90054-0600
TEL: (213) 937-1060
IN-STATE: (800) 431-6654
WWW.MERCURYINSURANCE.COM

TEXAS CLAIMS OFFICE
4484 WILSHIRE BLVD
PO BOX 54600
LOS ANGELES, CA 90054-0600
TEL: (213) 937-1060
IN-STATE: (800) 431-6654
WWW.MERCURYINSURANCE.COM

MERCYCARE HEALTH PLAN, INC

WISCONSIN CLAIMS OFFICE
3430 PALMER DR
PO BOX 2770
JANESVILLE, WI 53546
TEL: (608) 752-3431
FAX: (608) 752-3751
TOLL FREE: (800) 752-3431

MERIDIAN CITIZENS SECURITY MUTUAL INSURANCE CO

NATIONAL CLAIMS OFFICE
406 MAIN ST
PO BOX 3500
RED WING, MN 55066-2368
TEL: (612) 388-7171
FAX: (612) 388-0538
TOLL FREE: (800) 733-9464

MERIDIAN SECURITY

INDIANA CLAIMS OFFICE
2955 N MERIDIAN ST
PO BOX 6165
INDIANAPOLIS, IN 46206-6165
TEL: (317) 931-7709
FAX: (800) 688-7979
TOLL FREE: (800) 777-7324

MERIT LIFE INSURANCE CO

AMERICAN GENERAL FINANCE
601 NW 2ND ST
PO BOX 39
EVANSVILLE, IN 47701-0039
TEL: (812) 424-8031
FAX: (812) 468-5682
TOLL FREE: (800) 325-2147
IN-STATE: (800) 325-2147

MERRILL BOSTROM ASSOCIATES

UTAH CLAIMS OFFICE
M. B. A.
1121 E 3900 S, C101
PO BOX 651109
SALT LAKE CITY, UT 84124-1109
TEL: (801) 268-3334
FAX: (801) 266-2581
TOLL FREE: (800) 877-3727

MERRIMACK MUTUAL FIRE INSURANCE CO

MASSACHUSETTS CLAIMS OFFICE
95 OLD RIVER RD
PO BOX 9009
ANDOVER, MA 01810
TEL: (978) 475-3300
FAX: (800) 323-5112
TOLL FREE: (800) 225-0770

MERVYN'S HEALTH CARE PLAN

CALIFORNIA CLAIMS OFFICE
BLUE CROSS OF CALIFORNIA
PO BOX 3108
RANCHO CORDOVA, CA 95741-3108
FAX: (916) 636-2314
TOLL FREE: (800) 873-3039
WWW.BLUECROSSCA.COM

MET LIFE DISABILITY

NEW YORK CLAIMS OFFICE
5950 AIRPORT RD
PO BOX 3017
UTICA, NY 13504
FAX: (315) 792-2514
TOLL FREE: (800) 300-4296
WWW.METLIFE.COM

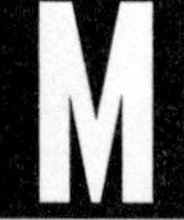

METRA HEALTHCARE NETWORK OF WISCONSIN, INC

WISCONSIN CLAIMS OFFICE
UNITED HEALTH CARE
330 E KILBOURN AVE- 11TH FL
PO BOX 3184
MILWAUKEE, WI 53210-3184
TEL: (414) 272-3735
TOLL FREE: (800) 357-1359

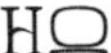

METROPOLITAN LIFE INSURANCE CO

CALIFORNIA CLAIMS OFFICE
UNITED HEALTH CARE
425 MARKET ST
SAN FRANCISCO, CA 94105-2406
TEL: (415) 546-3300

CONNECTICUT CLAIMS OFFICE
5950 AIRPORT RD
PO BOX 3015
UTICA, NY 13504
TEL: (315) 797-6000
FAX: (315) 736-1590
TOLL FREE: (800) 638-0900
WWW.METLIFE.COM

ILLINOIS CLAIMS OFFICE
177 S COMMONS DR
AURORA, IL 60505
TEL: (630) 820-7500
FAX: (630) 820-7997
WWW.METLIFE.COM

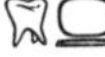

NEW YORK CLAIMS OFFICE
CORPORATE OFFICE
1 MADISON AVE 123RD ST
NEW YORK, NY 10010
TEL: (212) 578-2211
WWW.METLIFE.COM

UNITED HEALTH CARE
505 BOICES LN
PO BOX 1600
KINGSTON, NY 12401
TEL: (914) 382-7500
FAX: (914) 382-7995
TOLL FREE: (800) 942-4640
WWW.CS.STATE.NY.US

GE MEDICAL BENEFITS CLAIM CENTER
5950 AIRPORT RD
PO BOX 3023
UTICA, NY 13504
TEL: (315) 797-6000
TOLL FREE: (800) 552-3232
WWW.METLIFE.COM

RHODE ISLAND CLAIMS OFFICE
700 QUAKER LN
PO BOX 495
WARWICK, RI 02884
TEL: (401) 827-2482
TOLL FREE: (800) 854-6011

METROPOLITAN LIFE INSURANCE CO/AUTOMOBILE & HOME

OHIO CLAIMS OFFICE
9797 SPRINGBORO PIKE
PO BOX 48020
DAYTON, OH 45475
TEL: (937) 859-2400
FAX: (937) 859-2408
TOLL FREE: (800) 854-6011
IN-STATE: (800) 854-6011

METROPOLITAN PROPERTY & CASUALTY INSURANCE CO

RHODE ISLAND CLAIMS OFFICE
700 QUACKER LN
WARWICK, RI 02887
FAX: (401) 827-6098
TOLL FREE: (800) 422-4272
IN-STATE: (800) 854-6011

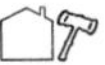

MGIS COMPANIES

UTAH CLAIMS OFFICE
MGIS P & C
1849 W NORTH TEMPLE- BLDG D
SALT LAKE CITY, UT 84116
TEL: (801) 990-2400
FAX: (801) 990-2401
TOLL FREE: (800) 969-6447
IN-STATE: (888) 918-1234

MHC EMPLOYEE BENEFITS TRUST

LOUISIANA CLAIMS OFFICE
2301 MILL ST
PO BOX 1110
ALEXANDRIA, LA 71309-1110
TEL: (318) 483-3875
FAX: (318) 487-1333
TOLL FREE: (800) 533-7169

MICHIGAN EMPLOYEE BENEFIT SERVICES

MICHIGAN CLAIMS OFFICE
25 JEFFERSON AVE SE
GRAND RAPIDS, MI 49503
TEL: (616) 458-6327
FAX: (616) 458-3495
TOLL FREE: (800) 968-6327
IN-STATE: (800) 968-9682
E-MAIL: CUSTSERV@MEBS.COM
WWW.MEBS.COM

MICHIGAN FARM BUREAU MUTUAL INSURANCE CO

7373 W SAGINAW
PO BOX 30100
LANSING, MI 48909
TEL: (517) 323-7000
FAX: (517) 323-6793
TOLL FREE: (800) 292-2680
WWW.FARMBUREAUINS/MI.COM

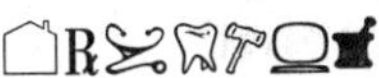

7971 MAIN
PO BOX 169
BIRCH RUN, MI 48415-0169
TEL: (517) 624-4777
FAX: (517) 624-4233
TOLL FREE: (800) 367-5343

3355 EAGLE PARK DR NE, STE 104
PO BOX 152100
GRAND RAPIDS, MI 49515-2100
TEL: (616) 956-1976
FAX: (616) 956-1981
TOLL FREE: (800) 332-9780
WWW.FARMBUREAUINSURANCE-MI.COM

9353 HAGGERTY RD
PO BOX 700980
PLYMOUTH, MI 48170
TEL: (734) 459-1414
TOLL FREE: (800) 322-7185

540 GARFIELD
PO BOX 929
TREVOR CITY, MI 49685-0929
TEL: (616) 947-6262
FAX: (616) 947-7555
TOLL FREE: (800) 782-1547

MICHIGAN MILLERS MUTUAL INSURANCE

2425 E GRAND RIVER
PO BOX 30060
LANSING, MI 48909-0060
TEL: (517) 482-6211
FAX: (517) 371-7733
TOLL FREE: (800) 888-1914
IN-STATE: (800) 457-0040

MICHIGAN MUTUAL INSURANCE CO

ALABAMA CLAIMS OFFICE
AMERISURE
2100 A SOUTHBRIDGE PKY, STE 450
PO BOX 59867
BIRMINGHAM, AL 35259-0867
TEL: (205) 879-3411
FAX: (205) 870-8768
TOLL FREE: (800) 421-7656
WWW.AMERISURE.COM

INDIANA CLAIMS OFFICE
AMERISURE
3600 WOODVIEW TRACE
PO BOX 68876
INDIANAPOLIS, IN 46268
TEL: (317) 872-8694
FAX: (317) 875-3515
IN-STATE: (800) 752-5929
WWW.AMERISURE.COM

MICHIGAN CLAIMS OFFICE
AMERISURE
26777 HALSTED RD
PO BOX 2060
FARMINGTON HILLS, MI 48333-2060
TEL: (248) 615-9000
TOLL FREE: (800) 437-5735
IN-STATE: (800) 257-1900
WWW.AMERISURE.COM

M

AMERISURE
207 E FULTON
PO BOX 116
GRAND RAPIDS, MI 49501-0116
TEL: (616) 451-2971
FAX: (616) 456-5610
TOLL FREE: (800) 632-4597
WWW.AMERISURE.COM

MISSOURI CLAIMS OFFICE
AMERISURE
701 EMERSON RD, STE 320
PO BOX 419058
SAINT LOUIS, MO 63141
TEL: (314) 994-3400
FAX: (314) 993-0791
TOLL FREE: (800) 325-1721
WWW.AMERISURE.COM

NORTH CAROLINA CLAIMS OFFICE
AMERISURE
301 S MCCULLULGH DR, STE 500
PO BOX 560769
CHARLOTTE, NC 28256-0769
TEL: (704) 510-1135
FAX: (704) 510-8327
TOLL FREE: (800) 532-6230
WWW.AMERISURE.COM

TENNESSEE CLAIMS OFFICE
AMERISURE- WHITE STA TWR
57 GERMAN TOWN CT, STE 100
CORDOVA, TN 38018
TEL: (901) 682-3341
FAX: (901) 683-6001
TOLL FREE: (800) 678-2637
WWW.AMERISURE.COM

TEXAS CLAIMS OFFICE
AMERISURE
7610 STEMMONS FWY, STE 350
PO BOX 569680
DALLAS, TX 75356
TEL: (214) 631-6370
FAX: (800) 531-9483
TOLL FREE: (800) 410-293

MID AMERICA MUTUAL LIFE INSURANCE CO

NEBRASKA CLAIMS OFFICE
WORLD INSURANCE
11808 GRANT ST
PO BOX 3160
OMAHA, NE 68103-0160
TEL: (605) 886-8363
TOLL FREE: (800) 995-9051
IN-STATE: (800) 786-7557

SOUTH DAKOTA CLAIMS OFFICE
WORLD INSURANCE
11808 GRANT ST
PO BOX 3160
OMAHA, NE 68103-0160
TEL: (605) 886-8363
TOLL FREE: (800) 995-9051
IN-STATE: (800) 786-7557

MID-AMERICAN INSURANCE GROUP, INC

NEBRASKA CLAIMS OFFICE
5310 N 99TH ST, STE 1
OMAHA, NE 68134-2565
TEL: (402) 571-6224
FAX: (402) 573-8058
TOLL FREE: (800) 364-9505

MID-ATLANTIC MEDICAL SERVICES, INC

DELAWARE CLAIMS OFFICE
4 TAFT CT
ROCKVILLE, MD 20850
TEL: (301) 294-5140
WWW.MAMSI.COM

DISTRICT OF COLUMBIA CLAIMS OFFICE
4 TAFT CT
ROCKVILLE, MD 20850
TEL: (301) 294-5140
WWW.MAMSI.COM

MARYLAND CLAIMS OFFICE
4 TAFT CT
ROCKVILLE, MD 20850
TEL: (301) 294-5140
FAX: (301) 738-1230
TOLL FREE: (800) 544-2853
WWW.MAMSI.COM

NORTH CAROLINA CLAIMS OFFICE
4 TAFT CT
ROCKVILLE, MD 20850
TEL: (301) 294-5140
WWW.MAMSI.COM

PENNSYLVANIA CLAIMS OFFICE
4 TAFT CT
ROCKVILLE, MD 20850
TEL: (301) 294-5140
WWW.MAMSI.COM

VIRGINIA CLAIMS OFFICE
4 TAFT CT
ROCKVILLE, MD 20850
TEL: (301) 294-5140
WWW.MAMSI.COM

WEST VIRGINIA CLAIMS OFFICE
4 TAFT CT
ROCKVILLE, MD 20850
TEL: (301) 294-5140
WWW.MAMSI.COM

MID-CONTINENT CASUALTY CO

OKLAHOMA CLAIMS OFFICE
1646 S BOULDER AVE
PO BOX 1409
TULSA, OK 74101
TEL: (918) 587-7221
FAX: (918) 585-3304
TOLL FREE: (800) 722-4994

MID-PLAINS INSURANCE

IOWA CLAIMS OFFICE
1300 WOODLAND AVE
PO BOX 65150
WEST DES MOINES, IA 50265
TEL: (515) 223-9438
FAX: (515) 223-8065
TOLL FREE: (800) 666-3226

MID-SOUTH BENEFIT PLANS, INC

NATIONAL CLAIMS OFFICE
PICA
110 WESTWOOD PL, STE 100
PO BOX 17208
BRENTWOOD, TN 37027
TEL: (615) 781-0720
FAX: (615) 331-4898
TOLL FREE: (800) 247-3694

MID-SOUTH INSURANCE CO

NORTH CAROLINA CLAIMS OFFICE
4317 RAMSEY ST
PO BOX 2547
FAYETTEVILLE, NC 28302-2069
TEL: (910) 822-1020
FAX: (910) 822-3018
TOLL FREE: (800) 822-9993

MIDA DENTAL PLANS

NATIONAL CLAIMS OFFICE
UNITED CONCORDIA
2000 TOWN CTR, STE 2200
PO BOX 2649
SOUTHFIELD, MI 48037-2649
TEL: (248) 353-6410
FAX: (248) 353-0727
TOLL FREE: (800) 937-6432

MIDDLESEX INSURANCE CO

MASSACHUSETTS CLAIMS OFFICE
CENTRY INSURANCE
3 CARLISLE RD
PO BOX 584
WESTFORD, MA 01886-0584
TEL: (978) 392-7000
FAX: (978) 392-7033
TOLL FREE: (800) 225-1390

MIDDLESEX MUTUAL ASSURANCE CO

CONNECTICUT CLAIMS OFFICE
213 COURT ST
PO BOX 891
MIDDLETOWN, CT 06457-0891
TEL: (860) 347-4621
FAX: (860) 638-5223
TOLL FREE: (800) 899-0032
IN-STATE: (800) 622-3780

Casualty/Liability Dental Disability EMC HCPCS Home Health HMO Medical

MIDLAND CO

OHIO CLAIMS OFFICE
7000 MIDLAND BLVD
PO BOX 5323
CINCINNATI, OH 45210-5323
TEL: (513) 943-7100
FAX: (513) 943-7363
TOLL FREE: (800) 543-2644
IN-STATE: (800) 375-2075

MIDWEST SECURITY ADMINISTRATORS

WISCONSIN CLAIMS OFFICE
MIDWEST SECURITY INSURANCE
1150 SPRINGHURST DR, STE 140
PO BOX 19035
GREEN BAY, WI 54307-9035
TEL: (920) 496-2500

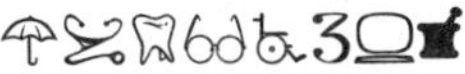

MIDWEST SECURITY INSURANCE CO

ILLINOIS CLAIMS OFFICE
2700 MIDWEST DR
ONALASKA, WI 54650-8764
TEL: (608) 783-7130
FAX: (608) 783-8581
TOLL FREE: (800) 542-6642

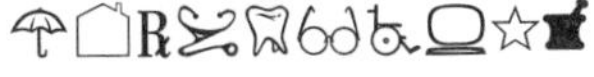

INDIANA CLAIMS OFFICE
2700 MIDWEST DR
ONALASKA, WI 54650-8764
TEL: (608) 783-7130
FAX: (608) 783-8581
TOLL FREE: (800) 542-6642

IOWA CLAIMS OFFICE
2700 MIDWEST DR
ONALASKA, WI 54650-8764
TEL: (608) 783-7130
FAX: (608) 783-8581
TOLL FREE: (800) 542-6642

MINNESOTA CLAIMS OFFICE
2700 MIDWEST DR
ONALASKA, WI 54650-8764
TEL: (608) 783-7130
FAX: (608) 783-8581
TOLL FREE: (800) 542-6642

OHIO CLAIMS OFFICE
2700 MIDWEST DR
ONALASKA, WI 54650-8764
TEL: (608) 783-7130
FAX: (608) 783-8581
TOLL FREE: (800) 542-6642

WISCONSIN CLAIMS OFFICE
2700 MIDWEST DR
ONALASKA, WI 54650-8764
TEL: (608) 783-7130
FAX: (608) 783-8581
TOLL FREE: (800) 542-6642

MILLENNIUM CARE ADMINISTRATORS (DBA MCA ADMINISTRATORS)

OHIO CLAIMS OFFICE
A DIVISION OF MANAGED CARE OF AMERICA
5900 ROCHE DR- 5TH FL
PO BOX 18245
COLUMBUS, OH 43218-0245
TEL: (614) 888-1212
FAX: (614) 888-2240
TOLL FREE: (800) 229-6786
IN-STATE: (800) 524-4426
WWW.MCOA.COM

MILLETTE ADMINISTRATORS, INC

MISSISSIPPI CLAIMS OFFICE
4619 MAIN ST, STE A
MOSS POINT, MS 39563
TEL: (228) 475-8687
TOLL FREE: (800) 456-8647

MILWAUKEE INSURANCE CO

WISCONSIN CLAIMS OFFICE
803 W MICHIGAN
PO BOX 1450
MILWAUKEE, WI 53201-1450
TEL: (414) 277-9175
TOLL FREE: (800) 733-7366

MINNEHOMA INSURANCE CO

NATIONAL CLAIMS OFFICE
OLD REPUBLIC ORDESCO
7050 S YALE AVE
PO BOX 470185
TULSA, OK 74147-0185
TEL: (918) 494-7000
FAX: (918) 494-3088
TOLL FREE: (800) 331-5554

MINNESOTA BENEFIT FIRE & CASUALTY INSURANCE CO

MINNESOTA CLAIMS OFFICE
10225 YELLOW CIR DR
PO BOX 1233
MINNEAPOLIS, MN 55440
TEL: (612) 939-7000
FAX: (612) 939-7117
TOLL FREE: (800) 237-1919

MINNESOTA MUTUAL LIFE INSURANCE CO

400 ROBERT ST N
SAINT PAUL, MN 55101
TEL: (651) 665-3500
FAX: (651) 665-3551

MISSISSIPPI FARM BUREAU MUTUAL INSURANCE CO

MISSISSIPPI CLAIMS OFFICE
MISSISSIPPI FARM FEDERATION
6310 I55 N
PO BOX 1972
JACKSON, MS 39215-1972
TEL: (601) 957-3200
FAX: (601) 977-4880
TOLL FREE: (800) 345-6682
IN-STATE: (800) 227-8244

MIT HEALTH PLAN

MASSACHUSETTS CLAIMS OFFICE
BLUE CROSS
77 MASSACHUSETTS AVE- BLDG E 23, STE 308
PO BOX E23-308 MIT
CAMBRIDGE, MA 02139-4307
TEL: (617) 253-1322
FAX: (617) 253-6558

MITSUBISHI MOTORS MANUFACTURING OF AMERICA INC

NATIONAL CLAIMS OFFICE
100 N MITSUBISHI MOTORWAY
NORMAL, IL 61761
TEL: (309) 888-8000
TOLL FREE: (800) 227-6592

MMA INSURANCE CO

INDIANA CLAIMS OFFICE
1110 N MAIN ST
PO BOX 483
GOSHEN, IN 46527
TEL: (219) 533-9511
FAX: (219) 533-5264
TOLL FREE: (800) 348-7468

MMI COMPANIES

NATIONAL CLAIMS OFFICE
AMERICAN CONTINENTAL LIFE INSURANCE CO
540 LAKE COOK RD
DEERFIELD, IL 60015
TEL: (847) 940-7550
FAX: (847) 940-2372
TOLL FREE: (800) 222-4774
WWW.MMICOMPANIES.COM

MONTGOMERY MUTUAL INSURANCE CO

DELAWARE CLAIMS OFFICE
4040 BLACKBURN RD
BURTONSVILLE, MD 20866
TEL: (301) 924-4700
FAX: (301) 924-5459
TOLL FREE: (800) 638-8933
IN-STATE: (800) 638-8933

DISTRICT OF COLUMBIA CLAIMS OFFICE
4040 BLACKBURN RD
BURTONSVILLE, MD 20866
TEL: (301) 924-4700
FAX: (301) 924-5459
TOLL FREE: (800) 638-8933
IN-STATE: (800) 638-8933

MARYLAND CLAIMS OFFICE
4040 BLACKBURN RD
BURTONSVILLE, MD 20866
TEL: (301) 924-4700
FAX: (301) 924-5459
TOLL FREE: (800) 638-8933
IN-STATE: (800) 638-8933

VIRGINIA CLAIMS OFFICE
4040 BLACKBURN RD
BURTONSVILLE, MD 20866
TEL: (301) 924-4700
FAX: (301) 924-5459
TOLL FREE: (800) 638-8933
IN-STATE: (800) 638-8933

WEST VIRGINIA CLAIMS OFFICE
4040 BLACKBURN RD
BURTONSVILLE, MD 20866
TEL: (301) 924-4700
FAX: (301) 924-5459
TOLL FREE: (800) 638-8933
IN-STATE: (800) 638-8933

MONUMENTAL AGENCY GROUP

NATIONAL CLAIMS OFFICE
CAPITAL SECURITY DIVISION
300 W MORGAN ST
PO BOX 61
DURHAM, NC 27702
TEL: (919) 687-8200
FAX: (919) 687-8534
TOLL FREE: (800) 933-4643
IN-STATE: (800) 544-9631

MONUMENTAL LIFE INSURANCE CO

GEORGIA CLAIMS OFFICE
3370 VINEVILLE AVE, STE 101
PO BOX 4585
MACON, GA 31208-4585
TEL: (912) 477-7183
FAX: (912) 477-7202
TOLL FREE: (800) 933-4643
IN-STATE: (800) 371-7183

NATIONAL CLAIMS OFFICE
2 E CHASE ST
BALTIMORE, MD 21202
TEL: (410) 685-2900
FAX: (410) 385-6903
TOLL FREE: (800) 638-3080
IN-STATE: (800) 753-4357

MOTEL 6 OPERATING LP HEADQUARTERS

TEXAS CLAIMS OFFICE
14651 DALLAS PKY, STE 405A
PO BOX 809092
DALLAS, TX 75240
TEL: (972) 386-6161
FAX: (972) 716-6575
TOLL FREE: (800) 558-5955

MOTOR CLUB OF AMERICA INSURANCE CO

NEW JERSEY CLAIMS OFFICE
95 RT 17 S
PARAMUS, NJ 07653-0931
TEL: (201) 291-2000
FAX: (201) 291-2125
TOLL FREE: (800) 833-3207
IN-STATE: (800) 242-0332
WWW.MOTOR.COM

MOUNT VERNON FIRE INSURANCE CO

NATIONAL CLAIMS OFFICE
US LIABILITY INSURANCE GROUP
1030 CONTINENTAL DR
KING OF PRUSSIA, PA 19406
TEL: (610) 688-2535
FAX: (610) 688-4391

MOUNTAIN STATES ADMINISTRATIVE SERVICE

7202 E ROSEWOOD ST
PO BOX 32702
TUCSON, AZ 85710
TEL: (520) 722-0811
FAX: (520) 722-7245
TOLL FREE: (800) 426-2756

MOUNTAIN STATES MUTUAL CASUALTY CO

NEW MEXICO CLAIMS OFFICE
501 SILVER SW
PO BOX 249
ALBUQUERQUE, NM 87103-0249
TEL: (505) 764-1400
FAX: (505) 247-8540

MOUNTAIN VIEW MEDICAL

UTAH CLAIMS OFFICE
4190 S HIGHLAND DR, STE 100
SALT LAKE CITY, UT 84124
TEL: (801) 272-9798
FAX: (801) 272-9809
TOLL FREE: (800) 336-2775

WYOMING CLAIMS OFFICE
4190 S HIGHLAND DR, STE 100
SALT LAKE CITY, UT 84124
TEL: (801) 272-9798
FAX: (801) 272-9809
TOLL FREE: (800) 336-2775

MOUNTAIN WEST FARM BUREAU MUTUAL INSURANCE CO

406 S 21ST
PO BOX 1348
LARAMIE, WY 82070-1348
TEL: (307) 745-4835
FAX: (307) 721-7738
TOLL FREE: (800) 814-9379

MS ADMINISTRATIVE SERVICES, INC

IDAHO CLAIMS OFFICE
2323 S VISTA, STE 205
PO BOX 45073
BOISE, ID 83705
TEL: (208) 343-2964
FAX: (208) 387-0151
WWW.MSADMIN.COM

MUTUAL ASSURANCE ADMINISTRATORS, INC

NATIONAL CLAIMS OFFICE
3015 UNITED FOUNDERS BLVD
PO BOX 42096
OKLAHOMA CITY, OK 73123-3096
TEL: (405) 848-1975
FAX: (405) 848-1284
TOLL FREE: (800) 825-3540

MUTUAL GROUP

IOWA CLAIMS OFFICE
7601 OFFICE PLZ DR, STE 155
PO BOX 65770
WEST DES MOINES, IA 50265
TOLL FREE: (800) 247-6716
IN-STATE: (800) 283-5433

MUTUAL LIFE INSURANCE CO OF NEW YORK

NEW YORK CLAIMS OFFICE
MONY
ONE MONY PLZ
PO BOX 4830
SYRACUSE, NY 13221
TEL: (315) 477-3336
FAX: (315) 477-3185
TOLL FREE: (800) 487-6669

MUTUAL MED BENEFIT ADMINISTRATORS

IOWA CLAIMS OFFICE
MUTUAL MED, INC
3216 E 35TH ST CT
DAVENPORT, IA 52807
TEL: (319) 344-2890
FAX: (319) 344-2891
TOLL FREE: (800) 747-4126
E-MAIL: MUTUAL@AOL.COM

MUTUAL OF AMERICA

NEW YORK CLAIMS OFFICE
320 PARK AVE
NEW YORK, NY 10022
TEL: (212) 224-1010
FAX: (212) 224-2502
TOLL FREE: (800) 872-6732

MUTUAL OF DETROIT INSURANCE CO

MICHIGAN CLAIMS OFFICE
333 PLYMOUTH RD
PO BOX 500
PLYMOUTH, MI 48170-0500
TEL: (734) 453-8500

Casualty/Liability Dental Disability EMC HCPCS Home Health HMO Medical

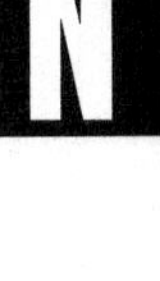

OHIO CLAIMS OFFICE
333 PLYMOUTH RD
PO BOX 500
PLYMOUTH, MI 48170-0500
TEL: (734) 453-8500

MUTUAL OF ENUMCLAW INSURANCE CO

WASHINGTON CLAIMS OFFICE
1460 WELLS ST
ENUMCLAW, WA 98022
TEL: (360) 825-2591
FAX: (360) 825-6507
TOLL FREE: (800) 366-5551

MUTUAL OF OMAHA

NATIONAL CLAIMS OFFICE
OMAHA GROUP PROCESSING CTR
MUTUAL OF OMAHA PLZ
OMAHA, NE 68175
TEL: (402) 342-7600
FAX: (402) 351-2683
TOLL FREE: (800) 775-6000
IN-STATE: (800) 335-5883

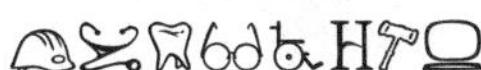

OKLAHOMA CLAIMS OFFICE
WOODWARD CLAIMS PROCESSING CTR
3200 OKLAHOMA AVE
PO BOX 9
WOODWARD, OK 73801
TEL: (580) 256-1717
FAX: (580) 256-2324
TOLL FREE: (800) 462-2877

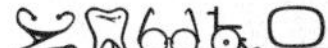

MUTUAL SAVINGS LIFE INSURANCE CO

ALABAMA CLAIMS OFFICE
2801 HWY 31 S
PO BOX 2222
DECATUR, AL 35609-2222
TEL: (256) 552-7011
FAX: (256) 552-7284
TOLL FREE: (800) 239-6754

GEORGIA CLAIMS OFFICE
2801 HWY 31 S
PO BOX 2222
DECATUR, AL 35609-2222
TEL: (256) 552-7011
FAX: (256) 552-7284
TOLL FREE: (800) 239-6754

MISSISSIPPI CLAIMS OFFICE
2801 HWY 31 S
PO BOX 2222
DECATUR, AL 35609-2222
TEL: (256) 552-7011
FAX: (256) 552-7284
TOLL FREE: (800) 239-6754

MUTUAL SERVICE INSURANCE CO

NATIONAL CLAIMS OFFICE
2 PINETREE DR
PO BOX 64035
ARDEN HILLS, MN 55112
TEL: (651) 631-7000
FAX: (651) 639-5400
TOLL FREE: (800) 544-3229
WWW.MSI-INSURANCE.COM

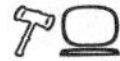

MVP HEALTH PLAN

NEW YORK CLAIMS OFFICE
MOHAWK VALLEY PHYSICIANS HEALTH PLAN
111 LIBERTY ST
PO BOX 2207
SCHENECTADY, NY 12301-2207
TEL: (518) 370-4793
FAX: (518) 370-0830
TOLL FREE: (800) 777-4793

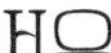

VERMONT CLAIMS OFFICE
MOHAWK VALLEY PHYSICIANS HEALTH PLAN
111 LIBERTY ST
PO BOX 2207
SCHENECTADY, NY 12301-2207
TEL: (518) 370-4793
FAX: (518) 370-0830
TOLL FREE: (800) 777-4793

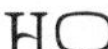

MYERS STEVENS

CALIFORNIA CLAIMS OFFICE
26101 MARGUERITE PKY
MISSION VIEJO, CA 92692
TEL: (949) 348-0656
FAX: (949) 348-2630
TOLL FREE: (800) 827-4695

NALC HEALTH BENEFIT PLAN

NATIONAL CLAIMS OFFICE
NATIONAL ASSOCIATION OF LETTER CARRIERS
20547 WAVERLY CT
ASHBURN, VA 20149-0001
TEL: (703) 729-4677
FAX: (703) 729-0076
TOLL FREE: (800) 548-8484
WWW.NALC.ORG/HBP

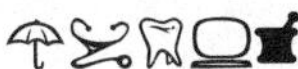

NAPUS HEALTH BENEFIT PLAN

BLUE CROSS & BLUE SHIELD
550 12TH ST SW
WASHINGTON, DC 20065-3520
TEL: (202) 479-8000
FAX: (202) 479-3520
TOLL FREE: (800) 424-7474
WWW.CAREFIRST.COM

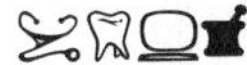

NATIONAL ACCIDENT INSURANCE UNDERWRITERS

85 W ALGONQUIN RD- 5TH FL
ARLINGTON HEIGHTS, IL 60005
TEL: (847) 981-9320
FAX: (847) 631-0139

NATIONAL AFFILIATED INVESTORS LIFE INSURANCE CO

LOUISIANA CLAIMS OFFICE
7228 ENGLAND DR, STE 24
PO BOX 12190
ALEXANDRIA, LA 71315
TEL: (318) 473-4355
FAX: (318) 442-3318
TOLL FREE: (800) 673-2220

NATIONAL ALLIANCE OF POSTAL & FEDERAL EMPLOYEES

NATIONAL CLAIMS OFFICE
AETNA U.S. HEALTH PLAN
655 S BAY RD ST 1A
PO BOX 7012
DOVER, DE 19903
TEL: (302) 674-7600
FAX: (302) 857-4808
TOLL FREE: (800) 572-9096
IN-STATE: (800) 572-9096
WWW.AETNA.COM

NATIONAL AMERICAN INSURANCE

1003 ALLISON AVE
PO BOX 38
CHANDLER, OK 74834-0038
TEL: (405) 258-0804
FAX: (405) 258-1329
TOLL FREE: (800) 332-2210

NATIONAL AMERICAN INSURANCE CO OF CALIFORNIA

ARIZONA CLAIMS OFFICE
DANIELSEN NATIONAL
19100 SUZANNA RD
PO BOX 5810
LONG BEACH, CA 90805-5810
TEL: (310) 605-3300
FAX: (310) 605-3273
TOLL FREE: (800) 624-4104
WWW.NAICC.COM

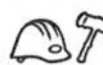

CALIFORNIA CLAIMS OFFICE
DANIELSEN NATIONAL
19100 SUZANNA RD
PO BOX 5810
LONG BEACH, CA 90805-5810
TEL: (310) 605-3300
FAX: (310) 605-3273
TOLL FREE: (800) 624-4104
WWW.NAICC.COM

NEVADA CLAIMS OFFICE
DANIELSEN NATIONAL
19100 SUZANNA RD
PO BOX 5810
LONG BEACH, CA 90805-5810
TEL: (310) 605-3300
FAX: (310) 605-3273
TOLL FREE: (800) 624-4104
WWW.NAICC.COM

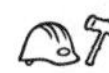

UTAH CLAIMS OFFICE
DANIELSEN NATIONAL
19100 SUZANNA RD
PO BOX 5810
LONG BEACH, CA 90805-5810
TEL: (310) 605-3300
FAX: (310) 605-3273
TOLL FREE: (800) 624-4104
WWW.NAICC.COM

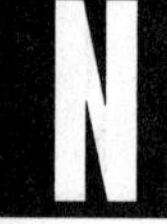

NATIONAL ASSOCIATION OF MUTUAL INSURANCE

NATIONAL CLAIMS OFFICE
3601 VINCENNES RD
PO BOX 68700
INDIANAPOLIS, IN 46268-0700
TEL: (317) 875-5250
FAX: (317) 879-8408
TOLL FREE: (800) 336-2642
WWW.NAMIC.ORG

NATIONAL AUTOMOBILE & CASUALTY INSURANCE CO

CALIFORNIA CLAIMS OFFICE
257 S FAIROAKS AVE
PO BOX 7040
PASADENA, CA 91105-7040
TEL: (626) 577-0600
FAX: (626) 356-0253
TOLL FREE: (800) 995-4449

NATIONAL BENEFIT LIFE INSURANCE CO

NATIONAL CLAIMS OFFICE
33 W 34TH ST
NEW YORK, NY 10116-5603
TEL: (212) 615-7500
FAX: (212) 615-7321
TOLL FREE: (800) 221-2554
IN-STATE: (800) 221-2554

NATIONAL BENEFIT PLANS, INC

VICARE ADMINISTRATIVE SERVICES
5 ROGER CTR, STE 127
PO BOX 13128
NORFOLK, VA 23506-0128
TEL: (757) 466-1940
FAX: (757) 466-7570
TOLL FREE: 800-582-2001

NATIONAL BENEFITS CORP

ILLINOIS CLAIMS OFFICE
AON SELECT
110 GIBRALTAR RD, STE 116
HORSHAM, PA 19044
TEL: (215) 443-0404
FAX: (215) 443-0435

PENNSYLVANIA CLAIMS OFFICE
AON SELECT
110 GIBRALTAR RD, STE 116
HORSHAM, PA 19044
TEL: (215) 443-0404
FAX: (215) 443-0435

NATIONAL CONTINENTAL PROGRESSIVE CASUALTY INSURANCE CO

CONNECTICUT CLAIMS OFFICE
100 CANAL PT BLVD, STE 210
PO BOX 7637
PRINCETON, NJ 08543
FAX: (609) 452-8812
TOLL FREE: (800) 444-0013

NEW JERSEY CLAIMS OFFICE
100 CANAL PT BLVD, STE 210
PO BOX 7637
PRINCETON, NJ 08543
FAX: (609) 452-8812
TOLL FREE: (800) 444-0013

NATIONAL EMPLOYEE BENEFIT ADMINISTRATORS

FLORIDA CLAIMS OFFICE
7950 NW 53RD ST, STE 202
MIAMI, FL 33166
TEL: (305) 591-0061
FAX: (305) 592-0093

NATIONAL CLAIMS OFFICE
505 S LENOLA RD, STE 217
MOORESTOWN, NJ 08057-1549
TEL: (609) 234-9086
FAX: (609) 727-3237
TOLL FREE: (800) 394-2524

OKLAHOMA CLAIMS OFFICE
7950 NW 53RD ST, STE 202
MIAMI, FL 33166
TEL: (305) 591-0061
FAX: (305) 592-0093

TEXAS CLAIMS OFFICE
7950 NW 53RD ST, STE 202
MIAMI, FL 33166
TEL: (305) 591-0061
FAX: (305) 592-0093

NATIONAL FAMILY CARE LIFE INSURANCE CO

13530 INWOOD RD
PO BOX 809043
DALLAS, TX 75380-9043
TEL: (972) 387-8553
FAX: (972) 788-1156
IN-STATE: (800) 527-0996

NATIONAL FARMERS UNION PROPERTY & CASUALTY CO

NATIONAL CLAIMS OFFICE
CLAIMS DEPARTMENT
11900 E CORNELL AVE
AURORA, CO 80014-3194
TEL: (303) 338-2216
FAX: (800) 496-4805
TOLL FREE: (800) 347-1961

NATIONAL FOUNDATION LIFE INSURANCE CO

KENTUCKY CLAIMS OFFICE
FREEDOM LIVES
110 W 7TH ST, STE 300
FT WORTH, TX 76102
TEL: (817) 878-3300
FAX: (817) 878-3480
TOLL FREE: (800) 221-9039

TEXAS CLAIMS OFFICE
FREEDOM LIVES
110 W 7TH ST, STE 300
FT WORTH, TX 76102
TEL: (817) 878-3300
FAX: (817) 878-3480
TOLL FREE: (800) 221-9039

NATIONAL GENERAL INSURANCE CO

NATIONAL CLAIMS OFFICE
1 NATIONAL GENERAL PLZ
EARTH CITY, MO 63045
TEL: (314) 298-0500
FAX: (314) 344-9988
TOLL FREE: (800) 325-1088
WWW.NGIC.COM

NATIONAL GRANGE MUTUAL INSURANCE CO

CONNECTICUT CLAIMS OFFICE
CLAIMS OFFICE
27 MIDSTATE DR
AUBURN, MA 01501
TEL: (508) 832-7171
FAX: (508) 832-4187
TOLL FREE: (800) 343-0562
IN-STATE: (800) 252-8704

MAINE CLAIMS OFFICE
55 WEST ST
PO BOX 2300
KEENE, NH 03431-3374
TEL: (603) 352-4000
FAX: (603) 358-1348
TOLL FREE: (800) 258-5340
IN-STATE: (800) 542-5396

CLAIMS OFFICE
27 MIDSTATE DR
AUBURN, MA 01501
TEL: (508) 832-7171
FAX: (508) 832-4187
TOLL FREE: (800) 343-0562
IN-STATE: (800) 252-8704

MASSACHUSETTS CLAIMS OFFICE
CLAIMS OFFICE
27 MIDSTATE DR
AUBURN, MA 01501
TEL: (508) 832-7171
FAX: (508) 832-4187
TOLL FREE: (800) 343-0562
IN-STATE: (800) 252-8704

NATIONAL CLAIMS OFFICE
PO BOX 4828
SYRACUSE, NY 13221
TEL: (800) 962-5515
FAX: (315) 434-1429
TOLL FREE: (800) 622-1282
IN-STATE: (800) 622-1282
WWW.MSAGROUP.COM

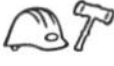

5010 CAMPAS DR
PO BOX 4828
SYRACUSE, NY 13221-4828
TEL: (315) 434-1400
FAX: (315) 434-1429
TOLL FREE: (800) 626-6020
IN-STATE: (800) 962-5515
WWW.MSAGROUP.COM

4186 INNSLAKE DR
PO BOX 6419
GLEN ALLEN, VA 23058-6419
TEL: (804) 270-6611
FAX: (888) 646-1005
TOLL FREE: (800) 446-7649
WWW.MSAGROUP.COM

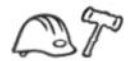

NEW HAMPSHIRE CLAIMS OFFICE
55 WEST ST
PO BOX 2300
KEENE, NH 03431-3374
TEL: (603) 352-4000
FAX: (603) 358-1348
TOLL FREE: (800) 258-5340
IN-STATE: (800) 542-5396

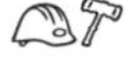

CLAIMS OFFICE
27 MIDSTATE DR
AUBURN, MA 01501
TEL: (508) 832-7171
FAX: (508) 832-4187
TOLL FREE: (800) 343-0562
IN-STATE: (800) 252-8704

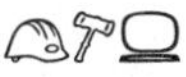

RHODE ISLAND CLAIMS OFFICE
CLAIMS OFFICE
27 MIDSTATE DR
AUBURN, MA 01501
TEL: (508) 832-7171
FAX: (508) 832-4187
TOLL FREE: (800) 343-0562
IN-STATE: (800) 252-8704

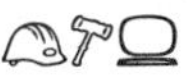

VERMONT CLAIMS OFFICE
55 WEST ST
PO BOX 2300
KEENE, NH 03431-3374
TEL: (603) 352-4000
FAX: (603) 358-1348
TOLL FREE: (800) 258-5340
IN-STATE: (800) 542-5396

CLAIMS OFFICE
27 MIDSTATE DR
AUBURN, MA 01501
TEL: (508) 832-7171
FAX: (508) 832-4187
TOLL FREE: (800) 343-0562
IN-STATE: (800) 252-8704

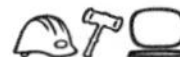

NATIONAL GUARDIAN LIFE INSURANCE CO

WISCONSIN CLAIMS OFFICE
2 E GILLMANN
PO BOX 1191
MADISON, WI 53701-1191
TEL: (608) 257-5611
FAX: (608) 257-4308
TOLL FREE: (800) 548-2962
WWW.NATIONALGUARDIAN.COM

NATIONAL HEALTH INSURANCE CO

TEXAS CLAIMS OFFICE
1901 N HWY 360
PO BOX 619999
DALLAS, TX 75261-9999
TEL: (817) 640-1900
FAX: (817) 640-3406
TOLL FREE: (800) 237-1900

NATIONAL HEALTH PLANS

CALIFORNIA CLAIMS OFFICE
NATIONAL-MED
1005 W ORANGEBURG, STE B
PO BOX 5356
MODESTO, CA 95352
TEL: (209) 527-3350
FAX: (209) 527-6773
TOLL FREE: (800) 468-8600
WWW.NATIONALHMO.COM

NATIONAL HOSPITAL NETWORK SYSTEM

NATIONAL CLAIMS OFFICE
ROBINSON HEALTH SERVICES
4458 S CLEVELAND AVE
FT MYERS, FL 33901
TEL: (941) 275-2666

H

NATIONAL INDEMNITY CO

NEBRASKA CLAIMS OFFICE
4016 FARNAM ST
OMAHA, NE 68131-3016
TEL: (402) 536-3000
FAX: (402) 536-3031
TOLL FREE: (800) 356-5750
E-MAIL: NICOCLAIMS@AOL.COM

NATIONAL MUTUAL BENEFIT

COLORADO CLAIMS OFFICE
6522 GRAND TETON PLZ
PO BOX 1527
MADISON, WI 53701-1527
TEL: (608) 833-1936
FAX: (608) 833-8714
TOLL FREE: (800) 779-1936

ILLINOIS CLAIMS OFFICE
6522 GRAND TETON PLZ
PO BOX 1527
MADISON, WI 53701-1527
TEL: (608) 833-1936
FAX: (608) 833-8714
TOLL FREE: (800) 779-1936

IOWA CLAIMS OFFICE
6522 GRAND TETON PLZ
PO BOX 1527
MADISON, WI 53701-1527
TEL: (608) 833-1936
FAX: (608) 833-8714
TOLL FREE: (800) 779-1936

MICHIGAN CLAIMS OFFICE
6522 GRAND TETON PLZ
PO BOX 1527
MADISON, WI 53701-1527
TEL: (608) 833-1936
FAX: (608) 833-8714
TOLL FREE: (800) 779-1936

MINNESOTA CLAIMS OFFICE
6522 GRAND TETON PLZ
PO BOX 1527
MADISON, WI 53701-1527
TEL: (608) 833-1936
FAX: (608) 833-8714
TOLL FREE: (800) 779-1936

MONTANA CLAIMS OFFICE
6522 GRAND TETON PLZ
PO BOX 1527
MADISON, WI 53701-1527
TEL: (608) 833-1936
FAX: (608) 833-8714
TOLL FREE: (800) 779-1936

NEBRASKA CLAIMS OFFICE
6522 GRAND TETON PLZ
PO BOX 1527
MADISON, WI 53701-1527
TEL: (608) 833-1936
FAX: (608) 833-8714
TOLL FREE: (800) 779-1936

NORTH DAKOTA CLAIMS OFFICE
6522 GRAND TETON PLZ
PO BOX 1527
MADISON, WI 53701-1527
TEL: (608) 833-1936
FAX: (608) 833-8714
TOLL FREE: (800) 779-1936

SOUTH DAKOTA CLAIMS OFFICE
6522 GRAND TETON PLZ
PO BOX 1527
MADISON, WI 53701-1527
TEL: (608) 833-1936
FAX: (608) 833-8714
TOLL FREE: (800) 779-1936

WISCONSIN CLAIMS OFFICE
6522 GRAND TETON PLZ
PO BOX 1527
MADISON, WI 53701-1527
TEL: (608) 833-1936
FAX: (608) 833-8714
TOLL FREE: (800) 779-1936

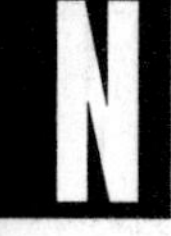

WYOMING CLAIMS OFFICE
6522 GRAND TETON PLZ
PO BOX 1527
MADISON, WI 53701-1527
TEL: (608) 833-1936
FAX: (608) 833-8714
TOLL FREE: (800) 779-1936

NATIONAL MUTUAL INSURANCE CO

NATIONAL CLAIMS OFFICE
CELINA GROUP
1 INSURANCE SQ
CELINA, OH 45822-1659
TEL: (419) 586-5181
FAX: (419) 586-6068
TOLL FREE: (800) 552-5181

NATIONAL RURAL LETTER CARRIERS' ASSOCIATION

UNION OF POSTAL WORKERS
2050 REMOUNT RD
GASTONIA, NC 28054
TEL: (704) 853-7900
FAX: (704) 853-7911
TOLL FREE: (800) 638-8432
WWW.MUTUALOFOMAHA.COM

NATIONAL SECURITY INSURANCE CO

ALABAMA CLAIMS OFFICE
661 E DAVIS ST
PO BOX 703
ELBA, AL 36323-9478
TEL: (334) 897-2273
TOLL FREE: (800) 239-2358

FLORIDA CLAIMS OFFICE
661 E DAVIS ST
PO BOX 703
ELBA, AL 36323-9478
TEL: (334) 897-2273
TOLL FREE: (800) 239-2358

GEORGIA CLAIMS OFFICE
661 E DAVIS ST
PO BOX 703
ELBA, AL 36323-9478
TEL: (334) 897-2273
TOLL FREE: (800) 239-2358

KENTUCKY CLAIMS OFFICE
661 E DAVIS ST
PO BOX 703
ELBA, AL 36323-9478
TEL: (334) 897-2273
TOLL FREE: (800) 239-2358

NATIONAL STATES INSURANCE CO

MISSOURI CLAIMS OFFICE
1830 CRAIG PARK CT
SAINT LOUIS, MO 63146-4146
TEL: (314) 878-0101
FAX: (314) 878-8118
TOLL FREE: (800) 868-6788

NATIONAL TRAVELERS LIFE INSURANCE CO

NATIONAL CLAIMS OFFICE
5700 WESTOWN PKY
PO BOX 9197
WEST DES MOINES, IA 50266-9197
TEL: (515) 221-0101
FAX: (515) 327-5830
TOLL FREE: 800-232-5818
WWW.NATIONALTRAVELERSLIFE.COM

NATIONWIDE HEALTH PLAN

OHIO CLAIMS OFFICE
ATTN: CLAIMS DEPT
525 PARK CTR CIR
PO BOX 182690
DUBLIN, OH 43218-2690
FAX: (614) 854-3401
TOLL FREE: (800) 826-9017
WWW.NATIONWIDEHEALTH.COM

H

NATIONWIDE INSURANCE ENTERPRISES

DELAWARE CLAIMS OFFICE
CLAIMS OFFICE
910 W BASIN RD
NEW CASTLE, DE 19720
TEL: (302) 325-8900
FAX: (302) 325-8930
TOLL FREE: (800) 431-3535

MARYLAND CLAIMS OFFICE
CLAIMS OFFICE
910 W BASIN RD
NEW CASTLE, DE 19720
TEL: (302) 325-8900
FAX: (302) 325-8930
TOLL FREE: (800) 431-3535

NATIONWIDE LIFE INSURANCE CO

NATIONAL CLAIMS OFFICE
ONE NATIONWIDE PLZ
PO BOX 2399
COLUMBUS, OH 43216-2399
TEL: (614) 249-7111
FAX: (614) 249-7705
TOLL FREE: (800) 772-9956
WWW.NATIONWIDEHEALTH.COM

NATIONWIDE MUTUAL INSURANCE CO

ALABAMA CLAIMS OFFICE
3300 WILLISTON RD
PO BOX 147081
GAINESVILLE, FL 32614-7081
TEL: (352) 377-8500
FAX: (352) 338-4815
TOLL FREE: (800) 421-3535
WWW.NATIONWIDEHEALTH.COM

CONNECTICUT CLAIMS OFFICE
10 RESEARCH PKY
WALLINGFORD, CT 06492
TEL: (203) 294-7600
FAX: (203) 294-7646
TOLL FREE: (800) 421-3535
WWW.NATIONWIDEHEALTH.COM

DELAWARE CLAIMS OFFICE
3300 WILLISTON RD
PO BOX 147081
GAINESVILLE, FL 32614-7081
TEL: (352) 377-8500
FAX: (352) 338-4815
TOLL FREE: (800) 421-3535
WWW.NATIONWIDEHEALTH.COM

DISTRICT OF COLUMBIA CLAIMS OFFICE
3300 WILLISTON RD
PO BOX 147081
GAINESVILLE, FL 32614-7081
TEL: (352) 377-8500
FAX: (352) 338-4815
TOLL FREE: (800) 421-3535
WWW.NATIONWIDEHEALTH.COM

FLORIDA CLAIMS OFFICE
3300 WILLISTON RD
PO BOX 147081
GAINESVILLE, FL 32614-7081
TEL: (352) 377-8500
FAX: (352) 338-4815
TOLL FREE: (800) 421-3535
WWW.NATIONWIDEHEALTH.COM

GEORGIA CLAIMS OFFICE
4500 N PT PKY
PO BOX 1612
ALPHARETTA, GA 30009
TEL: (770) 667-6600
FAX: (770) 667-6601
TOLL FREE: (800) 421-3535

3300 WILLISTON RD
PO BOX 147081
GAINESVILLE, FL 32614-7081
TEL: (352) 377-8500
FAX: (352) 338-4815
TOLL FREE: (800) 421-3535
WWW.NATIONWIDEHEALTH.COM

INDIANA CLAIMS OFFICE
11550 N MERIDIAN, STE 400
CARMEL, IN 46032
TEL: (317) 587-2600
FAX: (317) 587-0017
TOLL FREE: (800) 348-6632

MAINE CLAIMS OFFICE
10 RESEARCH PKY
WALLINGFORD, CT 06492
TEL: (203) 294-7600
FAX: (203) 294-7646
TOLL FREE: (800) 421-3535
WWW.NATIONWIDEHEALTH.COM

258 S RIVER RD
BEDFORD, NH 03110-6824
TEL: (603) 621-5310

Casualty/Liability Dental Disability EMC HCPCS Home Health H HMO Medical

MARYLAND CLAIMS OFFICE
3300 WILLISTON RD
PO BOX 147081
GAINESVILLE, FL 32614-7081
TEL: (352) 377-8500
FAX: (352) 338-4815
TOLL FREE: (800) 421-3535
WWW.NATIONWIDEHEALTH.COM

MICHIGAN CLAIMS OFFICE
901 TWR DR, STE 400
TROY, MI 48098
TEL: (248) 828-1200
FAX: (248) 828-1202
TOLL FREE: (800) 373-8769
WWW.NATIONWIDEHEALTH.COM

NATIONAL CLAIMS OFFICE
16410 HERITAGE BLVD
MITCHELLEVILLE, MD 20716-3109
TEL: (301) 352-5431
FAX: (301) 352-3467
TOLL FREE: (800) 421-3535

4401 CREEDMOOR RD
PO BOX 30000
RALEIGH, NC 27603-3000
TEL: (919) 781-3322
FAX: (919) 881-3335
TOLL FREE: (800) 421-3535
WWW.NATIONWIDE-HEALTH.COM

NATIONWIDE DIRECT
919 NE 19TH AVE
PO BOX 4114
PORTLAND, OR 97208-3100
TEL: (503) 238-4100
FAX: (503) 234-7575
TOLL FREE: (800) 243-7828
WWW.NDIRECT.COM

1000 NATIONWIDE DR
PO BOX 2655
HARRISBURG, PA 17105-2655
TEL: (717) 657-6400
FAX: (717) 657-6729
TOLL FREE: (800) 421-3535
WWW.NATIONWIDEHEALTH.COM

CALLE MEJICO 16
PO BOX 1899
HATO REY, PR 00918-1899
TEL: (787) 753-8600

100 GATEWAY BLVD
PO BOX 100276
COLUMBIA, SC 29202-3276
TEL: (803) 699-0051
FAX: (803) 699-8548
WWW.NATIONWIDEHEALTH.COM

NEW HAMPSHIRE CLAIMS OFFICE
258 S RIVER RD
BEDFORD, NH 03110-6824
TEL: (603) 621-5310

10 RESEARCH PKY
WALLINGFORD, CT 06492
TEL: (203) 294-7600
FAX: (203) 294-7646
TOLL FREE: (800) 421-3535
WWW.NATIONWIDEHEALTH.COM

OHIO CLAIMS OFFICE
1000 MARKET AVE N
PO BOX 8379
CANTON, OH 44712
TEL: (330) 489-5000
FAX: (330) 489-5797
TOLL FREE: (800) 421-3535
WWW.NATIONWIDE.COM

RHODE ISLAND CLAIMS OFFICE
10 RESEARCH PKY
WALLINGFORD, CT 06492
TEL: (203) 294-7600
FAX: (203) 294-7646
TOLL FREE: (800) 421-3535
WWW.NATIONWIDEHEALTH.COM

SOUTH CAROLINA CLAIMS OFFICE
4500 N PT PKY
PO BOX 1612
ALPHARETTA, GA 30009
TEL: (770) 667-6600
FAX: (770) 667-6601
TOLL FREE: (800) 421-3535

TENNESSEE CLAIMS OFFICE
5100 POPLAR AVE- CLOCK TWR, STE 2300
MEMPHIS, TN 38137-2301
TEL: (901) 821-5100
FAX: (901) 821-5127
TOLL FREE: (800) 421-3535
WWW.NATIONWIDEHEALTH.COM

TEXAS CLAIMS OFFICE
7990 INTERSTATE HWY 10 W
PO BOX 101517
SAN ANTONIO, TX 78201
TEL: (210) 949-6000
TOLL FREE: (800) 421-3535
IN-STATE: (800) 854-9265

VERMONT CLAIMS OFFICE
10 RESEARCH PKY
WALLINGFORD, CT 06492
TEL: (203) 294-7600
FAX: (203) 294-7646
TOLL FREE: (800) 421-3535
WWW.NATIONWIDEHEALTH.COM

258 S RIVER RD
BEDFORD, NH 03110-6824
TEL: (603) 621-5310

VIRGINIA CLAIMS OFFICE
800 GRAVES MILL RD
PO BOX 10338
LYNCHBURG, VA 24506-0338
TEL: (804) 237-7200
FAX: (804) 237-7475
TOLL FREE: (800) 446-0992
WWW.NATIONWIDEHEALTH.COM

WEST VIRGINIA CLAIMS OFFICE
2501 MOUNTAINEER BLVD
PO BOX 58220
SOUTH CHARLESTON, WV 25358
TEL: (304) 746-7600
FAX: (304) 746-7691
TOLL FREE: (800) 950-2959
WWW.NATIONWIDEHEALTH.COM

NAVISTAR

NATIONAL CLAIMS OFFICE
AETNA LIFE & CASUALTY
455 N CITYFRONT PLZ DR
PO BOX 5367
CHICAGO, IL 60611
TEL: (312) 836-2000
FAX: (312) 836-2227

NEIGHBORHOOD HEALTH PARTNERSHIP

FLORIDA CLAIMS OFFICE
7600 CORPORATE CTR DR
PO BOX 025680
MIAMI, FL 33102-5680
TEL: (305) 715-2200
FAX: (305) 715-2650
TOLL FREE: (800) 354-0222

H

NEIGHBORHOOD HEALTH PLAN, INC

NATIONAL CLAIMS OFFICE
253 SUMMER ST
BOSTON, MA 02210
TEL: (617) 772-5500
FAX: (617) 772-5513
TOLL FREE: (800) 433-5556
WWW.NHP.ORG

R H

NESTLE USA

ADMINISTRATORS
535 ANTON, STE 3300
PO BOX 5043
COSTA MESA, CA 92628
TEL: (714) 966-9131
TOLL FREE: (800) 315-3440

NETHERLANDS, PEERLESS, OR INDIANA INSURANCE CO

CONNECTICUT CLAIMS OFFICE
DIVISIONS OF LIBERTY MUTUAL
62 MAPLE AVE
KEENE, NH 03431-1625
TEL: (603) 358-3800
FAX: (603) 357-9995

3

ILLINOIS CLAIMS OFFICE
DIVISIONS OF LIBERTY MUTUAL
62 MAPLE AVE
KEENE, NH 03431-1625
TEL: (603) 358-3800
FAX: (603) 357-9995

3

INDIANA CLAIMS OFFICE
DIVISIONS OF LIBERTY MUTUAL
62 MAPLE AVE
KEENE, NH 03431-1625
TEL: (603) 358-3800
FAX: (603) 357-9995

3

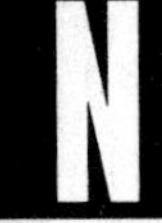

KENTUCKY CLAIMS OFFICE
DIVISIONS OF LIBERTY MUTUAL
62 MAPLE AVE
KEENE, NH 03431-1625
TEL: (603) 358-3800
FAX: (603) 357-9995

MAINE CLAIMS OFFICE
DIVISIONS OF LIBERTY MUTUAL
62 MAPLE AVE
KEENE, NH 03431-1625
TEL: (603) 358-3800
FAX: (603) 357-9995

MARYLAND CLAIMS OFFICE
DIVISIONS OF LIBERTY MUTUAL
62 MAPLE AVE
KEENE, NH 03431-1625
TEL: (603) 358-3800
FAX: (603) 357-9995

MICHIGAN CLAIMS OFFICE
DIVISIONS OF LIBERTY MUTUAL
62 MAPLE AVE
KEENE, NH 03431-1625
TEL: (603) 358-3800
FAX: (603) 357-9995

NEW HAMPSHIRE CLAIMS OFFICE
DIVISIONS OF LIBERTY MUTUAL
62 MAPLE AVE
KEENE, NH 03431-1625
TEL: (603) 358-3800
FAX: (603) 357-9995

NEW JERSEY CLAIMS OFFICE
DIVISIONS OF LIBERTY MUTUAL
62 MAPLE AVE
KEENE, NH 03431-1625
TEL: (603) 358-3800
FAX: (603) 357-9995

NEW YORK CLAIMS OFFICE
DIVISIONS OF LIBERTY MUTUAL
62 MAPLE AVE
KEENE, NH 03431-1625
TEL: (603) 358-3800
FAX: (603) 357-9995

NORTH CAROLINA CLAIMS OFFICE
DIVISIONS OF LIBERTY MUTUAL
62 MAPLE AVE
KEENE, NH 03431-1625
TEL: (603) 358-3800
FAX: (603) 357-9995

OHIO CLAIMS OFFICE
DIVISIONS OF LIBERTY MUTUAL
62 MAPLE AVE
KEENE, NH 03431-1625
TEL: (603) 358-3800
FAX: (603) 357-9995

RHODE ISLAND CLAIMS OFFICE
DIVISIONS OF LIBERTY MUTUAL
62 MAPLE AVE
KEENE, NH 03431-1625
TEL: (603) 358-3800
FAX: (603) 357-9995

TENNESSEE CLAIMS OFFICE
DIVISIONS OF LIBERTY MUTUAL
62 MAPLE AVE
KEENE, NH 03431-1625
TEL: (603) 358-3800
FAX: (603) 357-9995

VERMONT CLAIMS OFFICE
DIVISIONS OF LIBERTY MUTUAL
62 MAPLE AVE
KEENE, NH 03431-1625
TEL: (603) 358-3800
FAX: (603) 357-9995

VIRGINIA CLAIMS OFFICE
DIVISIONS OF LIBERTY MUTUAL
62 MAPLE AVE
KEENE, NH 03431-1625
TEL: (603) 358-3800
FAX: (603) 357-9995

WISCONSIN CLAIMS OFFICE
DIVISIONS OF LIBERTY MUTUAL
62 MAPLE AVE
KEENE, NH 03431-1625
TEL: (603) 358-3800
FAX: (603) 357-9995

NETWORK HEALTH PLAN OF WISCONSIN

1570 MIDWAY PL
PO BOX 120
MENASHA, WI 54952
TEL: (920) 727-0100
TOLL FREE: (800) 826-0940

NEW AIR LIFE

ALABAMA CLAIMS OFFICE
PO BOX 4884
HOUSTON, TX 77210-4884
TEL: (281) 368-7200
FAX: (281) 368-7329
TOLL FREE: (800) 552-7879

NEW CASTLE MUTUAL INSURANCE CO

DELAWARE CLAIMS OFFICE
31 E SOUTH ST
PO BOX 129
SMYRNA, DE 19977
TEL: (302) 653-5114
TOLL FREE: (800) 229-6164

MARYLAND CLAIMS OFFICE
31 E SOUTH ST
PO BOX 129
SMYRNA, DE 19977
TEL: (302) 653-5114
TOLL FREE: (800) 229-6164

NEW ENGLAND FINANCIAL

NATIONAL CLAIMS OFFICE
90 WOODRIDGE CTR DR
PO BOX 4015
ISELIN, NJ 08830
FAX: (732) 602-0657
TOLL FREE: (800) 685-4020

NEW ENGLAND GENERAL LIFE INSURANCE CO

GREAT WEST INSURANCE
PO BOX 88260
ATLANTA, GA 30356
FAX: (770) 394-5476
TOLL FREE: (800) 723-6991

900 2ND AVE S, STE 650
MINNEAPOLIS, MN 55402-3341
FAX: (612) 673-9738
TOLL FREE: (800) 374-2749

OHIO CLAIMS OFFICE
25145 COUNTRY CLUB BLVD
NORTH OLMSTED, OH 44070-5312
FAX: (440) 777-1474
TOLL FREE: (800) 944-6692

NEW ERA LIFE INSURANCE CO

NATIONAL CLAIMS OFFICE
200 WESTLAKE PARK BLVD
PO BOX 4884
HOUSTON, TX 77210-4884
TEL: (281) 368-7200
FAX: (281) 368-7382
TOLL FREE: (800) 552-7879

NEW HAMPSHIRE AUTO DEALERS TRUST

NEW HAMPSHIRE CLAIMS OFFICE
BLUE CROSS & BLUE SHIELD
507 S ST
PO BOX 2337
CONCORD, NH 03302-2337
TEL: (603) 224-2369
FAX: (603) 225-4895
TOLL FREE: (800) 852-3372

NEW INDEPENDENT LEATHER NOVELTY & PLASTIC WORKERS UNION

NEW YORK CLAIMS OFFICE
HEALTH & WELFARE FUND
1981 MARCUS AVE, STE C108
LAKE SUCCESS, NY 10042
TEL: (516) 355-0969
FAX: (516) 355-0668

NEW JERSEY HOSPITAL ASSOCIATION

NEW JERSEY CLAIMS OFFICE
760 ALEXANDER RD
PRINCETON, NJ 08543-0001
TEL: (609) 275-4000
FAX: (609) 452-2538

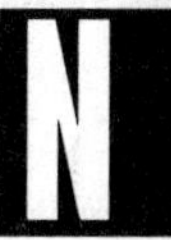

NEW JERSEY MANUFACTURERS INSURANCE CO

301 SULLIVAN WAY
WEST TRENTON, NJ 08628-3406
TEL: (609) 883-1300
FAX: (609) 771-9451
TOLL FREE: (800) 232-6600
IN-STATE: (800) 232-6600
WWW.NJM.COM

PENNSYLVANIA CLAIMS OFFICE
301 SULLIVAN WAY
WEST TRENTON, NJ 08628-3406
TEL: (609) 883-1300
FAX: (609) 771-9451
TOLL FREE: (800) 232-6600
IN-STATE: (800) 232-6600
WWW.NJM.COM

NEW LONDON COUNTY MUTUAL INSURANCE CO

CONNECTICUT CLAIMS OFFICE
101 HIGH ST
PO BOX 40
NORWICH, CT 06360
TEL: (860) 887-3553
FAX: (860) 887-2898

NEW MEXICO PHYSICIANS INSURANCE

NEW MEXICO CLAIMS OFFICE
MICOA
7770 JEFFERSON NE, STE 410
PO BOX 92890
ALBUQUERQUE, NM 87199-2890
TEL: (505) 821-9485
FAX: (505) 821-6202
TOLL FREE: (800) 880-9485
WWW.MICOA.COM

NEW WORLD SERVICES, LTD

NATIONAL CLAIMS OFFICE
2624 N 5TH ST
NILES, MI 49120-1030
TEL: (616) 684-6700
FAX: (616) 684-8138
TOLL FREE: (800) 624-0698

NEW YORK CASUALTY INSURANCE CO

NEW YORK CLAIMS OFFICE
HARLEYSVILLE INSURANCE CO
120 WASHINGTON ST
WATERTOWN, NY 13601-3330
TEL: (315) 782-1160
FAX: (315) 782-5819
TOLL FREE: (800) 962-1006

NEW YORK MARINE GENERAL INSURANCE CO

330 MADISON AVE- 7TH FL
NEW YORK, NY 10017
TEL: (212) 551-0600
FAX: (212) 986-1310
TOLL FREE: (800) 367-0224

NGS AMERICAN, INC

NATIONAL CLAIMS OFFICE
27575 HARPER AVE
PO BOX 7676
SAINT CLAIR SHORES, MI 48080-7676
TEL: (810) 779-7679
FAX: (810) 779-0117
WWW.NGSAMERICAN.COM

NOBEL INSURANCE CO

ALABAMA CLAIMS OFFICE
6923 N TRENHOLM RD
PO BOX 6108
COLUMBIA, SC 29260-6108
TEL: (803) 782-2373
FAX: (803) 782-5569
TOLL FREE: (800) 521-2675

CONNECTICUT CLAIMS OFFICE
6923 N TRENHOLM RD
PO BOX 6108
COLUMBIA, SC 29260-6108
TEL: (803) 782-2373
FAX: (803) 782-5569
TOLL FREE: (800) 521-2675

ILLINOIS CLAIMS OFFICE
6923 N TRENHOLM RD
PO BOX 6108
COLUMBIA, SC 29260-6108
TEL: (803) 782-2373
FAX: (803) 782-5569
TOLL FREE: (800) 521-2675

INDIANA CLAIMS OFFICE
6923 N TRENHOLM RD
PO BOX 6108
COLUMBIA, SC 29260-6108
TEL: (803) 782-2373
FAX: (803) 782-5569
TOLL FREE: (800) 521-2675

NEW HAMPSHIRE CLAIMS OFFICE
6923 N TRENHOLM RD
PO BOX 6108
COLUMBIA, SC 29260-6108
TEL: (803) 782-2373
FAX: (803) 782-5569
TOLL FREE: (800) 521-2675

NORTH CAROLINA CLAIMS OFFICE
6923 N TRENHOLM RD
PO BOX 6108
COLUMBIA, SC 29260-6108
TEL: (803) 782-2373
FAX: (803) 782-5569
TOLL FREE: (800) 521-2675

SOUTH CAROLINA CLAIMS OFFICE
6923 N TRENHOLM RD
PO BOX 6108
COLUMBIA, SC 29260-6108
TEL: (803) 782-2373
FAX: (803) 782-5569
TOLL FREE: (800) 521-2675

TENNESSEE CLAIMS OFFICE
6923 N TRENHOLM RD
PO BOX 6108
COLUMBIA, SC 29260-6108
TEL: (803) 782-2373
FAX: (803) 782-5569
TOLL FREE: (800) 521-2675

TEXAS CLAIMS OFFICE
8001 LBJ FWY, STE 300
DALLAS, TX 75251-1301
TEL: (972) 644-0434
FAX: (972) 644-0424
IN-STATE: (800) 766-6235

NOETICS

CALIFORNIA CLAIMS OFFICE
FIRM SOLUTIONS
15326 ALTON
PO BOX 19775
IRVINE, CA 92623
TEL: (949) 753-5900
FAX: (949) 753-5934
TOLL FREE: (800) 782-5888
IN-STATE: (800) 782-5888

NOITU INSURANCE TRUST FUND

CONNECTICUT CLAIMS OFFICE
148-06 HILLSIDE AVE
JAMAICA, NY 11435-3393
TEL: (718) 291-3434
FAX: (718) 291-0531

FLORIDA CLAIMS OFFICE
148-06 HILLSIDE AVE
JAMAICA, NY 11435-3393
TEL: (718) 291-3434
FAX: (718) 291-0531

NEW JERSEY CLAIMS OFFICE
148-06 HILLSIDE AVE
JAMAICA, NY 11435-3393
TEL: (718) 291-3434
FAX: (718) 291-0531

NEW YORK CLAIMS OFFICE
14806 HILLSIDE AVE
JAMAICA, NY 11435-3393
TEL: (718) 291-3434
FAX: (718) 291-0531

PENNSYLVANIA CLAIMS OFFICE
148-06 HILLSIDE AVE
JAMAICA, NY 11435-3393
TEL: (718) 291-3434
FAX: (718) 291-0531

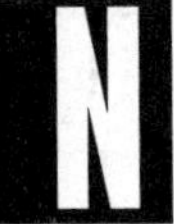

NORFOLK & DEDHAM GROUP

MASSACHUSETTS CLAIMS OFFICE
222 AMES ST
PO BOX 9109
DEDHAM, MA 02027-9109
TEL: (781) 326-4010
FAX: (781) 329-1818
TOLL FREE: (800) 688-1825

NORTH AMERICA ADMINISTRATORS, INC

ALABAMA CLAIMS OFFICE
1212 8TH AVE SOUTH
PO BOX 1984
NASHVILLE, TN 37202-1984
TEL: (615) 256-3561
FAX: (615) 256-1834
E-MAIL: NAA@WORLDNET.ATT.NET
WWW.NAAI.COM

GEORGIA CLAIMS OFFICE
1212 8TH AVE SOUTH
PO BOX 1984
NASHVILLE, TN 37202-1984
TEL: (615) 256-3561
FAX: (615) 256-1834
E-MAIL: NAA@WORLDNET.ATT.NET
WWW.NAAI.COM

ILLINOIS CLAIMS OFFICE
1212 8TH AVE SOUTH
PO BOX 1984
NASHVILLE, TN 37202-1984
TEL: (615) 256-3561
FAX: (615) 256-1834
E-MAIL: NAA@WORLDNET.ATT.NET
WWW.NAAI.COM

INDIANA CLAIMS OFFICE
1212 8TH AVE SOUTH
PO BOX 1984
NASHVILLE, TN 37202-1984
TEL: (615) 256-3561
FAX: (615) 256-1834
E-MAIL: NAA@WORLDNET.ATT.NET
WWW.NAAI.COM

KENTUCKY CLAIMS OFFICE
1212 8TH AVE SOUTH
PO BOX 1984
NASHVILLE, TN 37202-1984
TEL: (615) 256-3561
FAX: (615) 256-1834
E-MAIL: NAA@WORLDNET.ATT.NET
WWW.NAAI.COM

MISSISSIPPI CLAIMS OFFICE
1212 8TH AVE SOUTH
PO BOX 1984
NASHVILLE, TN 37202-1984
TEL: (615) 256-3561
FAX: (615) 256-1834
E-MAIL: NAA@WORLDNET.ATT.NET
WWW.NAAI.COM

OHIO CLAIMS OFFICE
1212 8TH AVE SOUTH
PO BOX 1984
NASHVILLE, TN 37202-1984
TEL: (615) 256-3561
FAX: (615) 256-1834
E-MAIL: NAA@WORLDNET.ATT.NET
WWW.NAAI.COM

PENNSYLVANIA CLAIMS OFFICE
1212 8TH AVE SOUTH
PO BOX 1984
NASHVILLE, TN 37202-1984
TEL: (615) 256-3561
FAX: (615) 256-1834
E-MAIL: NAA@WORLDNET.ATT.NET
WWW.NAAI.COM

TENNESSEE CLAIMS OFFICE
1212 8TH AVE S
PO BOX 1984
NASHVILLE, TN 37202-1984
TEL: (615) 256-3561
FAX: (615) 256-1834
E-MAIL: NAA@WORLDNET.ATT.NET
WWW.NAAI.COM

VIRGINIA CLAIMS OFFICE
1212 8TH AVE SOUTH
PO BOX 1984
NASHVILLE, TN 37202-1984
TEL: (615) 256-3561
FAX: (615) 256-1834
E-MAIL: NAA@WORLDNET.ATT.NET
WWW.NAAI.COM

NORTH CAROLINA FARM BUREAU MUTUAL INSURANCE CO

NORTH CAROLINA CLAIMS OFFICE
5301 GLENWOOD AVE
PO BOX 27427
RALEIGH, NC 27611-7427
TEL: (919) 782-1705
FAX: (919) 782-4921
TOLL FREE: (800) 849-2901

HWY 150 BYP
PO BOX 736
LINCOLNTON, NC 28093-0736
TEL: (704) 735-1483
FAX: (704) 732-2097
TOLL FREE: (800) 326-3599

NORTH CAROLINA MUTUAL LIFE INSURANCE CO

MUTUAL PLZ
411 W CHAPEL HILL ST
PO BOX 3616
DURHAM, NC 27701-3616
TEL: (919) 682-9201
FAX: (919) 683-1694
TOLL FREE: (800) 626-1849

301 S JAMES
PO BOX N
GOLDSBORO, NC 27530
TEL: (919) 734-3094
TOLL FREE: (800) 626-1899

411 W CHAPEL HILL ST
PO BOX 201
DURHAM, NC 27701
TEL: (919) 682-9201
FAX: (919) 683-1694
TOLL FREE: (800) 626-1899

PENNSYLVANIA CLAIMS OFFICE
411 W CHAPEL HILL ST
PO BOX 201
DURHAM, NC 27701
TEL: (919) 682-9201
FAX: (919) 683-1694
TOLL FREE: (800) 626-1899

VIRGINIA CLAIMS OFFICE
411 W CHAPEL HILL ST
PO BOX 201
DURHAM, NC 27701
TEL: (919) 682-9201
FAX: (919) 683-1694
TOLL FREE: (800) 626-1899

NORTH CENTRAL LIFE INSURANCE CO

MINNESOTA CLAIMS OFFICE
FINANCIAL LIFE
445 MINNESOTA ST
PO BOX 64139
SAINT PAUL, MN 55164
TEL: (651) 227-8000
FAX: (651) 292-1830
TOLL FREE: (800) 888-8625

NORTH DAKOTA WORKERS COMPENSATION BUREAU

NORTH DAKOTA CLAIMS OFFICE
500 E FRONT AVE
BISMARCK, ND 58504-5685
TEL: (701) 328-3800
FAX: (701) 328-3820
TOLL FREE: (800) 777-5033

NORTH PACIFIC INSURANCE CO

OREGON CLAIMS OFFICE
NORTH PACIFIC OREGON AUTO
1675 SW MARLOW AVE
PO BOX 74
PORTLAND, OR 97207-0074
TEL: (503) 643-7661
TOLL FREE: (800) 873-6742

NORTHEAST DELTA DENTAL

MAINE CLAIMS OFFICE
DELTA DENTAL PLAN OF MAINE
ONE DELTA DRIVE
PO BOX 2002
CONCORD, NH 03302-2002
TEL: (603) 223-1000
FAX: (603) 223-1199
TOLL FREE: (800) 537-1715
E-MAIL: NEDELTA@NEDELTA.COM
WWW.NEDELTA.COM

NEW HAMPSHIRE CLAIMS OFFICE
DELTA DENTAL PLAN OF NEW HAMPSHIRE
ONE DELTA DRIVE
PO BOX 2002
CONCORD, NH 03302-2002
TEL: (603) 223-1000
FAX: (603) 223-1199
TOLL FREE: (800) 537-1715
E-MAIL: NEDELTA@NEDELTA.COM
WWW.NEDELTA.COM

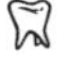

VERMONT CLAIMS OFFICE
DELTA DENTAL PLAN OF VERMONT
ONE DELTA DRIVE
PO BOX 2002
CONCORD, NH 03302-2002
TEL: (603) 223-1000
FAX: (603) 223-1199
TOLL FREE: (800) 537-1715
E-MAIL: NEDELTA@NEDELTA.COM
WWW.NEDELTA.COM

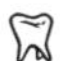

NORTHEAST INSURANCE CO

MAINE CLAIMS OFFICE
482 PAYNE RD- 4TH FL
PO BOX 1418
SCARBOROUGH, ME 04074-8929
TEL: (207) 883-2232
FAX: (207) 883-1501
TOLL FREE: (800) 456-1819

NORTHEAST MEDICAL CENTER

NORTH CAROLINA CLAIMS OFFICE
920 CHURCH ST N
CONCORD, NC 28025-2927
TEL: (704) 783-3000
FAX: (704) 783-1487
TOLL FREE: (800) 842-6868
WWW.NORTHEASTMEDICAL.ORG

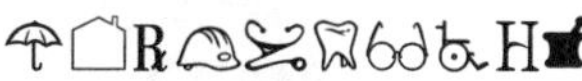

NORTHERN ADJUSTERS

ALASKA CLAIMS OFFICE
1401 RUDAKOF CIR
ANCHORAGE, AK 99508-3108
TEL: (907) 338-7484
FAX: (907) 338-6364
WWW.NADJ.COM

800 E DIAMOND BLVD, STE 3-470
ANCHORAGE, AK 99515
TEL: (907) 868-3999
FAX: (907) 868-3868
WWW.NADJ.COM

NORTHLAND INSURANCE CO

MINNESOTA CLAIMS OFFICE
1295 NORTHLAND DR
PO BOX 64816
SAINT PAUL, MN 55164-0816
TEL: (651) 688-4100
FAX: (651) 688-4170
TOLL FREE: (800) 328-5972
WWW.NORTHLANDINS.COM

NORTHWEST ADMINISTRATORS

CALIFORNIA CLAIMS OFFICE
2323 EASTLAKE AVE E
SEATTLE, WA 98102-3393
TEL: (206) 726-3277
FAX: (206) 726-3209
TOLL FREE: (800) 458-3053

IDAHO CLAIMS OFFICE
2323 EASTLAKE AVE E
SEATTLE, WA 98102-3393
TEL: (206) 726-3277
FAX: (206) 726-3229
TOLL FREE: (800) 458-3053

NEVADA CLAIMS OFFICE
2323 EASTLAKE AVE E
SEATTLE, WA 98102-3393
TEL: (206) 726-3277
FAX: (206) 726-3209
TOLL FREE: (800) 458-3053

OREGON CLAIMS OFFICE
2323 EASTLAKE AVE E
SEATTLE, WA 98102-3393
TEL: (206) 726-3277
FAX: (206) 726-3229
TOLL FREE: (800) 458-3053

WASHINGTON CLAIMS OFFICE
2323 EASTLAKE AVE E
SEATTLE, WA 98102-3393
TEL: (206) 726-3277
FAX: (206) 726-3209
TOLL FREE: (800) 458-3053

NORTHWEST LIFE ASSURANCE

BRITISH COLUMBIA CLAIMS OFFICE
2165 W BROADWAY
PO BOX 5900
VANCOUVER, BC V6B-5H6
TEL: (604) 734-1667
FAX: (604) 734-8221
TOLL FREE: (800) 663-9158

NORTHWEST WASHINGTON MEDICAL BUREAU

WASHINGTON CLAIMS OFFICE
3000 NORTHWEST AVE
PO BOX 9753
BELLINGHAM, WA 98227-9753
TEL: (360) 734-8000
FAX: (360) 734-6676
TOLL FREE: (800) 825-5962

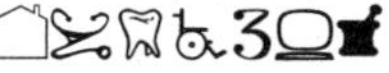

NORTHWESTERN MUTUAL LIFE INSURANCE CO

WISCONSIN CLAIMS OFFICE
DISABILITY BENEFITS DIVISION
720 E WISCONSIN AVE
PO BOX 2918
MILWAUKEE, WI 53201-9831
TEL: (414) 271-1444
FAX: (414) 299-1526
WWW.NORTHWESTERN.COM

NOVA HEALTHCARE ADMINISTRATORS

NEW YORK CLAIMS OFFICE
2680 GRAND ISLAND BLVD
PO BOX 308
GRAND ISLAND, NY 14072-0308
TEL: (716) 773-1143
FAX: (716) 773-1276
TOLL FREE: (800) 333-3195
IN-STATE: (800) 999-5703

NRECA

DISTRICT OF COLUMBIA CLAIMS OFFICE
HOME OFFICE FOR COOPERATIVE BENEFIT ADMINISTRATORS (CBA)
4301 WILSON BLVD
ARLINGTON, VA 22203-1860
TEL: (703) 907-5500
FAX: (703) 907-5525
WWW.NRECA.ORG

NYL CARE

NEW JERSEY CLAIMS OFFICE
NEW YORK LIFE INSURANCE CO
2337 LEMOINE
FORT LEE, NJ 07024
TEL: (201) 461-2668

TEXAS CLAIMS OFFICE
AETNA U.S. HEALTH CARE CO
4500 FULLER DR
PO BOX 972
IRVING, TX 75038
TEL: (972) 971-3900
FAX: (972) 650-5500
TOLL FREE: (800) 486-3040
WWW.AETNA.COM

2425 WEST LOOP S, STE 1000
PO BOX 56228
HOUSTON, TX 77027
TEL: (713) 624-5000
FAX: (713) 993-9462
TOLL FREE: (800) 833-5318

NYLIFE ADMINISTRATION CORP

98 SAN JACINTO BLVD STE 800
AUSTIN, TX 78701
TEL: (512) 703-5555
FAX: (512) 703-5566
TOLL FREE: (800) 723-5555

O'BRIEN, BOUCK & ASSOCIATES

KANSAS CLAIMS OFFICE
8340 MISSION RD STE 119
PO BOX 6826
LEAWOOD, KS 66206-0353
TEL: (913) 381-3444
FAX: (913) 381-3953

OAK AGENCY

ILLINOIS CLAIMS OFFICE
340 W BUTTERFIELD RD
ELMHURST, IL 60126-5024
TEL: (630) 833-9770
FAX: (630) 833-4484
TOLL FREE: (800) 441-4228

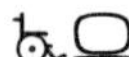

OAK CASUALTY CO

137 N OAK PARK AVE
PO BOX 4010
OAK PARK, IL 60303-4010
TEL: (708) 386-1646
FAX: (708) 386-1688

OAK CASUALTY INSURANCE CO

WEST VIRGINIA CLAIMS OFFICE
738 GASTON AVE
PO BOX 995
FAIRMONT, WV 26555-0995
TEL: (304) 366-6996
FAX: (304) 366-8305
TOLL FREE: (800) 462-5855

OCCIDENTAL FIRE & CASUALTY CO OF NORTH CAROLINA

NATIONAL CLAIMS OFFICE
702 OBERLIN RD
PO BOX 10800
RALEIGH, NC 27605
TEL: (919) 833-1600
FAX: (919) 834-0855
TOLL FREE: (800) 525-7486

ODS HEALTH PLAN

OREGON CLAIMS OFFICE
315 SW 5TH AVE
PO BOX 40384
PORTLAND, OR 97204
TEL: (503) 228-6554
FAX: (503) 243-5105
TOLL FREE: (800) 852-5195
WWW.ODSHP.COM

ODYSSEY REINSURANCE CO

NEW YORK CLAIMS OFFICE
ONE LIBERTY PLZ
NEW YORK, NY 10006-1404
TEL: (212) 978-4790
FAX: (212) 385-2169

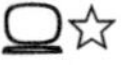

OHIO BUREAU OF WORKERS COMPENSATION

NATIONAL CLAIMS OFFICE
ZANESVILLE CUSTOMER SVC OFC
905 ZANE ST
PO BOX 37
ZANESVILLE, OH 43702-0037
TEL: (740) 450-5151
FAX: (740) 450-5150
TOLL FREE: (800) 898-6446
WWW.OHIOBWC.COM

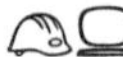

OHIO CLAIMS OFFICE
30 W SPRING ST
COLUMBUS, OH 43215
FAX: (614) 752-4732
TOLL FREE: (800) 644-6292
WWW.OHIOBWC.COM

161 S HIGH ST STE 300
AKRON, OH 44308-1617
TEL: (330) 643-3111
FAX: (330) 643-1369
TOLL FREE: (800) 644-6292
WWW.OHIOBWC.COM

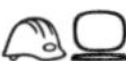

56104 NATIONAL RD STE 112
PO BOX 388-389
BRIDGEPORT, OH 43912-0388
TEL: (740) 635-1163
FAX: (740) 635-4808
TOLL FREE: (800) 635-1165
WWW.OHIOBWC.COM

125 E COURT ST- 9TH AND 10TH FLOOR
CINCINNATI, OH 45202-2196
TEL: (513) 852-3341
FAX: (513) 361-8474
TOLL FREE: (800) 644-6292
WWW.OHIOBWC.COM

8500 GOVERNOR'S HILL DR
CINCINNATI, OH 45249
TEL: (513) 583-4400
FAX: (513) 583-4827
TOLL FREE: (800) 644-6292
WWW.OHIOBWC.COM

615 W SUPERIOR AVE
CLEVELAND, OH 44113-1889
TEL: (216) 787-3050
FAX: (216) 787-3306
TOLL FREE: (800) 644-6292
WWW.OHIOBWC.COM

3401 PARK CENTER DR STE 100
PO BOX 13910
DAYTON, OH 45413-0910
TEL: (937) 264-5000
FAX: (937) 264-5088
TOLL FREE: (800) 6446292
WWW.OHIOBWC.COM

100 COMMERCIAL DR
FAIRFIELD, OH 45014
TEL: (513) 881-2000
FAX: (513) 881-2062
TOLL FREE: (800) 644-6292
WWW.OHIOBWC.COM

5990 W CREEK RD
PO BOX 318030
INDEPENDENCE, OH 44131-8030
TEL: (216) 573-7700
FAX: (216) 573-7709
TOLL FREE: (800) 644-6292
WWW.OHIOBWC.COM

2025 E FOURTH ST
PO BOX 780
LIMA, OH 45804-0780
TEL: (419) 227-3127
FAX: (419) 225-5399
WWW.OHIOBWC.COM

1225 W HUNTER
PO BOX 630
LOGAN, OH 43138-0630
TEL: (740) 385-5607
FAX: (740) 385-9048
TOLL FREE: (800) 644-6292
IN-STATE: (800) 385-5607
WWW.OHIOBWC.COM

240 TAPPAN DR N
PO BOX 8051
MANSFIELD, OH 44906-8051
TEL: (419) 747-4090
FAX: (419) 529-1307
TOLL FREE: (800) 644-6292
WWW.OHIOBWC.COM

1005 FOURTH ST
PO BOX 1307
PORTSMOUTH, OH 45662-4195
TEL: (740) 353-2187
FAX: (740) 354-4909
TOLL FREE: (800) 644-6292
WWW.OHIOBWC.COM

26301 CURTISSWRIGHT PKY
RICHMOND HEIGHTS, OH 44143-1433
TEL: (216) 289-4290
FAX: (216) 289-7120
TOLL FREE: (800) 644-6292
WWW.OHIOBWC.COM

ONE S LIMESTONE ST
PO BOX 1467
SPRINGFIELD, OH 45501-1467
TEL: (937) 327-1425
FAX: (937) 327-1485
TOLL FREE: (800) 644-6292
WWW.OHIOBWC.COM

ONE GOVERNMENT CTR STE 1236
PO BOX 794
TOLEDO, OH 43697-0794
TEL: (419) 245-2700
FAX: (419) 245-2666
TOLL FREE: (800) 644-2692
WWW.OHIOBWC.COM

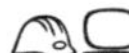

100 WESTCHESTER DR
PO BOX 4294
YOUNGSTOWN, OH 44515-0294
TEL: (330) 797-5500
FAX: (330) 797-6351
TOLL FREE: (800) 551-6446
WWW.OHIOBWC.COM

OHIO CASUALTY GROUP

MARYLAND CLAIMS OFFICE
11350 MCCORMICK RD, EXECUTIVE PLZ II, STE 806
HUNT VALLEY, MD 21031
TEL: (410) 584-0690
FAX: (410) 584-0670
TOLL FREE: (800) 793-6227

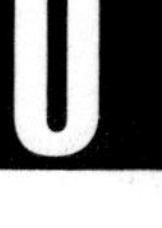

MINNESOTA CLAIMS OFFICE
7400 METRO BLVD, STE 350
PO BOX 583399
MINNEAPOLIS, MN 55458-3399
TEL: (612) 835-3755
FAX: (612) 835-7724
TOLL FREE: (800) 767-6446

MISSISSIPPI CLAIMS OFFICE
805 S WHITLY
PO BOX 1470
RIDGELAND, MS 39158-1470
TEL: (601) 956-0081
FAX: (601) 978-3279
TOLL FREE: (800) 597-6627

OHIO CLAIMS OFFICE
136 N 3RD ST
HAMILTON, OH 45025-0001
TEL: (513) 867-3000
FAX: (513) 867-3215
TOLL FREE: (800) 843-6446

1445 KEMPER MEADOW DR
PO BOX 405016
CINCINNATI, OH 45240-5016
TEL: (513) 742-8400
FAX: (513) 742-9185
TOLL FREE: (800) 742-8402
WWW.OCAS.COM

PENNSYLVANIA CLAIMS OFFICE
PO BOX 549
FOGELSVILLE, PA 18051-0549
TEL: (610) 398-8121
FAX: (610) 398-9204
TOLL FREE: (800) 743-5543

OHIO CASUALTY INSURANCE GROUP

COLORADO CLAIMS OFFICE
4380 S SYRACUSE
PO BOX 5620
DENVER, CO 80217-5620
TEL: (303) 221-1152
FAX: (303) 221-6067
TOLL FREE: (800) 326-6446

ILLINOIS CLAIMS OFFICE
ALL PAGE CORPORATE CENTER
1919 S HIGHLAND AVE, STE 300 B
LOMBARD, IL 60148-6119
TEL: (630) 629-6800
FAX: (630) 691-7431
TOLL FREE: (800) 624-6720

KENTUCKY CLAIMS OFFICE
3101 BEAUMONT CTR CIR
PO BOX 23203
LEXINGTON, KY 40523
TEL: (606) 223-3026
FAX: (606) 224-4381
TOLL FREE: (800) 735-5580

NEW JERSEY CLAIMS OFFICE
PO BOX 709
VINELAND, NJ 08362
TEL: (609) 692-4320
FAX: (609) 692-7015
TOLL FREE: (800) 692-4321

OHIO CLAIMS OFFICE
24500 CENTER RIDGE RD
PO BOX 450949
WESTLAKE, OH 44145
TEL: (440) 892-0800
TOLL FREE: (800) 326-3950

WEST AMERICAN INSURANCE
136 N 3RD ST
PO BOX 5001
HAMILTON, OH 45012-5001
TEL: (513) 867-3000
FAX: (513) 867-3215
TOLL FREE: (800) 366-6446
WWW.OCAS.COM

OREGON CLAIMS OFFICE
4380 S SYRACUSE, STE 600
DENVER, CO 80217-5620
TEL: (303) 221-1158
FAX: (888) 329-3730
TOLL FREE: (800) 366-6446
WWW.OCAS.COM

PENNSYLVANIA CLAIMS OFFICE
PO BOX 2035
SCRANTON, PA 18501-2035
TEL: (570) 342-7742
FAX: (570) 342-7737
TOLL FREE: (800) 726-6446

TENNESSEE CLAIMS OFFICE
PO BOX 172196
MEMPHIS, TN 38187-2196
TEL: (901) 766-7100
FAX: (901) 682-3838
TOLL FREE: (800) 669-5494

UTAH CLAIMS OFFICE
4380 S SYRACUSE
PO BOX 5620
DENVER, CO 80217-5620
TEL: (303) 221-1152
FAX: (303) 221-6067
TOLL FREE: (800) 326-6446
IN-STATE: (800) 843-6446

OHIO NATIONAL FINANCIAL SERVICE

OHIO CLAIMS OFFICE
ONE FINANCIAL WAY
PO BOX 237
CINCINNATI, OH 45242
TEL: (513) 794-6100
FAX: (513) 794-4521
TOLL FREE: (800) 366-6654

OHIO RETIREMENT SYSTEM

PUBLIC RETIREMENT SYSTEM
PO BOX 182332
COLUMBUS, OH 43215
TEL: (614) 466-2085

OKLAHOMA FARM BUREAU MUTUAL INSURANCE CO

OKLAHOMA CLAIMS OFFICE
AG SECURITY INSURANCE CO
2501 N STILES
OKLAHOMA CITY, OK 73105
TEL: (405) 523-2300
FAX: (405) 523-2362
WWW.SB.COM/OK501

2501 N STILES AVE
PO BOX 53332
OKLAHOMA CITY, OK 73152-3332
TEL: (405) 523-2300
FAX: (405) 523-2362

OLD AMERICAN INSURANCE CO

MISSOURI CLAIMS OFFICE
3520 BROADWAY
KANSAS CITY, MO 64111
TEL: (816) 753-4900
FAX: (816) 753-4902
TOLL FREE: (800) 733-6242

OLD RELIANCE INSURANCE CO

NATIONAL CLAIMS OFFICE
40 E VIRGINIA
PO BOX 13150
PHOENIX, AZ 85002-3150
TEL: (602) 604-9181
FAX: (602) 604-9171

OLD REPUBLIC INSURANCE CO

NEW YORK CLAIMS OFFICE
90 WILLIAM ST- 8TH FL
NEW YORK, NY 10038-4703
TEL: (212) 968-7899
FAX: (212) 509-6915

PENNSYLVANIA CLAIMS OFFICE
414 W PITTSBURGH ST
PO BOX 2200
GREENSBURG, PA 15601
TEL: (724) 834-5000
FAX: (724) 836-4909

OLD REPUBLIC INTERNATIONAL

ILLINOIS CLAIMS OFFICE
307 N MICHIGAN AVE
CHICAGO, IL 60601
TEL: (312) 346-8100
FAX: (312) 346-2050
TOLL FREE: (800) 621-0365

OLD REPUBLIC UNION INSURANCE

ALABAMA CLAIMS OFFICE
650 S MCDONOUGH
PO BOX 2031
MONTGOMERY, AL 36102-2031
TEL: (334) 263-0288
FAX: (334) 263-0186
TOLL FREE: (800) 239-7400

OLD SURETY LIFE INSURANCE CO

OKLAHOMA CLAIMS OFFICE
5235 N LINCOLN BLVD
PO BOX 54407
OKLAHOMA CITY, OK 73154-1407
TEL: (405) 523-2112
FAX: (405) 524-4011
TOLL FREE: (800) 272-5466

OLD UNITED LIFE INSURANCE CO

ARIZONA CLAIMS OFFICE
8500 SHAWNEE MISSION PKY, STE 210
PO BOX 795
SHAWNEE MISSION, KS 66201-0795
TEL: (913) 895-0259
FAX: (913) 789-1037
TOLL FREE: (800) 866-6090

ARKANSAS CLAIMS OFFICE
8500 SHAWNEE MISSION PKY, STE 210
PO BOX 795
SHAWNEE MISSION, KS 66201-0795
TEL: (913) 895-0259
FAX: (913) 789-1037
TOLL FREE: (800) 866-6090

ILLINOIS CLAIMS OFFICE
8500 SHAWNEE MISSION PKY, STE 210
PO BOX 795
SHAWNEE MISSION, KS 66201-0795
TEL: (913) 895-0259
FAX: (913) 789-1037
TOLL FREE: (800) 866-6090

INDIANA CLAIMS OFFICE
8500 SHAWNEE MISSION PKY, STE 210
PO BOX 795
SHAWNEE MISSION, KS 66201-0795
TEL: (913) 895-0259
FAX: (913) 789-1037
TOLL FREE: (800) 866-6090

KANSAS CLAIMS OFFICE
8500 SHAWNEE MISSION PKY, STE 210
PO BOX 795
SHAWNEE MISSION, KS 66201-0795
TEL: (913) 895-0259
FAX: (913) 789-1037
TOLL FREE: (800) 866-6090

MISSOURI CLAIMS OFFICE
8500 SHAWNEE MISSION PKY, STE 210
PO BOX 795
SHAWNEE MISSION, KS 66201-0795
TEL: (913) 895-0259
FAX: (913) 789-1037
TOLL FREE: (800) 866-6090

NEBRASKA CLAIMS OFFICE
8500 SHAWNEE MISSION PKY, STE 210
PO BOX 795
SHAWNEE MISSION, KS 66201-0795
TEL: (913) 895-0259
FAX: (913) 789-1037
TOLL FREE: (800) 866-6090

NEW MEXICO CLAIMS OFFICE
8500 SHAWNEE MISSION PKY, STE 210
PO BOX 795
SHAWNEE MISSION, KS 66201-0795
TEL: (913) 895-0259
FAX: (913) 789-1037
TOLL FREE: (800) 866-6090

TEXAS CLAIMS OFFICE
8500 SHAWNEE MISSION PKY, STE 210
PO BOX 795
SHAWNEE MISSION, KS 66201-0795
TEL: (913) 895-0259
FAX: (913) 789-1037
TOLL FREE: (800) 866-6090

OLYMPIC BENEFITS

WASHINGTON CLAIMS OFFICE
PO BOX 1077
BELLINGHAM, WA 98227-1077
TEL: (360) 734-9888
FAX: (360) 734-6199
TOLL FREE: (800) 533-3941
WWW.OHMSYSTEMS.COM

OMAHA PROPERTY & CASUALTY

NEBRASKA CLAIMS OFFICE
3102 FARNAM ST
OMAHA, NE 68131-3504
FAX: (402) 351-2650
TOLL FREE: (800) 788-9488

OMNI HEALTH CARE

CALIFORNIA CLAIMS OFFICE
1776 W MARCH LN, STE 240
STOCKTON, CA 95207
TEL: (209) 474-6664
FAX: (209) 955-7536
TOLL FREE: (800) 342-8462
WWW.OMNIHEALTHCARE.COM

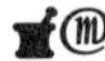

OMNICARE HEALTH PLAN

MICHIGAN CLAIMS OFFICE
1155 BREWERY PARK BLVD, STE 200
DETROIT, MI 48207-2402
TEL: (313) 259-4000
FAX: (313) 393-7944
TOLL FREE: (800) 380-3642
WWW.OMNIHEALTHCARE.COM

ON LOK SENIOR HEALTH SERVICES

CALIFORNIA CLAIMS OFFICE
1333 BUSH ST
SAN FRANCISCO, CA 94109-5611
TEL: (415) 550-2210

ONE BENEFIT SOURCE

NATIONAL CLAIMS OFFICE
FORMERLY PYRAMID BENEFIT SERVICES
107 W FRANKLIN ST
PO BOX 2775
ELKHART, IN 46515-2775
TEL: (219) 254-6000
FAX: (219) 254-6070
TOLL FREE: (800) 232-6437

OPTIMA HEALTH PLAN

VIRGINIA CLAIMS OFFICE
4417 CORPORATION LN
VIRGINIA BEACH, VA 23462-3114
TEL: (757) 552-7400
FAX: (757) 552-7397
TOLL FREE: (800) 736-8272

OPTIMUM CHOICE, INC

MARYLAND CLAIMS OFFICE
MID-ATLANTIC
4 TAFT COURT
PO BOX 6432
ROCKVILLE, MD 20850
TEL: (301) 762-8205
TOLL FREE: (800) 342-6141
WWW.MAMSI.COM

OPTIMUM REINSURANCE CO

TEXAS CLAIMS OFFICE
3434 FAIRMOUNT
PO BOX 660010
DALLAS, TX 75266-0010
TEL: (214) 528-2020
FAX: (214) 528-2777

ORAL HEALTH SERVICES

ALABAMA CLAIMS OFFICE
DNI- DENTAL NETWORK, INC
5775 BLUE LAGOON DR, STE 400
PO BOX 025779
MIAMI, FL 33102-5779
TEL: (305) 262-1333
FAX: (305) 262-6119
TOLL FREE: (800) 432-3376
IN-STATE: (800) 223-6447

ARKANSAS CLAIMS OFFICE
DNI- DENTAL NETWORK, INC
5775 BLUE LAGOON DR, STE 400
PO BOX 025779
MIAMI, FL 33102-5779
TEL: (305) 262-1333
FAX: (305) 262-6119
TOLL FREE: (800) 432-3376
IN-STATE: (800) 223-6447

FLORIDA CLAIMS OFFICE
DNI- DENTAL NETWORK, INC
5775 BLUE LAGOON DR, STE 400
PO BOX 025779
MIAMI, FL 33102-5779
TEL: (305) 262-1333
FAX: (305) 262-6119
TOLL FREE: (800) 432-3376
IN-STATE: (800) 223-6447

☂ H

GEORGIA CLAIMS OFFICE
DNI- DENTAL NETWORK, INC
5775 BLUE LAGOON DR, STE 400
PO BOX 025779
MIAMI, FL 33102-5779
TEL: (305) 262-1333
FAX: (305) 262-6119
TOLL FREE: (800) 432-3376
IN-STATE: (800) 223-6447

☂ H

LOUISIANA CLAIMS OFFICE
DNI- DENTAL NETWORK, INC
5775 BLUE LAGOON DR, STE 400
PO BOX 025779
MIAMI, FL 33102-5779
TEL: (305) 262-1333
FAX: (305) 262-6119
TOLL FREE: (800) 432-3376
IN-STATE: (800) 223-6447

☂ H

MISSISSIPPI CLAIMS OFFICE
DNI- DENTAL NETWORK, INC
5775 BLUE LAGOON DR, STE 400
PO BOX 025779
MIAMI, FL 33102-5779
TEL: (305) 262-1333
FAX: (305) 262-6119
TOLL FREE: (800) 432-3376
IN-STATE: (800) 223-6447

☂ H

TENNESSEE CLAIMS OFFICE
DNI- DENTAL NETWORK, INC
5775 BLUE LAGOON DR, STE 400
PO BOX 025779
MIAMI, FL 33102-5779
TEL: (305) 262-1333
FAX: (305) 262-6119
TOLL FREE: (800) 432-3376
IN-STATE: (800) 223-6447

☂ H

OREGON DENTAL SERVICE (ODS HEALTH PLANS)

OREGON CLAIMS OFFICE
601 SW 2ND AVE
PO BOX 40384
PORTLAND, OR 97240
TEL: (503) 228-6554
FAX: (503) 243-3895
TOLL FREE: (800) 852-5195
IN-STATE: (800) 452-1058
WWW.ODSHP.COM

OREGON MUTUAL AND WESTERN PROTECTORS

347 E FOURTH
PO BOX 808
MCMINNVILLE, OR 97128-0808
TEL: (503) 472-2141
FAX: (503) 434-3846
TOLL FREE: (800) 888-2141

OREGON QUALITY INSURANCE

12901 SE 97TH AVE
PO BOX 286
CLACKAMAS, OR 97015-0286
TEL: (503) 659-4212
FAX: (503) 652-4452
TOLL FREE: (800) 568-5628
WWW.PACC.COM

H

ORION AUTO

COLORADO CLAIMS OFFICE
9800 S MARIDIAN BLVD
PO BOX 3329
ENGLEWOOD, CO 80155-3329
TEL: (303) 754-8400
FAX: (303) 799-9626
TOLL FREE: (800) 456-4642

NORTH CAROLINA CLAIMS OFFICE
PO BOX 2027
GOLDSBORO, NC 27533-2027
TEL: (919) 751-1520
FAX: (919) 778-0728
TOLL FREE: (800) 443-8815

ORION AUTO INSURANCE CO

UNISUN & ATLANTIC CASUALTY
4194 MENDEN HALL OAKS PKY, STE 160
PO BOX 2206
HIGH POINT, NC 27261-2206
TEL: (336) 802-4200
FAX: (336) 812-8186
TOLL FREE: (800) 642-6342

SOUTH CAROLINA CLAIMS OFFICE
UNISUN & ATLANTIC CASUALTY
1 S PARK CIR
PO BOX 118090
CHARLESTON, SC 29423-8090
TEL: (843) 571-0510
FAX: (800) 774-6988
TOLL FREE: (888) 568-2886

ORION CAPITAL COMPANIES

NATIONAL CLAIMS OFFICE
NINE FARMSPRINGS RD
PO BOX 4310
FARMINGTON, CT 06032
TEL: (860) 674-6600
TOLL FREE: (800) 243-7060
WWW.ORIONCAPITAL.COM

ORION SPECIALTY, INC

CONNECTICUT CLAIMS OFFICE
9 FARM SPGS DR
PO BOX 4310
FARMINGTON, CT 06032
TEL: (860) 674-6600
FAX: (860) 674-6797
TOLL FREE: (800) 643-8587

ORIONAUTO INSURANCE CO

NATIONAL CLAIMS OFFICE
1224 DEMING WY
PO BOX 5365
MADISON, WI 53705-0365
TEL: (608) 836-3000
FAX: (608) 836-8931
TOLL FREE: (800) 322-2733

NORTH CAROLINA CLAIMS OFFICE
UNISUN & ATLANTIC CASUALTY
1 S PARK CIR
PO BOX 118090
CHARLESTON, SC 29423-8090
TEL: (843) 571-0510
FAX: (800) 774-6988
TOLL FREE: (8880) 568-2886

OSCHNER HEALTH PLAN

LOUISIANA CLAIMS OFFICE
1 GALLERIA BLVD, STE 1224
METAIRIE, LA 70001-2082
TEL: (504) 836-6600
FAX: (504) 836-6566
TOLL FREE: (800) 999-5979

☂ R H ☆

OSF HEALTH PLANS

ILLINOIS CLAIMS OFFICE
7915 N HALE AVE, STE D
PO BOX 5128
PEORIA, IL 61615
TEL: (309) 677-8200
FAX: (309) 677-8330
TOLL FREE: (800) 673-4699
WWW.OSFHEALTHCARE.ORG/HEALTHPLANS

H

OSHKOSH AREA HEALTH PROTECTION PLAN

WISCONSIN CLAIMS OFFICE
WAUSAU INSURANCE CO
2000 WESTWOOD DR
PO BOX 8013
WAUSAU, WI 54401-7881
TEL: (715) 842-0747
FAX: (715) 843-3882
TOLL FREE: (800) 826-9781

H

OXFORD HEALTH PLANS

CONNECTICUT CLAIMS OFFICE
PO BOX 7082
BRIDGEPORT, CT 06601
TEL: (203) 459-9100
TOLL FREE: (800) 444-6222
IN-STATE: (800) 201-7004

H

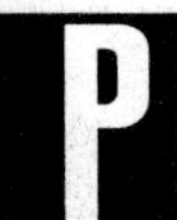

OXFORD LIFE INSURANCE CO

ARIZONA CLAIMS OFFICE
U-HAUL EMPLOYEES
2721 N CENTRAL AVE
PHOENIX, AZ 85004-1121
TEL: (602) 263-6666
FAX: (602) 277-5901
TOLL FREE: (888) 757-3732
WWW.OXFORDLIFE.COM

OZARK NATIONAL LIFE INSURANCE CO

ARKANSAS CLAIMS OFFICE
10201 W MARKUM ST, STE 300
LITTLE ROCK, AR 72205
TEL: (501) 227-4444
FAX: (501) 227-4520

PACIFIC ADMINISTRATORS

OREGON CLAIMS OFFICE
516 SE MORRISON, STE 420
PORTLAND, OR 97214-2344
TEL: (503) 230-2935
FAX: (503) 230-2974

PACIFIC COMPENSATION INSURANCE CO

CALIFORNIA CLAIMS OFFICE
500 N BRAND BLVD, STE 1100
PO BOX 29069
GLENDALE, CA 91209-9069
TEL: (818) 549-4500
FAX: (818) 502-5246

PACIFIC FIDELITY LIFE INSURANCE CO

NATIONAL CLAIMS OFFICE
4333 EDGEWOOD RD NE
CEDAR RAPIDS, IA 52499-0001
TEL: (319) 398-8511
FAX: (319) 369-2209
TOLL FREE: (800) 553-5957

PACIFIC GAS & ELECTRIC CO

CALIFORNIA CLAIMS OFFICE
123 MISSION
PO BOX 7779
SAN FRANCISCO, CA 94120-7779
TEL: (415) 973-3158
FAX: (415) 973-7828

PACIFIC HEALTH CARE

HAWAII CLAIMS OFFICE
1600 KAPIOLANI BLVD, STE 220
HONOLULU, HI 96814
TEL: (808) 973-3555
FAX: (808) 949-3259

PACIFIC HERITAGE ADMINISTRATORS

NATIONAL CLAIMS OFFICE
111 SW COLUMBIA, STE 600
PO BOX 1020
PORTLAND, OR 97207-1020
TEL: (503) 221-9410
FAX: (503) 228-1433
TOLL FREE: (800) 367-3721
IN-STATE: (800) 367-3721

PACIFIC INDEMNITY CO

CHUBB GROUP INSURANCE COMPANY
801 S FIGUROA ST
PO BOX 30850
LOS ANGELES, CA 90030-0850
TEL: (213) 612-0880
FAX: (213) 612-5731
TOLL FREE: (800) 262-4459

PACIFIC LIFE INSURANCE CO

CALIFORNIA CLAIMS OFFICE
PM GROUP
PO BOX 33699
PHOENIX, AZ 85067-3699
TOLL FREE: (800) 729-8545
WWW.PACIFICLIFE.COM

PACIFIC MUTUAL LIFE INSURANCE CO

ARIZONA CLAIMS OFFICE
PACIFIC LIFE
100 W CLARENDON, STE 2000
PO BOX 33699
PHOENIX, AZ 85067-3699
TEL: (602) 230-0680
FAX: (602) 263-0545
TOLL FREE: (800) 733-3227

PACIFIC NATIONAL INSURANCE CO

CALIFORNIA CLAIMS OFFICE
HIGHLAND INSURANCE GROUP
15661 RED HILL AVE, STE 100
PO BOX 2058
TUSTIN, CA 92781
TEL: (714) 259-5700
FAX: (714) 258-8311

PACIFIC SOURCE HEALTH PLANS

OREGON CLAIMS OFFICE
250 COUNTRY CLUB RD
PO BOX 7068
EUGENE, OR 97401-2224
TEL: (541) 686-1242
TOLL FREE: (800) 624-6052
WWW.PACIFIC-SOURCE.COM

PACIFICARE HEALTH SYSTEMS, INC

ARIZONA CLAIMS OFFICE
PACIFICARE OF ARIZONA, INC
4601 E HILTON AVE
PO BOX 52708
PHOENIX, AZ 85034
TEL: (602) 840-2520
FAX: (602) 303-7600
TOLL FREE: (800) 347-8600

PACIFICARE OF NEVADA, INC
4601 E HILTON AVE
PO BOX 52078
PHOENIX, AZ 85072-2078
TEL: (602) 244-2707
TOLL FREE: (800) 347-8600

CALIFORNIA CLAIMS OFFICE
PACIFICARE OF CALIFORNIA, INC
5701 KATELLA AVE
CYPRESS, CA 90630
TEL: (714) 952-1121
TOLL FREE: (800) 426-1065

5995 PLZ DR
PO BOX 6006
CYPRESS, CA 90630-6006
TEL: (714) 952-1121
FAX: (714) 226-5974
TOLL FREE: (800) 624-8822
WWW.PACIFICARE.COM

COLORADO CLAIMS OFFICE
PACIFICARE OF COLORADO, INC
6455 S YOSEMITE ST
ENGLEWOOD, CO 80111
TEL: (303) 220-5800
FAX: (303) 714-3998
TOLL FREE: (800) 877-9777
WWW.PACIFICARE.COM

NATIONAL CLAIMS OFFICE
PACIFICARE OF TEXAS, INC
1800 W LOOP S, STE 350
HOUSTON, TX 77027
TEL: (713) 621-9595
FAX: (713) 963-8318
TOLL FREE: (800) 933-1645

NEVADA CLAIMS OFFICE
PACIFICARE OF NEVADA, INC
4601 E HILTON AVE
PO BOX 52078
PHOENIX, AZ 85072-2078
TEL: (602) 244-2707
TOLL FREE: (800) 347-8600

OKLAHOMA CLAIMS OFFICE
PACIFICARE OF OKLAHOMA, INC
7666 EAST ST
TULSA, OK 74133
TEL: (405) 530-2200
FAX: (405) 521-8349
TOLL FREE: (800) 825-9355
IN-STATE: (800) 545-0389

PACIFICARE OF TEXAS, INC
PO BOX 29127
SAN ANTONIO, TX 78230
TEL: (210) 524-9800
TOLL FREE: (800) 825-9355
IN-STATE: (800) 474-5000

H

OREGON CLAIMS OFFICE
PACIFICARE OF OREGON, INC
5 CENTER PT DR, STE 600
LAKE OSWEGO, OR 97035
FAX: (503) 533-6335
TOLL FREE: (800) 922-1444

R 3H ☆

PACIFICARE OF WASHINGTON, INC
5 CENTER PT DR, STE 600
PO BOX 9005
LAKE OSWEGO, OR 98040
FAX: (503) 533-6335
TOLL FREE: (800) 922-1444

H

TEXAS CLAIMS OFFICE
PACIFICARE OF TEXAS, INC
PO BOX 29127
SAN ANTONIO, TX 78230
TEL: (210) 524-9800
TOLL FREE: (800) 825-9355
IN-STATE: (800) 474-5000

H

PACIFICARE OF OKLAHOMA, INC
7666 EAST ST
TULSA, OK 74133
TEL: (405) 530-2200
FAX: (405) 521-8349
TOLL FREE: (800) 825-9355
IN-STATE: (800) 545-0389

H

UTAH CLAIMS OFFICE
PACIFICARE OF UTAH, INC
35 W BROADWAY
SALT LAKE CITY, UT 84101-2020
TEL: (801) 355-1234
FAX: (801) 531-9003
TOLL FREE: (800) 337-4161

H

WASHINGTON CLAIMS OFFICE
PACIFICARE OF WASHINGTON, INC
5 CENTER PT DR, STE 600
PO BOX 9005
LAKE OSWEGO, OR 98040
FAX: (503) 533-6335
TOLL FREE: (800) 922-1444

H

PAFCO GENERAL INSURANCE CO

INDIANA CLAIMS OFFICE
4720 KINGSWAY DR
INDIANAPOLIS, IN 46205
TEL: (317) 259-6300
FAX: (317) 259-6353
TOLL FREE: (800) 342-5243
IN-STATE: (800) 899-4744
WWW.SIGINS.COM

PAID DENTAL ADMINISTRATORS, INC

NATIONAL CLAIMS OFFICE
7600 CHEVY CHASE DR, STE 30
PO BOX 9201
AUSTIN, TX 78766-9150
TEL: (512) 328-7979
FAX: (512) 459-1552
TOLL FREE: (800) 342-3279

PALMER & KAYE

GEORGIA CLAIMS OFFICE
6001 RIVER RD, STE 200
COLUMBUS, GA 31904
TEL: (706) 576-6990
FAX: (706) 576-6629

PAN AMERICAN LIFE INSURANCE CO

LOUISIANA CLAIMS OFFICE
601 POYDRAS ST
PO BOX 60219
NEW ORLEANS, LA 70130
TEL: (504) 566-1300
FAX: (504) 523-8584
TOLL FREE: (800) 227-3417

R ☆

PARAGON BENEFITS, INC

GEORGIA CLAIMS OFFICE
2202 FAIRBURN RD
PO BOX 1526
DOUGLASVILLE, GA 30133-1526
TEL: (770) 920-2086
FAX: (770) 489-8483
TOLL FREE: (800) 999-9094

PARAMOUNT HEALTH CARE

MICHIGAN CLAIMS OFFICE
1901 INDIAN WOOD CIR
PO BOX 928
MAUMEE, OH 43537-0928
TEL: (419) 887-2500
FAX: (419) 887-2014
TOLL FREE: (800) 462-3589

H

OHIO CLAIMS OFFICE
1901 INDIAN WOOD CIR
PO BOX 928
MAUMEE, OH 43537-0928
TEL: (419) 887-2500
FAX: (419) 887-2014
TOLL FREE: (800) 462-3589

H

PARTNERS MUTUAL INSURANCE CO

IOWA CLAIMS OFFICE
20935 SWENSON DR, STE 200
PO BOX 2003
MILWAUKEE, WI 53201-2003
TEL: (414) 798-5050
FAX: (414) 798-5040
TOLL FREE: (800) 551-5151
WWW.PARTNERSMUTUAL.COM

MICHIGAN CLAIMS OFFICE
20935 SWENSON DR, STE 200
PO BOX 2003
MILWAUKEE, WI 53201-2003
TEL: (414) 798-5050
FAX: (414) 798-5040
TOLL FREE: (800) 551-5151
WWW.PARTNERSMUTUAL.COM

WISCONSIN CLAIMS OFFICE
20935 SWENSON DR, STE 200
PO BOX 2003
MILWAUKEE, WI 53201-2003
TEL: (414) 798-5050
FAX: (414) 798-5040
TOLL FREE: (800) 551-5151
WWW.PARTNERSMUTUAL.COM

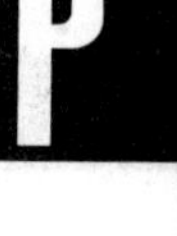

PARTNERS NATIONAL HEALTH PLANS

INDIANA CLAIMS OFFICE
1 MICHIANA SQ- 100 E WAYNE ST, STE 502
PO BOX 7600
SOUTH BEND, IN 46634
TEL: (219) 233-4899
FAX: (219) 234-7484
TOLL FREE: (800) 967-5439
WWW.PARTNERSINDIANA.COM

H

NORTH CAROLINA CLAIMS OFFICE
2085 FRONTIS PLZ BLVD
PO BOX 24907
WINSTON-SALEM, NC 27114
TEL: (336) 760-4822
FAX: (336) 760-3198
TOLL FREE: (800) 942-5695
IN-STATE: (800) 942-5695
WWW.PARTNERSHEALTH.COM

H ☆

SOUTH CAROLINA CLAIMS OFFICE
2085 FRONTIS PLZ BLVD
PO BOX 24907
WINSTON-SALEM, NC 27114
TEL: (336) 760-4822
FAX: (336) 760-3198
TOLL FREE: (800) 942-5695
IN-STATE: (800) 942-5695
WWW.PARTNERSHEALTH.COM

H ☆

VIRGINIA CLAIMS OFFICE
2085 FRONTIS PLZ BLVD
PO BOX 24907
WINSTON-SALEM, NC 27114
TEL: (336) 760-4822
FAX: (336) 760-3198
TOLL FREE: (800) 942-5695
IN-STATE: (800) 942-5695
WWW.PARTNERSHEALTH.COM

H ☆

PATUXENT MEDICAL GROUP

MARYLAND CLAIMS OFFICE
2 KNOLL N DR
COLUMBIA, MD 21045-2298
TEL: (410) 997-8500
FAX: (410) 964-4563
TOLL FREE: (800) 262-7526

H

PAUL BURKE & ASSOCIATES, INC

MINNESOTA CLAIMS OFFICE
DIRECT RESPONSE, INC
1300 FOSHAY TOWER
MINNEAPOLIS, MN 55402
TEL: (612) 332-6581
FAX: (612) 520-6711
TOLL FREE: (800) 421-0099
IN-STATE: (800) 328-3323

PAULA INSURANCE CO

ARIZONA CLAIMS OFFICE
PAN AMERICAN UNDERWRITERS (AGENCY)
5800 W GLENN DR, STE 315
PO BOX 1467
GLENDALE, AZ 85311-1467
TEL: (602) 939-3399
FAX: (602) 931-6917
TOLL FREE: (800) 245-2069

CALIFORNIA CLAIMS OFFICE
300 NORTHLAKE AVE, STE 300
PO BOX 7111
PASADENA, CA 91109-7211
TEL: (626) 304-0401
FAX: (626) 304-1249
TOLL FREE: (800) 252-2466

1780 E BULLARD, STE 101
PO BOX 40009
FRESNO, CA 93755-0009
TEL: (559) 439-3330
FAX: (559) 439-3505
WWW.TRWPICATALO.COM

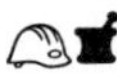

338 S "A" ST
PO BOX 1531
OXNARD, CA 93032-1531
TEL: (805) 486-4491
FAX: (805) 483-5787

PCA HEALTH PLANS OF FLORIDA, INC

FLORIDA CLAIMS OFFICE
HUMANA- PCA
6101 BLUE LAGOON DR, STE 300
PO BOX 025568
MIAMI, FL 33102
TEL: (305) 267-6633
FAX: (305) 266-6051
TOLL FREE: (800) 207-3078
IN-STATE: (800) 562-9262

H

PCS HEALTH SYSTEMS, INC

NATIONAL CLAIMS OFFICE
9501 E SHEA BLVD
SCOTTSDALE, AZ 85260-6719
TEL: (480) 391-4600

PEER REVIEW ORGANIZATIONS

ALABAMA CLAIMS OFFICE
ALABAMA QUALITY ASSURANCE FOUNDATION INC
1 PERIMETER PARK S, STE 220 N
BURMINGHAM, AL 35243-2354
TEL: (205) 970-1600
FAX: (205) 970-1624

ALASKA CLAIMS OFFICE
PRO-WEST
10700 MERIDIAN AVE N, STE 100
SEATTLE, WA 98133-9075
TEL: (206) 364-9700
FAX: (206) 368-2419

AMERICAN SAMOA CLAIMS OFFICE
HAWAII MEDICAL SERVICE ASSOCIATION
818 KEEAUMOKU ST
PO BOX 860
HONOLULU, HI 96808-0860
TEL: (808) 948-5110
FAX: (808) 948-6811
WWW.HMSA.COM

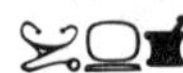

COLORADO CLAIMS OFFICE
COLORADO FOUNDATION FOR MEDICAL CARE
2851 S PARKER RD, STE 200
AURORA, CO 80014
TEL: (303) 695-3300
FAX: (303) 695-3350
WWW.CFMC.ORG

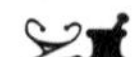

DISTRICT OF COLUMBIA CLAIMS OFFICE
DELMARVA FOUNDATION FOR MEDICAL CARE, INC
9240 CENTREVILLE RD
EASTON, MD 21601
TEL: (410) 822-0697
FAX: (410) 822-1997
TOLL FREE: (800) 999-3362
WWW.DFMC.ORG

FLORIDA CLAIMS OFFICE
FLORIDA MEDICAL QUALITY ASSURANCE, INC
4350 W CYPRESS ST #900
TAMPA, FL 33607
TEL: (813) 354-9111
FAX: (813) 354-0737
TOLL FREE: (800) 844-0795
WWW.FMQAI.COM

GEORGIA CLAIMS OFFICE
GEORGIA MEDICAL CARE FOUNDATION
57 EXECUTIVE PARK DR S, STE 200
ATLANTA, GA 30329
TEL: (404) 982-0411
FAX: (404) 982-7591
TOLL FREE: (800) 982-7581

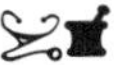

GUAM CLAIMS OFFICE
HAWAII MEDICAL SERVICE ASSOCIATION
818 KEEAUMOKU ST
PO BOX 860
HONOLULU, HI 96808-0860
TEL: (808) 948-5110
FAX: (808) 948-6811
WWW.HMSA.COM

HAWAII CLAIMS OFFICE
HAWAII MEDICAL SERVICE ASSOCIATION
818 KEEAUMOKU ST
PO BOX 860
HONOLULU, HI 96808-0860
TEL: (808) 948-5110
FAX: (808) 948-6811
WWW.HMSA.COM

IDAHO CLAIMS OFFICE
PRO-WEST
10700 MERIDIAN AVE N, STE 100
SEATTLE, WA 98133-9075
TEL: (206) 364-9700
FAX: (208) 343-4705

INDIANA CLAIMS OFFICE
HEALTH CARE EXCELL
2901 OHIO BLVD
PO BOX 3713
TERRE HAUTE, IN 47803
TEL: (812) 234-1499
FAX: (812) 232-6167

IOWA CLAIMS OFFICE
IOWA FOUNDATION FOR MEDICAL CARE
6000 WESTOWN PKY, STE 350 E
WEST DES MOINES, IA 50266-7771
TEL: (515) 223-2900
FAX: (515) 222-2407
TOLL FREE: (800) 383-2856
WWW.IFC.ORG

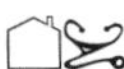

KENTUCKY CLAIMS OFFICE
HEALTH CARE EXCEL
9502 WILLIAMSBURG PLZ, STE 102
PO BOX 23540
LOUISVILLE, KY 40222
TEL: (502) 339-7442
FAX: (502) 339-8641

HEALTH CARE EXCELL
2901 OHIO BLVD
PO BOX 3713
TERRE HAUTE, IN 47803
TEL: (812) 234-1499
FAX: (812) 232-6167

MAINE CLAIMS OFFICE
NORTHEAST FOUNDATION FOR QUALITY FUND
15 OLD ROLLINSFORD RD, STE 302
DOVER, NH 03820-2830
TEL: (603) 749-1641
FAX: (603) 749-1195
TOLL FREE: (800) 772-0151

MARYLAND CLAIMS OFFICE
DELMARVA FOUNDATION FOR MEDICAL CARE, INC
9240 CENTREVILLE RD
EASTON, MD 21601
TEL: (410) 822-0697
FAX: (410) 822-1997
TOLL FREE: (800) 999-3362
WWW.DFMC.ORG

MASSACHUSETTS CLAIMS OFFICE
MASSACHUSETTS PEER REVIEW ORGANIZATION
235 WYMAN ST
WALTHAM, MA 02154-1231
TEL: (781) 890-0011
FAX: (781) 890-5485
TOLL FREE: (800) 334-6776

MICHIGAN CLAIMS OFFICE
MICHIGAN PEER REVIEW ORGANIZATION
40600 ANN ARBOR RD, STE 200
PLYMOUTH, MI 48170-4486
TEL: (734) 459-0900

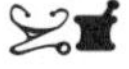

KEYSTONE PEER REVIEW ORGANIZATION, INC (KEPRO)
777 E PK DR
PO BOX 8310
HARRISBURG, PA 17105-8310
TEL: (717) 564-8288
FAX: (717) 564-4188

MONTANA CLAIMS OFFICE
MOUNTAIN PACIFIC QUALITY HEALTH FOUNDATION
400 N PARK- 2ND FL
HELENA, MT 59601
TEL: (406) 443-4020
FAX: (406) 443-4585

NATIONAL CLAIMS OFFICE
MISSOURI PATIENT CARE REVIEW FOUNDATION
505 HOBBS RD, STE 100
JEFFERSON CITY, MO 65109
TEL: (573) 893-7900
FAX: (573) 893-5827
TOLL FREE: (800) 735-6776
IN-STATE: (800) 347-1016

ISLAND PEER REVIEW ORGANIZATION, INC
1979 MARCUS AVE, STE 105
LAKE SUCCESS, NY 11042
TEL: (516) 326-7767
FAX: (516) 328-2310
TOLL FREE: (800) 852-3685
WWW.IPRO.ORG

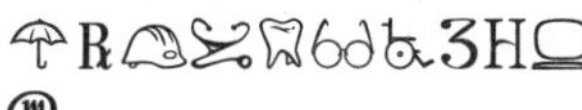

WEST VIRGINIA MEDICAL INSTITUTE, INC
3001 CHESTERFIELD PL
CHARLESTON, WV 25304
TEL: (304) 346-9864
FAX: (304) 346-9863
TOLL FREE: (800) 642-8686
WWW.WVMI.ORG

NEBRASKA CLAIMS OFFICE
IOWA FOUNDATION FOR MEDICAL CARE
6000 WESTOWN PKY, STE 350E
WEST DES MOINES, IA 50266-7771
TEL: (515) 223-2900
FAX: (402) 474-7410
TOLL FREE: (800) 383-2856
WWW.IFC.ORG

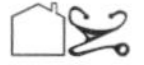

NEW HAMPSHIRE CLAIMS OFFICE
NORTHEAST FOUNDATION FOR QUALITY FUND
15 OLD ROLLINSFORD RD, STE 302
DOVER, NH 03820-2830
TEL: (603) 749-1641
FAX: (603) 749-1195
TOLL FREE: (800) 772-0151

NEW MEXICO CLAIMS OFFICE
NEW MEXICO MEDICAL REVIEW ASSOCIATION
2340 MENAUL ST, STE 300
PO BOX 3200
ALBUQUERQUE, NM 87190-3200
TEL: (505) 998-9898
FAX: (505) 998-9899

OHIO CLAIMS OFFICE
PEER REVIEW SYSTEMS, INC
757 BROOKSEDGE PLZ DR
WESTERVILLE, OH 43081-4913
TEL: (614) 895-9900
FAX: (614) 895-6784
IN-STATE: (800) 589-7337
WWW.PRSNET.ORG

PENNSYLVANIA CLAIMS OFFICE
KEYSTONE PEER REVIEW ORGANIZATION, INC (KEPRO)
777 E PK DR
PO BOX 8310
HARRISBURG, PA 17105-8310
TEL: (717) 564-8288
FAX: (717) 564-4188

SOUTH DAKOTA CLAIMS OFFICE
SOUTH DAKOTA FOUNDATION FOR MEDICAL CARE
1323 S MINNESOTA AVE
SIOUX FALLS, SD 57105
TEL: (605) 336-3505
FAX: (605) 336-0270
TOLL FREE: (800) 658-2285
WWW.SDFMC.ORG

VERMONT CLAIMS OFFICE
NORTHEAST FOUNDATION FOR QUALITY FUND
15 OLD ROLLINSFORD RD, STE 302
DOVER, NH 03820-2830
TEL: (603) 749-1641
FAX: (603) 749-1195
TOLL FREE: (800) 772-0151

VIRGINIA CLAIMS OFFICE
KEYSTONE PEER REVIEW ORGANIZATION, INC (KEPRO)
777 E PK DR
PO BOX 8310
HARRISBURG, PA 17105-8310
TEL: (717) 564-8288
FAX: (717) 564-4188

WASHINGTON CLAIMS OFFICE
PRO-WEST
10700 MERIDIAN AVE N, STE 100
SEATTLE, WA 98133-9075
TEL: (206) 364-9700
FAX: (208) 343-4705

WYOMING CLAIMS OFFICE
MOUNTAIN PACIFIC QUALITY HEALTH FOUNDATION
400 N PARK- 2ND FL
HELENA, MT 59601
TEL: (406) 443-4020
FAX: (406) 443-4585

PRO-WEST
10700 MERIDIAN AVE N, STE 100
SEATTLE, WA 98133-9075
TEL: (206) 364-9700
FAX: (208) 343-4705

PEERLESS

NEW JERSEY CLAIMS OFFICE
5062 BRITTAINFIELD PKY
PO BOX 4858
SYRACUSE, NY 13221
TEL: (315) 431-6100
FAX: (315) 431-6102
TOLL FREE: (800) 443-4000

NEW YORK CLAIMS OFFICE
5062 BRITTAINFIELD PKY
PO BOX 4858
SYRACUSE, NY 13221
TEL: (315) 431-6100
FAX: (315) 431-6102
TOLL FREE: (800) 443-4000

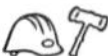

PEERLESS INSURANCE CO

CONNECTICUT CLAIMS OFFICE
NETHERLANDS
62 MAPLE AVE
KEENE, NH 03431
TEL: (603) 352-3221
FAX: (603) 352-4363
TOLL FREE: (800) 542-5385

NEW HAMPSHIRE CLAIMS OFFICE
NETHERLANDS
62 MAPLE AVE
KEENE, NH 03431
TEL: (603) 352-3221
FAX: (603) 352-4363
TOLL FREE: (800) 542-5385

NEW JERSEY CLAIMS OFFICE
NETHERLANDS
62 MAPLE AVE
KEENE, NH 03431
TEL: (603) 352-3221
FAX: (603) 352-4363
TOLL FREE: (800) 542-5385

NEW YORK CLAIMS OFFICE
NETHERLANDS
62 MAPLE AVE
KEENE, NH 03431
TEL: (603) 352-3221
FAX: (603) 352-4363
TOLL FREE: (800) 542-5385

RHODE ISLAND CLAIMS OFFICE
NETHERLANDS
62 MAPLE AVE
KEENE, NH 03431
TEL: (603) 352-3221
FAX: (603) 352-4363
TOLL FREE: (800) 542-5385

VERMONT CLAIMS OFFICE
NETHERLANDS
62 MAPLE AVE
KEENE, NH 03431
TEL: (603) 352-3221
FAX: (603) 352-4363
TOLL FREE: (800) 542-5385

PEKIN INSURANCE CO

ILLINOIS CLAIMS OFFICE
2505 COURT ST
PO BOX 129
PEKIN, IL 61558-0001
TEL: (309) 346-1161
FAX: (309) 346-8512
WWW.PEKININSURANCE.COM

INDIANA CLAIMS OFFICE
2505 COURT ST
PO BOX 129
PEKIN, IL 61558-0001
TEL: (309) 346-1161
FAX: (309) 346-8512
WWW.PEKININSURANCE.COM

IOWA CLAIMS OFFICE
2505 COURT ST
PO BOX 129
PEKIN, IL 61558-0001
TEL: (309) 346-1161
FAX: (309) 346-8512
WWW.PEKININSURANCE.COM

WISCONSIN CLAIMS OFFICE
2505 COURT ST
PO BOX 129
PEKIN, IL 61558-0001
TEL: (309) 346-1161
FAX: (309) 346-8512
WWW.PEKININSURANCE.COM

PEMBRIDGE GENERAL INSURANCE CO

ILLINOIS CLAIMS OFFICE
35 E WACKER DR, STE 2000
CHICAGO, IL 60601-2297
TEL: (312) 641-2000
FAX: (312) 641-6267
TOLL FREE: (800) 621-8320

PEMCO INSURANCE CO

WASHINGTON CLAIMS OFFICE
PEMCO FINANCIAL SERVICES
325 EASTLAKE AVE E
PO BOX 778
SEATTLE, WA 98111
TEL: (206) 628-4000
FAX: (206) 628-5976
TOLL FREE: (800) 552-7440
WWW.PEMCO.COM

PENINSULA INSURANCE CO

MARYLAND CLAIMS OFFICE
PO BOX 108
SALISBURY, MD 21803-0108
TEL: (410) 742-5132
FAX: (410) 546-1273
TOLL FREE: (800) 492-1205

PENN CORP FINANCIAL COMPANIES

NORTH CAROLINA CLAIMS OFFICE
TRANS-PACIFIC LIFE INSURANCE CO
2610 WYCLIFF RD
RALEIGH, NC 27607
TEL: (919) 786-8900
FAX: (919) 786-8095
TOLL FREE: (800) 275-7366

PENN CORP INSURANCE CO

NATIONAL CLAIMS OFFICE
PENN CORPORATION FINANCIAL COMPANIES
2610 WYCLIFF RD
PO BOX 10234
RALEIGH, NC 27605-0234
TEL: (919) 786-8900

PENN STATE GEISINGER HEALTH PLAN

PENNSYLVANIA CLAIMS OFFICE
1000 E MOUNTAIN ST
WILKES-BARRE, PA 18711
TEL: (570) 826-7300
TOLL FREE: (800) 447-4000

PENN TREATY AMERICAN COMPANIES

NATIONAL CLAIMS OFFICE
3440 LEHIGH ST
PO BOX 7066
ALLENTOWN, PA 18103
TEL: (610) 965-2222
FAX: (610) 967-4616
TOLL FREE: (800) 222-3469

PENN WESTERN BENEFITS, INC

NORTH CAROLINA CLAIMS OFFICE
36 TERRACE WAY
PO BOX 7834
GREENSBORO, NC 27417-0834
TEL: (336) 665-9400
FAX: (336) 664-1300

SOUTH CAROLINA CLAIMS OFFICE
36 TERRACE WAY
PO BOX 7834
GREENSBORO, NC 27417-0834
TEL: (336) 665-9400
FAX: (336) 664-1300

PENN-AMERICA INSURANCE CO

NATIONAL CLAIMS OFFICE
420 S YORK RD
HATBORO, PA 19040
TEL: (215) 443-3600
FAX: (215) 443-3604

PENNSYLVANIA LIFE

2610 WYCLIFF ST
PO BOX 10234
RALEIGH, NC 27605-0234
TEL: (919) 786-8900
TOLL FREE: (800) 275-7366

PENNSYLVANIA LUMBERMEN'S MUTUAL INSURANCE CO

PENNSYLVANIA CLAIMS OFFICE
THE CURTIS CTR
INDEPENDENCE SQ W
PHILADELPHIA, PA 19106
TEL: (215) 625-9233
FAX: (215) 625-9097
TOLL FREE: (800) 752-1895

PENNSYLVANIA MANUFACTURERS ASSOCIATION

NATIONAL CLAIMS OFFICE
PMA INSURANCE GROUP
380 CENTRY PKY
PO BOX 3031
BLUE BELL, PA 19422
TEL: (610) 397-5000

PENNSYLVANIA MILLERS MUTUAL INSURANCE CO

ALABAMA CLAIMS OFFICE
72 N FRANKLIN ST
PO BOX P
WILKES-BARRE, PA 18773-0016
TEL: (570) 822-8111
FAX: (570) 822-2165

ARKANSAS CLAIMS OFFICE
72 N FRANKLIN ST
PO BOX P
WILKES-BARRE, PA 18773-0016
TEL: (570) 822-8111
FAX: (570) 822-2165

CONNECTICUT CLAIMS OFFICE
72 N FRANKLIN ST
PO BOX P
WILKES-BARRE, PA 18773-0016
TEL: (570) 822-8111
FAX: (570) 822-2165

GEORGIA CLAIMS OFFICE
72 N FRANKLIN ST
PO BOX P
WILKES-BARRE, PA 18773-0016
TEL: (570) 822-8111
FAX: (570) 822-2165

LOUISIANA CLAIMS OFFICE
72 N FRANKLIN ST
PO BOX P
WILKES-BARRE, PA 18773-0016
TEL: (570) 822-8111
FAX: (570) 822-2165

MAINE CLAIMS OFFICE
72 N FRANKLIN ST
PO BOX P
WILKES-BARRE, PA 18773-0016
TEL: (570) 822-8111
FAX: (570) 822-2165

MASSACHUSETTS CLAIMS OFFICE
72 N FRANKLIN ST
PO BOX P
WILKES-BARRE, PA 18773-0016
TEL: (570) 822-8111
FAX: (570) 822-2165

MISSISSIPPI CLAIMS OFFICE
72 N FRANKLIN ST
PO BOX P
WILKES-BARRE, PA 18773-0016
TEL: (570) 822-8111
FAX: (570) 822-2165

NEW JERSEY CLAIMS OFFICE
72 N FRANKLIN ST
PO BOX P
WILKES-BARRE, PA 18773-0016
TEL: (570) 822-8111
FAX: (570) 822-2165

NEW YORK CLAIMS OFFICE
72 N FRANKLIN ST
PO BOX P
WILKES-BARRE, PA 18773-0016
TEL: (570) 822-8111
FAX: (570) 822-2165

NORTH CAROLINA CLAIMS OFFICE
72 N FRANKLIN ST
PO BOX P
WILKES-BARRE, PA 18773-0016
TEL: (570) 822-8111
FAX: (570) 822-2165

PENNSYLVANIA CLAIMS OFFICE
72 N FRANKLIN ST
PO BOX P
WILKES-BARRE, PA 18773-0016
TEL: (570) 822-8111
FAX: (570) 822-2165

SOUTH CAROLINA CLAIMS OFFICE
72 N FRANKLIN ST
PO BOX P
WILKES-BARRE, PA 18773-0016
TEL: (570) 822-8111
FAX: (570) 822-2165

VERMONT CLAIMS OFFICE
72 N FRANKLIN ST
PO BOX P
WILKES-BARRE, PA 18773-0016
TEL: (570) 822-8111
FAX: (570) 822-2165

VIRGINIA CLAIMS OFFICE
72 N FRANKLIN ST
PO BOX P
WILKES-BARRE, PA 18773-0016
TEL: (570) 822-8111
FAX: (570) 822-2165

PENNSYLVANIA NATIONAL MUTUAL CASUALTY INSURANCE CO

PENNSYLVANIA CLAIMS OFFICE
PENN NATIONAL INSURANCE
2 N 2ND ST
PO BOX 2361
HARRISBURG, PA 17101
TEL: (717) 234-4941
FAX: (717) 255-6852
TOLL FREE: (800) 388-4764

PEOPLES SECURITY INSURANCE CO

NATIONAL CLAIMS OFFICE
MONUMENTAL INSURANCE CO
300 W MORGON ST
PO BOX 61
DURHAM, NC 27702
TEL: (919) 687-8200
FAX: (919) 687-8391
TOLL FREE: (800) 444-5431

PERSONAL INSURANCE ADMINISTRATORS

CALIFORNIA CLAIMS OFFICE
PO BOX 5004
WOODLAND HILLS, CA 91359
TEL: (805) 777-0032
FAX: (805) 777-0033
TOLL FREE: (800) 468-4343

PERSONALCARE HEALTH MANAGEMENT

ILLINOIS CLAIMS OFFICE
ATTN: CLAIMS DEPT
210 BOX DR
CHAMPAIGN, IL 61820-7399
TEL: (217) 366-1226
FAX: (217) 366-5410
TOLL FREE: (800) 431-1211

INDIANA CLAIMS OFFICE
ATTN: CLAIMS DEPT
210 BOX DR
CHAMPAIGN, IL 61820-7399
TEL: (217) 366-1226
FAX: (217) 366-5410
TOLL FREE: (800) 431-1211

PFS INSURANCE GROUP

NATIONAL CLAIMS OFFICE
NATIONAL GROUP LIFE INSURANCE CO
PO BOX 1250
ROCKFORD, IL 61105-1250
TEL: (815) 965-8955
FAX: (815) 720-2990
TOLL FREE: (*00) 659-7374

PHARMACIST MUTUAL

IOWA CLAIMS OFFICE
808 U.S. HWY 18-W
PO BOX 370
ALGONA, IA 50511-0370
TEL: (515) 295-2461
FAX: (515) 295-9306
TOLL FREE: (800) 247-5930

PHICO

PENNSYLVANIA CLAIMS OFFICE
1 PHICO DR
PO BOX 85
MECHANICSBURG, PA 17055-0085
TEL: (717) 691-1600
FAX: (717) 766-2837
TOLL FREE: (800) 627-4626

PHILADELPHIA AMERICAN LIFE

NATIONAL CLAIMS OFFICE
PO BOX 4884
HOUSTON, TX 77210-4884
TOLL FREE: (800) 552-7879

PHILADELPHIA BENEFITS INSURANCE CO

NEW JERSEY CLAIMS OFFICE
1000 ATRIUM WAY, STE 203- ATRIUM #1
MT LAUREL, NJ 08054
TEL: (215) 467-8731
FAX: (215) 732-5898

PHILADELPHIA CONTRIBUTIONSHIP COMPANIES

212 S 4TH ST
PHILADELPHIA, PA 19106-3704
TEL: (215) 627-1752
FAX: (215) 627-8303
TOLL FREE: (800) 346-9229

PENNSYLVANIA CLAIMS OFFICE
212 S 4TH ST
PHILADELPHIA, PA 19106-3704
TEL: (215) 627-1752
FAX: (215) 627-8303
TOLL FREE: (800) 346-9229

PHILANTHROPIC MUTUAL LIFE INSURANCE CO

170 W GERMANTOWN PIKE, STE C-1
NORRISTOWN, PA 19401
TEL: (610) 270-2880
FAX: (610) 270-2889

P

PHN-HMO
MARYLAND CLAIMS OFFICE
1099 WINTERSAN RD
LINTHICUM HEIGHTS, MD 21090
TEL: (410) 850-7461
TOLL FREE: (800) 422-1996

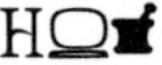

PHOENIX HOME LIFE MUTUAL INSURANCE CO
NATIONAL CLAIMS OFFICE
GROUP POLICIES
1011 MUNCHAN ST
PO BOX 677
GREENFIELD, MA 01302-0677
TEL: (413) 772-4000

INDIVIDUAL POLICIES
10 CRAY BLVD
RENSSELAER, NY 12144
TEL: (518) 479-8000
FAX: (518) 479-8057
TOLL FREE: (800) 628-1936

PHOENIX INDEMNITY INSURANCE CO
ARIZONA CLAIMS OFFICE
4041 N CENTRAL AVE STE 1900
PO BOX 52166
PHOENIX, AZ 85072
TEL: (602) 280-8200
FAX: (602) 280-8397
TOLL FREE: (800) 829-8298

PHYSICIANS BENEFITS TRUST
ILLINOIS CLAIMS OFFICE
150 S WACKER DR, STE 1200
PO BOX 8263
CHICAGO, IL 60680-8263
TEL: (312) 541-2711
FAX: (312) 541-4589
TOLL FREE: (800) 621-0748

PHYSICIANS CORPORATIONS OF AMERICA HEALTH PLAN
ALABAMA CLAIMS OFFICE
HEALTH PARTNERS OF ALABAMA
2 PERIMETER PLZ, STE 200 W
BIRMINGHAM, AL 35243
TEL: (205) 968-1000
TOLL FREE: (800) 826-0879

NATIONAL CLAIMS OFFICE
HUMANA PCA
8303 MOPAC, STE 450
PO BOX 9420
AUSTIN, TX 78766
TEL: (512) 338-6100
FAX: (512) 502-2627
TOLL FREE: (800) 318-4722

PHYSICIANS HEALTH PLAN, INC
MICHIGAN CLAIMS OFFICE
2405 WOOD LAKE DR
PO BOX 30377
LANSING, MI 48909-7877
TEL: (517) 349-2101
FAX: (517) 347-9280
TOLL FREE: (800) 832-9186
WWW.PHPMI.ORG

PHYSICIANS HEALTH PLAN OF NORTHERN INDIANA, INC
INDIANA CLAIMS OFFICE
8101 W JEFFERSON BLVD
PO BOX 2359
FT WAYNE, IN 46801
TEL: (219) 432-6690
FAX: (219) 432-0493
TOLL FREE: (800) 982-6257

PHYSICIANS HEALTH PLAN OF SOUTH CAROLINA
SOUTH CAROLINA CLAIMS OFFICE
201 EXECUTIVE CENTER DR, STE 300
COLUMBIA, SC 29210-8438
TEL: (803) 750-7400
FAX: (803) 750-7474
TOLL FREE: (800) 868-6734
WWW.PHPHEALTHPLAN.COM

PHYSICIANS HEALTH PLAN OF SOUTHWEST MICHIGAN
MICHIGAN CLAIMS OFFICE
UNITED HEALTHCARE
106 FARMER'S ALLEY, STE 400
PO BOX 50271
KALAMAZOO, MI 49005-0271
TEL: (616) 341-8000
FAX: (616) 341-6832
IN-STATE: (800) 722-3644

PHYSICIANS HEALTH SERVICES
CONNECTICUT CLAIMS OFFICE
MD HEALTH PLAN, INC
1 FARMILL CROSSING
PO BOX 904
SHELTON, CT 06484-0944
TEL: (203) 225-8000
FAX: (203) 225-4001
TOLL FREE: (800) 772-5869
IN-STATE: (800) 848-4747
WWW.PHSHMO.COM

PHYSICIANS HEALTH SERVICES OF CONNECTICUT, INC
EASTERN CONNECTICUT OFFICE
ONE FAR MILL CROSSING
PO BOX 904
SHELTON, CT 06484-0944
TEL: (860) 225-8000
FAX: (860) 225-4001
TOLL FREE: (800) 848-4747
WWW.PHSHMO.COM

NATIONAL CLAIMS OFFICE
CORPORATE HEADQUARTERS
1 FAR MILL XING
PO BOX 904
SHELTON, CT 06484-0944
TEL: (203) 225-8000
FAX: (203) 225-4001
TOLL FREE: (800) 772-5869
IN-STATE: (800) 848-4747
WWW.PHSHMO.COM

NEW JERSEY CLAIMS OFFICE
ONE FAR MILL CROSSING
PO BOX 904
SHELTON, CT 06484-0944
TEL: (203) 225-8000
FAX: (203) 225-4001
IN-STATE: (800) 848-4747
WWW.PHSHMO.COM

NEW YORK CLAIMS OFFICE
ONE FAR MILL CROSSING
PO BOX 904
SHELTON, CT 06484-0944
TEL: (203) 225-8000
FAX: (203) 225-4001
IN-STATE: (800) 848-4747
WWW.PHSHMO.COM

PHYSICIANS HEALTH SERVICES OF NEW JERSEY, INC
CONNECTICUT CLAIMS OFFICE
MACK CTR IV- S 61 PARAMUS RD
PARAMUS, NJ 07652
TEL: (201) 291-9300
FAX: (201) 291-1711
TOLL FREE: (800) 848-4747
WWW.PHSHMO.COM

NEW JERSEY CLAIMS OFFICE
MACK CTR IV- S 61 PARAMUS RD
PARAMUS, NJ 07652
TEL: (201) 291-9300
FAX: (201) 291-1711
TOLL FREE: (800) 848-4747
WWW.PHSHMO.COM

NEW YORK CLAIMS OFFICE
MACK CTR IV- S 61 PARAMUS RD
PARAMUS, NJ 07652
TEL: (201) 291-9300
FAX: (201) 291-1711
TOLL FREE: (800) 848-4747
WWW.PHSHMO.COM

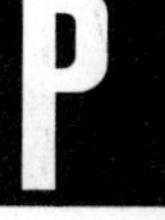

PHYSICIANS HEALTH SERVICES OF NEW YORK, INC

CONNECTICUT CLAIMS OFFICE
CROSSWEST OFFICE CENTER
399 KNOLLWOOD RD, STE 212
WHITE PLAINS, NY 10603-1900
TEL: (914) 682-8006
FAX: (914) 682-5692
TOLL FREE: (800) 848-4747
WWW.PHSHMO.COM

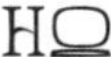

NEW JERSEY CLAIMS OFFICE
CROSSWEST OFFICE CENTER
399 KNOLLWOOD RD, STE 212
WHITE PLAINS, NY 10603-1900
TEL: (914) 682-8006
FAX: (914) 682-5692
TOLL FREE: (800) 848-4747
WWW.PHSHMO.COM

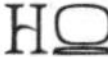

NEW YORK CLAIMS OFFICE
CROSSWEST OFFICE CENTER
399 KNOLLWOOD RD, STE 212
WHITE PLAINS, NY 10603-1900
TEL: (914) 682-8006
FAX: (914) 682-5692
TOLL FREE: (800) 848-4747
WWW.PHSHMO.COM

NASSAU COUNTY
LAKE SUCCESS PLZ- 1 HOLLOW LN, STE 101
LAKE SUCCESS, NY 11042
TEL: (516) 365-6962
FAX: (516) 365-6095
TOLL FREE: (800) 848-4747
WWW.PHSHMO.COM

CHRYSLER BLDG- 405 LEXINGTON AVE
NEW YORK, NY 10174
TEL: (212) 856-4500
FAX: (212) 661-8184
TOLL FREE: (800) 848-4747
WWW.PHSHMO.COM

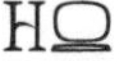

PHYSICIANS HEALTHCARE PLANS, INC

FLORIDA CLAIMS OFFICE
1410 N WEST SHORE BLVD, STE 200
TAMPA, FL 33607
TEL: (813) 273-7474
TOLL FREE: (800) 873-7474

PHYSICIANS MUTUAL

CALIFORNIA CLAIMS OFFICE
PHYSICIANS LIFE INSURANCE
2600 DODGE ST
PO BOX 2030
OMAHA, NE 68103-2018
TEL: (402) 633-1000
FAX: (402) 633-1088
TOLL FREE: (800) 228-9100
WWW.PMIC.COM

NEBRASKA CLAIMS OFFICE
PHYSICIANS LIFE INSURANCE
2600 DODGE ST
PO BOX 2018
OMAHA, NE 68103-2018
TEL: (402) 633-1000
FAX: (402) 633-1088
TOLL FREE: (800) 622-4642
WWW.PMIC.COM

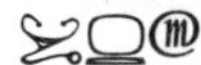

PILGRIM HEALTH CARE, INC

NATIONAL CLAIMS OFFICE
HARVARD
1200 CROWN COLONY DR
QUINCY, MA 02169
TEL: (617) 745-1000
FAX: (617) 745-1100
TOLL FREE: (800) 742-8326

PIONEER FINANCIAL

ILLINOIS CLAIMS OFFICE
CONSECO
11815 N PENNSYLVANIA ST
CARMEL, IN 46082
TEL: (317) 817-6100
FAX: (317) 817-6721
TOLL FREE: (800) 759-7007

INDIANA CLAIMS OFFICE
CONSECO
11815 N PENNSYLVANIA ST
CARMEL, IN 46082
TEL: (317) 817-6100
FAX: (317) 817-6721
TOLL FREE: (800) 759-7007

OKLAHOMA CLAIMS OFFICE
CONSECO
11815 N PENNSYLVANIA ST
CARMEL, IN 46082
TEL: (317) 817-6100
FAX: (317) 817-6721
TOLL FREE: (800) 759-7007

PIONEER LIFE

ILLINOIS CLAIMS OFFICE
PO BOX 1250
ROCKFORD, IL 61105
FAX: (815) 720-2931
TOLL FREE: (800) 950-0084
IN-STATE: (800) 659-7374

TEXAS CLAIMS OFFICE
PO BOX 1250
ROCKFORD, IL 61105
FAX: (815) 720-2931
TOLL FREE: (800) 950-0084
IN-STATE: (800) 659-7374

PIONEER MUTUAL INSURANCE CO

CONNECTICUT CLAIMS OFFICE
PO BOX 10
GREENVILLE, NY 12083
TEL: (518) 966-5311
FAX: (518) 966-5332
TOLL FREE: (800) 456-5311

NEW YORK CLAIMS OFFICE
PO BOX 10
GREENVILLE, NY 12083
TEL: (518) 966-5311
FAX: (518) 966-5332
TOLL FREE: (800) 456-5311

PITNEY BOWES, INC

NATIONAL CLAIMS OFFICE
WORLD HEADQUARTERS
1 ELMCROFT RD
STAMFORD, CT 06926-0700
TEL: (203) 356-5000
TOLL FREE: (800) 322-8000
WWW.PB.COM

PITTMAN & ASSOCIATES, INC

TENNESSEE CLAIMS OFFICE
1 PRESCOTT S
PO BOX 111047
MEMPHIS, TN 38111-1047
TEL: (901) 323-2140
FAX: (901) 327-9147
TOLL FREE: (800) 238-1344
E-MAIL: PITTMAN@LUNAWEB.NET

PLUMBERS & PIPEFITTERS LOCAL 190

MICHIGAN CLAIMS OFFICE
2320 WASHTENAW
ANN ARBOR, MI 48104
TEL: (313) 665-8022

POLICE & FIREMEN INSURANCE ASSOCIATION

NATIONAL CLAIMS OFFICE
101 E 116TH ST
PO BOX 1913
CARMEL, IN 46032
TEL: (317) 581-1913
FAX: (317) 571-5945
TOLL FREE: (800) 221-7342

POSTMASTERS BENEFIT PLAN

1019 N ROYAL ST
ALEXANDRIA, VA 22314-1596
TEL: (703) 683-1664
FAX: (703) 683-2937

PRAIRIE STATES LIFE INSURANCE CO

AMERICAN MEMORIAL
440 MT RUSHMORE RD
RAPID CITY, SD 57701
TEL: (605) 348-1262
FAX: (605) 348-6859
TOLL FREE: (800) 843-8810

PREFERRED CARE

NEW YORK CLAIMS OFFICE
259 MONROE AVE
ROCHESTER, NY 14607-3693
TEL: (716) 325-3920
FAX: (716) 325-3122
TOLL FREE: (800) 950-3224
WWW.PREFERREDCARE.ORG

PREFERRED CHOICE 65

OREGON CLAIMS OFFICE
3000 MARKET ST, STE 514
PO BOX 12625
SALEM, OR 97309
TEL: (503) 585-0560

PREFERRED HEALTH NETWORK

CALIFORNIA CLAIMS OFFICE
153 TECHNOLOGY
PO BOX 57009
IRVINE, CA 92619
TEL: (949) 788-6400
FAX: (949) 790-3360
TOLL FREE: (800) 334-5646

PREFERRED HEALTH NORTHWEST

OREGON CLAIMS OFFICE
BLUE CROSS & BLUE SHIELDS OF OREGON
100 SW MARKET
PO BOX 1271
PORTLAND, OR 97207-1271
TEL: (503) 274-0761
FAX: (503) 375-4293
TOLL FREE: (800) 452-7390
IN-STATE: (800) 452-7278
WWW.BCBSO.COM

PREFERRED HEALTH SYSTEMS INSURANCE CO

KANSAS CLAIMS OFFICE
355 N WACO
PO BOX 49288
WICHITA, KS 67201-5007
TEL: (316) 268-0345
FAX: (316) 268-0346
TOLL FREE: (800) 660-8114
WWW.PHSYSTEMS.COM

PREFERRED PLUS OF KANSAS
PO BOX 49218
WICHITA, KS 67202
TEL: (316) 268-0345
FAX: (316) 263-3673
TOLL FREE: (800) 660-8114
WWW.PHSYSTEMS.COM

PREFERRED MEDICAL PLAN, INC

FLORIDA CLAIMS OFFICE
4950 SW 8 ST
CORAL GABLES, FL 33134
TEL: (305) 669-1501
FAX: (305) 445-4525

PREFERRED MUTUAL INSURANCE CO

NEW YORK CLAIMS OFFICE
ONE PREFERRED WAY
NEW BERLIN, NY 13411
TEL: (607) 847-6161
FAX: (607) 847-6859
TOLL FREE: (800) 333-7642
WWW.PMINSCO.COM

PREFERRED RISK GROUP INSURANCE COMPANIES

KANSAS CLAIMS OFFICE
GUIDE ONE
17020 E 40 HWY, STE 12

INDEPENDENCE, MO 64055
TEL: (816) 478-6440
FAX: (816) 478-6226
TOLL FREE: (888) 748-4326

MISSOURI CLAIMS OFFICE
GUIDE ONE
17020 E 40 HWY, STE 12
INDEPENDENCE, MO 64055
TEL: (816) 478-6440
FAX: (816) 478-6226
TOLL FREE: (888) 748-4326

OKLAHOMA CLAIMS OFFICE
GUIDE ONE
PO BOX 4756
TULSA, OK 74159
TEL: (800) 777-0404
TOLL FREE: (888) 748-4326

WASHINGTON CLAIMS OFFICE
GUIDE ONE INSURANCE
15407 1ST AVE S
SEATTLE, WA 98148
TEL: (206) 433-8040
TOLL FREE: (888) 748-4326

PREMERA BLUE CROSS

ALASKA CLAIMS OFFICE
7001 220TH ST SW
PO BOX 327
MOUNTLAKE TERRACE, WA 98111
TEL: (425) 670-4700
FAX: (425) 670-5457
TOLL FREE: (800) 527-6675

IDAHO CLAIMS OFFICE
7001 220TH ST SW
PO BOX 327
MOUNTLAKE TERRACE, WA 98111
TEL: (425) 670-4700
FAX: (425) 670-5457
TOLL FREE: (800) 527-6675

OREGON CLAIMS OFFICE
7001 220TH ST SW
PO BOX 327
MOUNTLAKE TERRACE, WA 98111
TEL: (425) 670-4700
FAX: (425) 670-5457
TOLL FREE: (800) 527-6675

WASHINGTON CLAIMS OFFICE
7001 220TH ST SW
PO BOX 327
MOUNTLAKE TERRACE, WA 98111
TEL: (425) 670-4700
FAX: (425) 670-5457
TOLL FREE: (800) 527-6675

3900 E SPRAGUE
PO BOX 3048
SPOKANE, WA 99220-3048
TEL: (509) 536-4700
FAX: (509) 536-4771
TOLL FREE: (800) 835-3510
IN-STATE: (800) 572-0778
WWW.PREMERA.COM

PREMIER BLUE

KANSAS CLAIMS OFFICE
1133 SW TOPEKA AVE
PO BOX 3518
TOPEKA, KS 66601-3518
TEL: (785) 291-4010
FAX: (785) 291-8848
TOLL FREE: (800) 332-0028
WWW.BCBSKS.COM

PREPAID HEALTH PLAN

NEW YORK CLAIMS OFFICE
8278 WILLETT PKY
BALDWINSVILLE, NY 13027-1302
TEL: (315) 638-9162
FAX: (315) 635-7489
TOLL FREE: (800) 223-4780
WWW.PHPHMO.COM

PRESBYTERIAN HEALTH PLAN / FHP OF NEW MEXICO

NEW MEXICO CLAIMS OFFICE
PACIFICARE OF NEW MEXICO
PO BOX 27489
ALBUQUERQUE, NM 87125
TEL: (505) 923-5799
FAX: (505) 923-5277
TOLL FREE: (800) 356-2884
IN-STATE: (800) 356-2219

PRESIDIUM INC / CAMBRIDGE

MICHIGAN CLAIMS OFFICE
34820 HARPER AVE
PO BOX 2305
MT CLEMENS, MI 48046-2305
TEL: (810) 792-6355
FAX: (810) 792-9429
TOLL FREE: (800) 482-0615

PRIME CARE HEALTH PLAN, INC

WISCONSIN CLAIMS OFFICE
10701 W RESEARCH DR
PO BOX 3153
MILWAUKEE, WI 53201-3153
TEL: (414) 443-4000
FAX: (414) 443-4275
TOLL FREE: (800) 879-0071

PRIME HEALTH OF ALABAMA

ALABAMA CLAIMS OFFICE
MOBILE HEALTH PLAN DBA
1400 UNIVERSITY BLVD S
PO BOX 851239
MOBILE, AL 36685-1239
TEL: (334) 342-0022
FAX: (334) 380-3236
TOLL FREE: (800) 544-9449
WWW.PRIMEHEALTHONLINE.COM

MISSISSIPPI CLAIMS OFFICE
MOBILE HEALTH PLAN DBA
1400 UNIVERSITY BLVD S
PO BOX 851239
MOBILE, AL 36685-1239
TEL: (334) 342-0022
FAX: (334) 380-3236
TOLL FREE: (800) 544-9449
WWW.PRIMEHEALTHONLINE.COM

PRINCIPAL FINANCIAL GROUP

CALIFORNIA CLAIMS OFFICE
1360 E SPRUCE
FRESNO, CA 93711-3324
TEL: (559) 432-1277
TOLL FREE: (800) 523-5938
WWW.PRINCIPAL.COM

FLORIDA CLAIMS OFFICE
9428 BAYMEADOWS RD, STE 360
JACKSONVILLE, FL 32256-9933
TEL: (904) 731-8159
FAX: (904) 367-8444
TOLL FREE: (800) 445-6133
WWW.PRINCIPAL.COM

ILLINOIS CLAIMS OFFICE
PRINCIPAL LIFE INSURNACE CO
1245 CORPORATE BLVD, STE 200
AURORA, IL 60504-9955
TEL: (630) 978-5100
FAX: (630) 978-5117
WWW.PRINCIPAL.COM

INDIANA CLAIMS OFFICE
10985 CODY, STE 200
OVERLAND PARK, KS 66210
TEL: (913) 491-4833
FAX: (913) 491-5280
TOLL FREE: (800) 321-0123
WWW.PRINCIPAL.COM

IOWA CLAIMS OFFICE
CORPORATE HEADQUARTERS
711 HIGH ST
DES MOINES, IA 50392-0001
TEL: (515) 247-5111
TOLL FREE: (800) 247-4695
WWW.PRINCIPAL.COM

AMES SERVICE CENTER
414 S 17TH ST
PO BOX 3006
AMES, IA 50010-3006
TEL: (515) 232-0127
FAX: (515) 663-8900
TOLL FREE: (800) 443-9456
WWW.PRINCIPAL.COM

4050 RIVER RDG DR NE
PO BOX 28002
CEDAR RAPIDS, IA 52402
TEL: (319) 395-7987
FAX: (319) 395-7090
TOLL FREE: (319) 395-7987
WWW.PRINCIPAL.COM

PO BOX 65990
WEST DES MOINES, IA 50265-0990
TEL: (515) 247-6262
FAX: (515) 248-2445
TOLL FREE: (800) 422-4130
WWW.PRINCIPAL.COM

KANSAS CLAIMS OFFICE
10985 CODY, STE 200
OVERLAND PARK, KS 66210
TEL: (913) 491-4833
FAX: (913) 491-5280
TOLL FREE: (800) 321-0123
WWW.PRINCIPAL.COM

MICHIGAN CLAIMS OFFICE
PRINCIPAL MUTUAL LIFE
7330 SAN PEDRO #700
PO BOX 795014
SAN ANTONIO, TX 78279-5014
TEL: (210) 349-5454
FAX: (210) 524-9589
TOLL FREE: (800) 331-2557

MINNESOTA CLAIMS OFFICE
PRINCIPAL MUTUAL LIFE
7330 SAN PEDRO #700
PO BOX 795014
SAN ANTONIO, TX 78279-5014
TEL: (210) 349-5454
FAX: (210) 524-9589
TOLL FREE: (800) 331-2557

MISSOURI CLAIMS OFFICE
620 S GLENSTONE AVE, STE 300
PO BOX 2593
SPRINGFIELD, MO 65801-2593
TEL: (417) 877-0085
TOLL FREE: (800) 422-5002
WWW.PRINCIPAL.COM

NATIONAL CLAIMS OFFICE
1755 TELSTAR DR, STE 300
PO BOX 39710
COLORADO SPRINGS, CO 80949
TEL: (719) 548-4000
FAX: (719) 548-4001
TOLL FREE: (800) 273-2486
WWW.PRINCIPAL.COM

NEBRASKA CLAIMS OFFICE
330 N 117TH ST
PO BOX 542060
OMAHA, NE 68154
TEL: (402) 330-0800
FAX: (402) 330-1636
TOLL FREE: (800) 331-9443
WWW.PRINCIPAL.COM

OKLAHOMA CLAIMS OFFICE
620 S GLENSTONE AVE, STE 300
PO BOX 2593
SPRINGFIELD, MO 65801-2593
TEL: (417) 877-0085
TOLL FREE: (800) 422-5002
WWW.PRINCIPAL.COM

OREGON CLAIMS OFFICE
PRINCIPAL MUTUAL LIFE
7330 SAN PEDRO #700
PO BOX 795014
SAN ANTONIO, TX 78279-5014
TEL: (210) 349-5454
FAX: (210) 524-9589
TOLL FREE: (800) 331-2557

PENNSYLVANIA CLAIMS OFFICE
1 INTERNATIONAL PLZ, STE 100
PHILADELPHIA, PA 19113
TEL: (610) 668-2500
FAX: (610) 362-0930
TOLL FREE: (800) 522-1279
WWW.PRINCIPAL.COM

TEXAS CLAIMS OFFICE
PRINCIPAL MUTUAL LIFE
7330 SAN PEDRO #700
PO BOX 795014
SAN ANTONIO, TX 78279-5014
TEL: (210) 349-5454
FAX: (210) 524-9589
TOLL FREE: (800) 331-2557

UTAH CLAIMS OFFICE
4021 S 700 E, STE 500
PO BOX 57700
SALT LAKE CITY, UT 84157-7700
TEL: (801) 266-1490
FAX: (801) 288-0097
TOLL FREE: (800) 535-7212
WWW.PRINCIPAL.COM

WASHINGTON CLAIMS OFFICE
PRINCIPAL MUTUAL LIFE
7330 SAN PEDRO #700
PO BOX 795014
SAN ANTONIO, TX 78279-5014
TEL: (210) 349-5454
FAX: (210) 524-9589
TOLL FREE: (800) 331-2557

WISCONSIN CLAIMS OFFICE
PRINCIPAL MUTUAL LIFE
7330 SAN PEDRO #700
PO BOX 795014
SAN ANTONIO, TX 78279-5014
TEL: (210) 349-5454
FAX: (210) 524-9589
TOLL FREE: (800) 331-2557

PRINCIPAL HEALTH CARE, INC

FLORIDA CLAIMS OFFICE
1200 RIVERPLACE BLVD, STE 500
PO BOX 45076
JACKSONVILLE, FL 32232-5076
TEL: (904) 390-0935
FAX: (904) 390-0950
TOLL FREE: (800) 358-6205
H

P

Medigap Pharmacy 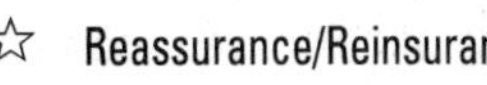 Reassurance/Reinsurance 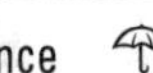 Self-Insured 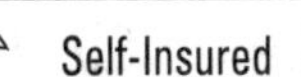 TPA 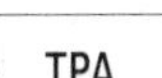 Vision 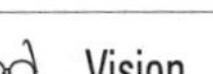 Workers Comp

1200 RIVERPLACE BLVD, STE 500
JACKSONVILLE, FL 32232
TEL: (904) 390-0935
FAX: (904) 390-0950
TOLL FREE: (800) 358-6205

H

KANSAS CLAIMS OFFICE
1001 E 101 TERRACE, STE 300
PO BOX 410976
KANSAS CITY, MO 64141
TEL: (816) 941-3030
FAX: (816) 941-8516
TOLL FREE: (800) 969-3343
WWW.PHCKC.COM

MISSOURI CLAIMS OFFICE
1001 E 101 TERRACE, STE 300
PO BOX 410976
KANSAS CITY, MO 64141
TEL: (816) 941-3030
FAX: (816) 941-8516
TOLL FREE: (800) 969-3343
WWW.PHCKC.COM

PRINCIPAL HEALTH CARE OF DELAWARE

DELAWARE CLAIMS OFFICE
2751 CENTERVILLE RD, STE 400
PO BOX 15294
WILMINGTON, DE 19850
TEL: (302) 995-6100
FAX: (302) 633-4044
TOLL FREE: (800) 833-7423

H

PRINCIPAL HEALTH CARE OF IOWA

IOWA CLAIMS OFFICE
4600 WESTOWN PKY- BLDG 6, STE 200
WEST DES MOINES, IA 50266
TEL: (515) 225-1234
FAX: (515) 223-0097
TOLL FREE: (800) 257-4692

H

PRINCIPAL HEALTH CARE OF LOUISIANA

LOUISIANA CLAIMS OFFICE
PO BOX 15294
WILMINGTON, LA 19850
TEL: (504) 834-0840
FAX: (504) 834-2694
TOLL FREE: (800) 341-6613

H

PRINCIPAL HEALTH CARE OF NEBRASKA, INC

NEBRASKA CLAIMS OFFICE
330 N 117 ST
PO BOX 541210
OMAHA, NE 68154
TEL: (402) 333-1720
FAX: (402) 333-1116
TOLL FREE: (800) 288-3343

PRINCIPAL HEALTHCARE OF FLORIDA

FLORIDA CLAIMS OFFICE
2203 N LOIS AVE, STE 900
PO BOX 31298
TAMPA, FL 33631-3298
TEL: (813) 875-3737
FAX: (813) 876-4572
TOLL FREE: (800) 443-5810

PRIORITY HEALTH

CALIFORNIA CLAIMS OFFICE
PACIFIC CARE
1111 E HERNDON, STE 202
PO BOX 25790
FRESNO, CA 93729-5790
TEL: (559) 435-8366
FAX: (559) 435-9718
TOLL FREE: (800) 350-8366

MICHIGAN CLAIMS OFFICE
1231 E BELTLINE NE
PO BOX 232
GRAND RAPIDS, MI 49505
TEL: (616) 942-0954
FAX: (616) 942-7916
TOLL FREE: (800) 942-0954
WWW.PRIORITY-HEALTH.COM

PRIORITY HEALTH CARE

VIRGINIA CLAIMS OFFICE
621 LYNNHAVEN PKY, STE 450
VIRGINIA BEACH, VA 23452-7330
TEL: (757) 463-4600
FAX: (757) 463-7172
TOLL FREE: (800) 640-0007
WWW.TRIGON.COM

PROCLAIM SERVICES

NEW YORK CLAIMS OFFICE
157 WOODRUFF ST
WATERTOWN, NY 13601
TEL: (315) 786-4935
FAX: (315) 786-4937
TOLL FREE: (800) 369-4325
IN-STATE: (800) 369-4325

PRODUCER'S EXCHANGE BENEFIT SERVICES, INC

TEXAS CLAIMS OFFICE
14665 MIDWAY RD, STE 110
ADDISON, TX 75001-3184
TEL: (972) 774-1100
FAX: (972) 774-1220
TOLL FREE: (800) 443-2595

PROFESSIONAL ADMINISTRATION GROUP

KANSAS CLAIMS OFFICE
PO BOX 13391
OVERLAND PARK, KS 66282-3391
TEL: (913) 327-7104
FAX: (913) 451-4762
E-MAIL: ADM-SVC@SWBELL.NET

PROFESSIONAL ADMINISTRATORS, INC

NATIONAL CLAIMS OFFICE
3751 MAGUIRE BLVD, STE 100
PO BOX 140415-0415
ORLANDO, FL 32803-0415
TEL: (407) 896-0521
FAX: (407) 897-6976
TOLL FREE: (800) 741-0521
IN-STATE: (800) 432-2686
E-MAIL: PA1001@AOL.COM

PROFESSIONAL BENEFIT ADMINISTRATORS, INC

ILLINOIS CLAIMS OFFICE
15 SPINNING WHEEL RD, STE 210
PO BOX 4687
OAKBROOK, IL 60522
TEL: (630) 655-3755
FAX: (630) 655-3781

PROFESSIONAL INSURANCE CORP

NORTH CAROLINA CLAIMS OFFICE
P. I. C.
2610 WYCLIFF
PO BOX 337
LANGHORNE, PA 19047
TOLL FREE: (800) 289-1122
IN-STATE: (800) 730-6484
WWW.PIC.COM

PENNSYLVANIA CLAIMS OFFICE
P. I. C.
2610 WYCLIFF
PO BOX 337
LANGHORNE, PA 19047
TOLL FREE: (800) 289-1122
IN-STATE: (800) 730-6484
WWW.PIC.COM

PROFESSIONAL RISK MANAGEMENT

CALIFORNIA CLAIMS OFFICE
2101 WEBSTER ST, STE 900
OAKLAND, CA 94612
TEL: (510) 452-9300
FAX: (510) 452-1479
WWW.APPLIEDRISK.COM

132 E ST, STE 3C
DAVIS, CA 95616
TEL: (530) 753-6500
FAX: (530) 757-1344
WWW.APPLIEDRISK.COM

444 MARKET ST, STE 1050
SAN FRANCISCO, CA 94111
TEL: (415) 398-3824
FAX: (415) 398-2214

OHIO CLAIMS OFFICE
7260 WEST BLVD
PO BOX 1049
BOARDMAN, OH 44512
TEL: (330) 726-5800
FAX: (330) 726-3786
TOLL FREE: (800) 331-7620

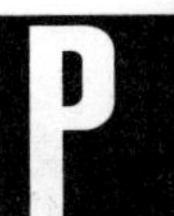

PENNSYLVANIA CLAIMS OFFICE
7260 WEST BLVD
PO BOX 1049
BOARDMAN, OH 44512
TEL: (330) 726-5800
FAX: (330) 726-3786
TOLL FREE: (800) 331-7620

WEST VIRGINIA CLAIMS OFFICE
7260 WEST BLVD
PO BOX 1049
BOARDMAN, OH 44512
TEL: (330) 726-5800
FAX: (330) 726-3786
TOLL FREE: (800) 331-7620

PROGRESSIVE CASUALTY INSURANCE CO

ALABAMA CLAIMS OFFICE
1025 OLD MONROVIA RD
HUNTSVILLE, AL 35806
TOLL FREE: (800) 274-4499
WWW.PROGRESSIVE.COM

2 E OFC CTR- 400 EASTERN BLVD, STE 305
MONTGOMERY, AL 36117
TOLL FREE: (800) 274-4499
WWW.PROGRESSIVE.COM

ALASKA CLAIMS OFFICE
8220 BRIARWOOD, STE 100
ANCHORAGE, AK 99518
TOLL FREE: (800) 274-4499
IN-STATE: (800) 478-4012
WWW.PROGRESSIVE.COM

8220 BRIARWOOD, STE 100
ANCHORAGE, AK 99518
TOLL FREE: (800) 274-4499
IN-STATE: (800) 478-4012
WWW.PROGRESSIVE.COM

ARIZONA CLAIMS OFFICE
PO BOX 47670
PHOENIX, AZ 85068-7670
TOLL FREE: (800) 274-4499
WWW.PROGRESSIVE.COM

3936 E FT LOWELL, STE 206
PO BOX 14045
TUCSON, AZ 85732
TOLL FREE: (800) 274-4499
IN-STATE: (800) 888-4543
WWW.PROGRESSIVE.COM

ARKANSAS CLAIMS OFFICE
4210-B FRONTAGE
FAYETTEVILLE, AR 72703
TEL: (501) 973-7800
FAX: (501) 521-8670
TOLL FREE: (800) 274-4499
WWW.PROGRESSIVE.COM

10810 EXECUTIVE CT DR, STE 308
LITTLE ROCK, AR 72212
FAX: (501) 223-9564
TOLL FREE: (800) 274-4499
WWW.PROGRESSIVE.COM

1121 JUDSON RD, STE 167
LONGVIEW, TX 75601
TEL: (903) 753-3821
FAX: (903) 753-1263
TOLL FREE: (800) 274-4499
WWW.PROGRESSIVE.COM

CALIFORNIA CLAIMS OFFICE
500 N STATE COLLEGE BLVD, STE 610
ORANGE, CA 92668
FAX: (714) 978-8366
TOLL FREE: (800) 274-4499
WWW.PROGRESSIVE.COM

11010 WHITE ROCK RD
PO BOX 1418
RANCHO CORDOVA, CA 95741
FAX: (916) 638-8342
TOLL FREE: (800) 274-4499
IN-STATE: (800) 888-7764
WWW.PROGRESSIVE.COM

658 BAIR ISLAND RD, STE 101
REDWOOD CITY, CA 94063
TOLL FREE: (800) 274-4499
WWW.PROGRESSIVE.COM

COLORADO CLAIMS OFFICE
2075 RESEARCH PKY, STE A
COLORADO SPRINGS, CO 80920
FAX: (719) 534-7818
TOLL FREE: (800) 274-4499
WWW.PROGRESSIVE.COM

12201 E ARAPAHOE RD, STE A-15
ENGLEWOOD, CO 80110
FAX: (303) 779-4704
TOLL FREE: (800) 274-4499
WWW.PROGRESSIVE.COM

CONNECTICUT CLAIMS OFFICE
185 PLAINS RD, STE 108E
MILFORD, CT 06460
FAX: (203) 877-8109
TOLL FREE: (800) 274-4499
WWW.PROGRESSIVE.COM

324 MAIN AVE
NORWALK, CT 06851
FAX: (203) 840-4869
TOLL FREE: (800) 274-4499
WWW.PROGRESSIVE.COM

SUMMIT EAST
300 CENTERVILLE RD, STE 220
WARWICK, RI 02886
TEL: (401) 732-5950
FAX: (401) 732-5954
TOLL FREE: (800) 274-4499
WWW.PROGRESSIVE.COM

1310 SILAS DEAN HWY
WETHERSFIELD, CT 06109
TOLL FREE: (800) 274-4499
WWW.PROGRESSIVE.COM

FLORIDA CLAIMS OFFICE
1609 W BRANDOM, STE 105
BRANDOM, FL 33511
FAX: (813) 651-2863
TOLL FREE: (800) 274-4499
IN-STATE: (800) 444-3909
WWW.PROGRESSIVE.COM

11081 US HWY 19 N, STE 206
CLEARWATER, FL 34624
TEL: (813) 572-5700
FAX: (813) 573-9212
TOLL FREE: (800) 274-4499
WWW.PROGRESSIVE.COM

1481 S NOVA RD
DAYTONA, FL 32114
FAX: (904) 258-7939
TOLL FREE: (800) 274-4499
WWW.PROGRESSIVE.COM

7265 NW 4TH BLVD
GAINESVILLE, FL 32607-1600
FAX: (352) 331-0099
TOLL FREE: (800) 274-4499
WWW.PROGRESSIVE.COM

3318 S FLORIDA AVE
LAKELAND, FL 33803
FAX: (941) 646-7019
TOLL FREE: (800) 274-4499
WWW.PROGRESSIVE.COM

1600 SARNO RD, STE 124
MELBOURNE, FL 32935
TOLL FREE: (800) 274-4499
WWW.PROGRESSIVE.COM

2506 PONCE DE LEON BLVD
CORAL GABLES, FL 33134
TEL: (305) 461-1604
FAX: (305) 461-6027
TOLL FREE: (800) 274-4499
IN-STATE: (800) 937-0103
WWW.PROGRESSIVE.COM

4292 BEE RIDGE RD
SARASOTA, FL 34233
TEL: (941) 342-5000
FAX: (941) 342-0406
TOLL FREE: (800) 274-4499
WWW.PROGRESSIVE.COM

2000 APALACHEE PKY, STE 202
TALLAHASSEE, FL 32301
TEL: (850) 656-8650
TOLL FREE: (800) 274-4499
WWW.PROGRESSIVE.COM

4619 OKEECHOBEE
PO BOX 17920
WEST PALM BEACH, FL 33417
TOLL FREE: (800) 274-4499
IN-STATE: (800) 999-0470
WWW.PROGRESSIVE.COM

GEORGIA CLAIMS OFFICE
2425 WESTGATE, STE 131
ALBANY, GA 31707
TEL: (912) 483-7480
FAX: (912) 436-3439
TOLL FREE: (800) 274-4499
WWW.PROGRESSIVE.COM

3720 ATLANTA HWY, STE 4
ATHENS, GA 30606
FAX: (706) 543-1249
TOLL FREE: (800) 274-4499
WWW.PROGRESSIVE.COM

380 INTERSTATE N PKY, STE 100
ATLANTA, GA 30339
FAX: (770) 988-3799
TOLL FREE: (800) 274-4499
IN-STATE: (800) 678-5670
WWW.PROGRESSIVE.COM

1054 CLAUSSEN RD, STE 311
AUGUSTA, GA 30907
TEL: (706) 729-2002
FAX: (706) 481-0910
TOLL FREE: (800) 274-4499
WWW.PROGRESSIVE.COM

1247 STARK AVE
COLUMBUS, GA 31906
TEL: (706) 660-0200
FAX: (706) 660-8822
TOLL FREE: (800) 274-4499
WWW.PROGRESSIVE.COM

316 S LEWIS ST- UNIT 5
PO BOX 3001
LA GRANGE, GA 30241
TEL: (706) 845-7519
FAX: (706) 845-7520
TOLL FREE: (800) 274-4499
WWW.PROGRESSIVE.COM

3200 RIVERSIDE DR- BLDG A, STE 300A
PO BOX 7929 (ZIP 31209)
MACON, GA 31210
TEL: (912) 475-6900
FAX: (912) 474-3269
TOLL FREE: (800) 274-4499
WWW.PROGRESSIVE.COM

808 AVE B, STE B
ROME, GA 30165-2746
FAX: (706) 234-4429
TOLL FREE: (800) 274-4499
WWW.PROGRESSIVE.COM

440 MALL BLVD, STE C
SAVANNAH, GA 31406
FAX: (912) 355-9864
TOLL FREE: (800) 274-4499
IN-STATE: (800) 999-7336
WWW.PROGRESSIVE.COM

1810 N ASHLEY ST, STE 3G
PO BOX 2185
VALDOSTA, GA 31604-2185
TEL: (912) 244-6869
FAX: (912) 244-7155
TOLL FREE: (800) 274-4499
WWW.PROGRESSIVE.COM

IDAHO CLAIMS OFFICE
1323 S MAPLE GROVE
BOISE, ID 83709
TEL: (208) 323-2035
FAX: (208) 376-0267
TOLL FREE: (800) 274-4499
IN-STATE: (800) 955-9789
WWW.PROGRESSIVE.COM

ILLINOIS CLAIMS OFFICE
2500 S HIGHLAND, STE 320
LOMBARD, IL 60148
TOLL FREE: (800) 274-4499
WWW.PROGRESSIVE.COM

3267 COURT ST
PEKIN, IL 61554
TEL: (309) 346-8007
FAX: (309) 346-6880
TOLL FREE: (800) 274-4499
WWW.PROGRESSIVE.COM

2435 KIMBERLY RD S120
BETTENDORF, IA 52722
TEL: (319) 359-4104
FAX: (319) 359-4363
TOLL FREE: (800) 274-4499
WWW.PROGRESSIVE.COM

INDIANA CLAIMS OFFICE
7222 SHADELAND AVE- 2ND FL
INDIANAPOLIS, IN 46050
TEL: (317) 585-7300
FAX: (317) 570-3918
TOLL FREE: (800) 274-4499
WWW.PROGRESSIVE.COM

618 W 81ST AVE
MERRILLVILLE, IN 46410
TEL: (219) 650-7001
FAX: (219) 736-8704
TOLL FREE: (800) 274-4499
WWW.PROGRESSIVE.COM

227 S MAIN ST, STE 201
SOUTH BEND, IN 46601
TOLL FREE: (800) 274-4499
WWW.PROGRESSIVE.COM

IOWA CLAIMS OFFICE
2435 KIMBERLY RD S120
BETTENDORF, IA 52722
TEL: (319) 359-4104
FAX: (319) 359-4363
TOLL FREE: (800) 274-4499
WWW.PROGRESSIVE.COM

1350 BOYSON RD- BLDG C
HIAWATHA, IA 52233
TEL: (319) 395-9787
FAX: (319) 395-9742
TOLL FREE: (800) 274-4499
WWW.PROGRESSIVE.COM

3636 W TOWN PKY, STE 104
WEST DES MOINES, IA 50266
FAX: (515) 224-6816
TOLL FREE: (800) 274-4499
WWW.PROGRESSIVE.COM

KANSAS CLAIMS OFFICE
10975 EL MONTE STE 180
OVERLAND PARK, KS 66211
TEL: (785) 776-8174
FAX: (785) 498-0105
TOLL FREE: (800) 274-4499
WWW.PROGRESSIVE.COM

400 N WOODLAWN, STE 205
WICHITA, KS 67208
FAX: (316) 686-3142
TOLL FREE: (800) 274-4499
WWW.PROGRESSIVE.COM

KENTUCKY CLAIMS OFFICE
230 SECOND ST
HENDERSON, KY 42420
TEL: (502) 827-4668
FAX: (502) 827-4716
TOLL FREE: (800) 274-4499
WWW.PROGRESSIVE.COM

2525 HARRODSBURG RD, STE 340
LEXINGTON, KY 40504
TEL: (606) 223-7755
FAX: (606) 223-5375
TOLL FREE: (800) 274-4499
IN-STATE: (800) 876-7040
WWW.PROGRESSIVE.COM

PO BOX 22366
LOUISVILLE, KY 40252
FAX: (502) 425-0952
TOLL FREE: (800) 274-4499
IN-STATE: (800) 876-8018
WWW.PROGRESSIVE.COM

4324 OLD SCIOTO TRL
PORTSMOUTH, OH 45662
TEL: (740) 355-0043
FAX: (740) 353-0143
TOLL FREE: (800) 274-4499
WWW.PROGRESSIVE.COM

LOUISIANA CLAIMS OFFICE
3636 S I-10 SERVICE RD W, STE 103
METAIRIE, LA 7001
FAX: (504) 837-8119
TOLL FREE: (800) 274-4499
WWW.PROGRESSIVE.COM

MAINE CLAIMS OFFICE
16 PENN PLAZA STILLWATER PROFESSIONAL PARK
BANGOR, ME 04401-3620
TEL: (207) 945-4003
FAX: (207) 945-5268
TOLL FREE: (800) 274-4499
WWW.PROGRESSIVE.COM

500 SOUTHBOROUGH DR
SOUTH PORTLAND, ME 04106
FAX: (207) 773-6187
TOLL FREE: (800) 274-4499
WWW.PROGRESSIVE.COM

MARYLAND CLAIMS OFFICE
21 GOVERNORS CT, STE 120
BALTIMORE, MD 21244
FAX: (410) 944-6837
TOLL FREE: (800) 274-4499
WWW.PROGRESSIVE.COM

18310 MONTGOMERY VLG AVE, STE 720
GAITHERSBURG, MD 20879
FAX: (301) 208-1436
TOLL FREE: (800) 274-4499
WWW.PROGRESSIVE.COM

8201 CORPORATE DR, STE 10
LANDOVER, MD 20705
FAX: (301) 577-9452
TOLL FREE: (800) 274-4499
WWW.PROGRESSIVE.COM

MICHIGAN CLAIMS OFFICE
1000 LONG BLVD, STE 7
LANSING, MI 48911
TOLL FREE: (800) 274-4499
WWW.PROGRESSIVE.COM

MINNESOTA CLAIMS OFFICE
8 PINE TREE DR, STE 200
ARDEN HILLS, MN 55112
TEL: (651) 766-2620
FAX: (651) 482-9414
TOLL FREE: (800) 274-4499
WWW.PROGRESSIVE.COM

606 25TH AVE S, STE 110
SAINT CLOUD, MN 55301
FAX: (320) 252-4289
TOLL FREE: (800) 274-4499
WWW.PROGRESSIVE.COM

MISSISSIPPI CLAIMS OFFICE
900 E COUNTY LINE RD, STE 150
RIDGELAND, MS 39157
FAX: (601) 956-3744
TOLL FREE: (800) 274-4499
IN-STATE: (800) 888-9421
WWW.PROGRESSIVE.COM

MISSOURI CLAIMS OFFICE
11457 OLDE CABIN LN, STE 235
SAINT LOUIS, MO 63141
TEL: (314) 812-5100
FAX: (314) 432-5265
TOLL FREE: (800) 274-4499
WWW.PROGRESSIVE.COM

6220 BLUE RDG CUT-OFF, STE 200
RAYTOWN, MO 64133
FAX: (816) 358-8290
TOLL FREE: (800) 274-4499
WWW.PROGRESSIVE.COM

NATIONAL CLAIMS OFFICE
4535 NORMAL BLVD, STE 295
LINCOLN, NE 68506
FAX: (402) 434-5324
TOLL FREE: (800) 274-4499
WWW.PROGRESSIVE.COM

PROGRESSIVE INSURANCE
6300 WILSON MILLS RD
MAYFIELD VILLAGE, OH 44143
TEL: (440) 461-5000
TOLL FREE: (800) 274-4499
WWW.PROGRESSIVE.COM

NEBRASKA CLAIMS OFFICE
PO BOX 213
GRAND ISLAND, NE 68801-0213
TOLL FREE: (800) 274-4499
WWW.PROGRESSIVE.COM

401 N 117TH ST, STE 110
OMAHA, NE 68154
TOLL FREE: (800) 274-4499
IN-STATE: (800) 274-4499
WWW.PROGRESSIVE.COM

NEVADA CLAIMS OFFICE
5250 S PECOS RD, STE 101
LAS VEGAS, NV 89120
TEL: (702) 547-5414
FAX: (702) 434-6313
TOLL FREE: (800) 274-4499
E-MAIL: PROGRESSIVE.COM
WWW.PROGRESSIVE.COM

NEW HAMPSHIRE CLAIMS OFFICE
3 EXECUTIVE PARK DR- UNIT 19
BEDFORD, NH 03110-6922
TEL: (603) 656-6300
FAX: (603) 624-4242
TOLL FREE: (800) 274-4499
WWW.PROGRESSIVE.COM

NEW JERSEY CLAIMS OFFICE
NATIONAL CONTINENTAL PROGRESSIVE CASUALTY INSURANCE CO
100 CANAL PT BLVD, STE 210
PO BOX 7637
PRINCETON, NJ 08540
FAX: (609) 452-8812
TOLL FREE: (800) 274-4499
WWW.PROGRESSIVE.COM

321 MAIN ST
WOODBRIDGE, NJ 07095
TEL: (732) 634-7788
FAX: (732) 634-4990
TOLL FREE: (800) 274-4499
WWW.PROGRESSIVE.COM

NATIONAL CONTINENTAL PROGRESSIVE CASUALTY INSURANCE CO
100 CANAL PT BLVD, STE 210
PO BOX 7637
PRINCETON, NJ 08543
FAX: (609) 452-8812
TOLL FREE: (800) 444-0013
WWW.PROGRESSIVE.COM

NEW MEXICO CLAIMS OFFICE
6739 ACADEMY NE, STE 380
PO BOX 37337
ALBUQUERQUE, NM 87176-7337
TEL: (505) 797-6930
FAX: (505) 821-1548
TOLL FREE: (800) 274-4499
IN-STATE: (800) 274-4499
WWW.PROGRESSIVE.COM

NEW YORK CLAIMS OFFICE
319 GREAT OAKS BLVD- OFFICE PARK
PO BOX 15102
ALBANY, NY 12212-5102
FAX: (518) 452-0204
TOLL FREE: (800) 274-4499
IN-STATE: (800) 627-4581
WWW.PROGRESSIVE.COM

3125 EMMONS AVENUE
BROOKLYN, NY 11235
TEL: (718) 368-7000
FAX: (718) 368-3874
TOLL FREE: (800) 274-4499
WWW.PROGRESSIVE.COM

TWO SUMMIT CT, STE 303
FISHKILL, NY 12524
FAX: (914) 896-7622
TOLL FREE: (800) 274-4499
WWW.PROGRESSIVE.COM

591 STEWART AVE, STE 400
GARDEN CITY, NY 11530
FAX: (516) 745-6234
TOLL FREE: (800) 274-4499
WWW.PROGRESSIVE.COM

941 RIVER RD
SCHENECTADY, NY 12306
TEL: (518) 899-3074
FAX: (518) 899-3352
TOLL FREE: (800) 274-4499
WWW.PROGRESSIVE.COM

251 SALINA MEADOWS PKY, STE 120
NORTH SYRACUSE, NY 13212
FAX: (315) 451-6383
TOLL FREE: (800) 274-4499
WWW.PROGRESSIVE.COM

207 E 94TH ST
NEW YORK, NY 10128
FAX: (212) 410-1589
TOLL FREE: (800) 274-4499
WWW.PROGRESSIVE.COM

560 WHITE PLAINS RD- 5TH FL
TARRYTOWN, NY 10591
FAX: (914) 332-4366
TOLL FREE: (800) 274-4499
WWW.PROGRESSIVE.COM

130 LOMOND CT
UTICA, NY 13502
FAX: (315) 733-2515
TOLL FREE: (800) 274-4499
WWW.PROGRESSIVE.COM

4100 OLD VESTAL RD, STE 205
VESTAL, NY 13850
TEL: (607) 729-6544
FAX: (607) 729-6546
TOLL FREE: (800) 274-4499
WWW.PROGRESSIVE.COM

NATIONAL CONTINENTAL PROGRESSIVE CASUALTY INSURANCE CO
100 CANAL PT BLVD, STE 210
PO BOX 7637
PRINCETON, NJ 08543
FAX: (609) 452-8812
TOLL FREE: (800) 444-0013
WWW.PROGRESSIVE.COM

NORTH CAROLINA CLAIMS OFFICE
7400 CARMEL EXECUTIVE PARK, STE 320
CHARLOTTE, NC 28226
TEL: (704) 541-4175
FAX: (704) 541-4199
TOLL FREE: (800) 274-4499
WWW.PROGRESSIVE.COM

4102 MARY AVE
ZEBULON, NC 27597
FAX: (919) 269-0440
TOLL FREE: (800) 274-4499
WWW.PROGRESSIVE.COM

OHIO CLAIMS OFFICE
3660 STUTZ DR STE 3
CANFIELD, OH 44406
TEL: (330) 533-7180
FAX: (330) 533-8969
TOLL FREE: (800) 274-4499
WWW.PROGRESSIVE.COM

4100 EXECUTIVE PARK DR, STE 300
CINCINNATI, OH 45241
FAX: (513) 733-3961
TOLL FREE: (800) 274-4499
WWW.PROGRESSIVE.COM

5595 TRANSPORTATION BLVD, STE 201
GARFIELD HEIGHTS, OH 44125
TEL: (216) 662-6210
FAX: (216) 662-0470
TOLL FREE: (800) 274-4499
WWW.PROGRESSIVE.COM

4480 REFUGEE RD, STE 303
PO BOX 32492
COLUMBUS, OH 43232
FAX: (614) 866-4030
TOLL FREE: (800) 274-4499
WWW.PROGRESSIVE.COM

190 MONTROSE WEST AVE, STE 150
COPLEY, OH 44321
TEL: (330) 665-7100
FAX: (330) 668-3804
TOLL FREE: (800) 274-4499
WWW.PROGRESSIVE.COM

SANDLAKE BLDG
6450 POE AVE, STE 409
DAYTON, OH 45414
TOLL FREE: (800) 274-4499
WWW.PROGRESSIVE.COM

2833 CRANSTON DR
DUBLIN, OH 43017
TEL: (614) 336-3100
FAX: (614) 766-4097
TOLL FREE: (800) 274-4499
WWW.PROGRESSIVE.COM

2166 ELIDA RD
PO BOX 727
LIMA, OH 45802
TEL: (419) 224-0177
FAX: (419) 229-4518
TOLL FREE: (800) 274-4499
WWW.PROGRESSIVE.COM

ONE MARION AVE, STE 303
MANSFIELD, OH 44903
FAX: (419) 526-0639
TOLL FREE: (800) 274-4499
WWW.PROGRESSIVE.COM

1789 INDIANWOOD CIR, STE 150
MAUMEE, OH 43537
TEL: (419) 893-1105
FAX: (419) 893-1665
TOLL FREE: (800) 274-4499
WWW.PROGRESSIVE.COM

4324 OLD SCIOTO TRL
PORTSMOUTH, OH 45662
TEL: (740) 355-0043
FAX: (740) 353-0143
TOLL FREE: (800) 274-4499
WWW.PROGRESSIVE.COM

2550 SOM CTR RD, STE 220
WILLOUGHBY HILLS, OH 44094
TOLL FREE: (800) 274-4499
WWW.PROGRESSIVE.COM

1300 BRANDYWINE
ZANESVILLE, OH 43701
FAX: (740) 452-9736
TOLL FREE: (800) 274-4499
WWW.PROGRESSIVE.COM

OKLAHOMA CLAIMS OFFICE
10830 E 45TH ST, STE 312
TULSA, OK 74146-3810
TOLL FREE: (800) 274-4499
IN-STATE: (800) 288-6776
WWW.PROGRESSIVE.COM

ONTARIO CLAIMS OFFICE
1550 ENTERPRISE RD, STE 101
MISSISSAUGA, ON L4W-4P4
FAX: (905) 670-0499
TOLL FREE: (800) 274-4499
WWW.PROGRESSIVE.COM

200 YORKLAND BLVD- 5TH FL
WILLOWDALE, ON M2J-5C1
TEL: (416) 499-9960
FAX: (416) 756-8021
WWW.PROGRESSIVE.COM

OREGON CLAIMS OFFICE
15605 SW 72ND AVE
PORTLAND, OR 97224
FAX: (503) 603-0329
TOLL FREE: (800) 274-4499
WWW.PROGRESSIVE.COM

PENNSYLVANIA CLAIMS OFFICE
5165 CAMPUS DR
WHITEMARSH TOWNSHIP, PA 19462
TEL: (215) 604-5000
FAX: (215) 639-5925
TOLL FREE: (800) 274-4499
WWW.PROGRESSIVE.COM

11279 PERRY HWY
WEXFORD, PA 15090
TEL: (724) 742-5000
FAX: (724) 776-1204
TOLL FREE: (800) 274-4499
WWW.PROGRESSIVE.COM

414 E DRINKER ST, STE 101
DUNMORE, PA 18512
TEL: (570) 963-2155
FAX: (570) 941-2777
TOLL FREE: (800) 274-4499
WWW.PROGRESSIVE.COM

3939 WESTRIDGE RD- 2ND FL
ERIE, PA 16506
TEL: (814) 836-5500
FAX: (814) 833-8406
TOLL FREE: (800) 274-4499
WWW.PROGRESSIVE.COM

417 LINCOLN ST
JOHNSTOWN, PA 15901
TEL: (814) 539-7538
FAX: (814) 535-8293
TOLL FREE: (800) 274-4499
WWW.PROGRESSIVE.COM

930 REDROSE CT, STE 301
LANCASTER, PA 17601-1981
TEL: (717) 481-5200
FAX: (717) 399-0221
TOLL FREE: (800) 274-4499
WWW.PROGRESSIVE.COM

ONE MONROEVILLE CTR
3824 NORTHERN PIKE STE 510
MONROEVILLE, PA 15146
TEL: (412) 380-5230
FAX: (412) 374-1502
TOLL FREE: (800) 274-4499
WWW.PROGRESSIVE.COM

2214 N ATHERTON ST- 2ND FL
STATE COLLEGE, PA 16803
FAX: (814) 231-1228
TOLL FREE: (800) 274-4499
WWW.PROGRESSIVE.COM

RHODE ISLAND CLAIMS OFFICE
SUMMIT EAST
300 CENTERVILLE RD, STE 220
WARWICK, RI 02886
TEL: (401) 732-5950
FAX: (401) 732-5954
TOLL FREE: (800) 274-4499
WWW.PROGRESSIVE.COM

SUMMIT EAST
300 CENTERVILLE RD, STE 220
WARWICK, RI 02886
TEL: (401) 732-5950
FAX: (401) 732-5954
TOLL FREE: (800) 274-4499
WWW.PROGRESSIVE.COM

TENNESSEE CLAIMS OFFICE
208 SUNSET DR, STE 103
JOHNSON CITY, TN 37604
TEL: (423) 283-5850
FAX: (423) 283-5864
TOLL FREE: (800) 274-4499
WWW.PROGRESSIVE.COM

412 EXECUTIVE TWR DR, STE 411
KNOXVILLE, TN 37923
FAX: (423) 539-3004
TOLL FREE: (800) 274-4499
WWW.PROGRESSIVE.COM

6555 QUINCE RD, STE 106
MEMPHIS, TN 38119
FAX: (901) 755-8655
TOLL FREE: (800) 274-4499
WWW.PROGRESSIVE.COM

555 MARRIOTT DR, STE 310
NASHVILLE, TN 37214
FAX: (615) 885-7354
TOLL FREE: (800) 274-4499
WWW.PROGRESSIVE.COM

208 SUNSET DR, STE 103
JOHNSON CITY, TN 37604
TEL: (423) 283-5850
FAX: (423) 283-5864
TOLL FREE: (800) 274-4499
WWW.PROGRESSIVE.COM

TEXAS CLAIMS OFFICE
3960 EASTEX FWY
BEAUMONT, TX 77703
FAX: (800) 876-8709
TOLL FREE: (800) 274-4499
WWW.PROGRESSIVE.COM

5000 S HULEN, STE 120
FT WORTH, TX 76132
FAX: (817) 346-7408
TOLL FREE: (800) 274-4499
WWW.PROGRESSIVE.COM

110 CYPRESS STA DR, STE 270
HOUSTON, TX 77090
FAX: (281) 586-9360
TOLL FREE: (800) 274-4499
WWW.PROGRESSIVE.COM

9800 NW FWY, STE 107
HOUSTON, TX 77092
TEL: (713) 975-7150
FAX: (713) 957-8465
TOLL FREE: (800) 274-4499
WWW.PROGRESSIVE.COM

1121 JUDSON RD, STE 167
LONGVIEW, TX 75601
TEL: (903) 753-3821
FAX: (903) 753-1263
TOLL FREE: (800) 274-4499
WWW.PROGRESSIVE.COM

4318 WOODCOCK, STE 217
SAN ANTONIO, TX 78228
FAX: (210) 732-6611
TOLL FREE: (800) 274-4499
WWW.PROGRESSIVE.COM

1121 JUDSON RD, STE 167
LONGVIEW, TX 75601
TEL: (903) 753-3821
FAX: (903) 753-1263
TOLL FREE: (800) 274-4499
WWW.PROGRESSIVE.COM

UTAH CLAIMS OFFICE
488 E WINCHESTER, STE 350
SALT LAKE CITY, UT 84107
TEL: (801) 281-5420
FAX: (801) 266-2166
TOLL FREE: (800) 274-4499
IN-STATE: (800) 950-1456
WWW.PROGRESSIVE.COM

VERMONT CLAIMS OFFICE
280 WILLISTON RD
PO BOX 923
WILLISTON, VT 05495
TEL: (802) 879-7143
FAX: (802) 879-7129
TOLL FREE: (800) 274-4499
WWW.PROGRESSIVE.COM

VIRGINIA CLAIMS OFFICE
10300 EATON PL, STE 260
FAIRFAX, VA 22030
TOLL FREE: (800) 274-4499
WWW.PROGRESSIVE.COM

ATTN: CLAIMS
4461 COX RD
GLEN ALLEN, VA 23060
FAX: (804) 527-6445
TOLL FREE: (800) 274-4499
WWW.PROGRESSIVE.COM

825 DILLIGENCE DR, STE 126
NEWPORT NEWS, VA 23606
TEL: (757) 873-0657
FAX: (757) 873-0295
TOLL FREE: (800) 274-4499
WWW.PROGRESSIVE.COM

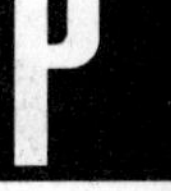

5115 BERNARD DR, STE 302
ROANOKE, VA 24018
FAX: (540) 989-7830
TOLL FREE: (800) 274-4499
WWW.PROGRESSIVE.COM

621 LYNNHAVEN PKY, STE 170
VIRGINIA BEACH, VA 23452
TEL: (757) 306-7660
FAX: (757) 486-4134
TOLL FREE: (800) 274-4499
WWW.PROGRESSIVE.COM

WASHINGTON CLAIMS OFFICE
N 300 MULLEN RD, STE 201
SPOKANE, WA 99206
TEL: (509) 928-7377
FAX: (509) 926-7388
TOLL FREE: (800) 274-4499
WWW.PROGRESSIVE.COM

WEST VIRGINIA CLAIMS OFFICE
4324 OLD SCIOTO TRL
PORTSMOUTH, OH 45662
TEL: (740) 355-0043
FAX: (740) 353-0143
TOLL FREE: (800) 274-4499
WWW.PROGRESSIVE.COM

WISCONSIN CLAIMS OFFICE
175 N CORPORATE DR, STE 160
PO BOX 0530
BROOKFIELD, WI 53045-5802
FAX: (414) 879-0371
TOLL FREE: (800) 274-4499
WWW.PROGRESSIVE.COM

4351 W COLLEGE AVE, STE 220
APPLETON, WI 54914
TEL: (920) 731-7765
FAX: (920) 731-8005
TOLL FREE: (800) 274-4499
WWW.PROGRESSIVE.COM

PROGRESSIVE DIVERSIFIED INSURANCE CO

NATIONAL CLAIMS OFFICE
747 ALPHA DR
PO BOX 94861
HIGHLAND HEIGHTS, OH 44143
TEL: (440) 473-3600
FAX: (440) 603-6584

PROGRESSIVE INSURANCE CO OF CANADA

ALBERTA CLAIMS OFFICE
200 YORKLAND BLVD- 5TH FL
WILLOWDALE, ON M2J-5C1
TEL: (416) 499-9960
FAX: (416) 756-8021
WWW.PROGRESSIVEINSURANCE.CA

BRITISH COLUMBIA CLAIMS OFFICE
200 YORKLAND BLVD- 5TH FL
WILLOWDALE, ON M2J-5C1
TEL: (416) 499-9960
FAX: (416) 756-8021
WWW.PROGRESSIVEINSURANCE.CA

MANITOBA CLAIMS OFFICE
200 YORKLAND BLVD- 5TH FL
WILLOWDALE, ON M2J-5C1
TEL: (416) 499-9960
FAX: (416) 756-8021
WWW.PROGRESSIVEINSURANCE.CA

NEW BRUNSWICK CLAIMS OFFICE
200 YORKLAND BLVD- 5TH FL
WILLOWDALE, ON M2J-5C1
TEL: (416) 499-9960
FAX: (416) 756-8021
WWW.PROGRESSIVEINSURANCE.CA

NEWFOUNDLAND CLAIMS OFFICE
200 YORKLAND BLVD- 5TH FL
WILLOWDALE, ON M2J-5C1
TEL: (416) 499-9960
FAX: (416) 756-8021
WWW.PROGRESSIVEINSURANCE.CA

NOVA SCOTIA CLAIMS OFFICE
200 YORKLAND BLVD- 5TH FL
WILLOWDALE, ON M2J-5C1
TEL: (416) 499-9960
FAX: (416) 756-8021
WWW.PROGRESSIVEINSURANCE.CA

PRINCE EDWARD ISLAND CLAIMS OFFICE
200 YORKLAND BLVD- 5TH FL
WILLOWDALE, ON M2J-5C1
TEL: (416) 499-9960
FAX: (416) 756-8021
WWW.PROGRESSIVEINSURANCE.CA

QUEBEC CLAIMS OFFICE
200 YORKLAND BLVD- 5TH FL
WILLOWDALE, ON M2J-5C1
TEL: (416) 499-9960
FAX: (416) 756-8021
WWW.PROGRESSIVEINSURANCE.CA

SASKATCHEWAN CLAIMS OFFICE
200 YORKLAND BLVD- 5TH FL
WILLOWDALE, ON M2J-5C1
TEL: (416) 499-9960
FAX: (416) 756-8021
WWW.PROGRESSIVEINSURANCE.CA

PROTECTED HOME MUTUAL LIFE INSURANCE CO

PENNSYLVANIA CLAIMS OFFICE
30 E STATE ST
SHARON, PA 16146
TEL: (724) 981-1520
FAX: (724) 981-2682
TOLL FREE: (800) 223-8821
IN-STATE: (800) 222-8894

PROTECTIVE INSURANCE CO

NATIONAL CLAIMS OFFICE
BALDWIN & LYONS, INC
1099 N MERIDIAN ST, STE 700
INDIANAPOLIS, IN 46204
TEL: (317) 636-9800
FAX: (317) 972-4735
TOLL FREE: (800) 231-6024
IN-STATE: (800) 845-2931

PROTECTIVE LIFE GUIDESTAR HEALTH SYSTEMS

ARKANSAS CLAIMS OFFICE
5900 MOSTELLER DR
PO BOX 57018
OKLAHOMA CITY, OK 73157-7018
TEL: (405) 843-4963
FAX: (405) 843-0316
TOLL FREE: (800) 873-5772
WWW.GUIDESTARHEALTH.COM

OKLAHOMA CLAIMS OFFICE
5900 MOSTELLER DR
PO BOX 57018
OKLAHOMA CITY, OK 73157-7018
TEL: (405) 843-4963
FAX: (405) 843-0316
TOLL FREE: (800) 873-5772
WWW.GUIDESTARHEALTH.COM

TEXAS CLAIMS OFFICE
5900 MOSTELLER DR
PO BOX 57018
OKLAHOMA CITY, OK 73157-7018
TEL: (405) 843-4963
FAX: (405) 843-0316
TOLL FREE: (800) 873-5772
WWW.GUIDESTARHEALTH.COM

PROTECTIVE NATIONAL INSURANCE CO

NEBRASKA CLAIMS OFFICE
CENTRAL NATIONAL
11128 JOHN GALT BLVD STE 200
OMAHA, NE 68137-2321
TEL: (402) 970-8600
FAX: (402) 970-8642

PROVIDENCE HEALTH PLANS

OREGON CLAIMS OFFICE
FORMERLY SELECT CARE HEALTH PLAN
PO BOX 3125
PORTLAND, OR 97208
TEL: (503) 574-7500
TOLL FREE: (800) 421-0544
WWW.PROVHEALTH.COM

WASHINGTON CLAIMS OFFICE
1501 FOURTH AVE, STE 600
SEATTLE, WA 98101
TEL: (206) 215-9000
TOLL FREE: (800) 443-0996
WWW.PROVHEALTH.COM

FORMERLY SELECT CARE HEALTH PLAN
PO BOX 3125
PORTLAND, OR 97208
TEL: (503) 574-7500
TOLL FREE: (800) 421-0544
WWW.PROVHEALTH.COM

PROVIDENCE MUTUAL FIRE INSURANCE CO

RHODE ISLAND CLAIMS OFFICE
340 E AVE
PO BOX 6066
PROVIDENCE, RI 02940
TEL: (401) 827-1800
FAX: (401) 822-1921
IN-STATE: (877) 763-1800

PROVIDENCE WASHINGTON INSURANCE

PW GROUP
88 BOYD AVE
PROVIDENCE, RI 02914-1231
TEL: (401) 453-7000
FAX: (401) 453-7354
TOLL FREE: (800) 556-3825
WWW.PROVWASH.COM

PROVIDENT AMERICAN INSURANCE CO

ARIZONA CLAIMS OFFICE
10501 N CENTRAL EXPY
PO BOX 679005
DALLAS, TX 75367-9005
TEL: (214) 696-9091
FAX: (214) 696-1681
TOLL FREE: (800) 933-9456
E-MAIL: PAIC@FLASH.NET

COLORADO CLAIMS OFFICE
10501 N CENTRAL EXPY
PO BOX 679005
DALLAS, TX 75367-9005
TEL: (214) 696-9091
FAX: (214) 696-1681
TOLL FREE: (800) 933-9456
E-MAIL: PAIC@FLASH.NET

LOUISIANA CLAIMS OFFICE
10501 N CENTRAL EXPY
PO BOX 679005
DALLAS, TX 75367-9005
TEL: (214) 696-9091
FAX: (214) 696-1681
TOLL FREE: (800) 933-9456
E-MAIL: PAIC@FLASH.NET

MONTANA CLAIMS OFFICE
10501 N CENTRAL EXPY
PO BOX 679005
DALLAS, TX 75367-9005
TEL: (214) 696-9091
FAX: (214) 696-1681
TOLL FREE: (800) 933-9456
E-MAIL: PAIC@FLASH.NET

NEVADA CLAIMS OFFICE
10501 N CENTRAL EXPY
PO BOX 679005
DALLAS, TX 75367-9005
TEL: (214) 696-9091
FAX: (214) 696-1681
TOLL FREE: (800) 933-9456
E-MAIL: PAIC@FLASH.NET

NEW MEXICO CLAIMS OFFICE
10501 N CENTRAL EXPY
PO BOX 679005
DALLAS, TX 75367-9005
TEL: (214) 696-9091
FAX: (214) 696-1681
TOLL FREE: (800) 933-9456
E-MAIL: PAIC@FLASH.NET

NORTH DAKOTA CLAIMS OFFICE
10501 N CENTRAL EXPY
PO BOX 679005
DALLAS, TX 75367-9005
TEL: (214) 696-9091
FAX: (214) 696-1681
TOLL FREE: (800) 933-9456
E-MAIL: PAIC@FLASH.NET

OKLAHOMA CLAIMS OFFICE
10501 N CENTRAL EXPY
PO BOX 679005
DALLAS, TX 75367-9005
TEL: (214) 696-9091
FAX: (214) 696-1681
TOLL FREE: (800) 933-9456
E-MAIL: PAIC@FLASH.NET

TEXAS CLAIMS OFFICE
10501 N CENTRAL EXPY
PO BOX 679005
DALLAS, TX 75367-9005
TEL: (214) 696-9091
FAX: (214) 696-1681
TOLL FREE: (800) 933-9456
E-MAIL: PAIC@FLASH.NET

UTAH CLAIMS OFFICE
10501 N CENTRAL EXPY
PO BOX 679005
DALLAS, TX 75367-9005
TEL: (214) 696-9091
FAX: (214) 696-1681
TOLL FREE: (800) 933-9456
E-MAIL: PAIC@FLASH.NET

PROVIDENT COMPANIES

NATIONAL CLAIMS OFFICE
ONE FOUNTAIN SQUARE
CHATTANOOGA, TN 37402-1330
TEL: (508) 799-4441
FAX: (508) 751-7079

PROVIDENT MUTUAL LIFE INSURANCE CO

300 CONTINENTAL DR
PO BOX 15750
NEWARK, DE 19713
TEL: (302) 452-4000
FAX: (302) 452-4255
TOLL FREE: (800) 523-4681
WWW.PROVIDENTMUTUAL.COM

PROVIDENTIAL LIFE INSURANCE CO

11815 N PENNSYLVANIA ST
PO BOX 2009
CARMEL, IN 46032
TEL: (317) 817-4075
FAX: (501) 666-3740
TOLL FREE: (800) 264-3300

PRUDENTIAL HEALTH CARE

NEW JERSEY CLAIMS OFFICE
200 WOOD AVE S
ISELIN, NJ 08830
TEL: (732) 632-7000
TOLL FREE: (800) 422-7399
WWW.PRUDENTIAL.COM

PRUDENTIAL HEALTH CARE OF TEXAS

TEXAS CLAIMS OFFICE
PRUCARE OF SAN ANTONIO
PO BOX 4710
HOUSTON, TX 77210
TEL: (713) 741-2273
FAX: (713) 663-0731
TOLL FREE: (800) 657-5959
WWW.PRUDENTIAL.COM

PRUDENTIAL HEALTH CARE PLAN, INC

FLORIDA CLAIMS OFFICE
PRUCARE OF TAMPA
841 PRUDENTIAL DR
PO BOX 2739
JACKSONVILLE, FL 32232
TEL: (904) 351-1000
FAX: (904) 351-1625
TOLL FREE: (800) 493-6845
WWW.PRUDENTIAL.COM

PRUDENTIAL HEALTHCARE- CENTRAL FLORIDA
2301 LUCIEN WAY, STE 200
MAITLAND, FL 32751
TEL: (407) 875-6600
FAX: (407) 660-0552
TOLL FREE: (800) 493-6845
WWW.PRUDENTIAL.COM

MISSOURI CLAIMS OFFICE
PRUCARE OF SAINT LOUIS
12312 OLIVE BLVD, STE 500- W VIEW PL
PO BOX 411340
SAINT LOUIS, MO 63141
TEL: (314) 542-4500
TOLL FREE: (800) 298-7625
WWW.PRUDENTIAL.COM

NEW JERSEY CLAIMS OFFICE
TRI-STATE PRUCARE
400 RELLA BLVD
PO BOX 4042
SUFFERN, NY 10901
TEL: (914) 368-4497
TOLL FREE: (800) 570-0300
WWW.PRUDENTIAL.COM

NEW YORK CLAIMS OFFICE
TRI-STATE PRUCARE
400 RELLA BLVD
PO BOX 4042
SUFFERN, NY 10901
TEL: (914) 368-4497
TOLL FREE: (800) 570-0300
WWW.PRUDENTIAL.COM

NORTH CAROLINA CLAIMS OFFICE
PRUCARE OF CHARLOTTE
841 PRUDENTIAL DR
PO BOX 45096
JACKSONVILLE, FL 32232
TEL: (904) 351-1000
FAX: (904) 351-3864
TOLL FREE: (800) 457-6903
IN-STATE: (800) 643-3610
WWW.PRUDENTIAL.COM

OKLAHOMA CLAIMS OFFICE
PRUCARE OF TULSA
7912 E 31 CT, STE 200
TULSA, OK 74145-1338
TEL: (918) 624-4600
FAX: (918) 624-5050
TOLL FREE: (800) 345-8310
WWW.PRUDENTIAL.COM

TENNESSEE CLAIMS OFFICE
PRUDENTIAL HEALTH CARE SYSTEMS
3150 LENOX PARK BLVD, STE 110
MEMPHIS, TN 38115
TEL: (901) 541-9400
FAX: (901) 368-0643
TOLL FREE: (800) 453-2391
WWW.PRUDENTIAL.COM

TEXAS CLAIMS OFFICE
PRUCARE OF AUSTIN
7700 CHEVY CHASE DR- BLDG 1, STE 500
PO BOX 26699
AUSTIN, TX 78755-0699
TEL: (512) 323-0440
FAX: (713) 663-0731
TOLL FREE: (800) 621-2645
WWW.PRUDENTIAL.COM

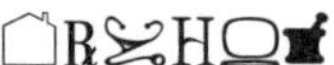

ONE PRUDENTIAL CIR
PO BOX 27718
HOUSTON, TX 77227
TEL: (713) 350-2150
FAX: (713) 663-0731
TOLL FREE: (800) 876-7778
WWW.PRUDENTIAL.COM

PRUDENTIAL HEALTH CARE PLAN OF MID-ATLANTIC

MARYLAND CLAIMS OFFICE
SETON COURT
2800 N CHARLES ST
BALTIMORE, MD 21218-4026
TEL: (410) 554-7000
FAX: (904) 351-3864
TOLL FREE: (800) 888-5447
WWW.PRUDENTIAL.COM

PRUDENTIAL HEALTH CARE SYSTEM

FLORIDA CLAIMS OFFICE
PRUDENTIAL HEALTH CARE- TAMPA BAY
6200 COURTNEY CAMPBELL CSWY, STE 200
TAMPA, FL 33607
TEL: (813) 288-0080
FAX: (813) 288-6181
TOLL FREE: (800) 367-2713
IN-STATE: (800) 284-4302
WWW.PRUDENTIAL.COM

PRUDENTIAL HEALTHCARE GROUP

1200 RIVERPLACE BLVD, STE 701
JACKSONVILLE, FL 32207
TEL: (904) 346-5800
FAX: (904) 346-5888
TOLL FREE: (800) 622-6084
WWW.PRUDENTIAL.COM

H

PRUDENTIAL HEALTHCARE OF CALIFORNIA

CALIFORNIA CLAIMS OFFICE
PRUDENTIAL HEALTHCARE
21261 BURBANK AVE
WOODLAND HILLS, CA 91367
TEL: (818) 992-2000
FAX: (818) 594-4266
TOLL FREE: (800) 433-3150

PRUDENTIAL INSURANCE CO OF AMERICA

FLORIDA CLAIMS OFFICE
H-POLICIES
701 SAN MARCO BLVD
PO BOX 44059
JACKSONVILLE, FL 32231-4059
FAX: (904) 313-4222
TOLL FREE: (800) 828-0153
WWW.PRUDENTIAL.COM

ILLINOIS CLAIMS OFFICE
PO BOX 540
MATTESON, IL 60443-0540
FAX: (708) 503-7308
TOLL FREE: (800) 352-5846
WWW.PRUDENTIAL.COM

LOUISIANA CLAIMS OFFICE
SMALL GROUP CLAIMS
PO BOX 2229
JACKSONVILLE, FL 32231-0077
TEL: (904) 351-2702
FAX: (904) 351-2988
TOLL FREE: (800) 622-6084
WWW.PRUDENTIAL.COM

PRUDENTIAL PROPERTY & CASUALTY INSURANCE CO

NEW JERSEY CLAIMS OFFICE
23 MAIN ST
PO BOX 419
HOLMDEL, NJ 07733-2136
TEL: (732) 946-5000
FAX: (732) 946-6118

PUBLIC EMPLOYEES HEALTH PROGRAM

UTAH CLAIMS OFFICE
560 E 200 S
SALT LAKE CITY, UT 84102-2020
TEL: (801) 366-7500
FAX: (801) 366-7596
TOLL FREE: (800) 933-7347

PUBLIC SERVICE MUTUAL INSURANCE CO

ARIZONA CLAIMS OFFICE
SOUTHWESTERN BRANCH
2425 E CAMELBACK RD, STE 840
PHOENIX, AZ 85016
TEL: (602) 954-6612
FAX: (602) 954-7518
TOLL FREE: (800) 309-5829

CALIFORNIA CLAIMS OFFICE
SOUTHERN CALIFORNIA BRANCH
11766 WILLSHIRE BLVD, STE 448
LOS ANGELES, CA 90025
TEL: (310) 479-8070
FAX: (310) 479-8866
TOLL FREE: (888) 239-7523

PACIFIC BRANCH
1990 N CALIFORNIA BLVD, STE 640
WALNUT CREEK, CA 94596
TEL: (510) 280-8260
FAX: (510) 280-8259
TOLL FREE: (800) 940-5981

COLORADO CLAIMS OFFICE
ROCKY MOUNTAIN BRANCH
5600 S QUEBEC ST, STE 319B
GREENWOOD VILLAGE, CO 80111
TEL: (303) 796-8102
FAX: (303) 796-8221
TOLL FREE: (800) 807-8639

CONNECTICUT CLAIMS OFFICE
MID-ATLANTIC BRANCH
TREEVIEW CORPORATE CTR, 2 MERIDIAN BLVD
WYOMISSING, PA 19610
TEL: (610) 396-0230
FAX: (610) 396-0240
TOLL FREE: (800) 988-6879

DELAWARE CLAIMS OFFICE
MID-ATLANTIC BRANCH
TREEVIEW CORPORATE CTR, 2 MERIDIAN BLVD
WYOMISSING, PA 19610
TEL: (610) 396-0230
FAX: (610) 396-0240
TOLL FREE: (800) 988-6879

IDAHO CLAIMS OFFICE
NORTHWESTERN BRANCH
700 NE MULTNOMAH, STE 470
PORTLAND, OR 97232
TEL: (503) 233-7045
FAX: (503) 233-7285
TOLL FREE: (800) 317-6775

MAINE CLAIMS OFFICE
MASSACHUSETTS BRANCH
220 FORBES RD
RAINTREE, MA 02184
TEL: (617) 848-9200
FAX: (617) 848-1085
TOLL FREE: (800) 972-5045

MASSACHUSETTS CLAIMS OFFICE
MASSACHUSETTS BRANCH
220 FORBES RD
BRAINTREE, MA 02184
TEL: (781) 848-9200
FAX: (781) 848-1085
TOLL FREE: (800) 972-5045

NEVADA CLAIMS OFFICE
PACIFIC BRANCH
1990 N CALIFORNIA BLVD, STE 640
WALNUT CREEK, CA 94596
TEL: (510) 280-8260
FAX: (510) 280-8259
TOLL FREE: (800) 940-5981

NEW MEXICO CLAIMS OFFICE
SOUTHWESTERN BRANCH
2425 E CAMELBACK RD, STE 840
PHOENIX, AZ 85016
TEL: (602) 954-6612
FAX: (602) 954-7518
TOLL FREE: (800) 309-5829

NEW YORK CLAIMS OFFICE
1 PARK AVENUE
NEW YORK, NY 10016
TEL: (212) 591-9500
FAX: (212) 947-4019
TOLL FREE: (800) 223-5213

OREGON CLAIMS OFFICE
NORTHWESTERN BRANCH
700 NE MULTNOMAH, STE 470
PORTLAND, OR 97232
TEL: (503) 233-7045
FAX: (503) 233-7285
TOLL FREE: (800) 317-6775

PENNSYLVANIA CLAIMS OFFICE
MID-ATLANTIC BRANCH
TREEVIEW CORPORATE CTR, 2 MERIDIAN BLVD
WYOMISSING, PA 19610
TEL: (610) 396-0230
FAX: (610) 396-0240
TOLL FREE: (800) 988-6879

UTAH CLAIMS OFFICE
ROCKY MOUNTAIN BRANCH
5600 S QUEBEC ST, STE 319B
GREENWOOD VILLAGE, CO 80111
TEL: (303) 796-8102
FAX: (303) 796-8221
TOLL FREE: (800) 807-8639

WASHINGTON CLAIMS OFFICE
NORTHWESTERN BRANCH
700 NE MULTNOMAH, STE 470
PORTLAND, OR 97232
TEL: (503) 233-7045
FAX: (503) 233-7285
TOLL FREE: (800) 317-6775

PYRAMID LIFE INSURANCE CO

NATIONAL CLAIMS OFFICE
6201 JOHNSON DR
PO BOX 772
MISSION, KS 66202
TEL: (913) 722-1110
FAX: (913) 722-3567
TOLL FREE: (800) 444-0321
WWW.PYRAMIDLIFE.COM

QUAKER OATS CO

ILLINOIS CLAIMS OFFICE
PO BOX 049001
CHICAGO, IL 60604-9001
TEL: (312) 222-7111
FAX: (312) 222-8392
WWW.QUAKEROATS.COM

QUAL MED OREGON HEALTH PLAN, INC

OREGON CLAIMS OFFICE
12901 SE 97TH AVE
PO BOX 286
CLACKAMAS, OR 97015-0286
TEL: (503) 802-7000
FAX: (503) 796-6366
TOLL FREE: (888) 802-7001
WWW.QUALMEDOREGON.COM

WASHINGTON CLAIMS OFFICE
12901 SE 97TH AVE
PO BOX 286
CLACKAMAS, OR 97015-0286
TEL: (503) 802-7000
FAX: (503) 796-6366
TOLL FREE: (888) 802-7001
WWW.QUALMEDOREGON.COM

QUAL MED WASHINGTON HEALTH PLAN, INC

IDAHO CLAIMS OFFICE
508 6TH AVE
PO BOX 2470
SPOKANE, WA 99204
TEL: (425) 869-3500
FAX: (425) 869-9234
TOLL FREE: (800) 869-7175
WWW.QUALMEDWA.COM

WASHINGTON CLAIMS OFFICE
2331 130TH AVE NE, #200
PO BOX 3387
BELLEVUE, WA 98009-3387
TEL: (425) 869-3500
FAX: (425) 869-9234
TOLL FREE: (800) 869-7175
WWW.QUALMEDWA.COM

508 6TH AVE
PO BOX 2470
SPOKANE, WA 99204
TEL: (425) 869-3500
FAX: (425) 869-9234
TOLL FREE: (800) 869-7175
WWW.QUALMEDWA.COM

QUAL-MED HEALTH PLAN

ARIZONA CLAIMS OFFICE
FOUNDATION HEALTH SYSTEMS
225 N MAIN ST
PO BOX 640
PUEBLO, CO 81002-0640
TEL: (719) 542-0500
FAX: (719) 585-8333
TOLL FREE: (800) 628-2287
WWW.QUALMED.COM

CALIFORNIA CLAIMS OFFICE
FOUNDATION HEALTH SYSTEMS
225 N MAIN ST
PO BOX 640
PUEBLO, CO 81002-0640
TEL: (719) 542-0500
FAX: (719) 585-8333
TOLL FREE: (800) 628-2287
WWW.QUALMED.COM

COLORADO CLAIMS OFFICE
FOUNDATION HEALTH SYSTEMS
225 N MAIN ST
PO BOX 640
PUEBLO, CO 81002-0640
TEL: (719) 542-0500
FAX: (719) 585-8333
TOLL FREE: (800) 628-2287
WWW.QUALMED.COM

CONNECTICUT CLAIMS OFFICE
FOUNDATION HEALTH SYSTEMS
225 N MAIN ST
PO BOX 640
PUEBLO, CO 81002-0640
TEL: (719) 542-0500
FAX: (719) 585-8333
TOLL FREE: (800) 628-2287
WWW.QUALMED.COM

NEW MEXICO CLAIMS OFFICE
FOUNDATION HEALTH SYSTEMS
225 N MAIN ST
PO BOX 640
PUEBLO, CO 81002-0640
TEL: (719) 542-0500
FAX: (719) 585-8333
TOLL FREE: (800) 628-2287
WWW.QUALMED.COM

OREGON CLAIMS OFFICE
OREGON HEALTH PLAN, INC
4800 SW MACADAM AVE, STE 400
PO BOX 69348
PORTLAND, OR 97201
TEL: (503) 222-5217
FAX: (503) 796-6366
TOLL FREE: (800) 388-8335
WWW.QUALMED.COM

FOUNDATION HEALTH SYSTEMS
225 N MAIN ST
PO BOX 640
PUEBLO, CO 81002-0640
TEL: (719) 542-0500
FAX: (719) 585-8333
TOLL FREE: (800) 628-2287
WWW.QUALMED.COM

WASHINGTON CLAIMS OFFICE
FOUNDATION HEALTH SYSTEMS
225 N MAIN ST
PO BOX 640
PUEBLO, CO 81002-0640
TEL: (719) 542-0500
FAX: (719) 585-8333
TOLL FREE: (800) 628-2287
WWW.QUALMED.COM

QUAL-MED PLANS FOR HEALTH

NEW JERSEY CLAIMS OFFICE
1835 MARKET ST- 9TH FL
PHILADELPHIA, PA 10913
TEL: (215) 209-6300
FAX: (215) 209-6922
IN-STATE: (800) 736-7931
WWW.QUALMED.COM

R

PENNSYLVANIA CLAIMS OFFICE
1835 MARKET ST- 9TH FL
PHILADELPHIA, PA 10913
TEL: (215) 209-6300
FAX: (215) 209-6622
IN-STATE: (800) 736-7931
WWW.QUALMED.COM

QUAL-MED WASHINGTON HEALTH PLAN

OREGON CLAIMS OFFICE
508 6TH AVE
PO BOX 2470
SPOKANE, WA 99204
TEL: (509) 459-6690
FAX: (509) 459-9298
TOLL FREE: (800) 423-9899

QUANTUM / EMPLOYEE ASSISTANCE

PENNSYLVANIA CLAIMS OFFICE
115 E WASHINGTON AVE
NEWTOWN, PA 18940
TEL: (215) 968-0844
FAX: (215) 579-9009

QUEEN'S ISLAND CARE/QUEEN'S HEALTH PLAN

HAWAII CLAIMS OFFICE
2 WATERFRONT PLAZA
500 ALA MOANA BLVD, STE 200
PO BOX 37549
HONOLULU, HI 96837
TEL: (808) 532-6900
FAX: (808) 522-8642
TOLL FREE: (800) 856-4668

R.E. MOULTON, INC

CONNECTICUT CLAIMS OFFICE
50 DOAKS LN
MARBLEHEAD, MA 01945
TEL: (781) 639-8501
FAX: (781) 631-2119

MASSACHUSETTS CLAIMS OFFICE
50 DOAKS LN
MARBLEHEAD, MA 01945
TEL: (781) 639-8501
FAX: (781) 631-2119

RANGER INSURANCE CO

TEXAS CLAIMS OFFICE
10777 WESTHEIMER
PO BOX 2807
HOUSTON, TX 77252-2807
TEL: (713) 954-8100
FAX: (713) 954-8803
TOLL FREE: (800) 392-1970
WWW.RANGERINSURANCE.COM

RAYTHEON CO

NATIONAL CLAIMS OFFICE
141 SPRING ST
LEXINGTON, MA 02173
TEL: (781) 862-6600
FAX: (781) 860-2172
TOLL FREE: (800) 843-4121

REASSURANCE CO OF HANNOVER

800 N MAGNOLIA AVE, STE 1000
ORLANDO, FL 32803
TEL: (407) 649-8411
FAX: (407) 649-8322
TOLL FREE: (800) 327-1910
WWW.RCH.NET

REDWOOD FIRE & CASUALTY INSURANCE CO

ARIZONA CLAIMS OFFICE
PO BOX 7008
PASADENA, CA 91109
TEL: (626) 351-1180
FAX: (626) 351-1622
TOLL FREE: (800) 339-9809

ARKANSAS CLAIMS OFFICE
PO BOX 7008
PASADENA, CA 91109
TEL: (626) 351-1180
FAX: (626) 351-1622
TOLL FREE: (800) 339-9809

CALIFORNIA CLAIMS OFFICE
PO BOX 7008
PASADENA, CA 91109
TEL: (626) 351-1180
FAX: (626) 351-1622
TOLL FREE: (800) 339-9809

CONNECTICUT CLAIMS OFFICE
PO BOX 7008
PASADENA, CA 91109
TEL: (626) 351-1180
FAX: (626) 351-1622
TOLL FREE: (800) 339-9809

GEORGIA CLAIMS OFFICE
PO BOX 7008
PASADENA, CA 91109
TEL: (626) 351-1180
FAX: (626) 351-1622
TOLL FREE: (800) 339-9809

IDAHO CLAIMS OFFICE
PO BOX 7008
PASADENA, CA 91109
TEL: (626) 351-1180
FAX: (626) 351-1622
TOLL FREE: (800) 339-9809

MISSISSIPPI CLAIMS OFFICE
PO BOX 7008
PASADENA, CA 91109
TEL: (626) 351-1180
FAX: (626) 351-1622
TOLL FREE: (800) 339-9809

NEW MEXICO CLAIMS OFFICE
PO BOX 7008
PASADENA, CA 91109
TEL: (626) 351-1180
FAX: (626) 351-1622
TOLL FREE: (800) 339-9809

NORTH CAROLINA CLAIMS OFFICE
PO BOX 7008
PASADENA, CA 91109
TEL: (626) 351-1180
FAX: (626) 351-1622
TOLL FREE: (800) 339-9809

SOUTH CAROLINA CLAIMS OFFICE
PO BOX 7008
PASADENA, CA 91109
TEL: (626) 351-1180
FAX: (626) 351-1622
TOLL FREE: (800) 339-9809

TENNESSEE CLAIMS OFFICE
PO BOX 7008
PASADENA, CA 91109
TEL: (626) 351-1180
FAX: (626) 351-1622
TOLL FREE: (800) 339-9809

VIRGINIA CLAIMS OFFICE
PO BOX 7008
PASADENA, CA 91109
TEL: (626) 351-1180
FAX: (626) 351-1622
TOLL FREE: (800) 339-9809

WISCONSIN CLAIMS OFFICE
PO BOX 7008
PASADENA, CA 91109
TEL: (626) 351-1180
FAX: (626) 351-1622
TOLL FREE: (800) 339-9809

REGAL LIFE OF AMERICA INSURANCE CO

TEXAS CLAIMS OFFICE
7001 GRAPEVINE HWY, STE 434
PO BOX 982005
NORTH RICHLAND HILLS, TX 76180
TEL: (817) 284-4888
FAX: (817) 284-4474
TOLL FREE: (800) 966-7491
IN-STATE: (800) 966-3712

REGENCE BLUE CROSS & BLUE SHIELD

IDAHO CLAIMS OFFICE
HMO OREGON, INC
201 HIGH ST SE
PO BOX 12625
SALEM, OR 97309
TEL: (503) 364-4868
FAX: (503) 588-4350
TOLL FREE: (800) 228-0978
WWW.BCBSOR.COM

OREGON CLAIMS OFFICE
REGENCE HMO OREGON
100 SW MARKET
PO BOX 100
PORTLAND, OR 97207
TEL: (503) 225-5227
TOLL FREE: (800) 452-7278
WWW.BCBSOR.COM

HMO OREGON, INC
201 HIGH ST SE
PO BOX 12625
SALEM, OR 97309
TEL: (503) 364-4868
FAX: (503) 588-4350
TOLL FREE: (800) 228-0978
WWW.BCBSOR.COM

WASHINGTON CLAIMS OFFICE
REGENCE HMO OREGON
100 SW MARKET
PO BOX 100
PORTLAND, OR 97207
TEL: (503) 225-5227
TOLL FREE: (800) 452-7278
WWW.BCBSOR.COM

HMO OREGON, INC
201 HIGH ST SE
PO BOX 12625
SALEM, OR 97309
TEL: (503) 364-4868
FAX: (503) 588-4350
TOLL FREE: (800) 228-0978
WWW.BCBSOR.COM

REGENCE BLUE CROSS & BLUE SHIELD OF UTAH

UTAH CLAIMS OFFICE
2870 E COTTONWOOD PKY
PO BOX 30270
SALT LAKE CITY, UT 84130-0270
TEL: (801) 333-2320
FAX: (801) 333-6523
TOLL FREE: (800) 662-0876
IN-STATE: (800) 624-6519

REGENCE BLUE SHIELD

WASHINGTON CLAIMS OFFICE
1800 NINTH AVE
PO BOX 21267
SEATTLE, WA 98111-3267
TEL: (206) 464-3600
TOLL FREE: (800) 544-4246
IN-STATE: (800) 458-3523
WWW.REGENCE.COM

1800 NINTH AVENUE
PO BOX 21267
SEATTLE, WA 98101-1322
TEL: (206) 464-6565
FAX: (206) 389-5669
TOLL FREE: (800) 732-9326
IN-STATE: (800) 322-1737
WWW.WA.REGENCE.COM

REGENCE BLUE SHIELD OF IDAHO

IDAHO CLAIMS OFFICE
1602 21ST AVE
PO BOX 1106
LEWISTON, ID 83501-1106
TEL: (208) 746-2671
FAX: (208) 798-2090
TOLL FREE: (800) 632-2022
WWW.ID.REGENCE.COM

REGENCE BLUESHIELD

WASHINGTON CLAIMS OFFICE
7600 EVERGREEN WAY
EVERETT, WA 98203-6413
TEL: (425) 348-8160
FAX: (425) 348-8167
TOLL FREE: (800) 328-7273
IN-STATE: (800) 548-8385
WWW.WA.REGENCE.COM

REGENCY EMPLOYEE BENEFITS

MICHIGAN CLAIMS OFFICE
ROBINS GROUP
330 SUPERIOR MALL
PO BOX 610609
PORT HURON, MI 48061-0609
TEL: (810) 987-7711
FAX: (810) 987-7603
TOLL FREE: (800) 369-3718

REGENT INSURANCE CO

WISCONSIN CLAIMS OFFICE
ONE GENERAL DR
SUN PRAIRIE, WI 53596
TEL: (608) 837-4440
FAX: (608) 837-0788
TOLL FREE: (800) 362-5448
WWW.GENCAS.COM

REGIONAL MEDICAL ADMINISTRATORS, INC

NORTH CAROLINA CLAIMS OFFICE
PO BOX 4128
GLEN RAVEN, NC 27215-0901
TEL: (336) 226-7950
FAX: (336) 570-0599
TOLL FREE: (800) 711-1507

SOUTH CAROLINA CLAIMS OFFICE
PO BOX 4128
GLEN RAVEN, NC 27215-0901
TEL: (336) 226-7950
FAX: (336) 570-0599
TOLL FREE: (800) 711-1507

REGIONS BLUE CROSS & BLUE SHIELD OF OREGON

IDAHO CLAIMS OFFICE
HMO OF OREGON
100 SW MARKET ST
PO BOX 900
PORTLAND, OR 97207
TEL: (503) 274-0761
FAX: (503) 375-4293
TOLL FREE: (800) 643-4512
IN-STATE: (800) 228-0978
WWW.BCBSO.COM

OREGON CLAIMS OFFICE
HMO OF OREGON
100 SW MARKET ST
PO BOX 900
PORTLAND, OR 97207
TEL: (503) 274-0761
FAX: (503) 375-4293
TOLL FREE: (800) 643-4512
IN-STATE: (800) 228-0978
WWW.BCBSO.COM

UTAH CLAIMS OFFICE
HMO OF OREGON
100 SW MARKET ST
PO BOX 900
PORTLAND, OR 97207
TEL: (503) 274-0761
FAX: (503) 375-4293
TOLL FREE: (800) 643-4512
IN-STATE: (800) 228-0978
WWW.BCBSO.COM

WASHINGTON CLAIMS OFFICE
HMO OF OREGON
100 SW MARKET ST
PO BOX 900
PORTLAND, OR 97207
TEL: (503) 274-0761
FAX: (503) 375-4293
TOLL FREE: (800) 643-4512
IN-STATE: (800) 228-0978
WWW.BCBSO.COM

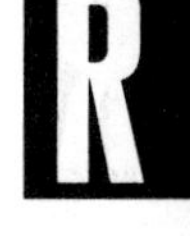

REHABILITATION NETWORK CORP

PENNSYLVANIA CLAIMS OFFICE
NOVAEON
1210 WARD AVE, STE 300
WEST CHESTER, PA 19380
TEL: (610) 719-6700
FAX: (610) 719-6774
WWW.NOVAEON.COM

REINSURANCE ALTERNATIVES

MINNESOTA CLAIMS OFFICE
7900 XERXES AVE S, STE 2030
MINNEAPOLIS, MN 55431-1105
TEL: (612) 832-3366
FAX: (612) 832-3379
TOLL FREE: (800) 541-5290

REINSURANCE MANAGEMENT, INC

NATIONAL CLAIMS OFFICE
MANAGED HEALTH FUNDING INSURANCE ADMINISTRATORS
9485 REGENCY SQ BLVD, STE 220
JACKSONVILLE, FL 32225
TEL: (904) 727-5088
FAX: (904) 727-7892
TOLL FREE: (800) 830-3856
WWW.RMIMHF.COM

MANAGED HEALTH FUNDING INSURANCE ADMINISTRATORS
21530 OXNARD ST
WOODLAND HILLS, CA 91367
TEL: (818) 227-6446
FAX: (818) 227-6465
TOLL FREE: (800) 828-8360

RELIABLE LIFE INSURANCE CO

231 W LOCKWOOD
SAINT LOUIS, MO 63119
TEL: (314) 968-4900
FAX: (314) 968-6795
TOLL FREE: (800) 325-9555

RELIANCE INSURANCE CO

ALBERTA CLAIMS OFFICE
RELIANCE NATIONAL
200 KING ST W, STE 1906
TORONTO, ON M5H-3T4
TEL: (416) 581-0101
FAX: (416) 581-1109
WWW.RELIANCE.COM

ARIZONA CLAIMS OFFICE
2901 N CENTRAL AVE, STE 400
PO BOX 16025
PHOENIX, AZ 85011
TEL: (602) 248-4330
FAX: (602) 248-7906
TOLL FREE: (800) 793-2322
WWW.RELIANCE.COM

PO BOX 16025
PHOENIX, AZ 85011
TEL: (602) 248-4330
FAX: (602) 230-8187
TOLL FREE: (800) 793-2322
IN-STATE: (800) 793-2322

BRITISH COLUMBIA CLAIMS OFFICE
RELIANCE NATIONAL
200 KING ST W, STE 1906
TORONTO, ON M5H-3T4
TEL: (416) 581-0101
FAX: (416) 581-1109
WWW.RELIANCE.COM

CALIFORNIA CLAIMS OFFICE
700 N BRAND BLVD, STE 1200
PO BOX 29008
GLENDALE, CA 91209-9008
TEL: (818) 507-9333
FAX: (818) 247-2447
TOLL FREE: (800) 252-5047
WWW.RELIANCE.COM

2882 PROSPECT PK PL, STE 300
RANCHO CORDOVA, CA 95670
TEL: (916) 638-8300
FAX: (916) 635-6431
TOLL FREE: (800) 597-7677
WWW.RELIANCE.COM

343 SANSOME ST, STE 900
PO BOX 2669
SAN FRANCISCO, CA 94126
TEL: (415) 623-3383
FAX: (415) 296-9522
TOLL FREE: (800) 831-9124
IN-STATE: (800) 231-2202
WWW.RELIANCE.COM

STERLING CLAIMS SERVICES
2601 MAIN ST, STE 800
IRVINE, CA 92614
TEL: (714) 553-0505
FAX: (949) 553-0779
TOLL FREE: (800) 995-1590
WWW.RELIANCE.COM

STERLING CLAIMS SERVICES
PO BOX 25099
SANTA ANA, CA 92799-5099
TEL: (949) 553-0505
FAX: (949) 553-0779
TOLL FREE: (800) 995-1590
WWW.RELIANCE.COM

COLORADO CLAIMS OFFICE
7600 E ORCHARD RD, STE 310S
ENGLEWOOD, CO 80111
TEL: (303) 770-1476
FAX: (303) 770-3395
TOLL FREE: (800) 497-4566
WWW.RELIANCE.COM

IDAHO CLAIMS OFFICE
700 NE MULTNOMAH, STE 600
PO BOX 5669
PORTLAND, OR 97228-5669
TEL: (503) 238-8700
FAX: (503) 238-9763
IN-STATE: (800) 775-5655

ILLINOIS CLAIMS OFFICE
233 S WACKER DR, STE 6120
PO BOX 06559
CHICAGO, IL 60606
TEL: (312) 655-1850
FAX: (312) 876-0923
WWW.RELIANCE.COM

MANITOBA CLAIMS OFFICE
RELIANCE NATIONAL
200 KING ST W, STE 1906
TORONTO, ON M5H-3T4
TEL: (416) 581-0101
FAX: (416) 581-1109
WWW.RELIANCE.COM

NEW BRUNSWICK CLAIMS OFFICE
RELIANCE NATIONAL
200 KING ST W, STE 1906
TORONTO, ON M5H-3T4
TEL: (416) 581-0101
FAX: (416) 581-1109
WWW.RELIANCE.COM

NEW YORK CLAIMS OFFICE
RELIANCE NATIONAL
77 WATER ST
NEW YORK, NY 10005
TEL: (212) 858-3600
FAX: (212) 858-3612
WWW.RELIANCE.COM

10 AIRLINE DR, STE 200
ALBANY, NY 12205
TEL: (518) 464-2900
FAX: (518) 464-2999
TOLL FREE: (800) 289-4565
WWW.RELIANCE.COM

NEWFOUNDLAND CLAIMS OFFICE
RELIANCE NATIONAL
200 KING ST W, STE 1906
TORONTO, ON M5H-3T4
TEL: (416) 581-0101
FAX: (416) 581-1109
WWW.RELIANCE.COM

NOVA SCOTIA CLAIMS OFFICE
RELIANCE NATIONAL
200 KING ST W, STE 1906
TORONTO, ON M5H-3T4
TEL: (416) 581-0101
FAX: (416) 581-1109
WWW.RELIANCE.COM

ONTARIO CLAIMS OFFICE
RELIANCE NATIONAL
200 KING ST W, STE 1906
TORONTO, ON M5H-3T4
TEL: (416) 581-0101
FAX: (416) 581-1109
WWW.RELIANCE.COM

OREGON CLAIMS OFFICE
700 NE MULTNOMAH, STE 600
PO BOX 5669
PORTLAND, OR 97228-5669
TEL: (503) 238-8700
FAX: (503) 238-9763
IN-STATE: (800) 775-5655

PENNSYLVANIA CLAIMS OFFICE
3 PARKWAY
PHILADELPHIA, PA 19102
TEL: (215) 864-4000
FAX: (215) 864-4477
TOLL FREE: (800) 441-1652
WWW.RELIANCE.COM

PRINCE EDWARD ISLAND CLAIMS OFFICE
RELIANCE NATIONAL
200 KING ST W, STE 1906
TORONTO, ON M5H-3T4
TEL: (416) 581-0101
FAX: (416) 581-1109
WWW.RELIANCE.COM

QUEBEC CLAIMS OFFICE
RELIANCE NATIONAL
200 KING ST W, STE 1906
TORONTO, ON M5H-3T4
TEL: (416) 581-0101
FAX: (416) 581-1109
WWW.RELIANCE.COM

SASKATCHEWAN CLAIMS OFFICE
RELIANCE NATIONAL
200 KING ST W, STE 1906
TORONTO, ON M5H-3T4
TEL: (416) 581-0101
FAX: (416) 581-1109
WWW.RELIANCE.COM

UTAH CLAIMS OFFICE
2901 N CENTRAL AVE, STE 400
PO BOX 16025
PHOENIX, AZ 85011
TEL: (602) 248-4330
FAX: (602) 230-8187
TOLL FREE: (800) 793-2322

WASHINGTON CLAIMS OFFICE
2505 S 320TH ST
PO BOX 9719
FEDERAL WAY, WA 98063-9719
TEL: (253) 952-5000
FAX: (253) 946-3247
TOLL FREE: (800) 859-5655
WWW.RELIANCE.COM

700 NE MULTNOMAH, STE 600
PO BOX 5669
PORTLAND, OR 97228-5669
TEL: (503) 238-8700
FAX: (503) 238-9763
IN-STATE: (800) 775-5655

RELIANCE STANDARD LIFE INSURANCE CO

PENNSYLVANIA CLAIMS OFFICE
2501 BEN FRANKLIN PKY
PHILADELPHIA, PA 19130
TEL: (215) 787-4000
FAX: (215) 787-4254
TOLL FREE: (800) 351-7500
WWW.RSL.COM

RELIASTAR

ALABAMA CLAIMS OFFICE
3480 PRESTON RIDGE RD, STE 550
ALPHARETTA, GA 30005
TEL: (770) 396-0788
FAX: (770) 399-9101
TOLL FREE: (800) 933-6965
WWW.RELIASTAR.COM

FLORIDA CLAIMS OFFICE
3480 PRESTON RIDGE RD, STE 550
ALPHARETTA, GA 30005
TEL: (770) 396-0788
FAX: (770) 399-9101
TOLL FREE: (800) 933-6965
WWW.RELIASTAR.COM

GEORGIA CLAIMS OFFICE
3480 PRESTON RIDGE RD, STE 550
ALPHARETTA, GA 30005
TEL: (770) 396-0788
FAX: (770) 399-9101
TOLL FREE: (800) 933-6965
WWW.RELIASTAR.COM

INDIANA CLAIMS OFFICE
3480 PRESTON RIDGE RD, STE 550
ALPHARETTA, GA 30005
TEL: (770) 396-0788
FAX: (770) 399-9101
TOLL FREE: (800) 933-6965
WWW.RELIASTAR.COM

RELIASTAR LIFE

MINNESOTA CLAIMS OFFICE
20 WASHINGTON AVE S
PO BOX 1195
MINNEAPOLIS, MN 55440-0020
TEL: (612) 372-5432
FAX: (612) 342-7592
TOLL FREE: (800) 444-6965

REPUBLIC AMERICAN LIFE INSURANCE CO

ARIZONA CLAIMS OFFICE
8200 BROOKRIVER DR, STE 600N
DALLAS, TX 75247-4069
TEL: (214) 631-6310
FAX: (214) 638-6431
TOLL FREE: (800) 876-8776

COLORADO CLAIMS OFFICE
8200 BROOKRIVER DR, STE 600N
DALLAS, TX 75247-4069
TEL: (214) 631-6310
FAX: (214) 638-6431
TOLL FREE: (800) 876-8776

FLORIDA CLAIMS OFFICE
8200 BROOKRIVER DR, STE 600N
DALLAS, TX 75247-4069
TEL: (214) 631-6310
FAX: (214) 638-6431
TOLL FREE: (800) 876-8776

GEORGIA CLAIMS OFFICE
8200 BROOKRIVER DR, STE 600N
DALLAS, TX 75247-4069
TEL: (214) 631-6310
FAX: (214) 638-6431
TOLL FREE: (800) 876-8776

INDIANA CLAIMS OFFICE
8200 BROOKRIVER DR, STE 600N
DALLAS, TX 75247-4069
TEL: (214) 631-6310
FAX: (214) 638-6431
TOLL FREE: (800) 876-8776

LOUISIANA CLAIMS OFFICE
8200 BROOKRIVER DR, STE 600N
DALLAS, TX 75247-4069
TEL: (214) 631-6310
FAX: (214) 638-6431
TOLL FREE: (800) 876-8776

NEW MEXICO CLAIMS OFFICE
8200 BROOKRIVER DR, STE 600N
DALLAS, TX 75247-4069
TEL: (214) 631-6310
FAX: (214) 638-6431
TOLL FREE: (800) 876-8776

OKLAHOMA CLAIMS OFFICE
8200 BROOKRIVER DR, STE 600N
DALLAS, TX 75247-4069
TEL: (214) 631-6310
FAX: (214) 638-6431
TOLL FREE: (800) 876-8776

TENNESSEE CLAIMS OFFICE
8200 BROOKRIVER DR, STE 600N
DALLAS, TX 75247-4069
TEL: (214) 631-6310
FAX: (214) 638-6431
TOLL FREE: (800) 876-8776

TEXAS CLAIMS OFFICE
8200 BROOKRIVER DR, STE 600N
DALLAS, TX 75247-4069
TEL: (214) 631-6310
FAX: (214) 638-6431
TOLL FREE: (800) 876-8776

UTAH CLAIMS OFFICE
8200 BROOKRIVER DR, STE 600N
DALLAS, TX 75247-4069
TEL: (214) 631-6310
FAX: (214) 638-6431
TOLL FREE: (800) 876-8776

REPUBLIC INDEMNITY CO OF AMERICA

CALIFORNIA CLAIMS OFFICE
15821 VENTURA BLVD, STE 370
ENCINO, CA 91436-2915
TEL: (818) 990-9860
FAX: (818) 986-6559
TOLL FREE: (800) 821-4520
WWW.REPUBLICINDEMNITY.COM

100 PINE ST, STE 1400
SAN FRANCISCO, CA 94111-5116
TEL: (415) 981-3200
FAX: (415) 954-1178
TOLL FREE: (800) 662-1485
WWW.REPUBLICINDEMNITY.COM

REPUBLIC UNDERWRITER'S INSURANCE

TEXAS CLAIMS OFFICE
2727 TURTLE CRK BLVD
PO BOX 660560
DALLAS, TX 75219
TEL: (214) 559-1222
FAX: (888) 224-5874
TOLL FREE: (800) 344-2275

R

REPUBLIC WESTERN INSURANCE CO

ARIZONA CLAIMS OFFICE
2721 N CENTRAL AVE
PO BOX 21748
PHOENIX, AZ 85036
TEL: (602) 263-6755
FAX: (602) 277-3538
TOLL FREE: (800) 528-7134
WWW.REPWEST.COM

RESERVE NATIONAL INSURANCE CO

NATIONAL CLAIMS OFFICE
6100 NW GRAND BLVD
PO BOX 18448
OKLAHOMA CITY, OK 73154-0448
TEL: (405) 848-7931
FAX: (405) 842-0499
TOLL FREE: (800) 654-9106

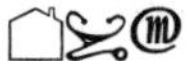

RESOURCE GROUP

TEXAS CLAIMS OFFICE
1345 RIVER BEND DR
PO BOX 191248
DALLAS, TX 75219
TEL: (214) 634-7014
FAX: (214) 630-8506
TOLL FREE: (800) 588-0455

RESOURCE PARTNER

OHIO CLAIMS OFFICE
180 E BROAD ST
PO BOX 189
COLUMBUS, OH 43216-0189
TEL: (614) 220-5001
FAX: (614) 220-5033
TOLL FREE: (800) 848-6181
WWW.RESOURCEPARTNER.COM

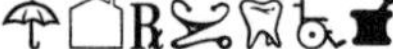

RISCO

MICHIGAN CLAIMS OFFICE
17187 N LAUREL PRK DR, STE 434
LIVONIA, MI 48152
TEL: (734) 953-4400
FAX: (734) 953-4600
WWW.RISCO.COM

RISK ENTERPRISE MANAGEMENT

NEW YORK CLAIMS OFFICE
59 MAIDEN LANE
NEW YORK, NY 10038
TEL: (212) 530-7000
FAX: (212) 530-3337
TOLL FREE: (800) 835-4663

RISK MANAGEMENT RESOURCES, INC

CALIFORNIA CLAIMS OFFICE
11161 ANDERSON ST, STE 200
PO BOX 1770
LOMA LINDA, CA 92354-0570
TEL: (909) 824-4386
FAX: (909) 824-4775

RITE AID CORP

CALIFORNIA CLAIMS OFFICE
30 HUNTER LN
PO BOX 3165
HARRISBURG, PA 17105
TEL: (717) 761-2633
WWW.RITEAID.COM

OREGON CLAIMS OFFICE
30 HUNTER LN
PO BOX 3165
HARRISBURG, PA 17105
TEL: (717) 761-2633
WWW.RITEAID.COM

PENNSYLVANIA CLAIMS OFFICE
30 HUNTER LN
PO BOX 3165
HARRISBURG, PA 17105
TEL: (717) 761-2633
WWW.RITEAID.COM

RIVERBEND GOVERNMENT BENEFITS ADMINISTRATOR

TENNESSEE CLAIMS OFFICE
730 CHESTNUT ST
CHATTANOOGA, TN 37402
TEL: (423) 755-5783
FAX: (423) 752-6518
WWW.RIVERBENDGBA.COM

RLI CORP

ILLINOIS CLAIMS OFFICE
9025 N LINDBERG DR
PEORIA, IL 61615-1431
TEL: (309) 692-1000
FAX: (309) 692-1068
TOLL FREE: (800) 331-4929
WWW.RLICORP.COM

RMSCO, INC

NEW YORK CLAIMS OFFICE
731 JAMES ST
PO BOX 6309
SYRACUSE, NY 13217
TEL: (315) 474-8200
FAX: (315) 476-8440

ROBERT PLAN CORP

NEW JERSEY CLAIMS OFFICE
NEWARK INSURANCE
200 METROPLEX DR
PO BOX 14000
NEW BRUNSWICK, NJ 08906
FAX: (609) 227-5093
TOLL FREE: (800) 526-4486
IN-STATE: (800) 526-4486

NEW YORK CLAIMS OFFICE
MATERIAL DAMAGE
999 STEWART AVE
PO BOX 9028
BETHPAGE, NY 11714
TEL: (516) 393-6700
FAX: (516) 393-6248

ROBERT S. WEISS & CO

CONNECTICUT CLAIMS OFFICE
SILVER HILLS BUS CTR- 500 S BROAD ST
PO BOX 1034
MERIDEN, CT 06450-1034
TEL: (203) 235-6882
FAX: (203) 639-7422
TOLL FREE: (800) 466-7900

ROBEY-BARBER INSURANCE SERVICES CORPOARTION

FLORIDA CLAIMS OFFICE
MANATEE SERVICE CENTER
PO BOX 1098
BRADENTON, FL 34206
TEL: (941) 742-5700
FAX: (941) 750-6970

ROCKFORD HEALTH PLANS

ILLINOIS CLAIMS OFFICE
3401 N PERRYVILLE RD
ROCKFORD, IL 61114
TEL: (815) 654-3600
FAX: (815) 282-0634
TOLL FREE: (800) 331-0424
WWW.RHSNET.ORG

ROCKWOOD CASUALTY INSURANCE CO

PENNSYLVANIA CLAIMS OFFICE
654 MAIN ST
ROCKWOOD, PA 15557
TEL: (814) 926-4661
FAX: (814) 926-4070
TOLL FREE: (800) 837-9062

ROCKY MOUNTAIN HMO

COLORADO CLAIMS OFFICE
HEALTH OPTIONS, INC
2775 CROSSROADS BLVD
PO BOX 10600
GRAND JUNCTION, CO 81506
TEL: (970) 244-7760
FAX: (970) 244-7880
TOLL FREE: (800) 843-0719
IN-STATE: (800) 843-0719
WWW.RMHMO.ORG

ROCKY MOUNTAIN LIFE INSURANCE CO OF COLORADO

700 BROADWAY, STE 1117
DENVER, CO 80273-0001
TEL: (303) 831-3085
FAX: (303) 831-3087
TOLL FREE: (800) 873-2257

ROYAL STATE GROUP

HAWAII CLAIMS OFFICE
819 S BERETANIA ST, STE 100
HONOLULU, HI 96813
TEL: (808) 539-1600
FAX: (808) 538-1458
WWW.HGEA.COM

ROYAL & SUNALLIANCE

CALIFORNIA CLAIMS OFFICE
801 N BRAND BLVD, STE 500
PO BOX 29035
GLENDALE, CA 91209-9035
TEL: (818) 241-5212
FAX: (818) 543-6393
TOLL FREE: (800) 252-0431
WWW.ROYALSUNALLIANCE.COM

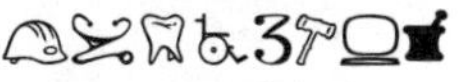

1600 RIVIERA AVE, STE 210
PO BOX 8194
WALNUT CREEK, CA 94596-8194
TEL: (510) 934-9660
FAX: (800) 671-4035
TOLL FREE: (800) 523-6269
WWW.ROYALSUNALLIANCE.COM

COLORADO CLAIMS OFFICE
7400 E ORCHARD RD, STE 4000
ENGLEWOOD, CO 80111
TEL: (303) 771-1970
FAX: (303) 930-6115
TOLL FREE: (800) 523-6235
WWW.ROYALSUNALLIANCE.COM

CONNECTICUT CLAIMS OFFICE
500 WINDING BRK DR
PO BOX 2912
HARTFORD, CT 06104-2912
TEL: (860) 659-4211
FAX: (860) 633-2428
TOLL FREE: (800) 842-1918
IN-STATE: (800) 525-5019
WWW.ROYALSUNALLIANCE.COM

80 WOLF RD, STE 606
PO BOX 15096
ALBANY, NY 12205
TEL: (518) 489-8331
TOLL FREE: (800) 553-2556
WWW.ROYALSUNALLIANCE.COM

FLORIDA CLAIMS OFFICE
4010 BOY SCOUT BLVD
PO BOX 22228
TAMPA, FL 33622-2228
TEL: (813) 872-6600
FAX: (813) 877-6171
TOLL FREE: (800) 282-2985
WWW.ROYALSUNALLIANCE.COM

GEORGIA CLAIMS OFFICE
5 CONCOURSE PKY, STE 500
PO BOX 105536
ATLANTA, GA 30348-5536
TEL: (770) 393-1300
FAX: (770) 393-9591
TOLL FREE: (800) 523-5431
WWW.ROYALSUNALLIANCE.COM

IDAHO CLAIMS OFFICE
PO BOX 57969
SALT LAKE CITY, UT 84157-0969
TEL: (801) 261-7700
FAX: (801) 268-3225
TOLL FREE: (800) 984-0939
WWW.ROYALSUNALLIANCE.COM

ILLINOIS CLAIMS OFFICE
1240 E DIEHL RD, STE 500
PO BOX 3144
NAPERVILLE, IL 60566
TEL: (630) 577-9200
FAX: (630) 577-9516
TOLL FREE: (800) 621-2297
WWW.ROYALSUNALLIANCE.COM

INDIANA CLAIMS OFFICE
255 E 5TH ST, STE 2100
CINCINNATI, OH 45202
TEL: (513) 421-2183
FAX: (513) 357-9580
TOLL FREE: (800) 843-5772
WWW.ROYALSUNALLIANCE.COM

KENTUCKY CLAIMS OFFICE
255 E 5TH ST, STE 2100
CINCINNATI, OH 45202
TEL: (513) 421-2183
FAX: (513) 357-9580
TOLL FREE: (800) 843-5772
WWW.ROYALSUNALLIANCE.COM

MAINE CLAIMS OFFICE
100 COMMERCIAL DR
PO BOX 4727
PORTLAND, ME 04112-4727
TEL: (207) 774-6286
FAX: (207) 774-1140
TOLL FREE: (800) 462-1921
WWW.ROYALSUNALLIANCE.COM

MARYLAND CLAIMS OFFICE
300 E LOMBARD ST, STE 700
BALTIMORE, MD 21202
TEL: (410) 685-5844
FAX: (410) 637-1699
TOLL FREE: (800) 482-4446
WWW.ROYALSUNALLIANCE.COM

MASSACHUSETTS CLAIMS OFFICE
25 NEW CHARDEN
PO BOX 8088
BOSTON, MA 02114-4774
TEL: (617) 742-7750
FAX: (617) 557-4252
TOLL FREE: (800) 367-7036
IN-STATE: (800) 367-7036
WWW.ROYALSUNALLIANCE.COM

255 PARK AVE, STE 601
WORCESTER, MA 01609
TEL: (508) 791-5563
FAX: (508) 791-0375
TOLL FREE: (800) 654-0070
WWW.ROYALSUNALLIANCE.COM

80 WOLF RD, STE 606
PO BOX 15096
ALBANY, NY 12205
TEL: (518) 489-8331
TOLL FREE: (800) 553-2556
WWW.ROYALSUNALLIANCE.COM

MICHIGAN CLAIMS OFFICE
255 E 5TH ST, STE 2100
CINCINNATI, OH 45202
TEL: (513) 421-2183
FAX: (513) 357-9580
TOLL FREE: (800) 843-5772
WWW.ROYALSUNALLIANCE.COM

MINNESOTA CLAIMS OFFICE
STATE AUTO INSURANCE
6465 WAYZATA BLVD, STE 810
SAINT LOUIS PARK, MN 55426
TEL: (612) 541-4744
FAX: (612) 544-6291
TOLL FREE: (800) 328-0710
WWW.ROYALSUNALLIANCE.COM

NATIONAL CLAIMS OFFICE
2 JERICHO PLZ
PO BOX 4002
JERICHO, NY 11753-0873
TEL: (516) 939-0600
FAX: (516) 937-3338
TOLL FREE: (800) 523-6273
WWW.ROYALSUNALLIANCE.COM

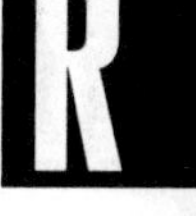

25800 NORTHWESTERN HWY, STE 701
PO BOX 5010
SOUTHFIELD, MI 48086-5010
TEL: (248) 746-6180
FAX: (248) 746-6190
IN-STATE: (800) 482-8772
WWW.ROYALSUNALLIANCE.COM

NEVADA CLAIMS OFFICE
PO BOX 57969
SALT LAKE CITY, UT 84157-0969
TEL: (801) 261-7700
FAX: (801) 268-3225
TOLL FREE: (800) 984-0939
WWW.ROYALSUNALLIANCE.COM

NEW HAMPSHIRE CLAIMS OFFICE
2 COMMERCE DR
PO BOX 4645
MANCHESTER, NH 03108-4645
TEL: (603) 669-3900
FAX: (603) 626-0714
TOLL FREE: (800) 258-5214
WWW.ROYALSUNALLIANCE.COM

NEW JERSEY CLAIMS OFFICE
4 GATEHALL DR
PO BOX 236
PARSIPPANY, NJ 07054-0432
TEL: (973) 829-6000
FAX: (973) 829-6130
TOLL FREE: (800) 222-0480
WWW.ROYALSUNALLIANCE.COM

NEW YORK CLAIMS OFFICE
80 WOLF RD, STE 606
PO BOX 15096
ALBANY, NY 12205
TEL: (518) 489-8331
TOLL FREE: (800) 553-2556
WWW.ROYALSUNALLIANCE.COM

555 TAXTER RD
PO BOX 1216
ELMSFORD, NY 10523-0916
TEL: (914) 789-7800
FAX: (914) 789-7885
IN-STATE: (800) 523-6253
WWW.ROYALSUNALLIANCE.COM

2351 N FOREST RD
GETZVILLE, NY 14068
TEL: (716) 636-1830
FAX: (716) 639-2095
TOLL FREE: (800) 523-6251
WWW.ROYALSUNALLIANCE.COM

1393 VETERANS HWY
HAUPPAUGE, NY 11788
TEL: (516) 382-5700
FAX: (516) 382-5725
TOLL FREE: (800) 221-3385
WWW.ROYALSUNALLIANCE.COM

ONE CHASE MANHATTAN PLZ- 38TH FL
NEW YORK, NY 10005
TEL: (212) 709-3600
TOLL FREE: (800) 221-5670
WWW.ROYALSUNALLIANCE.COM

400 W DIVISION ST
PO BOX 4701
SYRACUSE, NY 13221
TEL: (315) 426-4000
FAX: (315) 426-4095
TOLL FREE: (800) 524-4505
WWW.ROYALSUNALLIANCE.COM

PO BOX 1378
BUFFALO, NY 14240
TEL: (716) 636-1830
FAX: (716) 639-2095
TOLL FREE: (800) 523-6251
WWW.ROYALSUNALLIANCE.COM

NORTH CAROLINA CLAIMS OFFICE
9300 ARROW PT BLVD
PO BOX 1000
CHARLOTTE, NC 28201-1000
TEL: (704) 522-2000
FAX: (704) 522-3200
WWW.ROYALSUNALLIANCE.COM

1901 ROXBOROUGH RD
PO BOX 472488
CHARLOTTE, NC 28247-6488
TEL: (704) 543-3300
FAX: (800) 984-4515
TOLL FREE: (800) 426-4388
WWW.ROYALSUNALLIANCE.COM

OHIO CLAIMS OFFICE
255 E 5TH ST, STE 2100
CINCINNATI, OH 45202
TEL: (513) 421-2183
FAX: (513) 357-9580
TOLL FREE: (800) 843-5772
WWW.ROYALSUNALLIANCE.COM

PENNSYLVANIA CLAIMS OFFICE
1510 VLY CTR PKY, STE 130
BETHLEHEM, PA 18017
TEL: (610) 758-8414
FAX: (610) 758-8441
TOLL FREE: (800) 852-9282
WWW.ROYALSUNALLIANCE.COM

501 HOLIDAY DR, FOSTER PLZ 4
PITTSBURGH, PA 15220-2774
TEL: (412) 922-3740
FAX: (412) 920-9255
TOLL FREE: (800) 245-2232
E-MAIL: ROYAL-USA.COM
WWW.ROYALSUNALLIANCE.COM

SOUTH DAKOTA CLAIMS OFFICE
107 FLYNN DR, STE 500
PO BOX 7001
MILBANK, SD 57252
TEL: (605) 432-6468
FAX: (605) 432-4574
WWW.ROYALSUNALLIANCE.COM

TEXAS CLAIMS OFFICE
12750 MERIT DR, STE 400
PO BOX 809016
DALLAS, TX 75251
TEL: (972) 735-9941
TOLL FREE: (800) 523-6244
WWW.ROYALSUNALLIANCE.COM

UTAH CLAIMS OFFICE
PO BOX 57969
SALT LAKE CITY, UT 84157-0969
TEL: (801) 261-7700
FAX: (801) 268-3225
TOLL FREE: (800) 984-0939
WWW.ROYALSUNALLIANCE.COM

VIRGINIA CLAIMS OFFICE
720 MOORFIELD PRK DR, STE 300
RICHMOND, VA 23236
TEL: (804) 320-7800
FAX: (804) 560-8392
TOLL FREE: (800) 446-3826
WWW.ROYALSUNALLIANCE.COM

WASHINGTON CLAIMS OFFICE
999 3RD AVE, STE 2700
SEATTLE, WA 98104-4000
TEL: (206) 622-7791
FAX: (206) 689-0379
TOLL FREE: (800) 255-5469
WWW.ROYALSUNALLIANCE.COM

WISCONSIN CLAIMS OFFICE
1240 E DIEHL RD, STE 500
PO BOX 3144
NAPERVILLE, IL 60566
TEL: (630) 577-9200
FAX: (630) 577-9516
TOLL FREE: (800) 621-2297
WWW.ROYALSUNALLIANCE.COM

RSKCO CLAIM SERVICES

OREGON CLAIMS OFFICE
8625 SW CASCADE BLVD
BEAVERTON, OR 97008
TEL: (503) 526-6850
FAX: (503) 526-6810
TOLL FREE: (877) 894-1806

WASHINGTON CLAIMS OFFICE
8625 SW CASCADE BLVD
BEAVERTON, OR 97008
TEL: (503) 526-6850
FAX: (503) 526-6810
TOLL FREE: (877) 894-1806

RURAL MUTUAL INSURANCE CO

WISCONSIN CLAIMS OFFICE
1212 DEMINGWAY
PO BOX 5555
MADISON, WI 53705-0555
TEL: (608) 836-5525
FAX: (608) 828-5483
TOLL FREE: (800) 362-7881
WWW.RURALINS.COM

RTE 1, HIGHWAY 54 WEST
PO BOX 610
BLACK RIVER FALLS, WI 54615-0610
TEL: (715) 284-9416
FAX: (715) 284-2301
TOLL FREE: (800) 301-0490
WWW.RURALINS.COM

2417 SILVERNAIL RD
PEWAUKEE, WI 53072
TEL: (414) 544-4991
FAX: (414) 544-4335
TOLL FREE: (800) 801-9560

RUSH-PRUDENTIAL HEALTH PLAN

ILLINOIS CLAIMS OFFICE
233 S WACKER, STE 3900
CHICAGO, IL 60606
FAX: (312) 234-8005
TOLL FREE: (800) 234-7000

INDIANA CLAIMS OFFICE
233 S WACKER, STE 3900
CHICAGO, IL 60606
TEL: (312) 234-7000
FAX: (312) 234-8005
TOLL FREE: (800) 234-7000

S.E.I.U. LOCAL 36 BENEFIT FUNDS

PENNSYLVANIA CLAIMS OFFICE
42 S 15TH ST, STE 1500
PHILADELPHIA, PA 19102
TEL: (215) 568-3262
FAX: (215) 561-2382
TOLL FREE: (800) 338-9025

SAFE MATE LIFE INSURANCE CO

TEXAS CLAIMS OFFICE
2101 WHITCOMB
PO BOX 370710
EL PASO, TX 79925
TEL: (915) 779-3872
FAX: (915) 772-1907
TOLL FREE: (800) 443-9449

SAFECO INSURANCE CO OF AMERICA

CALIFORNIA CLAIMS OFFICE
AMERICAN STATES
330 N BRAND BLVD, STE 900
PO BOX 29082
GLENDALE, CA 91029-9082
TEL: (818) 956-4200
FAX: (818) 956-4259
TOLL FREE: (800) 826-8921
WWW.SAFECO.COM

3000 EXECUTIVE PKY STE 300
PO BOX 5152
SAN RAMON, CA 94583-5152
TEL: (925) 277-8600
TOLL FREE: (800) 847-5400
WWW.SAFECO.COM

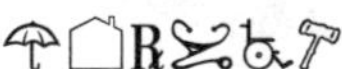

17570 BROOKHURST
PO BOX 25150
SANTA ANA, CA 92799-5150
TEL: (714) 963-0900
FAX: (714) 965-6543
TOLL FREE: (800) 637-4755
WWW.SAFECO.COM

1615 MURRAY CYN RD, STE 615
PO BOX 81425-92138-1425
SAN DIEGO, CA 92108
TEL: (619) 686-5460
FAX: (619) 686-5461
WWW.SAFECO.COM

COLORADO CLAIMS OFFICE
12499 W COLFAX
PO BOX 5687
DENVER, CO 80217
TEL: (303) 232-6622
FAX: (303) 679-5449
TOLL FREE: (800) 426-9963
IN-STATE: (800) 852-4288
WWW.SAFECO.COM

FLORIDA CLAIMS OFFICE
SAFECO AMERICAN STATES INSURANCE CO
2300 MAITLAND CTR PKY, STE 220
MAITLAND, FL 32751-7183
TEL: (407) 660-2185
FAX: (407) 875-7851
TOLL FREE: (888) 557-5010

GEORGIA CLAIMS OFFICE
1551 JULIET RD
PO BOX A
STONE MOUNTAIN, GA 30086
TEL: (770) 469-1111
FAX: (770) 879-3333
TOLL FREE: (800) 241-2279
WWW.SAFECO.COM

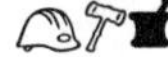

MICHIGAN CLAIMS OFFICE
900 E PARIS SE, STE 201
PO BOX 154
GRAND RAPIDS, MI 49501-0154
TEL: (616) 940-1200
FAX: (616) 940-1291
WWW.SAFECO.COM

MISSOURI CLAIMS OFFICE
3637 S GEYER RD
PO BOX 66783
SAINT LOUIS, MO 63127-6783
TEL: (314) 957-4500
FAX: (314) 957-4630
TOLL FREE: (800) 843-1487
WWW.SAFECO.COM

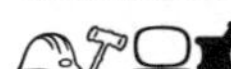

NORTH DAKOTA CLAIMS OFFICE
3217 FIETCHNER DR
PO BOX 10128
FARGO, ND 58106-0128
TEL: (701) 232-3717
FAX: (701) 232-2417
WWW.SAFECO.COM

OHIO CLAIMS OFFICE
5901 E GALBRAITH RD
PO BOX 36177
CINCINNATI, OH 45236-2251
TEL: (513) 745-5861
FAX: (513) 745-5810
TOLL FREE: (800) 543-7138
WWW.SAFECO.COM

OREGON CLAIMS OFFICE
4101 SW KRUSE WAY
PO BOX 1900
LAKE OSWEGO, OR 97035-0900
TEL: (503) 635-9111
FAX: (503) 697-0459
TOLL FREE: (800) 452-4970
WWW.SAFECO.COM

TENNESSEE CLAIMS OFFICE
SAFECO AMERICAN STATES INSURANCE CO
1101 KERMET DR, STE 400
PO BOX 305160
NASHVILLE, TN 37230-5160
TEL: (615) 360-1122
FAX: (615) 366-3600
TOLL FREE: (888) 557-5010
WWW.SAFECO.COM

TEXAS CLAIMS OFFICE
500 N CENTRAL, STE 300
PO BOX 869012
PLANO, TX 75086
TEL: (972) 516-8600
TOLL FREE: (800) 472-4455
WWW.SAFECO.COM

VIRGINIA CLAIMS OFFICE
ONE PARK W CIR, STE 200
PO BOX 2618
MIDLOTHIAN, VA 23113-8618
TEL: (804) 378-2150
FAX: (804) 378-2189
TOLL FREE: (888) 557-5010
WWW.SAFECO.COM

WASHINGTON CLAIMS OFFICE
14610 E SPRAGUE AVE
PO BOX 2726
SPOKANE, WA 99220-2726
TEL: (509) 928-6800
FAX: (509) 921-5027
TOLL FREE: (800) 833-6606
WWW.SAFECO.COM

SAFEGUARD HEALTH ENTERPRISES, INC

CALIFORNIA CLAIMS OFFICE
SAFEGUARD HEALTH PLAN
95 ENTERPRISE
PO BOX 30900
LAGUNA HILLS, CA 92654
TEL: (949) 425-4300
FAX: (949) 425-4588
TOLL FREE: (800) 352-4341

SAFETY NATIONAL CASUALTY CORP

MISSOURI CLAIMS OFFICE
2043 WOODLAND PKY, STE 200
SAINT LOUIS, MO 63146
TEL: (314) 995-5300
FAX: (314) 995-3897
TOLL FREE: (888) 995-5300
WWW.SNCC.COM

SAIF CORP

OREGON CLAIMS OFFICE
400 HIGH ST
SALEM, OR 97312
TEL: (503) 373-8383
FAX: (503) 373-8181
TOLL FREE: (800) 285-8525
WWW.SAIF.COM

SAN DIEGO ELECTRICAL HEALTH & WELFARE TRUST

CALIFORNIA CLAIMS OFFICE
4675 VIEW RDG, STE B
PO BOX 231219
SAN DIEGO, CA 92194-1219
TEL: (619) 569-6322
FAX: (619) 573-0830
TOLL FREE: (800) 632-2569

SAN FRANCISCO REINSURANCE CO

777 SAN MARIN DR
NOVATO, CA 94998-3452
TEL: (415) 899-4600
FAX: (415) 899-4696
TOLL FREE: (800) 227-1700
WWW.THE-FUND.COM

SCOR REINSURANCE
NEW YORK CLAIMS OFFICE
2 WORLD TRADE CTR- 23RD FL
NEW YORK, NY 10048
TEL: (212) 390-5200
FAX: (212) 390-5415

SCOTT & WHITE HEALTH PLAN
TEXAS CLAIMS OFFICE
2401 S 31ST ST
TEMPLE, TX 76508-0001
TEL: (254) 724-2111
TOLL FREE: (800) 321-7947
WWW.SW.ORG

H

SEABURY & SMITH
DISTRICT OF COLUMBIA CLAIMS OFFICE
1255 23RD ST NW, STE 300
WASHINGTON, DC 20037-1125
TEL: (202) 296-8030
FAX: (202) 296-8184
TOLL FREE: (800) 424-9883
IN-STATE: (800) 282-4495
WWW.SEABURY.COM

IOWA CLAIMS OFFICE
2615 NORTHGATE DR
PO BOX 1520
IOWA CITY, IA 52244-1520
TEL: (319) 351-2667
FAX: (319) 351-0603
TOLL FREE: (800) 562-4023

SECURITY HEALTH PLAN OF WISCONSIN, INC
WISCONSIN CLAIMS OFFICE
1000 N OAK AVE
MARSHFIELD, WI 54449-5703
TEL: (715) 387-5621
FAX: (715) 387-9399
TOLL FREE: (800) 472-2363
WWW.SECURITYHEALTH.ORG

H

SECURITY INDUSTRIAL INSURANCE CO
LOUISIANA CLAIMS OFFICE
110 RAILROAD AVE
PO BOX 609
DONALDSONVILLE, LA 70346-2520
TEL: (225) 473-8654

SECURITY LIFE INSURANCE CO OF AMERICA
MINNESOTA CLAIMS OFFICE
10901 RED CIRCLE DR
MINNETONKA, MN 55343-9137
TEL: (612) 544-2121
FAX: (612) 945-3409
TOLL FREE: (800) 328-4667

SECURITY NATIONAL LIFE INSURANCE CO
NATIONAL CLAIMS OFFICE
SECURITY NATIONAL FINANCIAL CORP
5300 S 360 W, STE 250
PO BOX 57220
SALT LAKE CITY, UT 84157-0220
TEL: (801) 264-1060
FAX: (801) 264-8430
TOLL FREE: (800) 574-7117

SEDGWICK
CALIFORNIA CLAIMS OFFICE
160 SPEAR ST
PO BOX 7601
SAN FRANCISCO, CA 94120
TEL: (415) 983-5600
FAX: (415) 398-1841
WWW.SEDGWICK.COM

TENNESSEE CLAIMS OFFICE
1000 RIDGEWAY LOOP RD
PO BOX 171377
MEMPHIS, TN 38120
TEL: (901) 761-1550
FAX: (901) 684-3858

SEIBELS BRUCE INSURANCE GROUP
KENTUCKY CLAIMS OFFICE
1501 LADY ST
PO BOX 1
COLUMBIA, SC 29202-0001
TEL: (803) 748-2000
FAX: (803) 748-2230
TOLL FREE: (800) 525-8835

SOUTH CAROLINA CLAIMS OFFICE
1501 LADY ST
PO BOX 1
COLUMBIA, SC 29202-0001
TEL: (803) 748-2000
FAX: (803) 748-8395
TOLL FREE: (800) 525-8835

SELECTCARE, INC
MICHIGAN CLAIMS OFFICE
2401 W BIG BEAVER RD
PO BOX 396
TROY, MI 48099-0396
TEL: (248) 637-5300
FAX: (248) 637-6701
TOLL FREE: (800) 332-2365

H

SELECTIVE INSURANCE CO
MARYLAND CLAIMS OFFICE
6 N PARK DR
HUNT VALLEY, MD 21030-1842
TEL: (410) 771-6500
FAX: (410) 771-8471
TOLL FREE: (800) 685-9656
WWW.SELECTIVEINSURANCE.COM

NEW JERSEY CLAIMS OFFICE
RT 130 AAA DR
PO BOX 7950
TRENTON, NJ 08650-7950
TEL: (609) 890-2200
FAX: (609) 586-3748
TOLL FREE: (800) 305-9656
WWW.SELECTIVEINSURANCE.COM

PENNSYLVANIA CLAIMS OFFICE
5050 TILGHMAN ST
PO BOX 25333
LEHIGH VALLEY, PA 18002-5333
TEL: (610) 481-9680
FAX: (610) 481-9538
TOLL FREE: (800) 374-9656
WWW.SELECTIVEINSURANCE.COM

VIRGINIA CLAIMS OFFICE
1100 BOULDERS PKY, STE 601
PO BOX 13325
RICHMOND, VA 23225-0325
TEL: (804) 272-7568
FAX: (804) 323-4017
TOLL FREE: (800) 568-9656
WWW.SELECTIVEINSURANCE.COM

SELECTIVE INSURANCE CO OF AMERICA
NEW JERSEY CLAIMS OFFICE
40 WANTAGE AVE
PO BOX 399
BRANCHVILLE, NJ 07890
TEL: (973) 948-3000
FAX: (973) 948-2089
TOLL FREE: (800) 777-9656
WWW.SELECTIVEINSURANCE.COM

NORTH CAROLINA CLAIMS OFFICE
40 WANTAGE AVE
PO BOX 399
BRANCHVILLE, NJ 07890
TEL: (973) 948-3000
FAX: (973) 948-2089
TOLL FREE: (800) 777-9656
WWW.SELECTIVEINSURANCE.COM

SELF FUNDING ADMINISTRATORS
MARYLAND CLAIMS OFFICE
339 BUSCHS FRONTAGE RD, STE 207
PO BOX 6596
ANNAPOLIS, MD 21401-0596
TEL: (410) 757-4200
FAX: (410) 349-9724
TOLL FREE: (800) 424-8611

SELF INSURED BENEFIT ADMINISTRATORS
FLORIDA CLAIMS OFFICE
18167 US HWY 19 N, STE 300
CLEARWATER, FL 33764
TEL: (727) 532-0400
FAX: (727) 530-0882
TOLL FREE: (800) 683-7422
WWW.ONESOURCEGROUP.COM

ILLINOIS CLAIMS OFFICE
18167 US HWY 19 N, STE 300
CLEARWATER, FL 33764
TEL: (727) 532-0400
FAX: (727) 530-0882
TOLL FREE: (800) 683-7422
WWW.ONESOURCEGROUP.COM

NEW JERSEY CLAIMS OFFICE
18167 US HWY 19 N, STE 300
CLEARWATER, FL 33764
TEL: (727) 532-0400
FAX: (727) 530-0882
TOLL FREE: (800) 683-7422
WWW.ONESOURCEGROUP.COM

OKLAHOMA CLAIMS OFFICE
18167 US HWY 19 N, STE 300
CLEARWATER, FL 33764
TEL: (727) 532-0400
FAX: (727) 530-0882
TOLL FREE: (800) 683-7422
WWW.ONESOURCEGROUP.COM

SELF INSURED SERVICES CO

NATIONAL CLAIMS OFFICE
SISCO
PO BOX 389
DUBUQUE, IA 52004-0389
TEL: (319) 583-7344
FAX: (319) 583-0439
WWW.CB-SISCO.COM

SELF-INSURED MANAGEMENT SERVICE

CALIFORNIA CLAIMS OFFICE
SIMS
9320 SW BARBUR BLVD #350
PO BOX 19990
PORTLAND, OR 97280-0990
TEL: (503) 245-9756
FAX: (503) 246-1581

OREGON CLAIMS OFFICE
SIMS
9320 SW BARBUR BLVD #350
PO BOX 19990
PORTLAND, OR 97280-0990
TEL: (503) 245-9756
FAX: (503) 246-1581

WASHINGTON CLAIMS OFFICE
SIMS
9320 SW BARBUR BLVD #350
PO BOX 19990
PORTLAND, OR 97280-0990
TEL: (503) 245-9756
FAX: (503) 246-1581

SELMAN & CO

NATIONAL CLAIMS OFFICE
6110 PARKLAND BLVD
CLEVELAND, OH 44124-4187
TEL: (440) 646-9336
FAX: (440) 646-9339
TOLL FREE: (800) 735-6262
WWW.SELCO.COM

SENATE INSURANCE CO

NEW YORK CLAIMS OFFICE
HUM HEALTHCARE SYSTEMS
2716 ALBANY ST
SCHENECTADY, NY 12304
TEL: (518) 370-3828
FAX: (518) 370-3890
TOLL FREE: (800) 833-3650

SENECA

NATIONAL CLAIMS OFFICE
160 WATER ST
NEW YORK, NY 10038-4922
TEL: (212) 344-3000
FAX: (212) 422-7541

SENTARA HEALTH PLAN

VIRGINIA CLAIMS OFFICE
4417 CORPORATION LN
VIRGINIA BEACH, VA 23462-3114
TEL: (757) 552-7100
FAX: (757) 552-7397
TOLL FREE: (800) 229-1199
IN-STATE: (800) 229-8822

SENTRY INSURANCE A MUTUAL CO

NATIONAL CLAIMS OFFICE
9060 E VIALINDA
PO BOX 29460
PHOENIX, AZ 85038
TEL: (602) 860-7000
FAX: (602) 860-7987
TOLL FREE: (800) 833-2244
WWW.SENTRYINSURANCE.COM

WISCONSIN CLAIMS OFFICE
1800 N POINT DR
STEVENS POINT, WI 54481
TEL: (715) 346-6000
FAX: (715) 346-6161
TOLL FREE: (800) 638-8763
WWW.SENTRYINSURANCE.COM

SENTRY INSURANCE GROUP

MASSACHUSETTS CLAIMS OFFICE
3 CARLISLE RD
PO BOX 584
WESTFORD, MA 01886-0584
TEL: (508) 392-7000
FAX: (978) 392-7033
TOLL FREE: (800) 225-1390

SENTRY INSURANCE MUTUAL CO

ARIZONA CLAIMS OFFICE
9060 E VIALINDA BLVD
SCOTTSDALE, AZ 85258
TEL: (602) 860-7000
FAX: (602) 860-7987
TOLL FREE: (800) 833-2244

SEQUOIA INSURANCE CO

CALIFORNIA CLAIMS OFFICE
4473 WILLOW RD, STE 105
PLEASANTON, CA 94588
TEL: (925) 416-8070
TOLL FREE: (888) 704-1384
IN-STATE: (800) 227-8642

SERVCO LIFE INSURANCE CO

ARKANSAS CLAIMS OFFICE
13201 NW FWY, STE 701
PO BOX 41194
HOUSTON, TX 77241-1194
TEL: (281) 552-2300
FAX: (713) 580-5080
TOLL FREE: (800) 444-2490

LOUISIANA CLAIMS OFFICE
13201 NW FWY, STE 701
PO BOX 41194
HOUSTON, TX 77241-1194
TEL: (281) 552-2300
FAX: (713) 580-5080
TOLL FREE: (800) 444-2490

MISSISSIPPI CLAIMS OFFICE
13201 NW FWY, STE 701
PO BOX 41194
HOUSTON, TX 77241-1194
TEL: (281) 552-2300
FAX: (713) 580-5080
TOLL FREE: (800) 444-2490

OKLAHOMA CLAIMS OFFICE
13201 NW FWY, STE 701
PO BOX 41194
HOUSTON, TX 77241-1194
TEL: (281) 552-2300
FAX: (713) 580-5080
TOLL FREE: (800) 444-2490

TEXAS CLAIMS OFFICE
13201 NW FWY, STE 701
PO BOX 41194
HOUSTON, TX 77241-1194
TEL: (281) 552-2300
FAX: (713) 580-5080
TOLL FREE: (800) 444-2490

SERVICE LIFE & CASUALTY

ARIZONA CLAIMS OFFICE
6907 CAPITOL OF TX HWY, STE 370
PO BOX 26800
AUSTIN, TX 78755-0800
TEL: (512) 343-0600
FAX: (512) 343-8673
TOLL FREE: (800) 299-6977

LOUISIANA CLAIMS OFFICE
6907 CAPITOL OF TX HWY, STE 370
PO BOX 26800
AUSTIN, TX 78755-0800
TEL: (512) 343-0600
FAX: (512) 343-8673
TOLL FREE: (800) 299-6977

NEW MEXICO CLAIMS OFFICE
6907 CAPITOL OF TX HWY, STE 370
PO BOX 26800
AUSTIN, TX 78755-0800
TEL: (512) 343-0600
FAX: (512) 343-8673
TOLL FREE: (800) 299-6977

SOUTH CAROLINA CLAIMS OFFICE
6907 CAPITOL OF TX HWY, STE 370
PO BOX 26800
AUSTIN, TX 78755-0800
TEL: (512) 343-0600
FAX: (512) 343-8673
TOLL FREE: (800) 299-6977

TEXAS CLAIMS OFFICE
6907 CAPITOL OF TX HWY, STE 370
PO BOX 26800
AUSTIN, TX 78755-0800
TEL: (512) 343-0600
FAX: (512) 343-8673
TOLL FREE: (800) 299-6977

SHAND MORHAN INSURANCE CO

NATIONAL CLAIMS OFFICE
EVANSTON INSURANCE
1007 CHURCH ST
EVANSTON, IL 60201
TEL: (847) 866-2800
FAX: (847) 866-0880
WWW.SHAND.COM

SHEFFIELD OLSON & MCQUEEN, INC

MINNESOTA CLAIMS OFFICE
2145 FORD PKY, STE 300
SAINT PAUL, MN 55116-1862
TEL: (651) 695-2555
FAX: (651) 695-1646
TOLL FREE: (800) 486-7664

SHELBY INSURANCE CO

ALABAMA CLAIMS OFFICE
3760 RIVER RUN DR
PO BOX 43360
BIRMINGHAM, AL 35243
TEL: (205) 970-7000
FAX: (800) 333-0315
TOLL FREE: (800) 443-1573

DELAWARE CLAIMS OFFICE
3760 RIVER RUN DR
PO BOX 43360
BIRMINGHAM, AL 35243
TEL: (205) 970-7000
FAX: (800) 333-0315
TOLL FREE: (800) 443-1573
IN-STATE: (800) 525-9591

INDIANA CLAIMS OFFICE
3760 RIVER RUN DR
PO BOX 43360
BIRMINGHAM, AL 35243
TEL: (205) 970-7000
FAX: (800) 333-0315
TOLL FREE: (800) 443-1573

MARYLAND CLAIMS OFFICE
3760 RIVER RUN DR
PO BOX 43360
BIRMINGHAM, AL 35243
TEL: (205) 970-7000
FAX: (800) 333-0315
TOLL FREE: (800) 443-1573
IN-STATE: (800) 525-9591

NORTH CAROLINA CLAIMS OFFICE
3760 RIVER RUN DR
PO BOX 43360
BIRMINGHAM, AL 35243
TEL: (205) 970-7000
FAX: (800) 333-0315
TOLL FREE: (800) 443-1573

OHIO CLAIMS OFFICE
3760 RIVER RUN DR
PO BOX 43360
BIRMINGHAM, AL 35243
TEL: (205) 970-7000
FAX: (800) 333-0315
TOLL FREE: (800) 443-1573

PENNSYLVANIA CLAIMS OFFICE
3760 RIVER RUN DR
PO BOX 43360
BIRMINGHAM, AL 35243
TEL: (205) 970-7000
FAX: (800) 333-0315
TOLL FREE: (800) 443-1573

TENNESSEE CLAIMS OFFICE
3760 RIVER RUN DR
PO BOX 43360
BIRMINGHAM, AL 35243
TEL: (205) 970-7000
FAX: (800) 333-0315
TOLL FREE: (800) 443-1573
IN-STATE: (800) 999-5246

VIRGINIA CLAIMS OFFICE
3760 RIVER RUN DR
PO BOX 43360
BIRMINGHAM, AL 35243
TEL: (205) 970-7000
FAX: (800) 333-0315
TOLL FREE: (800) 443-1573

WEST VIRGINIA CLAIMS OFFICE
3760 RIVER RUN DR
PO BOX 43360
BIRMINGHAM, AL 35243
TEL: (205) 970-7000
FAX: (800) 333-0315
TOLL FREE: (800) 443-1573
IN-STATE: (800) 525-9591

SHELBY INSURANCE GROUP

TENNESSEE CLAIMS OFFICE
3760 RIVER RUN DR
PO BOX 43360
BIRMINGHAM, AL 35243
TEL: (615) 859-8941
FAX: (800) 294-6867
IN-STATE: (800) 999-5246

SHELTER INSURANCE COMPANIES

ARKANSAS CLAIMS OFFICE
1817 W BROADWAY
COLUMBIA, MO 65218-0001
TEL: (573) 445-8441
FAX: (573) 445-3199
TOLL FREE: (800) 743-5837
WWW.SHELTERINS.COM

COLORADO CLAIMS OFFICE
1817 W BROADWAY
COLUMBIA, MO 65218-0001
TEL: (573) 445-8441
FAX: (573) 445-3199
TOLL FREE: (800) 743-5837
WWW.SHELTERINS.COM

ILLINOIS CLAIMS OFFICE
1817 W BROADWAY
COLUMBIA, MO 65218-0001
TEL: (573) 445-8441
FAX: (573) 445-3199
TOLL FREE: (800) 743-5837
WWW.SHELTERINS.COM

INDIANA CLAIMS OFFICE
1817 W BROADWAY
COLUMBIA, MO 65218-0001
TEL: (573) 445-8441
FAX: (573) 445-3199
TOLL FREE: (800) 743-5837
WWW.SHELTERINS.COM

IOWA CLAIMS OFFICE
1817 W BROADWAY
COLUMBIA, MO 65218-0001
TEL: (573) 445-8441
FAX: (573) 445-3199
TOLL FREE: (800) 743-5837
WWW.SHELTERINS.COM

KANSAS CLAIMS OFFICE
1817 W BROADWAY
COLUMBIA, MO 65218-0001
TEL: (573) 445-8441
FAX: (573) 445-3199
TOLL FREE: (800) 743-5837
WWW.SHELTERINS.COM

KENTUCKY CLAIMS OFFICE
1817 W BROADWAY
COLUMBIA, MO 65218-0001
TEL: (573) 445-8441
FAX: (573) 445-3199
TOLL FREE: (800) 743-5837
WWW.SHELTERINS.COM

LOUISIANA CLAIMS OFFICE
1817 W BROADWAY
COLUMBIA, MO 65218-0001
TEL: (573) 445-8441
FAX: (573) 445-3199
TOLL FREE: (800) 743-5837
WWW.SHELTERINS.COM

MISSISSIPPI CLAIMS OFFICE
1817 W BROADWAY
COLUMBIA, MO 65218-0001
TEL: (573) 445-8441
FAX: (573) 445-3199
TOLL FREE: (800) 743-5837
WWW.SHELTERINS.COM

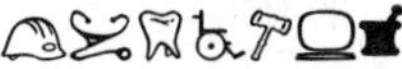

MISSOURI CLAIMS OFFICE
1817 W BROADWAY
COLUMBIA, MO 65218-0001
TEL: (573) 445-8441
FAX: (573) 445-3199
TOLL FREE: (800) 743-5837
WWW.SHELTERINS.COM

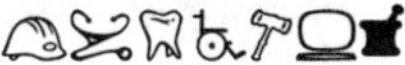

NEBRASKA CLAIMS OFFICE
1817 W BROADWAY
COLUMBIA, MO 65218-0001
TEL: (573) 445-8441
FAX: (573) 445-3199
TOLL FREE: (800) 743-5837
WWW.SHELTERINS.COM

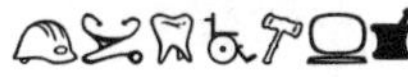

OKLAHOMA CLAIMS OFFICE
1817 W BROADWAY
COLUMBIA, MO 65218-0001
TEL: (573) 445-8441
FAX: (573) 445-3199
TOLL FREE: (800) 743-5837
WWW.SHELTERINS.COM

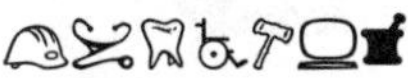

TENNESSEE CLAIMS OFFICE
1817 W BROADWAY
COLUMBIA, MO 65218-0001
TEL: (573) 445-8441
FAX: (573) 445-3199
TOLL FREE: (800) 743-5837
WWW.SHELTERINS.COM

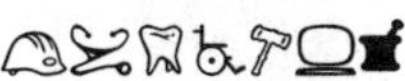

SHENANDOAH LIFE INSURANCE CO

VIRGINIA CLAIMS OFFICE
2301 BRAMBLETON AVE SW
PO BOX 12847
ROANOKE, VA 24029-2847
TEL: (540) 985-4400
FAX: (540) 985-4423
TOLL FREE: (800) 848-5433
WWW.SHENLIFE.COM

SID MURRAY CO

TEXAS CLAIMS OFFICE
4220 S.P.I.D.
PO BOX 270420
CORPUS CHRISTI, TX 78427-0420
TEL: (512) 814-0808
FAX: (512) 814-0824
TOLL FREE: (800) 368-1300

SIERRA HEALTH & LIFE INSURANCE CO, INC

NEVADA CLAIMS OFFICE
2720 N TENAYA WY
PO BOX 15645
LAS VEGAS, NV 89114-5645
TEL: (702) 646-8130
FAX: (702) 242-9350
IN-STATE: (800) 888-2264
WWW.SIERRAHEALTH.COM

SIGMA ADMINISTRATORS

UTAH CLAIMS OFFICE
SELF INSURED GROUP MARKETING & ADMINISTRATION, INC
111 E 5600 S, STE 305
PO BOX 57767
SALT LAKE CITY, UT 84157-0767
TEL: (801) 263-3300
FAX: (801) 263-3319

SIGNA HEALTH CARE/ COMED HMO

NEW JERSEY CLAIMS OFFICE
100 ENTERPRISE DR, STE 610
ROCKAWAY, NJ 07866
TEL: (201) 361-3444
TOLL FREE: (800) 462-6633
WWW.SIGNA.COM

SIGNA HEALTH CARE HEALTHSOURCE

SOUTH CAROLINA CLAIMS OFFICE
HEALTHSOURCE OF SOUTH CAROLINA
146 FAIRCHILD ST
PO BOX 190023
NORTH CHARLESTON, SC 29419-9023
TEL: (843) 884-4063
FAX: (843) 884-6211
TOLL FREE: (800) 962-8811
WWW.HLTHFRC.COM

SIGNA HEALTHCARE

MASSACHUSETTS CLAIMS OFFICE
HEALTHSOURCE OF MASSACHUSETTS
100 FRONT ST, STE 300
WORCESTER, MA 01608-1449
TEL: (508) 799-2642
FAX: (508) 849-4299
TOLL FREE: (800) 244-1870
IN-STATE: (800) 922-8380
WWW.SIGNAHEALTHCARE.COM

SIGNATURE GROUP

ILLINOIS CLAIMS OFFICE
200 N MARTINGALE
SCHAUMBURG, IL 60173
TEL: (847) 605-3000
FAX: (630) 787-8368
TOLL FREE: (800) 621-0393

SIGNET REINSURANCE CO

NEW JERSEY CLAIMS OFFICE
100 CAMPUS DR
PO BOX 0853
FLORHAM PARK, NJ 07932-0853
TEL: (973) 301-8000
FAX: (973) 301-8155
WWW.WRBC.COM

SILVER STATE MEDICAL ADMINISTRATORS

NEVADA CLAIMS OFFICE
PRIME SILVER STATE
2085 E SAHARA, STE B
PO BOX 14790
LAS VEGAS, NV 89114
TEL: (702) 732-0292
FAX: (800) 280-3782
TOLL FREE: (800) 230-3904

SM ADMINISTRATORS

OREGON CLAIMS OFFICE
PO BOX 695
EUGENE, OR 97440-0695
TEL: (541) 465-9322
FAX: (541) 465-9277
TOLL FREE: (800) 533-5513

SOCIETY'S INSURANCE

ILLINOIS CLAIMS OFFICE
SOCIETY'S INSURANCE: A MUTUAL COMPANY
PO BOX 1029
FOND DU LAC, WI 54936-1029
TEL: (920) 922-1220
FAX: (920) 922-9810
TOLL FREE: (800) 242-9703
IN-STATE: (888) 576-2438
WWW.SOCIETYINSURANCE.COM

INDIANA CLAIMS OFFICE
SOCIETY'S INSURANCE: A MUTUAL COMPANY
PO BOX 1029
FOND DU LAC, WI 54936-1029
TEL: (920) 922-1220
FAX: (920) 922-9810
TOLL FREE: (800) 242-9703
IN-STATE: (888) 576-2438
WWW.SOCIETYINSURANCE.COM

IOWA CLAIMS OFFICE
SOCIETY'S INSURANCE: A MUTUAL COMPANY
PO BOX 1029
FOND DU LAC, WI 54936-1029
TEL: (920) 922-1220
FAX: (920) 922-9810
TOLL FREE: (800) 242-9703
IN-STATE: (888) 576-2438
WWW.SOCIETYINSURANCE.COM

WISCONSIN CLAIMS OFFICE
SOCIETY'S INSURANCE: A MUTUAL COMPANY
PO BOX 1029
FOND DU LAC, WI 54936-1029
TEL: (920) 922-1220
FAX: (920) 922-9810
TOLL FREE: (800) 242-9703
IN-STATE: (888) 576-2438
WWW.SOCIETYINSURANCE.COM

SONS OF NORWAY

MINNESOTA CLAIMS OFFICE
1455 W LK ST
MINNEAPOLIS, MN 55408-2666
TEL: (612) 827-3611
FAX: (612) 827-0658
TOLL FREE: (800) 945-8851
WWW.SOFN.COM

S

SOUTH CAROLINA FARM BUREAU MUTUAL INSURANCE CO

SOUTH CAROLINA CLAIMS OFFICE
724 KNOX ABBOTT DR
PO BOX 2124
WEST COLUMBIA, SC 29171-2124
TEL: (803) 796-6700
FAX: (803) 791-4013
WWW.SCFBINS.COM

SOUTHEASTERN INDIANA HEALTH ORGANIZATION

INDIANA CLAIMS OFFICE
432 WASHINGTON ST
PO BOX 1787
COLUMBUS, IN 47202-1787
TEL: (812) 378-7000
FAX: (812) 378-7048
TOLL FREE: (800) 443-2980
WWW.SIHO.ORG

S

SOUTHERN BENEFIT ADMINISTRATORS, INC

TENNESSEE CLAIMS OFFICE
907 TWO MILE PKY, BLDG C
PO BOX 1449
GOODLETTSVILLE, TN 37070-1449
TEL: (615) 859-0131
FAX: (615) 859-0818
TOLL FREE: (800) 831-4914

TEXAS CLAIMS OFFICE
907 TWO MILE PKY, BLDG C
PO BOX 1449
GOODLETTSVILLE, TN 37070-1449
TEL: (615) 859-0131
FAX: (615) 859-0818
TOLL FREE: (800) 831-4914

SOUTHERN CALIFORNIA EDISON CO

CALIFORNIA CLAIMS OFFICE
8631 RUSH ST
PO BOX 800
ROSEMEAD, CA 91770-0900
TEL: (626) 302-1212
FAX: (626) 302-6988

WORKERS COMP
PO BOX 5038
ROSEMEAD, CA 91770
TEL: (626) 302-6890
FAX: (626) 302-4790

SOUTHERN CALIFORNIA PIPE TRADES TRUST FUND

501 SHATTO PL- 5TH FL
LOS ANGELES, CA 90020-1713
TEL: (213) 385-6161
FAX: (213) 487-3640
IN-STATE: (800) 595-7473

SOUTHERN GROUP ADMINISTRATORS, INC

NATIONAL CLAIMS OFFICE
200 S MARSHALL ST
WINSTON-SALEM, NC 27101-5251
TEL: (336) 723-7111
FAX: (336) 722-4748
TOLL FREE: (800) 334-8159

SOUTHERN GUARANTY INSURANCE CO

ALABAMA CLAIMS OFFICE
PO BOX 235004
MONTGOMERY, AL 36123-5004
TEL: (334) 270-6000
FAX: (334) 270-6115
TOLL FREE: (800) 633-5606
WWW.SGIC.COM

ARKANSAS CLAIMS OFFICE
PO BOX 235004
MONTGOMERY, AL 36123-5004
TEL: (334) 270-6000
FAX: (334) 270-6115
TOLL FREE: (800) 633-5606
WWW.SGIC.COM

FLORIDA CLAIMS OFFICE
PO BOX 235004
MONTGOMERY, AL 36123-5004
TEL: (334) 270-6000
FAX: (334) 270-6115
TOLL FREE: (800) 633-5606
WWW.SGIC.COM

GEORGIA CLAIMS OFFICE
1922 N LAKE PARKWAY
PO BOX 450409
ATLANTA, GA 31145-0409
TEL: (770) 493-1931
FAX: (770) 493-1220

MISSISSIPPI CLAIMS OFFICE
PO BOX 235004
MONTGOMERY, AL 36123-5004
TEL: (334) 270-6000
FAX: (334) 270-6115
TOLL FREE: (800) 633-5606
WWW.SGIC.COM

SOUTHERN HEALTH PLAN, INC

TENNESSEE CLAIMS OFFICE
APPLE PLAN
600 JEFFERSON AVE
PO BOX 97
MEMPHIS, TN 38101-0097
TEL: (901) 544-2636
FAX: (901) 544-2440
TOLL FREE: (800) 527-9206

SOUTHERN HEALTH SERVICES

VIRGINIA CLAIMS OFFICE
9881 MAYLAND DR
PO BOX 85603
RICHMOND, VA 23285-5603
TEL: (804) 747-3700
FAX: (804) 747-8723
TOLL FREE: (800) 627-4872
WWW.SOUTHERNHEALTH.COM

SOUTHERN INSURANCE MANAGEMENT ASSOCIATION

ALABAMA CLAIMS OFFICE
1812 UNIVERSITY BLVD
PO BOX 1250
TUSCALOOSA, AL 35403-1250
TEL: (205) 345-3505
TOLL FREE: (800) 476-9928

SOUTHERN RISK SERVICES, INC

2211 7TH AVE S
PO BOX 2408
BIRMINGHAM, AL 35201-2408
TEL: (205) 252-9870
FAX: (205) 581-9172
TOLL FREE: (800) 277-7500
WWW.SOUTHERNRISK.COM

ARKANSAS CLAIMS OFFICE
5333 WESTHEIMER, STE 600
HOUSTON, TX 77056
TEL: (713) 877-8975
FAX: (713) 629-9205
TOLL FREE: (800) 877-1449

LOUISIANA CLAIMS OFFICE
5333 WESTHEIMER, STE 600
HOUSTON, TX 77056
TEL: (713) 877-8975
FAX: (713) 629-9205
TOLL FREE: (800) 877-1449

MISSISSIPPI CLAIMS OFFICE
2093 LAKELAND DR
PO BOX 14248
JACKSON, MS 39236-4248
TEL: (601) 362-1973
FAX: (601) 366-3769
TOLL FREE: (800) 277-8127
WWW.SOUTHERNRISK.COM

NEW MEXICO CLAIMS OFFICE
1650 UNIVERSITY BLVD, STE 320
ALBUQUERQUE, NM 87102
TEL: (505) 244-1451
FAX: (505) 244-1479
TOLL FREE: (800) 787-8374

5333 WESTHEIMER, STE 600
HOUSTON, TX 77056
TEL: (713) 877-8975
FAX: (713) 629-9205
TOLL FREE: (800) 877-1449

NORTH CAROLINA CLAIMS OFFICE
PO BOX 19500
RALEIGH, NC 27619
TEL: (919) 845-8628
FAX: (919) 847-6192
TOLL FREE: (800) 258-0278

Casualty/Liability Dental Disability EMC HCPCS Home Health HMO Medical

OHIO CLAIMS OFFICE
1650 UNIVERSITY BLVD, STE 320
ALBUQUERQUE, NM 87102
TEL: (505) 244-1451
FAX: (505) 244-1479
TOLL FREE: (800) 787-8374

OKLAHOMA CLAIMS OFFICE
5333 WESTHEIMER, STE 600
HOUSTON, TX 77056
TEL: (713) 877-8975
FAX: (713) 629-9205
TOLL FREE: (800) 877-1449

SOUTH CAROLINA CLAIMS OFFICE
PO BOX 19500
RALEIGH, NC 27619
TEL: (919) 845-8628
FAX: (919) 847-6192
TOLL FREE: (800) 258-0278

TEXAS CLAIMS OFFICE
5333 WESTHEIMER, STE 600
HOUSTON, TX 77056
TEL: (713) 877-8975
FAX: (713) 629-9205
TOLL FREE: (800) 877-1449

1650 UNIVERSITY BLVD, STE 320
ALBUQUERQUE, NM 87102
TEL: (505) 244-1451
FAX: (505) 244-1479
TOLL FREE: (800) 787-8374

VIRGINIA CLAIMS OFFICE
PO BOX 19500
RALEIGH, NC 27619
TEL: (919) 845-8628
FAX: (919) 847-6192
TOLL FREE: (800) 258-0278

SOUTHERN TRUST INSURANCE CO

GEORGIA CLAIMS OFFICE
5444 RIVERSIDE DR
PO BOX 250
MACON, GA 31202-0250
TEL: (912) 743-7442
FAX: (912) 738-0457
TOLL FREE: (800) 476-5566

SOUTHLAND LIFE INSURANCE CO

5780 POWERS FERRY RD NW
PO BOX 105006
ATLANTA, GA 30348-5006
TEL: (770) 980-5100
FAX: (770) 980-5112
WWW.ING.COM

SOUTHLAND NATIONAL INSURANCE CORP

ALABAMA CLAIMS OFFICE
1812 UNIVERSITY BLVD
TUSCALOOSA, AL 35401
TEL: (205) 345-7410
FAX: (205) 343-1239
TOLL FREE: (800) 277-8762

SOUTHWEST ADMINISTRATORS

CALIFORNIA CLAIMS OFFICE
1000 S FREEMONT AVE
PO BOX 1121
ALHAMBRA, CA 91802-1121
TEL: (626) 284-4792

SOUTHWEST BUSINESS CORP

TEXAS CLAIMS OFFICE
9311 SAN PEDRO, STE 600
PO BOX 795027
SAN ANTONIO, TX 78279-5027
TEL: (210) 525-1241
FAX: (210) 525-9407
TOLL FREE: (800) 527-0066
WWW.SWBC.COM

SOUTHWEST HEALTH ALLIANCES

DBA FIRSTCARE
12940 RESEARCH BLVD
AUSTIN, TX 78750
TEL: (806) 356-5151
FAX: (806) 356-5278
TOLL FREE: (800) 431-7737

SOUTHWEST SERVICE ADMINISTRATORS, INC

NEW MEXICO CLAIMS OFFICE
4775 INDIAN SCHOOL RD NE, STE 105
ALBUQUERQUE, NM 87110
TEL: (505) 265-8422
FAX: (505) 266-9358
TOLL FREE: (800) 432-6636
IN-STATE: (800) 432-6636

SOUTHWIRE CO

NATIONAL CLAIMS OFFICE
ONE SOUTHWIRE DR
PO BOX 1000
CARROLLTON, GA 30119-0001
TEL: (770) 832-4242
FAX: (770) 832-4038
TOLL FREE: (800) 444-1700
WWW.SOUTHWIRE.COM

SPECIAL AGENTS MUTUAL BENEFIT ASSOCIATION

MARYLAND CLAIMS OFFICE
11301 OLD GEORGETOWN RD
ROCKVILLE, MD 20852-2800
TEL: (301) 984-1440
FAX: (301) 984-6224
TOLL FREE: (800) 638-6589
WWW.SAMBA-INSURANCE.COM

SPECTARA

2811 LORD BALTIMORE DR
BALTIMORE, MD 21244-2644
TEL: (410) 265-6033
FAX: (410) 944-5118
TOLL FREE: (800) 638-6265
IN-STATE: (800) 638-6265
WWW.SPECTARA.COM

SRC SERVICES, INC

SOUTH CAROLINA CLAIMS OFFICE
115 ATRIUM WAY, STE 210
PO BOX 23759
COLUMBIA, SC 29224-3759
TEL: (803) 736-1999
FAX: (803) 736-9952
TOLL FREE: (800) 869-0808

ST. FRANCIS HOME CARE

414 PETTIGRU ST
PO BOX 9312
GREENVILLE, SC 29605
TEL: (864) 233-5300
FAX: (864) 233-8473
WWW.STFRANCIS.COM

ST. LOUIS LABOR HEALTH INSTITUTE

MISSOURI CLAIMS OFFICE
300 S GRANDE BLVD
SAINT LOUIS, MO 63103-2430
TEL: (314) 658-5627
FAX: (314) 652-5022
TOLL FREE: (800) 466-5688

ST. PAUL COMPANIES

ILLINOIS CLAIMS OFFICE
PO BOX 706
SIKESTON, MO 63801-0706
TEL: (573) 472-4999
FAX: (573) 472-4116
TOLL FREE: (800) 873-2634

MISSOURI CLAIMS OFFICE
PO BOX 706
SIKESTON, MO 63801-0706
TEL: (573) 472-4999
FAX: (573) 472-4116
TOLL FREE: (800) 873-2634

VIRGINIA CLAIMS OFFICE
PO BOX 26267
RICHMOND, VA 23260
TEL: (804) 747-0300
FAX: (804) 965-1505
TOLL FREE: (800) 873-2634
IN-STATE: (800) 552-2140

PO BOX 20709
ROANOKE, VA 24018-0522
TEL: (540) 989-7156
FAX: (540) 989-1475
IN-STATE: (800) 552-6908

WEST VIRGINIA CLAIMS OFFICE
1409 GREENBRIER ST, STE 201
CHARLESTON, WV 25311-1005
TEL: (304) 344-1692
FAX: (304) 340-4314
TOLL FREE: (800) 242-8734
IN-STATE: (800) 242-8734

ST. PAUL/ ECONOMY FIRE & CASUALTY

ILLINOIS CLAIMS OFFICE
500 ECONOMY CT
PO BOX 441
FREEPORT, IL 61032-0441
TEL: (815) 266-5661
FAX: (815) 266-5623
TOLL FREE: (800) 608-2050

ST. PAUL FIRE & MARINE

MARYLAND CLAIMS OFFICE
NORTHBROOK INSURANCE
5801 CENTENNIAL WY
BALTIMORE, MD 21209
TEL: (410) 205-3000
TOLL FREE: (800) 877-3854
WWW.STPAUL.COM

ST. PAUL FIRE & MARINE INC

ALASKA CLAIMS OFFICE
700 FIFTH AVE, STE 4200
SEATTLE, WA 98104-5028
TEL: (206) 285-3636
FAX: (206) 286-2348
TOLL FREE: (800) 873-2634

IDAHO CLAIMS OFFICE
700 FIFTH AVE, STE 4200
SEATTLE, WA 98104-5028
TEL: (206) 285-3636
FAX: (206) 286-2348
TOLL FREE: (800) 873-2634

OREGON CLAIMS OFFICE
700 FIFTH AVE, STE 4200
SEATTLE, WA 98104-5028
TEL: (206) 285-3636
FAX: (206) 286-2348
TOLL FREE: (800) 873-2634

WASHINGTON CLAIMS OFFICE
700 FIFTH AVE, STE 4200
SEATTLE, WA 98104-5028
TEL: (206) 285-3636
FAX: (206) 286-2348
TOLL FREE: (800) 873-2634

ST. PAUL REINSURANCE MANAGEMENT CO

NEW YORK CLAIMS OFFICE
195 BROADWAY- 28TH FL
NEW YORK, NY 10007
TEL: (212) 238-9200
FAX: (212) 619-4092

STANDARD INSURANCE CO

NATIONAL CLAIMS OFFICE
1100 SW 6TH
PO BOX 711
PORTLAND, OR 97207
TEL: (503) 321-7000
FAX: (503) 321-6776
WWW.STANDARD.COM

STANDARD LIFE & ACCIDENT INSURANCE CO

TEXAS CLAIMS OFFICE
ONE MOODY PLZ
PO BOX 1800
GALVESTON, TX 77553
TEL: (405) 290-1000
FAX: (409) 766-6663
TOLL FREE: (800) 827-2524

STANDARD LIFE & CASUALTY INSURANCE CO OF FORT MILL, SC

SOUTH CAROLINA CLAIMS OFFICE
PO BOX 1514
FORT MILL, SC 29716
TEL: (803) 548-3657
FAX: (803) 548-3672
TOLL FREE: (800) 227-0251

STANDARD MUTUAL INSURANCE CO

ILLINOIS CLAIMS OFFICE
PO BOX 19267
SPRINGFIELD, IL 62794-9267
TEL: (217) 546-2894
FAX: (217) 793-1216
IN-STATE: (800) 252-8927
WWW.STANDARDMUTUAL.COM

INDIANA CLAIMS OFFICE
PO BOX 19267
SPRINGFIELD, IL 62794-9267
TEL: (217) 546-2894
FAX: (217) 793-1216
IN-STATE: (800) 252-8927
WWW.STANDARDMUTUAL.COM

STAR INSURANCE CO

MICHIGAN CLAIMS OFFICE
26600 TELEGRAPH RD
SOUTHFIELD, MI 48034-2438
TEL: (248) 358-4020
FAX: (248) 358-1614
TOLL FREE: (800) 482-2726
IN-STATE: (800) 482-0626
WWW.MEADOWBROOKINSGRP.COM

STATE AUTOMOBILE MUTUAL INSURANCE CO

ARKANSAS CLAIMS OFFICE
STATE AUTO INSURANCE COMPANIES
100 STATE AUTO BLVD
GOODLETTSVILLE, TN 37072-3130
TEL: (615) 851-6400
FAX: (615) 851-6664
TOLL FREE: (800) 234-1554

KENTUCKY CLAIMS OFFICE
STATE AUTO INSURANCE COMPANIES
100 STATE AUTO BLVD
GOODLETTSVILLE, TN 37072-3130
TEL: (615) 851-6400
FAX: (615) 851-6664
TOLL FREE: (800) 234-1554

MICHIGAN CLAIMS OFFICE
17197 N LAUREL PARK DR, STE 167
LIVONIA, MI 48152-2686
TEL: (734) 462-6100
FAX: (734) 462-6105
TOLL FREE: (800) 888-5469

MISSISSIPPI CLAIMS OFFICE
STATE AUTO INSURANCE COMPANIES
100 STATE AUTO BLVD
GOODLETTSVILLE, TN 37072-3130
TEL: (615) 851-6400
FAX: (615) 851-6664
TOLL FREE: (800) 234-1554

MISSOURI CLAIMS OFFICE
STATE AUTO INSURANCE COMPANIES
100 STATE AUTO BLVD
GOODLETTSVILLE, TN 37072-3130
TEL: (615) 851-6400
FAX: (615) 851-6664
TOLL FREE: (800) 234-1554

OHIO CLAIMS OFFICE
518 E BROAD ST
COLUMBUS, OH 43215-3976
TEL: (614) 464-5000
FAX: (614) 464-4868
TOLL FREE: (800) 444-9950
WWW.STATEAUTO.COM

OKLAHOMA CLAIMS OFFICE
STATE AUTO INSURANCE COMPANIES
100 STATE AUTO BLVD
GOODLETTSVILLE, TN 37072-3130
TEL: (615) 851-6400
FAX: (615) 851-6664
TOLL FREE: (800) 234-1554

PENNSYLVANIA CLAIMS OFFICE
STATE AUTO INSURANCE COMPANIES
4900 RITTER RD
PO BOX 2006
MECHANICSBURG, PA 17055-0733
TEL: (717) 697-1121
FAX: (717) 697-2803
TOLL FREE: (800) 288-1872

SOUTH CAROLINA CLAIMS OFFICE
STATE AUTO INSURANCE COMPANIES
112 S MAIN ST
PO BOX 199
GREER, SC 29652-0199
TEL: (864) 877-3311
FAX: (864) 968-2450
TOLL FREE: (800) 234-1878
WWW.STATE-AUTO-INS.COM

S

TENNESSEE CLAIMS OFFICE
STATE AUTO INSURANCE COMPANIES
100 STATE AUTO BLVD
GOODLETTSVILLE, TN 37072-3130
TEL: (615) 851-6400
FAX: (615) 851-6664
TOLL FREE: (800) 234-1554

STATE COMPENSATION INSURANCE FUND

CALIFORNIA CLAIMS OFFICE
STATE FUND
1504 4TH ST
PO BOX 7455
SAN FRANCISCO, CA 94103
TEL: (415) 974-8000
FAX: (415) 974-8090
WWW.SCIF.COM

900 CORP CENTER DR
MONTEREY PARK, CA 91754
TEL: (323) 266-5000
FAX: (323) 264-6129
TOLL FREE: (888) 222-3211
WWW.SCIF.COM

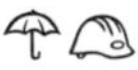

9801 CAMINO MEDIA
PO BOX 21810
BAKERSFIELD, CA 93390-1810
TEL: (805) 664-4000
FAX: (805) 664-4101
TOLL FREE: (888) 394-6262
WWW.SCIF.COM

10 RIVERPARK PLACE E
PO BOX 40000
FRESNO, CA 93755-4000
TEL: (559) 433-2700
FAX: (559) 433-2750
WWW.SCIF.COM

2955 PERALTA OAKS CT
PO BOX 12971
OAKLAND, CA 94604-2971
TEL: (510) 577-3000
FAX: (510) 729-7877
TOLL FREE: (888) 222-3211
WWW.SCIF.COM

2901 N VENTURA RD
PO BOX 9045
OXNARD, CA 93031-9045
TEL: (805) 988-5549
FAX: (805) 988-5528
TOLL FREE: (888) 222-3211
WWW.SCIF.COM

364 KNOLLCREST DR
PO BOX 496049
REDDING, CA 96049-6049
TEL: (530) 223-7000
FAX: (530) 223-7044
WWW.SCIF.COM

2275 GATEWAY OAKS
PO BOX 254700
SACRAMENTO, CA 95865-4700
TEL: (916) 924-5155
FAX: (916) 924-6888
WWW.SCIF.COM

375 W HOSPITALITY LN
PO BOX 1316
SAN BERNARDINO, CA 92402-1316
TEL: (909) 884-7281
FAX: (909) 384-4646
IN-STATE: (800) 342-7214
WWW.SCIF.COM

9444 WAPLES ST
PO BOX 85488
SAN DIEGO, CA 92186-5488
TEL: (619) 552-7100
FAX: (619) 552-7110
WWW.SCIF.COM

6203 SANIGNACIO AVE
PO BOX 530957
SAN JOSE, CA 95153-5357
TEL: (408) 363-7600
FAX: (408) 363-7866
WWW.SCIF.COM

1750 E 4TH ST
PO BOX 419
SANTA ANA, CA 92702-0419
TEL: (714) 565-5000
FAX: (714) 565-5801
WWW.SCIF.COM

1450 NEOTOMAS AVE
PO BOX 2407
SANTA ROSA, CA 95405-0407
TEL: (707) 573-6500
FAX: (707) 573-6504
WWW.SCIF.COM

3247 W MARCH LANE
PO BOX 8000
STOCKTON, CA 95208
TEL: (209) 476-2600
FAX: (209) 476-2750
IN-STATE: (800) 467-8437
WWW.SCIF.COM

21300 VICTORY BLVD, STE 500
PO BOX 1950
WOODLAND HILLS, CA 91365-1950
TEL: (818) 888-4750
FAX: (818) 713-2475
TOLL FREE: (888) 222-3211
WWW.SCIF.COM

STATE FARM INSURANCE CO

ALABAMA CLAIMS OFFICE
100 STATE FARM PKY
PO BOX 2661
BIRMINGHAM, AL 35297-0001
TEL: (205) 916-6000
WWW.STATEFARM.COM

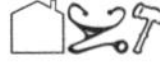

ARIZONA CLAIMS OFFICE
SUNLAND
1665 W ALAMEDA DR
TEMPE, AZ 85289-0001
TEL: (602) 784-3000
FAX: (602) 784-3870
WWW.STATEFARM.COM

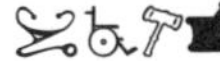

CALIFORNIA CLAIMS OFFICE
6400 STATE FARM DR
ROHNERT PARK, CA 94926-0002
TEL: (707) 588-6011
FAX: (707) 588-6100
WWW.STATEFARM.COM

31303 AGOURA RD
WESTLAKE VILLAGE, CA 91363-0001
TEL: (818) 707-5858
FAX: (818) 707-5346
WWW.STATEFARM.COM

COLORADO CLAIMS OFFICE
4645 W 18TH ST
GREELEY, CO 80634
TEL: (970) 339-1802
FAX: (970) 339-1898
WWW.STATEFARM.COM

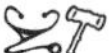

FLORIDA CLAIMS OFFICE
8001 BAYMEADOWS WAY
PO BOX 45061
JACKSONVILLE, FL 32232-5061
TEL: (904) 443-4000
FAX: (904) 443-5750
WWW.STATEFARM.COM

7401 CYPRESS GARDENS BLVD
WINTER HAVEN, FL 33888
TEL: (941) 318-3163
FAX: (941) 318-4081

ILLINOIS CLAIMS OFFICE
ONE STATE FARM PLZ
PO BOX 2700
BLOOMINGTON, IL 61710
TEL: (309) 766-2311
TOLL FREE: (800) 538-4643
WWW.STATEFARM.COM

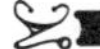

HEALTH CLAIM DEPARTMENT
2702 IRELAND GROVE RD
BLOOMINGTON, IL 61709-0001
TEL: (309) 763-0612
FAX: (309) 763-1346
WWW.STATEFARM.COM

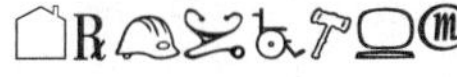

INDIANA CLAIMS OFFICE
3701 ROME DR
PO BOX 7620
LAFAYETTE, IN 47903
TEL: (765) 449-9500
FAX: (765) 449-9537
WWW.STATEFARM.COM

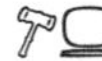

2550 NORTHWESTERN AVE
WEST LAFAYETTE, IN 47906-1332
TEL: (765) 463-8123
FAX: (765) 463-8446
WWW.STATEFARM.COM

1440 GRANVILLE RD
PO BOX 3020
NEWARK, OH 43093-0001
TEL: (740) 364-5972
FAX: (740) 364-3519
WWW.STATEFARM.COM

KENTUCKY CLAIMS OFFICE
2500 MEMORIAL BLVD
MURFREESBORO, TN 37131-0001
TEL: (615) 898-6000
FAX: (615) 898-6143
WWW.STATEFARM.COM

LOUISIANA CLAIMS OFFICE
100 STATE FARM PKY
PO BOX 2661
BIRMINGHAM, AL 35297-0001
TEL: (205) 916-6000
WWW.STATEFARM.COM

MARYLAND CLAIMS OFFICE
1715 GWYNN OAK AVE
BALTIMORE, MD 21207-5280
TEL: (410) 265-6600
FAX: (410) 455-4862
IN-STATE: (800) 492-7055
WWW.STATEFARM.COM

MICHIGAN CLAIMS OFFICE
410 E DR
MARSHALL, MI 49069-0002
TEL: (616) 789-5000
FAX: (616) 789-5619
WWW.STATEFARM.COM

1440 GRANVILLE RD
PO BOX 3020
NEWARK, OH 43093-0001
TEL: (740) 364-5972
FAX: (740) 364-3519
WWW.STATEFARM.COM

MINNESOTA CLAIMS OFFICE
8500 STATE FARM WAY
SAINT PAUL, MN 55125
TEL: (612) 631-4000
FAX: (612) 631-5823
WWW.STATEFARM.COM

MISSOURI CLAIMS OFFICE
HEALTH CLAIM DEPARTMENT
2702 IRELAND GROVE RD
BLOOMINGTON, IL 61709-0001
TEL: (309) 763-0612
FAX: (309) 763-1346
WWW.STATEFARM.COM

NEBRASKA CLAIMS OFFICE
222 S 84TH ST
PO BOX 82542
LINCOLN, NE 68510-2600
TEL: (402) 486-5000
WWW.STATEFARM.COM

OHIO CLAIMS OFFICE
1440 GRANVILLE RD
PO BOX 3020
NEWARK, OH 43093-0001
TEL: (740) 364-5972
FAX: (740) 364-3519
WWW.STATEFARM.COM

PENNSYLVANIA CLAIMS OFFICE
ONE STATE FARM DR
CONCORDVILLE, PA 19339-1000
TEL: (610) 358-7000
WWW.STATEFARM.COM

TENNESSEE CLAIMS OFFICE
2500 MEMORIAL BLVD
MURFREESBORO, TN 37131-0001
TEL: (615) 898-6000
FAX: (615) 898-6143
WWW.STATEFARM.COM

TEXAS CLAIMS OFFICE
8900 STATE FARM WAY
AUSTIN, TX 78729
TEL: (512) 918-4000
FAX: (512) 918-5298
WWW.STATEFARM.COM

17301 PRESTON RD
PO BOX 799100
DALLAS, TX 75252
TEL: (972) 732-5000
FAX: (972) 732-5625
WWW.STATEFARM.COM

UTAH CLAIMS OFFICE
4140 W PARRISH LN
PO BOX 369
CENTERVILLE, UT 84014
TEL: (801) 296-5000
FAX: (801) 296-5033
WWW.STATEFARM.COM

1245 E BRICKYARD RD, STE 70
SALT LAKE CITY, UT 84106
TEL: (801) 956-4000
FAX: (801) 485-2760
WWW.STATEFARM.COM

10585 S STATE
PO BOX 1159
SANDY, UT 84091-1159
TEL: (801) 576-4100
FAX: (801) 576-4139
WWW.STATEFARM.COM

VIRGINIA CLAIMS OFFICE
1500 STATE FARM BLVD
CHARLOTTESVILLE, VA 22909-0001
TEL: (804) 972-5000
FAX: (804) 972-5026
WWW.STATEFARM.COM

STATE LIFE INSURANCE CO

INDIANA CLAIMS OFFICE
141 E WASHINGTON ST
PO BOX 406
INDIANAPOLIS, IN 46206-0406
TEL: (317) 681-5300
FAX: (317) 681-5492
TOLL FREE: (800) 428-2316
WWW.AUL.COM

STATE LINE TPA

OHIO CLAIMS OFFICE
1718 INDIAN WOOD CIR, STE E
MAUMEE, OH 43537
TEL: (419) 897-1400
FAX: (419) 897-9648
TOLL FREE: (800) 428-8194

STATE OF ALASKA WORKERS COMP DIVISION

ALASKA CLAIMS OFFICE
3301 EAGLE
PO BOX 107019
ANCHORAGE, AK 99510-7019
TEL: (907) 269-4980
FAX: (907) 269-4975
WWW.LABOR.STATE.AK.US/WC/WC/HTM

STATE OF NEW YORK INSURANCE DEPARTMENT LIQUIDATION BUREAU

NEW YORK CLAIMS OFFICE
123 WILLIAM ST
NEW YORK, NY 10038-3804
TEL: (212) 341-6400
FAX: (212) 341-6104

STATES GENERAL INSURANCE CO

ALABAMA CLAIMS OFFICE
115 W 7TH ST, STE 1205
FT WORTH, TX 76102
TEL: (817) 338-4395
FAX: (817) 338-1076
TOLL FREE: (800) 782-8375

ARIZONA CLAIMS OFFICE
115 W 7TH ST, STE 1205
FT WORTH, TX 76102
TEL: (817) 338-4395
FAX: (817) 338-1076
TOLL FREE: (800) 782-8375

ARKANSAS CLAIMS OFFICE
115 W 7TH ST, STE 1205
FT WORTH, TX 76102
TEL: (817) 338-4395
FAX: (817) 338-1076
TOLL FREE: (800) 782-8375

FLORIDA CLAIMS OFFICE
115 W 7TH ST, STE 1205
FT WORTH, TX 76102
TEL: (817) 338-4395
FAX: (817) 338-1076
TOLL FREE: (800) 782-8375

KANSAS CLAIMS OFFICE
115 W 7TH ST, STE 1205
FT WORTH, TX 76102
TEL: (817) 338-4395
FAX: (817) 338-1076
TOLL FREE: (800) 782-8375

LOUISIANA CLAIMS OFFICE
115 W 7TH ST, STE 1205
FT WORTH, TX 76102
TEL: (817) 338-4395
FAX: (817) 338-1076
TOLL FREE: (800) 782-8375

MISSISSIPPI CLAIMS OFFICE
115 W 7TH ST, STE 1205
FT WORTH, TX 76102
TEL: (817) 338-4395
FAX: (817) 338-1076
TOLL FREE: (800) 782-8375

NEW MEXICO CLAIMS OFFICE
115 W 7TH ST, STE 1205
FT WORTH, TX 76102
TEL: (817) 338-4395
FAX: (817) 338-1076
TOLL FREE: (800) 782-8375

TEXAS CLAIMS OFFICE
CORPORATE OFFICE
115 W 7TH ST, STE 1205
FT WORTH, TX 76102
TEL: (817) 338-4395
FAX: (817) 338-1076
TOLL FREE: (800) 782-8375

UTAH CLAIMS OFFICE
115 W 7TH ST, STE 1205
FT WORTH, TX 76102
TEL: (817) 338-4395
FAX: (817) 338-1076
TOLL FREE: (800) 782-8375

STATES WEST LIFE INSURANCE CO

ALASKA CLAIMS OFFICE
7001-220TH ST SW
PO BOX 2272
SEATTLE, WA 98111-2272
TEL: (425) 670-4575
FAX: (425) 670-4485

ARIZONA CLAIMS OFFICE
7001-220TH ST SW
PO BOX 2272
SEATTLE, WA 98111-2272
TEL: (425) 670-4575
FAX: (425) 670-4485

CALIFORNIA CLAIMS OFFICE
7001-220TH ST SW
PO BOX 2272
SEATTLE, WA 98111-2272
TEL: (425) 670-4575
FAX: (425) 670-4485

IDAHO CLAIMS OFFICE
7001-220TH ST SW
PO BOX 2272
SEATTLE, WA 98111-2272
TEL: (425) 670-4575
FAX: (425) 670-4485

MONTANA CLAIMS OFFICE
7001-220TH ST SW
PO BOX 2272
SEATTLE, WA 98111-2272
TEL: (425) 670-4575
FAX: (425) 670-4485

NEW MEXICO CLAIMS OFFICE
7001-220TH ST SW
PO BOX 2272
SEATTLE, WA 98111-2272
TEL: (425) 670-4575
FAX: (425) 670-4485

NORTH DAKOTA CLAIMS OFFICE
7001-220TH ST SW
PO BOX 2272
SEATTLE, WA 98111-2272
TEL: (425) 670-4575
FAX: (425) 670-4485

OREGON CLAIMS OFFICE
7001-220TH ST SW
PO BOX 2272
SEATTLE, WA 98111-2272
TEL: (425) 670-4575
FAX: (425) 670-4485

UTAH CLAIMS OFFICE
7001-220TH ST SW
PO BOX 2272
SEATTLE, WA 98111-2272
TEL: (425) 670-4575
FAX: (425) 670-4485

WASHINGTON CLAIMS OFFICE
7001-220TH ST SW
PO BOX 2272
SEATTLE, WA 98111-2272
TEL: (425) 670-4575
FAX: (425) 670-4485

WYOMING CLAIMS OFFICE
7001-220TH ST SW
PO BOX 2272
SEATTLE, WA 98111-2272
TEL: (425) 670-4575
FAX: (425) 670-4485

STATEWIDE INSURANCE CO

NEW YORK CLAIMS OFFICE
20 MAIN ST
HEMPSTEAD, NY 11550
TEL: (516) 564-8000
FAX: (516) 564-8018
TOLL FREE: (800) 499-5646

STONE EAGLE INSURANCE CO

TEXAS CLAIMS OFFICE
14665 MIDWAY RD, STE 200
ADDISON, TX 75001
TEL: (972) 934-1751
FAX: (972) 934-8230
WWW.STONEEAGLE.COM

STUDENT INSURANCE

DIVISION OF UICI
4001 MCEWEN
PO BOX 809025
DALLAS, TX 75380-9025
TEL: (972) 233-8200
FAX: (972) 448-7199
TOLL FREE: (800) 767-0700
IN-STATE: (800) 251-0005
WWW.SID.COM

SUBURBAN HEALTH PLAN

CONNECTICUT CLAIMS OFFICE
680 BRIDGEPORT AVE
PO BOX 336
DERBY, CT 06418
TEL: (203) 734-4466
FAX: (203) 735-4930

H

SUN LIFE ASSURANCE OF CANADA

MASSACHUSETTS CLAIMS OFFICE
ONE SUN LIFE EXECUTIVE PARK
WELLESLEY HILLS, MA 02481
TEL: (781) 237-6030
FAX: (781) 431-7472
TOLL FREE: (800) 247-6875
WWW.SUNLIFE-USA.COM

SUN LIFE OF CANADA

ONTARIO CLAIMS OFFICE
225 KING ST W
PO BOX 4023 STA A
TORONTO, ON M5W-2P7
TEL: (416) 408-7500
FAX: (416) 595-0162

3

SUPERIOR NATIONAL INSURANCE CO

CALIFORNIA CLAIMS OFFICE
SUPERIOR SPECIFIC CASUALTY
26601 AGURA RD
PO BOX 10001
VAN NUYS, CA 91410-0001
TEL: (818) 880-1600
FAX: (818) 880-1654
TOLL FREE: (800) 859-4248
WWW.SUPERIOR.COM

SUPERMARKETS GENERAL CORP

CONNECTICUT CLAIMS OFFICE
PATH MARK STORES, INC
200 MILIK ST
PO BOX 5301
CARTERET, NJ 07095-0915
TEL: (732) 499-3000
FAX: (732) 499-4285
TOLL FREE: (800) 221-0507
WWW.PATHMARK.COM

S

DELAWARE CLAIMS OFFICE
PATH MARK STORES, INC
200 MILIK ST
PO BOX 5301
CARTERET, NJ 07095-0915
TEL: (732) 499-3000
FAX: (732) 499-4285
TOLL FREE: (800) 221-0507
WWW.PATHMARK.COM

NEW JERSEY CLAIMS OFFICE
PATH MARK STORES, INC
200 MILIK ST
PO BOX 5301
CARTERET, NJ 07095-0915
TEL: (732) 499-3000
FAX: (732) 499-4285
TOLL FREE: (800) 221-0507
WWW.PATHMARK.COM

NEW YORK CLAIMS OFFICE
PATH MARK STORES, INC
200 MILIK ST
PO BOX 5301
CARTERET, NJ 07095-0915
TEL: (732) 499-3000
FAX: (732) 499-4285
TOLL FREE: (800) 221-0507
WWW.PATHMARK.COM

PENNSYLVANIA CLAIMS OFFICE
PATH MARK STORES, INC
200 MILIK ST
PO BOX 5301
WOODBRIDGE, NJ 07095-0915
TEL: (908) 499-3000
FAX: (908) 499-4285
TOLL FREE: (800) 221-0507

SURETY AMERICAN LIFE INSURANCE

TEXAS CLAIMS OFFICE
UNITED MERCANTILE LIFE INS CO
5845 ONIX, STE 300
EL PASO, TX 79912-5552
TEL: (915) 585-0292
FAX: (915) 585-9925

SURETY LIFE INSURANCE CO

NEBRASKA CLAIMS OFFICE
206 S 13TH ST, STE 300
PO BOX 82599
LINCOLN, NE 68501
TEL: (402) 479-7845
TOLL FREE: (800) 669-7789
WWW.LDLWATS.COM

UTAH CLAIMS OFFICE
206 S 13TH ST, STE 300
PO BOX 82599
LINCOLN, NE 68501
TEL: (402) 479-7845
TOLL FREE: (800) 669-7789
WWW.LDLWATS.COM

SWANK INC GROUP INSURANCE

MASSACHUSETTS CLAIMS OFFICE
6 HAZEL ST
PO BOX 2962
ATTLEBORO, MA 02703-0962
TEL: (508) 222-3400
FAX: (508) 226-9598

SWISS RE AMERICA

NEW YORK CLAIMS OFFICE
175 KINGS ST
ARMONK, NY 10504
TEL: (914) 828-8000
FAX: (914) 828-7000
TOLL FREE: (800) 223-1919
IN-STATE: (800) 188-SWIS
WWW.SWISSREAMERICA.COM

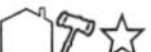

SWISS RE LIFE & HEALTH AMERICA

CONNECTICUT CLAIMS OFFICE
969 HIGH RDG RD
STAMFORD, CT 06905
TEL: (203) 321-3000
FAX: (203) 321-3200
TOLL FREE: (800) 292-2726
WWW.SWISSRE.COM

SWISS REASSURANCE

ONTARIO CLAIMS OFFICE
CANADA TRUST TOWER
161 BAY ST, STE 3000
TORONTO, ON M5J-2T6
TEL: (416) 947-3800
FAX: (416) 866-2112
TOLL FREE: (800) 268-9798
WWW.SWISSRE.COM

SYDNEY REINSURANCE CO

NEW YORK CLAIMS OFFICE
88 PINE ST, 16TH FL
NEW YORK, NY 10005
TEL: (212) 422-1212

T.I.G. INSURANCE

ALASKA CLAIMS OFFICE
2122 E HIGHLAND AVE, STE 300
PO BOX 52106
PHOENIX, AZ 85072-2106
TEL: (602) 808-5700
FAX: (800) 762-6384
TOLL FREE: (800) 336-5118
WWW.TIG1.COM

ARIZONA CLAIMS OFFICE
2122 E HIGHLAND AVE, STE 300
PO BOX 52106
PHOENIX, AZ 85072-2106
TEL: (602) 808-5700
FAX: (800) 762-6384
TOLL FREE: (800) 336-5118
WWW.TIG1.COM

CALIFORNIA CLAIMS OFFICE
1855 GATEWAY BLVD, STE 400
PO BOX 4131
CONCORD, CA 94524
TEL: (925) 603-5000
TOLL FREE: (800) 548-8475
WWW.TIG1.COM

COLORADO CLAIMS OFFICE
PO BOX 17005
DENVER, CO 80217
TEL: (303) 771-7150
FAX: (303) 741-4462
TOLL FREE: (800) 348-6767
IN-STATE: (800) 882-7600
WWW.TIG1.COM

2122 E HIGHLAND AVE, STE 300
PO BOX 52106
PHOENIX, AZ 85072-2106
TEL: (602) 808-5700
FAX: (800) 762-6384
TOLL FREE: (800) 336-5118
WWW.TIG1.COM

IDAHO CLAIMS OFFICE
2122 E HIGHLAND AVE, STE 300
PO BOX 52106
PHOENIX, AZ 85072-2106
TEL: (602) 808-5700
FAX: (800) 762-6384
TOLL FREE: (800) 336-5118
WWW.TIG1.COM

MONTANA CLAIMS OFFICE
2122 E HIGHLAND AVE, STE 300
PO BOX 52106
PHOENIX, AZ 85072-2106
TEL: (602) 808-5700
FAX: (800) 762-6384
TOLL FREE: (800) 336-5118
WWW.TIG1.COM

NEVADA CLAIMS OFFICE
2122 E HIGHLAND AVE, STE 300
PO BOX 52106
PHOENIX, AZ 85072-2106
TEL: (602) 808-5700
FAX: (800) 762-6384
TOLL FREE: (800) 336-5118
WWW.TIG1.COM

OREGON CLAIMS OFFICE
2122 E HIGHLAND AVE, STE 300
PO BOX 52106
PHOENIX, AZ 85072-2106
TEL: (602) 808-5700
FAX: (800) 762-6384
TOLL FREE: (800) 336-5118
WWW.TIG1.COM

WASHINGTON CLAIMS OFFICE
2122 E HIGHLAND AVE, STE 300
PO BOX 52106
PHOENIX, AZ 85072-2106
TEL: (602) 808-5700
FAX: (800) 762-6384
TOLL FREE: (800) 336-5118
WWW.TIG1.COM

T & M FINANCIAL

KANSAS CLAIMS OFFICE
3706 SW TOPEKA BLVD, STE 400
TOPEKA, KS 66609-1292
TEL: (785) 266-8333
FAX: (785) 266-7819

TAYLOR EMPLOYEES HEALTH & DENTAL PLAN

ALABAMA CLAIMS OFFICE
1725 ROE CREST
PO BOX 3728
NORTH MANKATO, MN 56002-3728
TEL: (507) 625-2828
FAX: (507) 625-7742
TOLL FREE: (800) 345-6954

CALIFORNIA CLAIMS OFFICE
1725 ROE CREST
PO BOX 3728
NORTH MANKATO, MN 56002-3728
TEL: (507) 625-2828
FAX: (507) 625-7742
TOLL FREE: (800) 345-6954

FLORIDA CLAIMS OFFICE
1725 ROE CREST
PO BOX 3728
NORTH MANKATO, MN 56002-3728
TEL: (507) 625-2828
FAX: (507) 625-7742
TOLL FREE: (800) 345-6954

GEORGIA CLAIMS OFFICE
1725 ROE CREST
PO BOX 3728
NORTH MANKATO, MN 56002-3728
TEL: (507) 625-2828
FAX: (507) 625-7742
TOLL FREE: (800) 345-6954

IDAHO CLAIMS OFFICE
1725 ROE CREST
PO BOX 3728
NORTH MANKATO, MN 56002-3728
TEL: (507) 625-2828
FAX: (507) 625-7742
TOLL FREE: (800) 345-6954

ILLINOIS CLAIMS OFFICE
1725 ROE CREST
PO BOX 3728
NORTH MANKATO, MN 56002-3728
TEL: (507) 625-2828
FAX: (507) 625-7742
TOLL FREE: (800) 345-6954

INDIANA CLAIMS OFFICE
1725 ROE CREST
PO BOX 3728
NORTH MANKATO, MN 56002-3728
TEL: (507) 625-2828
FAX: (507) 625-7742
TOLL FREE: (800) 345-6954

IOWA CLAIMS OFFICE
1725 ROE CREST
PO BOX 3728
NORTH MANKATO, MN 56002-3728
TEL: (507) 625-2828
FAX: (507) 625-7742
TOLL FREE: (800) 345-6954

MINNESOTA CLAIMS OFFICE
1725 ROE CREST
PO BOX 3728
NORTH MANKATO, MN 56002-3728
TEL: (507) 625-2828
FAX: (507) 625-7742
TOLL FREE: (800) 345-6954

NEW JERSEY CLAIMS OFFICE
1725 ROE CREST
PO BOX 3728
NORTH MANKATO, MN 56002-3728
TEL: (507) 625-2828
FAX: (507) 625-7742
TOLL FREE: (800) 345-6954

NEW YORK CLAIMS OFFICE
1725 ROE CREST
PO BOX 3728
NORTH MANKATO, MN 56002-3728
TEL: (507) 625-2828
FAX: (507) 625-7742
TOLL FREE: (800) 345-6954

PENNSYLVANIA CLAIMS OFFICE
1725 ROE CREST
PO BOX 3728
NORTH MANKATO, MN 56002-3728
TEL: (507) 625-2828
FAX: (507) 625-7742
TOLL FREE: (800) 345-6954

TEXAS CLAIMS OFFICE
1725 ROE CREST
PO BOX 3728
NORTH MANKATO, MN 56002-3728
TEL: (507) 625-2828
FAX: (507) 625-7742
TOLL FREE: (800) 345-6954

WASHINGTON CLAIMS OFFICE
1725 ROE CREST
PO BOX 3728
NORTH MANKATO, MN 56002-3728
TEL: (507) 625-2828
FAX: (507) 625-7742
TOLL FREE: (800) 345-6954

TC BILLING

FLORIDA CLAIMS OFFICE
921 37TH PLACE
VERO BEACH, FL 32960
TEL: (561) 778-6905
FAX: (561) 778-5437

TDC RANDMARK MANAGEMENT DENTAL SERVICES

WISCONSIN CLAIMS OFFICE
300 N MADISON
PO BOX 19049
GREEN BAY, WI 54307-9049
FAX: (920) 337-7331
TOLL FREE: (800) 955-0783
WWW.HUMANADENTAL.COM

TEACHERS INSURANCE & ANNUITY ASSOCIATION OF AMERICA

NEW YORK CLAIMS OFFICE
730 3RD AVE
NEW YORK, NY 10017-3206
TEL: (212) 490-9000
TOLL FREE: (800) 842-2733
WWW.TIAA/CREF.ORG

TEACHERS PROTECTIVE MUTUAL LIFE INSURANCE CO

MARYLAND CLAIMS OFFICE
116-118 N PRINCE ST
PO BOX 597
LANCASTER, PA 17608-0597
TEL: (717) 394-7156
TOLL FREE: (800) 555-3122
WWW.TPMINS.COM

NEW JERSEY CLAIMS OFFICE
116-118 N PRINCE ST
PO BOX 597
LANCASTER, PA 17608-0597
TEL: (717) 394-7156
TOLL FREE: (800) 555-3122
WWW.TPMINS.COM

OHIO CLAIMS OFFICE
116-118 N PRINCE ST
PO BOX 597
LANCASTER, PA 17608-0597
TEL: (717) 394-7156
TOLL FREE: (800) 555-3122
WWW.TPMINS.COM

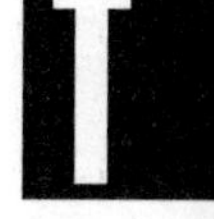

PENNSYLVANIA CLAIMS OFFICE
116-118 N PRINCE ST
PO BOX 597
LANCASTER, PA 17608-0597
TEL: (717) 394-7156
FAX: (717) 394-7024
TOLL FREE: (800) 555-3122
WWW.TPMINS.COM

VIRGINIA CLAIMS OFFICE
116-118 N PRINCE ST
PO BOX 597
LANCASTER, PA 17608-0597
TEL: (717) 394-7156
TOLL FREE: (800) 555-3122
WWW.TPMINS.COM

TEAMSTERS INDUSTRY WELFARE FUND

PENNSYLVANIA CLAIMS OFFICE
3025 WASHINGTON RD
MCMURRAY, PA 15317-3246
TEL: (724) 941-1124
FAX: (724) 941-1332

TEAMSTERS LOCAL 145 HEALTH SERVICES
CONNECTICUT CLAIMS OFFICE
2 RESEARCH DR-3RD FL
STRATFORD, CT 06615
TEL: (203) 375-6088
FAX: (203) 375-6106
TOLL FREE: (800) 291-6795
IN-STATE: (800) 291-6795

TELEDYNE CORP
CALIFORNIA CLAIMS OFFICE
2049 CENTURY PARK
LOS ANGELES, CA 90067-6001
TEL: (310) 277-3311
FAX: (310) 551-4369
WWW.ALLEGHENYTELEDYNE.COM

TENCO SERVICES
TENNESSEE CLAIMS OFFICE
3401 WEST END
PO BOX 129003
NASHVILLE, TN 37212
TEL: (615) 353-0357
FAX: (615) 292-0061
TOLL FREE: (800) 621-1313
E-MAIL: CLAIMS@TENCO.COM
WWW.TENCO.COM

TENCO SERVICES, INC
620 OLD HICKORY BLVD, STE 206
JACKSON, TN 38305-2977
TEL: (901) 668-4639
FAX: (901) 664-6960
E-MAIL: CLAIMS@TENCO.COM
WWW.TENCO.COM

5909 SHELBY OAKS DR, STE 146
MEMPHIS, TN 38134-7332
TEL: (901) 382-5821
FAX: (901) 382-5824
WWW.TENCO.COM

TENNESSEE FARM BUREAU MUTUAL INSURANCE CO
147 BEARCREEK PIKE
PO BOX 307
COLUMBIA, TN 38402-0307
TEL: (931) 388-7872
FAX: (931) 381-7571

TENNESSEE MANAGED CARE
210 ANTHENS WAY
NASHVILLE, TN 37208
TEL: (615) 329-2016
FAX: (615) 329-0250
TOLL FREE: (800) 523-3112

H

TETON NATIONAL INSURANCE CO
NATIONAL CLAIMS OFFICE
9777 S YOSEMITE
PO BOX 266007
HIGHLANDS RANCH, CO 80163
TEL: (303) 792-9507
FAX: (303) 792-9777
TOLL FREE: (800) 398-3866

TEXAS FARM BUREAU MUTUAL INSURANCE CO
TEXAS CLAIMS OFFICE
7420 FISH POND RD
PO BOX 2689
WACO, TX 76702-2689
TEL: (254) 772-3030
FAX: (254) 751-2463
TOLL FREE: (800) 772-6535

1703 E TOM GREEN
BRENHAM, TX 77833
TEL: (409) 836-5242
FAX: (409) 836-0687

TEXAS HEALTH CHOICE
12720 HILLCREST RD, STE 600
DALLAS, TX 75230-2010
TEL: (972) 458-5000
FAX: (972) 233-5281
TOLL FREE: (800) 324-8527

H

TEXAS LIFE INSURANCE CO
900 WASHINGTON AVE
PO BOX 830
WACO, TX 76703-0830
TEL: (254) 752-6521
FAX: (254) 752-8871
TOLL FREE: (800) 283-9233
WWW.TEXLIFE.COM

TEXAS SAVING LIFE INSURANCE
3636 EXECUTIVE CENTER DR, STE G22
AUSTIN, TX 78731
TEL: (512) 338-4397
FAX: (512) 338-0871
TOLL FREE: (800) 544-9242

TEXAS WORKER'S COMPENSATION COMMISSION
SOUTHFIELD BLDG- 4000 S INTERSTATE HWY 35
AUSTIN, TX 78704-7491
TEL: (512) 448-7900
FAX: (512) 707-5845
IN-STATE: (800) 252-7031
WWW.TWCC.STATE.TX.US

THE ALLIANCE
COLORADO CLAIMS OFFICE
A COMMUNITY HEALTH CARE PARTNERSHIP
650 S CHERRY ST, STE 300
DENVER, CO 80246
TEL: (303) 333-6767
FAX: (303) 322-3830
TOLL FREE: (800) 996-2447
E-MAIL: INFO@ALLIANCE-COLORADO.ORG
WWW.ALLIANCE-COLORADO.ORG

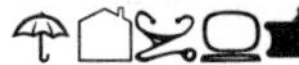

THE COMMERCE GROUP
OHIO CLAIMS OFFICE
PO BOX 900
ELYRIA, OH 44036
TEL: (440) 934-1033
FAX: (440) 934-1040
TOLL FREE: (800) 223-9941

THE DIAL CORPORATION
ARIZONA CLAIMS OFFICE
15501 N DIAL BLVD
SCOTTSDALE, AZ 85260-1619
TEL: (602) 754-3425
FAX: (602) 754-1098

THE GUARDIAN
NATIONAL CLAIMS OFFICE
2300 E CAPITAL DR
PO BOX 8007
APPLETON, WI 54913
FAX: (920) 749-5321
TOLL FREE: (800) 873-4542
WWW.THEGUARDIAN.COM

THE HARTFORD INSURANCE CO
CALIFORNIA CLAIMS OFFICE
PO BOX 7711
PLACENTIA, CA 92870
TEL: (714) 671-2811
FAX: (714) 256-1465
TOLL FREE: (800) 228-1320

ONE POINTE DR
BREA, CA 92821
TEL: (714) 671-2811
FAX: (714) 256-1465
TOLL FREE: (800) 228-1320

THE WHEELER COMPANIES
ALABAMA CLAIMS OFFICE
200 CAHABA PARK CIR, STE 250
PO BOX 43350
BIRMINGHAM, AL 35243-0350
TEL: (205) 995-8688
FAX: (940) 980-9047
TOLL FREE: (800) 741-8688

THIRD PARTY ASSOCIATES
OHIO CLAIMS OFFICE
614 SUPERIOR AVE NW, STE 605
CLEVELAND, OH 44113-1306
TEL: (216) 696-1448
FAX: (216) 696-1329
TOLL FREE: (800) 969-1448

THOMAS M. MURPHY & ASSOCIATES
CONNECTICUT CLAIMS OFFICE
79 BRIDGEPORT AVE
PO BOX 807
SHELTON, CT 06484-0807
TEL: (203) 924-2994
FAX: (203) 924-2644

T

THREE RIVERS BENEFIT CORP

IOWA CLAIMS OFFICE
PO BOX 3440
SIOUX CITY, IA 51102-3440
TEL: (712) 258-1525
FAX: (712) 255-3521
TOLL FREE: (800) 798-8115

MINNESOTA CLAIMS OFFICE
PO BOX 3440
SIOUX CITY, IA 51102-3440
TEL: (712) 258-1525
FAX: (712) 255-3521
TOLL FREE: (800) 798-8115

NEBRASKA CLAIMS OFFICE
PO BOX 3440
SIOUX CITY, IA 51102-3440
TEL: (712) 258-1525
FAX: (712) 255-3521
TOLL FREE: (800) 798-8115

SOUTH DAKOTA CLAIMS OFFICE
PO BOX 3440
SIOUX CITY, IA 51102-3440
TEL: (712) 258-1525
FAX: (712) 255-3521
TOLL FREE: (800) 798-8115

TIC INTERNATIONAL CORP

INDIANA CLAIMS OFFICE
11590 N MERIDIAN, STE 600
CARMEL, IN 46032-4529
TEL: (317) 580-8650
FAX: (317) 580-8699
IN-STATE: (800) 321-3856

TITAN INSURANCE CO

MICHIGAN CLAIMS OFFICE
901 WILSHIRE DR, STE 550
PO BOX 7024
TROY, MI 48007-7024
TEL: (248) 244-9770
FAX: (810) 244-6103
TOLL FREE: (800) 347-7930
IN-STATE: (800) 775-4642

TOPA INSURANCE CO

CALIFORNIA CLAIMS OFFICE
1800 AVE OF THE STARS- 12TH FL
PO BOX 67810
LOS ANGELES, CA 90067-0810
TEL: (310) 201-0451
FAX: (310) 286-7495

TOTAL HEALTH CARE, INC

MICHIGAN CLAIMS OFFICE
3011 W GRAND BLVD, STE 1600
DETROIT, MI 48202
TEL: (313) 871-2000
FAX: (313) 871-6409
IN-STATE: (800) 826-2862

MISSOURI CLAIMS OFFICE
BLUE CROSS & BLUE SHIELD OF KANSAS CITY
2301 MAIN ST
PO BOX 419169
KANSAS CITY, MO 64141-6169
TEL: (816) 395-2222
WWW.BCBSKC.COM

TOTAL HEALTH CARE PLAN, INC

OHIO CLAIMS OFFICE
12800 SHAKER BLVD
CLEVELAND, OH 44120
TEL: (216) 991-3000
FAX: (216) 991-3010
TOLL FREE: (800) 423-1615

TOWER LIFE INSURANCE CO

TEXAS CLAIMS OFFICE
400 TOWER LIFE BLDG
310 S ST MARY ST, STE 400
SAN ANTONIO, TX 78205-3164
TEL: (210) 554-4400
FAX: (210) 554-4401
TOLL FREE: (800) 880-4576

TPA

FLORIDA CLAIMS OFFICE
2500 MAITLAND CTR PKY, STE 100
PO BOX 945030
MAITLAND, FL 32794-5030
TEL: (407) 660-0202
FAX: (407) 660-0145
TOLL FREE: (800) 782-8103
WWW.THETPA.COM

NATIONAL CLAIMS OFFICE
2500 MAITLAND CTR PKY, STE 106
PO BOX 945030
MAITLAND, FL 32794-5030
TEL: (407) 660-0202
TOLL FREE: (800) 782-8103

7878 W 16TH ST, STE 140
PO BOX 52100
PHOENIX, AZ 85072-2100
TEL: (602) 866-1066
FAX: (602) 906-5070

TPA SERVICES, INC

ARIZONA CLAIMS OFFICE
820 E FORT LOWELL RD
PO BOX 42140
TUCSON, AZ 85733
TEL: (520) 670-0227
FAX: (520) 670-0229
TOLL FREE: (800) 448-0155

TR PAUL, INC

NATIONAL CLAIMS OFFICE
14 COMMERCE RD
PO BOX 5508
NEWTOWN, CT 06470-5508
TEL: (203) 426-8161
FAX: (203) 270-0927
TOLL FREE: (800) 678-8161

TRANS-NATIONAL LIFE INSURANCE CO

TEXAS CLAIMS OFFICE
4545 POST OAK PL DR, STE 302
HOUSTON, TX 77027-3105
TEL: (713) 622-1080
FAX: (713) 622-4060

TRANS-OCEANIC LIFE INSURANCE CO

FLORIDA CLAIMS OFFICE
GPO BOX 363467
SAN JUAN, PR 00936-3467
TEL: (787) 782-2680
FAX: (787) 793-6953
TOLL FREE: (800) 981-8662

PUERTO RICO CLAIMS OFFICE
GPO BOX 363467
SAN JUAN, PR 00936-3467
TEL: (787) 782-2680
FAX: (787) 793-6953
TOLL FREE: (800) 981-8662

VIRGIN ISLANDS CLAIMS OFFICE
GPO BOX 363467
SAN JUAN, PR 00936-3467
TEL: (787) 782-2680
FAX: (787) 793-6953
TOLL FREE: (800) 981-8662

TRANSATLANTIC REINSURANCE CO

NATIONAL CLAIMS OFFICE
80 PINE ST
NEW YORK, NY 10005
TEL: (212) 770-2000
FAX: (212) 809-4968

TRANSPORT INSURANCE CO

3191 TEMPLE AVE, STE 195
POMONA, CA 91768
TEL: (909) 468-0133
FAX: (909) 468-0725
TOLL FREE: (800) 274-0255

TEXAS CLAIMS OFFICE
4100 HARRY HINES BLVD
PO BOX 19706
DALLAS, TX 75219-3207
TEL: (214) 526-3876
FAX: (214) 520-4605
TOLL FREE: (800) 527-5412

TRAVELERS INSURANCE

MASSACHUSETTS CLAIMS OFFICE
NEW ENGLAND (MIDDLEBORO) CLAIM SERVICE CENTER
44 BEDFORD ST
PO BOX 1450
MIDDLEBORO, MA 02344-1450
TEL: (508) 946-4300
FAX: (508) 946-6572
TOLL FREE: (800) 422-3340
WWW.TRAVELERS.COM

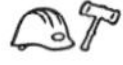

NEW ENGLAND (MIDDLEBORO) CLAIM SERVICE CENTER
44 BEDFORD ST
PO BOX 0111
MIDDLEBORO, MA 02344
TEL: (508) 946-4300
FAX: (508) 946-6382
TOLL FREE: (800) 422-3340
WWW.TRAVELERS.COM

NATIONAL CLAIMS OFFICE
INDIANAPOLIS, IN CLAIM SERVICE CENTER
6081 E 82ND ST, STE 300
PO BOX 50473
INDIANAPOLIS, IN 46250-0473
TEL: (317) 845-2855
FAX: (317) 845-2774
TOLL FREE: (800) 238-6210
WWW.TRAVELERS.COM

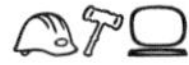

PO BOX 26985
MILWAUKEE, WI 53226
TEL: (414) 797-3100
FAX: (414) 797-3106
TOLL FREE: (800) 225-4144
WWW.TRAVELERS.COM

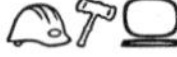

ONE TWR SQUARE
HARTFORD, CT 06183-0001
TEL: (860) 277-0111
WWW.TRAVELERS.COM

NEW YORK CLAIMS OFFICE
ALBANY, NY CLAIM SERVICE CENTER
80 WOLF RD
PO BOX 466
ALBANY, NY 12201
FAX: (518) 454-4757
TOLL FREE: (800) 223-4820
WWW.TRAVELERS.COM

ROCHESTER, NY WESTERN NY CLAIM SERVICE CENTER
100 MERIDIAN CENTRE
PO BOX 22986
ROCHESTER, NY 14692-2986
TEL: (716) 321-8000
FAX: (716) 321-8218
TOLL FREE: (800) 238-6216
WWW.TRAVELERS.COM

RHODE ISLAND CLAIMS OFFICE
NEW ENGLAND (MIDDLEBORO) CLAIM SERVICE CENTER
44 BEDFORD ST
PO BOX 1450
MIDDLEBORO, MA 02344-1450
TEL: (508) 946-4300
FAX: (508) 946-6572
TOLL FREE: (800) 422-3340
WWW.TRAVELERS.COM

NEW ENGLAND (MIDDLEBORO) CLAIM SERVICE CENTER
44 BEDFORD ST
PO BOX 0111
MIDDLEBORO, MA 02344
TEL: (508) 946-4300
FAX: (508) 946-6382
TOLL FREE: (800) 422-3340
WWW.TRAVELERS.COM

TRAVELERS PROPERTY & CASUALTY

ALASKA CLAIMS OFFICE
DENVER CLAIM SERVICE CENTER
7600 E ORCHARD RD
PO BOX 173798
DENVER, CO 80217
TOLL FREE: (800) 238-6225
IN-STATE: (800) 842-9488

ARIZONA CLAIMS OFFICE
DENVER CLAIM SERVICE CENTER
7600 E ORCHARD RD
PO BOX 173798
DENVER, CO 80217
TOLL FREE: (800) 238-6225
IN-STATE: (800) 842-9488

CALIFORNIA CLAIMS OFFICE
PO BOX 1903
VAN NUYS, CA 91408
TEL: (818) 778-0600
FAX: (800) 651-3746
TOLL FREE: (800) 238-6225

COLORADO CLAIMS OFFICE
DENVER CLAIM SERVICE CENTER
7600 E ORCHARD RD
PO BOX 173798
DENVER, CO 80217
TOLL FREE: (800) 238-6225
IN-STATE: (800) 842-9488

FLORIDA CLAIMS OFFICE
FIRST MERIDIAN AUTO & HOME INSURANCE
4890 W KENNEDY BLVD- 2 URBAN CTR, STE 700
PO BOX 30180
TAMPA, FL 33630-3180
TEL: (813) 890-4200
FAX: (813) 890-4200
TOLL FREE: (800) 238-6225
IN-STATE: (800) 842-6799

IDAHO CLAIMS OFFICE
DENVER CLAIM SERVICE CENTER
7600 E ORCHARD RD
PO BOX 173798
DENVER, CO 80217
TOLL FREE: (800) 238-6225
IN-STATE: (800) 842-9488

ILLINOIS CLAIMS OFFICE
215 SHUMAN BLVD
NAPERVILLE, IL 60563-8458
TOLL FREE: (800) 238-6225

LOUISIANA CLAIMS OFFICE
PO BOX 61124
NEW ORLEANS, LA 70161
TEL: (504) 832-7300

MONTANA CLAIMS OFFICE
DENVER CLAIM SERVICE CENTER
7600 E ORCHARD RD
PO BOX 173798
DENVER, CO 80217
TOLL FREE: (800) 238-6225
IN-STATE: (800) 842-9488

NEVADA CLAIMS OFFICE
PO BOX 1903
VAN NUYS, CA 91408
TEL: (818) 778-0600
FAX: (800) 651-3746
TOLL FREE: (800) 238-6225

NEW MEXICO CLAIMS OFFICE
DENVER CLAIM SERVICE CENTER
7600 E ORCHARD RD
PO BOX 173798
DENVER, CO 80217
TOLL FREE: (800) 238-6225
IN-STATE: (800) 842-9488

OHIO CLAIMS OFFICE
700 TWO CHATHAM CTR
PO BOX 1538
PITTSBURGH, PA 15230-1538
TEL: (412) 338-4200
TOLL FREE: (800) 238-6285

PENNSYLVANIA CLAIMS OFFICE
700 TWO CHATHAM CTR
PO BOX 1538
PITTSBURGH, PA 15230-1538
TEL: (412) 338-4200
TOLL FREE: (800) 238-6285

UTAH CLAIMS OFFICE
DENVER CLAIM SERVICE CENTER
7600 E ORCHARD RD
PO BOX 173798
DENVER, CO 80217
TOLL FREE: (800) 238-6225
IN-STATE: (800) 842-9488

WYOMING CLAIMS OFFICE
DENVER CLAIM SERVICE CENTER
7600 E ORCHARD RD
PO BOX 173798
DENVER, CO 80217
TOLL FREE: (800) 238-6225
IN-STATE: (800) 842-9488

TRAVELERS PROTECTIVE ASSOCIATION OF AMERICA

NATIONAL CLAIMS OFFICE
3755 LINDELL BLVD
SAINT LOUIS, MO 63108-3411
TEL: (314) 371-0533
FAX: (314) 371-0537

TRENWICK AMERICA REINSURANCE CORP

1 CANTERBURY GREEN
STAMFORD, CT 06901
TEL: (203) 353-5500
FAX: (203) 353-5555
TOLL FREE: (800) 873-6945
WWW.TRENWICK.COM

TRI-STATE INSURANCE CO OF MINNESOTA

MINNESOTA CLAIMS OFFICE
1 ROUNDWIND RD
PO BOX 500
LUVERNE, MN 56156-1361
TEL: (507) 283-9561
FAX: (507) 283-4324
TOLL FREE: (800) 533-0303
IN-STATE: (800) 533-0303

TRI-TEC EMPLOYEE BENEFITS, INC

NATIONAL CLAIMS OFFICE
2184 COMMONS PKY
PO BOX 804
OKEMOS, MI 48805-0804
TEL: (517) 349-8980
FAX: (517) 349-7615
TOLL FREE: (800) 782-0947

TRIBUS COMPANIES

NEW JERSEY CLAIMS OFFICE
65 WILLOW BROOK BLVD
WALDWICK, NJ 07470
TEL: (973) 890-1818
FAX: (973) 890-7841
TOLL FREE: (800) 333-9836
E-MAIL: TRIBUTE.COM

TRIGON

NATIONAL CLAIMS OFFICE
BLUE CROSS & BLUE SHIELD
PO BOX 27280
RICHMOND, VA 23261
TEL: (804) 358-1551
FAX: (804) 354-4340
IN-STATE: (800) 451-1527

VIRGINIA CLAIMS OFFICE
HEALTH KEEPERS
2015 STAPLES MILL RD
PO BOX 26623
RICHMOND, VA 23261-6623
TEL: (804) 354-3860
FAX: (804) 354-3936
TOLL FREE: (800) 451-1527
IN-STATE: (800) 421-1880
WWW.TRIGON.COM

H

TRIGON ADMINISTRATORS

MARYLAND CLAIMS OFFICE
7130 GLEN FOREST DR
PO BOX 85631
RICHMOND, VA 23285-5631
TEL: (804) 673-5900
FAX: (804) 673-5400
TOLL FREE: (800) 368-8002
WWW.TRIGONADMIN.COM

NORTH CAROLINA CLAIMS OFFICE
7130 GLEN FOREST DR
PO BOX 85631
RICHMOND, VA 23285-5631
TEL: (804) 673-5900
FAX: (804) 673-5400
TOLL FREE: (800) 368-8002
WWW.TRIGONADMIN.COM

VIRGINIA CLAIMS OFFICE
7130 GLEN FOREST DR
PO BOX 85631
RICHMOND, VA 23285-5631
TEL: (804) 673-5900
FAX: (804) 673-5400
TOLL FREE: (800) 368-8002
WWW.TRIGONADMIN.COM

TRIGON BLUE CROSS BLUE SHIELD

TRIGON HEALTHCARE INC
2221 EDWARD HOLLAND DR
RICHMOND, VA 23230
TEL: (804) 358-7390
FAX: (804) 354-3936
TOLL FREE: (800) 421-1880
WWW.TRIGON.COM

H

TRINITY UNIVERSAL INSURANCE CO

LOUISIANA CLAIMS OFFICE
3512 GOVERNMENT ST
PO BOX 5028
ALEXANDRIA, LA 71307-5028
TEL: (318) 445-9945
FAX: (318) 442-2912
TOLL FREE: (800) 456-6743

NATIONAL CLAIMS OFFICE
UNITURN
PO BOX 655028
DALLAS, TX 75265-5028
TEL: (214) 360-8000
FAX: (214) 360-8076
TOLL FREE: (800) 777-2249

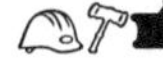

8200 I-10 W, STE 700
PO BOX 29839
SAN ANTONIO, TX 78229
TEL: (210) 525-8273
FAX: (800) 933-3707
TOLL FREE: (800) 766-6609

TRIPLE-S INC, OF PUERTO RICO

PUERTO RICO CLAIMS OFFICE
BLUE SHIELD OF PUERTO RICO
1441 ROOSEVELT AVE
PO BOX 363628
SAN JUAN, PR 00936-3628
TEL: (787) 749-4949
FAX: (787) 749-4190
WWW.SSSPR.COM

TRUCK INSURANCE EXCHANGE

ARIZONA CLAIMS OFFICE
FARMERS INSURANCE EXCHANGE
PO BOX 29054
PHOENIX, AZ 85038-9054
TEL: (602) 375-6800
FAX: (602) 375-6810

CALIFORNIA CLAIMS OFFICE
FARMERS INSURANCE EXCHANGE (WORKERS COMP OFFICE)
2200 GERARD AVE
PO BOX 3887
MERCED, CA 95344-1887
TEL: (209) 383-5333
FAX: (209) 383-5955

FARMERS INSURANCE EXCHANGE
PO BOX 10149
VAN NUYS, CA 91410-0149
TEL: (805) 583-7548
FAX: (805) 583-7554

NATIONAL CLAIMS OFFICE
FARMERS INSURANCE EXCHANGE
4680 WILSHIRE BLVD
PO BOX 2478
LOS ANGELES, CA 90051
TEL: (323) 932-3200
WWW.FARMERSINSURANCE.COM

NEVADA CLAIMS OFFICE
FARMERS INSURANCE EXCHANGE
PO BOX 29054
PHOENIX, AZ 85038-9054
TEL: (602) 375-6800
FAX: (602) 375-6810

NEW MEXICO CLAIMS OFFICE
FARMERS INSURANCE EXCHANGE
PO BOX 29054
PHOENIX, AZ 85038-9054
TEL: (602) 375-6800
FAX: (602) 375-6810

OREGON CLAIMS OFFICE
FARMERS INSURANCE EXCHANGE
13333 SW 68TH PKY
PO BOX 23306
TIGARD, OR 97281-3306
TEL: (503) 443-6451
FAX: (503) 443-6500

TRUST MARK

NATIONAL CLAIMS OFFICE
10777 SUNSET OFFICE DR, STE 300
SAINT LOUIS, MO 63127-1080
TEL: (314) 984-0666
FAX: (314) 984-9380
IN-STATE: (800) 325-8628

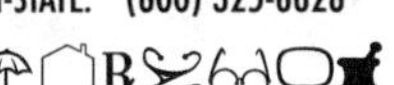

T

TRUSTED PLANS SERVICE CORP
6312 19TH ST W #200
PO BOX 1894
TACOMA, WA 98401-1894
TEL: (253) 564-5850
FAX: (253) 564-5881
TOLL FREE: (800) 426-9786

TRUSTMARK INSURANCE

ARIZONA CLAIMS OFFICE
8324 S AVE
BOARDMAN, OH 44512-6417
TEL: (330) 758-2212
FAX: (330) 758-3242
TOLL FREE: (800) 544-7312
WWW.TRUSTMARKINS.COM

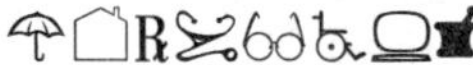

FLORIDA CLAIMS OFFICE
8324 S AVE
BOARDMAN, OH 44512-6417
TEL: (330) 758-2212
FAX: (330) 758-3242
TOLL FREE: (800) 544-7312
WWW.TRUSTMARKINS.COM

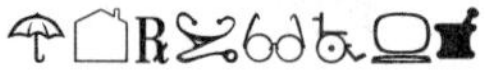

GEORGIA CLAIMS OFFICE
8324 S AVE
BOARDMAN, OH 44512-6417
TEL: (330) 758-2212
FAX: (330) 758-3242
TOLL FREE: (800) 544-7312
WWW.TRUSTMARKINS.COM

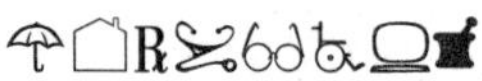

LOUISIANA CLAIMS OFFICE
8324 S AVE
BOARDMAN, OH 44512-6417
TEL: (330) 758-2212
FAX: (330) 758-3242
TOLL FREE: (800) 544-7312
WWW.TRUSTMARKINS.COM

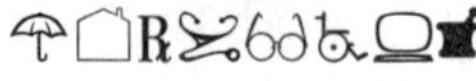

MASSACHUSETTS CLAIMS OFFICE
8324 S AVE
BOARDMAN, OH 44512-6417
TEL: (330) 758-2212
FAX: (330) 758-3242
TOLL FREE: (800) 544-7312
WWW.TRUSTMARKINS.COM

MISSISSIPPI CLAIMS OFFICE
8324 S AVE
BOARDMAN, OH 44512-6417
TEL: (330) 758-2212
FAX: (330) 758-3242
TOLL FREE: (800) 544-7312
WWW.TRUSTMARKINS.COM

NEW JERSEY CLAIMS OFFICE
8324 S AVE
BOARDMAN, OH 44512-6417
TEL: (330) 758-2212
FAX: (330) 758-3242
TOLL FREE: (800) 544-7312
WWW.TRUSTMARKINS.COM

NORTH CAROLINA CLAIMS OFFICE
8324 S AVE
BOARDMAN, OH 44512-6417
TEL: (330) 758-2212
FAX: (330) 758-3242
TOLL FREE: (800) 544-7312
WWW.TRUSTMARKINS.COM

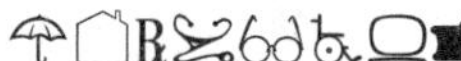

OHIO CLAIMS OFFICE
8324 S AVE
BOARDMAN, OH 44512-6417
TEL: (330) 758-2212
FAX: (330) 758-3242
TOLL FREE: (800) 544-7312
WWW.TRUSTMARKINS.COM

PENNSYLVANIA CLAIMS OFFICE
8324 S AVE
BOARDMAN, OH 44512-6417
TEL: (330) 758-2212
FAX: (330) 758-3242
TOLL FREE: (800) 544-7312
WWW.TRUSTMARKINS.COM

SOUTH CAROLINA CLAIMS OFFICE
8324 S AVE
BOARDMAN, OH 44512-6417
TEL: (330) 758-2212
FAX: (330) 758-3242
TOLL FREE: (800) 544-7312
WWW.TRUSTMARKINS.COM

TEXAS CLAIMS OFFICE
8324 S AVE
BOARDMAN, OH 44512-6417
TEL: (330) 758-2212
FAX: (330) 758-3242
TOLL FREE: (800) 544-7312
WWW.TRUSTMARKINS.COM

WEST VIRGINIA CLAIMS OFFICE
8324 S AVE
BOARDMAN, OH 44512-6417
TEL: (330) 758-2212
FAX: (330) 758-3242
TOLL FREE: (800) 544-7312
WWW.TRUSTMARKINS.COM

TRUSTMARK INSURANCE CO

ILLINOIS CLAIMS OFFICE
400 FIELD DR
LAKE FOREST, IL 60045-2586
TEL: (847) 615-1500
FAX: (847) 615-3910
WWW.TRUSTMARKINS.COM

NATIONAL CLAIMS OFFICE
1 MICHIANA SQ- 100 E WAYNE ST, STE 400
PO BOX 1467
SOUTH BEND, IN 46624-1467
TEL: (219) 288-2537
FAX: (219) 282-4825
IN-STATE: (800) 537-8275

TUCKER ADMINISTRATORS, INC
9140 ARROWPOINT BLVD, STE 200
CHARLOTTE, NC 28273-0001
TEL: (704) 525-9666
FAX: (704) 525-9534
TOLL FREE: (800) 342-1232

U.S. ABLE LIFE

ALABAMA CLAIMS OFFICE
320 W CAPITOL, STE 700
PO BOX 1650
LITTLE ROCK, AR 72203-1650
TEL: (501) 375-7200
FAX: (501) 378-3333
TOLL FREE: (800) 648-0271

ARIZONA CLAIMS OFFICE
320 W CAPITOL, STE 700
PO BOX 1650
LITTLE ROCK, AR 72203-1650
TEL: (501) 375-7200
FAX: (501) 378-3333
TOLL FREE: (800) 648-0271

ARKANSAS CLAIMS OFFICE
320 W CAPITOL, STE 700
PO BOX 1650
LITTLE ROCK, AR 72203-1650
TEL: (501) 375-7200
FAX: (501) 378-3333
TOLL FREE: (800) 648-0271

COLORADO CLAIMS OFFICE
320 W CAPITOL, STE 700
PO BOX 1650
LITTLE ROCK, AR 72203-1650
TEL: (501) 375-7200
FAX: (501) 378-3333
TOLL FREE: (800) 648-0271

DISTRICT OF COLUMBIA CLAIMS OFFICE
320 W CAPITOL, STE 700
PO BOX 1650
LITTLE ROCK, AR 72203-1650
TEL: (501) 375-7200
FAX: (501) 378-3333
TOLL FREE: (800) 648-0271

GEORGIA CLAIMS OFFICE
320 W CAPITOL, STE 700
PO BOX 1650
LITTLE ROCK, AR 72203-1650
TEL: (501) 375-7200
FAX: (501) 378-3333
TOLL FREE: (800) 648-0271

HAWAII CLAIMS OFFICE
320 W CAPITOL, STE 700
PO BOX 1650
LITTLE ROCK, AR 72203-1650
TEL: (501) 375-7200
FAX: (501) 378-3333
TOLL FREE: (800) 648-0271

IDAHO CLAIMS OFFICE
320 W CAPITOL, STE 700
PO BOX 1650
LITTLE ROCK, AR 72203-1650
TEL: (501) 375-7200
FAX: (501) 378-3333
TOLL FREE: (800) 648-0271

ILLINOIS CLAIMS OFFICE
320 W CAPITOL, STE 700
PO BOX 1650
LITTLE ROCK, AR 72203-1650
TEL: (501) 375-7200
FAX: (501) 378-3333
TOLL FREE: (800) 648-0271

IOWA CLAIMS OFFICE
320 W CAPITOL, STE 700
PO BOX 1650
LITTLE ROCK, AR 72203-1650
TEL: (501) 375-7200
FAX: (501) 378-3333
TOLL FREE: (800) 648-0271

KANSAS CLAIMS OFFICE
320 W CAPITOL, STE 700
PO BOX 1650
LITTLE ROCK, AR 72203-1650
TEL: (501) 375-7200
FAX: (501) 378-3333
TOLL FREE: (800) 648-0271

LOUISIANA CLAIMS OFFICE
320 W CAPITOL, STE 700
PO BOX 1650
LITTLE ROCK, AR 72203-1650
TEL: (501) 375-7200
FAX: (501) 378-3333
TOLL FREE: (800) 648-0271

MARYLAND CLAIMS OFFICE
320 W CAPITOL, STE 700
PO BOX 1650
LITTLE ROCK, AR 72203-1650
TEL: (501) 375-7200
FAX: (501) 378-3333
TOLL FREE: (800) 648-0271

MINNESOTA CLAIMS OFFICE
320 W CAPITOL, STE 700
PO BOX 1650
LITTLE ROCK, AR 72203-1650
TEL: (501) 375-7200
FAX: (501) 378-3333
TOLL FREE: (800) 648-0271

MISSISSIPPI CLAIMS OFFICE
320 W CAPITOL, STE 700
PO BOX 1650
LITTLE ROCK, AR 72203-1650
TEL: (501) 375-7200
FAX: (501) 378-3333
TOLL FREE: (800) 648-0271

MISSOURI CLAIMS OFFICE
320 W CAPITOL, STE 700
PO BOX 1650
LITTLE ROCK, AR 72203-1650
TEL: (501) 375-7200
FAX: (501) 378-3333
TOLL FREE: (800) 648-0271

MONTANA CLAIMS OFFICE
320 W CAPITOL, STE 700
PO BOX 1650
LITTLE ROCK, AR 72203-1650
TEL: (501) 375-7200
FAX: (501) 378-3333
TOLL FREE: (800) 648-0271

NEBRASKA CLAIMS OFFICE
320 W CAPITOL, STE 700
PO BOX 1650
LITTLE ROCK, AR 72203-1650
TEL: (501) 375-7200
FAX: (501) 378-3333
TOLL FREE: (800) 648-0271

NEVADA CLAIMS OFFICE
320 W CAPITOL, STE 700
PO BOX 1650
LITTLE ROCK, AR 72203-1650
TEL: (501) 375-7200
FAX: (501) 378-3333
TOLL FREE: (800) 648-0271

NEW MEXICO CLAIMS OFFICE
320 W CAPITOL, STE 700
PO BOX 1650
LITTLE ROCK, AR 72203-1650
TEL: (501) 375-7200
FAX: (501) 378-3333
TOLL FREE: (800) 648-0271

NORTH CAROLINA CLAIMS OFFICE
320 W CAPITOL, STE 700
PO BOX 1650
LITTLE ROCK, AR 72203-1650
TEL: (501) 375-7200
FAX: (501) 378-3333
TOLL FREE: (800) 648-0271

NORTH DAKOTA CLAIMS OFFICE
320 W CAPITOL, STE 700
PO BOX 1650
LITTLE ROCK, AR 72203-1650
TEL: (501) 375-7200
FAX: (501) 378-3333
TOLL FREE: (800) 648-0271

OKLAHOMA CLAIMS OFFICE
320 W CAPITOL, STE 700
PO BOX 1650
LITTLE ROCK, AR 72203-1650
TEL: (501) 375-7200
FAX: (501) 378-3333
TOLL FREE: (800) 648-0271

OREGON CLAIMS OFFICE
320 W CAPITOL, STE 700
PO BOX 1650
LITTLE ROCK, AR 72203-1650
TEL: (501) 375-7200
FAX: (501) 378-3333
TOLL FREE: (800) 648-0271

PENNSYLVANIA CLAIMS OFFICE
320 W CAPITOL, STE 700
PO BOX 1650
LITTLE ROCK, AR 72203-1650
TEL: (501) 375-7200
FAX: (501) 378-3333
TOLL FREE: (800) 648-0271

SOUTH DAKOTA CLAIMS OFFICE
320 W CAPITOL, STE 700
PO BOX 1650
LITTLE ROCK, AR 72203-1650
TEL: (501) 375-7200
FAX: (501) 378-3333
TOLL FREE: (800) 648-0271

TENNESSEE CLAIMS OFFICE
320 W CAPITOL, STE 700
PO BOX 1650
LITTLE ROCK, AR 72203-1650
TEL: (501) 375-7200
FAX: (501) 378-3333
TOLL FREE: (800) 648-0271

TEXAS CLAIMS OFFICE
320 W CAPITOL, STE 700
PO BOX 1650
LITTLE ROCK, AR 72203-1650
TEL: (501) 375-7200
FAX: (501) 378-3333
TOLL FREE: (800) 648-0271

UTAH CLAIMS OFFICE
320 W CAPITOL, STE 700
PO BOX 1650
LITTLE ROCK, AR 72203-1650
TEL: (501) 375-7200
FAX: (501) 378-3333
TOLL FREE: (800) 648-0271

VIRGINIA CLAIMS OFFICE
320 W CAPITOL, STE 700
PO BOX 1650
LITTLE ROCK, AR 72203-1650
TEL: (501) 375-7200
FAX: (501) 378-3333
TOLL FREE: (800) 648-0271

WASHINGTON CLAIMS OFFICE
320 W CAPITOL, STE 700
PO BOX 1650
LITTLE ROCK, AR 72203-1650
TEL: (501) 375-7200
FAX: (501) 378-3333
TOLL FREE: (800) 648-0271

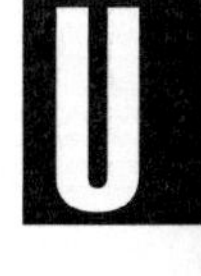

WISCONSIN CLAIMS OFFICE
320 W CAPITOL, STE 700
PO BOX 1650
LITTLE ROCK, AR 72203-1650
TEL: (501) 375-7200
FAX: (501) 378-3333
TOLL FREE: (800) 648-0271

WYOMING CLAIMS OFFICE
320 W CAPITOL, STE 700
PO BOX 1650
LITTLE ROCK, AR 72203-1650
TEL: (501) 375-7200
FAX: (501) 378-3333
TOLL FREE: (800) 648-0271

UCARE OF MINNESOTA

MINNESOTA CLAIMS OFFICE
2550 UNIVERSITY AVE W, STE 201 S
SAINT PAUL, MN 55114-1052
FAX: (651) 603-0650
TOLL FREE: (800) 203-7225
WWW.UCARE.ORG

H

UICI

NATIONAL CLAIMS OFFICE
501 W I-44 SERVICE RD, STE 400
PO BOX 548801
OKLAHOMA CITY, OK 73154-8801
TEL: (405) 848-0179
FAX: (405) 841-8758
TOLL FREE: (800) 725-7887

UIHMO, INC

ILLINOIS CLAIMS OFFICE
PLAN TRUST
2023 W OGDEN AVE, STE 205
CHICAGO, IL 60612-3741
TEL: (312) 913-1997
FAX: (312) 413-7872

H

UMAC, INC

NATIONAL CLAIMS OFFICE
1400 RENAISSANCE DR, STE 300
PARK RIDGE, IL 60068-1336
TEL: (847) 390-6606
FAX: (847) 390-8622
TOLL FREE: (800) 345-8622

UNDERWRITERS REINSURANCE CO

26050 MUREAU RD
PO BOX 4030
CALABASAS, CA 91302
TEL: (818) 878-9500
FAX: (818) 878-9535

UNDERWRITERS SAFETY & CLAIMS

PO BOX 23640
LOUISVILLE, KY 40223
TEL: (502) 244-1343
FAX: (502) 244-1411
TOLL FREE: (800) 678-1536

UNICARE

DISTRICT OF COLUMBIA CLAIMS OFFICE
MASS MUTUAL
220 RENINGTON BLVD
PO BOX 5033
BOLINGBROOK, IL 60440-5033
TEL: (630) 759-5055
TOLL FREE: (800) 444-3441

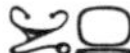

GEORGIA CLAIMS OFFICE
MASS MUTUAL
220 RENINGTON BLVD
PO BOX 5033
BOLINGBROOK, IL 60440-5033
TEL: (630) 759-5055
TOLL FREE: (800) 444-3441

ILLINOIS CLAIMS OFFICE
MASS MUTUAL
220 RENINGTON BLVD
PO BOX 5033
BOLINGBROOK, IL 60440-5033
TEL: (630) 759-5055
TOLL FREE: (800) 444-3441

INDIANA CLAIMS OFFICE
MASS MUTUAL
220 RENINGTON BLVD
PO BOX 5033
BOLINGBROOK, IL 60440-5033
TEL: (630) 759-5055
TOLL FREE: (800) 444-3441

NATIONAL CLAIMS OFFICE
SERVICE OFFICE
3820 AMERICAN DR
PLANO, TX 75070
TEL: (972) 599-6500
TOLL FREE: (800) 332-2060
WWW.WELLPOINT.COM

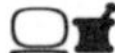

VIRGINIA CLAIMS OFFICE
MASS MUTUAL
220 RENINGTON BLVD
PO BOX 5033
BOLINGBROOK, IL 60440-5033
TEL: (630) 759-5055
TOLL FREE: (800) 444-3441

UNICARE ASSOCIATION SERVICES

NATIONAL CLAIMS OFFICE
13523 BARRET PKY, STE 250
PO BOX 120
BALLWIN, MO 63022-0120
TEL: (630) 679-4288
TOLL FREE: (800) 332-2060

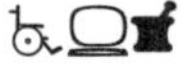

UNICARE LIFE & HEALTH

CALIFORNIA CLAIMS OFFICE
3179 TEMPLE AVE, STE 200
POMONA, CA 91768
TEL: (909) 444-6000
FAX: (909) 444-6161

NATIONAL CLAIMS OFFICE
PO BOX 4005
SCHAUMBURG, IL 60168-4005
TEL: (847) 706-4050

CLAIMS OFFICE
PO BOX 833947
RICHARDSON, TX 75083-3947
TEL: (972) 599-6500
TOLL FREE: (800) 332-2060
WWW.WELLPOINT.COM

3200 GREENFIELD RD
PO BOX 4479
DEARBORN, MI 48120
TEL: (313) 336-5550
TOLL FREE: (800) 332-2060
IN-STATE: (800) 843-8184

7025 ALBERTPICK RD- 5TH FL
GREENSBORO, NC 27409
TEL: (336) 665-1888
FAX: (336) 605-6406
TOLL FREE: (800) 597-6735

24650 CENTER RDG RD, STE 310
WESTLAKE, OH 44145-5680
TEL: (800) 543-4556
TOLL FREE: (800) 437-2277
IN-STATE: (800) 223-9940

UNIFIED LIFE INSURANCE CO

KANSAS CLAIMS OFFICE
7201 W 129TH ST, STE 300
PO BOX 25326
OVERLAND PARK, KS 66225-5326
TEL: (913) 685-2233
FAX: (913) 685-2204
TOLL FREE: (800) 237-4463

UNIGARD SECURITY INSURANCE CO

NATIONAL CLAIMS OFFICE
15805 NE 24TH ST
PO BOX 93000
BELLEVUE, WA 98009-3000
TEL: (425) 641-4321
FAX: (425) 562-5258
TOLL FREE: (800) 777-1757

3300 DOUGLAS BLVD, STE 155
PO BOX 13430
ROSEVILLE, CA 95813-4430
TEL: (916) 783-2930
FAX: (916) 783-7531
TOLL FREE: (800) 627-6320

UTAH CLAIMS OFFICE
UNIGARD
4444 S 700 E
PO BOX 57157
MURRAY, UT 84107-0157
TEL: (801) 266-1400
FAX: (801) 263-9131
TOLL FREE: (800) 777-4485
IN-STATE: (800) 662-6522

U

UNION BANKERS LIFE INSURANCE CO

NATIONAL CLAIMS OFFICE
717 N HARWOOD
PO BOX 655433
DALLAS, TX 75265-5433
TEL: (214) 954-7800
TOLL FREE: (800) 824-3577

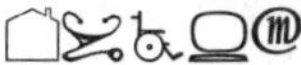

UNION CENTRAL INSURANCE & INVESTMENTS

1876 WAYCROSS RD
PO BOX 40888
CINCINNATI, OH 45240
TEL: (513) 595-2200
FAX: (513) 595-2218
TOLL FREE: (800) 825-1551

UNION FIDELITY INSURANCE CO

ILLINOIS CLAIMS OFFICE
FINANCIAL INSURANCE SERVICE CENTER
4890 STREET RD
TREVOSE, PA 19049-0002
TEL: (215) 953-4410
FAX: (215) 953-4494
TOLL FREE: (800) 626-6557

PENNSYLVANIA CLAIMS OFFICE
FINANCIAL INSURANCE SERVICE CENTER
4890 STREET RD
TREVOSE, PA 19049-0002
TEL: (215) 953-4410
FAX: (215) 953-4494
TOLL FREE: (800) 626-6557

UNION HEALTH SERVICE, INC

ILLINOIS CLAIMS OFFICE
1634 W POLK ST
CHICAGO, IL 60612-4352
TEL: (312) 829-4224
FAX: (312) 829-8241

H

UNION INSURANCE CO

COLORADO CLAIMS OFFICE
3641 VILLAGE DR
PO BOX 80439
LINCOLN, NE 68501
TEL: (402) 476-7688
FAX: (402) 421-4308
TOLL FREE: (800) 456-7688
WWW.UINS.COM

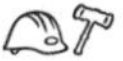

IOWA CLAIMS OFFICE
3641 VILLAGE DR
PO BOX 80439
LINCOLN, NE 68501
TEL: (402) 476-7688
FAX: (402) 421-4308
TOLL FREE: (800) 456-7688
WWW.UINS.COM

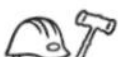

KANSAS CLAIMS OFFICE
3641 VILLAGE DR
PO BOX 80439
LINCOLN, NE 68501
TEL: (402) 476-7688
FAX: (402) 421-4308
TOLL FREE: (800) 456-7688
WWW.UINS.COM

NEBRASKA CLAIMS OFFICE
3641 VILLAGE DR
PO BOX 80439
LINCOLN, NE 68501
TEL: (402) 476-7688
FAX: (402) 421-4308
TOLL FREE: (800) 456-7688
WWW.UINS.COM

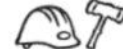

SOUTH CAROLINA CLAIMS OFFICE
3641 VILLAGE DR
PO BOX 80439
LINCOLN, NE 68501
TEL: (402) 476-7688
FAX: (402) 421-4308
TOLL FREE: (800) 456-7688
WWW.UINS.COM

UNION LABOR LIFE INSURANCE CO

CALIFORNIA CLAIMS OFFICE
ZENITH ADMIN, INC
301 MISSION ST, STE 600
PO BOX 422427
SAN FRANCISCO, CA 94142
TEL: (415) 546-7800
FAX: (415) 546-0600
TOLL FREE: (800) 387-9393
IN-STATE: (809) 388-0508

DISTRICT OF COLUMBIA CLAIMS OFFICE
111 MASSACHUSETTS AVE NW
WASHINGTON, DC 20001
TEL: (202) 682-0900
FAX: (202) 682-8795

MASSACHUSETTS CLAIMS OFFICE
111 MASSACHUSETTS AVE NW
WASHINGTON, DC 20001
TEL: (202) 682-0900
FAX: (202) 682-8795

NATIONAL CLAIMS OFFICE
161 FORBES RD, STE 204
BRAINTREE, MA 02184-2606
TEL: (781) 848-7474
FAX: (781) 849-6113
TOLL FREE: (800) 248-0029

NEW YORK CLAIMS OFFICE
111 MASSACHUSETTS AVE NW
WASHINGTON, DC 20001
TEL: (202) 682-0900
FAX: (202) 682-8795

UNION LIFE INSURANCE CO

NATIONAL CLAIMS OFFICE
424 W 4TH N
PO BOX 8006
LITTLE ROCK, AR 72203-8006
TEL: (501) 374-5715
FAX: (501) 374-3149
TOLL FREE: (800) 482-9260

UNION MUTUAL & NEW ENGLAND

VERMONT CLAIMS OFFICE
139 STATE ST
PO BOX 158
MONTPELIER, VT 05601
TEL: (802) 223-5261
FAX: (802) 229-2119
TOLL FREE: (800) 671-8550

UNION NATIONAL LIFE INSURANCE CO

LOUISIANA CLAIMS OFFICE
8282 GOODWOOD BLVD
PO BOX 4325
BATON ROUGE, LA 70821
TEL: (225) 927-3430
TOLL FREE: (800) 765-0550
IN-STATE: (800) 765-0550

MISSISSIPPI CLAIMS OFFICE
8282 GOODWOOD BLVD
PO BOX 4325
BATON ROUGE, LA 70821
TEL: (225) 927-3430
TOLL FREE: (800) 765-0550
IN-STATE: (800) 765-0550

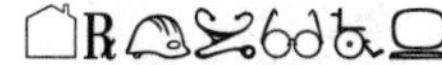

UNION SECURITY LIFE INSURANCE CO

GEORGIA CLAIMS OFFICE
260 INTERSTATE N CIR
ATLANTA, GA 30339
TEL: (770) 763-1000

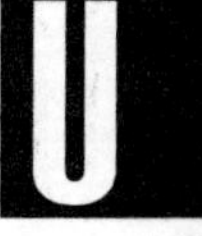

UNION STANDARD INSURANCE CO

ARKANSAS CLAIMS OFFICE
1501 N UNIVERSITY, STE 420
PO BOX 251758
LITTLE ROCK, AR 72225-1758
TEL: (501) 663-3888
FAX: (501) 663-8088
TOLL FREE: (800) 666-2452

NATIONAL CLAIMS OFFICE
122 W CARPENTER FWY, STE 350
PO BOX 152180
IRVING, TX 75015-2180
TEL: (972) 719-2400
FAX: (972) 719-2403
TOLL FREE: (800) 444-0049

TEXAS CLAIMS OFFICE
5368 FREDERICKSBURG RD, STE 300
SAN ANTONIO, TX 78229
TEL: (210) 979-9136
FAX: (210) 979-9157
TOLL FREE: (800) 206-0417

UNISYS

FLORIDA CLAIMS OFFICE
2525 S MONROE
TALLAHASSEE, FL 32301
TEL: (850) 671-0100
FAX: (850) 671-4528
TOLL FREE: (800) 289-7799

UNITE

PENNSYLVANIA CLAIMS OFFICE
BLUE CROSS & BLUE SHIELD
35 S FOURTH ST
PHILADELPHIA, PA 19106-2703
TEL: (215) 351-0750
IN-STATE: (800) 640-1136

UNITED AMERICAN HEALTHCARE CORP

NATIONAL CLAIMS OFFICE
1155 BREWERY PARK BLVD, STE 200
DETROIT, MI 48207
TEL: (313) 393-0200
FAX: (313) 393-7944
TOLL FREE: (800) 477-6664
WWW.OCHP.COM

UNITED AMERICAN INSURANCE

ALABAMA CLAIMS OFFICE
3700 S STONEBRIDGE DR
PO BOX 8080
MCKINNEY, TX 75070-8080
TEL: (972) 529-5085
FAX: (972) 569-3688
WWW.UNITEDAMERICAN.COM

UNITED AMERICAN INSURANCE CO

NATIONAL CLAIMS OFFICE
AMERICAN LIFE & ACCIDENT
3700 S STONEBRIDGE
PO BOX 8080
MCKINNEY, TX 75070
TEL: (972) 529-5085

UNITED BENEFIT MANAGED CARE CORP

3909 HULEN ST
FT WORTH, TX 76107
TEL: (817) 732-0399
FAX: (817) 377-5641
TOLL FREE: (800) 732-0657

UNITED CHAMBERS ADMINISTRATORS

1805 HIGH PT DR
PO BOX 3048
NAPERVILLE, IL 60566-7048
TEL: (630) 505-3100
FAX: (630) 577-2915
TOLL FREE: (800) 323-3529
E-MAIL: INFO@ACLIC.COM
WWW.ACLIC.COM

UNITED COMMERCIAL TRAVELERS OF AMERICA

632 N PARK ST
PO BOX 15919
COLUMBUS, OH 43215-8619
TEL: (614) 228-3276
FAX: (614) 228-1898
TOLL FREE: (800) 848-0123

UNITED EQUITABLE GROUP

ILLINOIS CLAIMS OFFICE
9833 WOODS DR
PO BOX 1091
SKOKIE, IL 60077
TEL: (847) 583-4600
FAX: (800) 996-7443
TOLL FREE: (800) 831-8330

UNITED FARM FAMILY MUTUAL INSURANCE

INDIANA CLAIMS OFFICE
225 S EAST ST
PO BOX 1250
INDIANAPOLIS, IN 46206-1250
TEL: (317) 692-7200
FAX: (317) 692-7641
TOLL FREE: (800) 723-3276

1104 BOYD BLVD
LA PORTE, IN 46350
TEL: (219) 326-6624
FAX: (219) 362-7622
TOLL FREE: (800) 627-1975

100 SAWMILL RUN DR
PO BOX 5889
LAFAYETTE, IN 47903-5889
TEL: (765) 471-8866
FAX: (765) 471-8877

3515 PARK PL W, STE 150
MISHAWAKA, IN 46545
TEL: (219) 271-3450
FAX: (219) 271-3464
TOLL FREE: (800) 730-5079
WWW.FARMBUREAU.COM

2676 CHARLESTOWN, STE 11
NEW ALBANY, IN 47150-2574
TEL: (812) 945-2337
FAX: (812) 945-7778

NATIONAL CLAIMS OFFICE
9135 BROADWAY
MARYVILLE, IN 46410
TEL: (219) 756-9650
FAX: (219) 756-9669
TOLL FREE: (800) 477-6767

500 E SPRINGHILL DR
PO BOX 2237
TERRE HAUTE, IN 47802-0237
TEL: (812) 234-0880
FAX: (812) 234-0888
TOLL FREE: (800) 477-6767
WWW.FARMBUREAU.COM

UNITED FIDELITY LIFE INSURANCE CO

MISSOURI CLAIMS OFFICE
FINANCIAL HOLDING CORP
300 W 11TH ST
KANSAS CITY, MO 64105
TEL: (816) 391-2000
FAX: (816) 391-2100
TOLL FREE: (800) 347-2825

UNITED FIRE & CASUALTY

ARKANSAS CLAIMS OFFICE
118 2ND AVE SE
PO BOX 73909
CEDAR RAPIDS, IA 52407-3909
TEL: (319) 399-5700
FAX: (319) 399-5400
TOLL FREE: (800) 343-9132
IN-STATE: (800) 343-9131
WWW.UNITEDFIREGROUP.COM

COLORADO CLAIMS OFFICE
118 2ND AVE SE
PO BOX 73909
CEDAR RAPIDS, IA 52407-3909
TEL: (319) 399-5700
FAX: (319) 399-5400
TOLL FREE: (800) 343-9132
IN-STATE: (800) 343-9131
WWW.UNITEDFIREGROUP.COM

ILLINOIS CLAIMS OFFICE
118 2ND AVE SE
PO BOX 73909
CEDAR RAPIDS, IA 52407-3909
TEL: (319) 399-5700
FAX: (319) 399-5400
TOLL FREE: (800) 343-9132
IN-STATE: (800) 343-9131
WWW.UNITEDFIREGROUP.COM

INDIANA CLAIMS OFFICE
118 2ND AVE SE
PO BOX 73909
CEDAR RAPIDS, IA 52407-3909
TEL: (319) 399-5700
FAX: (319) 399-5400
TOLL FREE: (800) 343-9132
IN-STATE: (800) 343-9131
WWW.UNITEDFIREGROUP.COM

IOWA CLAIMS OFFICE
118 2ND AVE SE
PO BOX 73909
CEDAR RAPIDS, IA 52407-3909
TEL: (319) 399-5700
FAX: (319) 399-5400
TOLL FREE: (800) 343-9132
IN-STATE: (800) 343-9131
WWW.UNITEDFIREGROUP.COM

KANSAS CLAIMS OFFICE
118 2ND AVE SE
PO BOX 73909
CEDAR RAPIDS, IA 52407-3909
TEL: (319) 399-5700
FAX: (319) 399-5400
TOLL FREE: (800) 343-9132
IN-STATE: (800) 343-9131
WWW.UNITEDFIREGROUP.COM

LOUISIANA CLAIMS OFFICE
118 2ND AVE SE
PO BOX 73909
CEDAR RAPIDS, IA 52407-3909
TEL: (319) 399-5700
FAX: (319) 399-5400
TOLL FREE: (800) 343-9132
IN-STATE: (800) 343-9131
WWW.UNITEDFIREGROUP.COM

MINNESOTA CLAIMS OFFICE
118 2ND AVE SE
PO BOX 73909
CEDAR RAPIDS, IA 52407-3909
TEL: (319) 399-5700
FAX: (319) 399-5400
TOLL FREE: (800) 343-9132
IN-STATE: (800) 343-9131
WWW.UNITEDFIREGROUP.COM

MISSISSIPPI CLAIMS OFFICE
118 2ND AVE SE
PO BOX 73909
CEDAR RAPIDS, IA 52407-3909
TEL: (319) 399-5700
FAX: (319) 399-5400
TOLL FREE: (800) 343-9132
IN-STATE: (800) 343-9131
WWW.UNITEDFIREGROUP.COM

MISSOURI CLAIMS OFFICE
118 2ND AVE SE
PO BOX 73909
CEDAR RAPIDS, IA 52407-3909
TEL: (319) 399-5700
FAX: (319) 399-5400
TOLL FREE: (800) 343-9132
IN-STATE: (800) 343-9131
WWW.UNITEDFIREGROUP.COM

NEBRASKA CLAIMS OFFICE
118 2ND AVE SE
PO BOX 73909
CEDAR RAPIDS, IA 52407-3909
TEL: (319) 399-5700
FAX: (319) 399-5400
TOLL FREE: (800) 343-9132
IN-STATE: (800) 343-9131
WWW.UNITEDFIREGROUP.COM

SOUTH DAKOTA CLAIMS OFFICE
118 2ND AVE SE
PO BOX 73909
CEDAR RAPIDS, IA 52407-3909
TEL: (319) 399-5700
FAX: (319) 399-5400
TOLL FREE: (800) 343-9132
IN-STATE: (800) 343-9131
WWW.UNITEDFIREGROUP.COM

UTAH CLAIMS OFFICE
118 2ND AVE SE
PO BOX 73909
CEDAR RAPIDS, IA 52407-3909
TEL: (319) 399-5700
FAX: (319) 399-5400
TOLL FREE: (800) 343-9132
IN-STATE: (800) 343-9131
WWW.UNITEDFIREGROUP.COM

WISCONSIN CLAIMS OFFICE
118 2ND AVE SE
PO BOX 73909
CEDAR RAPIDS, IA 52407-3909
TEL: (319) 399-5700
FAX: (319) 399-5400
TOLL FREE: (800) 343-9132
IN-STATE: (800) 343-9131
WWW.UNITEDFIREGROUP.COM

UNITED FIRE & LIFE INSURANCE CO

NATIONAL CLAIMS OFFICE
PO BOX 73909
CEDAR RAPIDS, IA 52407-3909
TEL: (319) 399-5700
FAX: (319) 399-5401
TOLL FREE: (800) 637-6318

UNITED FOOD & COMMERCIAL TRUST

CALIFORNIA CLAIMS OFFICE
SOUTHERN CALIFORNIA
6425 KATELLA
PO BOX 6010
CYPRESS, CA 90630-0010
TEL: (714) 220-2297
FAX: (714) 828-6573

UNITED GENERAL LIFE INSURANCE CO

NATIONAL CLAIMS OFFICE
WAKELY AND ASSOCIATES
PO BOX 10811
CLEARWATER, FL 33757-8811
TEL: (727) 584-8128
FAX: (727) 581-0578
TOLL FREE: (800) 226-6082

UNITED GOVERNMENT SERVICES

BLUE CROSS & BLUE SHIELD UNITED OF WISCONSIN
401 W MICHIGAN ST
MILWAUKEE, WI 53212
TEL: (414) 226-5000
FAX: (414) 226-5226
TOLL FREE: (800) 558-1584
WWW.UWSI.COM

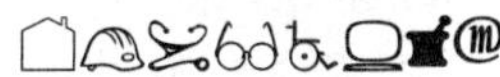

UNITED GROUP INSURANCE CO

TEXAS CLAIMS OFFICE
9151 GRAPEVINE HWY
PO BOX 982009
NORTH RICHLAND HILLS, TX 76180
TEL: (817) 656-6100
FAX: (800) 551-9939
TOLL FREE: (800) 527-2845

UNITED HEALTH

NATIONAL CLAIMS OFFICE
145 S STATE COLLEGE BLVD, STE 350
PO BOX 6101
BREA, CA 92821
TEL: (714) 257-3205
FAX: (714) 257-3204
TOLL FREE: (800) 553-7360

UNITED HEALTHCARE OF LOUISIANA

LOUISIANA CLAIMS OFFICE
2431 S ACADIAN THRUWAY, STE 350
BATON ROUGE, LA 70808-2387
TEL: (504) 923-0550
TOLL FREE: (800) 735-0559
IN-STATE: (800) 349-1000

UNITED HEALTH OF WISCONSIN INSURANCE CO, INC

WISCONSIN CLAIMS OFFICE
5 INNOVATION CT
PO BOX 507
APPLETON, WI 54912-0507
TEL: (920) 735-6300
TOLL FREE: (800) 236-6440

UNITED HEALTH PLAN

CALIFORNIA CLAIMS OFFICE
WATTS HEALTH FOUNDATION
3405 W IMPERIAL HWY
INGLEWOOD, CA 90303-2299
TEL: (310) 671-3465
FAX: (310) 673-9176

UNITED HEALTHCARE

ALABAMA CLAIMS OFFICE
3700 COLONNADE PKY
BIRMINGHAM, AL 35243
TEL: (205) 977-6300
FAX: (205) 977-6499
TOLL FREE: (800) 345-1520
WWW.UHC.COM

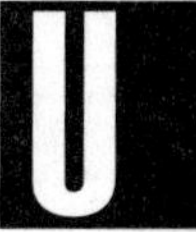

ARIZONA CLAIMS OFFICE
3141 N 3RD AVE
PHOENIX, AZ 85013
TEL: (602) 664-2600
FAX: (602) 664-2929
TOLL FREE: (880) 664-2779
WWW.UHC.COM

CALIFORNIA CLAIMS OFFICE
300 S PARK, #840
POMONA, CA 91766
TEL: (909) 620-1767
FAX: (909) 620-9119
TOLL FREE: (800) 421-9174
IN-STATE: (800) 842-7084
WWW.UHC.COM

Medicode, Inc.

COLORADO CLAIMS OFFICE
PO BOX 30555
SALT LAKE CITY, UT 84030-555
TEL: (303) 770-6050
WWW.UHC.COM

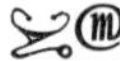

DELAWARE CLAIMS OFFICE
300 S PARK, #840
POMONA, CA 91766
TEL: (909) 620-1767
FAX: (909) 620-9119
TOLL FREE: (800) 421-9174
IN-STATE: (800) 842-7084
WWW.UHC.COM

H

FLORIDA CLAIMS OFFICE
UNITED HEALTH CARE OF FLORIDA
11140 N KENDALL DR
MIAMI, FL 33183
TEL: (305) 596-5696
FAX: (305) 275-4050
TOLL FREE: (800) 543-3145
IN-STATE: (888) 716-8787
WWW.UHC.COM

PO BOX 740800
ATLANTA, GA 33074
TEL: (813) 636-6990
WWW.UHC.COM

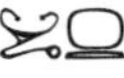

UNITED HEALTH CARE OF FLORIDA
75 VALENCIA AVE
PO BOX 149015
CORAL GABLES, FL 33134
TEL: (305) 441-1140
TOLL FREE: (800) 432-1141
IN-STATE: (800) 543-3145
WWW.UHC.COM

H

GEORGIA CLAIMS OFFICE
NETWORKS OF ALANTA, GA
2970 CLAIRMOUNT RD, STE 300
ATLANTA, GA 30329-1634
TEL: (404) 982-8800
FAX: (404) 982-3225
TOLL FREE: (800) 453-8440
WWW.UHC.COM

H

PO BOX 740800
ATLANTA, GA 33074
TEL: (813) 636-6990
WWW.UHC.COM

ILLINOIS CLAIMS OFFICE
UNITED HEALTH CARE OF ILLINOIS
ONE S WACKER DR
CHICAGO, IL 60606
TEL: (312) 424-4460
FAX: (312) 424-5620
TOLL FREE: (800) 826-9400
WWW.UHC.COM

INDIANA CLAIMS OFFICE
UNITED HEALTH CARE OF KENTUCKY, LTD.
2409 HARRODSBURG RD
LEXINGTON, KY 40504
TEL: (606) 296-6000
FAX: (606) 296-6196
TOLL FREE: (800) 495-5285
WWW.UHC.COM

IOWA CLAIMS OFFICE
UNITED HEALTH CARE OF THE MIDLAND
2717 N 118 CR
OMAHA, NE 68164-9672
TEL: (402) 445-5000
FAX: (402) 445-5502
TOLL FREE: (800) 641-1906
WWW.UHC.COM

KENTUCKY CLAIMS OFFICE
UNITED HEALTH CARE OF KENTUCKY, LTD.
2409 HARRODSBURG RD
LEXINGTON, KY 40504
TEL: (606) 296-6000
FAX: (602) 296-6196
TOLL FREE: (800) 495-5285
WWW.UHC.COM

MARYLAND CLAIMS OFFICE
UNITED HEALTH CARE OF THE MID-ATLANTIC
6300 SECURITY BLVD
PO BOX 25750
BALTIMORE, MD 21207
TEL: (410) 277-9449
TOLL FREE: (800) 625-6656
WWW.UHC.COM

MASSACHUSETTS CLAIMS OFFICE
99 HIGH ST- 32ND FL
BOSTON, MA 02110-2320
TEL: (617) 574-3945
FAX: (617) 426-4124
TOLL FREE: (800) 444-7855
WWW.UHC.COM

MINNESOTA CLAIMS OFFICE
MEDICARE- PART B
8120 PENN AVE S
BLOOMINGTON, MN 55431-1326
TEL: (612) 884-3030
FAX: (612) 885-2900
WWW.UHC.COM

MEDICAL CLAIMS
9900 BREN RD E
PO BOX 1459
MINNEAPOLIS, MN 55440-1459
TEL: (612) 936-6050
FAX: (612) 936-3095
TOLL FREE: (800) 325-6651
IN-STATE: (800) 554-5413
WWW.UHC.COM

MISSOURI CLAIMS OFFICE
UNITED HEALTH CARE OF THE MIDWEST
969 EXECUTIVE PKY, STE 100
PO BOX 419080
SAINT LOUIS, MO 63141-9080
TOLL FREE: (800) 535-9291
WWW.UHC.COM

NATIONAL CLAIMS OFFICE
UNITED HEALTH CARE OF THE MIDWEST, INC, PHYSICIANS HEALTH PLAN OF GREATER ST. LOUIS, INC
77 W PORT PLZ, STE 500
PO BOX 66867
SAINT LOUIS, MO 63146
TOLL FREE: (800) 554-9705
WWW.UHC.COM

NEBRASKA CLAIMS OFFICE
UNITED HEALTH CARE OF THE MIDLAND
2717 N 118 CR
OMAHA, NE 68164-9672
TEL: (402) 445-5000
FAX: (402) 445-5502
TOLL FREE: (800) 641-1906
WWW.UHC.COM

NORTH CAROLINA CLAIMS OFFICE
PHP, INC- UNITED HEALTH CARE OF NORTH CAROLINA, INC
2307 W CONE BLVD
GREENSBORO, NC 27408-4032
TOLL FREE: (800) 772-1180
WWW.UHC.COM

OHIO CLAIMS OFFICE
UNITED HEALTH CARE OF OHIO, INC
3650 OLENTANGY RIVER RD
PO BOX 182281
COLUMBUS, OH 43219
TEL: (614) 442-7100
FAX: (614) 442-3902
TOLL FREE: (800) 328-8835
IN-STATE: (800) 458-5346
WWW.UHC.COM

UNITED HEALTH CARE OF OHIO, INC
6601 CENTERVILLE BUSINESS PKY
DAYTON, OH 45459-9895
TEL: (937) 439-9355
FAX: (937) 439-8999
IN-STATE: (800) 231-2918
WWW.UHC.COM

TEXAS CLAIMS OFFICE
UNITED HEALTH CARE OF TEXAS
PO BOX 30555
SALT LAKE CITY, UT 84030-555
TEL: (303) 770-6050
WWW.UHC.COM

ADMINISTRATIVE SERVICES
555 N CARANCAHUA, STE 500
CORPUS CHRISTI, TX 78478
TEL: (512) 887-0101
FAX: (512) 887-8115
TOLL FREE: (800) 580-2247

UNITED HEALTH CARE OF TEXAS, INC, HOUSTON DIVISION
5 POST OAK PK, STE 505
HOUSTON, TX 77027
TEL: (713) 961-3286
TOLL FREE: (800) 548-1081
WWW.UHC.COM

UTAH CLAIMS OFFICE
UNITED HEALTH CARE OF UTAH
PO BOX 30555
SALT LAKE CITY, UT 84030-555
TEL: (303) 770-6050
WWW.UHC.COM

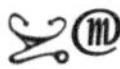

UNITED HEALTHCARE INSURANCE CO

MISSISSIPPI CLAIMS OFFICE
PO BOX 22545
JACKSON, MS 39225-2545
TEL: (601) 977-0208
FAX: (601) 977-5854

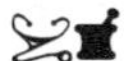

UNITED HEALTHCARE INSURANCE CO, PART A INTERMEDIARY

CONNECTICUT CLAIMS OFFICE
538 PRESTON AVE
PO BOX 1043
MERIDEN, CT 06450-1041
TEL: (203) 639-3230
FAX: (203) 639-3202

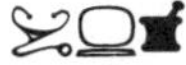

UNITED HEALTHCARE INSURANCE CO, PART B CARRIER

538 PRESTON AVE
PO BOX 1043
MERIDEN, CT 06450-1041
TEL: (203) 639-3124
FAX: (203) 639-3018

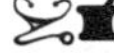

MINNESOTA CLAIMS OFFICE
8120 PENN AVE S
BLOOMINGTON, MN 55431-1394
TEL: (612) 884-3030
FAX: (612) 885-2839

VIRGINIA CLAIMS OFFICE
300 ARBORETUM PL- 4TH FL
PO BOX 26463
RICHMOND, VA 23261-3480
TEL: (804) 327-2211
FAX: (804) 327-2101

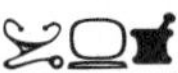

UNITED HEALTHCARE OF THE MIDWEST

MISSOURI CLAIMS OFFICE
13655 RIVERPORT DR
PO BOX 2560
MARYLAND HEIGHTS, MO 63043
TEL: (314) 592-7000
FAX: (314) 592-7200
TOLL FREE: (800) 627-0687

H

1949 E SUNSHINE ST, STE 300
PO BOX 2560
SPRINGFIELD, MO 65804
TEL: (417) 841-7100
FAX: (417) 841-7118
TOLL FREE: (800) 627-0687

H

UNITED HERITAGE MUTUAL LIFE INSURANCE CO

IDAHO CLAIMS OFFICE
1212 12TH AVE RD
PO BOX 48
NAMPA, ID 83653-0048
TEL: (208) 466-7856
FAX: (208) 466-0825
TOLL FREE: (800) 657-6351
E-MAIL: HERITAGE@UNITEDHERITAGE.COM
WWW.UNITEDHERITAGE.COM

UNITED INSURANCE CO OF AMERICA

ALABAMA CLAIMS OFFICE
UNION NATIONAL INSURANCE CO
PO BOX 4325
BATON ROUGE, LA 70821
TEL: (225) 927-3430
TOLL FREE: (800) 777-1195
IN-STATE: (800) 765-0550

DELAWARE CLAIMS OFFICE
ONE E WACKER DR
CHICAGO, IL 60601-4305
TEL: (312) 661-4500
FAX: (312) 424-5620
TOLL FREE: (800) 777-8467

DISTRICT OF COLUMBIA CLAIMS OFFICE
ONE E WACKER DR
CHICAGO, IL 60601-4305
TEL: (312) 661-4500
FAX: (312) 424-5620
TOLL FREE: (800) 777-8467

FLORIDA CLAIMS OFFICE
UNION NATIONAL INSURANCE CO
PO BOX 4325
BATON ROUGE, LA 70821
TEL: (225) 927-3430
TOLL FREE: (800) 777-1195
IN-STATE: (800) 765-0550

GEORGIA CLAIMS OFFICE
UNION NATIONAL INSURANCE CO
PO BOX 4325
BATON ROUGE, LA 70821
TEL: (225) 927-3430
TOLL FREE: (800) 777-1195
IN-STATE: (800) 765-0550

INDIANA CLAIMS OFFICE
ONE E WACKER DR
CHICAGO, IL 60601-4305
TEL: (312) 661-4500
FAX: (312) 424-5620
TOLL FREE: (800) 777-8467

KENTUCKY CLAIMS OFFICE
ONE E WACKER DR
CHICAGO, IL 60601-4305
TEL: (312) 661-4500
FAX: (312) 424-5620
TOLL FREE: (800) 777-8467

LOUISIANA CLAIMS OFFICE
UNION NATIONAL INSURANCE CO
PO BOX 4325
BATON ROUGE, LA 70821
TEL: (225) 927-3430
TOLL FREE: (800) 777-1195
IN-STATE: (800) 765-0550

MARYLAND CLAIMS OFFICE
ONE E WACKER DR
CHICAGO, IL 60601-4305
TEL: (312) 661-4500
FAX: (312) 424-5620
TOLL FREE: (800) 777-8467

MICHIGAN CLAIMS OFFICE
ONE E WACKER DR
CHICAGO, IL 60601-4305
TEL: (312) 661-4500
FAX: (312) 424-5620
TOLL FREE: (800) 777-8467

MISSISSIPPI CLAIMS OFFICE
UNION NATIONAL INSURANCE CO
PO BOX 4325
BATON ROUGE, LA 70821
TEL: (225) 927-3430
TOLL FREE: (800) 777-1195
IN-STATE: (800) 765-0550

MISSOURI CLAIMS OFFICE
ONE E WACKER DR
CHICAGO, IL 60601-4305
TEL: (312) 661-4500
FAX: (312) 424-5620
TOLL FREE: (800) 777-8467

NEW JERSEY CLAIMS OFFICE
ONE E WACKER DR
CHICAGO, IL 60601-4305
TEL: (312) 661-4500
FAX: (312) 424-5620
TOLL FREE: (800) 777-8467

NORTH CAROLINA CLAIMS OFFICE
ONE E WACKER DR
CHICAGO, IL 60601-4305
TEL: (312) 661-4500
FAX: (312) 424-5620
TOLL FREE: (800) 777-8467

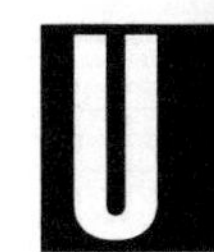

OHIO CLAIMS OFFICE
ONE E WACKER DR
CHICAGO, IL 60601-4305
TEL: (312) 661-4500
FAX: (312) 424-5620
TOLL FREE: (800) 777-8467

OKLAHOMA CLAIMS OFFICE
UNION NATIONAL INSURANCE CO
PO BOX 4325
BATON ROUGE, LA 70821
TEL: (225) 927-3430
TOLL FREE: (800) 777-1195
IN-STATE: (800) 765-0550

PENNSYLVANIA CLAIMS OFFICE
ONE E WACKER DR
CHICAGO, IL 60601-4305
TEL: (312) 661-4500
FAX: (312) 424-5620
TOLL FREE: (800) 777-8467

SOUTH CAROLINA CLAIMS OFFICE
ONE E WACKER DR
CHICAGO, IL 60601-4305
TEL: (312) 661-4500
FAX: (312) 424-5620
TOLL FREE: (800) 777-8467

TENNESSEE CLAIMS OFFICE
UNION NATIONAL INSURANCE CO
PO BOX 4325
BATON ROUGE, LA 70821
TEL: (225) 927-3430
TOLL FREE: (800) 777-1195
IN-STATE: (800) 765-0550

TEXAS CLAIMS OFFICE
UNION NATIONAL INSURANCE CO
PO BOX 4325
BATON ROUGE, LA 70821
TEL: (225) 927-3430
TOLL FREE: (800) 777-1195
IN-STATE: (800) 765-0550

VIRGINIA CLAIMS OFFICE
ONE E WACKER DR
CHICAGO, IL 60601-4305
TEL: (312) 661-4500
FAX: (312) 424-5620
TOLL FREE: (800) 777-8467

WEST VIRGINIA CLAIMS OFFICE
ONE E WACKER DR
CHICAGO, IL 60601-4305
TEL: (312) 661-4500
FAX: (312) 424-5620
TOLL FREE: (800) 777-8467

WISCONSIN CLAIMS OFFICE
ONE E WACKER DR
CHICAGO, IL 60601-4305
TEL: (312) 661-4500
FAX: (312) 424-5620
TOLL FREE: (800) 777-8467

UNITED LIFE & ACCIDENT INSURANCE CO

NATIONAL CLAIMS OFFICE
UNITED AMERICAN
3700 STONEBRIDGE DR
PO BOX 2390
MCKINNEY, TX 75070
TEL: (972) 540-6516
FAX: (972) 569-3709

UNITED MEDICAL RESOURCES, INC

KENTUCKY CLAIMS OFFICE
1329 E KEMPER RD, STE 4100
PO BOX 145804
CINCINNATI, OH 45250-5804
TEL: (513) 619-3000
FAX: (513) 619-3010
TOLL FREE: (800) 436-3100

OHIO CLAIMS OFFICE
1329 E KEMPER RD, STE 4100
PO BOX 145804
CINCINNATI, OH 45250-5804
TEL: (513) 619-3000
FAX: (513) 619-3010
TOLL FREE: (800) 436-3100

UNITED MEDICORP, INC

TEXAS CLAIMS OFFICE
10210 N CENTRAL EXPY, STE 400
DALLAS, TX 75231-3427
TEL: (214) 691-2140
FAX: (214) 361-2505
IN-STATE: (800) 468-5072

UNITED MERCANTILE LIFE INSURANCE CO

5845 ONIX, STE 300
EL PASO, TX 79912
TEL: (915) 585-0292
FAX: (915) 585-9925

UNITED METROPOLITAN LIFE INSURANCE CO

NATIONAL CLAIMS OFFICE
GENERAL MOTORS EMPLOYEES ONLY
2400 LAYTON PK DR, STE 800
PO BOX 2517
SMYRNA, GA 30081
TEL: (770) 437-5760
FAX: (770) 618-2217
TOLL FREE: (800) 241-9964

UNITED OHIO INSURANCE CO

OHIO CLAIMS OFFICE
1725 HOPLEY AVE
PO BOX 111
BUCYRUS, OH 44820-3569
TEL: (419) 562-3011
FAX: (419) 562-0995

UNITED PACIFIC INSURANCE CO

UTAH CLAIMS OFFICE
3995 S 700 E, STE 250
SALT LAKE CITY, UT 84107
TEL: (801) 263-2112
FAX: (801) 263-2266
TOLL FREE: (800) 892-5635
IN-STATE: (800) 892-5635

UNITED SECURITY LIFE INSURANCE CO OF ILLINOIS

ILLINOIS CLAIMS OFFICE
10275 W HIGGINS RD
ROSEMONT, IL 60018
TEL: (847) 298-1400
FAX: (847) 298-1407
TOLL FREE: (800) 875-4422
WWW.USOOFIL.COM

UNITED SERVICES AUTOMOBILE ASSOCIATION

TEXAS CLAIMS OFFICE
9800 FREDERICKSBURG RD
SAN ANTONIO, TX 78288
TEL: (210) 498-2211
FAX: (210) 498-6431
TOLL FREE: (800) 531-9017

UNITED STATES FIDELITY & GUARANTY CO

ALABAMA CLAIMS OFFICE
ST. PAUL COMPANIES
1200 CORPORATE DR, STE 300
PO BOX 385011
BIRMINGHAM, AL 35238-5011
TEL: (205) 995-2540
TOLL FREE: (800) 873-2634
IN-STATE: (800) 821-4880

ARIZONA CLAIMS OFFICE
ST. PAUL COMPANIES
2228 W NORTHERN AVE
PO BOX 37829
PHOENIX, AZ 85069-7829
TEL: (602) 678-3400
TOLL FREE: (800) 873-2634

CALIFORNIA CLAIMS OFFICE
ST. PAUL COMPANIES
500 S KRAMER BLVD, STE 200
PO BOX 5000
BREA, CA 92822-5000
TEL: (714) 993-4430
TOLL FREE: (800) 873-2634
IN-STATE: (800) 400-8734

COLORADO CLAIMS OFFICE
ST. PAUL COMPANIES
1670 BROADWAY, STE 2300
PO BOX 7
DENVER, CO 80201
TEL: (303) 812-9000
TOLL FREE: (800) 873-2634

CONNECTICUT CLAIMS OFFICE
ST. PAUL COMPANIES
175 CAPITOL BLVD
PO BOX 4013
ROCKY HILL, CT 06067-3578
TEL: (203) 874-2568
TOLL FREE: (800) 873-2634

GEORGIA CLAIMS OFFICE
ST. PAUL COMPANIES
9000 CENTRAL PRK W
PO BOX 105698
ATLANTA, GA 30348-5698
TEL: (770) 390-5500
FAX: (770) 390-5840
TOLL FREE: (800) 873-2634
IN-STATE: (800) 282-0404

ST. PAUL COMPANIES
100 CRESCENT CTR PKY, STE 1000
TUCKER, GA 30084
TOLL FREE: (800) 241-9245

IDAHO CLAIMS OFFICE
ST. PAUL COMPANIES
PO BOX 563
MERIDIAN, ID 83680
TEL: (208) 288-0071
FAX: (208) 288-0171
TOLL FREE: (800) 873-2634

ILLINOIS CLAIMS OFFICE
ST. PAUL COMPANIES
421 S PEORIA
DIXON, IL 61021
TEL: (815) 288-1017
TOLL FREE: (800) 873-2634

IOWA CLAIMS OFFICE
ST. PAUL COMPANIES
4201 WESTOWN PARKWAY #250
PO BOX 65459
WEST DES MOINES, IA 50306-4627
TEL: (515) 223-5700
FAX: (515) 222-4330
TOLL FREE: (800) 362-2480

KENTUCKY CLAIMS OFFICE
ST. PAUL COMPANIES
9911 SHELBYVILLE RD, STE 200
LOUISVILLE, KY 40223-2954
TEL: (502) 429-7000
FAX: (502) 429-7388
TOLL FREE: (800) 873-2634
IN-STATE: (800) 722-5026

LOUISIANA CLAIMS OFFICE
ST. PAUL COMPANIES
2450 SEVERN AVE, STE 302
PO BOX 6823
METAIRIE, LA 70009
TEL: (504) 837-6500
TOLL FREE: (800) 873-2634
IN-STATE: (800) 452-2126

MAINE CLAIMS OFFICE
ST. PAUL FIRE & CASUALTY
100 FODEN RD W
SOUTH PORTLAND, ME 04106
TEL: (207) 772-5515
TOLL FREE: (800) 442-6365

MARYLAND CLAIMS OFFICE
ST. PAUL COMPANIES
PO BOX 13576
BALTIMORE, MD 21203
TEL: (800) 638-5080
TOLL FREE: (800) 873-2634

MICHIGAN CLAIMS OFFICE
ST. PAUL MERCURY INSURANCE
1900 W BIG BEAVER RD
PO BOX 3704
TROY, MI 48007-3704
TEL: (248) 641-0200
FAX: (248) 641-1466
TOLL FREE: (800) 873-2634
IN-STATE: (800) 462-6157

MINNESOTA CLAIMS OFFICE
ST. PAUL COMPANIES
408 ST PETERS ST, STE 300
SAINT PAUL, MN 55102
TEL: (651) 310-5000
TOLL FREE: (800) 873-2634
IN-STATE: (800) 328-7152
WWW.THEST.PAUL.COM

MISSISSIPPI CLAIMS OFFICE
ST. PAUL COMPANIES
107 3RD AVE
PO BOX 1606
HATTIESBURG, MS 39403-1606
TEL: (601) 583-2631
FAX: (601) 583-2144
TOLL FREE: (800) 873-2634

ST. PAUL COMPANIES
143 LEFLUERS SQ
PO BOX 12224
JACKSON, MS 39236
TEL: (601) 987-8300
FAX: (601) 987-8397
TOLL FREE: (800) 873-2634

ST. PAUL COMPANIES
2680 N HILL ST
PO BOX 3097
MERIDIAN, MS 39303
TEL: (601) 693-1731
FAX: (601) 485-1029
TOLL FREE: (800) 873-2634
IN-STATE: (800) 222-6211

MISSOURI CLAIMS OFFICE
ST. PAUL COMPANIES
PO BOX 2954
OVERLAND PARK, KS 66201
TEL: (913) 451-1570
FAX: (913) 469-2787
TOLL FREE: (800) 873-2634
IN-STATE: (800) 821-2972
WWW.THEST.PAUL.COM

MONTANA CLAIMS OFFICE
ST. PAUL COMPANIES
1643 LEWIS AVE, STE 3
PO BOX 22237
BILLINGS, MT 59104-2237
TEL: (406) 248-5615
TOLL FREE: (800) 873-2634
IN-STATE: (800) 962-1148

ST. PAUL COMPANIES
910 E LYNDELL
PO BOX 6107
HELENA, MT 59604-6107
TEL: (406) 442-2270
FAX: (406) 447-1220
TOLL FREE: (800) 873-2634
IN-STATE: (800) 332-6112

NEBRASKA CLAIMS OFFICE
ST. PAUL COMPANIES
1010 S 1020 ST, STE 200
PO BOX 3728
OMAHA, NE 68103-0728
TEL: (402) 896-5534
TOLL FREE: (800) 873-2634
IN-STATE: (800) 642-9990

NEW HAMPSHIRE CLAIMS OFFICE
ST. PAUL COMPANIES
PO BOX 4767
MANCHESTER, NH 03108
TEL: (603) 669-3560
FAX: (603) 669-4254
TOLL FREE: (800) 873-2634
IN-STATE: (800) 873-8734

NEW MEXICO CLAIMS OFFICE
ST. PAUL COMPANIES
2201 SAN PEDRO NE- BLDG 2, STE 225
PO BOX 3566
ALBUQUERQUE, NM 87190-3566
TEL: (505) 889-5200
FAX: (505) 889-5209
TOLL FREE: (800) 873-2634
IN-STATE: (800) 432-6815

ST. PAUL COMPANIES
PO BOX 1353
ROSWELL, NM 88202-1353
TEL: (505) 622-2570
FAX: (505) 622-5608
TOLL FREE: (800) 873-2634
IN-STATE: (800) 628-8261

NEW YORK CLAIMS OFFICE
ST. PAUL COMPANIES
EXECUTIVE PARK- TOWER BLDG
ALBANY, NY 12203-3717
TEL: (518) 489-7446
FAX: (518) 489-5022
TOLL FREE: (800) 873-2634
IN-STATE: (800) 545-5854

ST. PAUL COMPANIES
ONE JERICHO PLZ
JERICHO, NY 11753
TEL: (516) 935-3700
FAX: (516) 935-4606
TOLL FREE: (800) 873-2634

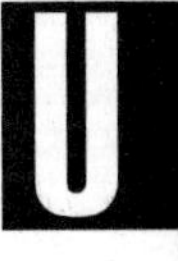

ST. PAUL COMPANIES
2500 WESTCHESTER AVE
PURCHASE, NY 10577-2515
TEL: (914) 251-2300
FAX: (914) 251-2424
TOLL FREE: (800) 873-2634
IN-STATE: (800) 248-8734

ST. PAUL COMPANIES
5786 WIDEWATERS PKY
PO BOX 4929
SYRACUSE, NY 13221-4929
TEL: (315) 449-5100
FAX: (315) 449-5220
TOLL FREE: (800) 873-2634
IN-STATE: (800) 962-5856

ST. PAUL COMPANIES
PO BOX 1770
WILLIAMSVILLE, NY 14231-1770
TEL: (716) 626-1880
FAX: (716) 626-0488
TOLL FREE: (800) 873-2634
IN-STATE: (800) 418-7268

NORTH CAROLINA CLAIMS OFFICE
ST. PAUL FIRE AND MARINE INSURANCE
5821 FAIRVIEW RD, STE 500
CHARLOTTE, NC 28209
TEL: (704) 544-1220
FAX: (704) 544-7194
TOLL FREE: (800) 873-2634
IN-STATE: (800) 432-6320

ST. PAUL COMPANIES
3117 POPLARWOOD CT, STE 300
RALEIGH, NC 27604
FAX: (919) 878-7355
TOLL FREE: (800) 873-2634
IN-STATE: (800) 662-7909

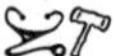

ST. PAUL FIRE AND MARINE INSURANCE
5821 FAIRVIEW RD, STE 500
CHARLOTTE, NC 28209
TEL: (423) 588-6506
FAX: (704) 544-7194
TOLL FREE: (800) 873-2634
IN-STATE: (800) 432-6320

U

OHIO CLAIMS OFFICE
ST. PAUL COMPANIES
24651 CENTER RIDGE RD
WEST LAKE, OH 44145
TEL: (440) 899-2300
TOLL FREE: (800) 873-2634
IN-STATE: (800) 362-8083

OKLAHOMA CLAIMS OFFICE
ST. PAUL COMPANIES
2601 NW EXPRESS WAY 500 E
OKLAHOMA CITY, OK 73112
TEL: (405) 843-7300
FAX: (405) 858-7475
TOLL FREE: (800) 873-2634
IN-STATE: (800) 522-6588

ST. PAUL COMPANIES
PO BOX 470288
TULSA, OK 74147-0288
TEL: (918) 664-8010
FAX: (918) 664-0530
TOLL FREE: (800) 873-2634

OREGON CLAIMS OFFICE
ST. PAUL COMPANIES
6650 SW REDWOOD LN, STE 250
PORTLAND, OR 97224
TEL: (503) 684-0880
FAX: (503) 624-5139
TOLL FREE: (800) 873-2634

PENNSYLVANIA CLAIMS OFFICE
ST. PAUL COMPANIES
2605 INTERSTATE DR, STE 200
PO BOX 9700
HARRISBURG, PA 17108-9700
TEL: (717) 671-8001
FAX: (717) 671-7351
TOLL FREE: (800) 873-2634

ST. PAUL COMPANIES
1 MELLON BANK CTR- 500 GRANT ST, STE 1110
PITTSBURGH, PA 15219-2510
TEL: (412) 261-2550
TOLL FREE: (800) 873-2634

SOUTH CAROLINA CLAIMS OFFICE
ST. PAUL FIRE AND MARINE INSURANCE
PO BOX 21800
COLUMBIA, SC 29221-1800
TEL: (803) 256-2325
TOLL FREE: (800) 873-2634

TENNESSEE CLAIMS OFFICE
ST. PAUL COMPANIES
564 CRAZY DOE RD
LEXINGTON, TN 38351
TEL: (901) 968-6747
FAX: (901) 968-6759
TOLL FREE: (800) 873-2634

ST. PAUL COMPANIES
5900 POPLAR, STE 210
MEMPHIS, TN 38119
TEL: (901) 761-6200
FAX: (901) 767-2031
TOLL FREE: (800) 873-2634

ST. PAUL MERCURY INSURANCE COMPANY
5409 MARYLAND WY, STE 320
PO BOX 5002
BRENTWOOD, TN 37027
TEL: (615) 377-0418
FAX: (615) 221-0295
TOLL FREE: (800) 873-2634
IN-STATE: (800) 342-5072

UTAH CLAIMS OFFICE
ST. PAUL COMPANIES
1100 E 6600 S
PO BOX 71100
SALT LAKE CITY, UT 84171
TEL: (801) 269-5656
FAX: (801) 269-5611
TOLL FREE: (800) 873-2634

VIRGINIA CLAIMS OFFICE
ST. PAUL COMPANIES
PO BOX 13108
NORFOLK, VA 23506-0108
TEL: (757) 461-1268
FAX: (757) 466-7114
TOLL FREE: (800) 873-2634
IN-STATE: (800) 845-2129

ST. PAUL COMPANIES
PO BOX 13576
BALTIMORE, MD 21203
TEL: (800) 638-5080
TOLL FREE: (800) 873-2634

WISCONSIN CLAIMS OFFICE
ST. PAUL FIRE AND MARINE INSURANCE
PO BOX 1313
APPLETON, WI 54911
TEL: (414) 454-0609
TOLL FREE: (800) 873-2634
IN-STATE: (800) 292-7674

UNITED STATES LIFE INSURANCE CO

NATIONAL CLAIMS OFFICE
AMERICAN GENERAL
3600 RTE 66
PO BOX 1581
NEPTUNE, NJ 07754-1581
TEL: (732) 922-7000
FAX: (732) 922-7136
TOLL FREE: (800) 221-3480
IN-STATE: (800) 346-7692

2101 CENTER AVE
PO BOX 15205
READING, PA 19612-5205
TEL: (610) 373-8232
FAX: (610) 373-1502
TOLL FREE: (800) 523-2767

UNITED TEACHER ASSOCIATES INSURANCE CO

5508 PARKCREST DR
PO BOX 26580
AUSTIN, TX 78755-0457
TEL: (512) 451-2224
FAX: (512) 467-7403
TOLL FREE: (800) 880-8824
WWW.UTAIC.COM

UNITED TRANSPORTATION UNION INSURANCE ASSOCIATION

14600 DETROIT AVE
CLEVELAND, OH 44107-4207
TEL: (216) 228-9400
FAX: (216) 228-0411
TOLL FREE: *00) 558-8842

UNITED WISCONSIN INSURANCE CO

WISCONSIN CLAIMS OFFICE
401 W MICHIGAN ST
PO BOX 2013
MILWAUKEE, WI 53201-2013
TEL: (414) 226-6300
FAX: (414) 226-6363
TOLL FREE: (800) 452-4250

UNITRON PROPERTY & CASUALTY GROUP

ILLINOIS CLAIMS OFFICE
301 S PROSPECT, STE 1
PO BOX 2170
BLOOMINGTON, IL 61702
TEL: (309) 664-8300
TOLL FREE: (800) 777-2034

INDIANA CLAIMS OFFICE
301 S PROSPECT, STE 1
PO BOX 2170
BLOOMINGTON, IL 61702
TEL: (309) 664-8300
TOLL FREE: (800) 777-2034

OHIO CLAIMS OFFICE
301 S PROSPECT, STE 1
PO BOX 2170
BLOOMINGTON, IL 61702
TEL: (309) 664-8300
TOLL FREE: (800) 777-2034

UNITY HEALTH PLANS
WISCONSIN CLAIMS OFFICE
840 CAROLINA ST
PO BOX 610
SAUK CITY, WI 53583
TEL: (608) 643-2491
FAX: (608) 643-2564
TOLL FREE: (800) 362-3308
WWW.UNITYHEALTH.COM

UNIVERSAL UNDERWRITERS GROUP
NATIONAL CLAIMS OFFICE
7045 COLLEGE BLVD
OVERLAND PARK, KS 66211-1551
TEL: (913) 339-1000
FAX: (913) 339-1026
TOLL FREE: (800) 821-7803

101 E PARK BLVD, STE 200
PLANO, TX 75074
TEL: (972) 422-3339
FAX: (972) 461-6075
TOLL FREE: (800) 622-6262

UNUM LIFE INSURANCE CO
2211 CONGRESS ST
PORTLAND, ME 04122
TEL: (207) 770-2211
FAX: (207) 770-9735
TOLL FREE: (800) 223-6937
WWW.UNUM.COM

US BENEFITS
OREGON CLAIMS OFFICE
906 NE 19TH
PO BOX 13190
PORTLAND, OR 97213-0190
TEL: (503) 233-3888
FAX: (503) 233-0904
TOLL FREE: (800) 797-3888

US HEALTHCARE, INC
RHODE ISLAND CLAIMS OFFICE
213 COURT ST- 7TH FL
MIDDLETOWN, CT 06457-3342
TEL: (860) 636-8300
TOLL FREE: (800) 872-3862

US LIABILITY INSURANCE CO
NATIONAL CLAIMS OFFICE
1030 CONTINENTAL DR
KING OF PRUSSIA, PA 19406-2808
TEL: (610) 688-2535
FAX: (610) 688-4391
TOLL FREE: (800) 523-5545
WWW.USLI.COM

USAA LIFE INSURANCE CO
9800 FREDERICKSBURG RD
SAN ANTONIO, TX 78288-0346
TEL: (210) 498-8000
FAX: (800) 531-6295
TOLL FREE: (800) 531-8000

USI ADMINISTRATORS
JONES, HILL & MERCER EMPLOYEE BENEFITS
7402 HODGSON MEMORIAL DR #210
PO BOX 9888
SAVANNAH, GA 31406
TEL: (912) 691-1551
FAX: (912) 352-8935
TOLL FREE: (800) 631-3441

UTAH FARM BUREAU MUTUAL INSURANCE CO
UTAH CLAIMS OFFICE
9865 S STATE ST
SANDY, UT 84070
TEL: (801) 233-3100
FAX: (801) 233-3135
TOLL FREE: (800) 388-7752

UTICA NATIONAL INSURANCE CO
NATIONAL CLAIMS OFFICE
180 GENESEE ST
PO BOX 530
UTICA, NY 13503-0530
TEL: (315) 734-2000
FAX: (315) 734-2010
TOLL FREE: (800) 274-1914

UTICA NATIONAL INSURANCE GROUP
2600 CORPORATE EXCHANGE DR, STE 200
PO BOX 29906
COLUMBUS, OH 43229-7506
TEL: (614) 823-5300
FAX: (614) 823-5319
TOLL FREE: (800) 955-1914

UTILITIES MUTUAL INSURANCE CO
NEW JERSEY CLAIMS OFFICE
4 GATEHALL DR, STE 215
PARSIPPANY, NJ 07054
TEL: (973) 539-4005
FAX: (973) 539-5997

VALERO ENERGY CORP
TEXAS CLAIMS OFFICE
HEALTH CARE ADMINISTRATION IF
PO BOX 500
SAN ANTONIO, TX 78292-0500
TEL: (210) 370-2100
FAX: (210) 370-2861
TOLL FREE: (800) 531-7911

SOUTH TEXAS HEALTH CARE ALLIANCE
7990 W IH 10
SAN ANTONIO, TX 78230-4715
TEL: (210) 370-2776
FAX: (210) 370-2861
TOLL FREE: (800) 531-7911
IN-STATE: (800) 292-7816

VALERO HEALTHCARE ADMISSION
ILLINOIS CLAIMS OFFICE
CCN (CHICAGO AREA)
2269 S UNIVERSITY DR, STE 308
FT LAUDERDALE, FL 33324
TEL: (210) 370-2100
TOLL FREE: (800) 531-7911
IN-STATE: (800) 292-7816

VANGUARD INSURANCE CO
TEXAS CLAIMS OFFICE
REPUBLIC
2727 TURTLE CRK BLVD
PO BOX 650358
DALLAS, TX 75265-0358
TEL: (214) 559-1222
TOLL FREE: (800) 344-2275

VANLINER INSURANCE CO
MISSOURI CLAIMS OFFICE
1 PREMIER DR
PO BOX 26352
FENTON, MO 63026-1552
TEL: (314) 343-9889
FAX: (314) 326-0403
TOLL FREE: (800) 325-3619

VIACHRISTI ST. FRANCIS
KANSAS CLAIMS OFFICE
929 N ST FRANCIS
WICHITA, KS 67214
TEL: (316) 268-5192
FAX: (316) 268-6985
TOLL FREE: (800) 362-0070

VIACHRISTI ST. JOSEPH MEDICAL CENTER
3600 E HARRY ST
WICHITA, KS 67218-3784
TEL: (316) 685-1111
TOLL FREE: (800) 851-0051

V

VIC BROTHERS-LMI
CALIFORNIA CLAIMS OFFICE
HIGHLANDS INSURANCE GROUP
6300 CANOGA AVE, 6TH FL
PO BOX 7709
VAN NUYS, CA 91409
TEL: (818) 992-5222
FAX: (818) 710-2050
TOLL FREE: (800) 553-5800
IN-STATE: (800) 553-5800

VIGILANT INSURANCE CO

NEW YORK CLAIMS OFFICE
55 WATER ST
NEW YORK, NY 10041
TEL: (212) 612-4000
FAX: (212) 612-4318
TOLL FREE: (800) 426-8938

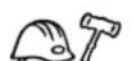

VIRGINIA FARM BUREAU MUTUAL INSURANCE CO

VIRGINIA CLAIMS OFFICE
PO BOX 27552
RICHMOND, VA 23261-7552
TEL: (804) 784-1234
FAX: (804) 784-2574
TOLL FREE: (800) 768-8323
WWW.VAFB.COM

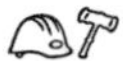

VIRGINIA HEALTH & ACCIDENT

710 N MAIN ST
PO BOX 1114
EMPORIA, VA 23847-1114
TEL: (804) 634-2513
FAX: (804) 634-2672
TOLL FREE: (800) 251-4347

VIRGINIA MASON MEDICAL CTR

WASHINGTON CLAIMS OFFICE
CUSTOMER & BUSINESS SERVICES
1100 OLIVE WAY, STE 1580
SEATTLE, WA 98101-1828
TEL: (206) 223-8844

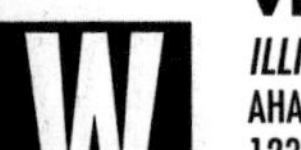

VIRGINIA SURETY CO

ILLINOIS CLAIMS OFFICE
AHAM
123 N WACKER DR
CHICAGO, IL 60606-1700
TEL: (312) 701-3700
FAX: (312) 701-4911
TOLL FREE: (800) 209-6206

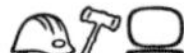

4850 STREET RD
TREVOSE, PA 19049
TEL: (215) 953-3000
FAX: (215) 953-3156
TOLL FREE: (800) 523-6599
IN-STATE: (800) 523-5758

PENNSYLVANIA CLAIMS OFFICE
4850 STREET RD
TREVOSE, PA 19049
TEL: (215) 953-3000
FAX: (215) 953-3156
TOLL FREE: (800) 523-6599
IN-STATE: (800) 523-5758

AHAM
123 N WACKER DR
CHICAGO, IL 60606-1700
TEL: (312) 701-3700
FAX: (312) 701-4911
TOLL FREE: (800) 209-6206

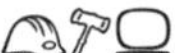

VIRGINIA CLAIMS OFFICE
AHAM
123 N WACKER DR
CHICAGO, IL 60606-1700
TEL: (312) 701-3700
FAX: (312) 701-4911
TOLL FREE: (800) 209-6206

VISION SERVICE PLAN

CALIFORNIA CLAIMS OFFICE
3333 QUALITY DR
PO BOX 997100
SACRAMENTO, CA 95899-7100
TEL: (916) 851-5000
FAX: (916) 851-5152
TOLL FREE: (800) 852-7600
E-MAIL: MEMBER@LAS.VSP.COM
WWW.VSP.COM

VOLUNTARY PLAN ADMINISTRATORS

PO BOX 9830
CALABASAS, CA 91372-0830
TEL: (818) 591-2772
FAX: (818) 591-7664

VYTRA HEALTH PLANS

NEW YORK CLAIMS OFFICE
395 N SERVICE RD
MELVILLE, NY 11747-3171
TEL: (516) 694-4000
FAX: (516) 249-6620
TOLL FREE: (800) 406-0806
WWW.VYTRA.COM

W.J. JONES ADMINISTRATIVE SERVICES, INC

CONNECTICUT CLAIMS OFFICE
SELECTPRO, INC (MANAGED CARE NETWORK)
1979 MARCUS AVE STE C101
LAKE SUCCESS, NY 11042-1312
TEL: (516) 775-5420
FAX: (516) 775-6601
TOLL FREE: (800) 831-7783
WWW.SELECTPRO.COM &
WWW.WJJONES.COM

NEW YORK CLAIMS OFFICE
SELECTPRO, INC (MANAGED CARE NETWORK)
1979 MARCUS AVE, STE C101
LAKE SUCCESS, NY 11042-1312
TEL: (516) 775-5420
FAX: (516) 775-6601
TOLL FREE: (800) 831-7783
WWW.SELECTPRO.COM &
WWW.WJJONES.COM

W. R. GIBBENS CO, INC

NEVADA CLAIMS OFFICE
GATES MCDONALD-GIBBENS
1610 MEADOW WOOD LN
PO BOX 71255
RENO, NV 89570
TEL: (775) 826-6600
FAX: (775) 826-6651

WAKELY & ASSOCIATES

FLORIDA CLAIMS OFFICE
1820 S HIGHLAND AVE
PO BOX 10811
CLEARWATER, FL 33757-8811
TEL: (727) 584-8128
FAX: (727) 581-0578
TOLL FREE: (888) 780-6388

WALDEN RISK MANAGEMENT GROUP

TENNESSEE CLAIMS OFFICE
712 SIGNAL MTN BLVD
PO BOX 15766
CHATTANOOGA, TN 37415
TEL: (423) 886-3033
FAX: (423) 886-6271
TOLL FREE: (800) 280-9764
E-MAIL: WRMGCW@AOL.COM

WALGREENS

ILLINOIS CLAIMS OFFICE
NATIONAL DISBURSING OFFICE
1517 N BOWMAN AVE
PO BOX 4007
DANVILLE, IL 61834-4007
TEL: (217) 443-0410
FAX: (217) 443-2456

WALMARK ADMINISTRATORS OF AMERICA, INC

IOWA CLAIMS OFFICE
500 WALNUT, STE 300
PO BOX 9120
DES MOINES, IA 50306
TEL: (515) 243-3210
FAX: (515) 282-0719
TOLL FREE: (800) 622-3339

WALMART BENEFITS

ARKANSAS CLAIMS OFFICE
922 W WALNUT, STE A
ROGERS, AR 72756-3206
TEL: (501) 621-2929
TOLL FREE: (800) 421-1362
WWW.WALMART.COM

WARD NORTH AMERICA

CALIFORNIA CLAIMS OFFICE
17862 E 17TH ST, STE 111
TUSTIN, CA 92780
TEL: (714) 544-0980
FAX: (714) 544-1979
TOLL FREE: (800) 677-3313
WWW.WARDNA.COM

WARD NORTH AMERICA, INC

ALASKA CLAIMS OFFICE
3330 ARCTIC BLVD, STE 206
ANCHORAGE, AK 99503
TEL: (907) 561-1725
FAX: (907) 562-6595
WWW.WARDNA.COM

WASATCH CREST INSURANCE CO

ARIZONA CLAIMS OFFICE
1600 W 2200 S- 4TH FL
PO BOX 27119
SALT LAKE CITY, UT 84127-0008
TEL: (801) 972-7555
FAX: (801) 972-7545
TOLL FREE: (800) 331-1686

IDAHO CLAIMS OFFICE
1600 W 2200 S- 4TH FL
PO BOX 27119
SALT LAKE CITY, UT 84127-0008
TEL: (801) 972-7555
FAX: (801) 972-7545
TOLL FREE: (800) 331-1686

NEVADA CLAIMS OFFICE
1600 W 2200 S- 4TH FL
PO BOX 27119
SALT LAKE CITY, UT 84127-0008
TEL: (801) 972-7555
FAX: (801) 972-7545
TOLL FREE: (800) 331-1686

UTAH CLAIMS OFFICE
1600 W 2200 S- 4TH FL
PO BOX 27119
SALT LAKE CITY, UT 84127-0008
TEL: (801) 972-7555
FAX: (801) 972-7545
TOLL FREE: (800) 331-1686

WASHINGTON DENTAL SERVICE

WASHINGTON CLAIMS OFFICE
9706 4TH AVE NE
PO BOX 75983
SEATTLE, WA 98125
TEL: (206) 522-1300
FAX: (206) 525-2330
TOLL FREE: (800) 367-4104
WWW.DDPWA.COM

WASHINGTON NATIONAL INSURANCE CO

ARIZONA CLAIMS OFFICE
2929 N CENTRAL AVE, STE 1500
PHOENIX, AZ 85012
TEL: (602) 263-4730

WATSON WYATT WORLDWIDE

DISTRICT OF COLUMBIA CLAIMS OFFICE
6707 DEMOCRACY BLVD, STE 800
BETHESDA, MD 20817-1129
TEL: (301) 581-4600
FAX: (301) 581-4937
WWW.WATSONWYATT.COM

MARYLAND CLAIMS OFFICE
6707 DEMOCRACY BLVD, STE 800
BETHESDA, MD 20817-1129
TEL: (301) 581-4600
FAX: (301) 581-4937
WWW.WATSONWYATT.COM

WAUSAU INSURANCE CO

ALASKA CLAIMS OFFICE
8905 SW NIMBUS, STE 300
PO BOX 4025
BEAVERTON, OR 97076-4025
TEL: (503) 626-4100
FAX: (503) 671-7217
TOLL FREE: (800) 424-0054

ARIZONA CLAIMS OFFICE
7600 N 16TH ST, STE 215
PHOENIX, AZ 85020-4499
TEL: (602) 997-2300
FAX: (602) 997-6753

CALIFORNIA CLAIMS OFFICE
PO BOX 7214
PASADENA, CA 91109-7314
TEL: (626) 440-0444
FAX: (626) 568-4499
TOLL FREE: (800) 252-9305
WWW.WAUSAU.COM

425 MARKET ST
PO BOX 7847
SAN FRANCISCO, CA 94120-7847
TEL: (415) 541-0144
FAX: (415) 733-8387
TOLL FREE: (800) 858-0880
WWW.WAUSAU.COM

5959 S MOONEY BLVD
VISALIA, CA 93277
FAX: (559) 730-4390
TOLL FREE: (800) 592-8728
WWW.WAUSAU.COM

COLORADO CLAIMS OFFICE
10975 EL MONTE, STE 225
PO BOX 419157
OVERLAND PARK, KS 64141
TEL: (303) 488-7483
FAX: (913) 344-2312
TOLL FREE: (800) 255-6740
WWW.WAUSAU.COM

FLORIDA CLAIMS OFFICE
PO BOX 140535
ORLANDO, FL 32814-0535
TEL: (407) 894-5151
FAX: (407) 895-3333
TOLL FREE: (800) 231-6165
WWW.WAUSAU.COM

GEORGIA CLAIMS OFFICE
2987 CLAIRMONT RD, STE 400
PO BOX 105067
ATLANTA, GA 30348-5067
TEL: (404) 633-1451
FAX: (404) 315-5350
TOLL FREE: (800) 223-1451
WWW.WAUSAU.COM

ILLINOIS CLAIMS OFFICE
1431 OPUS PL, STE 300
DOWNERS GROVE, IL 60515-1169
TEL: (630) 719-9700
FAX: (630) 719-0777
TOLL FREE: (800) 266-2800
WWW.WAUSAU.COM

INDIANA CLAIMS OFFICE
PO BOX 1187
INDIANAPOLIS, IN 46206-1187
TEL: (317) 576-9654
FAX: (317) 594-1212
TOLL FREE: (800) 782-2794
WWW.WAUSAU.COM

LOUISIANA CLAIMS OFFICE
PO BOX 7033
METAIRIE, LA 70010-7033
TEL: (504) 831-1106
FAX: (504) 841-3229
TOLL FREE: (800) 832-1106
WWW.WAUSAU.COM

MARYLAND CLAIMS OFFICE
8600 LA SALLE ST, STE 200
BALTIMORE, MD 21286
TEL: (410) 825-8060
FAX: (410) 512-0292
TOLL FREE: (800) 638-7887
WWW.WAUSAU.COM

MASSACHUSETTS CLAIMS OFFICE
34 CROSBY DR
PO BOX 9108
BEDFORD, MA 01730
TEL: (781) 275-6629
FAX: (781) 280-5498
TOLL FREE: (800) 343-5872
WWW.WAUSAU.COM

MICHIGAN CLAIMS OFFICE
PO BOX 994
SOUTHFIELD, MI 48037-0994
TEL: (248) 352-1500
FAX: (248) 948-0618
TOLL FREE: (800) 628-7236
IN-STATE: (800) 628-7236

MINNESOTA CLAIMS OFFICE
7450 FRANCE AVE S
PO BOX 1357
EDINA, MN 55435
TEL: (612) 830-1700
FAX: (612) 830-1778
TOLL FREE: (800) 862-6079

MISSOURI CLAIMS OFFICE
PO BOX 419157
KANSAS CITY, MO 64141-6157
TEL: (913) 345-1000
FAX: (913) 344-2312
TOLL FREE: (800) 255-6740
WWW.WAUSAU.COM

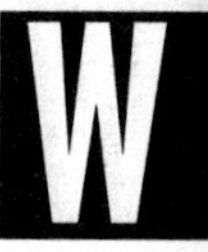

NATIONAL CLAIMS OFFICE
2000 WESTWOOD DR
WAUSAU, WI 54401-7881
TEL: (715) 847-7965
FAX: (715) 847-8402
TOLL FREE: (800) 472-1719
WWW.WAUSAU.COM

PO BOX 14319
SAINT LOUIS, MO 63178-4319
TEL: (314) 878-1030
FAX: (314) 542-8296
TOLL FREE: (800) 826-1661
E-MAIL: WAUSAU.COM/MAIL.MTM
WWW.WAUSAU.COM

NEW JERSEY CLAIMS OFFICE
300 EXECUTIVE DR
WEST ORANGE, NJ 07052
TEL: (973) 736-5000
FAX: (973) 736-6238
TOLL FREE: (800) 362-6920
WWW.WAUSAU.COM

NEW YORK CLAIMS OFFICE
NORTHEAST CLAIMS CENTER
PO BOX 4779
SYRACUSE, NY 13221
TEL: (315) 461-0092
FAX: (315) 461-3894
TOLL FREE: (800) 592-8728
WWW.WAUSAU.COM

NORTH CAROLINA CLAIMS OFFICE
10925 DAVID TAYLOR DR, STE 350
PO BOX 563982
CHARLOTTE, NC 28256-3982
TEL: (704) 510-1999
FAX: (704) 510-4333
TOLL FREE: (800) 447-1254
WWW.WAUSAU.COM

NORTH DAKOTA CLAIMS OFFICE
7450 FRANCE AVE S
PO BOX 1357
EDINA, MN 55435
TEL: (612) 830-1700
FAX: (612) 830-1778
TOLL FREE: (800) 862-6079

OREGON CLAIMS OFFICE
8905 SW NIMBUS, STE 300
PO BOX 4025
BEAVERTON, OR 97076-4025
TEL: (503) 626-4100
FAX: (503) 671-7217
TOLL FREE: (800) 424-0054

PENNSYLVANIA CLAIMS OFFICE
1818 MARKET ST, STE 3110
PHILADELPHIA, PA 19103-3999
TEL: (215) 568-2302
FAX: (215) 575-0392
TOLL FREE: (800) 222-2775
WWW.WAUSAU.COM

SOUTH DAKOTA CLAIMS OFFICE
7450 FRANCE AVE S
PO BOX 1357
EDINA, MN 55435
TEL: (612) 830-1700
FAX: (612) 830-1778
TOLL FREE: (800) 862-6079

TEXAS CLAIMS OFFICE
4828 LOOP CENTRAL DR, STE 700
PO BOX 27708
HOUSTON, TX 77227-7708
TEL: (713) 667-4242
FAX: (713) 295-4550
TOLL FREE: (800) 447-0102
WWW.WAUSAU.COM

106 DECKER CT, STE 600
PO BOX 152800
IRVING, TX 75015-2800
TEL: (972) 650-1955
FAX: (972) 650-5348
TOLL FREE: (800) 634-1955
WWW.WAUSAU.COM

UTAH CLAIMS OFFICE
8905 SW NIMBUS, STE 300
PO BOX 4025
BEAVERTON, OR 97076-4025
TEL: (503) 626-4100
FAX: (503) 671-7217
TOLL FREE: (800) 424-0054

WASHINGTON CLAIMS OFFICE
8905 SW NIMBUS, STE 300
PO BOX 4025
BEAVERTON, OR 97076-4025
TEL: (503) 626-4100
FAX: (503) 671-7217
TOLL FREE: (800) 424-0054

WISCONSIN CLAIMS OFFICE
200 WESTWOOD DR
PO BOX 8013
WAUSAU, WI 54401-7881
TEL: (715) 845-5211
FAX: (715) 847-7569
TOLL FREE: (800) 826-9781
WWW.WAUSAU.COM

WAUSAU INSURANCE COMPANY

NATIONAL CLAIMS OFFICE
115 W WAUSAU AVE
PO BOX 8013
WAUSAU, WI 54402-8013
TEL: (715) 847-7111
FAX: (715) 847-7569
TOLL FREE: (800) 826-9781
WWW.WAUSAU.COM

WEA INSURANCE GROUP

WISCONSIN CLAIMS OFFICE
45 NOB HILL RD
PO BOX 7338
MADISON, WI 53707-7330
TEL: (608) 276-4000
FAX: (608) 276-9119
TOLL FREE: (800) 279-4000

WELBORN HMO DIVISION OF WELBORN CLINIC

INDIANA CLAIMS OFFICE
421 CHESTNUT ST
EVANSVILLE, IN 47713
TEL: (812) 426-9710
FAX: (812) 426-9476
TOLL FREE: (800) 521-0265
WWW.WELBORNCLINIC.COM

H

WELL CARE HMO, INC

FLORIDA CLAIMS OFFICE
6800 N DALE MABRY HWY, STE 270-299
TAMPA, FL 33614
TEL: (813) 290-6200

H

WELL CARE MANAGEMENT GROUP, INC

NEW YORK CLAIMS OFFICE
PO BOX 4470
KINGSTON, NY 12402
TEL: (914) 334-4000
FAX: (914) 331-0041
TOLL FREE: (800) 334-4096

WELLMARK BLUE CROSS & BLUE SHIELD

IOWA CLAIMS OFFICE
HAMILTON BLVD & I-29
PO BOX 1677
SIOUX CITY, IA 51102
TEL: (712) 277-3081
FAX: (712) 279-8450
TOLL FREE: (800) 245-6105
WWW.BCBSIA.COM

SOUTH DAKOTA CLAIMS OFFICE
HAMILTON BLVD & I-29
PO BOX 1677
SIOUX CITY, IA 51102
TEL: (712) 277-3081
FAX: (712) 279-8450
TOLL FREE: (800) 245-6105
WWW.BCBSIA.COM

WELLMARK MEDICARE DIVISION

IOWA CLAIMS OFFICE
636 GRAND STATION 53
DES MOINES, IA 50309
TEL: (515) 245-4619
FAX: (515) 245-3984
WWW.BCBSIA.COM

W

Casualty/Liability Dental Disability 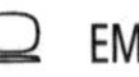 EMC  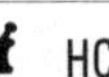 HCPCS 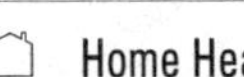 Home Health H HMO Medical

WELLNESS PLAN

MICHIGAN CLAIMS OFFICE
2875 W GRAND BLVD
PO BOX 02577
DETROIT, MI 48202
TEL: (313) 875-4200
TOLL FREE: (800) 875-9355
IN-STATE: (800) 323-3894

WESLEY MEDICAL CENTER

KANSAS CLAIMS OFFICE
550 N HILLSIDE ST
WICHITA, KS 67214-4910
TEL: (316) 688-2607
FAX: (316) 688-7931
WWW.WESLEYMC.COM

WEST BEND MUTUAL INSURANCE CO

WISCONSIN CLAIMS OFFICE
1900 S 18TH AVE
WEST BEND, WI 53095
TEL: (414) 334-5571
FAX: (414) 334-9109
TOLL FREE: (800) 236-5001
WWW.WESTBENDMUTUAL.COM

WESTCHESTER TEAMSTERS HEALTH & WELFARE

NEW YORK CLAIMS OFFICE
160 S CENTRAL AVE
ELMSFORD, NY 10523-3521
TEL: (914) 592-9330
FAX: (914) 592-1519

WESTCO CLAIMS MANAGEMENT

NATIONAL CLAIMS OFFICE
400 PARSON'S POND DR
PO BOX 607
FRANKLIN LAKES, NJ 07417-0607
TEL: (201) 847-8600
FAX: (201) 847-1780

WESTERN DIVERSIFIED LIFE INSURANCE CO

ILLINOIS CLAIMS OFFICE
510 LK COOK RD
PO BOX 770
DEERFIELD, IL 60015-0770
TEL: (847) 948-8988
FAX: (847) 948-1021

WESTERN MEDICAL CONSULTANTS, INC

OREGON CLAIMS OFFICE
350 MISSION ST SE, STE 102
SALEM, OR 97302
TEL: (503) 588-9323
FAX: (503) 796-0749
TOLL FREE: (800) 388-2775

WESTERN MUTUAL INSURANCE CO

IDAHO CLAIMS OFFICE
WESTERN PETROLEUM MARKETERS TRUST
310 E 4500 S, STE 560
PO BOX 572450
MURRAY, UT 84157-2450
TEL: (801) 263-8000
FAX: (801) 263-1247
TOLL FREE: (800) 748-5340

MONTANA CLAIMS OFFICE
WESTERN PETROLEUM MARKETERS TRUST
310 E 4500 S, STE 560
PO BOX 572450
MURRAY, UT 84157-2450
TEL: (801) 263-8000
FAX: (801) 263-1247
TOLL FREE: (800) 748-5340

NEVADA CLAIMS OFFICE
WESTERN PETROLEUM MARKETERS TRUST
310 E 4500 S, STE 560
PO BOX 572450
MURRAY, UT 84157-2450
TEL: (801) 263-8000
FAX: (801) 263-1247
TOLL FREE: (800) 748-5340

UTAH CLAIMS OFFICE
WESTERN PETROLEUM MARKETERS TRUST
310 E 4500 S, STE 560
PO BOX 572450
MURRAY, UT 84157-2450
TEL: (801) 263-8000
FAX: (801) 263-1247
TOLL FREE: (800) 748-5340

WESTERN NATIONAL MUTUAL INSURANCE CO

MINNESOTA CLAIMS OFFICE
PO BOX 1463
MINNEAPOLIS, MN 55440-1463
TEL: (612) 835-5350
FAX: (612) 921-3153
TOLL FREE: (800) 862-6070

WESTERN RESERVE GROUP

OHIO CLAIMS OFFICE
1685 CLEVELAND RD
PO BOX 36
WOOSTER, OH 44691
TEL: (330) 262-9060
FAX: (800) 392-7092

WESTERN UNION FINANCIAL SERVICES

NEW JERSEY CLAIMS OFFICE
1 MACK CTR DR- BLDG 2
PARAMUS, NJ 07652
TEL: (201) 986-5100
FAX: (201) 986-6702
WWW.WESTERNUNION.COM

WESTERN WORLD INSURANCE GROUP

400 PARSON'S POND DR
PO BOX 607
FRANKLIN LAKES, NJ 07417-0607
TEL: (201) 847-8600
FAX: (201) 847-1780

WESTFIELD COMPANIES

ILLINOIS CLAIMS OFFICE
1245 E DIEHL, STE 102
PO BOX 5250
NAPERVILLE, IL 60567-5250
TEL: (630) 955-9563
FAX: (630) 955-9574
TOLL FREE: (800) 414-4759

PO BOX 3499
PEORIA, IL 61612
TEL: (309) 693-7400
FAX: (309) 693-7414
TOLL FREE: (800) 414-4759

INDIANA CLAIMS OFFICE
7221 ENGLE RD, STE 220
FT WAYNE, IN 46804
TEL: (219) 432-3595
FAX: (219) 432-4989
TOLL FREE: (800) 243-0216

3905 VINCENNES RD
PO BOX 781078
INDIANAPOLIS, IN 46278-8078
TEL: (317) 879-1079
FAX: (317) 879-0287
TOLL FREE: (800) 243-0213

570 VALE PARK RD, STE A
VALPARAISO, IN 46385
TEL: (219) 548-3121
FAX: (219) 531-0818
TOLL FREE: (800) 243-0231

4220 EDISON LAKE PKY, STE 200
PO BOX 5128
MISHAWAKA, IN 46546
TEL: (219) 243-0710
FAX: (219) 243-0760
TOLL FREE: (800) 489-1220

KENTUCKY CLAIMS OFFICE
6040 DUTCHMANS LN, STE 320
LOUISVILLE, KY 40205
TEL: (502) 451-4198
FAX: (502) 451-4457
TOLL FREE: (800) 757-9245

MICHIGAN CLAIMS OFFICE
1120 GORNICK AVE
PO BOX 630
GAYLORD, MI 49734-0630
TEL: (517) 732-6719
FAX: (517) 732-3286
TOLL FREE: (800) 338-9096

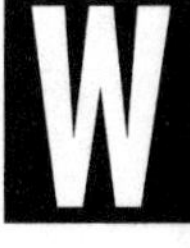

3350 EAGLE PARK DR NE, STE 104
PO BOX 151456
GRAND RAPIDS, MI 49515-1456
TEL: (616) 949-6510
FAX: (616) 949-6954
TOLL FREE: (800) 243-0247

38701 7 MILE RD, STE 255
PO BOX 531120
LIVONIA, MI 48153-1120
TEL: (734) 542-9170
FAX: (734) 542-9270
TOLL FREE: (800) 243-0237

MINNESOTA CLAIMS OFFICE
4940 VIKING DR, STE 404
EDINA, MN 55435-5312
TEL: (612) 831-6446
FAX: (612) 831-4015
TOLL FREE: (800) 757-9244

OHIO CLAIMS OFFICE
PO BOX 5001
WESTFIELD CENTER, OH 44251-5001
TEL: (330) 887-0101
FAX: (330) 887-0840
TOLL FREE: (800) 243-0210
E-MAIL: WEBMASTER@WESTFIELD-COS.COM
WWW.WESTFIELD-COS.COM

955 WINDHAM CT
PO BOX 5408
POLAND, OH 44514
TEL: (330) 726-4255
FAX: (330) 726-4270
TOLL FREE: (800) 358-7779

2000 POLARIS PKY
PO BOX 1690
COLUMBUS, OH 43216
TEL: (614) 431-4400
FAX: (614) 431-4424
TOLL FREE: (800) 283-2422

SOUTH DAKOTA CLAIMS OFFICE
4001 VALHALLA BLVD, STE 103
PO BOX 89707
SIOUX FALLS, SD 57109-9707
TEL: (605) 362-0054
FAX: (605) 362-9243
TOLL FREE: (800) 243-0249

WESTPORT BENEFITS

MISSOURI CLAIMS OFFICE
1600 S BRENTWOOD BLVD, STE 300
PO BOX 66743
SAINT LOUIS, MO 63166
TEL: (314) 918-2300
FAX: (314) 968-9589
TOLL FREE: (800) 548-2041

WESTWARD LIFE INSURANCE CO

CALIFORNIA CLAIMS OFFICE
PO BOX 6025
LAKEWOOD, CA 90714-6025
TEL: (562) 420-6103
FAX: (562) 425-7869
TOLL FREE: (800) 842-0875

HAWAII CLAIMS OFFICE
PO BOX 6025
LAKEWOOD, CA 90714-6025
TEL: (562) 420-6103
FAX: (562) 425-7869
TOLL FREE: (800) 842-0875

IOWA CLAIMS OFFICE
PO BOX 6025
LAKEWOOD, CA 90714-6025
TEL: (562) 420-6103
FAX: (562) 425-7869
TOLL FREE: (800) 842-0875

OREGON CLAIMS OFFICE
PO BOX 6025
LAKEWOOD, CA 90714-6025
TEL: (562) 420-6103
FAX: (562) 425-7869
TOLL FREE: (800) 842-0875

WEYCO, INC

NATIONAL CLAIMS OFFICE
PO BOX 30132
LANSING, MI 48909-7632
TEL: (517) 349-7010
FAX: (517) 349-7335
TOLL FREE: (800) 748-0003
WWW.WEYCOINC.COM

WEYERHAEUSER CO

WASHINGTON CLAIMS OFFICE
GROUP INSURANCE SERVICES
1145 BROADWAY, STE 600
PO BOX TF-C
TACOMA, WA 98402-3527
TEL: (253) 924-7381
FAX: (253) 924-3221
TOLL FREE: (800) 833-0030

WORKERS COMP SERVICES
2835 S 300 44TH ST
FEDERAL WAY, WA 98003
TEL: (253) 924-7676
FAX: (253) 924-4440
TOLL FREE: (800) 242-2331

WICHITA NATIONAL LIFE INSURANCE CO

OKLAHOMA CLAIMS OFFICE
711 "D" AVE
PO BOX 1709
LAWTON, OK 73502-1709
TEL: (580) 353-5776
FAX: (580) 353-6482
TOLL FREE: (800) 522-1625
E-MAIL: WNI@SIRINIT.NET

WILLIAM H. MCGEE CO, INC

NEW YORK CLAIMS OFFICE
2 WORLD TRADE CTR, 47TH FL
NEW YORK, NY 10048
TEL: (212) 775-1300
FAX: (212) 524-6805
WWW.WHMCGEE.COM

WILLIAM M. MERCER

1166 AVE OF THE AMERICAS
NEW YORK, NY 10036
TEL: (212) 574-9000
FAX: (212) 345-7414
WWW.WMMERCER.COM

WILLIAM M. MERCER, INC

CALIFORNIA CLAIMS OFFICE
10 ALMADEN BLVD, STE 1450
SAN JOSE, CA 95113-2239
TEL: (408) 291-6300
FAX: (408) 293-2923

WILLIAM PENN ASSOCIATION

PENNSYLVANIA CLAIMS OFFICE
709 BRIGHTON RD
PITTSBURGH, PA 15233-1821
TEL: (412) 231-2979
FAX: (412) 231-8535
TOLL FREE: (800) 848-7366

WILLIS CORROON CORP

ARIZONA CLAIMS OFFICE
300 W DOUGLAS- 800 R.H. GARVEY BLDG
PO BOX 2697
WICHITA, KS 67201-2697
TEL: (316) 264-5311
FAX: (316) 264-8077
TOLL FREE: (800) 235-7160

CALIFORNIA CLAIMS OFFICE
300 W DOUGLAS- 800 R.H. GARVEY BLDG
PO BOX 2697
WICHITA, KS 67201-2697
TEL: (316) 264-5311
FAX: (316) 264-8077
TOLL FREE: (800) 235-7160

COLORADO CLAIMS OFFICE
300 W DOUGLAS- 800 R.H. GARVEY BLDG
PO BOX 2697
WICHITA, KS 67201-2697
TEL: (316) 264-5311
FAX: (316) 264-8077
TOLL FREE: (800) 235-7160
E-MAIL: HALL_CP@WILCOR.COM

KANSAS CLAIMS OFFICE
300 W DOUGLAS- 800 R.H. GARVEY BLDG
PO BOX 2697
WICHITA, KS 67201-2697
TEL: (316) 264-5311
FAX: (316) 264-8077
TOLL FREE: (800) 235-7160

Insurance Directory

MINNESOTA CLAIMS OFFICE
300 W DOUGLAS- 800 R.H. GARVEY BLDG
PO BOX 2697
WICHITA, KS 67201-2697
TEL: (316) 264-5311
FAX: (316) 264-8077
TOLL FREE: (800) 235-7160
E-MAIL: HALL_CP@WILCOR.COM

MISSOURI CLAIMS OFFICE
300 W DOUGLAS- 800 R.H. GARVEY BLDG
PO BOX 2697
WICHITA, KS 67201-2697
TEL: (316) 264-5311
FAX: (316) 264-8077
TOLL FREE: (800) 235-7160

NEBRASKA CLAIMS OFFICE
300 W DOUGLAS- 800 R.H. GARVEY BLDG
PO BOX 2697
WICHITA, KS 67201-2697
TEL: (316) 264-5311
FAX: (316) 264-8077
TOLL FREE: (800) 235-7160
E-MAIL: HALL_CP@WILCOR.COM

NEW HAMPSHIRE CLAIMS OFFICE
95 S MAIN ST
ROCHESTER, NH 03867
TEL: (603) 332-5800
FAX: (603) 335-9290
TOLL FREE: (800) 288-5077

NEW MEXICO CLAIMS OFFICE
300 W DOUGLAS- 800 R.H. GARVEY BLDG
PO BOX 2697
WICHITA, KS 67201-2697
TEL: (316) 264-5311
FAX: (316) 264-8077
TOLL FREE: (800) 235-7160

OKLAHOMA CLAIMS OFFICE
300 W DOUGLAS- 800 R.H. GARVEY BLDG
PO BOX 2697
WICHITA, KS 67201-2697
TEL: (316) 264-5311
FAX: (316) 264-8077
TOLL FREE: (800) 235-7160

TENNESSEE CLAIMS OFFICE
1415 MURFREESBORO RD, STE 600
PO BOX 305154
NASHVILLE, TN 37230-5154
TEL: (615) 872-3000
FAX: (615) 360-2886
TOLL FREE: (800) 255-8109

TEXAS CLAIMS OFFICE
300 W DOUGLAS- 800 R.H. GARVEY BLDG
PO BOX 2697
WICHITA, KS 67201-2697
TEL: (316) 264-5311
FAX: (316) 264-8077
TOLL FREE: (800) 235-7160

WILLSE & ASSOCIATES

MARYLAND CLAIMS OFFICE
MEDICAL CLAIMS DEPARTMENT
100 S CHARLES- TWR 2, STE 9
PO BOX 1196
BALTIMORE, MD 21297-0417
TEL: (410) 347-1925
FAX: (410) 347-1924
TOLL FREE: (800) 423-9791

WILTON ADJUSTMENT SERVICES

ALASKA CLAIMS OFFICE
335 6TH AVE
PO BOX 70350
FAIRBANKS, AK 99707-0244
TEL: (907) 456-4342
FAX: (907) 456-4949
E-MAIL: WILTON@ALASKA.NET

625 E 34TH AVE, STE 401
PO BOX 92670
ANCHORAGE, AK 99509-2670
TEL: (907) 276-3311
FAX: (907) 276-7877

WINDSOR GROUP

NATIONAL CLAIMS OFFICE
1300 PARKWOOD CIR
PO BOX 105091
ATLANTA, GA 30348
TEL: (770) 951-5599
FAX: (770) 988-0290
TOLL FREE: (800) 428-2499
WWW.AUTOINSURANCE.COM

1300 PARKWOOD CIR
PO BOX 105091
ATLANTA, GA 30348-5091
TEL: (770) 951-5599
FAX: (770) 988-0290
TOLL FREE: (800) 428-2499
WWW.AUTOINSURANCE.COM

OKLAHOMA CLAIMS OFFICE
525 CENTRAL PARK DR, STE 600
PO BOX 268838
OKLAHOMA CITY, OK 73126
TEL: (405) 528-1900
FAX: (405) 530-7553
TOLL FREE: (800) 428-2499
WWW.AUTOINSURANCE.COM

WINNEBAGO INDUSTRIES, INC

IOWA CLAIMS OFFICE
605 W CRYSTAL LK RD
PO BOX 152
FOREST CITY, IA 50436-0152
TEL: (515) 582-3535
FAX: (515) 582-6966
WWW.WINNEBAGO-IND.COM

WINTERTHUR REINSURANCE CORP OF AMERICA

NEW YORK CLAIMS OFFICE
PARTNER REINSURANCE
2 WORLD TRADE CTR, 225 LIBERTY ST- 42ND FL
NEW YORK, NY 10281-1008
TEL: (212) 416-5700
FAX: (212) 524-6839

WISCONSIN NATIONAL LIFE INSURANCE CO

ALABAMA CLAIMS OFFICE
PROTECTIVE LIFE CO
PO BOX 12686
BIRMINGHAM, AL 35202-6686
TEL: (205) 879-9230
FAX: (205) 868-3684
TOLL FREE: (800) 955-4304
IN-STATE: (800) 866-3555

WISCONSIN PHYSICIAN SERVICE

WISCONSIN CLAIMS OFFICE
1717 W BROADWAY
PO BOX 8190
MADISON, WI 53713
TEL: (608) 221-4711
FAX: (608) 223-3626
TOLL FREE: (800) 765-4977
WWW.WPSIC.COM

WISCONSIN PHYSICIANS SERVICE INSURANCE CO (WPS)

CHAMPUS INTERMEDIARY FOR WISCONSIN
1717 W BROADWAY
PO BOX 1890
MADISON, WI 53703
TEL: (608) 221-4711
FAX: (608) 223-3626
TOLL FREE: (800) 828-2837
WWW.WPSIC.COM

WISCONSIN PUBLIC SERVICE CORP

2850 S ASHLAND AVE
GREEN BAY, WI 54304
TEL: (920) 448-7290
FAX: (920) 498-5201
WWW.PSR.COM

WISCONSIN SHEETMETAL HEALTH

PO BOX 3500
MADISON, WI 53704
TEL: (608) 277-0477
TOLL FREE: (800) 779-7577

W

WOLVERINE MUTUAL INSURANCE CO

INDIANA CLAIMS OFFICE
PO BOX 530
DOWAGIAC, MI 49047-0530
TEL: (616) 782-3451
FAX: (616) 782-7652
TOLL FREE: (800) 733-3320

MICHIGAN CLAIMS OFFICE
PO BOX 530
DOWAGIAC, MI 49047-0530
TEL: (616) 782-3451
FAX: (616) 782-7652
TOLL FREE: (800) 733-3320

WOODMEN ACCIDENT & LIFE CO

NEBRASKA CLAIMS OFFICE
1526 "K" ST
PO BOX 82288
LINCOLN, NE 68501-2288
TEL: (402) 476-6500
FAX: (402) 437-4592
TOLL FREE: (800) 869-0355
WWW.WALLO.COM

WOODMEN OF THE WORLD

COLORADO CLAIMS OFFICE
ASSURED LIFE ASSOCIATION
9777 S YOSEMITE ST, STE 200
PO BOX 266000
LITTLETON, CO 80124-6000
TEL: (303) 792-9777
FAX: (303) 792-9793
TOLL FREE: (800) 777-9777

WOODMEN OF THE WORLD LIFE INSURANCE SOCIETY

NEBRASKA CLAIMS OFFICE
OMAHA WOODMEN
1700 FARNAM ST
OMAHA, NE 68102-2078
TEL: (402) 342-1890
FAX: (402) 271-7852
TOLL FREE: (800) 582-0122
WWW.WOODMEN.COM

WORKMEN'S AUTO INSURANCE CO

CALIFORNIA CLAIMS OFFICE
714 W OLYMPIC BLVD, STE 800
LOS ANGELES, CA 90015-1472
TEL: (213) 747-6492
FAX: (213) 747-4699
TOLL FREE: (800) 697-6117

WORKMEN'S CIRCLE

NEW YORK CLAIMS OFFICE
45 E 33RD ST
NEW YORK, NY 10016-5336
TEL: (212) 889-6800
FAX: (212) 532-7518
TOLL FREE: (800) 922-2558
E-MAIL: WCFRIENDS@AOL.COM
WWW.CIRCLE.COM

WORLD INSURANCE CO

NEBRASKA CLAIMS OFFICE
11808 GRANT ST
PO BOX 3160
OMAHA, NE 68103-0160
TEL: (402) 496-8000
FAX: (402) 496-8040
TOLL FREE: (800) 786-7557

WORLD NET SERVICES

FLORIDA CLAIMS OFFICE
AMERICAN PIONEER LIFE
11 N BAYLEN ST
PO BOX 130
PENSACOLA, FL 32591-0130
TEL: (850) 469-8220
FAX: (850) 433-1186
TOLL FREE: (800) 999-2224
IN-STATE: (800) 825-3428

NEW YORK CLAIMS OFFICE
AMERICAN PIONEER LIFE
11 N BAYLEN ST
PO BOX 130
PENSACOLA, FL 32591-0130
TEL: (850) 469-8220
FAX: (850) 433-1186
TOLL FREE: (800) 999-2224
IN-STATE: (800) 825-3428

TEXAS CLAIMS OFFICE
AMERICAN PIONEER LIFE
11 N BAYLEN ST
PO BOX 130
PENSACOLA, FL 32591-0130
TEL: (850) 469-8220
FAX: (850) 433-1186
TOLL FREE: (800) 999-2224
IN-STATE: (800) 825-3428

XACT MEDICARE

PENNSYLVANIA CLAIMS OFFICE
PENNSYLVANIA BLUE SHIELD
1800 CTR ST
PO BOX 890413
CAMP HILL, PA 17089-0413
TEL: (717) 763-3601
FAX: (717) 760-9296
TOLL FREE: (800) 746-5680
IN-STATE: (800) 382-1274
WWW.XACT.ORG

XACT MEDICARE SERVICES — MEDICARE PART B CARRIER

1800 CENTER ST
PO BOX 890089
CAMP HILL, PA 17089-0089
TEL: (717) 763-5700
FAX: (717) 760-9296
WWW.XACT.ORG

YAKIMA INDIAN NATION TRIBAL INSURANCE

WASHINGTON CLAIMS OFFICE
PO BOX 151
TOPPENISH, WA 98948-0151
TEL: (509) 865-5121
FAX: (509) 865-5522

ZENITH ADMINISTRATORS, INC

ARIZONA CLAIMS OFFICE
4747 N 7TH ST, STE 308
PHOENIX, AZ 85014
TEL: (602) 248-8434
FAX: (602) 248-8301

CALIFORNIA CLAIMS OFFICE
6801 E WASHINGTON BLVD
PO BOX 22041
COMMERCE, CA 90022
TEL: (323) 724-1144

301 MISSION ST, STE 600
SAN FRANCISCO, CA 94105
TEL: (415) 546-7800
FAX: (415) 546-0600
TOLL FREE: (800) 388-0508

COLORADO CLAIMS OFFICE
8700 TURNPIKE DR, STE 200
WESTMINSTER, CO 80031
TEL: (303) 430-1118
FAX: (303) 430-0224

ILLINOIS CLAIMS OFFICE
303 E OHIO ST, STE 2600
CHICAGO, IL 60611
TEL: (312) 649-1200
FAX: (312) 649-1245

2873 N DIRKSEN PKY, STE 200
SPRINGFIELD, IL 62702
TEL: (217) 753-4531
FAX: (217) 753-3953
TOLL FREE: (800) 538-6466

INDIANA CLAIMS OFFICE
2601 FORTUNE CIR E, STE 103A
INDIANAPOLIS, IN 46241
TEL: (317) 247-7381
FAX: (317) 248-3279
TOLL FREE: (800) 382-1799

LOUISIANA CLAIMS OFFICE
2450 SEVERN AVE, STE 517
METAIRIE, LA 70001-1237
TEL: (504) 831-1544
FAX: (504) 831-1894
TOLL FREE: (800) 638-4855

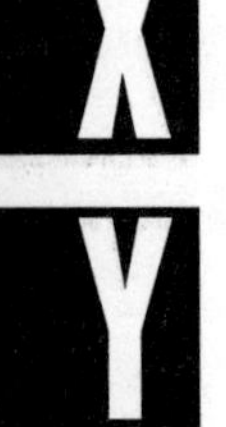

Casualty/Liability Dental Disability  EMC  HCPCS 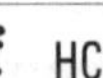 Home Health 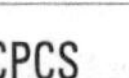 H HMO 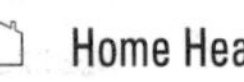 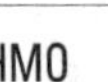 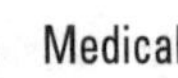 Medical

MARYLAND CLAIMS OFFICE
1320 PATUXTENT PKY, STE 610
PO BOX 1100
COLUMBIA, MD 21044
TEL: (410) 884-1440
FAX: (410) 997-3657
TOLL FREE: (800) 235-5805
E-MAIL: ZENITH TPA.COM
WWW.ZENITH TPA

MASSACHUSETTS CLAIMS OFFICE
100 GRANDVIEW RD, STE 402
BRAINTREE, MA 02184
TEL: (617) 849-1650
FAX: (617) 849-1652

MICHIGAN CLAIMS OFFICE
6011 W SAINT JOSEPH, STE 401
LANSING, MI 48917
TEL: (517) 323-9250
FAX: (517) 323-1093

MINNESOTA CLAIMS OFFICE
314 W SUPERIOR ST, STE 750
DULUTH, MN 55802
TEL: (218) 727-6668
FAX: (218) 727-5697
TOLL FREE: (800) 992-1465

7645 METRO BLVD
MINNEAPOLIS, MN 55436
TEL: (612) 835-7035
FAX: (612) 835-8373

MISSOURI CLAIMS OFFICE
4260 SHORELINE DR, STE 170
PO BOX 3016
EARTH CITY, MO 63044
TEL: (314) 344-8899
FAX: (314) 344-4407

3449 HOLLENBERG DR, STE 150
PO BOX 3016
EARTH CITY, MO 63044
TEL: (314) 739-2973
FAX: (314) 739-8059

3100 BROADWAY, STE 400
KANSAS CITY, MO 64111
TEL: (818) 756-0173
FAX: (816) 531-6518

NATIONAL CLAIMS OFFICE
33 EASTLAND ST
SPRINGFIELD, MA 01109
TEL: (413) 733-0177
FAX: (413) 733-3325

4380 SW MACADAN AVE, STE 300
PO BOX 1420
PORTLAND, OR 97201
TEL: (503) 226-6753
FAX: (503) 226-7900
TOLL FREE: (800) 547-5900

8207 CALLAGHAN RD, STE 300
SAN ANTONIO, TX 78230-4780
TEL: (210) 349-7774
FAX: (210) 349-0315
TOLL FREE: (800) 443-1606

TEXAS CLAIMS OFFICE
5430 L.B.J. FREEWAY, STE 270
DALLAS, TX 75240-2611
TEL: (972) 701-5700
FAX: (972) 701-5701
TOLL FREE: (800) 422-3342
WWW.THEZENITH.COM

4600 GULF FWY, STE 300
HOUSTON, TX 77023
TEL: (713) 926-2422
FAX: (713) 924-1299

410 HWY 69
PO BOX 1645
NEDERLAND, TX 77627
TEL: (409) 727-2343

8207 CALLAGHAN RD, STE 300
SAN ANTONIO, TX 78230-4780
TEL: (210) 349-7774
FAX: (210) 349-0315
TOLL FREE: (800) 443-1606

WASHINGTON CLAIMS OFFICE
201 QUEEN ANNE AVE N, STE 100
SEATTLE, WA 98109
TEL: (206) 282-4100
FAX: (206) 285-1701
TOLL FREE: (800) 426-5980

104 S FREYA, STE 220
SPOKANE, WA 99202
TEL: (509) 534-5625
TOLL FREE: (800) 522-2403

WISCONSIN CLAIMS OFFICE
2100 N MAYFAIR RD, STE 100
MILWAUKEE, WI 53226
TEL: (414) 476-1220
FAX: (414) 476-2997
TOLL FREE: (800) 242-4712
WWW.ZENITHTPA.COM

2801 COHO ST, STE 300
MADISON, WI 53713
TEL: (608) 274-4773
FAX: (608) 277-1088
TOLL FREE: (800) 397-3373

ZENITH INSURANCE CO

ALABAMA CLAIMS OFFICE
10 INVERNESS CTR PKY, STE 220
BIRMINGHAM, AL 35242
TEL: (205) 408-1836
FAX: (205) 408-6910
TOLL FREE: (800) 256-7477
WWW.ZENITH.COM

CALIFORNIA CLAIMS OFFICE
21255 CALIFA ST
PO BOX 9055
VAN NUYS, CA 91409-9055
TEL: (818) 713-1000
FAX: (818) 713-8296
TOLL FREE: (800) 448-4356
WWW.ZENITH.COM

575 E LOCUST, #101
PO BOX 12546
FRESNO, CA 93778-2546
TEL: (559) 226-0280
FAX: (559) 436-8839
WWW.ZENITH.COM

4309 HACIENDA DR, STE 200
PO BOX 8002
PLEASANTON, CA 94588-8602
TEL: (925) 460-0600
TOLL FREE: (800) 395-1124
WWW.ZENITH.COM

1660 N HOTEL CIR, STE 400
SAN DIEGO, CA 92108-2807
TEL: (619) 299-6252
FAX: (619) 542-0035
TOLL FREE: (800) 533-6212
WWW.ZENITH.COM

FLORIDA CLAIMS OFFICE
10 INVERNESS CTR PKY, STE 220
BIRMINGHAM, AL 35242
TEL: (205) 408-1836
FAX: (205) 408-6910
TOLL FREE: (800) 256-7477
WWW.ZENITH.COM

LOUISIANA CLAIMS OFFICE
10 INVERNESS CTR PKY, STE 220
BIRMINGHAM, AL 35242
TEL: (205) 408-1836
FAX: (205) 408-6910
TOLL FREE: (800) 256-7477
WWW.ZENITH.COM

MISSOURI CLAIMS OFFICE
10 INVERNESS CTR PKY, STE 220
BIRMINGHAM, AL 35242
TEL: (205) 408-1836
FAX: (205) 408-6910
TOLL FREE: (800) 256-7477
WWW.ZENITH.COM

NORTH CAROLINA CLAIMS OFFICE
10 INVERNESS CTR PKY, STE 220
BIRMINGHAM, AL 35242
TEL: (205) 408-1836
FAX: (205) 408-6910
TOLL FREE: (800) 256-7477
WWW.ZENITH.COM

OKLAHOMA CLAIMS OFFICE
10 INVERNESS CTR PKY, STE 220
BIRMINGHAM, AL 35242
TEL: (205) 408-1836
FAX: (205) 408-6910
TOLL FREE: (800) 256-7477
WWW.ZENITH.COM

ZURICH COMMERCIAL

LOUISIANA CLAIMS OFFICE
650 POYDRAS ST, STE 1210
NEW ORLEANS, LA 70130
TEL: (504) 561-8802
FAX: (504) 524-2360
TOLL FREE: (800) 727-1080

ZURICH GROUP COMPANIES

CONNECTICUT CLAIMS OFFICE
NE COMMERCIAL CLAIMS CENTER
PO BOX 1504010
HARTFORD, CT 06115-0410
TEL: (800) 239-4559
FAX: (800) 887-1335
TOLL FREE: (800) 243-3282
IN-STATE: (800) 922-4607

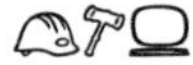

ZURICH U.S.

MARYLAND CLAIMS OFFICE
PO BOX 855
COCKEYSVILLE, 21030
TEL: (410) 527-3582
FAX: (410) 785-9624
TOLL FREE: (800) 262-6764
IN-STATE: (800) 262-6764

ZURICH-AMERICAN INSURANCE GROUP

ALABAMA CLAIMS OFFICE
2829 LAKELAND DR, STE 1503
JACKSON, MS 39208
TEL: (601) 939-0440
FAX: (601) 939-2674
TOLL FREE: (800) 366-8366
WWW.ZURICHAMERICAN.COM

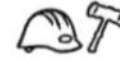

PO BOX 20791
ATLANTA, GA 30320
TEL: (770) 395-9241
FAX: (770) 395-6182
TOLL FREE: (800) 241-7570
WWW.ZURICHAMERICAN.COM

CALIFORNIA CLAIMS OFFICE
21300 VICTORY BLVD, 10TH FL
PO BOX 92566
LOS ANGELES, CA 90009-2566
TEL: (818) 227-1700
FAX: (818) 702-6179
TOLL FREE: (800) 338-3160
WWW.ZURICHAMERICAN.COM

44 MONTGOMERY ST, 27TH FL
SAN FRANCISCO, CA 94104-4801
TEL: (415) 986-4900
FAX: (415) 296-7368
TOLL FREE: (800) 701-4926
WWW.ZURICHAMERICAN.COM

CONNECTICUT CLAIMS OFFICE
200 UNICORN PARK
PO BOX 9217
BOSTON, MA 02205
TEL: (781) 939-0844
FAX: (781) 939-0825
TOLL FREE: (800) 225-1806
IN-STATE: (800) 818-5835
WWW.ZURICHAMERICAN.COM

DELAWARE CLAIMS OFFICE
10 LAKE CTR EXECUTIVE PRK, STE 200- 401
RTE 73 N
PO BOX 13761
PHILADELPHIA, PA 19104
TEL: (609) 596-2090
FAX: (609) 985-2960
TOLL FREE: (800) 257-8134
WWW.ZURICHAMERICAN.COM

FLORIDA CLAIMS OFFICE
1900 SUMMIT TWR BLVD, STE 900
PO BOX 628210
ORLANDO, FL 32862
TEL: (407) 660-9096
FAX: (407) 660-0339
TOLL FREE: (800) 340-8602
WWW.ZURICHAMERICAN.COM

GEORGIA CLAIMS OFFICE
PO BOX 20791
ATLANTA, GA 30320
TEL: (770) 395-9241
FAX: (770) 395-6182
TOLL FREE: (800) 241-7570
WWW.ZURICHAMERICAN.COM

ILLINOIS CLAIMS OFFICE
1400 AMERICAN LN
SCHAUMBURG, IL 60196-1056
TEL: (847) 605-6000
FAX: (847) 605-7811
TOLL FREE: (800) 382-2150
WWW.ZURICHAMERICAN.COM

ZURICH COMMERCIAL
200 W ADAMS, STE 1100
CHICAGO, IL 60606
TEL: (312) 332-7171
FAX: (312) 332-5417
TOLL FREE: (800) 783-0163
IN-STATE: (800) 981-8912
WWW.ZURICHAMERICAN.COM

KANSAS CLAIMS OFFICE
9225 INDIAN CRK PKY
PO BOX 20048
KANSAS CITY, MO 64195-0048
TEL: (913) 345-8600
FAX: (913) 491-5161
TOLL FREE: (800) 777-9005
WWW.ZURICHAMERICAN.COM

MAINE CLAIMS OFFICE
200 UNICORN PARK
PO BOX 9217
BOSTON, MA 02205
TEL: (781) 939-0844
FAX: (781) 939-0825
TOLL FREE: (800) 225-1806
IN-STATE: (800) 818-5835
WWW.ZURICHAMERICAN.COM

MARYLAND CLAIMS OFFICE
10 LAKE CTR EXECUTIVE PRK, STE 200- 401
RTE 73 N
PO BOX 13761
PHILADELPHIA, PA 19104
TEL: (609) 596-2090
FAX: (609) 985-2960
TOLL FREE: (800) 257-8134
WWW.ZURICHAMERICAN.COM

MASSACHUSETTS CLAIMS OFFICE
200 UNICORN PARK
PO BOX 9217
BOSTON, MA 02205
TEL: (781) 939-0844
FAX: (781) 939-0825
TOLL FREE: (800) 225-1806
IN-STATE: (800) 818-5835
WWW.ZURICHAMERICAN.COM

MICHIGAN CLAIMS OFFICE
ZURICH COMMERCIAL
28411 NORTHWESTERN HWY, STE 950
SOUTHFIELD, MI 48034
TEL: (248) 356-3569
FAX: (248) 350-9310
TOLL FREE: (800) 860-3628
WWW.ZURICHAMERICAN.COM

MINNESOTA CLAIMS OFFICE
PO BOX 3193
MILWAUKEE, WI 53201-3193
TEL: (414) 798-8920
FAX: (414) 798-8883
TOLL FREE: (800) 631-6074
WWW.ZURICHAMERICAN.COM

MISSISSIPPI CLAIMS OFFICE
2829 LAKELAND DR, STE 1503
JACKSON, MS 39208
TEL: (601) 939-0440
FAX: (601) 939-2674
TOLL FREE: (800) 366-8366
WWW.ZURICHAMERICAN.COM

MISSOURI CLAIMS OFFICE
9225 INDIAN CRK PKY
PO BOX 20048
KANSAS CITY, MO 64195-0048
TEL: (913) 345-8600
FAX: (913) 491-5161
TOLL FREE: (800) 777-9005
WWW.ZURICHAMERICAN.COM

NEW HAMPSHIRE CLAIMS OFFICE
200 UNICORN PARK
PO BOX 9217
BOSTON, MA 02205
TEL: (781) 939-0844
FAX: (781) 939-0825
TOLL FREE: (800) 225-1806
IN-STATE: (800) 818-5835
WWW.ZURICHAMERICAN.COM

NEW JERSEY CLAIMS OFFICE
25 VREELAND RD- BLDG A
PO BOX 905
NEWARK, NJ 07101-0905
TEL: (973) 765-0555
FAX: (973) 765-9444
TOLL FREE: (800) 255-3612
WWW.ZURICHAMERICAN.COM

NEW YORK CLAIMS OFFICE
1377 MOLDER PKY, STE 400
PO BOX ZZ
JAMAICA, NY 11430-0022
TEL: (516) 232-5800
FAX: (516) 234-4292
TOLL FREE: (800) 396-6677
WWW.ZURICHAMERICAN.COM

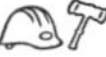

165 BROADWAY- 28TH FL
NEW YORK, NY 10006
TEL: (212) 238-3778
FAX: (212) 406-9536
WWW.ZURICHAMERICAN.COM

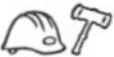

NORTH DAKOTA CLAIMS OFFICE
PO BOX 3193
MILWAUKEE, WI 53201-3193
TEL: (414) 798-8920
FAX: (414) 798-8883
TOLL FREE: (800) 631-6074
WWW.ZURICHAMERICAN.COM

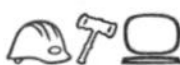

OHIO CLAIMS OFFICE
ZURICH GROUP
730 HOLIDAY DR- FOSTER PLZ, BLDG 8
PO BOX 1880
PITTSBURGH, PA 15230
TEL: (412) 928-9990
FAX: (412) 928-0101
TOLL FREE: (800) 888-8765
WWW.ZURICHAMERICAN.COM

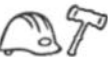

PENNSYLVANIA CLAIMS OFFICE
730 HOLIDAY DR- FOSTER PLZ #8
PO BOX 1880
PITTSBURGH, PA 15230-1880
TEL: (412) 928-9990
FAX: (412) 928-0543
TOLL FREE: (800) 888-8765
WWW.ZURICHAMERICAN.COM

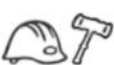

ZURICH GROUP
730 HOLIDAY DR- FOSTER PLZ #8
PO BOX 1880
PITTSBURGH, PA 15230
TEL: (412) 928-9990
FAX: (412) 928-0101
TOLL FREE: (800) 888-8765
WWW.ZURICHAMERICAN.COM

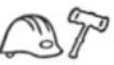

10 LAKE CTR EXECUTIVE PRK, STE 200- 401 RTE 73 N
PO BOX 13761
PHILADELPHIA, PA 19104
TEL: (609) 596-2090
FAX: (609) 985-2960
TOLL FREE: (800) 257-8134
WWW.ZURICHAMERICAN.COM

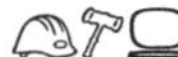

RHODE ISLAND CLAIMS OFFICE
200 UNICORN PARK
PO BOX 9217
BOSTON, MA 02205
TEL: (781) 939-0844
FAX: (781) 939-0825
TOLL FREE: (800) 225-1806
IN-STATE: (800) 818-5835
WWW.ZURICHAMERICAN.COM

SOUTH DAKOTA CLAIMS OFFICE
PO BOX 3193
MILWAUKEE, WI 53201-3193
TEL: (414) 798-8920
FAX: (414) 798-8883
TOLL FREE: (800) 631-6074
WWW.ZURICHAMERICAN.COM

TENNESSEE CLAIMS OFFICE
2829 LAKELAND DR, STE 1503
JACKSON, MS 39208
TEL: (601) 939-0440
FAX: (601) 939-2674
TOLL FREE: (800) 366-8366
WWW.ZURICHAMERICAN.COM

TEXAS CLAIMS OFFICE
9330 LBJ FWY, STE 1200
PO BOX 619507
DALLAS, TX 75261-9507
TEL: (972) 231-7001
FAX: (972) 783-0062
TOLL FREE: (800) 727-1080
WWW.ZURICHAMERICAN.COM

VERMONT CLAIMS OFFICE
200 UNICORN PARK
PO BOX 9217
BOSTON, MA 02205
TEL: (781) 939-0844
FAX: (781) 939-0825
TOLL FREE: (800) 225-1806
IN-STATE: (800) 818-5835
WWW.ZURICHAMERICAN.COM

WISCONSIN CLAIMS OFFICE
PO BOX 3193
MILWAUKEE, WI 53201-3193
TEL: (414) 798-8920
FAX: (414) 798-8883
TOLL FREE: (800) 631-6074
WWW.ZURICHAMERICAN.COM

X Y Z

State-by-State Index

ALABAMA

ALABAMA— cont

ALASKA

ALBERTA

AMERICAN SAMOA

ARIZONA

ARKANSAS

CALIFORNIA— *cont*

COLORADO

CONNECTICUT

CONNECTICUT— cont

DELAWARE

DISTRICT OF COLUMBIA

FLORIDA

GUAM

HAWAII

IDAHO

IDAHO— cont

ILLINOIS

ILLINOIS— cont

INDIANA

IOWA

IOWA— cont

KANSAS

KENTUCKY

MAINE

MANITOBA

MARYLAND

MARYLAND— cont

MASSACHUSETTS

MEXICO

MICHIGAN

MISSISSIPPI

MISSOURI

MISSOURI— cont

MONTANA

NATIONAL

NATIONAL— cont

NATIONAL— cont

NEBRASKA

NEBRASKA— cont

NEVADA

NEW BRUNSWICK

NEW HAMPSHIRE

NEW JERSEY

NEW JERSEY— cont

NEW MEXICO

NEW YORK

NEW YORK— cont

NEWFOUNDLAND

NORTH CAROLINA

NORTH DAKOTA

OKLAHOMA

OKLAHOMA— cont

ONTARIO

OREGON

PENNSYLVANIA

PENNSYLVANIA— cont

PRINCE EDWARD ISLAND

PUERTO RICO

QUEBEC

RHODE ISLAND

SASKATCHEWAN

SOUTH CAROLINA

SOUTH CAROLINA— cont

SOUTH DAKOTA

TENNESSEE

TEXAS

TEXAS— cont

UTAH

UTAH— cont

VERMONT

VIRGIN ISLANDS

WASHINGTON— cont

WEST VIRGINIA

WISCONSIN

WISCONSIN— cont

WYOMING

Appendix A

Companies Verifying HCPCS Level II Codes

Note: Although companies within the *2000 Insurance Directory* have indicated that they process HCPCS Level II codes, it is important to check that the particular plan being billed processes these claims.

ACS CLAIMS SERVICE

TEXAS CLAIMS OFFICE
PO BOX 296
DALLAS, TX 75221
TEL: (214) 826-8148
FAX: (214) 826-8239
TOLL FREE: (800) 456-9653

ADMINISTRATION SYSTEMS RESEARCH CORP

MICHIGAN CLAIMS OFFICE
3033 ORCHARD VISTA DR SE
GRAND RAPIDS, MI 49546-7000
TEL: (616) 957-1751
FAX: (616) 957-8986
TOLL FREE: (800) 968-2449
WWW.ASRCORP.COM,
WWW.PHYSICIANSCARE.COM

ADMINISTRATIVE CONSULTANTS, INC

CONNECTICUT CLAIMS OFFICE
92 BROOKSIDE RD
PO BOX 1471
WATERBURY, CT 06721
TEL: (203) 756-8061
FAX: (203) 754-3941

ADMINISTRATIVE SERVICE CONSULTANTS

NATIONAL CLAIMS OFFICE
3301 E ROYALTON RD
BROADVIEW HEIGHTS, OH 44147
TEL: (440) 526-2730
FAX: (440) 526-1608
TOLL FREE: (800) 634-8816
WWW.ASCOFOHIO.COM

ADMINISTRATIVE SERVICES, INC

FLORIDA CLAIMS OFFICE
7990 SW 117TH AVE
PO BOX 839000
MIAMI, FL 33283
TEL: (305) 595-4040
FAX: (305) 596-6820
TOLL FREE: (800) 749-1858
E-MAIL: INFO@ADMINSERV.COM
WWW.ADMINSERV.COM

ADMIRAL INSURANCE CO

NEW JERSEY CLAIMS OFFICE
1255 CALDWELL RD
PO BOX 5725
CHERRY HILL, NJ 08034-3220
TEL: (609) 429-9200
FAX: (609) 428-3390
WWW.ADMIRALINS.COM

ADVANCED BENEFIT ADMINISTRATORS

IDAHO CLAIMS OFFICE
6420 SW MACADAM AVE, STE 380
PORTLAND, OR 97201-3519
TEL: (503) 245-3770
FAX: (503) 245-4122
TOLL FREE: (800) 443-6531

OREGON CLAIMS OFFICE
6420 SW MACADAM AVE, STE 380
PORTLAND, OR 97201-3519
TEL: (503) 245-3770
FAX: (503) 245-4122
TOLL FREE: (800) 443-6531

WASHINGTON CLAIMS OFFICE
6420 SW MACADAM AVE, STE 380
PORTLAND, OR 97201-3519
TEL: (503) 245-3770
FAX: (503) 245-4122
TOLL FREE: (800) 443-6531

ADVANCED INSURANCE SERVICES

TENNESSEE CLAIMS OFFICE
600 JEFFERSON AVE
PO BOX 19
MEMPHIS, TN 38101-0019
TEL: (901) 544-2344
FAX: (901) 544-2328
TOLL FREE: (800) 772-1352

AETNA / U.S. HEALTHCARE

CALIFORNIA CLAIMS OFFICE
6795 N PALM AVE
FRESNO, CA 93704
TEL: (209) 241-1000
FAX: (209) 241-1226
TOLL FREE: (800) 756-7039
WWW.AETNAUSHC.COM

CONNECTICUT CLAIMS OFFICE
151 FARMINGTON AVE
PO BOX 150417
HARTFORD, CT 06156
TEL: (860) 273-0123
TOLL FREE: (800) 872-3862
WWW.AETNAUSHEALTHCARE.COM

1000 MIDDLE ST
MIDDLETOWN, CT 06457-4621
TEL: (860) 636-8300
FAX: (860) 638-6599
TOLL FREE: (800) 445-3184
WWW.AETNAUSHC.COM

FLORIDA CLAIMS OFFICE
4300 W CYPRESS ST
PO BOX 31450
TAMPA, FL 33631-3450
TEL: (813) 870-6670
TOLL FREE: (800) 872-3862
WWW.AETNAUSHC.COM

PO BOX 30167
TAMPA, FL 33630-3167
TEL: (813) 870-7940
FAX: (813) 878-7839
TOLL FREE: (800) 323-9930
IN-STATE: (800) 282-3517
WWW.AETNAUSHC.COM

MASSACHUSETTS CLAIMS OFFICE
400-1 TOTTEN POND RD
WALTHAM, MA 02154
TEL: (781) 273-5600
FAX: (781) 902-3871
TOLL FREE: (800) 448-8742
WWW.AETNAUSHC.COM

400-1 TOTTEN POND RD
WALTHAM, MA 02154
TEL: (781) 273-5600
FAX: (781) 902-3871
TOLL FREE: (800) 448-8742
WWW.AETNAUSHC.COM

NEW JERSEY CLAIMS OFFICE
55 LANE RD
FAIRFIELD, NJ 07004
TEL: (973) 575-5600
FAX: (973) 244-3911
TOLL FREE: (800) 852-0629
WWW.AETNAUSHC.COM

PENNSYLVANIA CLAIMS OFFICE
1425 UNION MEETING RD
PO BOX 1125
BLUE BELL, PA 19422
TEL: (215) 775-4800
TOLL FREE: (800) 233-3105
WWW.AETNAUSHC.COM

VIRGINIA CLAIMS OFFICE
AETNA HEALTH PLANS OF THE MID-ATLANTIC, INC
7600 A LEESBURG PIKE, STE 300
FALLS CHURCH, VA 22043-2413
TEL: (703) 903-7100
FAX: (703) 903-0316
TOLL FREE: (800) 231-8415
WWW.AETNAUSHC.COM

AETNA / U.S. HEALTHCARE CO

NATIONAL CLAIMS OFFICE
7601 ORA GLEN DR
GREENBELT, MD 20770-3647
TEL: (301) 441-1600
FAX: (301) 489-5284
TOLL FREE: (800) 635-3121
IN-STATE: (800) 635-3121

AIG CLAIM SERVICES, INC

FLORIDA CLAIMS OFFICE
PO BOX 25477
TAMPA, FL 33622-5477
TEL: (813) 218-3000
FAX: (813) 272-1122
IN-STATE: (800) 647-4767
WWW.AIG.COM

KANSAS CLAIMS OFFICE
120 S CENTRAL AVE, STE 300
CLAYTON, MO 63105
TEL: (314) 719-4000
FAX: (314) 863-5939
TOLL FREE: (888) 745-7819
WWW.AIG.COM

NEW YORK CLAIMS OFFICE
70 PINE ST
NEW YORK, NY 10270-0002
TEL: (212) 770-7000
FAX: (212) 943-1125
WWW.AIG.COM

PENNSYLVANIA CLAIMS OFFICE
1700 CNG TWR, 625 LIBERTY AVE
PITTSBURGH, PA 15222
TEL: (412) 393-3960
FAX: (412) 288-5959
TOLL FREE: (800) 892-9779
IN-STATE: (800) 258-7152
WWW.AIG.COM

ALL RISK ADMINISTRATORS

FLORIDA CLAIMS OFFICE
PO BOX 66237
SAINT PETERSBURG BEACH, FL 33736-6210
TEL: (727) 367-3315
FAX: (727) 367-4510
TOLL FREE: (800) 338-4485

ALLIED GROUP INSURANCE CO

MINNESOTA CLAIMS OFFICE
PO BOX 1420
MINNEAPOLIS, MN 55440-1420
TEL: (612) 896-1774
FAX: (612) 896-6640
TOLL FREE: (800) 862-6024

ALPHA DATA SYSTEMS, INC

TEXAS CLAIMS OFFICE
1545 W MOCKINGBIRD LN, STE 6000
DALLAS, TX 75235
TEL: (214) 638-1485
TOLL FREE: (800) 342-5248

AMERICAN COMMERCIAL LINES

INDIANA CLAIMS OFFICE
1701 E MARKET ST
PO BOX 610
JEFFERSONVILLE, IN 47131-0610
TEL: (812) 288-0100
FAX: (812) 288-1720
TOLL FREE: (800) 548-7689

AMERICAN FAMILY INSURANCE

INNESOTA CLAIMS OFFICE
PO BOX 59173
MINNEAPOLIS, MN 55459
TEL: (612) 933-4446
FAX: (612) 933-7268
TOLL FREE: (800) 374-1111
WWW.AMFAM.COM

AMERICAN HEALTH CARE

NATIONAL CLAIMS OFFICE
PO BOX 7000
RICHTON, IL 60471
TEL: (630) 916-8400
FAX: (630) 261-7988
TOLL FREE: (800) 624-8568

AMERICAN HEALTH CARE PROVIDERS, INC

ARKANSAS CLAIMS OFFICE
900 S SHACKLEFORD RD, STE 110
LITTLE ROCK, AR 72211-3845
TEL: (501) 221-3534
FAX: (501) 221-3049
TOLL FREE: (800) 333-3534

AMERICAN OCCUPATIONAL HEALTH SERVICES
4601 SAUK TRAIL
PO BOX 7000
RICHTON PARK, IL 60471
TEL: (708) 503-5000
FAX: (708) 503-5001
TOLL FREE: (800) 242-7460

ILLINOIS CLAIMS OFFICE
AMERICAN OCCUPATIONAL HEALTH SERVICES
4601 SAUK TRAIL
PO BOX 7000
RICHTON PARK, IL 60471
TEL: (708) 503-5000
FAX: (708) 503-5001
TOLL FREE: (800) 242-7460

INDIANA CLAIMS OFFICE
AMERICAN OCCUPATIONAL HEALTH SERVICES
4601 SAUK TRAIL
PO BOX 7000
RICHTON PARK, IL 60471
TEL: (708) 503-5000
FAX: (708) 503-5001
TOLL FREE: (800) 242-7460

AMERICAN HERITAGE LIFE INSURANCE CO

FLORIDA CLAIMS OFFICE
1776 AMERICAN HERITAGE LIFE DR
JACKSONVILLE, FL 32224-3492
TEL: (904) 992-1776
FAX: (904) 992-2695
TOLL FREE: (800) 535-8086

AMERICAN LIFE INSURANCE CO

ILLINOIS CLAIMS OFFICE
208 S LA SALLE ST, STE 2070
CHICAGO, IL 60604
TEL: (312) 372-5722
FAX: (312) 372-5727

AMERICAN MEDICAL & LIFE INSURANCE CO

NEW YORK CLAIMS OFFICE
35 N BROADWAY
HICKSVILLE, NY 11801-4236
TEL: (516) 822-8700
FAX: (516) 931-1010
TOLL FREE: (800) 822-0004

AMERICAN MINING INSURANCE CO, INC

ALABAMA CLAIMS OFFICE
CGH INSURANCE GROUP
550 MONTGOMERY HWY
PO BOX 660847
BIRMINGHAM, AL 35266-0847
TEL: (205) 823-4496
FAX: (205) 823-6177
TOLL FREE: (800) 448-5621
WWW.CGHINSURANCE.COM

AMERICAN NATIONAL INSURANCE CO

TEXAS CLAIMS OFFICE
1 MOODY PLZ
PO BOX 1520
GALVESTON, TX 77550-1520
TEL: (409) 763-4661
FAX: (409) 766-6694
TOLL FREE: (800) 899-6805
WWW.ANICO.COM

AMERICAN PIONEER LIFE

FLORIDA CLAIMS OFFICE
11 N BAYLEN ST
PO BOX 130
PENSACOLA, FL 32591-0130
TEL: (850) 469-8220
FAX: (850) 433-1186
TOLL FREE: (800) 999-2224

AMERICAN POSTAL WORKERS UNION HEALTH PLAN

NATIONAL CLAIMS OFFICE
12345 NEW COLUMBIA PIKE
PO BOX 967
SILVER SPRING, MD 20910-0967
TEL: (301) 622-1700
FAX: (301) 622-6074
TOLL FREE: (800) 222-2798
IN-STATE: (800) 222-2798
WWW.APWUHP.COM

AMERICAN REPUBLIC INSURANCE CO

IOWA CLAIMS OFFICE
NATIONAL HEADQUARTERS
601 6TH AVE
PO BOX 10
DES MOINES, IA 50301-0001
TEL: (515) 245-2000
FAX: (515) 245-4282
TOLL FREE: (800) 247-2190

AMERICAN RESOURCES INSURANCE CO

ALABAMA CLAIMS OFFICE
1111 HILLCREST RD
PO BOX 91149
MOBILE, AL 36691
TEL: (334) 639-0985
FAX: (334) 633-2944
TOLL FREE: (800) 826-6570

KENTUCKY CLAIMS OFFICE
1111 HILLCREST RD
PO BOX 91149
MOBILE, AL 36691
TEL: (334) 639-0985
FAX: (334) 633-2944
TOLL FREE: (800) 826-6570

AMERICAN SERVICE LIFE INSURANCE CO

TEXAS CLAIMS OFFICE
9151 GRAPEVINE HWY
PO BOX 982017
NORTH RICHLAND HILLS, TX 76182
FAX: (817) 255-8101
TOLL FREE: (800) 733-8880
IN-STATE: (800) 733-1110

AMERICAN TRUST ADMINISTRATORS, INC

KANSAS CLAIMS OFFICE
CLAIMS DEPT
7101 COLLEGE BLVD, STE 1505
PO BOX 87
SHAWNEE MISSION, KS 66201
TEL: (913) 451-4900
FAX: (913) 451-0598
TOLL FREE: (800) 843-4121

AMERICAN UNION LIFE INSURANCE CO

ILLINOIS CLAIMS OFFICE
303 E WASHINGTON
PO BOX 2814
BLOOMINGTON, IL 61701-2814
TEL: (309) 829-1061
FAX: (309) 827-0303

AMERIHEALTH

TEXAS CLAIMS OFFICE
10151 DEERWOOD PRK BLVD- BLDG 200, STE 400
PO BOX 40238
JACKSONVILLE, FL 32203
TEL: (904) 998-6700
FAX: (904) 998-5411
TOLL FREE: (800) 274-5466

AMERIHEALTH HMO, INC

DELAWARE CLAIMS OFFICE
AMERIHEALTH INSURANCE CO
919 N MARKET ST
WILMINGTON, DE 19801-3021
FAX: (302) 777-6444
TOLL FREE: (800) 444-6282

NEW JERSEY CLAIMS OFFICE
AMERIHEALTH INSURANCE CO
919 N MARKET ST
WILMINGTON, DE 19801-3021
FAX: (302) 777-6444
TOLL FREE: (800) 444-6282

PENNSYLVANIA CLAIMS OFFICE
AMERIHEALTH INSURANCE CO
919 N MARKET ST
WILMINGTON, DE 19801-3021
FAX: (302) 777-6444
TOLL FREE: (800) 444-6282

AMERITAS LIFE INSURANCE CORP

NATIONAL CLAIMS OFFICE
5900 O ST
PO BOX 81889
LINCOLN, NE 68501
TEL: (402) 467-1122
FAX: (402) 467-7935
TOLL FREE: (800) 487-5553
E-MAIL: GROUP@AMERITAS.COM
WWW.AMERITAS.COM

AMOCO INSURANCE PLANS

PENNSYLVANIA CLAIMS OFFICE
COMBINED INSURANCE COMPANY OF AMERICA
4850 STREET RD
TREVOSE, PA 19049-8000
TEL: (215) 953-3000
FAX: (215) 953-3156
TOLL FREE: (800) 626-0038

AMWAY CORP

MICHIGAN CLAIMS OFFICE
7575 E FULTON RD
ADA, MI 49355-0001
TEL: (616) 787-6000
FAX: (616) 787-6177
TOLL FREE: (800) 528-5748

ANTHEM BLUE CROSS & BLUE SHIELD

KENTUCKY CLAIMS OFFICE
ANTHEM BLUE CROSS & BLUE SHIELD OF SOUTHWEST OHIO
PO BOX 37180
LOUISVILLE, KY 40233
TEL: (513) 872-8100
FAX: (513) 872-8174
TOLL FREE: (800) 442-1832

OHIO CLAIMS OFFICE
2400 MARKET ST
YOUNGSTOWN, OH 44507
TEL: (330) 492-2151

ANTHEM BLUE CROSS & BLUE SHIELD OF CONNECTICUT

CONNECTICUT CLAIMS OFFICE
370 BASSETT RD
HAVEN, CT 06473
TEL: (203) 239-4911
FAX: (203) 985-7834
TOLL FREE: (800) 922-4670
WWW.ANTHEMBCBSCT.COM

ANTHEM BLUE CROSS & BLUE SHIELD OF SOUTHWEST OHIO

OHIO CLAIMS OFFICE
PO BOX 37180
LOUISVILLE, KY 40233
TEL: (513) 872-8100
FAX: (513) 872-8174
TOLL FREE: (800) 442-1832

ARIZONA PHYSICIANS, IPA, INC

ARIZONA CLAIMS OFFICE
3141 N 3RD AVE
PHOENIX, AZ 85013
TEL: (602) 274-6102
FAX: (602) 664-5466
IN-STATE: (800) 348-4058

ARIZONA PUBLIC SERVICE CO

STA 8482
PO BOX 53970
PHOENIX, AZ 85072-3970
TEL: (602) 250-3578
FAX: (602) 250-2453

ARKANSAS BEST CORP

ARKANSAS CLAIMS OFFICE
BENEFIT DEPARTMENT
3801 OLD GREENWOOD RD
PO BOX 10048
FORT SMITH, AR 72917-0048
TEL: (501) 785-6178
FAX: (501) 785-6011

ARTHUR J. GALLAGAR & CO

NATIONAL CLAIMS OFFICE
A. J. GALLAGAR & CO
2345 GRAND BLVD, STE 800
KANSAS CITY, MO 64108
TEL: (816) 421-7788
FAX: (816) 472-5517
TOLL FREE: (800) 279-7500

ASH GROVE CEMENT CO

KANSAS CLAIMS OFFICE
EMPLOYEE HEALTH CARE PLAN
8900 INDIAN CRK PKY
PO BOX 25900
OVERLAND PARK, KS 66225-5900
TEL: (913) 451-8900
FAX: (913) 451-8324
TOLL FREE: (800) 545-1822

ASSOCIATED ADMINISTRATORS, INC

OREGON CLAIMS OFFICE
2929 NW 31ST AVE
PO BOX 5096
PORTLAND, OR 97210-1721
TEL: (503) 223-3185
FAX: (503) 727-7444
TOLL FREE: (800) 888-9603

ASSOCIATION & SOCIETY INSURANCE CORP

NATIONAL CLAIMS OFFICE
ASI
11300 ROCKVILLE PIKE, STE 500
PO BOX 2510
ROCKVILLE, MD 20852
TEL: (301) 816-0045
FAX: (301) 816-1125
TOLL FREE: (800) 638-2610
WWW.ASICORPORATION.COM

ASSUMPTION MUTUAL LIFE INSURANCE CO

NEW BRUNSWICK CLAIMS OFFICE
770 MAIN ST
PO BOX 160
MONCTON, NB E1C-8L1
TEL: (506) 853-6040
FAX: (506) 853-5459
TOLL FREE: (800) 455-7337

ASSURE CARE

MICHIGAN CLAIMS OFFICE
4660 S HAGADORN RD, STE 210
EAST LANSING, MI 48823
TEL: (517) 351-6616
FAX: (517) 351-6633
TOLL FREE: (800) 968-6616

ATLANTIC MUTUAL / CENTENNIAL INSURANCE CO

CONNECTICUT CLAIMS OFFICE
628 HEBORN AVE- BLDG 2
PO BOX 6510
GLASTONBURY, CT 06033-6510
TEL: (860) 657-9966
FAX: (860) 657-7962
TOLL FREE: (800) 289-2299
WWW.ATLANTICMUTUAL.COM

MASSACHUSETTS CLAIMS OFFICE
628 HEBORN AVE- BLDG 2
PO BOX 6510
GLASTONBURY, CT 06033-6510
TEL: (860) 657-9966
FAX: (860) 657-7962
TOLL FREE: (800) 289-2299
WWW.ATLANTICMUTUAL.COM

NEW HAMPSHIRE CLAIMS OFFICE
628 HEBORN AVE- BLDG 2
PO BOX 6510
GLASTONBURY, CT 06033-6510
TEL: (860) 657-9966
FAX: (860) 657-7962
TOLL FREE: (800) 289-2299
WWW.ATLANTICMUTUAL.COM

RHODE ISLAND CLAIMS OFFICE
628 HEBORN AVE- BLDG 2
PO BOX 6510
GLASTONBURY, CT 06033-6510
TEL: (860) 657-9966
FAX: (860) 657-7962
TOLL FREE: (800) 289-2299
WWW.ATLANTICMUTUAL.COM

AUTOMOBILE MECHANICS LOCAL NO 701

ILLINOIS CLAIMS OFFICE
HEALTH & WELFARE FUND
500 W PLAINFIELD RD
COUNTRYSIDE, IL 60525
TEL: (708) 482-0110
FAX: (708) 482-9140
TOLL FREE: (800) 704-6270

AUTOMOTIVE PETROLEUM & ALLIED

MISSOURI CLAIMS OFFICE
300 S GRAND AVE, RM 232
SAINT LOUIS, MO 63103-2430
TEL: (314) 531-3052
FAX: (314) 531-5285

BABB, INC

PENNSYLVANIA CLAIMS OFFICE
850 RIDGE AVE
PITTSBURGH, PA 15212
TEL: (412) 237-2020
FAX: (412) 322-1756
TOLL FREE: (800) 245-6102
IN-STATE: (800) 892-1015

BASHAS', INC

ARIZONA CLAIMS OFFICE
FOOD CITY, A.J.'S MERCADO BARGAIN BASKET
22402 S BASHA RD
PO BOX 488
CHANDLER, AZ 85244
TEL: (602) 895-5247
FAX: (602) 802-5497
TOLL FREE: (800) 755-7292
WWW.BASHAS.COM

BELLSOUTH ADMINISTRATORS

LOUISIANA CLAIMS OFFICE
3616 S I-10 SERVICE RD
PO BOX 8570
METAIRIE, LA 70011-8570
TEL: (504) 849-1459
FAX: (504) 849-1347
TOLL FREE: (800) 366-2475

BENEFIT ADMINISTRATORS, INC

NATIONAL CLAIMS OFFICE
1111 S GLENSTONE, STE 2-203
PO BOX 10868
SPRINGFIELD, MO 65808
TEL: (417) 866-8913
FAX: (417) 866-2103
TOLL FREE: (800) 375-8913
E-MAIL: CLAIMS@BATPA.COM
WWW.BATPA.COM

SOUTH CAROLINA CLAIMS OFFICE
JOHNSON INSURANCE
PO BOX 21308
COLUMBIA, SC 29221-1308
TEL: (803) 739-0001
FAX: (803) 739-2200

BENEFIT CLAIMS PAYERS, INC

ARIZONA CLAIMS OFFICE
1717 W NORTHERN AVE, STE 200
PO BOX 37400
PHOENIX, AZ 85069
TEL: (602) 861-6868
FAX: (602) 861-6878
TOLL FREE: (800) 266-6868
WWW.DHSNYU.COM

BENEFIT COORDINATORS CORP

PENNSYLVANIA CLAIMS OFFICE
200 FLEET ST- 5TH FL
PITTSBURGH, PA 15220-2910
TEL: (412) 920-2200
FAX: (412) 920-2279
TOLL FREE: (800) 685-6100

BENEFIT MANAGEMENT, INC

ARKANSAS CLAIMS OFFICE
628 W BROADWAY, STE 100
PO BOX 5989
LITTLE ROCK, AR 72119
TEL: (501) 375-5500
FAX: (501) 375-4718

BENEFIT PLAN ADMINISTRATORS, INC

KENTUCKY CLAIMS OFFICE
101 S JEFFERSON ST
PO BOX 11746
ROANOKE, VA 24022-1746
TEL: (540) 345-2721
FAX: (540) 342-0282
TOLL FREE: (800) 277-8973
WWW.BPATPA.COM

MARYLAND CLAIMS OFFICE
101 S JEFFERSON ST
PO BOX 11746
ROANOKE, VA 24022-1746
TEL: (540) 345-2721
FAX: (540) 342-0282
TOLL FREE: (800) 277-8973
WWW.BPATPA.COM

NEW YORK CLAIMS OFFICE
ONE HUNTINGTON QUANDRANGLE, STE 4N
PO BOX 8911
MELVILLE, NY 11747
TEL: (516) 694-4900
FAX: (516) 694-5650

NORTH CAROLINA CLAIMS OFFICE
101 S JEFFERSON ST
PO BOX 11746
ROANOKE, VA 24022-1746
TEL: (540) 345-2721
FAX: (540) 342-0282
TOLL FREE: (800) 277-8973
WWW.BPATPA.COM

SOUTH CAROLINA CLAIMS OFFICE
101 S JEFFERSON ST
PO BOX 11746
ROANOKE, VA 24022-1746
TEL: (540) 345-2721
FAX: (540) 342-0282
TOLL FREE: (800) 277-8973
WWW.BPATPA.COM

TENNESSEE CLAIMS OFFICE
101 S JEFFERSON ST
PO BOX 11746
ROANOKE, VA 24022-1746
TEL: (540) 345-2721
FAX: (540) 342-0282
TOLL FREE: (800) 277-8973
WWW.BPATPA.COM

VIRGINIA CLAIMS OFFICE
101 S JEFFERSON ST
PO BOX 11746
ROANOKE, VA 24022-1746
TEL: (540) 345-2721
FAX: (540) 342-0282
TOLL FREE: (800) 277-8973
WWW.BPATPA.COM

WEST VIRGINIA CLAIMS OFFICE
101 S JEFFERSON ST
PO BOX 11746
ROANOKE, VA 24022-1746
TEL: (540) 345-2721
FAX: (540) 342-0282
TOLL FREE: (800) 277-8973
WWW.BPATPA.COM

BENEFIT PLANNERS, INC

TEXAS CLAIMS OFFICE
PO BOX 690450
SAN ANTONIO, TX 78269-0450
TEL: (210) 699-1872
FAX: (210) 697-3108
TOLL FREE: (800) 292-5386
E-MAIL: SERVICE@BENPLAN.COM
WWW.BENPLAN.COM

194 S MAIN
BOERNE, TX 78006
TEL: (210) 699-1872
FAX: (210) 697-3108
TOLL FREE: (800) 292-5386
E-MAIL: SERVICE@BENPLAN.COM
WWW.BENPLAN.COM

BENEFIT & RISK MANAGEMENT SERVICES

CALIFORNIA CLAIMS OFFICE
3610 AMERICAN RIVER DR, STE 150
SACRAMENTO, CA 95864
TEL: (916) 974-2626
FAX: (916) 974-2653
TOLL FREE: (800) 476-0218
WWW.BEST-ONLINE.COM

BENICORP INSURANCE CO

INDIANA CLAIMS OFFICE
5285 W LAKEVIEW PKY S DR
PO BOX 68917
INDIANAPOLIS, IN 46268-4111
TEL: (317) 290-1205
FAX: (317) 216-7877
TOLL FREE: (800) 837-1205
E-MAIL: CLAIMS@BENICORP.COM
WWW.BENICORP.COM

BERWANGER OVERMYER ASSOCIATES

OHIO CLAIMS OFFICE
2245 NORTHBANK DR
PO BOX 20945
COLUMBUS, OH 43220
TEL: (614) 457-7000
FAX: (614) 457-1507
TOLL FREE: (800) 837-0503
IN-STATE: (800) 837-0503
E-MAIL: BOA@BOA-INS.COM
WWW.BOA-INS.COM

BLUE CROSS & BLUE SHIELD

ALABAMA CLAIMS OFFICE
BLUE CROSS & BLUE SHIELD OF ALABAMA
450 RIVERCHASE PKY E
PO BOX 995
BIRMINGHAM, AL 35298-0001
TEL: (205) 988-2100
FAX: (205) 988-2949
E-MAIL: WEBINPUT@BCBSAL.ORG
WWW.BCBSAL

ARIZONA CLAIMS OFFICE
BLUE CROSS & BLUE SHIELD OF ARIZONA
PO BOX 2924
PHOENIX, AZ 85062-2924
TEL: (602) 864-4400
FAX: (602) 864-4242
TOLL FREE: (800) 232-2345

COLORADO CLAIMS OFFICE
BLUE CROSS & BLUE SHIELD OF COLORADO
700 BROADWAY
DENVER, CO 80273
TEL: (303) 831-2131
TOLL FREE: (800) 433-5447
WWW.BCBSCO.COM

DELAWARE CLAIMS OFFICE
BLUE CROSS & BLUE SHIELD OF DELAWARE
ONE BRANDYWINE GTWY
PO BOX 1991
WILMINGTON, DE 19899-1991
TEL: (302) 421-3000
FAX: (302) 421-2089
TOLL FREE: (800) 633-2563
IN-STATE: (800) 292-7865
WWW.BCBSDE.COM

DISTRICT OF COLUMBIA CLAIMS OFFICE
BLUE CROSS & BLUE SHIELD OF MARYLAND
550 12TH ST SW
WASHINGTON, DC 20065
TEL: (202) 479-8000
FAX: (202) 479-3520
TOLL FREE: (800) 424-7474

FLORIDA CLAIMS OFFICE
BLUE CROSS & BLUE SHIELD OF FLORIDA
532 RIVERSIDE AVE
PO BOX 1798
JACKSONVILLE, FL 32231-0014
TEL: (904) 791-6111
FAX: (904) 791-8738

GEORGIA CLAIMS OFFICE
BLUE CROSS & BLUE SHIELD OF GEORGIA
PO BOX 4445
ATLANTA, GA 30302-4445
TEL: (404) 842-8000
FAX: (404) 842-8010
TOLL FREE: (800) 441-2273
WWW.BCBSGA.COM

BLUE CROSS & BLUE SHIELD OF GEORGIA
2357 WARM SPRINGS RD
PO BOX 9907
COLUMBUS, GA 31908-9907
TEL: (706) 571-5371
FAX: (706) 571-5487
TOLL FREE: (800) 241-7475
WWW.BCBSGA.COM

HAWAII CLAIMS OFFICE
HAWAII MEDICAL SERVICE ASSOCIATION
818 KEEAUMOKU ST
PO BOX 860
HONOLULU, HI 96808-0860
TEL: (808) 948-5110
FAX: (808) 948-6555
IN-STATE: (800) 790-4672

ILLINOIS CLAIMS OFFICE
BLUE CROSS & BLUE SHIELD OF ILLINOIS
PO BOX 1364
CHICAGO, IL 60690-1364
TEL: (312) 653-6000
FAX: (312) 819-1220
WWW.BCBSIL.COM

KENTUCKY CLAIMS OFFICE
ANTHEM BLUE CROSS & BLUE SHIELD- DELTA DENTAL
9901 LINN STATION RD
LOUISVILLE, KY 40223
TEL: (502) 423-2011
FAX: (502) 423-2627
TOLL FREE: (800) 880-2583
WWW.ANTHEM.COM

MAINE CLAIMS OFFICE
BLUE CROSS & BLUE SHIELD OF MAINE
2 GANNETT DR
SOUTH PORTLAND, ME 04106-6911
TEL: (207) 822-7000
FAX: (207) 822-7375
TOLL FREE: (800) 482-0966
IN-STATE: (800) 482-0966
WWW.MAINEBLUE.COM

MISSOURI CLAIMS OFFICE
ALLIANCE BLUE CROSS & BLUE SHIELD OF MISSOURI
1831 CHESTNUT ST
SAINT LOUIS, MO 63103-2275
TEL: (314) 923-4444
FAX: (417) 888-9075
TOLL FREE: (800) 392-8740
WWW.ABCBS.COM

MONTANA CLAIMS OFFICE
BLUE CROSS & BLUE SHIELD OF MONTANA, INC
404 FULLER
PO BOX 4309
HELENA, MT 59604-4309
TEL: (406) 444-8200
FAX: (406) 442-6946
TOLL FREE: (800) 447-7828
E-MAIL: GENERAL@BCBSMT.COM
WWW.BCBSMT.COM

NATIONAL CLAIMS OFFICE
BLUE CROSS & BLUE SHIELD OF NEBRASKA
7261 MERCY RD
PO BOX 3248
OMAHA, NE 68180-0001
TEL: (402) 390-1800
FAX: (402) 392-2141
TOLL FREE: (800) 642-8980
WWW.BCBSNE.COM

NEW JERSEY CLAIMS OFFICE
HORIZON BLUE CROSS & BLUE SHIELD OF NEW JERSEY, INC
3 PENN PLZ E
NEWARK, NJ 07105
TEL: (973) 466-4000
TOLL FREE: (800) 355-2583
WWW.HORIZONBCBSNJ.COM

NEW MEXICO CLAIMS OFFICE
BLUE CROSS & BLUE SHIELD OF NEW MEXICO
PO BOX 27630
ALBUQUERQUE, NM 87125-7630
TEL: (505) 291-3500
FAX: (505) 291-3541
TOLL FREE: (800) 432-0750

NEW YORK CLAIMS OFFICE
EMPIRE BLUE CROSS & BLUE SHIELD
622 3RD AVE
PO BOX 345
NEW YORK, NY 10017
TEL: (212) 476-1000
TOLL FREE: (800) 261-5962
WWW.EMPIREBCBS.COM

BLUE CROSS & BLUE SHIELD OF UTICA-WATERTOWN
12 RHOADS DR- UTICA BUSINESS PARK
UTICA, NY 13502-6398
TEL: (315) 798-4200
FAX: (315) 792-9752
TOLL FREE: (800) 765-5226

BLUE CROSS & BLUE SHIELD OF ROCHESTER
165 COURT ST
ROCHESTER, NY 14647-0001
TEL: (716) 454-1700
FAX: (716) 238-4400
TOLL FREE: (800) 847-1200

NORTH CAROLINA CLAIMS OFFICE
BLUE CROSS & BLUE SHIELD OF NORTH CAROLINA
800 S DUKE ST
PO BOX 2291
DURHAM, NC 27702
TEL: (919) 489-7431
FAX: (919) 765-4837
TOLL FREE: (800) 222-2783
IN-STATE: (800) 222-5028
WWW.BCBSNC.COM

OHIO CLAIMS OFFICE
ANTHEM BLUE CROSS & BLUE SHIELD OF OHIO- HOME OFFICE
1351 WILLIAM HOWARD TAFT RD
CINCINNATI, OH 45206
TEL: (513) 872-8100
FAX: (513) 872-8174
TOLL FREE: (800) 442-1832
WWW.AICI.COM

MUTUAL MEDICAL OF OHIO
3737 W SALVANIA AVE
PO BOX 943
TOLEDO, OH 43656-0001
TEL: (419) 473-7100
FAX: (419) 473-6200
WWW.MMOH.COM

ANTHEM BLUE CROSS & BLUE SHIELD-CUSTOMER SERVICE OFFICE
3530 VELMONT
YOUNGSTOWN, OH 44505
TEL: (330) 759-0771
TOLL FREE: (800) 458-6813
WWW.MMOH.COM

OKLAHOMA CLAIMS OFFICE
BLUE CROSS & BLUE SHIELD OF OKLAHOMA
1215 S BOULDER
PO BOX 3283
TULSA, OK 74102-3283
TEL: (918) 560-3500
WWW.BCBSOK.COM

SOUTH CAROLINA CLAIMS OFFICE
BLUE CROSS & BLUE SHIELD OF SOUTH CAROLINA
I-20 E AT ALPINE RD
COLUMBIA, SC 29219-0001
TEL: (803) 788-3860
FAX: (803) 736-3420
TOLL FREE: (800) 868-2500
IN-STATE: (800) 288-2227
WWW.BCBSSC.COM

UTAH CLAIMS OFFICE
REGENTS BLUE CROSS & BLUE SHIELD OF UTAH
2890 E COTTONWOOD PKY
PO BOX 30270
SALT LAKE CITY, UT 84121-0270
TEL: (801) 333-2000
FAX: (801) 333-6523
TOLL FREE: (800) 624-6519
E-MAIL: UT.CUSTSERV@REGENTS.COM
WWW.BCBSUTAH.COM

VERMONT CLAIMS OFFICE
BLUE CROSS & BLUE SHIELD OF VERMONT
PO BOX 186
MONTPELIER, VT 05601-0186
TEL: (802) 223-6131
FAX: (802) 223-1077
TOLL FREE: (800) 457-6648
IN-STATE: (800) 247-2583
WWW.BCBSVT.COM

VIRGINIA CLAIMS OFFICE
TRIGON BLUE CROSS & BLUE SHIELD
PO BOX 27401
RICHMOND, VA 23279-7401
TEL: (804) 354-7000
FAX: (804) 354-7600
TOLL FREE: (800) 451-1527
WWW.TRIGON.COM

TRIGON BLUE CROSS & BLUE SHIELD
PO BOX 27401
RICHMOND, VA 23279
TEL: (804) 342-0010
TOLL FREE: (800) 533-1120
WWW.TRIGON.COM

WASHINGTON CLAIMS OFFICE
REGENCE BLUE CROSS & BLUE SHIELD - KING COUNTY MEDICAL
1800 9TH AVE
PO BOX 21267
SEATTLE, WA 98111-3267
TEL: (206) 464-3600
FAX: (206) 389-6778
TOLL FREE: (800) 464-3663
IN-STATE: (800) 458-3523

MEDICAL SERVICE CORPORATION PREMERA BLUE CROSS
EAST 3900 SPRAGUE
PO BOX 3048
SPOKANE, WA 99220-3048
TEL: (509) 536-4700
TOLL FREE: (800) 835-3510
IN-STATE: (800) 572-0778
WWW.PREMERA.COM

WISCONSIN CLAIMS OFFICE
BLUE CROSS & BLUE SHIELD UNITED OF WISCONSIN
401 W MICHIGAN ST
PO BOX 2025
MILWAUKEE, WI 53201-2025
TEL: (414) 226-5000
FAX: (414) 226-5040
TOLL FREE: (800) 558-1584
WWW.BCBSUW.ORG

WYOMING CLAIMS OFFICE
BLUE CROSS & BLUE SHIELD OF WYOMING
PO BOX 2266
CHEYENNE, WY 82003-2266
TEL: (307) 634-1393
FAX: (307) 778-8582
TOLL FREE: (800) 442-2376
IN-STATE: (800) 442-2376

BLUE PLUS

MINNESOTA CLAIMS OFFICE
BLUE CROSS & BLUE SHIELD OF MINNESOTA BLUE PLUS & AFFILIATES
PO BOX 64179
SAINT PAUL, MN 55164-0179
TEL: (651) 456-8501
FAX: (651) 456-1004
TOLL FREE: (800) 382-2000
WWW.BCBSMN.COM

BLUE RIDGE ADMINISTRATORS

VIRGINIA CLAIMS OFFICE
COMMONWEALTH HEALTH ALLIANCE, INC
105 S PANTOPS DR, STE C3
PO BOX 1067
CHARLOTTESVILLE, VA 22902
TEL: (804) 977-3500
FAX: (804) 979-5626
TOLL FREE: (800) 677-1867
WWW.COMCLIN.NET

BLUE SHIELD OF CALIFORNIA

CALIFORNIA CLAIMS OFFICE
CARE AMERICA
103 WOOD MERE
PO BOX 272550
FOLSOM, CA 95630
TOLL FREE: (800) 424-6521
IN-STATE: (800) 424-6521
WWW.BLUESHIELDCA.COM

SENIOR PLANS
129 N GUILD AVE
PO BOX 241004
LODI, CA 95241-9504
TEL: (209) 367-2800
TOLL FREE: (800) 248-2341
WWW.BLUESHIELDCA.COM

PERS CARE SERVICE CENTER
129 N GUILD AVE
PO BOX 272530
CHICO, CA 95927-2530
TEL: (209) 367-2800
TOLL FREE: (800) 444-2595
WWW.BLUESHIELDCA.COM

CLAIMS CENTER FOR GENERAL ELECTRIC
40 NE ST
PO BOX 769028
WOODLAND, CA 95776-9028
TEL: (530) 674-0504
FAX: (530) 668-2801
TOLL FREE: (800) 688-0327
WWW.GEOACCESS.COM

BLUE SHIELD OF NORTHEASTERN NEW YORK
NEW YORK CLAIMS OFFICE
187 WOLF RD
PO BOX 15013
ALBANY, NY 12212
TEL: (518) 453-5700
FAX: (518) 438-1837
TOLL FREE: (800) 888-1238
WWW.BLUECARES.COM/BLUECARD

BOON-CHAPMAN
TEXAS CLAIMS OFFICE
7600 CHEVY CHASE DR, STE 300
PO BOX 9201
AUSTIN, TX 78766-9201
TEL: (512) 454-2681
FAX: (512) 459-1552
TOLL FREE: (800) 252-9653
WWW.BOONCHAPMAN.COM

BPS INC
NATIONAL CLAIMS OFFICE
145 N CHURCH ST, STE 300
PO BOX 1227
SPARTANBURG, SC 29304-1227
TEL: (864) 585-4338
FAX: (864) 573-7709
TOLL FREE: (800) 868-7526
WWW.BPSINC.COM

BROKERAGE CONCEPTS, INC
PENNSYLVANIA CLAIMS OFFICE
BENEFIT CONCEPTS
651 ALLENDALE RD
PO BOX 60608
KING OF PRUSSIA, PA 19406-0608
TEL: (610) 337-2600
FAX: (610) 491-4992
TOLL FREE: (800) 220-2600

BROKERAGE SERVICES, INC
NEW MEXICO CLAIMS OFFICE
11200 LOOMAS BLVD NE
PO BOX 11020
ALBUQUERQUE, NM 87192-0020
TEL: (505) 292-5533
FAX: (505) 293-7725
TOLL FREE: (800) 274-5533

BUFFALO ROCK CO, INC
ALABAMA CLAIMS OFFICE
103 OXMOOR RD
PO BOX 10048
BIRMINGHAM, AL 35202-0048
TEL: (205) 942-3435
FAX: (205) 940-7768

BUILDERS TRANSPORT, INC
SOUTH CAROLINA CLAIMS OFFICE
PO BOX 24949
COLUMBIA, SC 29223
TEL: (803) 699-9940
FAX: (803) 699-6673

BUNZL DISTRIBUTION USA, INC
MISSOURI CLAIMS OFFICE
701 EMERSON RD, STE 500
PO BOX 419111
SAINT LOUIS, MO 63141-9111
TEL: (314) 997-5959
FAX: (314) 997-0247

BUSINESS ADMINISTRATORS & CONSULTANTS, INC
OHIO CLAIMS OFFICE
6331 E LIVINGSTON AVE
PO BOX 107
REYNOLDSBURG, OH 43068-0107
TEL: (614) 863-8780
FAX: (614) 863-9137
TOLL FREE: (800) 521-2654

C.F.S. HEALTH GROUP
MARYLAND CLAIMS OFFICE
BLUE CROSS & BLUE SHIELD OF MARYLAND SUBSIDIARY
10455 MILL RUN CIR
PO BOX 819
OWINGS MILLS, MD 21117-0819
TEL: (410) 654-9394
FAX: (410) 998-5177
TOLL FREE: (800) 553-3745

C & O EMPLOYEES' HOSPITAL ASSOCIATION
ILLINOIS CLAIMS OFFICE
543 CHURCH ST
CLIFTON FORGE, VA 24422-1199
TEL: (540) 862-5728
FAX: (540) 862-3552

INDIANA CLAIMS OFFICE
543 CHURCH ST
CLIFTON FORGE, VA 24422-1199
TEL: (540) 862-5728
FAX: (540) 862-3552

KENTUCKY CLAIMS OFFICE
543 CHURCH ST
CLIFTON FORGE, VA 24422-1199
TEL: (540) 862-5728
FAX: (540) 862-3552

OHIO CLAIMS OFFICE
543 CHURCH ST
CLIFTON FORGE, VA 24422-1199
TEL: (540) 862-5728
FAX: (540) 862-3552

VIRGINIA CLAIMS OFFICE
543 CHURCH ST
CLIFTON FORGE, VA 24422-1199
TEL: (540) 862-5728
FAX: (540) 862-3552

WEST VIRGINIA CLAIMS OFFICE
543 CHURCH ST
CLIFTON FORGE, VA 24422-1199
TEL: (540) 862-5728
FAX: (540) 862-3552

CABOT SAFETY CORP
NATIONAL CLAIMS OFFICE
AEARO CO
90 MECHANIC ST
SOUTHBRIDGE, MA 01550-2555
TEL: (508) 764-5705
FAX: (508) 764-5648
WWW.AEARO.COM

CALIFORNIA MOTOR CAR DEALERS ASSOCIATION
CALIFORNIA CLAIMS OFFICE
420 CULVER BLVD
PLAYA DEL REY, CA 90293-7706
TEL: (310) 306-6232
FAX: (310) 822-6733
TOLL FREE: (800) 445-8290
IN-STATE: (800) 262-6232
WWW.CMCDA.COM

CAM ADMINISTRATIVE SERVICES, INC
MICHIGAN CLAIMS OFFICE
25800 NORTHWESTERN HWY, STE 700
PO BOX 5131
SOUTHFIELD, MI 48086-5131
TEL: (248) 827-1050
FAX: (248) 827-2112
TOLL FREE: (800) 732-8906

CAPITAL BLUE CROSS & PENNSYLVANIA BLUE SHIELD
PENNSYLVANIA CLAIMS OFFICE
2500 ELMERTON AVE
HARRISBURG, PA 17110
TEL: (717) 541-7000
FAX: (717) 541-6072
TOLL FREE: (800) 958-5558
WWW.CAPBLUECROSS.COM

CAPITAL DISTRICT PHYSICIANS' HEALTH PLAN, INC
NEW YORK CLAIMS OFFICE
17 COLUMBIA CIR
ALBANY, NY 12203-5190
TEL: (518) 862-3700
FAX: (518) 452-0003
TOLL FREE: (800) 777-CARE
E-MAIL: INFO@CDPHP.COM
WWW.CDPHP.COM

CAPITAL HEALTH PLAN
FLORIDA CLAIMS OFFICE
2140 CENTERVILLE PL
PO BOX 15349
TALLAHASSEE, FL 32317-5349
TEL: (850) 383-3377
FAX: (850) 383-3441

CARE AMERICA HEALTH PLANS
CALIFORNIA CLAIMS OFFICE
CARE AMERICA/ BLUE SHIELD
6300 CANOGA AVE
PO BOX 946
WOODLAND HILLS, CA 91365
TEL: (818) 228-5050
FAX: (818) 228-5103
TOLL FREE: (800) 827-2273
WWW.CAREAMERICA.COM

CARE CHOICES HEALTH PLANS
IOWA CLAIMS OFFICE
PREFERRED CHOICE
522 4TH ST- TERRE CENTRE, STE 250
SIOUX CITY, IA 51101-1748
TEL: (712) 252-2344
FAX: (712) 294-7018
TOLL FREE: (800) 535-6252

CAREMARK MEDICAL & DENTAL PLAN
NATIONAL CLAIMS OFFICE
MED PARTNERS, INC
2211 SANDERS RD
NORTHBROOK, IL 60062-6126
TEL: (847) 559-4700
FAX: (847) 559-3905

CARETON HEALTH CARE
PO BOX 22987
KNOXVILLE, TN 37933
FAX: (423) 778-4620
TOLL FREE: (800) 976-7747

CARILION HEALTH PLANS
VIRGINIA CLAIMS OFFICE
110 W CAMPBELL AVE
PO BOX 1531
ROANOKE, VA 24007
TEL: (540) 343-6101
FAX: (540) 343-0748
WWW.CARILION.COM

CARNEGIE-MELLON UNIVERSITY
PENNSYLVANIA CLAIMS OFFICE
WHITFIELD HALL
143 N CRAIG ST
PITTSBURGH, PA 15213
TEL: (412) 268-4747
FAX: (412) 268-1524
WWW.CMU.EDU/BA/HR/

CAROLINA BENEFIT ADMINISTRATORS OF SOUTH CAROLINA
SOUTH CAROLINA CLAIMS OFFICE
291 S PINE ST
PO BOX 3257
SPARTANBURG, SC 29304
TEL: (864) 573-6937
FAX: (864) 582-2265
TOLL FREE: (800) 476-2295

CARPENTERS COMBINED FUNDS

PENNSYLVANIA CLAIMS OFFICE
495 MANSFIELD AVE- 1ST FL
PITTSBURGH, PA 15205-4376
TEL: (412) 922-5330
FAX: (412) 922-3420
IN-STATE: (800) 242-2539

CELTIC LIFE INSURANCE CO

ILLINOIS CLAIMS OFFICE
CELTIC INDIVIDUAL HEALTH
200 S WACKER DR, STE 900
PO BOX 06410
CHICAGO, IL 60606-5802
TEL: (312) 332-5401
TOLL FREE: (800) 477-7870
WWW.CELTIC_NET.COM

CEMARA ADMINISTRATORS INC

KANSAS CLAIMS OFFICE
3450 N ROCK RD, STE 605
PO BOX 8902
WICHITA, KS 67208-0902
TEL: (316) 631-3939
FAX: (316) 631-3788
TOLL FREE: (800) 285-1551

CEMETERY WORKERS WELFARE FUND

NEW YORK CLAIMS OFFICE
2409 38TH AVE
LONG ISLAND CITY, NY 11101
TEL: (718) 729-7400
FAX: (718) 729-0253

CENTRAL DATA SERVICES, INC

PENNSYLVANIA CLAIMS OFFICE
503 MARTINDALE ST, 5TH FL
PITTSBURGH, PA 15212
TEL: (412) 321-6172
FAX: (412) 237-1444

CENTRAL ILLINOIS CARPENTERS

ILLINOIS CLAIMS OFFICE
2400 N MAIN ST, STE 100
EAST PEORIA, IL 61611-1735
TEL: (309) 699-7200
FAX: (309) 699-7032

CENTRAL PENNSYLVANIA TEAMSTERS HEALTH & WELFARE FUND

NATIONAL CLAIMS OFFICE
1055 SPRING ST
PO BOX 15224
READING, PA 19612-5224
TEL: (610) 320-5500
FAX: (610) 320-9209
TOLL FREE: (800) 331-0420
IN-STATE: (800) 422-8330

CENTURY FURNITURE

NORTH CAROLINA CLAIMS OFFICE
401 11TH ST NW
PO BOX 608
HICKORY, NC 28603
TEL: (828) 328-1851
FAX: (828) 328-2176
WWW.CENTURYFURNITURE.COM

CHAMPUS

ALABAMA CLAIMS OFFICE
PALMETTO GOVERNMENT BENEFIT ADMINISTRATORS, REGIONS 3 & 4
PO BOX 202000
FLORENCE, SC 29502-2000
TEL: (843) 665-7822
TOLL FREE: (800) 403-3950
WWW.HUMANAMILITARY.COM

CONNECTICUT CLAIMS OFFICE
TRICARE - REGION 1 CLAIMS
PO BOX 7011
CAMDEN, SC 29020-7011
TOLL FREE: (800) 578-1294
WWW.OCHAMPUS.MIL

DELAWARE CLAIMS OFFICE
TRICARE - REGION 1 CLAIMS
PO BOX 7011
CAMDEN, SC 29020-7011
TOLL FREE: (800) 578-1294
WWW.OCHAMPUS.MIL

DISTRICT OF COLUMBIA CLAIMS OFFICE
TRICARE - REGION 1 CLAIMS
PO BOX 7011
CAMDEN, SC 29020-7011
TOLL FREE: (800) 578-1294
WWW.OCHAMPUS.MIL

FLORIDA CLAIMS OFFICE
PALMETTO GOVERNMENT BENEFIT ADMINISTRATORS, REGIONS 3 & 4
PO BOX 202000
FLORENCE, SC 29502-2000
TEL: (843) 665-7822
TOLL FREE: (800) 403-3950
WWW.HUMANAMILITARY.COM

GEORGIA CLAIMS OFFICE
PALMETTO GOVERNMENT BENEFIT ADMINISTRATORS, REGIONS 3 & 4
PO BOX 202000
FLORENCE, SC 29502-2000
TEL: (843) 665-7822
TOLL FREE: (800) 403-3950
WWW.HUMANAMILITARY.COM

IDAHO CLAIMS OFFICE
PALMETTO GOVERNMENT BENEFIT ADMINISTRATORS, REGIONS 3 & 4
PO BOX 100598
FLORENCE, SC 29501-0598
TEL: (843) 665-7822
TOLL FREE: (800) 403-3950
WWW.HUMANAMILITARY.COM

ILLINOIS CLAIMS OFFICE
TRICARE - REGIONS 2 & 5 CLAIMS
PO BOX 7021
CAMDEN, SC 29020-7021
TOLL FREE: (800) 613-7124
WWW.ANTHEM-INC.COM

INDIANA CLAIMS OFFICE
TRICARE - REGIONS 2 & 5 CLAIMS
PO BOX 7021
CAMDEN, SC 29020-7021
TOLL FREE: (800) 613-7124
WWW.ANTHEM-INC.COM

IOWA CLAIMS OFFICE
PALMETTO GOVERNMENT BENEFIT ADMINISTRATORS, REGIONS 3 & 4
PO BOX 100598
FLORENCE, SC 29501-0598
TEL: (843) 665-7822
TOLL FREE: (800) 403-3950
WWW.HUMANAMILITARY.COM

KENTUCKY CLAIMS OFFICE
PALMETTO GOVERNMENT BENEFIT ADMINISTRATORS, REGIONS 3 & 4
PO BOX 100598
FLORENCE, SC 29501-0598
TEL: (843) 665-7822
TOLL FREE: (800) 403-3950
WWW.HUMANAMILITARY.COM

MAINE CLAIMS OFFICE
TRICARE - REGION 1 CLAIMS
PO BOX 7011
CAMDEN, SC 29020-7011
TOLL FREE: (800) 578-1294
WWW.OCHAMPUS.MIL

MARYLAND CLAIMS OFFICE
TRICARE - REGION 1 CLAIMS
PO BOX 7011
CAMDEN, SC 29020-7011
TOLL FREE: (800) 578-1294
WWW.OCHAMPUS.MIL

MASSACHUSETTS CLAIMS OFFICE
TRICARE - REGION 1 CLAIMS
PO BOX 7011
CAMDEN, SC 29020-7011
TOLL FREE: (800) 578-1294
WWW.OCHAMPUS.MIL

MICHIGAN CLAIMS OFFICE
TRICARE - REGIONS 2 & 5 CLAIMS
PO BOX 7021
CAMDEN, SC 29020-7021
TOLL FREE: (800) 578-1294
WWW.ANTHEM-INC.COM

MINNESOTA CLAIMS OFFICE
PALMETTO GOVERNMENT BENEFIT ADMINISTRATORS, REGIONS 3 & 4
PO BOX 100598
FLORENCE, SC 29501-0598
TEL: (843) 665-7822
TOLL FREE: (800) 403-3950
WWW.HUMANAMILITARY.COM

MISSISSIPPI CLAIMS OFFICE
PALMETTO GOVERNMENT BENEFIT ADMINISTRATORS, REGIONS 3 & 4
PO BOX 202000
FLORENCE, SC 29502-2000
TEL: (843) 665-7822
TOLL FREE: (800) 403-3950
WWW.HUMANAMILITARY.COM

NEW HAMPSHIRE CLAIMS OFFICE
TRICARE - REGION 1 CLAIMS
PO BOX 7011
CAMDEN, SC 29020-7011
TOLL FREE: (800) 578-1294
WWW.OCHAMPUS.MIL

NEW JERSEY CLAIMS OFFICE
TRICARE - REGION 1 CLAIMS
PO BOX 7011
CAMDEN, SC 29020-7011
TOLL FREE: (800) 578-1294
WWW.OCHAMPUS.MIL

NEW YORK CLAIMS OFFICE
TRICARE - REGION 1 CLAIMS
PO BOX 7011
CAMDEN, SC 29020-7011
TOLL FREE: (800) 578-1294
WWW.OCHAMPUS.MIL

NORTH CAROLINA CLAIMS OFFICE
TRICARE - REGIONS 2 & 5 CLAIMS
PO BOX 7021
CAMDEN, SC 29020-7021
TOLL FREE: (800) 613-7124
WWW.ANTHEM-INC.COM

OHIO CLAIMS OFFICE
TRICARE - REGION 1 CLAIMS
PO BOX 7021
CAMDEN, SC 29020-7021
TOLL FREE: (800) 613-7124
WWW.ANTHEM-INC.COM

PENNSYLVANIA CLAIMS OFFICE
TRICARE - REGION 1 CLAIMS
PO BOX 7011
CAMDEN, SC 29020-7011
TOLL FREE: (800) 578-1294
WWW.OCHAMPUS.MIL

RHODE ISLAND CLAIMS OFFICE
TRICARE - REGION 1 CLAIMS
PO BOX 7011
CAMDEN, SC 29020-7011
TOLL FREE: (800) 578-1294
WWW.OCHAMPUS.MIL

SOUTH CAROLINA CLAIMS OFFICE
PALMETTO GOVERNMENT BENEFIT ADMINISTRATORS, REGIONS 3 & 4
PO BOX 202000
FLORENCE, SC 29502-2000
TEL: (843) 665-7822
TOLL FREE: (800) 403-3950
WWW.HUMANAMILITARY.COM

TENNESSEE CLAIMS OFFICE
PALMETTO GOVERNMENT BENEFIT ADMINISTRATORS, REGIONS 3 & 4
PO BOX 202000
FLORENCE, SC 29502-2000
TEL: (843) 665-7822
TOLL FREE: (800) 403-3950
WWW.HUMANAMILITARY.COM

VERMONT CLAIMS OFFICE
TRICARE - REGION 1 CLAIMS
PO BOX 7011
CAMDEN, SC 29020-7011
TOLL FREE: (800) 578-1294
WWW.OCHAMPUS.MIL

VIRGIN ISLANDS CLAIMS OFFICE
WPS TRICARE SERVICES OVERSEAS
1717 W BROADWAY
PO BOX 7985
MADISON, WI 53707-7985
TEL: (608) 259-4848
WWW.WPSIC.COM/TRICARE

VIRGINIA CLAIMS OFFICE
TRICARE - REGIONS 2 & 5 CLAIMS
PO BOX 7021
CAMDEN, SC 29020-7021
TOLL FREE: (800) 613-7124
WWW.ANTHEM-INC.COM

TRICARE - REGION 1 CLAIMS
PO BOX 7011
CAMDEN, SC 29020-7011
TOLL FREE: (800) 578-1294
WWW.OCHAMPUS.MIL

WEST VIRGINIA CLAIMS OFFICE
TRICARE - REGIONS 2 & 5 CLAIMS
PO BOX 7021
CAMDEN, SC 29020-7021
TOLL FREE: (800) 613-7124
WWW.ANTHEM-INC.COM

TRICARE - REGION 1 CLAIMS
PO BOX 7011
CAMDEN, SC 29020-7011
TOLL FREE: (800) 578-1294
WWW.OCHAMPUS.MIL

WISCONSIN CLAIMS OFFICE
TRICARE - REGIONS 2 & 5 CLAIMS
PO BOX 7021
CAMDEN, SC 29020-7021
TOLL FREE: (800) 613-7124
WWW.ANTHEM-INC.COM

CHER BUMPS & ASSOCIATES

OKLAHOMA CLAIMS OFFICE
6100 N ROBINSON, STE 204
PO BOX 548805
OKLAHOMA CITY, OK 73154-8805
TEL: (405) 840-6022
FAX: (405) 858-7361
TOLL FREE: (888) 840-8924

CHOICECARE HEALTH PLANS, INC

OHIO CLAIMS OFFICE
CHOICECARE HUMANA
655 EDEN PARK DR, STE 400
PO BOX 3188
CINCINNATI, OH 45201
TEL: (513) 784-5200
FAX: (513) 784-5310
TOLL FREE: (800) 543-7158
WWW.CHOICECARE.COM

CHURCHILL ADMINISTRATIVE PLANS, INC

NEW JERSEY CLAIMS OFFICE
270 SYLVAN AVE
ENGLEWOOD CLIFFS, NJ 07632
TEL: (201) 871-8400

CIGNA CORPORATION

FLORIDA CLAIMS OFFICE
CIGNA HEALTHCARE OF SOUTH FLORIDA
2220 PARK LAKE DR, STE 100
PO BOX 49400
ATLANTA, GA 30359
TEL: (770) 723-7894
FAX: (770) 723-7890
TOLL FREE: (800) 942-2471
IN-STATE: (800) 526-7431

GEORGIA CLAIMS OFFICE
CIGNA HEALTHCARE OF SOUTH FLORIDA
2220 PARK LAKE DR, STE 100
PO BOX 49400
ATLANTA, GA 30359
TEL: (770) 723-7894
FAX: (770) 723-7890
TOLL FREE: (800) 942-2471
IN-STATE: (800) 526-7431

NATIONAL CLAIMS OFFICE
1601 CHESTNUT ST- TWO LIBERTY PL
PHILADELPHIA, PA 19192-1550
TEL: (215) 761-1000

CIGNA HEALTHCARE OF ARIZONA, TUCSON
600 E TAYLOR
PO BOX 9328
SHERMAN, TX 75091-9328
TEL: (903) 892-8167
FAX: (903) 892-6271
TOLL FREE: (800) 525-5803
IN-STATE: (800) 238-8801
WWW.CIGNA.COM

9740 APPALOOSA DR
PO BOX 85490
SAN DIEGO, CA 92121
TEL: (619) 693-4600
FAX: (619) 693-4881
TOLL FREE: (800) 822-2994
WWW.CIGNA.COM

CIGNA HEALTHCARE CONNECTICUT GENERAL SERVICE CENTER
4025 W MINERAL KING
PO BOX 5038
VISALIA, CA 93278-5038
TEL: (209) 738-2000
FAX: (209) 738-2050
TOLL FREE: (800) 272-2471
WWW.CIGNA.COM

MEDICARE
2 VANTAGE WY
PO BOX 22599
NASHVILLE, TN 37202
TEL: (615) 244-5650
FAX: (615) 782-4651
IN-STATE: (800) 627-2782
WWW.CIGNA.COM

CONNECTICUT GENERAL (UNITED AIRLINE EMPLOYEE DEPT)
21 HERITAGE DR
BOURBONNAIS, IL 60914
TEL: (815) 939-4566
FAX: (815) 935-3499
TOLL FREE: (800) 654-8777
WWW.CIGNA.COM

CIGNA HEALTHCARE OF KANSAS
600 E TAYLOR
PO BOX 9303
SHERMAN, TX 75091-9303
TEL: (903) 892-8167
FAX: (903) 892-6271
TOLL FREE: (800) 525-5803
IN-STATE: (800) 238-8801
WWW.CIGNA.COM

CIGNA HEALTHCARE OF LOUISIANA, BATON ROUGE
600 E TAYLOR
PO BOX 9022
SHERMAN, TX 75091-9022
TEL: (903) 892-8167
FAX: (903) 892-6271
TOLL FREE: (800) 525-5803
IN-STATE: (800) 238-8801
WWW.CIGNA.COM

CIGNA HEALTHCARE OF LOUISIANA, SHREVEPORT
600 E TAYLOR
PO BOX 9305
SHERMAN, TX 75091-9305
TEL: (903) 892-8167
FAX: (903) 892-6271
TOLL FREE: (800) 525-5803
IN-STATE: (800) 238-8801
WWW.CIGNA.COM

CIGNA HEALTHCARE OF MISSISSIPPI
600 E TAYLOR
PO BOX 9338
SHERMAN, TX 75091-9338
TEL: (903) 892-8167
FAX: (903) 892-6271
TOLL FREE: (800) 525-5803
IN-STATE: (800) 238-8801
WWW.CIGNA.COM

CIGNA HEALTHCARE OF OKLAHOMA
600 E TAYLOR
PO BOX 9336
SHERMAN, TX 75091-9336
TEL: (903) 892-8167
FAX: (903) 892-6271
TOLL FREE: (800) 525-5803
IN-STATE: (800) 238-8801
WWW.CIGNA.COM

CIGNA HEALTHCARE OF OREGON / WASHINGTON
1630 E SHAW AVE, STE 106
PO BOX 24022
FRESNO, CA 93779-4022
TEL: (209) 222-2500
TOLL FREE: (800) 245-2471
IN-STATE: (800) 428-8891
WWW.CIGNA.COM/HEALTHCARE

CIGNA HEALTHCARE
PO BOX 2300
PITTSBURGH, PA 15230
TEL: (412) 562-2960
TOLL FREE: (800) 338-7691
WWW.CIGNA.COM

CIGNA HEALTHCARE OF MEMPHIS, TENNESSEE
600 E TAYLOR
PO BOX 9337
SHERMAN, TX 75091-9337
TEL: (903) 892-8167
FAX: (903) 892-6271
TOLL FREE: (800) 525-5803
IN-STATE: (800) 238-8801
WWW.CIGNA.COM

CIGNA HEALTHCARE OF TEXAS, INC
600 E TAYLOR
PO BOX 2546
SHERMAN, TX 75091-2546
TEL: (903) 892-8167
FAX: (903) 892-6271
TOLL FREE: (800) 525-5803
IN-STATE: (800) 238-8801
WWW.CIGNA.COM

CIGNA HEALTHCARE OF VIRGINIA
4050 INNSLAKE DR, STE 300
PO BOX 31353
RICHMOND, VA 23294
TEL: (804) 273-1100
FAX: (804) 273-1219
TOLL FREE: (800) 533-1708
WWW.CIGNA.COM

CIGNA HEALTHPLAN OF LOUISIANA, NEW ORLEANS
3838 N CSWY BLVD #2800-B
METAIRIE, LA 70002
TEL: (504) 832-1994
FAX: (504) 831-7499
TOLL FREE: (800) 654-3106
IN-STATE: (800) 238-8801
WWW.CIGNA.COM

CIGNA WORLDWIDE INSURANCE CO
1 BEAVER VALLEY RD
PO BOX 15408
WILMINGTON, DE 19850
TEL: (302) 324-1841
TOLL FREE: (800) 441-7150
WWW.CIGNA.COM

CIGNA HEALTHCARE OF TENNESSEE
ONE CORP CTR DR, STE 500-472-50
PO BOX 9339
SHERMAN, TX 75091
TEL: (903) 892-8167
TOLL FREE: (800) 492-2224
WWW.CIGNA.COM

CIGNA HEALTHCARE OF ILLINOIS INC
1700 HIGGINS, STE 600
DES PLAINES, IL 60018
TEL: (815) 939-4566
FAX: (815) 939-0473
TOLL FREE: (800) 541-7526
WWW.CIGNA.COM

OKLAHOMA CLAIMS OFFICE
CIGNA HEALTHCARE
5100 N BROOKLINE- 9TH FL
OKLAHOMA CITY, OK 73112
TOLL FREE: (800) 245-2471
IN-STATE: (800) 245-2471

CINCINNATI INSURANCE CO

ALABAMA CLAIMS OFFICE
3150 HOLCOMB BRDIGE RD, STE 350
PO BOX 920338
NORCROSS, GA 30092-0338
TEL: (770) 662-8753
FAX: (770) 417-4635
WWW.CINFIN.COM

GEORGIA CLAIMS OFFICE
3150 HOLCOMB BRDIGE RD, STE 350
PO BOX 920338
NORCROSS, GA 30092-0338
TEL: (770) 662-8753
FAX: (770) 417-4635
WWW.CINFIN.COM

SOUTH CAROLINA CLAIMS OFFICE
3150 HOLCOMB BRDIGE RD, STE 350
PO BOX 920338
NORCROSS, GA 30092-0338
TEL: (770) 662-8753
FAX: (770) 417-4635
WWW.CINFIN.COM

TENNESSEE CLAIMS OFFICE
3150 HOLCOMB BRDIGE RD, STE 350
PO BOX 920338
NORCROSS, GA 30092-0338
TEL: (770) 662-8753
FAX: (770) 417-4635
WWW.CINFIN.COM

CITY OF AMARILLO GROUP HEALTH PLAN

TEXAS CLAIMS OFFICE
909 E 7TH
PO BOX 1971
AMARILLO, TX 79105-1971
TEL: (806) 378-4209
FAX: (806) 378-9488

CITY OF EULESS EMPLOYEE BENEFITS PLAN

201 N ECTOR DR
EULESS, TX 76039-3543
TEL: (817) 685-1475
FAX: (817) 685-1819

CITY PUBLIC SERVICE GROUP HEALTH PLAN

145 NAVARRO
PO BOX 1771
SAN ANTONIO, TX 78296-1771
TEL: (210) 978-2900
FAX: (210) 978-3351

COAST BENEFITS

NEVADA CLAIMS OFFICE
3850 S VALLEY VIEW BLVD
PO BOX 80040
LAS VEGAS, NV 89180-0040
TEL: (702) 889-1155
FAX: (702) 889-1284

COLLIN COUNTY COURTHOUSE

TEXAS CLAIMS OFFICE
HUMAN RESOURCE OFFICE
210 S MCDONALD ST, STE 612
MCKINNEY, TX 75069-5667
TEL: (972) 548-4604
WWW.CO.COLLIN.TX.US.COM

COLUMBIA UNIVERSAL LIFE INSURANCE CO

NATIONAL CLAIMS OFFICE
11211 TAYLOR DRAPER LN
PO BOX 200225
AUSTIN, TX 78720-0225
TEL: (512) 345-3200
FAX: (512) 343-7599
TOLL FREE: (800) 880-1370
WWW.COLUMBIA-UNIVERSAL.COM

COMCAR INDUSTRIES, INC

FLORIDA CLAIMS OFFICE
111 HAVENDALE BLVD
PO BOX 67
AUBURNDALE, FL 33823
TEL: (941) 967-1101
FAX: (941) 551-1442
TOLL FREE: (800) 524-1101

COMMUNITY HEALTH PLAN OF OHIO

OHIO CLAIMS OFFICE
1915 TAMARACK RD
NEWARK, OH 43055-1300
TEL: (740) 348-1400
FAX: (740) 348-1500
TOLL FREE: (800) 806-2756

COMPREHENSIVE CARE SERVICES

MINNESOTA CLAIMS OFFICE
AFFILIATE OF BLUE CROSS & BLUE SHIELD OF MINNESOTA
1200 YANKEE DOODLE RD
PO BOX 64668
EGAN, MN 55122
TEL: (612) 456-5940
FAX: (612) 456-1582
TOLL FREE: (800) 365-2735

COMPREHENSIVE HEALTH SERVICES INC

NATIONAL CLAIMS OFFICE
THE WELLNESS PLAN
2875 W GRAND BLVD
DETROIT, MI 48202
TEL: (313) 875-4200
TOLL FREE: (800) 875-9355

COMPUTER SCIENCE CORP

800 N PEARL ST
PO BOX 4444
ALBANY, NY 12204-0444
TEL: (518) 447-9200
FAX: (518) 447-9240
IN-STATE: (800) 522-5518

CONSECO

INDIANA CLAIMS OFFICE
JEFFERSON NATIONAL LIFE INSURANCE
11815 N PENN ST
PO BOX 1951
CARMEL, IN 46032
TEL: (317) 817-3700
FAX: (317) 817-3345
TOLL FREE: (800) 824-2726
WWW.CONSECO.COM

CONSOLIDATED ASSOCIATION OF RAILROAD EMPLOYEES CARE

NATIONAL CLAIMS OFFICE
4912 MIDWAY DR
PO BOX 6130
TEMPLE, TX 76503
TEL: (254) 773-1330
FAX: (254) 774-8029
TOLL FREE: (800) 334-1330

CONTINENTAL GENERAL INSURANCE CO

NEBRASKA CLAIMS OFFICE
8901 INDIAN HILLS DR
PO BOX 247007
OMAHA, NE 68124-7007
TEL: (402) 397-3200
FAX: (402) 392-7771
TOLL FREE: (800) 545-8905
IN-STATE: (800) 397-3200
WWW.CONTINENTALGENERAL.COM

CONTINENTAL LIFE & ACCIDENT

ILLINOIS CLAIMS OFFICE
CONSECO
304 N MAIN ST
PO BOX 1300
ROCKFORD, IL 61105-1300
TEL: (815) 987-5000
FAX: (815) 720-2829
TOLL FREE: (800) 221-3770

COOPERATIVE BENEFIT ADMINISTRATORS

NATIONAL CLAIMS OFFICE
PO BOX 6249
LINCOLN, NE 68506-0249
TEL: (402) 483-9200
FAX: (402) 483-9201

CORESOURCE

NORTH CAROLINA CLAIMS OFFICE
6100 FAIRVIEW RD, STE 1000
CHARLOTTE, NC 28210-3291
TEL: (704) 552-0900
FAX: (704) 552-8635
TOLL FREE: (800) 327-5462
IN-STATE: (800) 821-0345

CORESOURCE, INC

NATIONAL CLAIMS OFFICE
4940 CAMPBELL BLVD, STE 200
BALTIMORE, MD 21236
TEL: (410) 931-5060
FAX: (410) 931-3653
TOLL FREE: (800) 624-7130

229 HUBER VLG BLVD
PO BOX 6118
WESTERVILLE, OH 43081-6118
TEL: (614) 890-0070
FAX: (614) 794-0736
TOLL FREE: (800) 282-3920

NEW JERSEY CLAIMS OFFICE
940 W VALLEY RD
PO BOX 6994
WAYNE, PA 19087
TEL: (610) 687-5924
FAX: (610) 687-1959
TOLL FREE: (800) 345-1166

PENNSYLVANIA CLAIMS OFFICE
940 W VALLEY RD
PO BOX 6994
WAYNE, PA 19087
TEL: (610) 687-5924
FAX: (610) 687-1959
TOLL FREE: (800) 345-1166

CORESTAR

ILLINOIS CLAIMS OFFICE
JACKSON CLAIM CENTER
146 INDUSTRIAL PARK
JACKSON, MN 56143-9511
TEL: (507) 847-5740
FAX: (507) 847-2358
TOLL FREE: (800) 274-6965

MINNESOTA CLAIMS OFFICE
JACKSON CLAIM CENTER
146 INDUSTRIAL PARK
JACKSON, MN 56143-9511
TEL: (507) 847-5740
FAX: (507) 847-2358
TOLL FREE: (800) 274-6965

CORPORATE DIVERSIFIED SERVICES

NEBRASKA CLAIMS OFFICE
2401 S 73RD ST, STE 1
PO BOX 2835
OMAHA, NE 68103-2835
TEL: (402) 393-3133
FAX: (402) 398-3773
TOLL FREE: (800) 642-4089

CORVEL CORP

NATIONAL CLAIMS OFFICE
10260 SW GREENBERG RD, STE 1165
PORTLAND, OR 97223
TEL: (503) 244-2093
FAX: (503) 244-2189
WWW.CORVEL.COM

COUNTY OF LOS ANGELES

CALIFORNIA CLAIMS OFFICE
1436 GOODRICH BLVD
COMMERCE, CA 90022
TEL: (213) 738-2279

COVENANT ADMINISTRATORS, INC

NATIONAL CLAIMS OFFICE
11330 LAKEFIELD DR, STE 100
PO BOX 740042
ATLANTA, GA 30374
TEL: (770) 242-6100
FAX: (770) 239-3989
TOLL FREE: (800) 374-6101

CPIC LIFE

CALIFORNIA CLAIMS OFFICE
PO BOX 3007
LODI, CA 95241-1911
TEL: (209) 367-3415
FAX: (209) 367-3450
TOLL FREE: (800) 642-5599
IN-STATE: (800) 537-0666

CRAWFORD & CO

ALASKA CLAIMS OFFICE
4341 B ST, STE 301
ANCHORAGE, AK 99503
TEL: (907) 561-5222
FAX: (907) 561-7383
IN-STATE: (888) 549-5222
WWW.CRAWFORDANDCOMPANY.COM

DAKOTACARE

SOUTH DAKOTA CLAIMS OFFICE
1323 S MINNESOTA AVE
SIOUX FALLS, SD 57105-0624
TEL: (605) 334-4000
FAX: (605) 336-0270
TOLL FREE: (800) 628-3778
IN-STATE: (800) 325-5598
WWW.DAKOTACARE.COM

DC CHARTERED HEALTH PLAN, INC

DISTRICT OF COLUMBIA CLAIMS OFFICE
820 FIRST ST NE, STE LL100
WASHINGTON, DC 20002
TEL: (202) 408-4710
FAX: (202) 408-4730
TOLL FREE: (800) 799-4710
WWW.CHARTER-HEALTH.COM

DCA HEALTHCARE MANAGEMENT GROUP

NORTH DAKOTA CLAIMS OFFICE
13100 WAYZATA BLVD
MINNETONKA, MN 55305-1840
TEL: (612) 541-7500
FAX: (612) 541-5999
TOLL FREE: (800) 284-4464

DCA INC

NATIONAL CLAIMS OFFICE
3405 ANNAPOLIS LN N, STE 100
PLYMOUTH, MN 55447
TEL: (612) 278-4000
FAX: (612) 278-4601
TOLL FREE: (800) 284-4464

DELMARVA HEALTH PLAN, INC

DELAWARE CLAIMS OFFICE
301 BAY ST, STE 401
PO BOX 2410
EASTON, MD 21601
TEL: (410) 822-7223
FAX: (410) 822-8152
TOLL FREE: (800) 334-3427
IN-STATE: (800) 334-3427
WWW.CAREFIRST.COM

MARYLAND CLAIMS OFFICE
301 BAY ST, STE 401
PO BOX 2410
EASTON, MD 21601
TEL: (410) 822-7223
FAX: (410) 822-8152
TOLL FREE: (800) 334-3427
IN-STATE: (800) 334-3427
WWW.CAREFIRST.COM

DELTA DENTAL PLAN OF NEW JERSEY INC

NATIONAL CLAIMS OFFICE
DELTA DENTAL OF NEW JERSEY
1639 RT 10
PO BOX 222
PARSIPPANY, NJ 07054
TEL: (973) 285-4000
FAX: (973) 285-4141
TOLL FREE: (800) 321-0142
WWW.DELTADENTALNJ.COM

DISTRICT 6 HEALTH FUND

18 E 31ST ST
NEW YORK, NY 10016-6702
TEL: (212) 696-5545
FAX: (212) 696-5556
TOLL FREE: (800) 331-1070

DIVERSIFIED GROUP ADMINISTRATORS

311 S CENTRAL
PO BOX 330
CANONSBURG, PA 15317-0330
TEL: (724) 746-8700
FAX: (724) 746-8508
TOLL FREE: (800) 221-8490
IN-STATE: (800) 222-2322

EASTERN BENEFIT SYSTEMS OF CENTENNIAL FINANCIAL GROUP

NEW JERSEY CLAIMS OFFICE
200 FREEWAY DR E
EAST ORANGE, NJ 07018
TEL: (973) 676-6100
FAX: (973) 676-6794
TOLL FREE: (800) 524-0227
IN-STATE: (800) 772-3610

EAU CLAIRE HEALTH PROTECTION PLAN

NATIONAL CLAIMS OFFICE
3430 OAKWOOD MALL DR
PO BOX 1060
EAU CLAIRE, WI 54702
TEL: (715) 835-6174
FAX: (715) 838-0220
TOLL FREE: (800) 835-6174

EDUCATORS MUTUAL LIFE INSURANCE CO

MASSACHUSETTS CLAIMS OFFICE
202 N PRINCE ST
PO BOX 83888
LANCASTER, PA 17608-3888
TEL: (717) 397-2751
FAX: (717) 397-1821
TOLL FREE: (800) 233-0307
E-MAIL: CALLCENTER@EMLIFE.COM

PENNSYLVANIA CLAIMS OFFICE
202 N PRINCE ST
PO BOX 83888
LANCASTER, PA 17608-3888
TEL: (717) 397-2751
FAX: (717) 397-1821
TOLL FREE: (800) 233-0307
E-MAIL: CALLCENTER@EMLIFE.COM

RHODE ISLAND CLAIMS OFFICE
202 N PRINCE ST
PO BOX 83888
LANCASTER, PA 17608-3888
TEL: (717) 397-2751
FAX: (717) 397-1821
TOLL FREE: (800) 233-0307
E-MAIL: CALLCENTER@EMLIFE.COM

SOUTH CAROLINA CLAIMS OFFICE
202 N PRINCE ST
PO BOX 83888
LANCASTER, PA 17608-3888
TEL: (717) 397-2751
FAX: (717) 397-1821
TOLL FREE: (800) 233-0307
E-MAIL: CALLCENTER@EMLIFE.COM

ELCA BOARD OF PENSIONS

NATIONAL CLAIMS OFFICE
800 MARQUETTE AVE, STE 1050
PO BOX 59093
MINNEAPOLIS, MN 55459-0093
TEL: (612) 333-7651
FAX: (612) 334-5407
IN-STATE: (800) 352-2876
WWW.ELCABOP.ORG

ELECTRONIC DATA SYSTEMS

EDS
PO BOX 15508
SACRAMENTO, CA 95852
TEL: (916) 636-1100
FAX: (916) 636-1056
IN-STATE: (800) 541-5555

EMERALD HEALTH NETWORK, INC

OHIO CLAIMS OFFICE
1100 SUPERIOR AVE- 16TH FL
PO BOX 94808
CLEVELAND, OH 44101-4808
TEL: (216) 479-2030
FAX: (216) 241-4158
TOLL FREE: (800) 683-6830
WWW.EMERALDHEALTH.COM

EMPIRE BLUE CROSS & BLUE SHIELD

NEW YORK CLAIMS OFFICE
11 CORPORATE WOODS BLVD
PO BOX 11800
ALBANY, NY 12211-0800
TEL: (518) 367-4737
FAX: (518) 367-5373
WWW.EMPIREHEALTHCARE.COM

EMPIRE MEDICARE SERVICES

PO BOX 4846
SYRACUSE, NY 13221-4846
TEL: (315) 442-4400
FAX: (315) 442-4815
TOLL FREE: (800) 442-8430

EMPLOYEE BENEFIT ASSOCIATION

OHIO CLAIMS OFFICE
2858 W MARKET ST, STE N
PO BOX 5427
AKRON, OH 44333
TEL: (330) 867-9050
FAX: (330) 867-7029
TOLL FREE: (800) 624-2564

EMPLOYEE BENEFIT CLAIMS, INC

NATIONAL CLAIMS OFFICE
820 PARISH ST
PITTSBURGH, PA 15220-3405
TEL: (412) 922-0780
FAX: (412) 922-3071
TOLL FREE: (800) 922-4966

EMPLOYEE BENEFIT PLAN ADMINISTRATORS

CONNECTICUT CLAIMS OFFICE
CT PIPE TRADES BENEFIT FUNDS ADMINISTRATORS INC
210 MAIN ST
MANCHESTER, CT 06040
TEL: (860) 643-6401
FAX: (860) 643-6818
TOLL FREE: (800) 848-2129

EMPLOYEE BENEFIT SYSTEMS CORP

IOWA CLAIMS OFFICE
1701 MT PLEASANT ST, STE 1
PO BOX 1053
BURLINGTON, IA 52601-2799
TEL: (319) 752-3200
FAX: (319) 754-4480
TOLL FREE: (800) 373-1327
E-MAIL: EBS4BENEFITS@LISCO.NET

EQUITABLE PLAN SERVICES, INC

OKLAHOMA CLAIMS OFFICE
12312 SAINT ANDREWS DR
PO BOX 770466
OKLAHOMA CITY, OK 73177
TEL: (405) 755-2929
FAX: (405) 755-1185
TOLL FREE: (800) 749-2631

ERISA ADMINISTRATIVE SERVICES, INC

ARIZONA CLAIMS OFFICE
3108 N 24TH ST- BLDG B
PHOENIX, AZ 85016-7313
TEL: (602) 956-3516
FAX: (602) 956-1943
WWW.CSERISA.COM

COLORADO CLAIMS OFFICE
10520 E BETHANY DR- BLDG 7
AURORA, CO 80014
TEL: (303) 745-0147
FAX: (303) 745-7010
WWW.CSERISA.COM

NEW MEXICO CLAIMS OFFICE
1200 SAN PEDRO NE
ALBUQUERQUE, NM 87110
TEL: (505) 262-1821
FAX: (505) 262-1822
WWW.CSERISA.COM

1429 SECOND ST
SANTA FE, NM 87505
TEL: (505) 988-4974
FAX: (505) 988-8943
WWW.CSERISA.COM

TEXAS CLAIMS OFFICE
12325 HYMEADOW DR- BLDG 4
AUSTIN, TX 78750-0001
TEL: (512) 250-9397
FAX: (512) 335-7298
TOLL FREE: (800) 933-7472
WWW.CSERISA.COM

UTAH CLAIMS OFFICE
2156 W 2200 S
SALT LAKE CITY, UT 84119-1326
TEL: (801) 973-1001
FAX: (801) 973-1007
WWW.CSERISA.COM

FARM BUREAU MUTUAL INSURANCE CO

IDAHO CLAIMS OFFICE
194 E COMMERCIAL
WEISER, ID 83672-2511
TEL: (208) 549-1414
FAX: (208) 549-1433

FARM BUREAU MUTUAL INSURANCE CO OF IDAHO

WESTERN FARM BUREAU LIFE INSURANCE CO
444 E 5TH N
PO BOX 1148
BURLEY, ID 83318-1148
TEL: (208) 678-0431
FAX: (208) 678-5368

345 MAIN
PO BOX 428
GRAND VIEW, ID 83624-0428
TEL: (208) 834-2766
FAX: (208) 834-2526

WESTERN COMMUNITY INSURANCE CO
170 S 2ND E
PO BOX 506
SODA SPRINGS, ID 83276-0506
TEL: (208) 547-3315
FAX: (208) 547-3316

FARMERS AUTO INSURANCE ASSOCIATION

ILLINOIS CLAIMS OFFICE
PEKIN INSURANCE CO
2505 COURT ST
PO BOX 129
PEKIN, IL 61558-0001
TEL: (309) 346-1161
FAX: (309) 346-8265
TOLL FREE: (800) 322-0160
WWW.PEKININSURANCE.COM

INDIANA CLAIMS OFFICE
PEKIN INSURANCE CO
2505 COURT ST
PO BOX 129
PEKIN, IL 61558-0001
TEL: (309) 346-1161
FAX: (309) 346-8265
TOLL FREE: (800) 322-0160
WWW.PEKININSURANCE.COM

IOWA CLAIMS OFFICE
PEKIN INSURANCE CO
2505 COURT ST
PO BOX 129
PEKIN, IL 61558-0001
TEL: (309) 346-1161
FAX: (309) 346-8265
TOLL FREE: (800) 322-0160
WWW.PEKININSURANCE.COM

WISCONSIN CLAIMS OFFICE
PEKIN INSURANCE CO
2505 COURT ST
PO BOX 129
PEKIN, IL 61558-0001
TEL: (309) 346-1161
FAX: (309) 346-8265
TOLL FREE: (800) 322-0160
WWW.PEKININSURANCE.COM

FEDERATED MUTUAL INSURANCE CO

ALABAMA CLAIMS OFFICE
2701 N ROCKY PT DR, STE 1200
PO BOX 31716
TAMPA, FL 33631-3716
TEL: (813) 287-0155
FAX: (813) 287-0785
IN-STATE: (800) 237-8292
WWW.FEDERATEDINS.COM

FLORIDA CLAIMS OFFICE
2701 N ROCKY PT DR, STE 1200
PO BOX 31716
TAMPA, FL 33631-3716
TEL: (813) 287-0155
FAX: (813) 287-0785
IN-STATE: (800) 237-8292
WWW.FEDERATEDINS.COM

GEORGIA CLAIMS OFFICE
2701 N ROCKY PT DR, STE 1200
PO BOX 31716
TAMPA, FL 33631-3716
TEL: (813) 287-0155
FAX: (813) 287-0785
IN-STATE: (800) 237-8292
WWW.FEDERATEDINS.COM

MISSISSIPPI CLAIMS OFFICE
2701 N ROCKY PT DR, STE 1200
PO BOX 31716
TAMPA, FL 33631-3716
TEL: (813) 287-0155
FAX: (813) 287-0785
IN-STATE: (800) 237-8292
WWW.FEDERATEDINS.COM

NORTH CAROLINA CLAIMS OFFICE
2701 N ROCKY PT DR, STE 1200
PO BOX 31716
TAMPA, FL 33631-3716
TEL: (813) 287-0155
FAX: (813) 287-0785
IN-STATE: (800) 237-8292
WWW.FEDERATEDINS.COM

SOUTH CAROLINA CLAIMS OFFICE
2701 N ROCKY PT DR, STE 1200
PO BOX 31716
TAMPA, FL 33631-3716
TEL: (813) 287-0155
FAX: (813) 287-0785
IN-STATE: (800) 237-8292
WWW.FEDERATEDINS.COM

TENNESSEE CLAIMS OFFICE
2701 N ROCKY PT DR, STE 1200
PO BOX 31716
TAMPA, FL 33631-3716
TEL: (813) 287-0155
FAX: (813) 287-0785
IN-STATE: (800) 237-8292
WWW.FEDERATEDINS.COM

VIRGINIA CLAIMS OFFICE
2701 N ROCKY PT DR, STE 1200
PO BOX 31716
TAMPA, FL 33631-3716
TEL: (813) 287-0155
FAX: (813) 287-0785
IN-STATE: (800) 237-8292
WWW.FEDERATEDINS.COM

FIDELITY SECURITY LIFE INSURANCE CO

NATIONAL CLAIMS OFFICE
PO BOX 418131
KANSAS CITY, MO 64141-9131
TEL: (816) 756-1060
FAX: (816) 968-0560
TOLL FREE: (800) 821-7303

FIRST HEALTH

ALASKA CLAIMS OFFICE
4411 BUSINESS PARK BLVD, STE 16
ANCHORAGE, AK 99503
TEL: (907) 561-5650
FAX: (907) 563-1082

FIRST INTEGRATED HEALTH

CALIFORNIA CLAIMS OFFICE
19191 S VERMONT, STE 700
PO BOX 5279
TORRANCE, CA 90510-5279
TEL: (310) 532-8887
FAX: (310) 532-2824
TOLL FREE: (800) 433-3554
WWW.FIH.COM

FORTIS BENEFITS INSURANCE CO

GEORGIA CLAIMS OFFICE
FORTIS BENEFIT
1950 SPECTRUM CIR, STE B100
MARIETTA, GA 30067-6052
FAX: (770) 916-0905
TOLL FREE: (800) 955-1586

FOX-EVERETT, INC

MISSISSIPPI CLAIMS OFFICE
3780 I-55 N FRONTAGE RD, STE 200
PO BOX 23096
JACKSON, MS 39225-3095
TEL: (601) 981-6000
FAX: (601) 718-5399

FREMONT COMPENSATION INSURANCE CO

CALIFORNIA CLAIMS OFFICE
INDUSTRIAL INDEMNITY CO
255 CALIFORNIA ST
PO BOX 7468
SAN FRANCISCO, CA 94111
TEL: (415) 627-5000
FAX: (415) 296-3099
IN-STATE: (800) 464-0556
WWW.INSWEB.COM

FRINGE BENEFIT COORDINATORS

FLORIDA CLAIMS OFFICE
1239 NW 10TH AVE
GAINESVILLE, FL 32601-4154
TEL: (352) 372-2028
FAX: (352) 372-9805
IN-STATE: (800) 654-1452

GALLATIN MEDICAL CLINICS

CALIFORNIA CLAIMS OFFICE
10720 PARAMOUNT BLVD
PO BOX 868
DOWNEY, CA 90241-3306
TEL: (562) 923-6511
FAX: (562) 861-6884

GARDNER & WHITE

INDIANA CLAIMS OFFICE
8902 N MERIDIAN ST, STE 202
PO BOX 40619
INDIANAPOLIS, IN 46260-5307
TEL: (317) 581-1580
FAX: (317) 587-0780
TOLL FREE: (800) 347-5737

GEM INSURANCE CO

ARIZONA CLAIMS OFFICE
525 E 100 S
PO BOX 115
PUEBLO, CO 81002-0115
FAX: (888) 359-5304
TOLL FREE: (800) 888-7164

NEVADA CLAIMS OFFICE
525 E 100 S
PO BOX 115
PUEBLO, CO 81002-0115
FAX: (888) 359-5304
TOLL FREE: (800) 888-7164

NEW MEXICO CLAIMS OFFICE
525 E 100 S
PO BOX 115
PUEBLO, CO 81002-0115
FAX: (888) 359-5304
TOLL FREE: (800) 888-7164

TEXAS CLAIMS OFFICE
525 E 100 S
PO BOX 115
PUEBLO, CO 81002-0115
FAX: (888) 359-5304
TOLL FREE: (800) 888-7164

UTAH CLAIMS OFFICE
525 E 100 S
PO BOX 115
PUEBLO, CO 81002-0115
FAX: (888) 359-5304
TOLL FREE: (800) 888-7164

GENERAL AMERICAN LIFE INSURANCE CO

NATIONAL CLAIMS OFFICE
719 TEACO RD
PO BOX 882
KENNETT, MO 63857-3749
TEL: (314) 843-8700
FAX: (314) 525-5740
TOLL FREE: (800) 633-8989

GENERAL INSURANCE EXCHANGE AGENCY, INC

OHIO CLAIMS OFFICE
4301 DARROW RD
PO BOX 1849
STOW, OH 44224-0849
TEL: (330) 688-4322
FAX: (330) 688-4904
TOLL FREE: (800) 968-7222
WWW.CHANDLER-GROUP.COM

GEORGIA BANKERS ASSOCIATION INSURANCE

GEORGIA CLAIMS OFFICE
50 HURT PLZ, STE 1050
ATLANTA, GA 30303-2916
TEL: (404) 522-1501
FAX: (404) 522-9848
WWW.GABANKERS.COM

GILBERT-MAGILL CO

MISSOURI CLAIMS OFFICE
920 MAIN ST, STE 1800
PO BOX 410249
KANSAS CITY, MO 64141-0249
TEL: (816) 474-3535
FAX: (816) 842-5795
TOLL FREE: (800) 522-2460

GOLDEN RULE LIFE INSURANCE CO

ILLINOIS CLAIMS OFFICE
712 11TH ST
LAWRENCEVILLE, IL 62439-2395
TEL: (618) 943-8000
FAX: (618) 943-8031

NATIONAL CLAIMS OFFICE
7440 WOODLAND DR
INDIANAPOLIS, IN 46278-1719
TEL: (317) 297-4123
FAX: (317) 298-4410
IN-STATE: (800) 265-7791
WWW.GOLDENRULE.COM

GOLDEN STATE MUTUAL LIFE INSURANCE CO

1999 W ADAMS BLVD
PO BOX 512332
LOS ANGELES, CA 90051-0332
TEL: (323) 731-1131
TOLL FREE: (800) 225-5476
WWW.GSMLIFE.COM

GOULD MEDICAL FOUNDATION

CALIFORNIA CLAIMS OFFICE
PO BOX 254708
SACRAMENTO, CA 95865
TEL: (209) 524-2221
FAX: (209) 524-4562
IN-STATE: (800) 564-6853

GRAND VALLEY CORP

MICHIGAN CLAIMS OFFICE
829 FOREST HILLS AVE SE
GRAND RAPIDS, MI 49546-2325
TEL: (616) 949-2410
FAX: (616) 949-4978

GRANGE INSURANCE ASSOCIATION

KENTUCKY CLAIMS OFFICE
2425 REGENCY RD
PO BOX 8035
LEXINGTON, KY 40533-8035
TEL: (606) 278-5481
FAX: (800) 837-0802
TOLL FREE: (800) 837-0801

GRAY INSURANCE CO

LOUISIANA CLAIMS OFFICE
3601 N I-10 SERVICE RD W
PO BOX 6202
METAIRIE, LA 70009-6202
TEL: (504) 888-7790
FAX: (504) 887-5658
WWW.GRAYINSCO.COM

GREAT WEST LIFE

NATIONAL CLAIMS OFFICE
1740 TECHNOLOGY DR, STE 300
PO BOX 1120
SAN JOSE, CA 95108
FAX: (408) 453-7963
TOLL FREE: (800) 685-1050
WWW.1HEALTHPLAN.COM

1511 N WEST SHORE BLVD, STE 850
PO BOX 31251
TAMPA, FL 33631-3251
FAX: (813) 281-0019
TOLL FREE: (800) 333-5251
WWW.1HEALTHPLAN.COM

NEW ENGLAND
10000 N CENTRAL EXPY, STE 800
DALLAS, TX 75231
FAX: (214) 987-0827
TOLL FREE: (800) 685-3020
WWW.GWL.COM

1802 DEL RANGE BLVD, STE 200
CHEYENNE, WY 82001
TOLL FREE: (800) 288-9575

GREAT-WEST LIFE & ANNUITY

PO BOX 950
DENVER, CO 80201
FAX: (303) 790-1998
TOLL FREE: (800) 685-2020
WWW.GWLA.COM

OREGON CLAIMS OFFICE
1800 S W 1ST AVE, STE 410
PO BOX 429
PORTLAND, OR 97207-0429
FAX: (503) 224-2202
TOLL FREE: (800) 685-1020

GREAT-WEST LIFE ASSURANCE CO

CALIFORNIA CLAIMS OFFICE
455 MARKET ST, STE 2000
SAN FRANCISCO, CA 94105-2403
TEL: (415) 777-4646
FAX: (415) 957-9842
TOLL FREE: (800) 685-1040

GROCER'S INSURANCE GROUP

NATIONAL CLAIMS OFFICE
6605 SE LAKE RD
PO BOX 22146
PORTLAND, OR 97269
TEL: (503) 833-1600
FAX: (503) 833-1699
TOLL FREE: (800) 777-3602
WWW.GROCINS.COM

GROUP BENEFIT SERVICES, INC

6 N PARK, STE 310
HUNT VALLEY, MD 21030
TEL: (410) 832-1300
FAX: (410) 832-1315
TOLL FREE: (800) 638-6085
WWW.G-B-S.COM

GROUP BENEFITS UNLIMITED

ILLINOIS CLAIMS OFFICE
1000 PLAZA DR, STE 300
CHAMBERG, IL 60173
TEL: (847) 330-6000
FAX: (847) 330-9400
TOLL FREE: (800) 772-0666

GROUP HEALTH MANAGERS

MICHIGAN CLAIMS OFFICE
26205 FIVE-MILE RD
REDFORD, MI 48239-3154
TEL: (313) 535-7100
FAX: (313) 535-8472
TOLL FREE: (800) 992-2508

GROUP HEALTH NORTHWEST

NATIONAL CLAIMS OFFICE
CORP CTR- 5615 W SUNSET HWY
PO BOX 204
SPOKANE, WA 99210
TEL: (509) 838-9100
FAX: (509) 838-3292
TOLL FREE: (800) 497-2210
IN-STATE: (800) 377-8853
WWW.GHNW.ORG

WASHINGTON CLAIMS OFFICE
5615 W SUNSET HIGH
PO BOX 204
SPOKANE, WA 99210-0204
TEL: (509) 838-9100
FAX: (509) 458-0368
TOLL FREE: (800) 767-4670
IN-STATE: (800) 838-9100
WWW.GHNW.ORG

GROUP HEALTH PLAN OF ST. LOUIS

ILLINOIS CLAIMS OFFICE
111 CORPERATE OFFICE DR, STE 400
EARTH CITY, MO 63145
TEL: (314) 453-1700
FAX: (314) 506-1958
TOLL FREE: (800) 743-3901
WWW.GHP.COM

GROUP HEALTH PLAN OF ST LOUIS

MISSOURI CLAIMS OFFICE
111 CORPERATE OFFICE DR, STE 400
EARTH CITY, MO 63145
TEL: (314) 453-1700
FAX: (314) 506-1555
TOLL FREE: (800) 743-3901
WWW.GHP.COM

GROUP INSURANCE PLAN CHATTANOOGA

FLORIDA CLAIMS OFFICE
1500 N DALE MABRY HWY E 6
PO BOX 31601
TAMPA, FL 33631-3601
TEL: (813) 871-4664
FAX: (813) 871-4601

GROUP MAJOR MEDICAL EXPENSE

MISSOURI CLAIMS OFFICE
PO BOX 6614
SAINT LOUIS, MO 63166-6149
TEL: (314) 554-6490

GROUP SERVICES & ADMINISTRATION, INC

KANSAS CLAIMS OFFICE
3113 CLASSEN BLVD
OKLAHOMA CITY, OK 73118-3818
TEL: (405) 528-4400
FAX: (405) 528-5558
TOLL FREE: (800) 475-4445

MISSOURI CLAIMS OFFICE
3113 CLASSEN BLVD
OKLAHOMA CITY, OK 73118-3818
TEL: (405) 528-4400
FAX: (405) 528-5558
TOLL FREE: (800) 475-4445

OKLAHOMA CLAIMS OFFICE
3113 CLASSEN BLVD
OKLAHOMA CITY, OK 73118-3818
TEL: (405) 528-4400
FAX: (405) 528-5558
TOLL FREE: (800) 475-4445

TEXAS CLAIMS OFFICE
3113 CLASSEN BLVD
OKLAHOMA CITY, OK 73118-3818
TEL: (405) 528-4400
FAX: (405) 528-5558
TOLL FREE: (800) 475-4445

GUARANTEE RESERVE LIFE INSURANCE CO

ILLINOIS CLAIMS OFFICE
530 RIVER OAKS W
CALUMET CITY, IL 60409
TEL: (708) 868-4232
FAX: (708) 891-8886
TOLL FREE: (800) 323-8764

GUARDIAN LIFE INSURANCE CO OF AMERICA

NATIONAL CLAIMS OFFICE
THE GUARDIAN
777 E MAGNESIUM
PO BOX 2467
SPOKANE, WA 99210
TEL: (509) 468-6000
FAX: (509) 468-6420
TOLL FREE: (800) 695-4542
WWW.THEGUARDIAN.COM

GULF GUARANTY EMPLOYEE BENEFIT SERVICES, INC

MISSISSIPPI CLAIMS OFFICE
4785 I-55 N, STE 106
PO BOX 14977
JACKSON, MS 39236-4977
TEL: (601) 981-9505
FAX: (601) 981-6805
TOLL FREE: (800) 890-7337

GULFCO LIFE INSURANCE CO

LOUISIANA CLAIMS OFFICE
660 N MAIN
PO BOX 157
MARKSVILLE, LA 71351-0157
TEL: (318) 253-7564
FAX: (318) 253-4903

H.E.R.E.I.U. WELFARE FUNDS

NATIONAL CLAIMS OFFICE
HOTEL EMPLOYEES & RESTAURANT EMPLOYEES INT'L UNION
711 N COMMONS DR
PO BOX 6020
AURORA, IL 60598
TEL: (630) 236-5100
FAX: (630) 236-4394

HARRINGTON BENEFIT SERVICES

OHIO CLAIMS OFFICE
HEALTHPLAN SERVICES, INC
3041 MORSE XING
PO BOX 16789
COLUMBUS, OH 43216-6789
TEL: (614) 470-7000
FAX: (614) 470-7171
TOLL FREE: (800) 848-4623
IN-STATE: (800) 848-2664

HARRIS METHODIST HEALTH PLAN

TEXAS CLAIMS OFFICE
611 RYAN PLZ DR, STE 900
PO BOX 90100
ARLINGTON, TX 76011
TEL: (817) 878-5800
FAX: (817) 462-7235
TOLL FREE: (800) 633-8598
WWW.HMHP.COM

HAWAII MEDICAL SERVICE ASSOCIATION

HAWAII CLAIMS OFFICE
BLUE CROSS & BLUE SHIELD OF HAWAII
818 KEEAUMOKU ST
PO BOX 860
HONOLULU, HI 96808
TEL: (808) 948-6111
FAX: (808) 948-6555
TOLL FREE: (800) 776-4672
WWW.HMSA.COM

HEALTH ALLIANCE MEDICAL PLANS

NATIONAL CLAIMS OFFICE
102 MAIN ST
URBANA, IL 61801
TEL: (217) 337-8100
FAX: (217) 337-8008
TOLL FREE: (800) 851-3379
WWW.HEALTHALLIANCE.ORG

HEALTH ALLIANCE PLAN OF MICHIGAN

MICHIGAN CLAIMS OFFICE
HAP
2850 W GRAND BLVD
DETROIT, MI 48202-2692
TEL: (313) 872-8100
FAX: (313) 874-7496
TOLL FREE: (800) 422-4641
IN-STATE: (800) 367-3292
WWW.HAPCORP.ORG

HEALTH AMERICA

PENNSYLVANIA CLAIMS OFFICE
2575 INTERSTATE DR
HARRISBURG, PA 17110
TEL: (412) 553-7300
FAX: (412) 553-7384
TOLL FREE: (800) 735-2202
WWW.HEALTHAMERICA.CVTY.COM

HEALTH CARE ADMINISTRATORS

OKLAHOMA CLAIMS OFFICE
HEALTH CARE SOLUTIONS
2401 CHANDLER RD, STE 300
PO BOX 1309
MUSKOGEE, OK 74402
TEL: (918) 687-1261
FAX: (918) 682-7984
TOLL FREE: (800) 749-1422

HEALTH CARE ADMINISTRATORS, INC

INDIANA CLAIMS OFFICE
ARNET HEALTH PLANS
415 N 26TH ST, STE 101
PO BOX 6108
LAFAYETTE, IN 47903-6108
TEL: (765) 474-5455
FAX: (765) 448-7799
TOLL FREE: (888) 448-7447

HEALTH CARE SERVICE CORP

ILLINOIS CLAIMS OFFICE
BLUE CROSS & BLUE SHIELD
300 E RANDOLPH ST
PO BOX 1364
CHICAGO, IL 60690
TEL: (312) 938-6000

MICHIGAN CLAIMS OFFICE
BLUE CROSS & BLUE SHIELD
300 E RANDOLPH ST
PO BOX 1364
CHICAGO, IL 60690
TEL: (312) 938-6000

TEXAS CLAIMS OFFICE
BLUE CROSS & BLUE SHIELD
300 E RANDOLPH ST
PO BOX 1364
CHICAGO, IL 60690
TEL: (312) 938-6000

HEALTH FIRST

OHIO CLAIMS OFFICE
278 BARKS RD W
PO BOX 1820
MARION, OH 43301-1820
TEL: (740) 387-6355
FAX: (740) 383-3840
TOLL FREE: (800) 858-1472
E-MAIL: HFIRSTDP@ACC-NET.COM

HEALTH FIRST, INC

TEXAS CLAIMS OFFICE
HEALTH PLAN
821 E SE LOOP 323, II AMERICAN CTR, STE 200
PO BOX 130217
TYLER, TX 75713
TEL: (903) 581-2600
FAX: (903) 509-5726
TOLL FREE: (800) 477-2287
IN-STATE: (800) 477-2287

HEALTH GUARD

PENNSYLVANIA CLAIMS OFFICE
280 GRANITE RUN DR, STE 105
LANCASTER, PA 17601-6810
TEL: (717) 560-9049
FAX: (717) 560-9413
TOLL FREE: (800) 269-4606
WWW.HGUARD.COM

HEALTH MANAGEMENT ASSOCIATES

NATIONAL CLAIMS OFFICE
1600 W BROADWAY RD, STE 385
TEMPE, AZ 85282
TEL: (480) 921-8944
FAX: (480) 894-5230
TOLL FREE: (800) 331-9562
E-MAIL: HMA@VERDINET.COM

HEALTH NET

CALIFORNIA CLAIMS OFFICE
FOUNDATION HEALTH SYSTEMS
21600 OXIDE ST
PO BOX 9103
WOODLAND HILLS, CA 91367-9103
TEL: (818) 676-6775
FAX: (818) 676-8755
TOLL FREE: (800) 522-0088
WWW.HEALTHNET.COM

KANSAS CLAIMS OFFICE
2300 MAIN ST, STE 700
KANSAS CITY, MO 64108
TEL: (816) 221-8400
FAX: (816) 221-7709
TOLL FREE: (800) 468-1442
WWW.HEALTH NET_KC.COM

MISSOURI CLAIMS OFFICE
2300 MAIN ST, STE 700
KANSAS CITY, MO 64108
TEL: (816) 221-8400
FAX: (816) 221-7709
TOLL FREE: (800) 468-1442
WWW.HEALTH NET_KC.COM

HEALTH NET HMO, INC

TENNESSEE CLAIMS OFFICE
44 VANTAGE WAY, STE 300
PO BOX 20000
NASHVILLE, TN 37202
TEL: (615) 291-7022
FAX: (615) 401-4647
TOLL FREE: (800) 881-9466
IN-STATE: (800) 314-3258

HEALTH PARTNERS

MINNESOTA CLAIMS OFFICE
PO BOX 1309
MINNEAPOLIS, MN 55440-1309
TEL: (612) 883-6000
FAX: (612) 883-6100
TOLL FREE: (800) 828-1159
WWW.HEALTHPARTNER.COM

HEALTH PLAN

OHIO CLAIMS OFFICE
52160 NATIONAL RD E
ST. CLAIRSVILLE, OH 43950-9306
TEL: (740) 695-7605
FAX: (740) 695-8103
TOLL FREE: (800) 624-6961
WWW.HEALTHPLAN.ORG

WEST VIRGINIA CLAIMS OFFICE
52160 NATIONAL RD E
ST. CLAIRSVILLE, OH 43950-9306
TEL: (740) 695-7605
FAX: (740) 695-8103
TOLL FREE: (800) 624-6961
WWW.HEALTHPLAN.ORG

HEALTH PLAN OF NEVADA, INC

NEVADA CLAIMS OFFICE
SIERRA HEALTH SERVICES
2724 TENAYA
PO BOX 15645
LAS VEGAS, NV 89114-5645
TEL: (702) 242-7444
FAX: (702) 242-9038

HEALTH PLAN OF THE REDWOODS

CALIFORNIA CLAIMS OFFICE
3033 CLEVELAND AVE
SANTA ROSA, CA 95403-2126
TEL: (707) 544-2273
FAX: (707) 525-4261
IN-STATE: (800) 248-2070
WWW.HPR.ORG

HEALTH RISK MANAGEMENT

MICHIGAN CLAIMS OFFICE
5250 LOVERS LN
PO BOX 4022
KALAMAZOO, MI 49002-1564
TEL: (616) 381-7995
FAX: (616) 382-1525
TOLL FREE: (800) 253-0966
IN-STATE: (800) 632-5674

NATIONAL CLAIMS OFFICE
10900 HAMPSHIRE AVE S
PO BOX 226
MINNEAPOLIS, MN 55440-0226
TEL: (612) 829-3500
FAX: (612) 829-3622
TOLL FREE: (800) 642-4456

HEALTH SERVICES MEDICAL CORP

NEW YORK CLAIMS OFFICE
UNIVERA
8278 WILLETT PKY
BALDWINSVILLE, NY 13027
TEL: (315) 638-2133
FAX: (315) 638-0985
TOLL FREE: (800) 388-3264
WWW.PHPHMO.COM

HEALTHCARE AMERICA PLANS, INC

KANSAS CLAIMS OFFICE
453 S WEBB RD, STE 200
PO BOX 780467
WICHITA, KS 67278-0467
TEL: (316) 687-1600
FAX: (316) 616-2076
TOLL FREE: (800) 475-4274

HEALTHCARE PARTNERS MEDICAL GROUP, INC

CALIFORNIA CLAIMS OFFICE
PO BOX 6099
TORRANCE, CA 90504
TEL: (310) 965-1100
FAX: (310) 352-6219

HEALTHFIRST, INC

SOUTH CAROLINA CLAIMS OFFICE
PO BOX 17709
GREENVILLE, SC 29606
TEL: (864) 289-3000
FAX: (864) 289-3053
TOLL FREE: (800) 832-7713
WWW.HEALTHFIRST.COM

HEALTHSOURCE

MASSACHUSETTS CLAIMS OFFICE
HEALTHSOURCE OF NEW HAMPSHIRE
2 COLLEGE PARK DR
HOOKSETT, NH 03106
TEL: (603) 225-5077
FAX: (603) 268-7981
TOLL FREE: (800) 531-3121
IN-STATE: (800) 531-3121
WWW.CIGNA.COM

NEW HAMPSHIRE CLAIMS OFFICE
HEALTHSOURCE OF NEW HAMPSHIRE
2 COLLEGE PARK DR
HOOKSETT, NH 03106
TEL: (603) 225-5077
FAX: (603) 268-7981
TOLL FREE: (800) 531-3121
IN-STATE: (800) 531-3121
WWW.CIGNA.COM

NEW YORK CLAIMS OFFICE
5794 WIDEWATERS PKY- 2ND FL
PO BOX 1498
SYRACUSE, NY 13201-1498
TEL: (315) 449-1100
FAX: (315) 449-2200
TOLL FREE: (800) 999-0874
WWW.SIGNA.COM

HELLER ASSOCIATES

NATIONAL CLAIMS OFFICE
2755 BRISTOL ST, STE 250
COSTA MESA, CA 92626-5956
TEL: (714) 549-7052
FAX: (714) 549-4816
IN-STATE: (800) 552-2929
E-MAIL: CLAIMS@HELLERTPA.COM
WWW.HELLERTPA.COM

2235 FLAMINGO RD #406
LAS VEGAS, NV 89119
TEL: (714) 549-7052
FAX: (714) 549-4816
E-MAIL: CLAIMS@HELLERTPA.COM
WWW.HELLERTPA.COM

8228 MAYFIELD RD, STE 5-B
CHESTERLAND, OH 44026
TEL: (714) 549-7052
FAX: (714) 549-4816
E-MAIL: CLAIMS@HELLERTPA.COM
WWW.HELLERTPA.COM

HERITAGE INSURANCE MANAGERS, INC

TEXAS CLAIMS OFFICE
PO BOX 659570
SAN ANTONIO, TX 78265-9570
TEL: (210) 829-7467
FAX: (210) 822-4113
TOLL FREE: (800) 456-7480
E-MAIL: SALES@HERITAGE-INS.COM
WWW.HERITAGE-INS.COM

HMA, INC

ARIZONA CLAIMS OFFICE
DBA HEALTH MANAGEMENT ASSOCIATES, INC
PO BOX 2069
COTTONWOOD, AZ 86326
TEL: (602) 921-8944
FAX: (602) 894-5230
TOLL FREE: (800) 448-3585

COLORADO CLAIMS OFFICE
DBA HEALTH MANAGEMENT ASSOCIATES, INC
PO BOX 2069
COTTONWOOD, AZ 86326
TEL: (602) 921-8944
FAX: (602) 894-5230
TOLL FREE: (800) 448-3585

NEVADA CLAIMS OFFICE
DBA HEALTH MANAGEMENT ASSOCIATES, INC
PO BOX 2069
COTTONWOOD, AZ 86326
TEL: (602) 921-8944
FAX: (602) 894-5230
TOLL FREE: (800) 448-3585

HMO COLORADO, INC

COLORADO CLAIMS OFFICE
BLUE CROSS BLUE SHIELD OF COLORADO
700 BROADWAY
DENVER, CO 80273
TEL: (303) 831-0801
FAX: (303) 861-9018
TOLL FREE: (800) 544-3879
IN-STATE: (800) 533-5643
WWW.BCBSCO.COM

HMO MONTANA

MONTANA CLAIMS OFFICE
PLAN OF BLUE CROSS AND BLUE SHIELD OF MT
404 FULLER AVE
PO BOX 5004
GREAT FALLS, MT 59403
TEL: (406) 447-8600
TOLL FREE: (800) 447-7828
WWW.BCBSMT.COM

HMO NEBRASKA

IOWA CLAIMS OFFICE
2401 S 73RD ST, STE 2
PO BOX 241739
OMAHA, NE 68124-5739
TEL: (402) 392-2800
FAX: (402) 392-2761
TOLL FREE: (800) 843-2373

NEBRASKA CLAIMS OFFICE
2401 S 73RD ST, STE 2
PO BOX 241739
OMAHA, NE 68124-5739
TEL: (402) 392-2800
FAX: (402) 392-2761
TOLL FREE: (800) 843-2373

HMO NEW MEXICO, INC

COLORADO CLAIMS OFFICE
12800 INDIAN SCHOOL NE
PO BOX 11968
ALBUQUERQUE, NM 87112
TEL: (505) 291-6945
TOLL FREE: (800) 423-1630
IN-STATE: (800) 423-1630

NEVADA CLAIMS OFFICE
12800 INDIAN SCHOOL NE
PO BOX 11968
ALBUQUERQUE, NM 87112
TEL: (505) 291-6945
TOLL FREE: (800) 423-1630
IN-STATE: (800) 423-1630

NEW MEXICO CLAIMS OFFICE
12800 INDIAN SCHOOL NE
PO BOX 11968
ALBUQUERQUE, NM 87112
TEL: (505) 291-6945
TOLL FREE: (800) 423-1630
IN-STATE: (800) 423-1630

HMO REGENCE CARE

WASHINGTON CLAIMS OFFICE
1800 9TH AVE
PO BOX 91005
SEATTLE, WA 98111-9105
TEL: (206) 340-6600
FAX: (206) 389-6719
TOLL FREE: (800) 222-6129

HOLY CROSS RESOURCES, INC

INDIANA CLAIMS OFFICE
ST MARY'S LOURDES HALL
3575 MOREAU CT
SOUTH BEND, IN 46628-4320
TEL: (219) 283-4600
FAX: (219) 283-4709
TOLL FREE: (800) 348-2616
WWW.HCRI.ORG

HOMETOWN HEALTH NETWORK

OHIO CLAIMS OFFICE
100 LILLIAN GISH BLVD, STE 301
MASSILLON, OH 44647
TEL: (330) 837-6880
FAX: (330) 837-6869
IN-STATE: (800) 426-9013
WWW.HOMETOWNHEALTHNET.COM

HOMETOWN HEALTH PLAN

NEVADA CLAIMS OFFICE
400 S WELLS AVE
RENO, NV 89502-1823
TEL: (775) 325-3000
FAX: (775) 982-3160
TOLL FREE: (800) 336-0123
IN-STATE: (800) 336-0123
WWW.WASHOEHEALTH.COM

HUMANA

WISCONSIN CLAIMS OFFICE
PO BOX 12359
MILWAUKEE, WI 53212-0359
TEL: (414) 223-3300
FAX: (414) 223-7777
TOLL FREE: (800) 289-0260
WWW.HUMANA.COM

HUMANA HEALTH CARE PLAN, INC

KENTUCKY CLAIMS OFFICE
500 W MAIN
LOUISVILLE, KY 40202
TEL: (502) 580-5251
FAX: (502) 580-3127
TOLL FREE: (800) 448-6262
WWW.HUMANA.COM

HUMANA, INC

ALABAMA CLAIMS OFFICE
500 W MAIN ST
LOUISVILLE, KY 40202-1438
TEL: (502) 580-1000
FAX: (502) 580-3127
TOLL FREE: (800) 448-6262
IN-STATE: (800) 486-2620
WWW.HUMANA.COM

ARIZONA CLAIMS OFFICE
500 W MAIN ST
LOUISVILLE, KY 40202-1438
TEL: (502) 580-1000
FAX: (502) 580-3127
TOLL FREE: (800) 448-6262
IN-STATE: (800) 486-2620
WWW.HUMANA.COM

CALIFORNIA CLAIMS OFFICE
500 W MAIN ST
LOUISVILLE, KY 40202-1438
TEL: (502) 580-1000
FAX: (502) 580-3127
TOLL FREE: (800) 448-6262
IN-STATE: (800) 486-2620
WWW.HUMANA.COM

COLORADO CLAIMS OFFICE
500 W MAIN ST
LOUISVILLE, KY 40202-1438
TEL: (502) 580-1000
FAX: (502) 580-3127
TOLL FREE: (800) 448-6262
IN-STATE: (800) 486-2620
WWW.HUMANA.COM

DISTRICT OF COLUMBIA CLAIMS OFFICE
500 W MAIN ST
LOUISVILLE, KY 40202-1438
TEL: (502) 580-1000
FAX: (502) 580-3127
TOLL FREE: (800) 448-6262
IN-STATE: (800) 486-2620
WWW.HUMANA.COM

FLORIDA CLAIMS OFFICE
500 W MAIN ST
LOUISVILLE, KY 40202-1438
TEL: (502) 580-1000
FAX: (502) 580-3127
TOLL FREE: (800) 448-6262
IN-STATE: (800) 486-2620
WWW.HUMANA.COM

GEORGIA CLAIMS OFFICE
500 W MAIN ST
LOUISVILLE, KY 40202-1438
TEL: (502) 580-1000
FAX: (502) 580-3127
TOLL FREE: (800) 448-6262
IN-STATE: (800) 486-2620
WWW.HUMANA.COM

ILLINOIS CLAIMS OFFICE
500 W MAIN ST
LOUISVILLE, KY 40202-1438
TEL: (502) 580-1000
FAX: (502) 580-3127
TOLL FREE: (800) 448-6262
IN-STATE: (800) 486-2620
WWW.HUMANA.COM

INDIANA CLAIMS OFFICE
500 W MAIN ST
LOUISVILLE, KY 40202-1438
TEL: (502) 580-1000
FAX: (502) 580-3127
TOLL FREE: (800) 448-6262
IN-STATE: (800) 486-2620
WWW.HUMANA.COM

KANSAS CLAIMS OFFICE
500 W MAIN ST
LOUISVILLE, KY 40202-1438
TEL: (502) 580-1000
FAX: (502) 580-3127
TOLL FREE: (800) 448-6262
IN-STATE: (800) 486-2620
WWW.HUMANA.COM

KENTUCKY CLAIMS OFFICE
500 W MAIN ST
LOUISVILLE, KY 40202-1438
TEL: (502) 580-1000
FAX: (502) 580-3127
TOLL FREE: (800) 448-6262
IN-STATE: (800) 486-2620
WWW.HUMANA.COM

MARYLAND CLAIMS OFFICE
500 W MAIN ST
LOUISVILLE, KY 40202-1438
TEL: (502) 580-1000
FAX: (502) 580-3127
TOLL FREE: (800) 448-6262
IN-STATE: (800) 486-2620
WWW.HUMANA.COM

MICHIGAN CLAIMS OFFICE
500 W MAIN ST
LOUISVILLE, KY 40202-1438
TEL: (502) 580-1000
FAX: (502) 580-3127
TOLL FREE: (800) 448-6262
IN-STATE: (800) 486-2620
WWW.HUMANA.COM

MINNESOTA CLAIMS OFFICE
500 W MAIN ST
LOUISVILLE, KY 40202-1438
TEL: (502) 580-1000
FAX: (502) 580-3127
TOLL FREE: (800) 448-6262
IN-STATE: (800) 486-2620
WWW.HUMANA.COM

MISSOURI CLAIMS OFFICE
10450 HOLMES RD, STE 200
KANSAS CITY, MO 64131
TEL: (816) 941-8900
FAX: (816) 942-6782
WWW.HUMANA.COM

NEBRASKA CLAIMS OFFICE
500 W MAIN ST
LOUISVILLE, KY 40202-1438
TEL: (502) 580-1000
FAX: (502) 580-3127
TOLL FREE: (800) 448-6262
IN-STATE: (800) 486-2620
WWW.HUMANA.COM

NORTH CAROLINA CLAIMS OFFICE
500 W MAIN ST
LOUISVILLE, KY 40202-1438
TEL: (502) 580-1000
FAX: (502) 580-3127
TOLL FREE: (800) 448-6262
IN-STATE: (800) 486-2620
WWW.HUMANA.COM

OHIO CLAIMS OFFICE
500 W MAIN ST
LOUISVILLE, KY 40202-1438
TEL: (502) 580-1000
FAX: (502) 580-3127
TOLL FREE: (800) 448-6262
IN-STATE: (800) 486-2620
WWW.HUMANA.COM

TENNESSEE CLAIMS OFFICE
500 W MAIN ST
LOUISVILLE, KY 40202-1438
TEL: (502) 580-1000
FAX: (502) 580-3127
TOLL FREE: (800) 448-6262
IN-STATE: (800) 486-2620
WWW.HUMANA.COM

TEXAS CLAIMS OFFICE
500 W MAIN ST
LOUISVILLE, KY 40202-1438
TEL: (502) 580-1000
FAX: (502) 580-3127
TOLL FREE: (800) 448-6262
IN-STATE: (800) 486-2620
WWW.HUMANA.COM

VIRGINIA CLAIMS OFFICE
500 W MAIN ST
LOUISVILLE, KY 40202-1438
TEL: (502) 580-1000
FAX: (502) 580-3127
TOLL FREE: (800) 448-6262
IN-STATE: (800) 486-2620
WWW.HUMANA.COM

WISCONSIN CLAIMS OFFICE
500 W MAIN ST
LOUISVILLE, KY 40202-1438
TEL: (502) 580-1000
FAX: (502) 580-3127
TOLL FREE: (800) 448-6262
IN-STATE: (800) 486-2620
WWW.HUMANA.COM

HUMANA/ WISCONSIN HEALTH ORGANIZATION

111 W PLEASANT ST
MILWAUKEE, WI 53212
TEL: (414) 223-3300
TOLL FREE: (800) 289-0906
IN-STATE: (800) 777-0184

IDAHO FARM BUREAU MUTUAL INSURANCE CO

IDAHO CLAIMS OFFICE
435 LINCOLN
PO BOX 239
AMERICAN FALLS, ID 83211-0239
TEL: (208) 226-5066
FAX: (208) 226-7929

225 W GRAND
PO BOX 824
ARCO, ID 83213-0824
TEL: (208) 527-3431
FAX: (208) 527-3432

WESTERN COMMUNITY INSURANCE CO
124 N OAK
PO BOX 668
BLACKFOOT, ID 83221-0668
TEL: (208) 785-2410
FAX: (208) 785-2422

6426 KOOTENAI ST
PO BOX 1387
BONNERS FERRY, ID 83805-1387
TEL: (208) 267-5502
FAX: (208) 267-5503

6912 N GOVERNMENT WY
DALTON GARDENS, ID 83815-8747
TEL: (208) 772-6662
FAX: (208) 772-2553

906 S WASHINGTON
PO BOX 156
EMMETT, ID 83617-0156
TEL: (208) 365-5382
FAX: (208) 365-2465

131 3RD AVE E
GOODING, ID 83330-1101
TEL: (208) 934-8405
FAX: (208) 934-8406

711 N MAIN
PO BOX 609
HAILEY, ID 83333-0609
TEL: (208) 788-3529
FAX: (208) 788-3619

118 W IDAHO
PO BOX 1197
HOMEDALE, ID 83620-1197
TEL: (208) 337-4041
FAX: (208) 337-4042

BONNEVILLE COUNTY FARM BUREAU
956 LINCOLN
PO BOX 2948
IDAHO FALLS, ID 83403-2948
TEL: (208) 522-2652
FAX: (208) 522-2675

200 E AVE A
PO BOX C
JEROME, ID 83338-0326
TEL: (208) 324-4378
FAX: (208) 324-4393

2007 14TH AVE
LEWISTON, ID 83501-3019
TEL: (208) 743-5533
FAX: (208) 743-5535

34 N MAIN
MALAD, ID 83252-1247
TEL: (208) 766-2259
FAX: (208) 766-4211

470 WASHINGTON ST
MONTPELIER, ID 83254-1545
TEL: (208) 847-0851
FAX: (208) 847-0856

140 E 2ND N
PO BOX 673
MOUNTAIN HOME, ID 83647-0673
TEL: (208) 587-8484
FAX: (208) 587-8121

1501 26TH ST, STE C
OROFINO, ID 83544
TEL: (208) 476-4722
FAX: (208) 476-7348

235 N MAIN
PAYETTE, ID 83661-2852
TEL: (208) 642-4414
FAX: (208) 642-4415

200 W ALAMEDA
PO BOX 4848
POCATELLO, ID 83205
TEL: (208) 233-9442
FAX: (208) 233-4167

112 CENTER ST
PO BOX 1924
SALMON, ID 83467-1924
TEL: (208) 756-3335
FAX: (208) 756-3357

325 E MAIN
PO BOX 528
SAINT ANTHONY, ID 83445-0528
TEL: (208) 624-3171
FAX: (208) 624-3173

414 MAIN AVE
SAINT MARIES, ID 83861-2059
TEL: (208) 245-5568
FAX: (208) 245-5569

435 LINCOLN
PO BOX 239
AMERICAN FALLS, ID 83211-0239
TEL: (208) 226-5066
FAX: (208) 226-7929

225 W GRAND
PO BOX 824
ARCO, ID 83213-0824
TEL: (208) 527-3431
FAX: (208) 527-3432

IHC HEALTH PLANS

INTERMOUNTAIN HEALTH CARE
4646 W LAKE PARK BLVD
SALT LAKE CITY, UT 84120-8212
TEL: (801) 442-5000
FAX: (801) 442-5003
TOLL FREE: (800) 538-5038
IN-STATE: (800) 442-5038
E-MAIL: WEBMASTER@IHC.COM
WWW.IHC.COM

UTAH CLAIMS OFFICE
INTERMOUNTAIN HEALTH CARE
4646 W LAKE PARK BLVD
SALT LAKE CITY, UT 84120-8212
TEL: (801) 442-5000
FAX: (801) 442-5003
TOLL FREE: (800) 538-5038
IN-STATE: (800) 442-5038
E-MAIL: WEBMASTER@IHC.COM
WWW.IHC.COM

INTERMOUNTAIN HEALTH CARE
4646 W LAKE PARK BLVD
PO BOX 30192
SALT LAKE CITY, UT 84130-0192
TEL: (801) 442-5000
FAX: (801) 442-5752
TOLL FREE: (800) 442-5038
IN-STATE: (800) 442-5038

WYOMING CLAIMS OFFICE
INTERMOUNTAIN HEALTH CARE
4646 W LAKE PARK BLVD
SALT LAKE CITY, UT 84120-8212
TEL: (801) 442-5000
FAX: (801) 442-5003
TOLL FREE: (800) 538-5038
IN-STATE: (800) 442-5038
E-MAIL: WEBMASTER@IHC.COM
WWW.IHC.COM

ILLINOIS MASONIC COMMUNITY HEALTH PLAN

ILLINOIS CLAIMS OFFICE
836 W WELLINGTON
CHICAGO, IL 60657-5147
TEL: (773) 296-7167
FAX: (773) 296-5598

INSURANCE CO OF THE WEST

CALIFORNIA CLAIMS OFFICE
ICW GROUP
11455 EL CAMINO REAL
PO BOX 85563
SAN DIEGO, CA 92186-5563
TEL: (619) 350-2400
FAX: (619) 350-2543
TOLL FREE: (800) 877-1111

INSURANCE MANAGEMENT ADMINISTRATORS OF LOUISIANA

LOUISIANA CLAIMS OFFICE
1325 BARKSDALE BLVD, STE 300
PO BOX 71120
BOSSIER, LA 71171
TEL: (318) 868-0600
FAX: (318) 747-5074

INSURANCE MANAGEMENT ASSOCIATES, INC

KANSAS CLAIMS OFFICE
250 N WATER ST, STE 600
PO BOX 2992
WICHITA, KS 67201
TEL: (316) 267-9221
FAX: (316) 266-6385
TOLL FREE: (800) 288-6732
WWW.IMACORP.COM

INSURANCE & PERSONNEL SERVICES

NEBRASKA CLAIMS OFFICE
2121 N WEBB RD
PO BOX 2160
GRAND ISLAND, NE 68802-2160
TEL: (308) 384-8700
FAX: (308) 384-8423

INSURERS ADMINISTRATIVE CORP

ARIZONA CLAIMS OFFICE
2101 W PEORIA AVE, STE 100
PO BOX 39119
PHOENIX, AZ 85029-9119
TEL: (602) 870-1400
FAX: (602) 395-0496
TOLL FREE: (800) 843-3106

INSUREX BENEFITS ADMINISTRATORS

TENNESSEE CLAIMS OFFICE
1835 UNION AVE, STE 400
PO BOX 41779
MEMPHIS, TN 38174-1779
TEL: (901) 725-6435
FAX: (901) 725-6437

INTEGON CORP

NORTH CAROLINA CLAIMS OFFICE
P & C CLAIMS
500 W 5TH ST
PO BOX 3199
WINSTON-SALEM, NC 27102-3199
TEL: (336) 770-2000
FAX: (336) 770-2122
TOLL FREE: (800) 642-0506
WWW.INTEGON.COM

INTEGRATED HEALTH SERVICES

NEW MEXICO CLAIMS OFFICE
SOUTHWEST EMPLOYEE BENEFITS
235 ELM ST NE
PO BOX 30278
ALBUQUERQUE, NM 87190
TEL: (505) 222-8260

INTER VALLEY HEALTH PLAN

CALIFORNIA CLAIMS OFFICE
300 S PARK AVE
PO BOX 6002
POMONA, CA 91769-6002
TEL: (909) 623-6333
FAX: (909) 622-2907
TOLL FREE: (800) 251-8191
WWW.IVHP.COM

INTERACTIVE MEDICAL SYSTEMS, INC

NORTH CAROLINA CLAIMS OFFICE
4505 FALLS OF NEUSE, STE 550
PO BOX 19108
RALEIGH, NC 27619
TEL: (919) 877-9933
FAX: (919) 846-8887

SOUTH CAROLINA CLAIMS OFFICE
4505 FALLS OF NEUSE, STE 550
PO BOX 19108
RALEIGH, NC 27619
TEL: (919) 877-9933
FAX: (919) 846-8887

INTERCARE BENEFIT SYSTEMS, INC

COLORADO CLAIMS OFFICE
INTERCARE HEALTH PLAN
5500 GREENWOOD PLZ BLVD
PO BOX 3559
ENGLEWOOD, CO 80111-3559
TEL: (303) 770-5710
FAX: (303) 770-2743
TOLL FREE: (800) 426-7453

INTERCONTINENTAL CORP

INDIANA CLAIMS OFFICE
135 N PENNSYLVANIA ST, STE 770
INDIANAPOLIS, IN 46204
TEL: (317) 238-5700
FAX: (317) 637-6634
TOLL FREE: (800) 962-6831
WWW.INTERCONTINENTALCORP.COM

INTERGROUP OF ARIZONA

ARIZONA CLAIMS OFFICE
930 N FINANCE CTR DR
TUCSON, AZ 85710
TEL: (520) 751-6111
FAX: (520) 290-5176
TOLL FREE: (800) 289-2818

INTERGROUP OF UTAH, INC

UTAH CLAIMS OFFICE
127 S 500 E
SALT LAKE CITY, UT 84102
TEL: (801) 532-7665

INTERMOUNTAIN ADMINISTRATORS, INC

MONTANA CLAIMS OFFICE
2806 GARFIELD
PO BOX 3018
MISSOULA, MT 59806
TEL: (406) 721-2222
FAX: (406) 721-2252
TOLL FREE: (800) 877-1122
WWW.IAI-TPA.COM

J.P. FARLEY CORP

NATIONAL CLAIMS OFFICE
22021 BROOKPARK RD, STE 100
PO BOX 268000
CLEVELAND, OH 44126-8000
TEL: (440) 734-6800
FAX: (440) 734-1668
TOLL FREE: (800) 634-0173
E-MAIL: BENEFITS@JPFARLEY.COM
WWW.JPFARLEY.COM

JARDINE GROUP SERVICES CORP

13 CORNELL RD
LATHAM, NY 12110
TEL: (518) 782-3000
FAX: (518) 782-3157
TOLL FREE: (800) 366-5273
WWW.JGSC.COM

JEFFERSON LIFE INSURANCE CO

TEXAS CLAIMS OFFICE
9304 FOREST LN N, STE 256
PO BOX 749008
DALLAS, TX 75374-9008
TEL: (214) 340-8995
FAX: (214) 340-6114
TOLL FREE: (800) 343-5542

JEFFERSON-PILOT LIFE INSURANCE CO

NORTH CAROLINA CLAIMS OFFICE
JEFFERSON-PILOT FINANCIAL
100 N GREEN ST
PO BOX 21008
GREENSBORO, NC 27420-1008
TEL: (336) 691-3000
FAX: (336) 691-4500
TOLL FREE: (800) 458-1419
IN-STATE: (800) 792-2268

JENSEN ADMINISTRATIVE SERVICES

ARIZONA CLAIMS OFFICE
4885 S 9TH E, STE 202
SALT LAKE CITY, UT 84117-5725
TEL: (801) 266-3256
FAX: (801) 266-4383
TOLL FREE: (800) 345-3248

IDAHO CLAIMS OFFICE
4885 S 9TH E, STE 202
SALT LAKE CITY, UT 84117-5725
TEL: (801) 266-3256
FAX: (801) 266-4383
TOLL FREE: (800) 345-3248

NEVADA CLAIMS OFFICE
4885 S 9TH E, STE 202
SALT LAKE CITY, UT 84117-5725
TEL: (801) 266-3256
FAX: (801) 266-4383
TOLL FREE: (800) 345-3248

UTAH CLAIMS OFFICE
4885 S 9TH E, STE 202
SALT LAKE CITY, UT 84117-5725
TEL: (801) 266-3256
FAX: (801) 266-4383
TOLL FREE: (800) 345-3248

JFP BENEFIT MANAGEMENT

MICHIGAN CLAIMS OFFICE
100 S JACKSON ST, STE 200
PO BOX 189
JACKSON, MI 49201
TEL: (517) 784-0535
FAX: (517) 784-0821
IN-STATE: (800) 589-7660
E-MAIL: DPELHAM@IBM.NET

JM FAMILY ENTERPRISES

FLORIDA CLAIMS OFFICE
8019 BAYBERRY RD
JACKSONVILLE, FL 32256-7411
TEL: (904) 443-6650
FAX: (904) 443-6670
TOLL FREE: (800) 736-3936

KAISER PERMANENTE

HAWAII CLAIMS OFFICE
711 KAPIOLANI BLVD
PO BOX 31000
HONOLULU, HI 96849-5086
TEL: (808) 597-5340
FAX: (808) 597-5300
TOLL FREE: (800) 596-5955
IN-STATE: (800) 596-5955
WWW.KAISERPERMANENTE.ORG

NATIONAL CLAIMS OFFICE
PO BOX 40669
RALEIGH, NC 27629
TEL: (919) 981-6000
FAX: (919) 981-6052
TOLL FREE: (800) 221-5347
WWW.KAISERPERMANENTE.ORG

OREGON CLAIMS OFFICE
500 NE MULTNOMAH, STE 100
PORTLAND, OR 97232-2099
TEL: (503) 813-2800
FAX: (503) 813-2710
TOLL FREE: (800) 813-2000
WWW.KAISERPERMANENTE.ORG

KEENAN & ASSOCIATES

CALIFORNIA CLAIMS OFFICE
2105 S BASCOM AVE, STE 310
CAMPBELL, CA 95008-3271
TEL: (408) 377-3338
FAX: (408) 371-1796
TOLL FREE: (800) 334-6554
WWW.KEENANASSOCIATES.COM

3610 CENTRAL, STE 400
RIVERSIDE, CA 92506-2405
TEL: (909) 788-0330
FAX: (909) 788-8013
TOLL FREE: (800) 654-8347

KENTUCKY FARM BUREAU MUTUAL INSURANCE CO

KENTUCKY CLAIMS OFFICE
2909 RING RD
PO BOX 958
ELIZABETHTOWN, KY 42702-0958
TEL: (270) 765-4400
FAX: (270) 765-7756
TOLL FREE: (800) 782-3811

3036 PARRISH AVE
PO BOX 21369
OWENSBORO, KY 42304-1369
TEL: (502) 684-2165
FAX: (502) 684-4019
TOLL FREE: (800) 538-8655

KEYSTONE MERCY HEALTH PLAN

PENNSYLVANIA CLAIMS OFFICE
CLAIMS PROCESSING CTR
200 STEVENS DR
LESTER, PA 19113-1570
TEL: (215) 937-7300
FAX: (215) 937-5300
IN-STATE: (800) 521-6007

KITSAP PHYSICIANS SERVICE

WASHINGTON CLAIMS OFFICE
400 WARREN AVE
PO BOX 339
BREMERTON, WA 98337
TEL: (360) 377-5576
FAX: (360) 415-6514
TOLL FREE: (800) 552-7114

KLAIS & CO

OHIO CLAIMS OFFICE
1867 W MARKET ST
AKRON, OH 44313
TEL: (330) 867-8443
FAX: (330) 867-0827
TOLL FREE: (800) 331-1096

LANCER CLAIM SERVICE CORP

CALIFORNIA CLAIMS OFFICE
333 CITY BLVD W
PO BOX 7048
ORANGE, CA 92863
TEL: (714) 939-0700
FAX: (714) 978-8023
TOLL FREE: (800) 821-0540
IN-STATE: (800) 645-5324

LANDMARK HEALTH CARE

1750 HOWE AVE, STE 300
SACRAMENTO, CA 95825
TEL: (916) 646-3477
FAX: (916) 929-8350
TOLL FREE: (800) 638-4557
WWW.LANDMARKHEALTHCARE.COM

LEWER AGENCY, INC

NATIONAL CLAIMS OFFICE
4534 WORNALL RD
KANSAS CITY, MO 64111-3211
TEL: (816) 753-4390
FAX: (816) 561-6840
TOLL FREE: (800) 821-7715
WWW.LEWER.COM

LIFE INSURANCE CO OF GEORGIA

ALABAMA CLAIMS OFFICE
ADMINISTRATIVE OFFICES
4850 STREET RD
PO BOX 3013
LANGHORNE, PA 19047-9113
TOLL FREE: (800) 877-7756

LOCALS 302 & 612 INTERNATIONAL

WASHINGTON CLAIMS OFFICE
WELFARE & PENSION ADMIN SERV
2815 SECOND AVE #300
PO BOX 34684
SEATTLE, WA 98124-1203
TEL: (206) 441-7574
FAX: (206) 441-9110
TOLL FREE: (800) 331-6158
IN-STATE: (800)732-1121
WWW.WPAS-INC.COM

LOMA LINDA UNIVERSITY ADVENTIST HEALTH SCIENCES CENTER

CALIFORNIA CLAIMS OFFICE
11161 ANDERSON ST, STE 200
PO BOX 1770
LOMA LINDA, CA 92354-0570
TEL: (909) 824-4386
FAX: (909) 824-4775

M-PLAN

INDIANA CLAIMS OFFICE
8802 N MERIDIAN ST, STE 100
INDIANAPOLIS, IN 46260-5318
TEL: (317) 571-5300
FAX: (317) 705-3119
TOLL FREE: (800) 878-8802

MANAGED HEALTH, INC

NEW YORK CLAIMS OFFICE
25 BROADWAY, STE 900
NEW YORK, NY 10004
FAX: (212) 801-1799
TOLL FREE: (888) 260-1010

MASSACHUSETTS MUTUAL LIFE INSURANCE CO

MASSACHUSETTS CLAIMS OFFICE
UNICARE LIFE AND HEALTH
1350 MAIN ST
PO BOX 51130
SPRINGFIELD, MA 01151-5130
TOLL FREE: (800) 288-8630

MAYO HEALTH PLAN

MINNESOTA CLAIMS OFFICE
MAYO MANAGEMENT SERVICES, INC
21 1ST ST SW, STE 401
ROCHESTER, MN 55902
TEL: (507) 284-8274
FAX: (507) 284-0528
TOLL FREE: (800) 635-6671

MED-PAY, INC

MISSOURI CLAIMS OFFICE
1650 E BATTLEFIELD, STE 300
PO BOX 10909
SPRINGFIELD, MO 65808
TEL: (417) 886-6886
FAX: (417) 886-2276
TOLL FREE: (800) 777-9087

MEDICAID FISCAL AGENTS

ALABAMA CLAIMS OFFICE
1460 ANN ST
MONTGOMERY, AL 36107
TEL: (334) 834-3330
FAX: (334) 834-5301
IN-STATE: (800) 688-7989

ARIZONA CLAIMS OFFICE
AHCCCS ADMINISTRATION
701 E JEFFERSON
PO BOX 25520
PHOENIX, AZ 85002-9949
TEL: (602) 417-4000
FAX: (602) 253-5472
TOLL FREE: (800) 523-0231
WWW.AHCCCS.STATE.AZ.US

ARKANSAS CLAIMS OFFICE
EDS FEDERAL CORP
PO BOX 8036
LITTLE ROCK, AR 72203-2501
TEL: (501) 374-6608
FAX: (501) 374-0549
IN-STATE: (800) 457-4454
WWW.MEDICAID.STATE.AR.US.COM

COLORADO CLAIMS OFFICE
HEALTHCARE FINANCE & POLICY
700 BROADWAY
PO BOX 173300
DENVER, CO 80217-3300
TEL: (303) 831-0504
TOLL FREE: (800) 443-5747
IN-STATE: (800) 443-5747

CONNECTICUT CLAIMS OFFICE
EDS FEDERAL CORP
PO BOX 2941
HARTFORD, CT 06104-2941
TEL: (860) 832-9259
IN-STATE: (800) 842-8440

DELAWARE CLAIMS OFFICE
EDS
MANOR BRANCH
PO BOX 908
NEW CASTLE, DE 19720
TEL: (302) 454-7154
FAX: (302) 454-7603
IN-STATE: (800) 999-3371

ILLINOIS CLAIMS OFFICE
DEPARTMENT OF PUBLIC AID
201 S GRAND AVE E- PRESCOTT BLOOM BLDG
PO BOX 19105
SPRINGFIELD, IL 62794-9105
TEL: (217) 782-5567
FAX: (217) 524-7194

KANSAS CLAIMS OFFICE
EDS FEDERAL CORP
PO BOX 3571
TOPEKA, KS 66601
TOLL FREE: (800) 933-6593

KENTUCKY CLAIMS OFFICE
DEPT FOR MEDICAID SERVICES
275 E MAIN ST
FRANKFORT, KY 40621-0001
TEL: (502) 564-4321

LOUISIANA CLAIMS OFFICE
UNISYS CORP
8591 UNITED PLZ BLVD
PO BOX 91024
BATON ROUGE, LA 70821-9024
TEL: (504) 237-3200
TOLL FREE: (800) 473-2783

MAINE CLAIMS OFFICE
MEDICAL ASSISTANCE CLAIMS PROCESSING M500
BUREAU OF MED SVCS- 249 WESTERN AVE
AUGUSTA, ME 04333-0001
TEL: (207) 287-3081
IN-STATE: (800) 321-5557

MARYLAND CLAIMS OFFICE
201 W PRESTON ST, RM L9
PO BOX 1935
BALTIMORE, MD 21203
TEL: (410) 767-5503
FAX: (410) 333-7118
TOLL FREE: (800) 445-1159

MASSACHUSETTS CLAIMS OFFICE
UNISYS CORP
5 MIDDLESEX AVE
PO BOX 9101
SOMMERVILLE, MA 02145-9101
TEL: (617) 625-0120
FAX: (617) 576-4087
TOLL FREE: (800) 325-5231

MINNESOTA CLAIMS OFFICE
DEPT OF HUMAN SERVICES
444 LAFAYETTE
PO BOX 3849
SAINT PAUL, MN 55155-3849
TEL: (612) 296-3598
FAX: (612) 282-6744
TOLL FREE: (800) 366-5411

MISSISSIPPI CLAIMS OFFICE
EDS FEDERAL CORP
111 E CAPITOL ST, STE 400
PO BOX 23077
JACKSON, MS 39225-3077
TEL: (601) 960-2800
FAX: (601) 960-2807
TOLL FREE: (800) 884-3222

MISSOURI CLAIMS OFFICE
MISSOURI MEDICAID
PO BOX 5600
JEFFERSON CITY, MO 65102
TEL: (573) 751-2896
TOLL FREE: (800) 392-0938

MONTANA CLAIMS OFFICE
CONSULTEC, INC
PO BOX 8000
HELENA, MT 59604-8000
TEL: (406) 442-1837
FAX: (406) 442-4402
IN-STATE: (800) 624-3958
E-MAIL: CONSULTEC-IIX.COM/

NEBRASKA CLAIMS OFFICE
NEBRASKA DEPT OF HEALTH & HUMAN SVCS
PO BOX 95026
LINCOLN, NE 68509-5026
TEL: (402) 471-9147
FAX: (402) 471-9092
TOLL FREE: (800) 430-3244

NEW HAMPSHIRE CLAIMS OFFICE
EDS FEDERAL CORP
7 EAGLE SQ
PO BOX 2001
CONCORD, NH 03302-2001
TEL: (603) 224-1747
FAX: (603) 225-7964
IN-STATE: (800) 423-8303

NEW JERSEY CLAIMS OFFICE
UNISYS CORP
3705 QUAKERBRIDGE RD, STE 101
TRENTON, NJ 08619-1209
TEL: (609) 584-0200
FAX: (609) 584-8270
TOLL FREE: (800) 776-6334

NEW MEXICO CLAIMS OFFICE
CONSULTEC, I NC
1720 RANDOLPH RD, STE A
PO BOX 25700
ALBUQUERQUE, NM 87125
TEL: (505) 246-9988
FAX: (505) 246-8485
IN-STATE: (800) 282-4477

NORTH CAROLINA CLAIMS OFFICE
EDS FEDERAL CORP OF NORTH CAROLINA
4905 WATEREDGE DR
RALEIGH, NC 27606
TEL: (919) 851-8888
FAX: (919) 851-4014
TOLL FREE: (800) 688-6696

NORTH DAKOTA CLAIMS OFFICE
DEPT OF HUMAN SERVICES, MEDICAL SERVICES
600 E BLVD AVE
BISMARCK, ND 58505-0261
TEL: (701) 328-2321
FAX: (701) 328-1544
TOLL FREE: (800) 755-2604

OKLAHOMA CLAIMS OFFICE
UNISYS CORP
201 NW 63RD, STE 100
OKLAHOMA CITY, OK 73116
TEL: (405) 841-3400
FAX: (405) 841-3510

PENNSYLVANIA CLAIMS OFFICE
DEPT OF PUBLIC WELFARE
PO BOX 2675
HARRISBURG, PA 17105-2675
TEL: (717) 787-1870
FAX: (717) 787-4639
TOLL FREE: (800) 537-8862

RHODE ISLAND CLAIMS OFFICE
STATE OF RHODE ISLAND MEDICAL SERVICES
600 NEW LONDON AVE
CRANSTON, RI 02920-3037
TEL: (401) 464-3575

SOUTH DAKOTA CLAIMS OFFICE
DEPT OF SOCIAL SERVICES- OFFICE OF MEDICAL SERVICES
700 GOVERNORS DR- KNIEP BLDG
PIERRE, SD 57501-2291
TEL: (605) 945-5006
FAX: (605) 773-5246
IN-STATE: (800) 452-7691

UTAH CLAIMS OFFICE
UTAH STATE DEPT MEDICAID PROCESSING
PO BOX 143106
SALT LAKE CITY, UT 84114-3106
TEL: (801) 538-6451
FAX: (801) 538-6952
TOLL FREE: (800) 662-9651
IN-STATE: (800) 662-9651

VIRGINIA CLAIMS OFFICE
FIRST HEALTH SERVICES CORP
4300 COX RD
PO BOX 3900
GLEN ALLEN, VA 23060
TEL: (804) 965-7400
FAX: (804) 965-7416
TOLL FREE: (800) 884-2822
IN-STATE: (800) 884-2822
WWW.FHSC.COM

WASHINGTON CLAIMS OFFICE
DEPT OF SOCIAL & HEALTH SERVICES
5000 CAPITAL BLVD
PO BOX 45080
DUMWATER, WA 98501
TEL: (360) 753-1777
FAX: (360) 586-6787
TOLL FREE: (800) 562-3022
IN-STATE: (800) 321-6787

MEDICAL MUTUAL OF OHIO

OHIO CLAIMS OFFICE
PO BOX 6018
CLEVELAND, OH 44101-1355
TEL: (216) 522-8622
FAX: (216) 694-2910
TOLL FREE: (800) 233-2058

MEDICARE PART A

WYOMING CLAIMS OFFICE
PO BOX 908
CHEYENNE, WY 82003
TEL: (307) 432-2860
FAX: (307) 632-1654
IN-STATE: (800) 442-2376

MEDICARE — PART A HORIZON BLUE CROSS BLUE SHIELD OF NEW JERSEY

NEW JERSEY CLAIMS OFFICE
33 WASHINGTON ST
PO BOX 1236
NEWARK, NJ 07101-1236
TEL: (973) 456-2112
FAX: (973) 456-2086

MEDICARE — PART A INTERMEDIARIES

ARIZONA CLAIMS OFFICE
BLUE CROSS & BLUE SHIELD OF ARIZONA, INC
2444 W LAS PAMARITAS DR
PO BOX 13466
PHOENIX, AZ 85002-3466
TEL: (602) 864-4100
FAX: (602) 864-4653
WWW.BCBSAZ.COM

ARKANSAS CLAIMS OFFICE
ARKANSAS BLUE CROSS & BLUE SHIELD
601 GAINES ST
PO BOX 2181
LITTLE ROCK, AR 72203-2181
TEL: (501) 378-2000
FAX: (501) 378-2576
TOLL FREE: (800) 813-8868

CALIFORNIA CLAIMS OFFICE
BLUE CROSS OF CALIFORNIA (WELLPOINT HEALTH NETWORKS)
21555 OXNARD ST
PO BOX 70000
VAN NUYS, CA 91470
TEL: (818) 703-2345
FAX: (818) 703-2848
TOLL FREE: (800) 234-0111
WWW.BLUECROSSCA.COM

DELAWARE CLAIMS OFFICE
MEDICAL SERVICES ASSOCIATION OF PENNSYLVANIA
1800 CENTER ST
PO BOX 890089
CAMP HILL, PA 17089-0089
TEL: (717) 763-3151
FAX: (717) 763-3544

DISTRICT OF COLUMBIA CLAIMS OFFICE
MEDICAL SERVICES ASSOCIATION OF PENNSYLVANIA
1800 CENTER ST
PO BOX 890089
CAMP HILL, PA 17089-0089
TEL: (717) 763-3151
FAX: (717) 763-3544

GEORGIA CLAIMS OFFICE
BLUE CROSS & BLUE SHIELD OF GEORGIA, INC
2357 WARM SPGS RD
PO BOX 9048
COLUMBUS, GA 31908-9048
TEL: (706) 571-5371
FAX: (706) 571-5431

INDIANA CLAIMS OFFICE
ADMINISTER FEDERAL, INC
8115 KNUE RD
INDIANAPOLIS, IN 46250-2804
TEL: (317) 841-4400
FAX: (317) 841-4691
TOLL FREE: (800) 999-7608

IOWA CLAIMS OFFICE
WELLMARK BLUE CROSS & BLUE SHIELD OF IOWA
636 GRAND AVE
STATION 120
DES MOINES, IA 50309
TEL: (515) 245-4834
FAX: (515) 245-3984
WWW.WELLMEDICARE.COM

KANSAS CLAIMS OFFICE
SEE BLUE CROSS & BLUE SHEILD OF KANSAS
133 S TOPEKA
TOPEKA, KS 66601-1712
TEL: (785) 291-7000
FAX: (785) 291-6924

KENTUCKY CLAIMS OFFICE
ADMINASTAR FEDERAL - KENTUCKY
9901 LINN STATION RD
PO BOX 23711
LOUISVILLE, KY 40223-0711
TEL: (502) 425-7776
FAX: (502) 329-8559

LOUISIANA CLAIMS OFFICE
SOCIAL SECURITY
346 HOLMER RD
MENDON, LA 71055
TEL: (318) 377-7387
TOLL FREE: (800) 772-1213

MAINE CLAIMS OFFICE
ASSOC HOSP SVC OF MAINE- DBA BLUE CROSS & BLUE SHIELD OF MAINE
2 GANNETT DR
SOUTH PORTLAND, ME 04106-6911
TEL: (207) 822-8484
FAX: (207) 822-7926
TOLL FREE: (888) 896-4997
E-MAIL: MEDICARE@BCBSME.COM
WWW.AHSMEDICARE.COM

MASSACHUSETTS CLAIMS OFFICE
ASSOC HOSP SVC OF MAINE- DBA BLUE CROSS & BLUE SHIELD OF MAINE
2 GANNETT DR
SOUTH PORTLAND, ME 04106-6911
TEL: (207) 822-8484
FAX: (207) 822-7926
TOLL FREE: (888) 896-4997
E-MAIL: MEDICARE@BCBSME.COM
WWW.AHSMEDICARE.COM

MINNESOTA CLAIMS OFFICE
BLUE CROSS & BLUE SHIELD OF MINNESOTA
PO BOX 64357
SAINT PAUL, MN 55164-0357
TEL: (651) 662-8000
FAX: (651) 662-2745
TOLL FREE: (800) 382-2000

METRAHEALTH INSURANCE CO
450 COLOUMBUS BLVD - 5GB
PO BOX 150450
HARTFORD, CT 06115-0450
TEL: (860) 702-6668
FAX: (860) 702-6587

NORIDIAN MUTUAL INSURANCE CO
4305 13TH AVE SW
FARGO, ND 58103-3309
TEL: (701) 277-2655
FAX: (701) 277-2196

MISSISSIPPI CLAIMS OFFICE
BLUE CROSS & BLUE SHIELD OF MISSISSIPPI, INC
1064 FLINT DR
PO BOX 23035
JACKSON, MS
TEL: (601) 936-0105
FAX: (601) 932-9233

METRAHEALTH INSURANCE CO
450 COLOUMBUS BLVD - 5GB
PO BOX 150450
HARTFORD, CT 06115-0450
TEL: (860) 702-6669
FAX: (860) 702-6587

MISSOURI CLAIMS OFFICE
SEE BLUE CROSS & BLUE SHEILD OF KANSAS
133 S TOPEKA
TOPEKA, KS 66601-1712
TEL: (785) 291-7000
FAX: (785) 291-6924

MONTANA CLAIMS OFFICE
BLUE CROSS & BLUE SHIELD OF MONTANA, INC
340 N LAST CHANCE GULCH
PO BOX 4309
HELENA, MT 59604
TEL: (406) 791-4000
FAX: (406) 791-4119
TOLL FREE: (800) 447-7828
WWW.BCBSMT.COM

NATIONAL CLAIMS OFFICE
FIRST COAST SERVICE OPTIONS, INC / BLUE CROSS & BLUE SHIELD OF FLORIDA, INC
532 RIVERSIDE AVENUE- 17TH & 18TH FLS
PO BOX 2711
JACKSONVILLE, FL 32231-0021
TEL: (904) 355-8899
FAX: (904) 791-8296
IN-STATE: (800) 333-7586

NEBRASKA CLAIMS OFFICE
BLUE CROSS & BLUE SHIELD OF NEBRASKA ALSO PROCESSED AT BLUE CROSS AND BLUE SHEILD OF KANSAS
7261 MERCY RD
PO BOX 24563
OMAHA, NE 68124-0563
TEL: (402) 390-1850
FAX: (402) 398-3640

NEW HAMPSHIRE CLAIMS OFFICE
NH- VT HEALTH SERVICE- DBA BLUE CROSS & BLUE SHIELD OF NEW HAMPSHIRE
3000 GOFF FALLS RD
MANCHESTER, NH 03111-0001
TEL: (603) 695-7204
FAX: (603) 695-7741

NEW HAMPSHIRE-VERMONT HEALTH SERVICES- DBA BCBS OF NEW HAMPSHIRE
3000 GOFFS FALLS RD
MANCHESTER, NH 03111-0001
TEL: (603) 695-7204
FAX: (603) 695-7741

NEW YORK CLAIMS OFFICE
BLUE CROSS & BLUE SHIELD OF WESTERN NEW YORK
1901 MAIN ST
PO BOX 80
BUFFALO, NY 14208
TEL: (716) 887-6900
FAX: (716) 887-8981
TOLL FREE: (800) 252-6550
IN-STATE: (800) 695-2583

EMPIRE BLUE CROSS AND BLUE SHIELD MEDICARE SERVICES
ONE WORLD TRADE CENTER
PO BOX 1407
NEW YORK, NY 10048
TEL: (212) 476-1000
TOLL FREE: (800) 442-8430

NORTH DAKOTA CLAIMS OFFICE
NORIDIAN MUTUAL INSURANCE CO
4305 13TH AVE SW
FARGO, ND 58103-3309
TEL: (701) 277-2655
FAX: (701) 277-2196

BLUE CROSS BLUE SHIELD OF NORTH DAKOTA
4510 13TH AVE SW
PO BOX 6706
FARGO, ND 58108-6706
TEL: (701) 277-1100
FAX: (701) 282-1002
TOLL FREE: (800) 874-2656
WWW.NORIDIAN.COM

OHIO CLAIMS OFFICE
ANTHEM- DBA COMMUNITY MUTUAL BLUE CROSS & BLUE SHIELD
4361 ERWIN SIMPSON RD
MASON, OH 45050
TEL: (513) 872-8100
FAX: (513) 852-4562

OKLAHOMA CLAIMS OFFICE
GROUP HEALTH SVC OF OK, INC- DBA BLUE CROSS & BLUE SHIELD OF OK
1215 S BOULDER AVE
PO BOX 3404
TULSA, OK 74101
TEL: (918) 560-2090
FAX: (918) 560-3506

PENNSYLVANIA CLAIMS OFFICE
MEDICAL SERVICES ASSOCIATION OF PENNSYLVANIA
1800 CENTER ST
PO BOX 890089
CAMP HILL, PA 17089-0089
TEL: (717) 763-3151
FAX: (717) 763-3544

RHODE ISLAND CLAIMS OFFICE
BLUE CROSS & BLUE SHIELD OF RHODE ISLAND
444 WESTMINSTER ST
PROVIDENCE, RI 02903
TEL: (401) 455-0177
FAX: (401) 459-1709
TOLL FREE: (800) 662-5170

TENNESSEE CLAIMS OFFICE
730 CHESTNUT ST
CHATTANOOGA, TN 37402-1790
TEL: (423) 755-5950

VERMONT CLAIMS OFFICE
NEW HAMPSHIRE-VERMONT HEALTH SERVICES- DBA BCBS OF NH
3000 GOFFS FALLS RD
MANCHESTER, NH 03111-0001
TEL: (603) 695-7204
FAX: (603) 695-7741

NH- VT HEALTH SERVICE- DBA BLUE CROSS & BLUE SHIELD OF NH
3000 GOFF FALLS RD
MANCHESTER, NH 03111-0001
TEL: (603) 695-7204
FAX: (603) 695-7741

WASHINGTON CLAIMS OFFICE
730 CHESTNUT ST
CHATTANOOGA, TN 37402-1790
TEL: (423) 755-5950

WEST VIRGINIA CLAIMS OFFICE
NATIONAL MUTUAL INSURANCE COMPANY
PO BOX 57
COLUMBUS, OH 43216-0057
TEL: (614) 249-7111
FAX: (614) 249-4467
IN-STATE: (800) 848-0106
WWW.NATIONWIDE-MEDICARE.COM

MEDICARE — PART B CARRIERS

ALABAMA CLAIMS OFFICE
BLUE CROSS & BLUE SHEILD OF ALABAMA
PO BOX 830140
BIRMINGHAM, AL 35283-0140
TEL: (205) 981-4842
FAX: (205) 981-4965
TOLL FREE: (800) 292-8855
WWW.BCBSAL.ORG

ARIZONA CLAIMS OFFICE
BLUE CROSS & BLUE SHIELD OF NORTH DAKOTA
4305 16TH AVE S
PO BOX 6704
FARGO, ND 58108-6704
TOLL FREE: (800) 444-4606
IN-STATE: (800) 332-6681

CALIFORNIA CLAIMS OFFICE
TRANSAMERICA OCCIDENTAL LIFE INSURANCE
1149 SOUTH BROADWAY
PO BOX 54905
LOS ANGELES, CA 90054-0905
TEL: (213) 748-2311
FAX: (213) 741-6803
TOLL FREE:
WWW.MEDICARE.TRANSAMERICA.COM

STATE OF CALIFORNIA NATIONAL HERITAGE INSURANCE CO - NORTHERN CALIFORNIA CLAIMS OFFICE
450 W EAST AVE
CHICO, CA 95926
TEL: (530) 896-7025
FAX: (530) 896-7182

COLORADO CLAIMS OFFICE
BLUE CROSS & BLUE SHIELD OF NORTH DAKOTA
4305 16TH AVE S
PO BOX 6028
FARGO, ND 58108-6028
TOLL FREE: (800) 444-4606
IN-STATE: (800) 332-6681

DISTRICT OF COLUMBIA CLAIMS OFFICE
PENNSYLVANIA BLUE SHIELD
1800 CENTER ST
PO BOX 890101
CAMP HILL, PA 17089-0101
TEL: (717) 731-2333

FLORIDA CLAIMS OFFICE
BLUE CROSS & BLUE SHIELD OF FLORIDA
532 RIVERSIDE AVE
PO BOX 2525
JACKSONVILLE, FL 32231-0019
TEL: (904) 634-4994
FAX: (904) 791-8378
IN-STATE: (800) 333-7586

HAWAII CLAIMS OFFICE
BLUE CROSS & BLUE SHIELD OF HAWAII
818 KEEAUMOKU ST
PO BOX 860
HONOLULU, HI 96808
TEL: (808) 948-6247
FAX: (808) 948-6555

INDIANA CLAIMS OFFICE
ADMINISTAR FEDERAL, INC
8115 KNUE RD
INDIANAPOLIS, IN 46250-2804
TEL: (317) 841-4400
FAX: (317) 841-4691
TOLL FREE: (800) 999-7608

IOWA CLAIMS OFFICE
WELLMARK, INC
636 GRAND AVE, STATION 28
DES MOINES, IA 50309
TEL: (515) 245-4618
FAX: (515) 245-3984
WWW.WELLMEDICARE.COM

KANSAS CLAIMS OFFICE
BLUE CROSS & BLUE SHIELD OF KANSAS
1133 TOPEKA AVE
PO BOX 239
TOPEKA, KS 66601
TEL: (816) 756-1601
FAX: (913) 291-8532

BLUE CROSS & BLUE SHIELD OF KANSAS
1133 SW TOPEKA BLVD
PO BOX 239
TOPEKA, KS 66629
TEL: (785) 291-4003
FAX: (785) 291-8532

KENTUCKY CLAIMS OFFICE
ADMINISTAR FEDERAL INC
8115 KNUE RD
PO BOX 37630
INDIANAPOLIS, IN 46250-2804
TEL: (317) 841-4400
FAX: (317) 841-4691
TOLL FREE: (800) 999-7608

MISSOURI CLAIMS OFFICE
BLUE CROSS & BLUE SHIELD OF KANSAS
1133 SW TOPEKA BLVD
PO BOX 239
TOPEKA, KS 66629
TEL: (816) 756-1601
FAX: (785) 291-8532

NEBRASKA CLAIMS OFFICE
BLUE CROSS & BLUE SHIELD OF KANSAS, INC
1133 TOPEKA AVE
PO BOX 239
TOPEKA, KS 66601
TEL: (785) 291-4155
FAX: (785) 291-8532

NEW YORK CLAIMS OFFICE
BLUE CROSS & BLUE SHIELD OF WESTERN NEW YORK, INC
1901 MAIN ST
PO BOX 80
BUFFALO, NY 14240-0080
TEL: (716) 887-6900
TOLL FREE: (800) 950-0051

NORTH DAKOTA CLAIMS OFFICE
BLUE CROSS & BLUE SHIELD OF TEXAS
4305 16TH AVE S
PO BOX 6701
FARGO, ND 58103-3373
TOLL FREE: (800) 444-4606
IN-STATE: (800) 332-6681

OHIO CLAIMS OFFICE
WEST VA- NATIONWIDE
PO BOX 16788 OR 57
COLUMBUS, OH 43216-0057
TEL: (614) 249-7111
FAX: (616) 249-4467
IN-STATE: (800) 282-0530
WWW.NATIONWIDE-MEDICARE.COM

OREGON CLAIMS OFFICE
BLUE CROSS & BLUE SHIELD OF NORTH DAKOTA
4510 13TH AVE SW
FARGO, ND 58121-0001
TEL: (701) 277-1100
FAX: (701) 282-1002
TOLL FREE: (800) 874-2656
IN-STATE: (800) 247-2267
WWW.NORIDIAN.COM

BLUE CROSS & BLUE SHIELD OF TEXAS
4305 16TH AVE S
PO BOX 6702
FARGO, ND 58108-6702
TOLL FREE: (800) 444-4606
IN-STATE: (800) 332-6681

RHODE ISLAND CLAIMS OFFICE
BLUE CROSS & BLUE SHIELD OF RHODE ISLAND
444 WESTMINSTER ST
PROVIDENCE, RI 02903
TEL: (401) 272-3131

SOUTH CAROLINA CLAIMS OFFICE
BLUE CROSS & BLUE SHIELD OF SOUTH CAROLINA
300 ARBOR LK DR, STE 1300
COLUMBIA, SC 29223
TEL: (803) 788-5568
FAX: (803) 691-2188

SOUTH DAKOTA CLAIMS OFFICE
BLUE CROSS & BLUE SHIELD OF NORTH DAKOTA
4305 16TH AVE S
PO BOX 6707
FARGO, ND 58108-6707
TOLL FREE: (800) 444-4606
IN-STATE: (800) 332-6681

TENNESSEE CLAIMS OFFICE
CONNECTICUT GENERAL LIFE INSURANCE CO (CGLIC)
TWO VANTAGE WAY
PO BOX 1465
NASHVILLE, TN 37228
TEL: (615) 782-4576
FAX: (615) 782-4662
TOLL FREE: (800) 342-8900
WWW.CIGNAMEDICARE.COM

UTAH CLAIMS OFFICE
BLUE CROSS & BLUE SHIELD OF UTAH
2890 COTTONWOOD PKY
PO BOX 30269
SALT LAKE CITY, UT 84130-0269
TEL: (801) 333-2440
FAX: (801) 333-6505
IN-STATE: (800) 426-3477

WASHINGTON CLAIMS OFFICE
BLUE CROSS & BLUE SHIELD OF NORTH DAKOTA
4305 16TH AVE S
PO BOX 6700
FARGO, ND 58108-6700
TOLL FREE: (800) 444-4606
IN-STATE: (800) 332-6681

WEST VIRGINIA CLAIMS OFFICE
NATIONAL MUTUAL INSURANCE CO
PO BOX 57
COLUMBUS, OH 43216-0057
TEL: (614) 249-7111
FAX: (614) 249-4467
IN-STATE: (800) 848-0106
WWW.NATIONWIDE-MEDICARE.COM

WISCONSIN CLAIMS OFFICE
WISCONSIN PHYSICIANS' SERVICE INSURANCE CORP
PO BOX 1787
MADISON, WI 53701-1787
TEL: (608) 221-3218
IN-STATE: (800) 944-0051
WWW.WPSIC.COM/MEDICARE/INDEX

WYOMING CLAIMS OFFICE
BLUE CROSS & BLUE SHIELD OF NORTH DAKOTA
4305 16TH AVE S
PO BOX 6708
FARGO, ND 58108-6708
TOLL FREE: (800) 444-4606
IN-STATE: (800) 332-6681

MEMORIAL SISTERS OF CHARITY HEALTH NETWORK INC

TEXAS CLAIMS OFFICE
MSCH HEALTH NETWORK
9494 SOUTHWEST FWY, STE 300
HOUSTON, TX 77074-1419
TEL: (713) 430-1400
FAX: (713) 778-2375
TOLL FREE: (800) 776-2885
WWW.MSCH.COM

MENNONITE MUTUAL AID ASSOCIATION

INDIANA CLAIMS OFFICE
1110 N MAIN ST
PO BOX 483
GOSHEN, IN 46526-0483
TEL: (219) 533-9511
FAX: (219) 533-5264
TOLL FREE: (800) 348-7468

MERVYN'S HEALTH CARE PLAN

CALIFORNIA CLAIMS OFFICE
BLUE CROSS OF CALIFORNIA
PO BOX 3108
RANCHO CORDOVA, CA 95741-3108
FAX: (916) 636-2314
TOLL FREE: (800) 873-3039
WWW.BLUECROSSCA.COM

MICHIGAN FARM BUREAU MUTUAL INSURANCE CO

MICHIGAN CLAIMS OFFICE
7373 W SAGINAW
PO BOX 30100
LANSING, MI 48909
TEL: (517) 323-7000
FAX: (517) 323-6793
TOLL FREE: (800) 292-2680
WWW.FARMBUREAUINS/MI.COM

MID AMERICA MUTUAL LIFE INSURANCE CO

NEBRASKA CLAIMS OFFICE
WORLD INSURANCE
11808 GRANT ST
PO BOX 3160
OMAHA, NE 68103-0160
TEL: (605) 886-8363
TOLL FREE: (800) 995-9051
IN-STATE: (800) 786-7557

SOUTH DAKOTA CLAIMS OFFICE
WORLD INSURANCE
11808 GRANT ST
PO BOX 3160
OMAHA, NE 68103-0160
TEL: (605) 886-8363
TOLL FREE: (800) 995-9051
IN-STATE: (800) 786-7557

MID-SOUTH INSURANCE CO

NORTH CAROLINA CLAIMS OFFICE
4317 RAMSEY ST
PO BOX 2547
FAYETTEVILLE, NC 28302-2069
TEL: (910) 822-1020
FAX: (910) 822-3018
TOLL FREE: (800) 822-9993

MIDWEST SECURITY ADMINISTRATORS

WISCONSIN CLAIMS OFFICE
MIDWEST SECURITY INSURANCE
1150 SPRINGHURST DR, STE 140
PO BOX 19035
GREEN BAY, WI 54307-9035
TEL: (920) 496-2500

MIDWEST SECURITY INSURANCE CO

ILLINOIS CLAIMS OFFICE
2700 MIDWEST DR
ONALASKA, WI 54650-8764
TEL: (608) 783-7130
FAX: (608) 783-8581
TOLL FREE: (800) 542-6642

INDIANA CLAIMS OFFICE
2700 MIDWEST DR
ONALASKA, WI 54650-8764
TEL: (608) 783-7130
FAX: (608) 783-8581
TOLL FREE: (800) 542-6642

IOWA CLAIMS OFFICE
2700 MIDWEST DR
ONALASKA, WI 54650-8764
TEL: (608) 783-7130
FAX: (608) 783-8581
TOLL FREE: (800) 542-6642

MINNESOTA CLAIMS OFFICE
2700 MIDWEST DR
ONALASKA, WI 54650-8764
TEL: (608) 783-7130
FAX: (608) 783-8581
TOLL FREE: (800) 542-6642

OHIO CLAIMS OFFICE
2700 MIDWEST DR
ONALASKA, WI 54650-8764
TEL: (608) 783-7130
FAX: (608) 783-8581
TOLL FREE: (800) 542-6642

WISCONSIN CLAIMS OFFICE
2700 MIDWEST DR
ONALASKA, WI 54650-8764
TEL: (608) 783-7130
FAX: (608) 783-8581
TOLL FREE: (800) 542-6642

MILLENNIUM CARE ADMINISTRATORS (DBA MCA ADMINISTRATORS)

OHIO CLAIMS OFFICE
A DIVISION OF MANAGED CARE OF AMERICA
5900 ROCHE DR- 5TH FL
PO BOX 18245
COLUMBUS, OH 43218-0245
TEL: (614) 888-1212
FAX: (614) 888-2240
TOLL FREE: (800) 229-6786
IN-STATE: (800) 524-4426
WWW.MCOA.COM

MILLETTE ADMINISTRATORS, INC

MISSISSIPPI CLAIMS OFFICE
4619 MAIN ST, STE A
MOSS POINT, MS 39563
TEL: (228) 475-8687
TOLL FREE: (800) 456-8647

MIT HEALTH PLAN

MASSACHUSETTS CLAIMS OFFICE
BLUE CROSS
77 MASSACHUSETTS AVE- BLDG E 23, STE 308
PO BOX E23-308 MIT
CAMBRIDGE, MA 02139-4307
TEL: (617) 253-1322
FAX: (617) 253-6558

MMA INSURANCE CO

INDIANA CLAIMS OFFICE
1110 N MAIN ST
PO BOX 483
GOSHEN, IN 46527
TEL: (219) 533-9511
FAX: (219) 533-5264
TOLL FREE: (800) 348-7468

MUTUAL MED BENEFIT ADMINISTRATORS

IOWA CLAIMS OFFICE
MUTUAL MED, INC
3216 E 35TH ST CT
DAVENPORT, IA 52807
TEL: (319) 344-2890
FAX: (319) 344-2891
TOLL FREE: (800) 747-4126
E-MAIL: MUTUAL@AOL.COM

NALC HEALTH BENEFIT PLAN

NATIONAL CLAIMS OFFICE
NATIONAL ASSOCIATION OF LETTER CARRIERS
20547 WAVERLY CT
ASHBURN, VA 20149-0001
TEL: (703) 729-4677
FAX: (703) 729-0076
TOLL FREE: (800) 548-8484
WWW.NALC.ORG/HBP

NAPUS HEALTH BENEFIT PLAN

BLUE CROSS & BLUE SHIELD
550 12TH ST SW
WASHINGTON, DC 20065-3520
TEL: (202) 479-8000
FAX: (202) 479-3520
TOLL FREE: (800) 424-7474
WWW.CAREFIRST.COM

NATIONAL HEALTH PLANS

CALIFORNIA CLAIMS OFFICE
NATIONAL-MED
1005 W ORANGEBURG, STE B
PO BOX 5356
MODESTO, CA 95352
TEL: (209) 527-3350
FAX: (209) 527-6773
TOLL FREE: (800) 468-8600
WWW.NATIONALHMO.COM

NATIONAL TRAVELERS LIFE INSURANCE CO

NATIONAL CLAIMS OFFICE
5700 WESTOWN PKY
PO BOX 9197
WEST DES MOINES, IA 50266-9197
TEL: (515) 221-0101
FAX: (515) 327-5830
TOLL FREE: 800-232-5818
WWW.NATIONALTRAVELERSLIFE.COM

NATIONWIDE LIFE INSURANCE CO

ONE NATIONWIDE PLZ
PO BOX 2399
COLUMBUS, OH 43216-2399
TEL: (614) 249-7111
FAX: (614) 249-7705
TOLL FREE: (800) 772-9956
WWW.NATIONWIDEHEALTH.COM

NAVISTAR

AETNA LIFE & CASUALTY
455 N CITYFRONT PLZ DR
PO BOX 5367
CHICAGO, IL 60611
TEL: (312) 836-2000
FAX: (312) 836-2227

NEW AIR LIFE

ALABAMA CLAIMS OFFICE
PO BOX 4884
HOUSTON, TX 77210-4884
TEL: (281) 368-7200
FAX: (281) 368-7329
TOLL FREE: (800) 552-7879

NORTH DAKOTA WORKERS COMPENSATION BUREAU

NORTH DAKOTA CLAIMS OFFICE
500 E FRONT AVE
BISMARCK, ND 58504-5685
TEL: (701) 328-3800
FAX: (701) 328-3820
TOLL FREE: (800) 777-5033

NORTHEAST MEDICAL CENTER

NORTH CAROLINA CLAIMS OFFICE
920 CHURCH ST N
CONCORD, NC 28025-2927
TEL: (704) 783-3000
FAX: (704) 783-1487
TOLL FREE: (800) 842-6868
WWW.NORTHEASTMEDICAL.ORG

NORTHWEST WASHINGTON MEDICAL BUREAU

WASHINGTON CLAIMS OFFICE
3000 NORTHWEST AVE
PO BOX 9753
BELLINGHAM, WA 98227-9753
TEL: (360) 734-8000
FAX: (360) 734-6676
TOLL FREE: (800) 825-5962

NYL CARE

TEXAS CLAIMS OFFICE
2425 WEST LOOP S, STE 1000
PO BOX 56228
HOUSTON, TX 77027
TEL: (713) 624-5000
FAX: (713) 993-9462
TOLL FREE: (800) 833-5318

O'BRIEN, BOUCK & ASSOCIATES

KANSAS CLAIMS OFFICE
8340 MISSION RD STE 119
PO BOX 6826
LEAWOOD, KS 66206-0353
TEL: (913) 381-3444
FAX: (913) 381-3953

ODS HEALTH PLAN

OREGON CLAIMS OFFICE
315 SW 5TH AVE
PO BOX 40384
PORTLAND, OR 97204
TEL: (503) 228-6554
FAX: (503) 243-5105
TOLL FREE: (800) 852-5195
WWW.ODSHP.COM

OLYMPIC BENEFITS

WASHINGTON CLAIMS OFFICE
PO BOX 1077
BELLINGHAM, WA 98227-1077
TEL: (360) 734-9888
FAX: (360) 734-6199
TOLL FREE: (800) 533-3941
WWW.OHMSYSTEMS.COM

OMNI HEALTH CARE

CALIFORNIA CLAIMS OFFICE
1776 W MARCH LN, STE 240
STOCKTON, CA 95207
TEL: (209) 474-6664
FAX: (209) 955-7536
TOLL FREE: (800) 342-8462
WWW.OMNIHEALTHCARE.COM

PACIFIC INDEMNITY CO

NATIONAL CLAIMS OFFICE
CHUBB GROUP INSURANCE COMPANY
801 S FIGUROA ST
PO BOX 30850
LOS ANGELES, CA 90030-0850
TEL: (213) 612-0880
FAX: (213) 612-5731
TOLL FREE: (800) 262-4459

PACIFICARE HEALTH SYSTEMS, INC

OREGON CLAIMS OFFICE
PACIFICARE OF OREGON, INC
5 CENTER PT DR, STE 600
LAKE OSWEGO, OR 97035
FAX: (503) 533-6335
TOLL FREE: (800) 922-1444

PAN AMERICAN LIFE INSURANCE CO

LOUISIANA CLAIMS OFFICE
601 POYDRAS ST
PO BOX 60219
NEW ORLEANS, LA 70130
TEL: (504) 566-1300
FAX: (504) 523-8584
TOLL FREE: (800) 227-3417

PARTNERS NATIONAL HEALTH PLANS

NORTH CAROLINA CLAIMS OFFICE
2085 FRONTIS PLZ BLVD
PO BOX 24907
WINSTON-SALEM, NC 27114
TEL: (336) 760-4822
FAX: (336) 760-3198
TOLL FREE: (800) 942-5695
IN-STATE: (800) 942-5695
WWW.PARTNERSHEALTH.COM

SOUTH CAROLINA CLAIMS OFFICE
2085 FRONTIS PLZ BLVD
PO BOX 24907
WINSTON-SALEM, NC 27114
TEL: (336) 760-4822
FAX: (336) 760-3198
TOLL FREE: (800) 942-5695
IN-STATE: (800) 942-5695
WWW.PARTNERSHEALTH.COM

VIRGINIA CLAIMS OFFICE
2085 FRONTIS PLZ BLVD
PO BOX 24907
WINSTON-SALEM, NC 27114
TEL: (336) 760-4822
FAX: (336) 760-3198
TOLL FREE: (800) 942-5695
IN-STATE: (800) 942-5695
WWW.PARTNERSHEALTH.COM

PAULA INSURANCE CO

CALIFORNIA CLAIMS OFFICE
1780 E BULLARD, STE 101
PO BOX 40009
FRESNO, CA 93755-0009
TEL: (559) 439-3330
FAX: (559) 439-3505
WWW.TRWPICATALO.COM

PEER REVIEW ORGANIZATIONS

AMERICAN SAMOA CLAIMS OFFICE
HAWAII MEDICAL SERVICE ASSOCIATION
818 KEEAUMOKU ST
PO BOX 860
HONOLULU, HI 96808-0860
TEL: (808) 948-5110
FAX: (808) 948-6811
WWW.HMSA.COM

COLORADO CLAIMS OFFICE
COLORADO FOUNDATION FOR MEDICAL CARE
2851 S PARKER RD, STE 200
AURORA, CO 80014
TEL: (303) 695-3300
FAX: (303) 695-3350
WWW.CFMC.ORG

GEORGIA CLAIMS OFFICE
GEORGIA MEDICAL CARE FOUNDATION
57 EXECUTIVE PARK DR S, STE 200
ATLANTA, GA 30329
TEL: (404) 982-0411
FAX: (404) 982-7591
TOLL FREE: (800) 982-7581

GUAM CLAIMS OFFICE
HAWAII MEDICAL SERVICE ASSOCIATION
818 KEEAUMOKU ST
PO BOX 860
HONOLULU, HI 96808-0860
TEL: (808) 948-5110
FAX: (808) 948-6811
WWW.HMSA.COM

HAWAII CLAIMS OFFICE
HAWAII MEDICAL SERVICE ASSOCIATION
818 KEEAUMOKU ST
PO BOX 860
HONOLULU, HI 96808-0860
TEL: (808) 948-5110
FAX: (808) 948-6811
WWW.HMSA.COM

IDAHO CLAIMS OFFICE
PRO-WEST
10700 MERIDIAN AVE N, STE 100
SEATTLE, WA 98133-9075
TEL: (206) 364-9700
FAX: (208) 343-4705

MICHIGAN CLAIMS OFFICE
MICHIGAN PEER REVIEW ORGANIZATION
40600 ANN ARBOR RD, STE 200
PLYMOUTH, MI 48170-4486
TEL: (734) 459-0900

PERSONAL INSURANCE ADMINISTRATORS

CALIFORNIA CLAIMS OFFICE
PO BOX 5004
WOODLAND HILLS, CA 91359
TEL: (805) 777-0032
FAX: (805) 777-0033
TOLL FREE: (800) 468-4343

PERSONALCARE HEALTH MANAGEMENT

ILLINOIS CLAIMS OFFICE
ATTN: CLAIMS DEPT
210 BOX DR
CHAMPAIGN, IL 61820-7399
TEL: (217) 366-1226
FAX: (217) 366-5410
TOLL FREE: (800) 431-1211

INDIANA CLAIMS OFFICE
ATTN: CLAIMS DEPT
210 BOX DR
CHAMPAIGN, IL 61820-7399
TEL: (217) 366-1226
FAX: (217) 366-5410
TOLL FREE: (800) 431-1211

PFS INSURANCE GROUP

NATIONAL CLAIMS OFFICE
NATIONAL GROUP LIFE INSURANCE CO
PO BOX 1250
ROCKFORD, IL 61105-1250
TEL: (815) 965-8955
FAX: (815) 720-2990
TOLL FREE: (*00) 659-7374

PHARMACIST MUTUAL

IOWA CLAIMS OFFICE
808 U.S. HWY 18-W
PO BOX 370
ALGONA, IA 50511-0370
TEL: (515) 295-2461
FAX: (515) 295-9306
TOLL FREE: (800) 247-5930

PHICO

PENNSYLVANIA CLAIMS OFFICE
1 PHICO DR
PO BOX 85
MECHANICSBURG, PA 17055-0085
TEL: (717) 691-1600
FAX: (717) 766-2837
TOLL FREE: (800) 627-4626

PHN-HMO

MARYLAND CLAIMS OFFICE
1099 WINTERSAN RD
LINTHICUM HEIGHTS, MD 21090
TEL: (410) 850-7461
TOLL FREE: (800) 422-1996

PHYSICIANS BENEFITS TRUST

ILLINOIS CLAIMS OFFICE
150 S WACKER DR, STE 1200
PO BOX 8263
CHICAGO, IL 60680-8263
TEL: (312) 541-2711
FAX: (312) 541-4589
TOLL FREE: (800) 621-0748

PHYSICIANS HEALTH PLAN OF NORTHERN INDIANA, INC

INDIANA CLAIMS OFFICE
8101 W JEFFERSON BLVD
PO BOX 2359
FT WAYNE, IN 46801
TEL: (219) 432-6690
FAX: (219) 432-0493
TOLL FREE: (800) 982-6257

PHYSICIANS HEALTH SERVICES

CONNECTICUT CLAIMS OFFICE
MD HEALTH PLAN, INC
1 FARMILL CROSSING
PO BOX 904
SHELTON, CT 06484-0944
TEL: (203) 225-8000
FAX: (203) 225-4001
TOLL FREE: (800) 772-5869
IN-STATE: (800) 848-4747
WWW.PHSHMO.COM

PREFERRED HEALTH NORTHWEST

OREGON CLAIMS OFFICE
BLUE CROSS & BLUE SHIELDS OF OREGON
100 SW MARKET
PO BOX 1271
PORTLAND, OR 97207-1271
TEL: (503) 274-0761
FAX: (503) 375-4293
TOLL FREE: (800) 452-7390
IN-STATE: (800) 452-7278
WWW.BCBSO.COM

PREFERRED HEALTH SYSTEMS INSURANCE CO

KANSAS CLAIMS OFFICE
355 N WACO
PO BOX 49288
WICHITA, KS 67201-5007
TEL: (316) 268-0345
FAX: (316) 268-0346
TOLL FREE: (800) 660-8114
WWW.PHSYSTEMS.COM

PREFERRED PLUS OF KANSAS
PO BOX 49218
WICHITA, KS 67202
TEL: (316) 268-0345
FAX: (316) 263-3673
TOLL FREE: (800) 660-8114
WWW.PHSYSTEMS.COM

PREMERA BLUE CROSS

ALASKA CLAIMS OFFICE
7001 220TH ST SW
PO BOX 327
MOUNTLAKE TERRACE, WA 98111
TEL: (425) 670-4700
FAX: (425) 670-5457
TOLL FREE: (800) 527-6675

IDAHO CLAIMS OFFICE
7001 220TH ST SW
PO BOX 327
MOUNTLAKE TERRACE, WA 98111
TEL: (425) 670-4700
FAX: (425) 670-5457
TOLL FREE: (800) 527-6675

OREGON CLAIMS OFFICE
7001 220TH ST SW
PO BOX 327
MOUNTLAKE TERRACE, WA 98111
TEL: (425) 670-4700
FAX: (425) 670-5457
TOLL FREE: (800) 527-6675

WASHINGTON CLAIMS OFFICE
7001 220TH ST SW
PO BOX 327
MOUNTLAKE TERRACE, WA 98111
TEL: (425) 670-4700
FAX: (425) 670-5457
TOLL FREE: (800) 527-6675

3900 E SPRAGUE
PO BOX 3048
SPOKANE, WA 99220-3048
TEL: (509) 536-4700
FAX: (509) 536-4771
TOLL FREE: (800) 835-3510
IN-STATE: (800) 572-0778
WWW.PREMERA.COM

PREMIER BLUE

KANSAS CLAIMS OFFICE
1133 SW TOPEKA AVE
PO BOX 3518
TOPEKA, KS 66601-3518
TEL: (785) 291-4010
FAX: (785) 291-8848
TOLL FREE: (800) 332-0028
WWW.BCBSKS.COM

PRESBYTERIAN HEALTH PLAN / FHP OF NEW MEXICO

NEW MEXICO CLAIMS OFFICE
PACIFICARE OF NEW MEXICO
PO BOX 27489
ALBUQUERQUE, NM 87125
TEL: (505) 923-5799
FAX: (505) 923-5277
TOLL FREE: (800) 356-2884
IN-STATE: (800) 356-2219

PRIME HEALTH OF ALABAMA

ALABAMA CLAIMS OFFICE
MOBILE HEALTH PLAN DBA
1400 UNIVERSITY BLVD S
PO BOX 851239
MOBILE, AL 36685-1239
TEL: (334) 342-0022
FAX: (334) 380-3236
TOLL FREE: (800) 544-9449
WWW.PRIMEHEALTHONLINE.COM

MISSISSIPPI CLAIMS OFFICE
MOBILE HEALTH PLAN DBA
1400 UNIVERSITY BLVD S
PO BOX 851239
MOBILE, AL 36685-1239
TEL: (334) 342-0022
FAX: (334) 380-3236
TOLL FREE: (800) 544-9449
WWW.PRIMEHEALTHONLINE.COM

PRINCIPAL FINANCIAL GROUP

FLORIDA CLAIMS OFFICE
9428 BAYMEADOWS RD, STE 360
JACKSONVILLE, FL 32256-9933
TEL: (904) 731-8159
FAX: (904) 367-8444
TOLL FREE: (800) 445-6133
WWW.PRINCIPAL.COM

ILLINOIS CLAIMS OFFICE
PRINCIPAL LIFE INSURANCE CO
1245 CORPORATE BLVD, STE 200
AURORA, IL 60504-9955
TEL: (630) 978-5100
FAX: (630) 978-5117
WWW.PRINCIPAL.COM

MISSOURI CLAIMS OFFICE
620 S GLENSTONE AVE, STE 300
PO BOX 2593
SPRINGFIELD, MO 65801-2593
TEL: (417) 877-0085
TOLL FREE: (800) 422-5002
WWW.PRINCIPAL.COM

NATIONAL CLAIMS OFFICE
1755 TELSTAR DR, STE 300
PO BOX 39710
COLORADO SPRINGS, CO 80949
TEL: (719) 548-4000
FAX: (719) 548-4001
TOLL FREE: (800) 273-2486
WWW.PRINCIPAL.COM

NEBRASKA CLAIMS OFFICE
330 N 117TH ST
PO BOX 542060
OMAHA, NE 68154
TEL: (402) 330-0800
FAX: (402) 330-1636
TOLL FREE: (800) 331-9443
WWW.PRINCIPAL.COM

OKLAHOMA CLAIMS OFFICE
620 S GLENSTONE AVE, STE 300
PO BOX 2593
SPRINGFIELD, MO 65801-2593
TEL: (417) 877-0085
TOLL FREE: (800) 422-5002
WWW.PRINCIPAL.COM

PRINCIPAL HEALTHCARE OF FLORIDA

FLORIDA CLAIMS OFFICE
2203 N LOIS AVE, STE 900
PO BOX 31298
TAMPA, FL 33631-3298
TEL: (813) 875-3737
FAX: (813) 876-4572
TOLL FREE: (800) 443-5810

PRIORITY HEALTH

CALIFORNIA CLAIMS OFFICE
PACIFIC CARE
1111 E HERNDON, STE 202
PO BOX 25790
FRESNO, CA 93729-5790
TEL: (559) 435-8366
FAX: (559) 435-9718
TOLL FREE: (800) 350-8366

PROFESSIONAL ADMINISTRATION GROUP

KANSAS CLAIMS OFFICE
PO BOX 13391
OVERLAND PARK, KS 66282-3391
TEL: (913) 327-7104
FAX: (913) 451-4762
E-MAIL: ADM-SVC@SWBELL.NET

PROFESSIONAL ADMINISTRATORS, INC

NATIONAL CLAIMS OFFICE
3751 MAGUIRE BLVD, STE 100
PO BOX 140415-0415
ORLANDO, FL 32803-0415
TEL: (407) 896-0521
FAX: (407) 897-6976
TOLL FREE: (800) 741-0521
IN-STATE: (800) 432-2686
E-MAIL: PA1001@AOL.COM

PROFESSIONAL BENEFIT ADMINISTRATORS, INC

ILLINOIS CLAIMS OFFICE
15 SPINNING WHEEL RD, STE 210
PO BOX 4687
OAKBROOK, IL 60522
TEL: (630) 655-3755
FAX: (630) 655-3781

PROFESSIONAL RISK MANAGEMENT

CALIFORNIA CLAIMS OFFICE
2101 WEBSTER ST, STE 900
OAKLAND, CA 94612
TEL: (510) 452-9300
FAX: (510) 452-1479
WWW.APPLIEDRISK.COM

PROTECTED HOME MUTUAL LIFE INSURANCE CO

PENNSYLVANIA CLAIMS OFFICE
30 E STATE ST
SHARON, PA 16146
TEL: (724) 981-1520
FAX: (724) 981-2682
TOLL FREE: (800) 223-8821
IN-STATE: (800) 222-8894

PROVIDENCE HEALTH PLANS

WASHINGTON CLAIMS OFFICE
1501 FOURTH AVE, STE 600
SEATTLE, WA 98101
TEL: (206) 215-9000
TOLL FREE: (800) 443-0996
WWW.PROVHEALTH.COM

PRUDENTIAL HEALTH CARE PLAN, INC

OKLAHOMA CLAIMS OFFICE
PRUCARE OF TULSA
7912 E 31 CT, STE 200
TULSA, OK 74145-1338
TEL: (918) 624-4600
FAX: (918) 624-5050
TOLL FREE: (800) 345-8310
WWW.PRUDENTIAL.COM

TEXAS CLAIMS OFFICE
PRUCARE OF AUSTIN
7700 CHEVY CHASE DR- BLDG 1, STE 500
PO BOX 26699
AUSTIN, TX 78755-0699
TEL: (512) 323-0440
FAX: (713) 663-0731
TOLL FREE: (800) 621-2645
WWW.PRUDENTIAL.COM

ONE PRUDENTIAL CIR
PO BOX 27718
HOUSTON, TX 77227
TEL: (713) 350-2150
FAX: (713) 663-0731
TOLL FREE: (800) 876-7778
WWW.PRUDENTIAL.COM

PRUDENTIAL HEALTHCARE OF CALIFORNIA

CALIFORNIA CLAIMS OFFICE
PRUDENTIAL HEALTHCARE
21261 BURBANK AVE
WOODLAND HILLS, CA 91367
TEL: (818) 992-2000
FAX: (818) 594-4266
TOLL FREE: (800) 433-3150

PUBLIC EMPLOYEES HEALTH PROGRAM

UTAH CLAIMS OFFICE
560 E 200 S
SALT LAKE CITY, UT 84102-2020
TEL: (801) 366-7500
FAX: (801) 366-7596
TOLL FREE: (800) 933-7347

PYRAMID LIFE INSURANCE CO

NATIONAL CLAIMS OFFICE
6201 JOHNSON DR
PO BOX 772
MISSION, KS 66202
TEL: (913) 722-1110
FAX: (913) 722-3567
TOLL FREE: (800) 444-0321
WWW.PYRAMIDLIFE.COM

QUAL-MED HEALTH PLAN

ARIZONA CLAIMS OFFICE
FOUNDATION HEALTH SYSTEMS
225 N MAIN ST
PO BOX 640
PUEBLO, CO 81002-0640
TEL: (719) 542-0500
FAX: (719) 585-8333
TOLL FREE: (800) 628-2287
WWW.QUALMED.COM

CALIFORNIA CLAIMS OFFICE
FOUNDATION HEALTH SYSTEMS
225 N MAIN ST
PO BOX 640
PUEBLO, CO 81002-0640
TEL: (719) 542-0500
FAX: (719) 585-8333
TOLL FREE: (800) 628-2287
WWW.QUALMED.COM

COLORADO CLAIMS OFFICE
FOUNDATION HEALTH SYSTEMS
225 N MAIN ST
PO BOX 640
PUEBLO, CO 81002-0640
TEL: (719) 542-0500
FAX: (719) 585-8333
TOLL FREE: (800) 628-2287
WWW.QUALMED.COM

CONNECTICUT CLAIMS OFFICE
FOUNDATION HEALTH SYSTEMS
225 N MAIN ST
PO BOX 640
PUEBLO, CO 81002-0640
TEL: (719) 542-0500
FAX: (719) 585-8333
TOLL FREE: (800) 628-2287
WWW.QUALMED.COM

NEW MEXICO CLAIMS OFFICE
FOUNDATION HEALTH SYSTEMS
225 N MAIN ST
PO BOX 640
PUEBLO, CO 81002-0640
TEL: (719) 542-0500
FAX: (719) 585-8333
TOLL FREE: (800) 628-2287
WWW.QUALMED.COM

OREGON CLAIMS OFFICE
FOUNDATION HEALTH SYSTEMS
225 N MAIN ST
PO BOX 640
PUEBLO, CO 81002-0640
TEL: (719) 542-0500
FAX: (719) 585-8333
TOLL FREE: (800) 628-2287
WWW.QUALMED.COM

WASHINGTON CLAIMS OFFICE
FOUNDATION HEALTH SYSTEMS
225 N MAIN ST
PO BOX 640
PUEBLO, CO 81002-0640
TEL: (719) 542-0500
FAX: (719) 585-8333
TOLL FREE: (800) 628-2287
WWW.QUALMED.COM

QUEEN'S ISLAND CARE/QUEEN'S HEALTH PLAN

HAWAII CLAIMS OFFICE
2 WATERFRONT PLAZA
500 ALA MOANA BLVD, STE 200
PO BOX 37549
HONOLULU, HI 96837
TEL: (808) 532-6900
FAX: (808) 522-8642
TOLL FREE: (800) 856-4668

RAYTHEON CO

NATIONAL CLAIMS OFFICE
141 SPRING ST
LEXINGTON, MA 02173
TEL: (781) 862-6600
FAX: (781) 860-2172
TOLL FREE: (800) 843-4121

REGENCE BLUE CROSS & BLUE SHIELD

IDAHO CLAIMS OFFICE
HMO OREGON, INC
201 HIGH ST SE
PO BOX 12625
SALEM, OR 97309
TEL: (503) 364-4868
FAX: (503) 588-4350
TOLL FREE: (800) 228-0978
WWW.BCBSOR.COM

OREGON CLAIMS OFFICE
REGENCE HMO OREGON
100 SW MARKET
PO BOX 100
PORTLAND, OR 97207
TEL: (503) 225-5227
TOLL FREE: (800) 452-7278
WWW.BCBSOR.COM

HMO OREGON, INC
201 HIGH ST SE
PO BOX 12625
SALEM, OR 97309
TEL: (503) 364-4868
FAX: (503) 588-4350
TOLL FREE: (800) 228-0978
WWW.BCBSOR.COM

WASHINGTON CLAIMS OFFICE
REGENCE HMO OREGON
100 SW MARKET
PO BOX 100
PORTLAND, OR 97207
TEL: (503) 225-5227
TOLL FREE: (800) 452-7278
WWW.BCBSOR.COM

HMO OREGON, INC
201 HIGH ST SE
PO BOX 12625
SALEM, OR 97309
TEL: (503) 364-4868
FAX: (503) 588-4350
TOLL FREE: (800) 228-0978
WWW.BCBSOR.COM

REGENCE BLUE CROSS & BLUE SHIELD OF UTAH

UTAH CLAIMS OFFICE
2870 E COTTONWOOD PKY
PO BOX 30270
SALT LAKE CITY, UT 84130-0270
TEL: (801) 333-2320
FAX: (801) 333-6523
TOLL FREE: (800) 662-0876
IN-STATE: (800) 624-6519

REGENCE BLUE SHIELD

WASHINGTON CLAIMS OFFICE
1800 NINTH AVE
PO BOX 21267
SEATTLE, WA 98111-3267
TEL: (206) 464-3600
TOLL FREE: (800) 544-4246
IN-STATE: (800) 458-3523
WWW.REGENCE.COM

REGENCE BLUE SHIELD OF IDAHO

IDAHO CLAIMS OFFICE
1602 21ST AVE
PO BOX 1106
LEWISTON, ID 83501-1106
TEL: (208) 746-2671
FAX: (208) 798-2090
TOLL FREE: (800) 632-2022
WWW.ID.REGENCE.COM

REGENCE BLUESHIELD

WASHINGTON CLAIMS OFFICE
7600 EVERGREEN WAY
EVERETT, WA 98203-6413
TEL: (425) 348-8160
FAX: (425) 348-8167
TOLL FREE: (800) 328-7273
IN-STATE: (800) 548-8385
WWW.WA.REGENCE.COM

REGENCY EMPLOYEE BENEFITS

MICHIGAN CLAIMS OFFICE
ROBINS GROUP
330 SUPERIOR MALL
PO BOX 610609
PORT HURON, MI 48061-0609
TEL: (810) 987-7711
FAX: (810) 987-7603
TOLL FREE: (800) 369-3718

REGIONS BLUE CROSS & BLUE SHIELD OF OREGON

IDAHO CLAIMS OFFICE
HMO OF OREGON
100 SW MARKET ST
PO BOX 900
PORTLAND, OR 97207
TEL: (503) 274-0761
FAX: (503) 375-4293
TOLL FREE: (800) 643-4512
IN-STATE: (800) 228-0978
WWW.BCBSO.COM

OREGON CLAIMS OFFICE
HMO OF OREGON
100 SW MARKET ST
PO BOX 900
PORTLAND, OR 97207
TEL: (503) 274-0761
FAX: (503) 375-4293
TOLL FREE: (800) 643-4512
IN-STATE: (800) 228-0978
WWW.BCBSO.COM

UTAH CLAIMS OFFICE
HMO OF OREGON
100 SW MARKET ST
PO BOX 900
PORTLAND, OR 97207
TEL: (503) 274-0761
FAX: (503) 375-4293
TOLL FREE: (800) 643-4512
IN-STATE: (800) 228-0978
WWW.BCBSO.COM

WASHINGTON CLAIMS OFFICE
HMO OF OREGON
100 SW MARKET ST
PO BOX 900
PORTLAND, OR 97207
TEL: (503) 274-0761
FAX: (503) 375-4293
TOLL FREE: (800) 643-4512
IN-STATE: (800) 228-0978
WWW.BCBSO.COM

REINSURANCE MANAGEMENT, INC

NATIONAL CLAIMS OFFICE
MANAGED HEALTH FUNDING INSURANCE ADMINISTRATORS
9485 REGENCY SQ BLVD, STE 220
JACKSONVILLE, FL 32225
TEL: (904) 727-5088
FAX: (904) 727-7892
TOLL FREE: (800) 830-3856
WWW.RMIMHF.COM

RESOURCE PARTNER

OHIO CLAIMS OFFICE
180 E BROAD ST
PO BOX 189
COLUMBUS, OH 43216-0189
TEL: (614) 220-5001
FAX: (614) 220-5033
TOLL FREE: (800) 848-6181
WWW.RESOURCEPARTNER.COM

RIVERBEND GOVERNMENT BENEFITS ADMINISTRATOR

TENNESSEE CLAIMS OFFICE
730 CHESTNUT ST
CHATTANOOGA, TN 37402
TEL: (423) 755-5783
FAX: (423) 752-6518
WWW.RIVERBENDGBA.COM

RMSCO, INC

NEW YORK CLAIMS OFFICE
731 JAMES ST
PO BOX 6309
SYRACUSE, NY 13217
TEL: (315) 474-8200
FAX: (315) 476-8440

ROBERT S. WEISS & CO

CONNECTICUT CLAIMS OFFICE
SILVER HILLS BUS CTR- 500 S BROAD ST
PO BOX 1034
MERIDEN, CT 06450-1034
TEL: (203) 235-6882
FAX: (203) 639-7422
TOLL FREE: (800) 466-7900

ROCKFORD HEALTH PLANS

ILLINOIS CLAIMS OFFICE
3401 N PERRYVILLE RD
ROCKFORD, IL 61114
TEL: (815) 654-3600
FAX: (815) 282-0634
TOLL FREE: (800) 331-0424
WWW.RHSNET.ORG

ROCKY MOUNTAIN HMO

COLORADO CLAIMS OFFICE
HEALTH OPTIONS, INC
2775 CROSSROADS BLVD
PO BOX 10600
GRAND JUNCTION, CO 81506
TEL: (970) 244-7760
FAX: (970) 244-7880
TOLL FREE: (800) 843-0719
IN-STATE: (800) 843-0719
WWW.RMHMO.ORG

ROYAL STATE GROUP

HAWAII CLAIMS OFFICE
819 S BERETANIA ST, STE 100
HONOLULU, HI 96813
TEL: (808) 539-1600
FAX: (808) 538-1458
WWW.HGEA.COM

ROYAL & SUNALLIANCE

CALIFORNIA CLAIMS OFFICE
801 N BRAND BLVD, STE 500
PO BOX 29035
GLENDALE, CA 91209-9035
TEL: (818) 241-5212
FAX: (818) 543-6393
TOLL FREE: (800) 252-0431
WWW.ROYALSUNALLIANCE.COM

CONNECTICUT CLAIMS OFFICE
80 WOLF RD, STE 606
PO BOX 15096
ALBANY, NY 12205
TEL: (518) 489-8331
TOLL FREE: (800) 553-2556
WWW.ROYALSUNALLIANCE.COM

INDIANA CLAIMS OFFICE
255 E 5TH ST, STE 2100
CINCINNATI, OH 45202
TEL: (513) 421-2183
FAX: (513) 357-9580
TOLL FREE: (800) 843-5772
WWW.ROYALSUNALLIANCE.COM

KENTUCKY CLAIMS OFFICE
255 E 5TH ST, STE 2100
CINCINNATI, OH 45202
TEL: (513) 421-2183
FAX: (513) 357-9580
TOLL FREE: (800) 843-5772
WWW.ROYALSUNALLIANCE.COM

MARYLAND CLAIMS OFFICE
300 E LOMBARD ST, STE 700
BALTIMORE, MD 21202
TEL: (410) 685-5844
FAX: (410) 637-1699
TOLL FREE: (800) 482-4446
WWW.ROYALSUNALLIANCE.COM

MASSACHUSETTS CLAIMS OFFICE
25 NEW CHARDEN
PO BOX 8088
BOSTON, MA 02114-4774
TEL: (617) 742-7750
FAX: (617) 557-4252
TOLL FREE: (800) 367-7036
IN-STATE: (800) 367-7036
WWW.ROYALSUNALLIANCE.COM

80 WOLF RD, STE 606
PO BOX 15096
ALBANY, NY 12205
TEL: (518) 489-8331
TOLL FREE: (800) 553-2556
WWW.ROYALSUNALLIANCE.COM

MICHIGAN CLAIMS OFFICE
255 E 5TH ST, STE 2100
CINCINNATI, OH 45202
TEL: (513) 421-2183
FAX: (513) 357-9580
TOLL FREE: (800) 843-5772
WWW.ROYALSUNALLIANCE.COM

NATIONAL CLAIMS OFFICE
2 JERICHO PLZ
PO BOX 4002
JERICHO, NY 11753-0873
TEL: (516) 939-0600
FAX: (516) 937-3338
TOLL FREE: (800) 523-6273
WWW.ROYALSUNALLIANCE.COM

25800 NORTHWESTERN HWY, STE 701
PO BOX 5010
SOUTHFIELD, MI 48086-5010
TEL: (248) 746-6180
FAX: (248) 746-6190
IN-STATE: (800) 482-8772
WWW.ROYALSUNALLIANCE.COM

NEW YORK CLAIMS OFFICE
80 WOLF RD, STE 606
PO BOX 15096
ALBANY, NY 12205
TEL: (518) 489-8331
TOLL FREE: (800) 553-2556
WWW.ROYALSUNALLIANCE.COM

OHIO CLAIMS OFFICE
255 E 5TH ST, STE 2100
CINCINNATI, OH 45202
TEL: (513) 421-2183
FAX: (513) 357-9580
TOLL FREE: (800) 843-5772
WWW.ROYALSUNALLIANCE.COM

SAFECO INSURANCE CO OF AMERICA

CALIFORNIA CLAIMS OFFICE
AMERICAN STATES
330 N BRAND BLVD, STE 900
PO BOX 29082
GLENDALE, CA 91029-9082
TEL: (818) 956-4200
FAX: (818) 956-4259
TOLL FREE: (800) 826-8921
WWW.SAFECO.COM

GEORGIA CLAIMS OFFICE
1551 JULIET RD
PO BOX A
STONE MOUNTAIN, GA 30086
TEL: (770) 469-1111
FAX: (770) 879-3333
TOLL FREE: (800) 241-2279
WWW.SAFECO.COM

MISSOURI CLAIMS OFFICE
3637 S GEYER RD
PO BOX 66783
SAINT LOUIS, MO 63127-6783
TEL: (314) 957-4500
FAX: (314) 957-4630
TOLL FREE: (800) 843-1487
WWW.SAFECO.COM

OHIO CLAIMS OFFICE
5901 E GALBRAITH RD
PO BOX 36177
CINCINNATI, OH 45236-2251
TEL: (513) 745-5861
FAX: (513) 745-5810
TOLL FREE: (800) 543-7138
WWW.SAFECO.COM

SAN DIEGO ELECTRICAL HEALTH & WELFARE TRUST

CALIFORNIA CLAIMS OFFICE
4675 VIEW RDG, STE B
PO BOX 231219
SAN DIEGO, CA 92194-1219
TEL: (619) 569-6322
FAX: (619) 573-0830
TOLL FREE: (800) 632-2569

SEABURY & SMITH

IOWA CLAIMS OFFICE
2615 NORTHGATE DR
PO BOX 1520
IOWA CITY, IA 52244-1520
TEL: (319) 351-2667
FAX: (319) 351-0603
TOLL FREE: (800) 562-4023

SECURITY HEALTH PLAN OF WISCONSIN, INC

WISCONSIN CLAIMS OFFICE
1000 N OAK AVE
MARSHFIELD, WI 54449-5703
TEL: (715) 387-5621
FAX: (715) 387-9399
TOLL FREE: (800) 472-2363
WWW.SECURITYHEALTH.ORG

SEDGWICK

TENNESSEE CLAIMS OFFICE
1000 RIDGEWAY LOOP RD
PO BOX 171377
MEMPHIS, TN 38120
TEL: (901) 761-1550
FAX: (901) 684-3858

SELF INSURED SERVICES CO

NATIONAL CLAIMS OFFICE
SISCO
PO BOX 389
DUBUQUE, IA 52004-0389
TEL: (319) 583-7344
FAX: (319) 583-0439
WWW.CB-SISCO.COM

SENTARA HEALTH PLAN

VIRGINIA CLAIMS OFFICE
4417 CORPORATION LN
VIRGINIA BEACH, VA 23462-3114
TEL: (757) 552-7100
FAX: (757) 552-7397
TOLL FREE: (800) 229-1199
IN-STATE: (800) 229-8822

SENTRY INSURANCE A MUTUAL CO

WISCONSIN CLAIMS OFFICE
1800 N POINT DR
STEVENS POINT, WI 54481
TEL: (715) 346-6000
FAX: (715) 346-6161
TOLL FREE: (800) 638-8763
WWW.SENTRYINSURANCE.COM

SENTRY INSURANCE GROUP

MASSACHUSETTS CLAIMS OFFICE
3 CARLISLE RD
PO BOX 584
WESTFORD, MA 01886-0584
TEL: (508) 392-7000
FAX: (978) 392-7033
TOLL FREE: (800) 225-1390

SHELTER INSURANCE COMPANIES

ARKANSAS CLAIMS OFFICE
1817 W BROADWAY
COLUMBIA, MO 65218-0001
TEL: (573) 445-8441
FAX: (573) 445-3199
TOLL FREE: (800) 743-5837
WWW.SHELTERINS.COM

COLORADO CLAIMS OFFICE
1817 W BROADWAY
COLUMBIA, MO 65218-0001
TEL: (573) 445-8441
FAX: (573) 445-3199
TOLL FREE: (800) 743-5837
WWW.SHELTERINS.COM

ILLINOIS CLAIMS OFFICE
1817 W BROADWAY
COLUMBIA, MO 65218-0001
TEL: (573) 445-8441
FAX: (573) 445-3199
TOLL FREE: (800) 743-5837
WWW.SHELTERINS.COM

INDIANA CLAIMS OFFICE
1817 W BROADWAY
COLUMBIA, MO 65218-0001
TEL: (573) 445-8441
FAX: (573) 445-3199
TOLL FREE: (800) 743-5837
WWW.SHELTERINS.COM

IOWA CLAIMS OFFICE
1817 W BROADWAY
COLUMBIA, MO 65218-0001
TEL: (573) 445-8441
FAX: (573) 445-3199
TOLL FREE: (800) 743-5837
WWW.SHELTERINS.COM

KANSAS CLAIMS OFFICE
1817 W BROADWAY
COLUMBIA, MO 65218-0001
TEL: (573) 445-8441
FAX: (573) 445-3199
TOLL FREE: (800) 743-5837
WWW.SHELTERINS.COM

KENTUCKY CLAIMS OFFICE
1817 W BROADWAY
COLUMBIA, MO 65218-0001
TEL: (573) 445-8441
FAX: (573) 445-3199
TOLL FREE: (800) 743-5837
WWW.SHELTERINS.COM

LOUISIANA CLAIMS OFFICE
1817 W BROADWAY
COLUMBIA, MO 65218-0001
TEL: (573) 445-8441
FAX: (573) 445-3199
TOLL FREE: (800) 743-5837
WWW.SHELTERINS.COM

MISSISSIPPI CLAIMS OFFICE
1817 W BROADWAY
COLUMBIA, MO 65218-0001
TEL: (573) 445-8441
FAX: (573) 445-3199
TOLL FREE: (800) 743-5837
WWW.SHELTERINS.COM

MISSOURI CLAIMS OFFICE
1817 W BROADWAY
COLUMBIA, MO 65218-0001
TEL: (573) 445-8441
FAX: (573) 445-3199
TOLL FREE: (800) 743-5837
WWW.SHELTERINS.COM

NEBRASKA CLAIMS OFFICE
1817 W BROADWAY
COLUMBIA, MO 65218-0001
TEL: (573) 445-8441
FAX: (573) 445-3199
TOLL FREE: (800) 743-5837
WWW.SHELTERINS.COM

OKLAHOMA CLAIMS OFFICE
1817 W BROADWAY
COLUMBIA, MO 65218-0001
TEL: (573) 445-8441
FAX: (573) 445-3199
TOLL FREE: (800) 743-5837
WWW.SHELTERINS.COM

TENNESSEE CLAIMS OFFICE
1817 W BROADWAY
COLUMBIA, MO 65218-0001
TEL: (573) 445-8441
FAX: (573) 445-3199
TOLL FREE: (800) 743-5837
WWW.SHELTERINS.COM

SIGMA ADMINISTRATORS

UTAH CLAIMS OFFICE
SELF INSURED GROUP MARKETING & ADMINISTRATION, INC
111 E 5600 S, STE 305
PO BOX 57767
SALT LAKE CITY, UT 84157-0767
TEL: (801) 263-3300
FAX: (801) 263-3319

SIGNA HEALTHCARE

MASSACHUSETTS CLAIMS OFFICE
HEALTHSOURCE OF MASSACHUSETTS
100 FRONT ST, STE 300
WORCESTER, MA 01608-1449
TEL: (508) 799-2642
FAX: (508) 849-4299
TOLL FREE: (800) 244-1870
IN-STATE: (800) 922-8380
WWW.SIGNAHEALTHCARE.COM

SILVER STATE MEDICAL ADMINISTRATORS

NEVADA CLAIMS OFFICE
PRIME SILVER STATE
2085 E SAHARA, STE B
PO BOX 14790
LAS VEGAS, NV 89114
TEL: (702) 732-0292
FAX: (800) 280-3782
TOLL FREE: (800) 230-3904

SOUTHERN BENEFIT ADMINISTRATORS, INC

TENNESSEE CLAIMS OFFICE
907 TWO MILE PKY, BLDG C
PO BOX 1449
GOODLETTSVILLE, TN 37070-1449
TEL: (615) 859-0131
FAX: (615) 859-0818
TOLL FREE: (800) 831-4914

TEXAS CLAIMS OFFICE
907 TWO MILE PKY, BLDG C
PO BOX 1449
GOODLETTSVILLE, TN 37070-1449
TEL: (615) 859-0131
FAX: (615) 859-0818
TOLL FREE: (800) 831-4914

SOUTHERN CALIFORNIA PIPE TRADES TRUST FUND

CALIFORNIA CLAIMS OFFICE
501 SHATTO PL- 5TH FL
LOS ANGELES, CA 90020-1713
TEL: (213) 385-6161
FAX: (213) 487-3640
IN-STATE: (800) 595-7473

SOUTHERN GROUP ADMINISTRATORS, INC

NATIONAL CLAIMS OFFICE
200 S MARSHALL ST
WINSTON-SALEM, NC 27101-5251
TEL: (336) 723-7111
FAX: (336) 722-4748
TOLL FREE: (800) 334-8159

SOUTHERN GUARANTY INSURANCE CO

ALABAMA CLAIMS OFFICE
PO BOX 235004
MONTGOMERY, AL 36123-5004
TEL: (334) 270-6000
FAX: (334) 270-6115
TOLL FREE: (800) 633-5606
WWW.SGIC.COM

ARKANSAS CLAIMS OFFICE
PO BOX 235004
MONTGOMERY, AL 36123-5004
TEL: (334) 270-6000
FAX: (334) 270-6115
TOLL FREE: (800) 633-5606
WWW.SGIC.COM

FLORIDA CLAIMS OFFICE
PO BOX 235004
MONTGOMERY, AL 36123-5004
TEL: (334) 270-6000
FAX: (334) 270-6115
TOLL FREE: (800) 633-5606
WWW.SGIC.COM

MISSISSIPPI CLAIMS OFFICE
PO BOX 235004
MONTGOMERY, AL 36123-5004
TEL: (334) 270-6000
FAX: (334) 270-6115
TOLL FREE: (800) 633-5606
WWW.SGIC.COM

SOUTHERN HEALTH PLAN, INC

TENNESSEE CLAIMS OFFICE
APPLE PLAN
600 JEFFERSON AVE
PO BOX 97
MEMPHIS, TN 38101-0097
TEL: (901) 544-2636
FAX: (901) 544-2440
TOLL FREE: (800) 527-9206

SOUTHERN HEALTH SERVICES

VIRGINIA CLAIMS OFFICE
9881 MAYLAND DR
PO BOX 85603
RICHMOND, VA 23285-5603
TEL: (804) 747-3700
FAX: (804) 747-8723
TOLL FREE: (800) 627-4872
WWW.SOUTHERNHEALTH.COM

SOUTHERN INSURANCE MANAGEMENT ASSOCIATION

ALABAMA CLAIMS OFFICE
1812 UNIVERSITY BLVD
PO BOX 1250
TUSCALOOSA, AL 35403-1250
TEL: (205) 345-3505
TOLL FREE: (800) 476-9928

SOUTHWEST ADMINISTRATORS

CALIFORNIA CLAIMS OFFICE
1000 S FREEMONT AVE
PO BOX 1121
ALHAMBRA, CA 91802-1121
TEL: (626) 284-4792

SPECIAL AGENTS MUTUAL BENEFIT ASSOCIATION

MARYLAND CLAIMS OFFICE
11301 OLD GEORGETOWN RD
ROCKVILLE, MD 20852-2800
TEL: (301) 984-1440
FAX: (301) 984-6224
TOLL FREE: (800) 638-6589
WWW.SAMBA-INSURANCE.COM

SPECTARA

2811 LORD BALTIMORE DR
BALTIMORE, MD 21244-2644
TEL: (410) 265-6033
FAX: (410) 944-5118
TOLL FREE: (800) 638-6265
IN-STATE: (800) 638-6265
WWW.SPECTARA.COM

ST. FRANCIS HOME CARE

SOUTH CAROLINA CLAIMS OFFICE
414 PETTIGRU ST
PO BOX 9312
GREENVILLE, SC 29605
TEL: (864) 233-5300
FAX: (864) 233-8473
WWW.STFRANCIS.COM

ST. LOUIS LABOR HEALTH INSTITUTE

MISSOURI CLAIMS OFFICE
300 S GRANDE BLVD
SAINT LOUIS, MO 63103-2430
TEL: (314) 658-5627
FAX: (314) 652-5022
TOLL FREE: (800) 466-5688

STANDARD LIFE & ACCIDENT INSURANCE CO

TEXAS CLAIMS OFFICE
ONE MOODY PLZ
PO BOX 1800
GALVESTON, TX 77553
TEL: (405) 290-1000
FAX: (409) 766-6663
TOLL FREE: (800) 827-2524

STATE FARM INSURANCE CO

ARIZONA CLAIMS OFFICE
SUNLAND
1665 W ALAMEDA DR
TEMPE, AZ 85289-0001
TEL: (602) 784-3000
FAX: (602) 784-3870
WWW.STATEFARM.COM

ILLINOIS CLAIMS OFFICE
ONE STATE FARM PLZ
PO BOX 2700
BLOOMINGTON, IL 61710
TEL: (309) 766-2311
TOLL FREE: (800) 538-4643
WWW.STATEFARM.COM

TEXAS CLAIMS OFFICE
8900 STATE FARM WAY
AUSTIN, TX 78729
TEL: (512) 918-4000
FAX: (512) 918-5298
WWW.STATEFARM.COM

STATE OF NEW YORK INSURANCE DEPARTMENT LIQUIDATION BUREAU

NEW YORK CLAIMS OFFICE
123 WILLIAM ST
NEW YORK, NY 10038-3804
TEL: (212) 341-6400
FAX: (212) 341-6104

TAYLOR EMPLOYEES HEALTH & DENTAL PLAN

ALABAMA CLAIMS OFFICE
1725 ROE CREST
PO BOX 3728
NORTH MANKATO, MN 56002-3728
TEL: (507) 625-2828
FAX: (507) 625-7742
TOLL FREE: (800) 345-6954

CALIFORNIA CLAIMS OFFICE
1725 ROE CREST
PO BOX 3728
NORTH MANKATO, MN 56002-3728
TEL: (507) 625-2828
FAX: (507) 625-7742
TOLL FREE: (800) 345-6954

FLORIDA CLAIMS OFFICE
1725 ROE CREST
PO BOX 3728
NORTH MANKATO, MN 56002-3728
TEL: (507) 625-2828
FAX: (507) 625-7742
TOLL FREE: (800) 345-6954

GEORGIA CLAIMS OFFICE
1725 ROE CREST
PO BOX 3728
NORTH MANKATO, MN 56002-3728
TEL: (507) 625-2828
FAX: (507) 625-7742
TOLL FREE: (800) 345-6954

IDAHO CLAIMS OFFICE
1725 ROE CREST
PO BOX 3728
NORTH MANKATO, MN 56002-3728
TEL: (507) 625-2828
FAX: (507) 625-7742
TOLL FREE: (800) 345-6954

ILLINOIS CLAIMS OFFICE
1725 ROE CREST
PO BOX 3728
NORTH MANKATO, MN 56002-3728
TEL: (507) 625-2828
FAX: (507) 625-7742
TOLL FREE: (800) 345-6954

INDIANA CLAIMS OFFICE
1725 ROE CREST
PO BOX 3728
NORTH MANKATO, MN 56002-3728
TEL: (507) 625-2828
FAX: (507) 625-7742
TOLL FREE: (800) 345-6954

IOWA CLAIMS OFFICE
1725 ROE CREST
PO BOX 3728
NORTH MANKATO, MN 56002-3728
TEL: (507) 625-2828
FAX: (507) 625-7742
TOLL FREE: (800) 345-6954

MINNESOTA CLAIMS OFFICE
1725 ROE CREST
PO BOX 3728
NORTH MANKATO, MN 56002-3728
TEL: (507) 625-2828
FAX: (507) 625-7742
TOLL FREE: (800) 345-6954

NEW JERSEY CLAIMS OFFICE
1725 ROE CREST
PO BOX 3728
NORTH MANKATO, MN 56002-3728
TEL: (507) 625-2828
FAX: (507) 625-7742
TOLL FREE: (800) 345-6954

NEW YORK CLAIMS OFFICE
1725 ROE CREST
PO BOX 3728
NORTH MANKATO, MN 56002-3728
TEL: (507) 625-2828
FAX: (507) 625-7742
TOLL FREE: (800) 345-6954

PENNSYLVANIA CLAIMS OFFICE
1725 ROE CREST
PO BOX 3728
NORTH MANKATO, MN 56002-3728
TEL: (507) 625-2828
FAX: (507) 625-7742
TOLL FREE: (800) 345-6954

TEXAS CLAIMS OFFICE
1725 ROE CREST
PO BOX 3728
NORTH MANKATO, MN 56002-3728
TEL: (507) 625-2828
FAX: (507) 625-7742
TOLL FREE: (800) 345-6954

WASHINGTON CLAIMS OFFICE
1725 ROE CREST
PO BOX 3728
NORTH MANKATO, MN 56002-3728
TEL: (507) 625-2828
FAX: (507) 625-7742
TOLL FREE: (800) 345-6954

TEACHERS PROTECTIVE MUTUAL LIFE INSURANCE CO

MARYLAND CLAIMS OFFICE
116-118 N PRINCE ST
PO BOX 597
LANCASTER, PA 17608-0597
TEL: (717) 394-7156
TOLL FREE: (800) 555-3122
WWW.TPMINS.COM

NEW JERSEY CLAIMS OFFICE
116-118 N PRINCE ST
PO BOX 597
LANCASTER, PA 17608-0597
TEL: (717) 394-7156
TOLL FREE: (800) 555-3122
WWW.TPMINS.COM

OHIO CLAIMS OFFICE
116-118 N PRINCE ST
PO BOX 597
LANCASTER, PA 17608-0597
TEL: (717) 394-7156
TOLL FREE: (800) 555-3122
WWW.TPMINS.COM

PENNSYLVANIA CLAIMS OFFICE
116-118 N PRINCE ST
PO BOX 597
LANCASTER, PA 17608-0597
TEL: (717) 394-7156
FAX: (717) 394-7024
TOLL FREE: (800) 555-3122
WWW.TPMINS.COM

VIRGINIA CLAIMS OFFICE
116-118 N PRINCE ST
PO BOX 597
LANCASTER, PA 17608-0597
TEL: (717) 394-7156
TOLL FREE: (800) 555-3122
WWW.TPMINS.COM

THE ALLIANCE

COLORADO CLAIMS OFFICE
A COMMUNITY HEALTH CARE PARTNERSHIP
650 S CHERRY ST, STE 300
DENVER, CO 80246
TEL: (303) 333-6767
FAX: (303) 322-3830
TOLL FREE: (800) 996-2447
E-MAIL: INFO@ALLIANCE-COLORADO.ORG
WWW.ALLIANCE-COLORADO.ORG

THE WHEELER COMPANIES

ALABAMA CLAIMS OFFICE
200 CAHABA PARK CIR, STE 250
PO BOX 43350
BIRMINGHAM, AL 35243-0350
TEL: (205) 995-8688
FAX: (940) 980-9047
TOLL FREE: (800) 741-8688

TOWER LIFE INSURANCE CO

TEXAS CLAIMS OFFICE
400 TOWER LIFE BLDG
310 S ST MARY ST, STE 400
SAN ANTONIO, TX 78205-3164
TEL: (210) 554-4400
FAX: (210) 554-4401
TOLL FREE: (800) 880-4576

TRAVELERS PROPERTY & CASUALTY

ILLINOIS CLAIMS OFFICE
215 SHUMAN BLVD
NAPERVILLE, IL 60563-8458
TOLL FREE: (800) 238-6225

TRIGON

NATIONAL CLAIMS OFFICE
BLUE CROSS & BLUE SHIELD
PO BOX 27280
RICHMOND, VA 23261
TEL: (804) 358-1551
FAX: (804) 354-4340
IN-STATE: (800) 451-1527

TRINITY UNIVERSAL INSURANCE CO

UNITURN
PO BOX 655028
DALLAS, TX 75265-5028
TEL: (214) 360-8000
FAX: (214) 360-8076
TOLL FREE: (800) 777-2249

TRUST MARK

10777 SUNSET OFFICE DR, STE 300
SAINT LOUIS, MO 63127-1080
TEL: (314) 984-0666
FAX: (314) 984-9380
IN-STATE: (800) 325-8628

TRUSTMARK INSURANCE

ARIZONA CLAIMS OFFICE
8324 S AVE
BOARDMAN, OH 44512-6417
TEL: (330) 758-2212
FAX: (330) 758-3242
TOLL FREE: (800) 544-7312
WWW.TRUSTMARKINS.COM

FLORIDA CLAIMS OFFICE
8324 S AVE
BOARDMAN, OH 44512-6417
TEL: (330) 758-2212
FAX: (330) 758-3242
TOLL FREE: (800) 544-7312
WWW.TRUSTMARKINS.COM

GEORGIA CLAIMS OFFICE
8324 S AVE
BOARDMAN, OH 44512-6417
TEL: (330) 758-2212
FAX: (330) 758-3242
TOLL FREE: (800) 544-7312
WWW.TRUSTMARKINS.COM

LOUISIANA CLAIMS OFFICE
8324 S AVE
BOARDMAN, OH 44512-6417
TEL: (330) 758-2212
FAX: (330) 758-3242
TOLL FREE: (800) 544-7312
WWW.TRUSTMARKINS.COM

MASSACHUSETTS CLAIMS OFFICE
8324 S AVE
BOARDMAN, OH 44512-6417
TEL: (330) 758-2212
FAX: (330) 758-3242
TOLL FREE: (800) 544-7312
WWW.TRUSTMARKINS.COM

MISSISSIPPI CLAIMS OFFICE
8324 S AVE
BOARDMAN, OH 44512-6417
TEL: (330) 758-2212
FAX: (330) 758-3242
TOLL FREE: (800) 544-7312
WWW.TRUSTMARKINS.COM

NEW JERSEY CLAIMS OFFICE
8324 S AVE
BOARDMAN, OH 44512-6417
TEL: (330) 758-2212
FAX: (330) 758-3242
TOLL FREE: (800) 544-7312
WWW.TRUSTMARKINS.COM

NORTH CAROLINA CLAIMS OFFICE
8324 S AVE
BOARDMAN, OH 44512-6417
TEL: (330) 758-2212
FAX: (330) 758-3242
TOLL FREE: (800) 544-7312
WWW.TRUSTMARKINS.COM

OHIO CLAIMS OFFICE
8324 S AVE
BOARDMAN, OH 44512-6417
TEL: (330) 758-2212
FAX: (330) 758-3242
TOLL FREE: (800) 544-7312
WWW.TRUSTMARKINS.COM

PENNSYLVANIA CLAIMS OFFICE
8324 S AVE
BOARDMAN, OH 44512-6417
TEL: (330) 758-2212
FAX: (330) 758-3242
TOLL FREE: (800) 544-7312
WWW.TRUSTMARKINS.COM

SOUTH CAROLINA CLAIMS OFFICE
8324 S AVE
BOARDMAN, OH 44512-6417
TEL: (330) 758-2212
FAX: (330) 758-3242
TOLL FREE: (800) 544-7312
WWW.TRUSTMARKINS.COM

TEXAS CLAIMS OFFICE
8324 S AVE
BOARDMAN, OH 44512-6417
TEL: (330) 758-2212
FAX: (330) 758-3242
TOLL FREE: (800) 544-7312
WWW.TRUSTMARKINS.COM

WEST VIRGINIA CLAIMS OFFICE
8324 S AVE
BOARDMAN, OH 44512-6417
TEL: (330) 758-2212
FAX: (330) 758-3242
TOLL FREE: (800) 544-7312
WWW.TRUSTMARKINS.COM

TRUSTMARK INSURANCE CO

ILLINOIS CLAIMS OFFICE
400 FIELD DR
LAKE FOREST, IL 60045-2586
TEL: (847) 615-1500
FAX: (847) 615-3910
WWW.TRUSTMARKINS.COM

UNICARE

NATIONAL CLAIMS OFFICE
SERVICE OFFICE
3820 AMERICAN DR
PLANO, TX 75070
TEL: (972) 599-6500
TOLL FREE: (800) 332-2060
WWW.WELLPOINT.COM

UNICARE ASSOCIATION SERVICES

13523 BARRET PKY, STE 250
PO BOX 120
BALLWIN, MO 63022-0120
TEL: (630) 679-4288
TOLL FREE: (800) 332-2060

UNICARE LIFE & HEALTH

CALIFORNIA CLAIMS OFFICE
3179 TEMPLE AVE, STE 200
POMONA, CA 91768
TEL: (909) 444-6000
FAX: (909) 444-6161

NATIONAL CLAIMS OFFICE
CLAIMS OFFICE
PO BOX 833947
RICHARDSON, TX 75083-3947
TEL: (972) 599-6500
TOLL FREE: (800) 332-2060
WWW.WELLPOINT.COM

3200 GREENFIELD RD
PO BOX 4479
DEARBORN, MI 48120
TEL: (313) 336-5550
TOLL FREE: (800) 332-2060
IN-STATE: (800) 843-8184

7025 ALBERTPICK RD- 5TH FL
GREENSBORO, NC 27409
TEL: (336) 665-1888
FAX: (336) 605-6406
TOLL FREE: (800) 597-6735

24650 CENTER RDG RD, STE 310
WESTLAKE, OH 44145-5680
TEL: (800) 543-4556
TOLL FREE: (800) 437-2277
IN-STATE: (800) 223-9940

UNION LABOR LIFE INSURANCE CO

DISTRICT OF COLUMBIA CLAIMS OFFICE
111 MASSACHUSETTS AVE NW
WASHINGTON, DC 20001
TEL: (202) 682-0900
FAX: (202) 682-8795

MASSACHUSETTS CLAIMS OFFICE
111 MASSACHUSETTS AVE NW
WASHINGTON, DC 20001
TEL: (202) 682-0900
FAX: (202) 682-8795

NATIONAL CLAIMS OFFICE
161 FORBES RD, STE 204
BRAINTREE, MA 02184-2606
TEL: (781) 848-7474
FAX: (781) 849-6113
TOLL FREE: (800) 248-0029

NEW YORK CLAIMS OFFICE
111 MASSACHUSETTS AVE NW
WASHINGTON, DC 20001
TEL: (202) 682-0900
FAX: (202) 682-8795

UNISYS

FLORIDA CLAIMS OFFICE
2525 S MONROE
TALLAHASSEE, FL 32301
TEL: (850) 671-0100
FAX: (850) 671-4528
TOLL FREE: (800) 289-7799

UNITED AMERICAN INSURANCE

ALABAMA CLAIMS OFFICE
3700 S STONEBRIDGE DR
PO BOX 8080
MCKINNEY, TX 75070-8080
TEL: (972) 529-5085
FAX: (972) 569-3688
WWW.UNITEDAMERICAN.COM

UNITED CHAMBERS ADMINISTRATORS

NATIONAL CLAIMS OFFICE
1805 HIGH PT DR
PO BOX 3048
NAPERVILLE, IL 60566-7048
TEL: (630) 505-3100
FAX: (630) 577-2915
TOLL FREE: (800) 323-3529
E-MAIL: INFO@ACLIC.COM
WWW.ACLIC.COM

UNITED FARM FAMILY MUTUAL INSURANCE

9135 BROADWAY
MARYVILLE, IN 46410
TEL: (219) 756-9650
FAX: (219) 756-9669
TOLL FREE: (800) 477-6767

UNITED GOVERNMENT SERVICES

BLUE CROSS & BLUE SHIELD UNITED OF WISCONSIN
401 W MICHIGAN ST
MILWAUKEE, WI 53212
TEL: (414) 226-5000
FAX: (414) 226-5226
TOLL FREE: (800) 558-1584
WWW.UWSI.COM

UNITED HEALTH CARE

TEXAS CLAIMS OFFICE
ADMINISTRATIVE SERVICES
555 N CARANCAHUA, STE 500
CORPUS CHRISTI, TX 78478
TEL: (512) 887-0101
FAX: (512) 887-8115
TOLL FREE: (800) 580-2247

UNITED HEALTHCARE

FLORIDA CLAIMS OFFICE
UNITED HEALTH CARE OF FLORIDA
11140 N KENDALL DR
MIAMI, FL 33183
TEL: (305) 596-5696
FAX: (305) 275-4050
TOLL FREE: (800) 543-3145
IN-STATE: (888) 716-8787
WWW.UHC.COM

ILLINOIS CLAIMS OFFICE
UNITED HEALTH CARE OF ILLINOIS
ONE S WACKER DR
CHICAGO, IL 60606
TEL: (312) 424-4460
FAX: (312) 424-5620
TOLL FREE: (800) 826-9400
WWW.UHC.COM

MISSOURI CLAIMS OFFICE
UNITED HEALTH CARE OF THE MIDWEST
969 EXECUTIVE PKY, STE 100
PO BOX 419080
SAINT LOUIS, MO 63141-9080
TOLL FREE: (800) 535-9291
WWW.UHC.COM

OHIO CLAIMS OFFICE
UNITED HEALTH CARE OF OHIO, INC
3650 OLENTANGY RIVER RD
PO BOX 182281
COLUMBUS, OH 43219
TEL: (614) 442-7100
FAX: (614) 442-3902
TOLL FREE: (800) 328-8835
IN-STATE: (800) 458-5346
WWW.UHC.COM

UNITED HEALTHCARE INSURANCE CO

MISSISSIPPI CLAIMS OFFICE
PO BOX 22545
JACKSON, MS 39225-2545
TEL: (601) 977-0208
FAX: (601) 977-5854

UNITED HEALTHCARE INSURANCE CO, PART A INTERMEDIARY

CONNECTICUT CLAIMS OFFICE
538 PRESTON AVE
PO BOX 1043
MERIDEN, CT 06450-1041
TEL: (203) 639-3230
FAX: (203) 639-3202

UNITED HEALTHCARE INSURANCE CO, PART B CARRIER
538 PRESTON AVE
PO BOX 1043
MERIDEN, CT 06450-1041
TEL: (203) 639-3124
FAX: (203) 639-3018

MINNESOTA CLAIMS OFFICE
8120 PENN AVE S
BLOOMINGTON, MN 55431-1394
TEL: (612) 884-3030
FAX: (612) 885-2839

VIRGINIA CLAIMS OFFICE
300 ARBORETUM PL- 4TH FL
PO BOX 26463
RICHMOND, VA 23261-3480
TEL: (804) 327-2211
FAX: (804) 327-2101

UNITED HERITAGE MUTUAL LIFE INSURANCE CO
IDAHO CLAIMS OFFICE
1212 12TH AVE RD
PO BOX 48
NAMPA, ID 83653-0048
TEL: (208) 466-7856
FAX: (208) 466-0825
TOLL FREE: (800) 657-6351
E-MAIL: HERITAGE@UNITEDHERITAGE.COM
WWW.UNITEDHERITAGE.COM

USI ADMINISTRATORS
NATIONAL CLAIMS OFFICE
JONES, HILL & MERCER EMPLOYEE BENEFITS
7402 HODGSON MEMORIAL DR #210
PO BOX 9888
SAVANNAH, GA 31406
TEL: (912) 691-1551
FAX: (912) 352-8935
TOLL FREE: (800) 631-3441

VALERO ENERGY CORP
TEXAS CLAIMS OFFICE
SOUTH TEXAS HEALTH CARE ALLIANCE
7990 W IH 10
SAN ANTONIO, TX 78230-4715
TEL: (210) 370-2776
FAX: (210) 370-2861
TOLL FREE: (800) 531-7911
IN-STATE: (800) 292-7816

VALERO HEALTHCARE ADMISSION
ILLINOIS CLAIMS OFFICE
CCN (CHICAGO AREA)
2269 S UNIVERSITY DR, STE 308
FT LAUDERDALE, FL 33324
TEL: (210) 370-2100
TOLL FREE: (800) 531-7911
IN-STATE: (800) 292-7816

VIACHRISTI ST. FRANCIS
KANSAS CLAIMS OFFICE
929 N ST FRANCIS
WICHITA, KS 67214
TEL: (316) 268-5192
FAX: (316) 268-6985
TOLL FREE: (800) 362-0070

VIACHRISTI ST. JOSEPH MEDICAL CENTER
3600 E HARRY ST
WICHITA, KS 67218-3784
TEL: (316) 685-1111
TOLL FREE: (800) 851-0051

VIRGINIA SURETY CO
ILLINOIS CLAIMS OFFICE
4850 STREET RD
TREVOSE, PA 19049
TEL: (215) 953-3000
FAX: (215) 953-3156
TOLL FREE: (800) 523-6599
IN-STATE: (800) 523-5758

PENNSYLVANIA CLAIMS OFFICE
4850 STREET RD
TREVOSE, PA 19049
TEL: (215) 953-3000
FAX: (215) 953-3156
TOLL FREE: (800) 523-6599
IN-STATE: (800) 523-5758

WARD NORTH AMERICA, INC
ALASKA CLAIMS OFFICE
3330 ARCTIC BLVD, STE 206
ANCHORAGE, AK 99503
TEL: (907) 561-1725
FAX: (907) 562-6595
WWW.WARDNA.COM

WAUSAU INSURANCE CO
WISCONSIN CLAIMS OFFICE
200 WESTWOOD DR
PO BOX 8013
WAUSAU, WI 54401-7881
TEL: (715) 845-5211
FAX: (715) 847-7569
TOLL FREE: (800) 826-9781
WWW.WAUSAU.COM

WEA INSURANCE GROUP
45 NOB HILL RD
PO BOX 7338
MADISON, WI 53707-7330
TEL: (608) 276-4000
FAX: (608) 276-9119
TOLL FREE: (800) 279-4000

WESTCHESTER TEAMSTERS HEALTH & WELFARE
NEW YORK CLAIMS OFFICE
160 S CENTRAL AVE
ELMSFORD, NY 10523-3521
TEL: (914) 592-9330
FAX: (914) 592-1519

WEYCO, INC
NATIONAL CLAIMS OFFICE
PO BOX 30132
LANSING, MI 48909-7632
TEL: (517) 349-7010
FAX: (517) 349-7335
TOLL FREE: (800) 748-0003
WWW.WEYCOINC.COM

WEYERHAEUSER CO
WASHINGTON CLAIMS OFFICE
GROUP INSURANCE SERVICES
1145 BROADWAY, STE 600
PO BOX TF-C
TACOMA, WA 98402-3527
TEL: (253) 924-7381
FAX: (253) 924-3221
TOLL FREE: (800) 833-0030

WILLSE & ASSOCIATES
MARYLAND CLAIMS OFFICE
MEDICAL CLAIMS DEPARTMENT
100 S CHARLES- TWR 2, STE 9
PO BOX 1196
BALTIMORE, MD 21297-0417
TEL: (410) 347-1925
FAX: (410) 347-1924
TOLL FREE: (800) 423-9791

WISCONSIN PHYSICIANS SERVICE INSURANCE CO (WPS)
WISCONSIN CLAIMS OFFICE
CHAMPUS INTERMEDIARY FOR WISCONSIN
1717 W BROADWAY
PO BOX 1890
MADISON, WI 53703
TEL: (608) 221-4711
FAX: (608) 223-3626
TOLL FREE: (800) 828-2837
WWW.WPSIC.COM

WISCONSIN SHEETMETAL HEALTH
PO BOX 3500
MADISON, WI 53704
TEL: (608) 277-0477
TOLL FREE: (800) 779-7577

XACT MEDICARE SERVICES — MEDICARE PART B CARRIER
PENNSYLVANIA CLAIMS OFFICE
1800 CENTER ST
PO BOX 890089
CAMP HILL, PA 17089-0089
TEL: (717) 763-5700
FAX: (717) 760-9296
WWW.XACT.ORG

ZENITH ADMINISTRATORS, INC
CALIFORNIA CLAIMS OFFICE
6801 E WASHINGTON BLVD
PO BOX 22041
COMMERCE, CA 90022
TEL: (323) 724-1144

ILLINOIS CLAIMS OFFICE
2873 N DIRKSEN PKY, STE 200
SPRINGFIELD, IL 62702
TEL: (217) 753-4531
FAX: (217) 753-3953
TOLL FREE: (800) 538-6466

MARYLAND CLAIMS OFFICE
1320 PATUXTENT PKY, STE 610
PO BOX 1100
COLUMBIA, MD 21044
TEL: (410) 884-1440
FAX: (410) 997-3657
TOLL FREE: (800) 235-5805
E-MAIL: ZENITH TPA.COM
WWW.ZENITH TPA

MISSOURI CLAIMS OFFICE
3100 BROADWAY, STE 400
KANSAS CITY, MO 64111
TEL: (818) 756-0173
FAX: (816) 531-6518

NATIONAL CLAIMS OFFICE
4380 SW MACADAN AVE, STE 300
PO BOX 1420
PORTLAND, OR 97201
TEL: (503) 226-6753
FAX: (503) 226-7900
TOLL FREE: (800) 547-5900

WISCONSIN CLAIMS OFFICE
2100 N MAYFAIR RD, STE 100
MILWAUKEE, WI 53226
TEL: (414) 476-1220
FAX: (414) 476-2997
TOLL FREE: (800) 242-4712
WWW.ZENITHTPA.COM

2801 COHO ST, STE 300
MADISON, WI 53713
TEL: (608) 274-4773
FAX: (608) 277-1088
TOLL FREE: (800) 397-3373

Appendix B

Abbreviations

State and Province Abbreviations

ALABAMA .... AL
ALASKA .... AK
AMERICAN SAMOA .... AS
ARIZONA .... AZ
ARKANSAS .... AR
CALIFORNIA .... CA
COLORADO .... CO
CONNECTICUT .... CT
DELAWARE .... DE
DISTRICT OF COLUMBIA .... DC
FEDERATED STATES OF MICRONESIA .... FM
FLORIDA .... FL
GEORGIA .... GA
GUAM .... GU
HAWAII .... HI
IDAHO .... ID
ILLINOIS IL
INDIANA .... IN
IOWA .... IA
KANSAS .... KS
KENTUCKY .... KY
LOUISIANA .... LA
MAINE .... ME
MARSHALL ISLANDS .... MH
MARYLAND .... MD
MASSACHUSETTS .... MA
MICHIGAN .... MI
MINNESOTA .... MN
MISSISSIPPI .... MS
MISSOURI .... MO
MONTANA .... MT
NEBRASKA .... NE
NEVADA .... NV
NEW HAMPSHIRE .... NH
NEW JERSEY .... NJ
NEW MEXICO .... NM
NEW YORK .... NY
NORTH CAROLINA .... NC
NORTH DAKOTA .... ND
NORTHERN MARIANA ISLANDS .... MP
OHIO .... OH
OKLAHOMA .... OK
OREGON .... OR
PALAU .... PW
PENNSYLVANIA .... PA
PEURTO RICO .... PR
RHODE ISLAND .... RI
SOUTH CAROLINA .... SC
SOUTH DAKOTA .... SD
TENNESSEE .... TN
TEXAS .... TX
UTAH .... UT
VERMONT .... VT
VIRGIN ISLANDS VI
VIRGINIA .... VA
WASHINGTON .... WA
WEST VIRGINIA .... WV
WISCONSIN .... WI
WYOMING .... WY

Geographic Directional Abbreviations

NORTH .... N
EAST .... E
SOUTH .... S
WEST .... W
NORTHEAST .... NE
SOUTHEAST .... SE
SOUTHWEST .... SW
NORTHWEST .... NW

Regional Abbreviations

ALL REGIONS .... NATL
CENTRAL REGION .... CR
EASTERN REGION .... ER
NORTHEAST REGION .... NE
SOUTHERN REGION .... SR
WESTERN REGION .... WR

Abbreviations for Street Designators

Street Suffix or Suffix Abbrev.	USPS Suffix Abbrev
ALLEE	ALY
ALLEY	ALY
ALLY	ALY
ANEX	ANX
ANNEX	ANX
ANNX	ANX
ARCADE	ARC
AV	AVE
AVEN	AVE
AVENU	AVE
AVENUE	AVE
AVN	AVE
AVNUE	AVE
BAYOO	BYU
BAYOU	BYU
BEACH	BCH
BEND	BND
BLUF	BLF
BLUFF	BLF
BLUFFS	BLF
BOT	BTM
BOTTM	BTM
BOTTOM	BTM
BOUL	BLVD
BOULEVARD	BLVD
BOULV	BLVD
BRANCH	BR
BRDGE	BRG
BRIDGE	BRG
BRNCH	BR
BROOK	BRK
BROOKS	BRK
BURG	BG
BURGS	BG
BYPA	BYP
BYPAS	BYP
BYPASS	BYP
BYPS	BYP
CAMP	CP
CANYN	CYN
CANYON	CYN
CAPE	CPE
CAUSEWAY	CSWY
CAUSWAY	CSWY
CEN	CTR
CENT	CTR
CENTER	CTR
CENTERS	CTR
CENTR	CTR
CIRC	CIR
CIRCL	CIR
CIRCLE	CIR

Street Suffix or Suffix Abbrev.	USPS Suffix Abbrev
CRCLES	CIR
CLF	CLFS
CLIFF	CLFS
CLIFFS	CLFS
CLUB	CLB
CMP	CP
CNTER	CTR
CNTR	CTR
CNYN	CYN
CORNER	COR
CORNERS	CORS
COURSE	CRSE
COURT	CT
COURTS	CTS
COVE	CV
COVES	CV
CRCL	CIR
CIRCLE	CIR
CRECENT	CRES
CREEK	CRK
CREST	CRES
CRESCENT	CRES
CRESENT	CRES
CROSSING	XING
CRSCENT	CRES
CRSENT	CRES
CRSNT	CRES
CRSSNG	XING
DALE	DL
DAM	DM
DIV	DV
DIVIDE	DV
DRIV	DR
DRIVE	DR
DRIVES	DR
DRV	DR
DVD	DV
ESTATE	EST
ESTATES	EST
ESTS	EST
EXP	EXPY
EXPR	EXPY
EXPRESS	EXPY
EXPRESSWAY	EXPY
EXPW	EXP
EXTENSION	EXT
EXTN	EXT
EXTNSN	EXT
EXTS	EXT
FALLS	FLS
FERRY	FRY
FIELD	FLD
FIELDS	FLDS
FLAT	FLT
FLATS	FLT
FLTS	FLT

Street Suffix or Suffix Abbrev.	USPS Suffix Abbrev
FORD	FRD
FORDS	FRD
FOREST	FRST
FORESTS	FRST
FORG	FRG
FORGE	FRG
FORGES	FRG
FORK	FRK
FORKS	FRKS
FORT	FT
FREEWAY	FWY
FREEWY	FWY
FRRY	FRY
FRT	FT
FRWAY	FWY
FRWY	FWY
GARDEN	GDNS
GARDENS	GDNS
GARDN	GDNS
GATEWAY	GTWY
GATEWY	GTWY
GATWAY	GTWY
GDN	GDNS
GLEN	GLN
GLENS	GLN
GRDEN	GDNS
GRDN	GDNS
GRDNS	GDNS
GREEN	GRN
GREENS	GRN
GROV	GRV
GROVE	GRV
GTWAY	GTWY
HARB	HBR
HARBOR	HBR
HARBORS	HBR
HARBR	HBR
HAVEN	HVN
HAVN	HVN
HEIGHT	HTS
HEIGHTS	HTS
HIGHWAY	HWY
HIGHWY	HWY
HILL	HL
HILLS	HLS
HIWAY	HWY
HIWY	HWY
HLLW	HOLW
HOLLOW	HOLW
HOLWS	HOLW
HRBOR	HBR
HT	HTS
HWAY	HWY
INLET	INLT
ISLAND	IS
ISLANDS	ISS

Street Suffix or Suffix Abbrev.	USPS Suffix Abbrev
ISLES	ISLE
ISLND	IS
ISLNDS	ISS
JCTION	JCT
JCTN	JCT
JCTNS	JCT
JCTS	JCT
JUNCTION	JCT
JUNCTN	JCT
JUNCTON	JCT
KEY	KY
KEYS	KY
KNL	KNLS
KNOL	KNLS
KNOLL	KNLS
KNOLLS	KNLS
KYS	KY
LAKE	LK
LAKES	LKS
LANDING	LNDG
LANE	LN
LANES	LN
LDGE	LDG
LIGHT	LGT
LIGHTS	LGT
LNDNG	LNDG
LOAF	LF
LOCK	LCKS
LOCKS	LCKS
LODG	LDG
LODGE	LDG
LOOPS	LOOP
MANOR	MNR
MANORS	MNR
MDW	MDWS
MEADOW	MDWS
MEADOWS	MDWS
MEDOWS	MDWS
MILL	ML
MILLS	MLS
MISSION	MSN
MISSN	MSN
MNRS	MNR
MNT	MT
MNTAIN	MTN
MNTN	MTN
MNTNS	MTN
MOUNT	MT
MOUNTAIN	MTN
MOUNTIN	MTN
MSSN	MSN
MTIN	MTN
NECK	NCK
ORCHARD	ORCH
ORCHRD	ORCH
OVL	OVAL

Street Suffix or Suffix Abbrev.	USPS Suffix Abbrev
PARKS	PARK
PARKWAY	PKY
PARKWY	PKY
PATHS	PATH
PIKES	PIKE
PINE	PNES
PINES	PNES
PKWAY	PKY
PKWY	PKY
PKWYS	PKY
PLACE	PL
PLAIN	PLN
PLAINES	PLNS
PLAZA	PLZ
PLZA	PLZ
POINT	PT
POINTS	PT
PORT	PRT
PORTS	PRT
PRARIE	PR
PRK	PARK
PRR	PR
PRTS	PRT
PTS	PT
RAD	RADL
RADIAL	RADL
RADIEL	RADL
RANCHES	RNCH
RAPID	RPDS
RAPIDS	RPDS
RDGE	RDG
RDGS	RDG
RDS	RD
REST	RST
RIDGE	RDG
RIDGES	RDG
RIVER	RIV
RIVR	RIV
RNCHS	RNCH
ROAD	RD
ROADS	RD
RPD	RPDS
RVR	RIV
SHOAL	SHL
SHOALS	SHLS
SHOAR	SHR
SHOARS	SHRS
SHORE	SHR
SHORES	SHRS
SPNG	SPG
SPNGS	SPGS
SPRING	SPG
SPRINGS	SPGS
SPRNG	SPG
SPRNGS	SPGS
SPURS	SPUR
SQR	SQ
SQRE	SQ
SQU	SQ
SQUARE	SQ
SQUARES	SQ
STATION	STA
STATN	STA
STN	STA
STR	ST
STRAV	STRA
STRAVE	STRA
STRAVEN	STRA
STRAVENUE	STRA
STRAVN	STRA
STREAM	STRM
STREET	ST
STREETS	ST
STREME	STRM
STRT	ST
STRVN	STRA
STRVNUE	STRA
SUMIT	SMT
SUMITT	SMT
SUMMIT	SMT
TERR	TER
TERRACE	TER
TPK	TPKE
TRACE	TRCE
TRACES	TRCE
TRACK	TRAK
TRACKS	TRAK
TRAIL	TRL
TRAILER	TRLR
TRAILS	TRL
TRK	TRAK
TRKS	TRAK
TRLRS	TRLR
TRLS	TRL
TRNPK	TPKE
TUNEL	TUNL
TUNLS	TUNL
TUNNEL	TUNL
TUNNL	TUNL
TURNPIKE	TPKE
TURNPK	TPKE
UNION	UN
UNIONS	UN
VALLEY	VLY
VALLEYS	VLY
VALLY	VLY
VDCT	VIA
VIADCT	VIA
VIADUCT	VIA
VIEW	VW
VIEWS	VW
VILL	VLG

Street Suffix or Suffix Abbrev.	USPS Suffix Abbrev
VILLAG	VLG
VILLAGE	VLG
VILLE	VL
VILLG	VLG
VILLIAGE	VLG
VIST	VIS
VISTA	VIS
VLG	VLG
VLGS	VLG
VLLY	VLY
VLYS	VLY
VST	VIS
VSTA	VIS
VWS	VW
WALKS	WALK
WAYS	WAY
WELL	WLS
WELLS	WLS
WY	WAY

USPS Approved Envelope Addressing Formats

MISS JANICE SMITH
PO BOX 34
DULUTH MN 55803-0034

336543M 80V
MS LOIS SMITH
4653 GEORGIA AVE NW
WASHINGTON DC 22001-7128

H E BROWN
RR 3 BOX 9
CANTON OH 44730-9521

MR STANLEY DOE
LAST NATIONAL BANK
PO BOX 345
NEW YORK NY 10163-0345

MR JAMES F JONES
4417 BROOKS ST NE
WASHINGTON DC 20019-4649

ACME INSURANCE CO
CAREW TOWERS
300 E MAIN ST RM 1121
MEMPHIS TN 38166-1121

B G LIGHT CO
HC 2 BOX 293A
DULUTH MN 55811-9702

PVT WILLARD J SMITH
COMPANY F
167TH INFANTRY REGT
APO NEW YORK NY 09801-1087

MR THOMAS CLARK
17 RUSSELL DRIVE
LONDON WIP 6HQ
ENGLAND

MS HELEN SANDERS
1010 CLEAR ST
OTTAWA ON K1AOB1
CANADA

Appendix C

Mergers and Acquisitions

The companies listed were involved in a merger or acquisition during the past year.

ACACIA MUTUAL LIFE INSURANCE CO

ACS NORTH AMERICAN

AEGON INSURANCE GROUP

AETNA / U.S. HEALTHCARE

AETNA / U.S. HEALTHCARE CO

ALLIANZ LIFE INSURANCE CO OF NORTH AMERICA

ALLIED GROUP INSURANCE CO

ALLIED INSURANCE CO

ALLSTATE INSURANCE CO

AMERICA RE-INSURANCE

AMERICAN COMMERCIAL LINES

AMERICAN POLICY HOLDERS LIQUIDATING TRUST

AMERICAN TRAVEL, INC

AMERIHEALTH

ANTHEM INSURANCE

ANTHEM SERVICES ADMINISTRATORS

ARTHUR J. GALLAGAR & CO

BALBOA INSURANCE

BANKERS LIFE & CASUALTY CO

BEECH STREET, INC

BETTER BRANDS & AFFILIATES

BITUMINOUS CASUALTY CORP

BLUE CROSS & BLUE SHIELD

CERTIFIED LIFE INSURANCE CO

CGU

CGU INSURANCE / GENERAL ACCIDENT

CGU INTERNS CO

CHUBB GROUP OF INSURANCE COMPANIES

CNA

COLUMBIA INSURANCE GROUP

COMBINED INSURANCE

COMMERCIAL GENERAL UNION

COMMERCIAL UNION INSURANCE CO OF AMERICA

COMPANION LIFE INSURANCE CO

CONSECO

CONSECO DIRECT LIFE INSURANCE CO

CONSOLIDATED NATURAL GAS CO

CONTECH CONSTRUCTION PRODUCTS INC

CONTINENTAL WESTERN INSURANCE CO

CORESOURCE, INC

CORESTAR

COVENTRY HEALTHCARE

CPIC LIFE

CRUM & FORSTER INSURANCE

EAGLE PACIFIC INSURANCE CO

EAU CLAIRE HEALTH PROTECTION PLAN

FARMERS CASUALTY INSURANCE CO

FARMERS INSURANCE GROUP

FARMLAND INSURANCE CO

FIREMAN'S FUND INSURANCE CO

FIREMAN'S INSURANCE CO OF WASHINGTON, DC

FREMONT COMPENSATION INSURANCE CO

GEM INSURANCE CO

GENERAL REINSURANCE CORP

GERLING GLOBAL REINSURANCE CORP

GRE INSURANCE GROUP

GREAT AMERICAN INSURANCE COMPANIES

GREAT WEST LIFE

GREAT-WEST LIFE & ANNUITY

GREAT-WEST LIFE ASSURANCE CO

GROCER'S INSURANCE GROUP

GROUP HEALTH PLAN OF ST. LOUIS

GROUP HEALTH PLAN OF ST LOUIS

HEALTH CARE PLAN

HEALTH CARE SERVICE CORP

HEALTH GUARD SERVICES, INC

HEALTH NET

HEALTH SERVICES MEDICAL CORP

HIGHLANDS INSURANCE

HIGHLANDS NORTHWESTERN NATIONAL INSURANCE CO

HMO ILLINOIS

HOMETOWN HEALTH NETWORK

IBA HEALTH & LIFE ASSURANCE CO

INDIANA INSURANCE CO

INDIANAPOLIS LIFE

INTERGROUP OF UTAH, INC

INTERNATIONAL BENEFIT SERVICES CORP

IU MEDICAL GROUP PRIMARY CARE

JEFFERSON PILOT FINANCIAL

JOHN ALDEN LIFE INSURANCE CO

KAISER PERMANENTE

KEMPER INSURANCE COMPANIES

LIFE INSURANCE CO OF NORTH AMERICA

LIFE INVESTORS

MERIDIAN CITIZENS SECURITY MUTUAL INSURANCE CO

MERIT LIFE INSURANCE CO

METRA HEALTHCARE NETWORK OF WISCONSIN, INC

METROPOLITAN LIFE INSURANCE CO

MICHIGAN MILLERS MUTUAL INSURANCE

MICHIGAN MUTUAL INSURANCE CO

NEW MEXICO PHYSICIANS INSURANCE

NOVA HEALTHCARE ADMINISTRATORS

NYL CARE

OHIO CASUALTY GROUP

ONE BENEFIT SOURCE

PREFERRED HEALTH NETWORK

PRINCIPAL HEALTH CARE, INC

PROFESSIONAL RISK MANAGEMENT

SELF-INSURED MANAGEMENT SERVICE

SIGNA HEALTHCARE

TEXAS SAVING LIFE INSURANCE

UNITED HEALTHCARE

WARD NORTH AMERICA

WASATCH CREST INSURANCE CO

WAUSAU INSURANCE COMPANY

Appendix D

Email and Web Site Addresses

EMAIL ADDRESSES

ADMINISTRATION SERVICES, INC . . . . ASI@ADMIN-SERV.COM

ADMINISTRATIVE SERVICES, INC . . . . INFO@ADMINSERV.COM

AMERITAS LIFE INSURANCE CORP . . . . GROUP@AMERITAS.COM

BEAR RIVER MUTUAL INSURANCE CO . . . . BRMUTUAL.COM

BENEFIT ADMINISTRATIVE SYSTEMS, LTD . . . . ADMIN@BENADMINSYS.COM

BENEFIT ADMINISTRATORS, INC . . . . CLAIMS@BATPA.COM

BENEFIT PLANNERS, INC . . . . SERVICE@BENPLAN.COM

BENICOMP, INC . . . . BENICOMP@BENICOMP.COM

BENICORP INSURANCE CO . . . . CLAIMS@BENICORP.COM

BERWANGER OVERMYER ASSOCIATES . . . . BOA@BOA-INS.COM

BEST LIFE ASSURANCE CO OF CALIFORNIA . . . . BASSURANCE@EARTHLINK.NET

BLUE CROSS & BLUE SHIELD . . . . WEBINPUT@BCBSAL.ORG

BRADFORD FINANCIAL CENTER . . . . BRADFORD@NETINS.NET

CALENDS GROUP . . . . CALENDS1@AOL.COM

CALIFORNIA ASSOCIATION OF EMPLOYERS . . . . INFO@EMPLOYERS.ORG

CANADA LIFE ASSURANCE CO . . . . INFO@CANADALIFE.COM

CANON COCHRAN MANAGEMENT SERVICES, INC . . . . CCMSI@CCMSI.COM

CAPITAL DISTRICT PHYSICIANS' HEALTH PLAN, INC . . . INFO@CDPHP.COM

CARE MANAGEMENT 2000, INC . . . . CM2000INC@AOL.COM

CENTRAL RESERVE LIFE INSURANCE CO OF NORTH AMERICA . . . . CLAIMS@CENTRALRESERVE.COM

CENTURY PLANNERS, LLC .... CPLLTD@ANET-STL.COM

CLAIMS ADMINISTRATION SERVICES, INC .... INFO@CASI.COM

COLUMBUS LIFE INSURANCE CO .... CLIENT.SERVICES@COLUMBUSLIFE.COM

COMPANION LIFE INSURANCE CO .... C.LIFECOMPANIONGROUP.COM

CONSOLIDATED HEALTH PLANS .... CHP@VGERNET.NET

CONSUMER HEALTH NETWORK .... MARKETING@4CHN.COM

CORPORATE BENEFIT SERVICES OF AMERICA, INC .... CUSTOMER.SERVICE@CBSAINC.COM

DELTA DENTAL INSURANCE CO .... DDPSD@DTGNET.COM

DELTA DENTAL OF CALIFORNIA .... CMS@DELTA.ORG

DELTA DENTAL PLAN OF WISCONSIN .... OPERATIONS@DELTADENTALWI.COM

EDUCATORS MUTUAL LIFE INSURANCE CO .... CALLCENTER@EMLIFE.COM

EMPLOYEE BENEFIT SYSTEMS CORP .... EBS4BENEFITS@LISCO.NET

EQUITABLE LIFE & CASUALTY INSURANCE CO .... INFO@EQUILIFE.COM

ERIE INSURANCE CO .... ERIE-INSURANCE.COM

EXCESS REINSURANCE UNDERWRITERS AGENCY, INC . ACCESS@WORLDNET.ATT.NET

FARM BUREAU MUTUAL INSURANCE CO OF IDAHO ... IDFBHA@MICRON.NET

FOREIGN SERVICE BENEFIT PLAN .... AFSPA@AFSPA.ORG

GAB ROBINS NORTH AMERICA .... ANSWERS@GABROBINS.COM

GAINSCO, INC .... CLAIMS@GAINSCO.COM

GILSBAR, INC .... GILSBAR@GILSBAR.COM

GREAT REPUBLIC LIFE INSURANCE CO .... GRLIC@AOL.COM

HEALTH AGENCIES OF THE WEST, INC .... HAWADMIN@AOL.COM

HEALTH FIRST .... HFIRSTDP@ACC-NET.COM

HEALTH MANAGEMENT ASSOCIATES .... HMA@VERDINET.COM

HEALTH PLAN SERVICES .... HEALTHCARE.COM

HEALTH SPECIAL RISK, INC .... HSRTEXAS@COMPETEK.NET

HEALTHPLEX, INC .... HEALTHPLEX@AOL.COM

HELLER ASSOCIATES .... CLAIMS@HELLERTPA.COM

HERITAGE INSURANCE MANAGERS, INC .... SALES@HERITAGE-INS.COM

HOLYOKE MUTUAL INSURANCE CO .... INFO@HOLYOKEMUTUAL.COM

IHC HEALTH PLANS .... WEBMASTER@IHC.COM

INDIANAPOLIS LIFE .... CORPCOMMSG.INDIANAPOLISLIFE.COM

INTERNATIONAL BENEFIT SERVICES CORP	IBSTX@AOL.COM
J.P. FARLEY CORP	BENEFITS@JPFARLEY.COM
JENKINS & ATHENS INSURANCE SERVICES	INFO@JENKINS-ATHENS.COM
JFP BENEFIT MANAGEMENT	DPELHAM@IBM.NET
KEMPER INSURANCE COMPANIES	KEMPERINSURANCE.COM
L.I.U. OF NORTH AMERICA LOCAL 415	BENEFIT415@AOL.COM
LONE STAR LIFE INSURANCE CO	LSLCLMS2@DFW.NET
LOOMIS CO	LOOMIS@LOOMISCO.COM
MADISON NATIONAL LIFE INSURANCE CO, INC	MNLMADISN#@AOL.COM
MAKSIN MANAGEMENT CORP	MAKSIN@MAKSIN.COM
MEDEX ASSISTANCE CORP	MEDEXASST@AOL.COM
MEDICAID FISCAL AGENTS	CONSULTEC-IIX.COM/
MEDICARE — PART A INTERMEDIARIES	MEDICARE@BCBSME.COM
MICHIGAN EMPLOYEE BENEFIT SERVICES	CUSTSERV@MEBS.COM
MUTUAL MED BENEFIT ADMINISTRATORS	MUTUAL@AOL.COM
NATIONAL INDEMNITY CO	NICOCLAIMS@AOL.COM
NORTH AMERICA ADMINISTRATORS, INC	NAA@WORLDNET.ATT.NET
NORTHEAST DELTA DENTAL	NEDELTA@NEDELTA.COM
PITTMAN & ASSOCIATES, INC	PITTMAN@LUNAWEB.NET
PROFESSIONAL ADMINISTRATION GROUP	ADM-SVC@SWBELL.NET
PROFESSIONAL ADMINISTRATORS, INC	PA1001@AOL.COM
PROGRESSIVE CASUALTY INSURANCE CO	PROGRESSIVE.COM
PROVIDENT AMERICAN INSURANCE CO	PAIC@FLASH.NET
ROYAL & SUNALLIANCE	ROYAL-USA.COM
TENCO SERVICES	CLAIMS@TENCO.COM
THE ALLIANCE	INFO@ALLIANCE-COLORADO.ORG
TRIBUS COMPANIES	TRIBUTE.COM
UNITED CHAMBERS ADMINISTRATORS	INFO@ACLIC.COM
UNITED HERITAGE MUTUAL LIFE INSURANCE CO	HERITAGE@UNITEDHERITAGE.COM
VISION SERVICE PLAN	MEMBER@LAS.VSP.COM
WALDEN RISK MANAGEMENT GROUP	WRMGCW@AOL.COM
WAUSAU INSURANCE CO	WAUSAU.COM/MAIL.MTM

WESTFIELD COMPANIES .... WEBMASTER@WESTFIELD-COS.COM
WICHITA NATIONAL LIFE INSURANCE CO .... WNI@SIRINIT.NET
WILLIS CORROON CORP .... HALL_CP@WILCOR.COM
WILTON ADJUSTMENT SERVICES .... WILTON@ALASKA.NET
WORKMEN'S CIRCLE .... WCFRIENDS@AOL.COM
ZENITH ADMINISTRATORS, INC .... ZENITH TPA.COM

WEB SITES

20TH CENTURY INSURANCE CO WWW.20THCENTINS.COM
AARP CLAIMS UNIT .... WWW.AARPHEALTHCARE.COM
ACACIA MUTUAL LIFE INSURANCE CO .... WWW.ACACIAGROUP.COM
ACORDIA NATIONAL .... WWW.ACORDIA.COM
ADMAR CORP .... WWW.ADMARINC.COM
ADMINISTRATION SYSTEMS RESEARCH CORP .... WWW.ASRCORP.COM
ADMINISTRATION SYSTEMS RESEARCH CORP .... WWW.PHYSICIANSCARE.COM
ADMINISTRATIVE SERVICE CONSULTANTS .... WWW.ASCOFOHIO.COM
ADMINISTRATIVE SERVICES, INC .... WWW.ADMINSERV.COM
ADMIRAL INSURANCE CO .... WWW.ADMIRALINS.COM
AEGON INSURANCE GROUP .... WWW.AEGON.COM
AETNA LIFE INSURANCE CO OF CANADA .... WWW.AETNA.COM
AETNA / U.S. HEALTHCARE .... WWW.AETNAUSHC.COM
AFLAC .... WWW.AFLAC.COM
AGENCY SERVICES, INC .... WWW.AGENCYSERVICES.COM
AGIA, INC .... WWW.AGIA.COM
AIG CLAIM SERVICES, INC .... WWW.AIG.COM
ALFA INSURANCE CORP .... WWW.ALFAINS.COM
ALL AMERICA FINANCIAL .... WWW.ALLMERICA.COM
ALLIANCE BLUE CROSS & BLUE SHIELD .... WWW.BCBSMO.COM
ALLIANCE UNDERWRITERS, LLC .... WWW.ALLIANCEU.COM

ALLIANZ LIFE INSURANCE CO OF NORTH AMERICA . . . . WWW.ALLIANZLIFE.COM

ALLIED BENEFIT SYSTEMS, INC . . . . WWW.ALLIEDBENEFIT.COM

ALLIED GROUP INSURANCE CO . . . . WWW.ALLIEDGROUP.COM

ALLMERICA FINANCIAL . . . . WWW.ALLMERICA.COM

ALLSTATE INSURANCE CO . . . . WWW.ALLSTATE.COM

ALTERNATIVE HEALTH CARE . . . . WWW.AICI.COM

AM CASTLE & CO NON-BARGAINING . . . . WWW.AMCASTLE.COM

AMERAPLAN, INC . . . . WWW.AMERIPLAN.COM

AMERICAN AGRICULTURAL INSURANCE CO . . . . WWW.AAIC.FB.COM

AMERICAN COMMUNITY MUTUAL INSURANCE CO . . . WWW.AMERICAN-COMMUNITY.COM

AMERICAN FAMILY INSURANCE . . . . WWW.AMFAM.COM

AMERICAN FAMILY LIFE ASSURANCE CO . . . . WWW.AFLAC.COM

AMERICAN FAMILY MUTUAL INSURANCE . . . . WWW.AMFAM.COM

AMERICAN FIDELITY ASSURANCE CO . . . . WWW.AF-GROUP.COM

AMERICAN GROUP ADMINISTRATORS, INC . . . . WWW.AGA+AHSA.COM

AMERICAN INCOME LIFE INSURANCE CO . . . . WWW.AILINS.COM

AMERICAN MEDICAL SECURITY . . . . WWW.AMSCHOICES.COM

AMERICAN MINING INSURANCE CO, INC . . . . WWW.CGHINSURANCE.COM

AMERICAN MODERN INSURANCE GROUP . . . . WWW.MIDLANDCOMPANY.COM

AMERICAN NATIONAL INSURANCE CO . . . . WWW.ANICO.COM

AMERICAN NATIONAL PROPERTY & CASUALTY CO . . . WWW.ANPAC.COM

AMERICAN POSTAL WORKERS UNION HEALTH PLAN . . WWW.APWUHP.COM

AMERICAN SKANDIA LIFE REINSURANCE CORP . . . . . . WWW.AMERICAN_SKANDIA.COM

AMERICAN STATES INSURANCE CO . . . . WWW.SAFECO.COM

AMERICAN TRAVEL, INC . . . . WWW.CONSECO.COM

AMERIHEALTH . . . . WWW.AMERIHEALTHTPA.COM

AMERISURE COMPANIES . . . . WWW.AMERISUE.COM

AMERITAS LIFE INSURANCE CORP . . . . WWW.AMERITAS.COM

ANTHEM BLUE CROSS & BLUE SHIELD OF CONNECTICUT . . . . WWW.ANTHEMBCBSCT.COM

ANTHEM, INC . . . . WWW.ANTHEM-INC.COM

ANTHEM INSURANCE . . . . WWW.AHLIC.COM

ANTHEM LIFE .... WWW.ANTHEM-INC.COM

ARGONAUT INSURANCE CO .... WWW.CHI.ARGONAUTGROUP.COM

ARKANSAS FARM BUREAU MUTUAL INSURANCE ..... WWW.ARFB.COM

ASSOCIATION & SOCIETY INSURANCE CORP .... WWW.ASICORPORATION.COM

ATLANTIC MUTUAL / CENTENNIAL INSURANCE CO ... WWW.ATLANTICMUTUAL.COM

AUTO OWNERS INSURANCE CO .... WWW.AUTO-OWNERS.COM

AV-MED HEALTH PLAN .... WWW.ABNET.COM

BALBOA INSURANCE .... WWW.BALBOAINSURANCE.COM

BANKERS INSURANCE GROUP .... WWW.BANKERSINSURANCE.COM

BANKERS LIFE & CASUALTY CO .... WWW.BANKLIFE.COM

BASHAS', INC .... WWW.BASHAS.COM

BEAR RIVER MUTUAL INSURANCE CO .... WWW.BRMUTUAL.COM

BENEFIT ADMINISTRATIVE SYSTEMS, LTD .... WWW.BENADMINSYS.COM

BENEFIT ADMINISTRATORS, INC .... WWW.BATPA.COM

BENEFIT CLAIMS PAYERS, INC .... WWW.DHSNYU.COM

BENEFIT PLAN ADMINISTRATORS, INC .... WWW.BPATPA.COM

BENEFIT PLANNERS, INC .... WWW.BENPLAN.COM

BENEFIT & RISK MANAGEMENT SERVICES .... WWW.BEST-ONLINE.COM

BENEFITSOURCE, INC .... WWW.BENEFITSOURCEINC.COM

BENICOMP, INC .... WWW.BENICOMP.COM

BENICORP INSURANCE CO .... WWW.BENICORP.COM

BERWANGER OVERMYER ASSOCIATES .... WWW.BOA-INS.COM

BITUMINOUS FIRE & MARINE INSURANCE CO .... WWW.BITUMINOUSINSURANCE.COM

BLUE CARE NETWORK .... WWW.BCBSM.COM

BLUE CROSS & BLUE SHIELD .... WWW.BCBSAL

BLUE CROSS & BLUE SHIELD OF MAINE .... WWW.MAINEBLUECROSS.COM

BLUE CROSS OF IDAHO HEALTH SERVICE, INC .... WWW.BCIDAHO.COM

BLUE PLUS .... WWW.BCBSMN.COM

BLUE RIDGE ADMINISTRATORS .... WWW.COMCLIN.NET

BLUE RIDGE INSURANCE CO .... WWW.BLUERIDGEINS.COM

BLUE SHIELD OF CALIFORNIA .... WWW.BLUESHIELDCA.COM

BLUE SHIELD OF CALIFORNIA HEADQUARTERS .... WWW.BLUESHIELOFCALIFORNIA.COM

BLUE SHIELD OF NORTHEASTERN NEW YORK . . . . WWW.BLUECARES.COM/BLUECARD

BLUELINCS HMO . . . . WWW.BCBSOK.COM

BOON-CHAPMAN . . . . WWW.BOONCHAPMAN.COM

BOSTON MUTUAL LIFE INSURANCE CO . . . . WWW.BOSTONMUTUAL.COM

BPS INC . . . . WWW.BPSINC.COM

BRETHREN MUTUAL INSURANCE CO . . . . WWW.BMICONLINE.COM

BRISTOL WEST INSURANCE SERVICES . . . . WWW.BRISTOLWEST.COM

BURLINGTON MOTOR CARRIERS . . . . WWW.BMTR.COM

BUSINESS COUNCIL OF NEW YORK . . . . WWW.BCYS.ORG

BUSINESSMEN'S ASSURANCE CO OF AMERICA . . . . . . WWW.BMA.COM

C. L. FRATES INSURANCE CO . . . . WWW.BANKINSURE.COM

CABELL HUNTINGTON HOSPITAL INC . . . . WWW.CABELL HUNTINGTON.ORG

CABOT SAFETY CORP . . . . WWW.AEARO.COM

CADBURY BEVERAGES, INC . . . . WWW.MOTTS.COM

CADENCE GROUP LIFE HEALTH & DISABILITY . . . . WWW.CADENCE.COM

CAHABA GBA - GEORGIA MEDICARE OPERATIONS . . . WWW.GAMEDICARE.COM

CAL FARM INSURANCE CO . . . . WWW.CALFARM.COM

CALIFORNIA CASUALTY INSURANCE CO . . . . WWW.CALCAS.COM

CALIFORNIA CEDAR PRODUCTS CO . . . . WWW.CALCEDAR.COM

CALIFORNIA COMPENSATION INSURANCE CO . . . . . . WWW.SUPERIOR.COM

CALIFORNIA MOTOR CAR DEALERS ASSOCIATION . . . . WWW.CMCDA.COM

CALMAR, INC . . . . WWW.CALMAR.COM

CAMELOT MUSIC INC . . . . WWW.CAMELOTMUSIC.COM

CAMPBELL SOUP CO . . . . WWW.CAMPBELLSOUP.COM

CANADA LIFE ASSURANCE CO . . . . WWW.CANADALIFE.COM

CANON COCHRAN MANAGEMENT SERVICES, INC . . . . WWW.CCMSI.COM

CAPITAL BLUE CROSS . . . . WWW.CAPBLUECROSS.COM

CAPITAL DISTRICT PHYSICIANS' HEALTH PLAN, INC . . . WWW.CDPHP.COM

CARE AMERICA HEALTH PLANS . . . . WWW.CAREAMERICA.COM

CAREFIRST BLUE CROSS & BLUE SHIELD . . . . WWW.CAREFIRST.COM

CARILION HEALTH PLANS . . . . WWW.CARILION.COM

CARNEGIE-MELLON UNIVERSITY . . . . WWW.CMU.EDU/BA/HR/

CAROLINA CASUALTY INSURANCE CO, INC . . . . WWW.CAROLINACAS.COM

CASUALTY INSURANCE CO . . . . WWW.FREMONTCOMP.COM

CASUALTY RECIPROCAL EXCHANGE . . . . WWW.DODSONGROUP.COM

CAVALIER FORD . . . . WWW.CAVFORD.COM

CELTIC LIFE INSURANCE CO . . . . WWW.CELTIC_NET.COM

CENTRAL BENEFITS MUTUAL INSURANCE CO . . . . WWW.CENTRALBENEFITS.COM

CENTRAL INSURANCE CO . . . . WWW.CENTRAL-INSURANCE.COM

CENTRAL MAINE POWER . . . . WWW.CMPCO.COM

CENTRAL MUTUAL INSURANCE CO . . . . WWW.CENTRAL-INSURANCE.COM

CENTRAL RESERVE LIFE INSURANCE CO OF NORTH AMERICA . . . . WWW.CENTRALRESERVE.COM

CENTRAL VALLEY SCHOOL TRUST . . . . WWW.CVTRUST.ORG

CENTURY FURNITURE . . . . WWW.CENTURYFURNITURE.COM

CENTURY PLANNERS, LLC . . . . WWW.CENTURYPLANNERS.COM

CGU . . . . WWW.CUUSA.COM

CGU HAWKEYE UNITED SECURITY INSURANCE CO . . . . WWW.CGU-HAWKEYE.COM

CHAMPUS . . . . WWW.HUMANAMILITARY.COM

CHARTER BENEFIT ADMINISTRATORS . . . . WWW.CHARTERBENEFITS.COM

CHILDREN'S HOSPITAL OF ORANGE COUNTY . . . . WWW.CHOC.ORG

CHOICECARE HEALTH PLANS, INC . . . . WWW.CHOICECARE.COM

CHUBB CORPORATION . . . . WWW.CHUBB.COM

CHURCH MUTUAL INSURANCE CO . . . . WWW.CHURCHHILL-MUTUAL.COM

CIGNA CORPORATION . . . . WWW.CIGNAHEALTHCARE.COM

CINCINNATI INSURANCE CO . . . . WWW.CINFIN.COM

CITIZENS INSURANCE CO OF AMERICA . . . . WWW.ALLMERICA.COM

CITRUS INSURANCE TRUST . . . . WWW.APASCO.COM

CIVIL SERVICE EMPLOYEES INSURANCE CO . . . . WWW.CSE-INSURANCE.COM

CNA . . . . WWW.CNA.COM

COLLIN COUNTY COURTHOUSE . . . . WWW.CO.COLLIN.TX.US.COM

COLUMBIA INSURANCE GROUP . . . . WWW.COLINSGRP.COM

COLUMBIA UNIVERSAL LIFE INSURANCE CO . . . . WWW.COLUMBIA-UNIVERSAL.COM

COLUMBUS LIFE INSURANCE CO . . . . WWW.COLUMBUSLIFE.COM

COMBINED INSURANCE CO OF AMERICA . . . . WWW.COMBINEDINSURANCE.COM

COMMERCE INSURANCE CO	WWW.COMMERCEINSURANCE.COM
COMMERCIAL UNION INSURANCE CO OF AMERICA	WWW.CGU.COM
COMPANION HEALTH CARE CORP	WWW.BCBSSC
COMPDENT	WWW.COMPDENT.COM
CONCENTRA MANAGED CARE, INC	WWW.CONCENTRAMC.COM
CONESTOGA LIFE ASSURANCE CO	WWW.CONESTOGALIFEANDHEALTH.COM
CONNECTICARE INC & AFFILIATES	WWW.CONNECTICARE.COM
CONSECO	WWW.CONSECO.COM
CONSOLIDATED NATURAL GAS CO	WWW.CNG.COM
CONSUMER HEALTH NETWORK	WWW.4CHN.COM
CONTECH CONSTRUCTION PRODUCTS INC	WWW.CONTECH-CPI.COM
CONTINENTAL GENERAL INSURANCE CO	WWW.CONTINENTALGENERAL.COM
CONTINENTAL WESTERN INSURANCE CO	WWW.CONTWESTINS.COM
COOK & CO INC	WWW.COOKANDCOMPANY.COM
COORDINATED HEALTH PARTNERS, INC	WWW.BCBSRI.COM
COPPS CORP.	WWW.COPPS.COM
CORESOURCE, INC	WWW.TRUSTMARKINSURANCE.COM
CORPORATE BENEFIT SERVICES OF AMERICA, INC	WWW.CBSAINC.COM
CORPORATE SYSTEMS ADMINISTRATION, INC	WWW.CSABENEFITS.COM
CORVEL CORP	WWW.CORVEL.COM
COVENTRY HEALTHCARE	WWW.CZTY.COM
CRAWFORD & CO	WWW.CRAWFORDANDCOMPANY.COM
CRUM & FORSTER INSURANCE	WWW.CFINS.COM
CUMBERLAND MUTUAL FIRE INSURANCE CO	WWW.CUMBERLAND GROUP.COM
CUNA MUTUAL GROUP	WWW.CUNAMUTUAL.COM
CUNNINGHAM LINDSEY INC	WWW.CUNNINGHAMLINDSEY.COM
DAKOTACARE	WWW.DAKOTACARE.COM
DC CHARTERED HEALTH PLAN, INC	WWW.CHARTER-HEALTH.COM
DEAN HEALTH PLAN HMO	WWW.DEANCARE.COM
DELMARVA HEALTH PLAN, INC	WWW.CAREFIRST.COM
DELOITTE & TOUCHE	WWW.US.DELOIT.COM
DELTA DENTAL INSURANCE CO	WWW.DELTADENTALIN.COM

DELTA DENTAL OF CALIFORNIA .... WWW.DELTADENTALCA.ORG

DELTA DENTAL OF KANSAS, INC .... WWW.DELTADENTALKS.COM

DELTA DENTAL OF RHODE ISLAND .... WWW.DELTADENTALRI.COM

DELTA DENTAL OF WEST VIRGINIA .... WWW.DELTADENTAL.COM

DELTA DENTAL PLAN OF ILLINOIS .... WWW.DELTADENTALIL.COM

DELTA DENTAL PLAN OF KENTUCKY .... WWW.DDPKY.COM

DELTA DENTAL PLAN OF MASSACHUSETTS .... WWW.DELTAMASS.COM

DELTA DENTAL PLAN OF MICHIGAN .... WWW.DELTADENTALOH.COM

DELTA DENTAL PLAN OF NEW JERSEY INC .... WWW.DELTADENTALNJ.COM

DELTA DENTAL PLAN OF OHIO .... WWW.DELTADENTALOH.COM

DELTA DENTAL PLAN OF OKLAHOMA .... WWW.DELTADENTALOK.COM

DELTA DENTAL PLAN OF WISCONSIN .... WWW.DELTADENTALWI.COM

DENTALCOMP, INC .... WWW.DENTALCOMP.COM

DESERET MUTUAL .... WWW.DMBA.COM

DIVERSIFIED GROUP ADMINISTRATORS, INC .... WWW.DGATPA.COM

DIVISION OF HEALTH CARE FINANCING .... WWW.HLUNIX.EX.STATE.UT.US/MEDICAID

DODSON INSURANCE GROUP .... WWW.DODSONGROUP.COM

DONEGAL MUTUAL INSURANCE CO .... WWW.DONEGAL.COM

DUNCANSON & HOLT GROUP(S) .... WWW.DHGROUP.COM

EBI COMPANIES .... WWW.EBICO.COM

ELCA BOARD OF PENSIONS .... WWW.ELCABOP.ORG

EMERALD HEALTH NETWORK, INC .... WWW.EMERALDHEALTH.COM

EMPIRE BLUE CROSS & BLUE SHIELD .... WWW.EMPIREHEALTHCARE.COM

EMPLOYEE BENEFIT INSURANCE .... WWW.EBICO.COM

EMPLOYEE BENEFIT MANAGEMENT SERVICES INC .... WWW.EBMSTPA.COM

EMPLOYER PLAN SERVICES, INC .... WWW.ETSIBENEFITSINC.COM

EMPLOYERS INSURANCE CO OF NEVADA .... WWW.EMPLOYERSINSCO.COM

EMPLOYERS REINSURANCE CORP .... WWW.ERCGROUP.COM

EPIC LIFE INSURANCE CO, INC .... WWW.WPS.COM

ERIE INSURANCE CO .... WWW.ERIE-INSURANCE.COM

ERISA ADMINISTRATIVE SERVICES, INC .... WWW.CSERISA.COM

EXCLUSIVE HEALTHCARE, INC .... WWW.MUTUALOFOMAHA.COM

FALLON COMMUNITY HEALTH PLAN, INC	WWW.FCHP.ORG
FAMILY HEALTH PLAN COOPERATIVE	WWW.FAMILYHP.ORG
FAMILY HEALTH PLAN OF OHIO	WWW.FAMILYHEALTHPLAN.ORG
FARM BUREAU MUTUAL INSURANCE CO OF IDAHO	WWW.FBINSURANCE.COM
FARM FAMILY CASUALTY	WWW.FARMFAMILY.COM
FARMERS ALLIANCE MUTUAL INSURANCE CO	WWW.FAMI.COM
FARMERS AUTO INSURANCE ASSOCIATION	WWW.PEKININSURANCE.COM
FARMERS INSURANCE GROUP	WWW.FARMERSINSURANCE.COM
FBD CONSULTING, INC	WWW.FBDCONSULT.COM
FEDERATED MUTUAL INSURANCE CO	WWW.FEDERATEDINS.COM
FIC INSURANCE	WWW.FICGROUP.COM
FIRE & CASUALTY INSURANCE CO OF CONNECTICUT	WWW.ORIONCAPITAL.COM
FIREMAN'S FUND INSURANCE CO	WWW.THE-FUND.COM
FIRST AMERICAN INSURANCE CO	WWW.FAIC.COM
FIRST ASSURANCE LIFE INSURANCE CO	WWW.THELDSGROUP.COM
FIRST EXCESS & REINSURANCE CORP	WWW.GEREINSURANCE.COM
FIRST INSURANCE CO OF HAWAII	WWW.FICOH.COM
FIRST INTEGRATED HEALTH	WWW.FIH.COM
FIRST RELIANCE STANDARD LIFE INSURANCE CO	WWW.RSL.COM
FLORISTS MUTUAL INSURANCE CO	WWW.PLANTNET.COM
FOREIGN SERVICE BENEFIT PLAN	WWW.AFSPA.ORG
FOREMOST CORP OF AMERICA	WWW.FOREMOST.COM
FORTIS BENEFITS INSURANCE CO	WWW.FORTIS.COM
FOUNDATION HEALTH	WWW.FHS.COM
FREE STATE HEALTH PLAN	WWW.CAREFIRST.COM
FREMONT COMPENSATION INSURANCE CO	WWW.FREMONTCOMP.COM
FREMONT MUTUAL INSURANCE CO	WWW.FMIC.COM
FRONTIER INSURANCE GROUP	WWW.FTR.COM
GAB ROBINS NORTH AMERICA	WWW.GABROBINS.COM
GAINSCO, INC	WWW.GAINSCO.COM
GALILEO INTERNATIONAL	WWW.GALILEO.COM
GENENTECH INC GROUP	WWW.GENE.COM

GENERAL AMERICAN LIFE INSURANCE CO	WWW.GENM.COM
GENERAL INSURANCE EXCHANGE AGENCY, INC	WWW.CHANDLER-GROUP.COM
GEORGIA BANKERS ASSOCIATION INSURANCE	WWW.GABANKERS.COM
GERLING AMERICA INSURANCE CO	WWW.GERLING.COM
GILSBAR, INC	WWW.GILSBAR.COM
GOLDEN RULE LIFE INSURANCE CO	WWW.GOLDENRULE.COM
GOLDEN STATE MUTUAL LIFE INSURANCE CO	WWW.GSMLIFE.COM
GOOD SAMARITAN WOUND CENTER	WWW.CURITIVE.COM
GOVERNMENT EMPLOYEES HOSPITAL ASSOCIATION . .	WWW.GEHA.COM
GRAIN DEALERS MUTUAL INSURANCE CO	WWW.GRAINDEALERS.COM
GRAND PACIFIC LIFE INSURANCE CO, LTD	WWW.GPLI.COM
GRANGE MUTUAL CASUALTY CO	WWW.GRANGEINSURANCE.COM
GRAY INSURANCE CO	WWW.GRAYINSCO.COM
GRE INSURANCE GROUP	WWW.GRE-INSURANCE.COM
GREAT AMERICAN INSURANCE COMPANIES	WWW.OCAS.COM
GREAT NORTHERN INSURANCE CO	WWW.CHUBB.COM
GREAT WEST CASUALTY CO	WWW.GWCCNET.COM
GREAT WEST LIFE	WWW.1HEALTHPLAN.COM
GREAT-WEST LIFE & ANNUITY	WWW.GWLA.COM
GREAT-WEST LIFE ASSURANCE CO	WWW.1HEALTHPLAN.COM
GREATER GEORGIA LIFE INSURANCE CO	WWW.BCBSGA.COM
GROCER'S INSURANCE GROUP	WWW.GROCINS.COM
GROUP BENEFIT SERVICES, INC	WWW.G-B-S.COM
GROUP HEALTH COOPERATIVE OF PUGET SOUND	WWW.GHC.ORG
GROUP HEALTH NORTHWEST	WWW.GHNW.COM
GROUP HEALTH PLAN OF ST. LOUIS	WWW.GHP.COM
GUARANTEE TRUST LIFE INSURANCE CO	WWW.GTLIC.COM
GUARDIAN LIFE INSURANCE CO OF AMERICA	WWW.THEGUARDIAN.COM
GUIDEONE INSURANCE	WWW.GUIDEONE.COM
GULF SOUTH HEALTH PLANS, INC	WWW.GENERALHEALTH.ORG
HALLMARK INSURANCE ADMINISTRATORS, INC	WWW.BCBSIL.COM
HANOVER INSURANCE CO	WWW.ALLMERICA.COM

HARLEYSVILLE INSURANCE CO .... WWW.HARLEYSVILLEGROUP.COM

HARRIS METHODIST HEALTH PLAN .... WWW.HMHP.COM

HARTFORD FINANCIAL GROUP INC .... WWW.ATTHEHARTFORD.COM

HARTFORD LIFE .... WWW.THEHARTFORD.COM

HARVARD INDUSTRIES .... WWW.HARVARDIND.COM

HARVARD PILGRIM HEALTH CARE .... WWW.HARVARDPILGRIM.ORG

HARVARD UNIVERSITY GROUP HEALTH PLAN .... WWW.UHF.HARVARD.EDU

HAWAII MEDICAL SERVICE ASSOCIATION .... WWW.HMSA.COM

HAWORTH, INC .... WWW.HAWORTH.COM

HEALTH ALLIANCE MEDICAL PLANS .... WWW.HEALTHALLIANCE.ORG

HEALTH ALLIANCE PLAN OF MICHIGAN .... WWW.HAPCORP.ORG

HEALTH AMERICA .... WWW.HEALTHAMERICA.CVTY.COM

HEALTH BENEFIT TRUST FUND LOCAL 94 .... WWW.LOCAL94.COM

HEALTH BENEFITS FUND .... WWW.INSTABN.COM

HEALTH CARE PLAN .... WWW.UNIVERAHEALTHCARE.ORG

HEALTH FUTURE, INC .... WWW.HEALTHFUTURELLC.COM

HEALTH GUARD .... WWW.HGUARD.COM

HEALTH INSURANCE PLAN OF GREATER NEW YORK .. WWW.HIPUSA.COM

HEALTH NET .... WWW.HEALTHNET.COM

HEALTH NETWORK AMERICA, INC .... WWW.HEALTHNETWORKAMERICA.COM

HEALTH PARTNERS .... WWW.HEALTHPARTNERS.COM

HEALTH PLAN .... WWW.HEALTHPLAN.ORG

HEALTH PLAN OF THE REDWOODS .... WWW.HPR.ORG

HEALTH PLAN SERVICES .... WWW.HPS.COM

HEALTH PLAN SOUTHEAST .... WWW.HPSE.COM

HEALTH PLUS OF MICHIGAN .... WWW.HEALTHPLUS.COM

HEALTH SERVICES MEDICAL CORP .... WWW.PHPHMO.COM

HEALTH SPECIAL RISK, INC .... WWW.HEALTHSPECIALRISK.COM

HEALTHFIRST, INC .... WWW.HEALTHFIRST.COM

HEALTHNOW .... WWW.HEALTHNOWNY.COM

HEALTHPLEX, INC .... WWW.HEALTHPLEX.COM

HEALTHSOURCE .... WWW.CIGNA.COM

HELLER ASSOCIATES	WWW.HELLERTPA.COM
HELMSMAN MANAGEMENT SERVICES	WWW.LIBERTYMUTUAL.COM
HERBERT L. JAMISON & CO LLC	WWW.JAMISONGROUP.COM
HERITAGE INSURANCE MANAGERS, INC	WWW.HERITAGE-INS.COM
HERITAGE MUTUAL INSURANCE CO	WWW.HERITAGEINSURANCE.COM
HIGHLANDS INSURANCE GROUP	WWW.HIGHLANDSINSURANCE.COM
HMO COLORADO, INC	WWW.BCBSCO.COM
HMO ILLINOIS	WWW.BCBSIL.COM
HMO MONTANA	WWW.BCBSMT.COM
HOLY CROSS RESOURCES, INC	WWW.HCRI.ORG
HOLYOKE MUTUAL INSURANCE CO	WWW.HOLYOKEMUTUAL.COM
HOMETOWN HEALTH NETWORK	WWW.HOMETOWNHEALTHNET.COM
HOMETOWN HEALTH PLAN	WWW.WASHOEHEALTH.COM
HORACE MANN COMPANIES	WWW.HORACEMANN.COM
HUMANA	WWW.HUMANA.COM
IBA HEALTH & LIFE ASSURANCE CO	WWW.IBAHEALTH.COM
IDAHO STATE INSURANCE FUND	WWW.STATE.ID.US/ISIF
IHC HEALTH PLANS	WWW.IHC.COM
INDEPENDENCE BLUE CROSS	WWW.IBX.COM
INDEPENDENT HEALTH	WWW.INDEPENDENTHEALTH.COM
INDIANAPOLIS LIFE	WWW.INDIANAPOLISLIFE.COM
INFINITY GROUP	WWW.INFINITY-INSURANCE.COM
INSURANCE MANAGEMENT ASSOCIATES, INC	WWW.IMACORP.COM
INSURANCE & RISK MANAGEMENT	WWW.INSURANCERISKMGMT.COM
INTEGON	WWW.INTEGON.COM
INTEGRITY MUTUAL INSURANCE CO	WWW.INTEGRITY.INSURANCE.COM
INTER VALLEY HEALTH PLAN	WWW.IVHP.COM
INTERCONTINENTAL CORP	WWW.INTERCONTINENTALCORP.COM
INTERMOUNTAIN ADMINISTRATORS, INC	WWW.IAI-TPA.COM
INTERNATIONAL BENEFIT SERVICES CORP	WWW.IBSUSI.COM
IU MEDICAL GROUP PRIMARY CARE	WWW.IHUC.COM
J. C. PENNEY INSURANCE	WWW.JCPENNEYINSURANCEGROUP.COM

J & H, MARSH & MCLENNAN . . . . WWW.MARSHMAC.COM

J.P. FARLEY CORP . . . . WWW.JPFARLEY.COM

JARDINE GROUP SERVICES CORP . . . . WWW.JGSC.COM

JEFFERSON PILOT FINANCIAL . . . . WWW.CHUBB.COM

JENKINS & ATHENS INSURANCE SERVICES . . . . WWW.JENKINS-ATHENS.COM

JEWELERS MUTUAL INSURANCE CO . . . . WWW.JEWELERSMUTUAL.COM

JOHN P. PEARL & ASSOCIATES . . . . WWW.PEARLINS.COM

K & K INSURANCE GROUP . . . . WWW.K&KINSURANCE.COM

KAISER FOUNDATION HEALTH PLAN OF CALIFORNIA . WWW.KAIPERM.ORG

KAISER / GROUP HEALTH . . . . WWW.GHC.ORG

KAISER PERMANENTE . . . . WWW.KAISERPERMANENTE.ORG

KANSAS FARM BUREAU & AFFILIATED SERVICES . . . . . WWW.KFBF.COM

KEENAN & ASSOCIATES . . . . WWW.KEENANASSOC.COM

KEMPER INSURANCE . . . . WWW.KEMPERINSURANCE.COM

KEMPTON GROUP . . . . WWW.KEMPTONGROUP.COM

KENTUCKY FARM BUREAU MUTUAL INSURANCE CO . . WWW.KYFB.COM

KEYSTONE HEALTH PLAN CENTRAL . . . . WWW.KHPC.COM

LANDMARK HEALTH CARE . . . . WWW.LANDMARKHEALTHCARE.COM

LEWER AGENCY, INC . . . . WWW.LEWER.COM

LIBERTY LIFE INSURANCE CO . . . . WWW.LIBERTY.COM

LIBERTY MUTUAL GROUP . . . . WWW.LIBERTYMUTUAL.COM

LIBERTY NORTHWEST . . . . WWW.LIBERTYNORTHWEST.COM

LIFE & HEALTH INSURANCE CO OF AMERICA . . . . WWW.LIFE-HEALTHAMERICA.COM

LIFE OF THE SOUTH SERVICE CO . . . . WWW.LIFE-SOUTH.COM

LIFEGUARD, INC . . . . WWW.LIFEGUARD.COM

LIFEWISE A PREMERA HEALTH PLAN, INC . . . . WWW.PREMERA.COM/LIFEWISE

LINCOLN MUTUAL LIFE & CASUALTY INSURANCE CO . . WWW.LML.COM

LOCALS 302 & 612 INTERNATIONAL . . . . WWW.WPAS-INC.COM

LONDON LIFE REINSURANCE . . . . WWW.LONDONLIFE.COM

LOOMIS CO . . . . WWW.LOOMISCO.COM

LOVE BOX CO . . . . WWW.LOVEBOX.COM

LOVELACE HEALTH PLAN, INC . . . . WWW.LOVELACE.COM

LUFKIN INDUSTRIES, INC . . . . WWW.LUFKIN.COM

LUMBER INSURANCE COMPANIES . . . . WWW.LUMBERINS.COM

LUMBERMEN'S MUTUAL CASUALTY CO . . . . WWW.KEMPERINSURANCE.COM

LUTHERAN BROTHERHOOD INSURANCE CO . . . . WWW.LUTHBRO.COM

M.S.I. INSURANCE . . . . WWW.MSI-INSURANCE.COM

MAGINNIS & ASSOCIATES, INC . . . . WWW.MAGINNIS.COM

MAIL HANDLERS BENEFIT PLAN . . . . WWW.MHBP.COM

MAKSIN MANAGEMENT CORP . . . . WWW.MAKSIN.COM

MANULIFE FINANCIAL . . . . WWW.MANULIFE.COM

MARRIOTT INTERNATIONAL, INC . . . . WWW.MARRIOTT.COM

MARTIN'S POINT HEALTH CARE . . . . WWW.MARTINSPOINT.COM

MASSACHUSETTS MUTUAL LIFE INSURANCE CO . . . . . . WWW.MASSINSURANCE.COM

MASSMUTUAL LIFE INSURANCE . . . . WWW.MASSMUTUAL.COM

MAXICARE HEALTH INSURANCE CO OF WISCONSIN . . WWW.MAXICARE.COM

MCC BEHAVIORAL CARE . . . . WWW.MCC/CARE.COM

MD INDIVIDUAL PRACTICE ASSOCIATION . . . . WWW.MAMSI.COM

MEAD CORP . . . . WWW.MEAD.COM

MEDEX ASSISTANCE CORP . . . . WWW.MEDEXASSIST.COM

MEDICAID FISCAL AGENTS . . . . WWW.AHCCCS.STATE.AZ.US

MEDICAL CENTER OF OCEAN COUNTY . . . . WWW.MERIDIANHEALTH.COM

MEDICAL LIFE INSURANCE CO . . . . WWW.MED-LIFE.COM

MEDICARE — PART A INTERMEDIARIES . . . . WWW.BCBSAZ.COM

MEDICARE — PART B CARRIER . . . . WWW.MEDICARE.BCBSMT.COM

MEDICARE — PART B CARRIERS . . . . WWW.BCBSAL.ORG

MEMORIAL SISTERS OF CHARITY HEALTH NETWORK INC . . . . WWW.MSCH.COM

MERCURY CASUALTY CO . . . . WWW.MERCURYINSURANCE.COM

MERVYN'S HEALTH CARE PLAN . . . . WWW.BLUECROSSCA.COM

MET LIFE DISABILITY . . . . WWW.METLIFE.COM

MICHIGAN EMPLOYEE BENEFIT SERVICES . . . . WWW.MEBS.COM

MICHIGAN FARM BUREAU MUTUAL INSURANCE CO . . WWW.FARMBUREAUINS/MI.COM

MICHIGAN MUTUAL INSURANCE CO . . . . WWW.AMERISURE.COM

MID-ATLANTIC MEDICAL SERVICES, INC . . . . WWW.MAMSI.COM

MILLENNIUM CARE ADMINISTRATORS (DBA MCA ADMINISTRATORS) . . . . WWW.MCOA.COM

MMI COMPANIES . . . . WWW.MMICOMPANIES.COM

MOTOR CLUB OF AMERICA INSURANCE CO . . . . WWW.MOTOR.COM

MS ADMINISTRATIVE SERVICES, INC . . . . WWW.MSADMIN.COM

MUTUAL SERVICE INSURANCE CO . . . . WWW.MSI-INSURANCE.COM

NALC HEALTH BENEFIT PLAN . . . . WWW.NALC.ORG/HBP

NAPUS HEALTH BENEFIT PLAN . . . . WWW.CAREFIRST.COM

NATIONAL ALLIANCE OF POSTAL & FEDERAL EMPLOYEES . . . . WWW.AETNA.COM

NATIONAL AMERICAN INSURANCE CO OF CALIFORNIA . . . . WWW.NAICC.COM

NATIONAL ASSOCIATION OF MUTUAL INSURANCE . . . WWW.NAMIC.ORG

NATIONAL GENERAL INSURANCE CO . . . . WWW.NGIC.COM

NATIONAL GRANGE MUTUAL INSURANCE CO . . . . WWW.MSAGROUP.COM

NATIONAL GUARDIAN LIFE INSURANCE CO . . . . WWW.NATIONALGUARDIAN.COM

NATIONAL HEALTH PLANS . . . . WWW.NATIONALHMO.COM

NATIONAL RURAL LETTER CARRIERS' ASSOCIATION . . . WWW.MUTUALOFOMAHA.COM

NATIONAL TRAVELERS LIFE INSURANCE CO . . . . WWW.NATIONALTRAVELERSLIFE.COM

NATIONWIDE HEALTH PLAN . . . . WWW.NATIONWIDEHEALTH.COM

NEIGHBORHOOD HEALTH PLAN, INC . . . . WWW.NHP.ORG

NEW JERSEY MANUFACTURERS INSURANCE CO . . . . . WWW.NJM.COM

NEW MEXICO PHYSICIANS INSURANCE . . . . WWW.MICOA.COM

NGS AMERICAN, INC . . . . WWW.NGSAMERICAN.COM

NORTH AMERICA ADMINISTRATORS, INC . . . . WWW.NAAI.COM

NORTHEAST DELTA DENTAL . . . . WWW.NEDELTA.COM

NORTHEAST MEDICAL CENTER . . . . WWW.NORTHEASTMEDICAL.ORG

NORTHERN ADJUSTERS . . . . WWW.NADJ.COM

NORTHLAND INSURANCE CO . . . . WWW.NORTHLANDINS.COM

NORTHWESTERN MUTUAL LIFE INSURANCE CO . . . . . . WWW.NORTHWESTERN.COM

NRECA . . . . WWW.NRECA.ORG

NYL CARE . . . . WWW.AETNA.COM

ODS HEALTH PLAN . . . . WWW.ODSHP.COM

OHIO BUREAU OF WORKERS COMPENSATION ...... WWW.OHIOBWC.COM

OHIO CASUALTY GROUP .... WWW.OCAS.COM

OKLAHOMA FARM BUREAU MUTUAL INSURANCE CO . WWW.SB.COM/OK501

OLYMPIC BENEFITS .... WWW.OHMSYSTEMS.COM

OMNI HEALTH CARE .... WWW.OMNIHEALTHCARE.COM

OPTIMUM CHOICE, INC .... WWW.MAMSI.COM

OREGON DENTAL SERVICE (ODS HEALTH PLANS) ..... WWW.ODSHP.COM

OREGON QUALITY INSURANCE .... WWW.PACC.COM

ORION CAPITAL COMPANIES .... WWW.ORIONCAPITAL.COM

OSF HEALTH PLANS .... WWW.OSFHEALTHCARE.ORG/HEALTHPLANS

OXFORD LIFE INSURANCE CO .... WWW.OXFORDLIFE.COM

PACIFIC LIFE INSURANCE CO .... WWW.PACIFICLIFE.COM

PACIFIC SOURCE HEALTH PLANS .... WWW.PACIFIC-SOURCE.COM

PACIFICARE HEALTH SYSTEMS, INC .... WWW.PACIFICARE.COM

PAFCO GENERAL INSURANCE CO .... WWW.SIGINS.COM

PARTNERS MUTUAL INSURANCE CO .... WWW.PARTNERSMUTUAL.COM

PARTNERS NATIONAL HEALTH PLANS .... WWW.PARTNERSINDIANA.COM

PAULA INSURANCE CO .... WWW.TRWPICATALO.COM

PEER REVIEW ORGANIZATIONS .... WWW.HMSA.COM

PEKIN INSURANCE CO .... WWW.PEKININSURANCE.COM

PEMCO INSURANCE CO .... WWW.PEMCO.COM

PHYSICIANS HEALTH PLAN, INC .... WWW.PHPMI.ORG

PHYSICIANS HEALTH PLAN OF SOUTH CAROLINA .... WWW.PHPHEALTHPLAN.COM

PHYSICIANS HEALTH SERVICES .... WWW.PHSHMO.COM

PHYSICIANS MUTUAL .... WWW.PMIC.COM

PITNEY BOWES, INC .... WWW.PB.COM

PREFERRED CARE .... WWW.PREFERREDCARE.ORG

PREFERRED HEALTH NORTHWEST .... WWW.BCBSO.COM

PREFERRED HEALTH SYSTEMS INSURANCE CO .... WWW.PHSYSTEMS.COM

PREFERRED MUTUAL INSURANCE CO .... WWW.PMINSCO.COM

PREMERA BLUE CROSS .... WWW.PREMERA.COM

PREMIER BLUE .... WWW.BCBSKS.COM

PREPAID HEALTH PLAN .... WWW.PHPHMO.COM

PRIME HEALTH OF ALABAMA .... WWW.PRIMEHEALTHONLINE.COM

PRINCIPAL FINANCIAL GROUP .... WWW.PRINCIPAL.COM

PRINCIPAL HEALTH CARE, INC .... WWW.PHCKC.COM

PRIORITY HEALTH .... WWW.PRIORITY-HEALTH.COM

PRIORITY HEALTH CARE .... WWW.TRIGON.COM

PROFESSIONAL INSURANCE CORP .... WWW.PIC.COM

PROFESSIONAL RISK MANAGEMENT .... WWW.APPLIEDRISK.COM

PROGRESSIVE CASUALTY INSURANCE CO .... WWW.PROGRESSIVE.COM

PROGRESSIVE INSURANCE CO OF CANADA .... WWW.PROGRESSIVEINSURANCE.CA

PROTECTIVE LIFE GUIDESTAR HEALTH SYSTEMS ...... WWW.GUIDESTARHEALTH.COM

PROVIDENCE HEALTH PLANS .... WWW.PROVHEALTH.COM

PROVIDENCE WASHINGTON INSURANCE .... WWW.PROVWASH.COM

PROVIDENT MUTUAL LIFE INSURANCE CO .... WWW.PROVIDENTMUTUAL.COM

PRUDENTIAL HEALTH CARE .... WWW.PRUDENTIAL.COM

PYRAMID LIFE INSURANCE CO .... WWW.PYRAMIDLIFE.COM

QUAKER OATS CO .... WWW.QUAKEROATS.COM

QUAL MED OREGON HEALTH PLAN, INC .... WWW.QUALMEDOREGON.COM

QUAL MED WASHINGTON HEALTH PLAN, INC .... WWW.QUALMEDWA.COM

QUAL-MED HEALTH PLAN .... WWW.QUALMED.COM

RANGER INSURANCE CO .... WWW.RANGERINSURANCE.COM

REASSURANCE CO OF HANNOVER .... WWW.RCH.NET

REGENCE BLUE CROSS & BLUE SHIELD .... WWW.BCBSOR.COM

REGENCE BLUE SHIELD .... WWW.REGENCE.COM

REGENCE BLUE SHIELD OF IDAHO .... WWW.ID.REGENCE.COM

REGENCE BLUESHIELD .... WWW.WA.REGENCE.COM

REGENT INSURANCE CO .... WWW.GENCAS.COM

REGIONS BLUE CROSS & BLUE SHIELD OF OREGON .... WWW.BCBSO.COM

REHABILITATION NETWORK CORP .... WWW.NOVAEON.COM

REINSURANCE MANAGEMENT, INC .... WWW.RMIMHF.COM

RELIANCE INSURANCE CO .... WWW.RELIANCE.COM

RELIANCE STANDARD LIFE INSURANCE CO .... WWW.RSL.COM

RELIASTAR . . . . WWW.RELIASTAR.COM
REPUBLIC INDEMNITY CO OF AMERICA . . . . WWW.REPUBLICINDEMNITY.COM
REPUBLIC WESTERN INSURANCE CO . . . . WWW.REPWEST.COM
RESOURCE PARTNER . . . . WWW.RESOURCEPARTNER.COM
RISCO . . . . WWW.RISCO.COM
RITE AID CORPORATION . . . . WWW.RITEAID.COM
RIVERBEND GOVERNMENT BENEFITS ADMINISTRATOR . WWW.RIVERBENDGBA.COM
RLI CORP . . . . WWW.RLICORP.COM
ROCKFORD HEALTH PLANS . . . . WWW.RHSNET.ORG
ROCKY MOUNTAIN HMO . . . . WWW.RMHMO.ORG
ROYAL STATE GROUP . . . . WWW.HGEA.COM
ROYAL & SUNALLIANCE . . . . WWW.ROYALSUNALLIANCE.COM
RURAL MUTUAL INSURANCE CO . . . . WWW.RURALINS.COM
SAFECO INSURANCE CO OF AMERICA . . . . WWW.SAFECO.COM
SAFETY NATIONAL CASUALTY CORP . . . . WWW.SNCC.COM
SAIF CORP . . . . WWW.SAIF.COM
SAN FRANCISCO REINSURANCE CO . . . . WWW.THE-FUND.COM
SCOTT & WHITE HEALTH PLAN . . . . WWW.SW.ORG
SEABURY & SMITH . . . . WWW.SEABURY.COM
SECURITY HEALTH PLAN OF WISCONSIN, INC . . . . WWW.SECURITYHEALTH.ORG
SEDGWICK . . . . WWW.SEDGWICK.COM
SELECTIVE INSURANCE CO . . . . WWW.SELECTIVEINSURANCE.COM
SELF INSURED BENEFIT ADMINISTRATORS . . . . WWW.ONESOURCEGROUP.COM
SELF INSURED SERVICES CO . . . . WWW.CB-SISCO.COM
SELMAN & CO . . . . WWW.SELCO.COM
SENTRY INSURANCE A MUTUAL CO . . . . WWW.SENTRYINSURANCE.COM
SHAND MORHAN INSURANCE CO . . . . WWW.SHAND.COM
SHELTER INSURANCE COMPANIES . . . . WWW.SHELTERINS.COM
SHENANDOAH LIFE INSURANCE CO . . . . WWW.SHENLIFE.COM
SIERRA HEALTH & LIFE INSURANCE CO, INC . . . . WWW.SIERRAHEALTH.COM
SIGNA HEALTH CARE / COMED HMO . . . . WWW.SIGNA.COM
SIGNA HEALTH CARE HEALTHSOURCE . . . . WWW.HLTHFRC.COM

SIGNA HEALTHCARE . . . . WWW.SIGNAHEALTHCARE.COM

SIGNET REINSURANCE CO . . . . WWW.WRBC.COM

SOCIETY'S INSURANCE . . . . WWW.SOCIETYINSURANCE.COM

SONS OF NORWAY . . . . WWW.SOFN.COM

SOUTH CAROLINA FARM BUREAU MUTUAL INSURANCE CO . . . . WWW.SCFBINS.COM

SOUTHEASTERN INDIANA HEALTH ORGANIZATION . . . WWW.SIHO.ORG

SOUTHERN GUARANTY INSURANCE CO . . . . WWW.SGIC.COM

SOUTHERN HEALTH SERVICES . . . . WWW.SOUTHERNHEALTH.COM

SOUTHERN RISK SERVICES, INC . . . . WWW.SOUTHERNRISK.COM

SOUTHLAND LIFE INSURANCE CO . . . . WWW.ING.COM

SOUTHWEST BUSINESS CORP . . . . WWW.SWBC.COM

SOUTHWIRE CO . . . . WWW.SOUTHWIRE.COM

SPECIAL AGENTS MUTUAL BENEFIT ASSOCIATION . . . . WWW.SAMBA-INSURANCE.COM

SPECTARA . . . . WWW.SPECTARA.COM

ST. FRANCIS HOME CARE . . . . WWW.STFRANCIS.COM

ST. PAUL FIRE & MARINE . . . . WWW.STPAUL.COM

STANDARD INSURANCE CO . . . . WWW.STANDARD.COM

STANDARD MUTUAL INSURANCE CO . . . . WWW.STANDARDMUTUAL.COM

STAR INSURANCE CO . . . . WWW.MEADOWBROOKINSGRP.COM

STATE AUTOMOBILE MUTUAL INSURANCE CO . . . . . . WWW.STATEAUTO.COM

STATE COMPENSATION INSURANCE FUND . . . . WWW.SCIF.COM

STATE FARM INSURANCE CO . . . . WWW.STATEFARM.COM

STATE LIFE INSURANCE CO . . . . WWW.AUL.COM

STATE OF ALASKA WORKERS COMP DIVISION . . . . . . WWW.LABOR.STATE.AK.US/WC/WC/HTM

STONE EAGLE INSURANCE CO . . . . WWW.STONEEAGLE.COM

STUDENT INSURANCE . . . . WWW.SID.COM

SUN LIFE ASSURANCE OF CANADA . . . . WWW.SUNLIFE-USA.COM

SUPERIOR NATIONAL INSURANCE CO . . . . WWW.SUPERIOR.COM

SUPERMARKETS GENERAL CORP . . . . WWW.PATHMARK.COM

SURETY LIFE INSURANCE CO . . . . WWW.LDLWATS.COM

SWISS RE AMERICA . . . . WWW.SWISSREAMERICA.COM

SWISS RE LIFE & HEALTH AMERICA . . . . WWW.SWISSRE.COM

T.I.G. INSURANCE WWW.TIG1.COM

TDC RANDMARK MANAGEMENT DENTAL SERVICES . . . WWW.HUMANADENTAL.COM

TEACHERS INSURANCE & ANNUITY ASSOCIATION OF AMERICA . . . . WWW.TIAA/CREF.ORG

TEACHERS PROTECTIVE MUTUAL LIFE INSURANCE CO . . WWW.TPMINS.COM

TELEDYNE CORP . . . . WWW.ALLEGHENYTELEDYNE.COM

TENCO SERVICES . . . . WWW.TENCO.COM

TEXAS LIFE INSURANCE CO . . . . WWW.TEXLIFE.COM

TEXAS WORKER'S COMPENSATION COMMISSION . . . . WWW.TWCC.STATE.TX.US

THE ALLIANCE . . . . WWW.ALLIANCE-COLORADO.ORG

THE GUARDIAN . . . . WWW.THEGUARDIAN.COM

TOTAL HEALTH CARE, INC . . . . WWW.BCBSKC.COM

TPA . . . . WWW.THETPA.COM

TRAVELERS INSURANCE . . . . WWW.TRAVELERS.COM

TRENWICK AMERICA REINSURANCE CORP . . . . WWW.TRENWICK.COM

TRIGON . . . . WWW.TRIGON.COM

TRIGON ADMINISTRATORS . . . . WWW.TRIGONADMIN.COM

TRIGON BLUE CROSS BLUE SHIELD . . . . WWW.TRIGON.COM

TRIPLE-S INC, OF PUERTO RICO . . . . WWW.SSSPR.COM

TRUCK INSURANCE EXCHANGE . . . . WWW.FARMERSINSURANCE.COM

TRUSTMARK INSURANCE . . . . WWW.TRUSTMARKINS.COM

UCARE OF MINNESOTA . . . . WWW.UCARE.ORG

UNICARE . . . . WWW.WELLPOINT.COM

UNION INSURANCE CO . . . . WWW.UINS.COM

UNITED AMERICAN HEALTHCARE CORP . . . . WWW.OCHP.COM

UNITED AMERICAN INSURANCE . . . . WWW.UNITEDAMERICAN.COM

UNITED CHAMBERS ADMINISTRATORS . . . . WWW.ACLIC.COM

UNITED FARM FAMILY MUTUAL INSURANCE . . . . WWW.FARMBUREAU.COM

UNITED FIRE & CASUALTY . . . . WWW.UNITEDFIREGROUP.COM

UNITED GOVERNMENT SERVICES . . . . WWW.UWSI.COM

UNITED HEALTHCARE . . . . WWW.UHC.COM

UNITED HERITAGE MUTUAL LIFE INSURANCE CO . . . . . WWW.UNITEDHERITAGE.COM

UNITED SECURITY LIFE INSURANCE CO OF ILLINOIS . . . WWW.USOOFIL.COM

UNITED STATES FIDELITY & GUARANTY CO . . . . WWW.THEST.PAUL.COM

UNITED TEACHER ASSOCIATES INSURANCE CO . . . . . . WWW.UTAIC.COM

UNITY HEALTH PLANS . . . . WWW.UNITYHEALTH.COM

UNUM LIFE INSURANCE CO . . . . WWW.UNUM.COM

US LIABILITY INSURANCE CO . . . . WWW.USLI.COM

VIRGINIA FARM BUREAU MUTUAL INSURANCE CO . . . WWW.VAFB.COM

VISION SERVICE PLAN . . . . WWW.VSP.COM

VYTRA HEALTH PLANS . . . . WWW.VYTRA.COM

W.J. JONES ADMINISTRATIVE SERVICES, INC . . . . WWW.SELECTPRO.COM

W.J. JONES ADMINISTRATIVE SERVICES, INC . . . . WWW.WJJONES.COM

WALMART BENEFITS . . . . WWW.WALMART.COM

WARD NORTH AMERICA . . . . WWW.WARDNA.COM

WASHINGTON DENTAL SERVICE . . . . WWW.DDPWA.COM

WATSON WYATT WORLDWIDE . . . . WWW.WATSONWYATT.COM

WAUSAU INSURANCE CO . . . . WWW.WAUSAU.COM

WELBORN HMO DIVISION OF WELBORN CLINIC . . . . . WWW.WELBORNCLINIC.COM

WELLMARK BLUE CROSS & BLUE SHIELD . . . . WWW.BCBSIA.COM

WESLEY MEDICAL CENTER . . . . WWW.WESLEYMC.COM

WEST BEND MUTUAL INSURANCE CO . . . . WWW.WESTBENDMUTUAL.COM

WESTERN UNION FINANCIAL SERVICES . . . . WWW.WESTERNUNION.COM

WESTFIELD COMPANIES . . . . WWW.WESTFIELD-COS.COM

WEYCO, INC . . . . WWW.WEYCOINC.COM

WILLIAM H. MCGEE CO, INC . . . . WWW.WHMCGEE.COM

WILLIAM M. MERCER . . . . WWW.WMMERCER.COM

WINDSOR GROUP . . . . WWW.AUTOINSURANCE.COM

WINNEBAGO INDUSTRIES, INC . . . . WWW.WINNEBAGO-IND.COM

WISCONSIN PHYSICIAN SERVICE . . . . WWW.WPSIC.COM

WISCONSIN PUBLIC SERVICE CORP . . . . WWW.PSR.COM

WOODMEN ACCIDENT & LIFE CO . . . . WWW.WALLO.COM

WOODMEN OF THE WORLD LIFE INSURANCE SOCIETY . WWW.WOODMEN.COM

WORKMEN'S CIRCLE . . . . WWW.CIRCLE.COM

XACT MEDICARE . . . . WWW.XACT.ORG

ZENITH ADMINISTRATORS, INC . . . . WWW.ZENITH TPA

ZENITH INSURANCE CO . . . . WWW.ZENITH.COM

ZURICH-AMERICAN INSURANCE GROUP . . . . WWW.ZURICHAMERICAN.COM

Appendix E

Central Claims Offices

ACS NORTH AMERICAN
NORTH AMERICAN HEALTH PLANS
PO BOX 9501
AMHERST, NY 14226

ADMINISTRATIVE SERVICES, INC
7990 SW 117TH AVE
MIAMI, FL 33283

AETNA / U.S. HEALTHCARE
PO BOX 1125
BLUE BELL, PA 19422

AGIA, INC
1155 EUGENIA PL
CARPINTERIA, CA 93013-2062

AIG CLAIM SERVICES, INC
400 INTERPLACE PKWY, BLDG A 2ND FL
PARSIPPANY, NY 07054

111 JOHN ST
NEW YORK, NY 10038

ALFA INSURANCE CORP
2108 E SOUTH BLVD
PO BOX 11000
MONTGOMERY, AL 36191

ALLIED GROUP INSURANCE CO
3820 109TH ST
DES MOINES, IA 50391

ALLSTATE INSURANCE CO
2775 SANDERS RD, STE B-7
NORTHBROOK, IL 60062-6127

10135 SE SUNNYSIDE RD, STE 200
CLACKAMAS, OR 97015

33801 FIRST WAY S, STE 111
FEDERAL WAY, WA 98003

PO BOX 39
MARYSVILLE, WA 98270

ALPHA DATA SYSTEMS, INC
1545 W MOCKINGBIRD LN, STE 6000
DALLAS, TX 75235

ALTERNATIVE RISK MANAGEMENT, INC
3275 N ARLINGTON HTS RD, STE 401
ARLINGTON HEIGHTS, IL 60004

AM CASTLE & CO NON-BARGAINING
3400 N WOLF RD
FRANKLIN PARK, IL 60131-1319

AMALGAMATED LIFE & HEALTH INSURANCE CO
333 S ASHLAND AVE
CHICAGO, IL 60607-2702

AMERAPLAN, INC
22500 METROPOLITAN PKY, STE 100
CLINTON, MI 48035

AMERICA RE-INSURANCE
555 COLLEGE RD E
PO BOX 5241
PRINCETON, NJ 08543-5241

AMERICAID AMERIGROUP CO
617 7TH AVE- 2ND FL
FT WORTH, TX 76112

AMERICAN AMBASSADOR CASUALTY CO
1501 E WOODFIELD RD, STE 300 E
SCHAUMBURG, IL 60173-6000

AMERICAN BANKERS INSURANCE GROUP
11222 QUAIL ROOST DR
MIAMI, FL 33157-6543

AMERICAN BENEFIT MANAGEMENT
6520 WHIPPLE AVE NW
PO BOX 35008
NORTH CANTON, OH 44735

AMERICAN CENTENNIAL INSURANCE CO
FOULKSTONE PLZ- 1415 FOULK RD, STE 202
WILMINGTON, DE 19803-2766

AMERICAN COMMERCIAL LINES
1701 E MARKET ST
PO BOX 610
JEFFERSONVILLE, IN 47131-0610

AMERICAN COMMUNITY MUTUAL INSURANCE CO
39201 SEVEN-MILE RD
LIVONIA, MI 48152-1056

AMERICAN DENTAL EXAMINERS, INC
370 7TH AVE, STE 1206
NEW YORK, NY 10001-3907

AMERICAN FAMILY INSURANCE
6000 AMERICAN PKWY
MADISON, WI 53783

AMERICAN FREIGHTWAYS, INC
2200 FORWARD DR
PO BOX 840
HARRISON, AR 72602-0840

AMERICAN MEDICAL SECURITY
3100 AMS BLVD
GREEN BAY, WI 54313

AMERICAN MODERN INSURANCE GROUP
7000 MIDLAND BLVD
CINCINNATI, OH 45102-2607

AMERICAN NATIONAL PROPERTY & CASUALTY CO
CORPORATE CENTER, 1949 E SUNSHINE ST
SPRINGFIELD, MO 65899-0001

AMERICAN PUBLIC LIFE INSURANCE CO
2305 LAKELAND DR
JACKSON, MS 39208

AMERICAN REPUBLIC INSURANCE CO
601 6TH AVE
DES MOINES, IA 50301

AMERICAN SKANDIA LIFE REINSURANCE CORP
1 CORPORATE DR
SHELTON, CT 06484

AMERICAN TRAVEL, INC
PO BOX 66949
CHICAGO, IL 60666-0949

AMERICAN UNDERWRITERS LIFE INSURANCE CO
1035 S 18300 ST W
PO BOX 9510
WICHITA, KS 67277-0510

AMERICAN UNION LIFE INSURANCE CO
303 E WASHINGTON
PO BOX 2814
BLOOMINGTON, IL 61701-2814

AMERIHEALTH
720 BLAIR MILL RD
HORSHAM, PA 19044-2269

AMERIHEALTH HMO, INC
919 N MARKET ST
WILMINGTON, DE 19801-3021

AMERISURE COMPANIES
207 E FULTON
PO BOX 116
GRAND RAPIDS, MI 49501-0116

AMOCO INSURANCE PLANS
4850 STREET RD
TREVOSE, PA 19049-8000

ANDREW JERGENS CO
2535 SPRING GROVE AVE
CINCINNATI, OH 45214-1729

ANTHEM HEALTH & LIFE INSURANCE AGENCY
3575 KOGER BLVD, STE 400
DULUTH, GA 30136

ANTHEM SERVICES ADMINISTRATORS
1650 WATERMARK DR
PO BOX 528
COLUMBUS, OH 43216

APPALACHIAN LIFE INSURANCE CO
1124 4TH AVE
HUNTINGTON, WV 25707

ARGONAUT GREAT CENTRAL INSURANCE CO
3625 N SHERIDAN RD
PEORIA, IL 61633-1434

ARGUS SERVICES CORP
9500 FOREST LN, STE 300
DALLAS, TX 75243-5938

ARKANSAS FARM BUREAU MUTUAL INSURANCE
WARDEN RD 5051
NORTH LITTLE ROCK, AR 72231

ASSOCIATES FINANCIAL LIFE
290 E JOHN CARPENTER FWY
DALLAS, TX 75222

ATLANTIC MUTUAL / CENTENNIAL INSURANCE CO
7557 RAMBLER RD, STE 1000
DALLAS, TX 75231-2304

AUTO OWNERS INSURANCE CO
6101 ANACAPRI BLVD
LANSING, MI 48917

AUTOMATED BENEFITS SERVICES, INC
8220 IRVING
STERLING HEIGHTS, MI 48312

AUTOMOBILE CLUB INSURANCE CO
3590 TWIN CREEKS DR
COLUMBUS, OH 43218

AUTOMOTIVE PETROLEUM & ALLIED
300 S GRAND AVE, RM 232
SAINT LOUIS, MO 63103

AV-MED HEALTH PLAN
4300 NW 89TH BLVD
GAINSVILLE, FL 32606

9400 S DADELAND BLVD
MIAMI, FL 33256-9000

BABB, INC
850 RIDGE AVE
PITTSBURGH, PA 15212

BADGER MUTUAL INSURANCE CO
1635 W NATIONAL AVE
MILWAUKEE, WI 53204

BAKERY & CONFECTIONARY UNION
10401 CONNECTICUT AVE
KENSINGTON, MD 20895

BALBOA INSURANCE
PO BOX 19702
IRVINE, CA 92623-9702

BANC ONE KENTUCKY INSURANCE CO
312 S FOUR ST, STE 402
LOUISVILLE, KY 40232

BANK OF AMERICA
231 S LASALLE ST
CHICAGO, IL 60697

BANKERS FIDELITY LIFE INSURANCE
4370 PEACHTREE RD NE
ATLANTA, GA 31119

BANKERS INSURANCE GROUP
360 CENTRAL AVE
SAINT PETERSBURG, FL 33701

BANKERS LIFE & CASUALTY CO
222 MERCHANDISE MART PLZ
PO BOX 66927
CHICAGO, IL 60654

BASHAS', INC
2255 N 44TH ST, STE 220
PHOENIX, AZ 85008

BEECH STREET, INC
173 TECHNOLOGY
IRVINE, CA 92618

BENEFIT ADMINISTRATION CORP
770 E SHAW AVE, STE 1200
FRESNO, CA 93794

BENEFIT PLANNERS, INC
194 S MAIN
BOERNE, TX 78006

BENEFIT SUPPORT, INC
305 GREEN ST
GAINESVILLE, GA 30501

BENEFIT SYSTEMS & SERVICES, INC
760 PASQUINELLI DR, STE 320
WESTMONT, IL 60559-5555

BITUMINOUS CASUALTY CORP
600 VESTAVIA PKY, STE 121
PO BOX 360865
BIRMINGHAM, AL 35236-0865

320 18TH ST
ROCK ISLAND, IL 61201-8744

10800 FINANCIAL CTR PKY, STE 400
PO BOX 25326
LITTLE ROCK, AR 72221-5326

2310 PARKLAKE DR NE, STE 550
ATLANTA, GA 30345-2904

234 MADISON AVE, BUSINESS STE 102
PEORIA, IL 61602-8600

PO BOX 718
SHAWNEE, MO 66201-0718

312 WHITTINGTON PKY
PO BOX 7567
LOUISVILLE, KY 40257-0567

1301 YORK RD
PO BOX 509
LUTHERVILLE, MD 21094-0509

10733 SUNSET OFFICE DR, STE 430
SAINT LOUIS, MO 63127-1033

4801 EINDEPENDENCE BLVD, STE 505
CHARLOTTE, NC 28212-5400

234 MADISON AVE, BUSINESS STE 102
PEORIA, IL 61602

222 W LAS COLINAS BLVD, STE 1720
PO BOX 167968
IRVING, TX 75016-7968

BLUE CARE NETWORK
25925 TELEGRAPH RD
SOUTHFIELD, MI 48086-5043

BLUE CROSS & BLUE SHIELD
601 GAINES ST
PO BOX 2181
LITTLE ROCK, AR 72203-2181

21555 OXNARD ST
PO BOX 70000
WOODLAND HILLS, CA 91367-4943

532 RIVERSIDE AVE
PO BOX 1798
JACKSONVILLE, FL 32231-0014

PO BOX 4445
ATLANTA, GA 30302-4445

2357 WARM SPRINGS RD
COLUMBUS, GA 31908

818 KEEAUMOKU ST
PO BOX 860
HONOLULU, HI 96808-0860

636 GRAND AVE STATION 39
DES MOINES, IA 50309

1133 SW TOPEKA BLVD
PO BOX 239
TOPEKA, KS 66629-0001

2301 MAIN ST
PO BOX 419169
KANSAS CITY, MO 64141-6169

560 N PARK AVE
HELENA, MT 59604

7261 MERCY RD
OMAHA, NE 68180

PO BOX 2291
DURHAM, NC 27702-2291

PO BOX 7368
COLUMBUS, GA 31908

7261 MERCY RD
OMAHA, NE 68180

4510 13TH AVE SW
FARGO, ND 58121

165 COURT ST
ROCHESTER, NY 14647-0001

PO BOX 35
DURHAM, NC 27702

PO BOX 37180
LOUISVILLE, KY 40233

1215 S BOULDER
PO BOX 3283
TULSA, OK 74102-3283

PO BOX 10
MEMPHIS, TN 38101

PO BOX 660044
DALLAS, TX 75266-0044

PO BOX 91080
SEATTLE, WA 98111-9180

BLUE RIDGE INSURANCE CO
86 HOPMEADOW ST
SIMSBURY, CT 06074

BOSTON MUTUAL LIFE INSURANCE CO
120 ROYALL ST
CANTON, MA 02021-1098

BRETHREN MUTUAL INSURANCE CO
149 N EDGEWOOD DR
HAGERSTOWN, MD 21740-6599

BROTHERHOOD MUTUAL INSURANCE CO
6400 BROTHERHOOD WY
FT WAYNE, IN 46801

BURNHAM SERVICE CORP
1630 PHOENIX BLVD
PO BOX 100541
ATLANTA, GA 30384-0541

C.F.S. HEALTH GROUP
PO BOX 820 (MEDICARE CLAIMS)
OWINGS MILLS, MD 27117-0820

CAL FARM INSURANCE CO
PO BOX 15016
SACRAMENTO, CA 95851-1016

CALIFORNIA BENEFITS DENTAL PLAN
3611 S HARBOR BLVD, STE 150
SANTA ANA, CA 92704

CALIFORNIA CASUALTY INSURANCE CO
PO BOX 42630
PHOENIX, AZ 85080

CASUALTY INSURANCE CO
500 N BRAND BLVD
GLENDALE, CA 91203-3392

CGU
707 SABLE OAKS DR
SOUTH PORTLAND, ME 04106

2455 CORPORATE WEST DR
LISLE, IL 60532

1 BEACON ST
PO BOX 9003
BOSTON, MA 02108

100 CORPORATE CTR DR
CAMP HILL, PA 17011

801 N BRAND BLVD- 8TH FL
PO BOX 29037
GLENDALE, CA 91209-9037

504 S SERVICE RD E
RUSTON, LA 71273

178 MAIN ST
WATERVILLE, ME 04901

175 DWIGHT RD
LONGMEADOW, MA 01106

8 ESSEX CTR DR
PEABODY, MA 01961

PO BOX 302
BUFFALO, NY 14240-0302

CGU HAWKEYE UNITED SECURITY INSURANCE CO
10303 E DRY CREEK RD, STE 300
ENGLEWOOD, CO 80112

CGU INSURANCE / GENERAL ACCIDENT
8282 S MEMORIAL
TULSA, OK 74102

CHAMPUS
PO BOX 202000
FLORENCE, SC 29502-2000

CHUBB GROUP OF INSURANCE COMPANIES
6200 COURTNEY CAMPBELL CSWY, STE 700
TAMPA, FL 33607

25 INDEPENDENCE BLVD, 1ST FL
WARREN, NJ 07059

600 INDEPENDENCE PKY
PO BOX 4700
CHESAPEAKE, VA 23327

5050 HOPYARD RD, STE 400
PLEASANTON, CA 94588-3321

3445 PIEDMONT RD NE, STE 900
ATLANTA, GA 30326-1276

SEARS TWR- 233 S WACKER DR, STE 4700
CHICAGO, IL 60606

6200 COURTNEY CAMPBELL CSWY, STE 700
TAMPA, FL 33607

3445 PIEDMONT RD NE, STE 900
ATLANTA, GA 30326-1276

5750 NEW KING ST, STE 200
TROY, MI 48098

10 PETTICOAT LN- 3RD FL
PO BOX 13167
KANSAS CITY, MO 64199-3167

111 WINNER'S CIR
ALBANY, NY 12212

OLYMPIC TWRS- 300 PEARL ST, STE 900
BUFFALO, NY 14202

55 WATER ST
NEW YORK, NY 10041

1221 AVE OF THE AMERICAS- 25TH FL
NEW YORK, NY 10020

333 EARLE OVINGTON BLVD
UNIONDALE, NY 11553

2200 1ST UNION CTR- 301 S COLLEGE ST
CHARLOTTE, NC 28202

312 WALNUT ST- 18TH FL
CINCINNATI, OH 45202

BANK ONE CTR- 600 SUPERIOR AVE E- 11TH FL
CLEVELAND, OH 44114

PIONEER TWR- 888 SW 5TH AVE, STE 400
PORTLAND, OR 97204

2 WARREN PL- 6120 S YALE, STE 450
TULSA, OK 74136

5TH AVE PL- 120 5TH AVE
PITTSBURGH, PA 15222

NATIONS BANK PLZ- 300 CONVENT ST, STE 2300
SAN ANTONIO, TX 78205

2 PLZ E- 330 E KILBOURNE AVE, STE 1450
MILWAUKEE, WI 53202

15 MOUNTAINVIEW RD
WARREN, NJ 07059

1445 ROSS AVE, STE 4200
DALLAS, TX 75202-2785

CHURCH MUTUAL INSURANCE CO
3000 SCHUSTER LN
MERRILL, WI 54452-3098

CHURCHILL ADMINISTRATIVE PLANS, INC
270 SYLVAN AVE
ENGLEWOOD CLIFFS, NJ 07632

CIGNA CORPORATION
1 BEAVER VALLEY RD
WILMINGTON, DE 19850

1601 CHESTNUT ST- TWO LIBERTY PL
PHILADELPHIA, PA 19192-1550

600 E TAYLOR
SHERMAN, TX 75091

PO BOX 152035
IRVING, TX 75015

10860 GOLD CTR DR, STE 455
RANCHO CORDOVA, CA 95670

9740 APPALOOSA DR
SAN DIEGO, CA 92121

4025 W MINERAL KING
VISALIA, CA 93278-5038

100 PEACHTREE ST NW, STE 700
ATLANTA, GA 30303

2 VANTAGE WY
PO BOX 22599
NASHVILLE, TN 37202

21 HERITAGE DR
BOURBONNAIS, IL 60914

13300 HICKMAN RD
CLIVE, IA 50325

9700 PATUXENT WOOD DR
COLUMBIA, MD 21046

24750 LAHSER DR
SOUTHFIELD, MI 48086

26913 NORTHWESTERN HWY, STE 300
SOUTHFIELD, MI 48037

PO BOX 64143
SAINT PAUL, MN 55164-0143

PO BOX 3316 STA DR
ALBUQUERQUE, NM 87190-3310

32 VALLEY ST
BRISTOL, CT 06010

263 RT 17K
NEWBURGH, NY 12550

255 EAST AVE
ROCHESTER, NY 14604

4198 COX RD- 2ND FL
GLEN ALLEN, VA 23060

1000 POLARIS PKY
COLUMBUS, OH 43240

1630 E SHAW AVE, STE 106
PO BOX 24022
FRESNO, CA 93779-4022

PO BOX 2300
PITTSBURGH, PA 15230

250 YOUNGS ST, STE 1400
TORONTO, ON M5B-2L7

12225 GREENVILLE AVE
PO BOX 9384
DALLAS, TX 75243-9384

PO BOX 13088
SACRAMENTO, CA 95813-4088

3838 N CSWY BLVD #2800-B
METAIRIE, LA 70002

600 E LAS COLINAS BLVD
IRVING, TX 75039

8310 N CAPITOL TX HWY, STE 175
AUSTIN, TX 78731

7555 GOODWIN RD
PO BOX 188002
CHATTANOOGA, TN 37421

ONE CORP CTR DR, STE 500-472-50
SHERMAN, TX

1700 HIGGINS, STE 600
DES PLAINES, IL 60018

CINCINNATI EQUITABLE
525 VINE ST, STE 2100
CINCINNATI, OH 45201

CINCINNATI INSURANCE CO
6200 S GILMORE
FAIRFIELD, OH 45014

CITGO PETROLEUM CORP
PO BOX 3758
TULSA, OK 74102-3758

CITIZENS INSURANCE CO OF AMERICA
3950 PRIORITY WAY S DR, STE 200
INDIANAPOLIS, IN 46240

2501 14TH AVE S
PO BOX 1028
ESCANABA, MI 49829-1028

814 S OTSEGO
GAYLORD, MI 49734

645 W GRAND RIVER AVE
HOWELL, MI 48843

8101 N HIGH ST, STE 40
COLUMBUS, OH 43235

CITRUS INSURANCE TRUST
25060 AVE STANFORD, STE 200
VALENCIA, CA 91355-3446

CITY OF AMARILLO GROUP HEALTH PLAN
909 E 7TH
AMARILLO, TX 79105

CITY OF LONG BEACH
333 W OCEAN BLVD- 8TH FL
LONG BEACH, CA 90802-4664

CIVIL SERVICE EMPLOYEES INSURANCE CO
989 MARKET ST
SAN FRANCISCO, CA 94103

CIVIL SERVICE EMPLOYEES INSURANCE GROUP
2720 GATEWAY OAK DR #300
SACRAMENTO, CA 95835

CLARK UNITED PROVIDERS
505 NE 87TH AVE, STE 1147
VANCOUVER, WA 98664

CMS CAP MANAGEMENT SYSTEMS
12966 EUCLID ST, STE 500
GARDEN GROVE, CA 92840

CNA
CNA PLZ- 333 S WABASH AVE
CHICAGO, IL 60685

1800 E IMPERIAL HWY
BREA, CA 92821

3075 E IMPERIAL HWY
PO BOX 6500
BREA, CA 92822

10333 E DRY CREEK RD, STE 300
ENGLEWOOD, CO 80217

707 ORLANDO CENTRAL PKY
ORLANDO, FL 32809

200 S WACKER DR
CHICAGO, IL 60606

1411 OPUS PL
PO BOX 1562
DOWNERS GROVE, IL 60515

8403 COLESVILLE RD
SILVER SPRING, MD 20910

1250 HANCOCK ST
PO BOX 9167
QUINCY, MA 02269-9167

400 GALLERIA OFC CTR, STE 300
PO BOX 5159
SOUTHFIELD, MI 48086-5159

175 PINELAWN RD
MELVILLE, NY 11747

333 GLEN ST
PO BOX 5000
GLENS FALLS, NY 12801

ONE TELERGY PKY
SYRACUSE, NY 13057

PO BOX 182644
COLUMBUS, OH 43218-2644

1111 E BROAD ST
COLUMBUS, OH 43205

2 CHATHAM CTR- 112 WASHINGTON PL
PITTSBURGH, PA 15219

600 N PEARL ST, STE 1400F
DALLAS, TX 75381

PO BOX 27537
HOUSTON, TX 77227-7537

6805 CAPITOL OF TX HWY, STE 260
HOUSTON, TX 78731

CO-OP INSURANCE COMPANIES
292 COLONIAL DR
MIDDLEBURY, VT 05735

COASTCAST CORP
3025 E VICTORIA ST
RANCHO DOMINGUEZ, CA 90224

COLLIN COUNTY COURTHOUSE
210 S MCDONALD ST, STE 612
MCKINNEY, TX 75069

COLONIAL INSURANCE CO
5525 PARKCENTER CIR
DUBLIN, OH 43017

COLONIAL LIFE & ACCIDENT INSURANCE CO
1200 COLONIAL LIFE BLVD
PO BOX 1365
COLUMBIA, SC 29202-1365

COLORADO FARM BUREAU MUTUAL INSURANCE CO
9177 E MINERAL CIR
ENGLEWOOD, CO 80112

COLUMBIA INSURANCE GROUP, INC
2102 WHITE GATE DR
PO BOX 618
COLUMBIA, MO 65205

COMAIR INC
2258 TOWER DR
ERLANGER, KY 41818

COMBINED INSURANCE CO OF AMERICA
5050 N BROADWAY
CHICAGO, IL 60640

COMMERCIAL UNION INSURANCE CO OF AMERICA
108 MYRTLE ST
NORTH QUINCY, MA 02171

COMMONWEALTH HEALTH ALLIANCE
1650 STATE FARM BLVD
CHARLOTTESVILLE, VA 22902

COMPANION HEALTH CARE CORP
200 ARBOR LAKE DR, STE 200
COLUMBIA, SC 29260

COMPCARE HEALTH SERVICES INSURANCE CO
401 W MICHIGAN ST
PO BOX 1581
MILWAUKEE, WI 53201

COMPDENT
100 MANSELL CT E, STE 400
ROSWELL, GA 30076

COMPENSATION PROGRAMS OF OHIO, INC
1123 N CANFIELD NILES RD
PO BOX 230
AUSTINTOWN, OH 44515

COMPREHENSIVE BENEFITS ADMINISTRATORS, INC
30 AIRPORT RD
PO BOX 2365
SOUTH BURLINGTON, VT 05407-2365

COMPREHENSIVE CARE SERVICES
1200 YANKEE DOODLE RD
EGAN, MN 55122

COMPUTER SCIENCE CORP
800 N PEARL ST
ALBANY, NY 12204

CONCORD GENERAL
510 S ST
PO BOX 2048
CONCORD, NH 03302-2048

CONCORD GROUP INSURANCE
AIRPORT RD
PO BOX 870
MONTPELIER, VT 05601

CONCORD GROUP INSURANCE CO
4 BOUTON ST
CONCORD, NH 03301

308 CENTER ST
PO BOX 300
AUBURN, ME 04212

CONESTOGA LIFE ASSURANCE CO
1871 SANTA BARBARA DR, PO BOX 7777
LANCASTER, PA 17604-7777

CONSECO DIRECT LIFE INSURANCE CO
399 MARKET ST
PHILADELPHIA, PA 19181

CONSOLIDATED AMERICAN INSURANCE CO
1501 LADY ST
PO BOX 1
COLUMBIA, SC 29202

CONSOLIDATED HEALTH PLANS
195 STAFFORD ST
SPRINGFIELD, MA 01104-3503

CONSOLIDATED INTERNATIONAL, INC
1415 FOULK RD, STE 205
WILMINGTON, DE 19803

CONSOLIDATED NATURAL GAS CO
625 LIBERTY AVE- CNG TWR
PITTSBURGH, PA 15222-3199

CONTAINER SUPPLY CO
12571 WESTERN
PO BOX 5367
GARDEN GROVE, CA 92841

CONTINENTAL GENERAL INSURANCE CO
8901 INDIAN HILLS DR
OMAHA, NE 68124

CONTINENTAL LIFE & ACCIDENT
304 N MAIN ST
ROCKFORD, IL 61105

CONTINENTAL WESTERN INSURANCE CO
3641 S WEST PLZ
TOPEKA, KS 66604

100 N 84TH ST
LINCOLN, NE 68501

CONTRA COSTA HEALTH PLAN
595 CENTER AVE, STE 100
MARTINEZ, CA 94553

COOK GROUP HEALTH PLAN TRUST
PO BOX 489
BLOOMINGTON, IN 47402

COOPERATIVA DE SEGUROS
DE VIDA DE PUERTO RICO
PO BOX 363428
SAN JUAN, PR 00936-3428

CORESOURCE
14440 MYERLAKE CIR
CLEARWATER, FL 33760

400 FIELD DR
LAKE FOREST, IL 60045

CORESOURCE, INC
4801 SOUTHWICK DR, STE 400
MATTESON, IL 60443

410 FIELD DRIVE
LAKE FOREST, IL 60045

4210 SHAWNEE MISSION PKY, STE 302A
SHAWNEE MISSION, KS 66205

3717 NATIONAL DR, STE 217
RALEIGH, NC 27622

229 HUBER VLG BLVD
PO BOX 6118
WESTERVILLE, OH 43081-6118

CORPORATE BENEFIT SERVICE, INC
145 SCALEY BARK, STE B
CHARLOTTE, NC 28209

COTTON STATES INSURANCE COMPANIES
244 PERIMETER CENTER PKY
ATLANTA, GA 30346

COUNTRY MUTUAL & COUNTRY CASUALTY
PO BOX 2100
BLOOMINGTON, IL 61702

2150 COUNTRY DR S
PO BOX 2209
SALEM, OR 97308

COVENTRY HEALTHCARE
6705 ROCKLEDGE DR, STE 900
BETHESDA, MD 20817

COX INSURANCE GROUP, INC
5170 COMMERCE CIR
INDIANAPOLIS, IN 46237

CPIC LIFE
PO BOX 3007
LODI, CA 95241-1911

CRAWFORD & CO
5620 GLENRIDGE DR NE
PO BOX 5047
ATLANTA, GA 30302

10802 EXECUTIVE CTR DR, STE 208
LITTLE ROCK, AR 72211

562 MANZANITA AVE, STE 9
CHICO, CA 95926

400 CORPORATE PT
CULVER CITY, CA 90230

10411 OLD PLACERVILLE RD, STE 200
SACRAMENTO, CA 95827-2508

3870 MURPHY CANYON RD, STE 100
SAN DIEGO, CA 92123

711 KAPIOLANI BLVD, STE 900
HONOLULU, OAHU, HI

625 CENTRAL AVE W, STE 100
GREAT FALLS, MT 59403

CRUM & FORSTER INSURANCE
305 MADISON AVE
MORRISTOWN, NJ 07960

27710 NORTHWESTERN HWY, STE 200
SOUTHFIELD, MI 48034

275 BATTERY ST- 7TH FL
SAN FRANCISCO, CA 94120

201 MERCHANT ST, STE 1960
HONOLULU, HI 96813

111 W 22ND ST
OAK BROOK, IL 60523

4445 LK FOREST DR, STE 700
CINCINNATI, OH 45242

89 S ST- LINCOLN PLZ- 5TH FL
BOSTON, MA 02111

55 S LAKE AVE, STE 700
PASADENA, CA 91101

305 MADISON AVE
MORRISTOWN, NJ 07960

225 GREENFIELD PKY
LIVERPOOL, NY 13088

400 N EXECUTIVE DR
BROOKFIELD, WI 53008

7900 INTERNATIONAL DR, STE 700
BLOOMINGTON, MN 55425

PO BOX 7791
SAN FRANCISCO, CA 94111

1601 5TH AVE, STE 1450
SEATTLE, WA 98101

QUADRANT, STE 500, 5445 DTC PKY
DENVER, CO 80217

CSA BENEFIT
4625 S WENDLER DR, STE 211
TEMPE, AZ 85282

CTI ADMINISTRATIORS, INC
100 COURT AVE, STE 306
DES MOINES, IA 50309-2200

CUNA MUTUAL GROUP
5190 MINERAL POINT RD
MADISON, WI 53705

5910 MINERAL POINT RD
MADISON, WI 53701

CUNNINGHAM LINDSEY INC
PO BOX 6030
TYLER, TX 75711

CYPRESS INSURANCE CO
PO BOX 7008
PASADENA, CA 91109

DBL SERVICES, INC
PO BOX 66714
SAINT LOUIS, MO 63166-6714

DC CHARTERED HEALTH PLAN, INC
820 FIRST ST NE, STE LL100
WASHINGTON, DC 20002

DEACONESS MEDICAL CENTER
PO BOX 37000
BILLINGS, MT 59107-7000

DEAN HEALTH PLAN HMO
1277 DEMING WAY
MADISON, WI 53705

DEEP SOUTH SURPLUS OF TEXAS
PO BOX 143-0099
IRVING, TX 75014

DELMARVA HEALTH PLAN, INC
PO BOX 2410
EASTON, MD 21601

DELOITTE & TOUCHE
10 WESTPORT RD
WILTON, CT 06897

DELTA CASUALTY CO
4711 N CLARK ST
CHICAGO, IL 60640-4632

DELTA DENTAL INSURANCE CO
ONE DELTA DR
MECHANICSBURG, PA 17055-6999

PO BOX 1809
ALPHARETTA, GA 30023-1809

ONE DELTA DR
MECHANICSBURG, PA 17055-6999

AVE DE DIEGO ESQ LOIZA ST, STE 75
SAN JUAN, PR 00902-0992

PO BOX 29
CHEYENNE, WY 82003

DELTA DENTAL OF CALIFORNIA
PO BOX 7736
SAN FRANCISCO, CA 94120

DELTA DENTAL OF RHODE ISLAND
PO BOX 1517
PROVIDENCE, RI 02901-1517

DELTA DENTAL OF WEST VIRGINIA
ONE DELTA DR
MECHANICSBURG, PA 17055-6999

DELTA DENTAL PLAN OF KENTUCKY
PO BOX 242810
LOUISVILLE, KY 40224-2810

DELTA DENTAL PLAN OF MASSACHUSETTS
PO BOX 9695
BOSTON, MA 02114

DELTA DENTAL PLAN OF MICHIGAN
PO BOX 9085
FARMINGTON HILLS, MT 48333-9085

DELTA DENTAL PLAN OF NEBRASKA
PO BOX 245
MINNEAPOLIS, MN 55440-0330

DELTA DENTAL PLAN OF NEW JERSEY INC
1639 RT 10
PARSIPPANY, NJ 07054

DELTA DENTAL PLAN OF NEW MEXICO
2500 LOUISIANA BLVD NE, STE 600
ALBUQUERQUE, NM 87110

DELTA DENTAL PLAN OF NORTH CAROLINA
333 SIX FORKS RD, STE 180
RALEIGH, NC 27609

DELTA DENTAL PLAN OF OHIO
PO BOX 9085
FARMINGTON HILLS, MT 48333-9085

DELTA DENTAL PLAN OF OKLAHOMA
PO BOX 16175
LITTLE ROCK, AR 72231

DELTA DENTAL PLAN OF VIRGINIA
4818 STARKEY RD SW
ROANOKE, VA 24014-4010

DENTAL BENEFIT PROVIDERS
PO BOX 30640
BETHESDA, MD 20814

311 CALIFORNIA ST, STE 550
SAN FRANCISCO, CA 94104

DEPARTMENT OF WATER & POWER CITY OF LOS ANGELES
PO BOX 5111
LOS ANGELES, CA 90051

DESERET MUTUAL
60 E SOUTH TEMPLE
SALT LAKE CITY, UT 84145-0530

DIAMOND G EMPLOYEE BENEFIT PLAN
102 COILE ST
GREENEVILLE, TN 37744-0877

DIRECT RESPONSE INSURANCE ADMINISTRATIVE SERVICES, INC
PO BOX 96
MINNEAPOLIS, MN 55440

DISTRICT 6 HEALTH FUND
18 E 31ST ST
NEW YORK, NY 10016-6702

DIVISION 1181 ATU NEW YORK WELFARE
10149 WOODHAVEN BLVD
OZONE PARK, NY 11416-2300

DODSON INSURANCE GROUP
PO BOX 419497
KANSAS CITY, MO 64141-6497

DOLLAR GENERAL CORP
427 BEACH ST
SCOTTSVILLE, TN 42164

DONEGAL MUTUAL INSURANCE CO
1195 RIVER RD
MARIETTA, PA 17547

DONOVAN BENEFIT SYSTEMS, INC
440 LOUISIANA ST, STE 1600
HOUSTON, TX 77002-1634

DUNCANSON & HOLT GROUP(S)
100 WALL ST, 5TH FL
NEW YORK, NY 10005

E.B.A. & M. CORP
30501 AGOURA RD, STE 102
AGOURA, CA 91301

EAGLE INSURANCE GROUP
4025 DELRIDGE WAY SW, STE 300
SEATTLE, WA 98106

EAGLE PACIFIC INSURANCE CO
4300 B ST, STE 403
ANCHORAGE, AK 99503-5929

EASTERN SHORE TEAMSTERS
1323 N SALISBURY BLVD
SALISBURY, MD 21801-3674

EAU CLAIRE HEALTH PROTECTION PLAN
2000 WESTWOOD DR
WAUSAU, WI 55401

EBI CO
10 WATERSIDE
FARMINGTON, CT 06032

EBI COMPANIES
PO BOX 4322
WOODLAND HILLS, CA 91365-4322

2443 WARRENVILLE RD, STE 115
LISLE, IL 60532

PO BOX 3725
PORTLAND, OR 97208

EDUCATORS HEALTH CARE, INC
852 E ARROWHEAD LN
MURRAY, UT 84107-5298

EDUCATORS MUTUAL LIFE INSURANCE CO
PO BOX 83888
LANCASTER, PA 17608-3888

ELECTRIC INSURANCE CO
152 CONANT ST
BEVERLY, MA

ELECTRONIC DATA SYSTEMS
PO BOX 15508
SACRAMENTO, CA 95852

EMERALD HEALTH NETWORK, INC
PO BOX 94808
CLEVELAND, OH 44101-4808

EMPIRE BLUE CROSS & BLUE SHIELD
PO BOX 11800
ALBANY, NY 12211-0800

EMPIRE FIRE & MARINE INSURANCE CO
13810 SMB PKY
OMAHA, NE 68154-5202

EMPIRE INSURANCE GROUP/ ALL CITY INSURANCE CO
35 STREET ADAM ST
BROOKLYN, NY 11201

EMPIRE MEDICARE SERVICES
PO BOX 4846
SYRACUSE, NY 13221-4846

EMPLOYEE BENEFIT ASSOCIATION
2858 W MARKET ST, STE N
AKRON, OH 44333

EMPLOYEE BENEFIT CLAIMS, INC
820 PARISH ST
PITTSBURGH, PA 15220-3405

EMPLOYEE BENEFIT INSURANCE
PO BOX 4322
WOODLAND HILLS, CA 91365-4322

EMPLOYEE BENEFIT MANAGEMENT SERVICES INC
PO BOX 21367
BILLINGS, MT 59104-1367

EMPLOYEE BENEFIT TRUST
PO BOX 6279
SPRINGFIELD, IL 62708-6279

EMPLOYEE SECURITY, INC
5565 STERRETT PL, STE 300
COLUMBIA, MD 21044-2608

EMPLOYER PLAN SERVICES, INC
2180 N LOOP W, STE 400
HOUSTON, TX 77018

EMPLOYERS REINSURANCE CORP
PO BOX 2991
OVERLAND PARK, KS 66202-1296

EMS ADMINISTRATIVE SERVICE CORP
1115 W LANCASTER AVE
FT WORTH, TX 76102-4509

ENTERPRISE LIFE INSURANCE CO
PO BOX 167667
IRVING, TX 75016

EPIC LIFE INSURANCE CO, INC
6801 SOUTH TOWNE DR
MADISON, WI 53708-8924

EQUAFAX HEALTH CORP
PO BOX 6000
HOUSTON, TX 73534

EQUITABLE LIFE & CASUALTY INSURANCE CO
PO BOX 2460
SALT LAKE CITY, UT 84110-2460

EQUITABLE PLAN SERVICES, INC
PO BOX 770466
OKLAHOMA CITY, OK 73177

EQUITY MUTUAL INSURANCE CO
PO BOX 419497
KANSAS CITY, MO 64141-6497

ERIE INSURANCE CO
PO BOX 9031
CANTON, 44711-9031

PO BOX 9326
FT WAYNE, IN 46899-0326

PO BOX 4286
BETHLEHEM, PA 18018-0286

PO BOX 1699
ERIE, PA 16530

PO BOX 999
JOHNSTOWN, PA 15907

100 ERIE INSURANCE PL
ERIE, PA 16530

PO BOX 598
PARKERSBURG, WV 26102-0598

1400 N PROVIDENCE RD
MEDIA, PA 19063-2094

100 ERIE INSURANCE PLACE
ERIE, PA 16530

ERIE INSURANCE GROUP
PO BOX 80129
INDIANAPOLIS, IN 46280-0129

PO BOX 28120
RICHMOND, VA 23228-0120

PO BOX 20769
ROANOKE, VA 24018-0524

PO BOX 4158
HAGERSTOWN, MD 21741-4158

PO BOX 730
CORY, NC 27512-0730

PO BOX 2013
MECHANICSBURG, PA 17055-0710

ERIN GROUP ADMINISTRATORS, INC
PO BOX 7777
LANCASTER, PA 17604-7777

ERISA ADMINISTRATIVE SERVICES, INC
12325 HYMEADOW DR- BLDG 4
AUSTIN, TX 78750-0001

ESIS CO
PO BOX 5025
FREMONT, CA 94537-5025

EVEREADY INSURANCE CO
59 MAIDEN LN
NEW YORK, NY 10038-4510

EXCESS REINSURANCE UNDERWRITERS AGENCY, INC
PO BOX 667
WOODBURY, NJ 08096-7667

EXCLUSIVE HEALTHCARE, INC
PO BOX 31488
OMAHA, NE 68131-0488

EXECUTIVE RESOURCES, INC
3140 CAHABA HTS RD, STE 102
BIRMINGHAM, AL 35243

EYE CARE OF WISCONSIN, INC
8633 N PORT WASHINGTON RD
FOX POINT, WI 53217-2213

FALLON COMMUNITY HEALTH PLAN, INC
10 CHESTNUT ST- ONE CHESTNUT PL
WORCESTER, MA 01608

FAMILY FINANCIAL LIFE INSURANCE CO
2555 SEVERN AVE
METAIRIE, LA 70002

FAMILY HEALTH PLAN COOPERATIVE
11524 W THEO TRECKER WY
MILWAUKEE, WI 53214

FAMILY HEALTH PLAN OF OHIO
PO BOX 4708
TOLEDO, OH 43610

FARM BUREAU MUTUAL INSURANCE CO
194 E COMMERCIAL
WEISER, ID 83672-2511

FARM BUREAU MUTUAL INSURANCE CO OF IDAHO
1250 S ALLANTE AVE
BOISE, ID 83709

PO BOX 4848
POCATELLO, ID 83205

FARM BUREAU TOWN & COUNTRY INSURANCE CO OF MISSOURI
701 S COUNTRY CLUB DR
JEFFERSON CITY, 65101-0658

FARM FAMILY CASUALTY
PO BOX 656
ALBANY, NY 12201-0656

FARM FAMILY CASUALTY INSURANCE
41 LIBERTY ST, STE 2
BATAVIA, NY 14020

FARMERS ALLIANCE MUTUAL INSURANCE CO
PO BOX 1401
MC PHERSON, KS 67460-1401

FARMERS CASUALTY INSURANCE CO
PO BOX 65150
WEST DES MOINES, IA 50265-0150

FARMERS HOME GROUP
PO BOX 9420
MINNEAPOLIS, MN 55440-9420

PO BOX 17347
SALT LAKE CITY, UT 84117

10536 JUSTIN DR
URBANDALE, IA 50322

FARMERS INSURANCE EXCHANGE
PO BOX 9075
VAN NUYS, CA 91409

FARMERS INSURANCE GROUP
9135 S REDWOOD RD
WEST JORDAN, UT 84088

PO BOX 3887
MERCED, CA 95344-3887

4680 WILSHIRE BLVD
LOS ANGELES, CA 90010

PO BOX 9756
OGDEN, UT 84409

FARMINGTON MEDICAL ASSOCIATES
95 GLASTONBURY BLVD
GLASTONBURY , MA 06033

FARMLAND INSURANCE CO
PO BOX 2660
BLOOMINGTON, IL 61702-2660

PO BOX 2650
HUTCHINSON, KS 67504-2650

1963 BELL AVE
DES MOINES, IA 50315

PO BOX 15445
AMARILLO, TX 79105-5445

FARMLAND MUTUAL
PO BOX 6065
LINCOLN, NE 68506-0065

FARMLAND MUTUAL/ NATIONWIDE AGRA BUSINESS
1963 BELL AVE
DES MOINES, IA 50315-1000

FEDERATED AMERICAN INSURANCE CO
15300 BOTHELL WAY NE
SEATTLE, WA 98155-7699

FEDERATED GUARANTY LIFE INSURANCE COMPANIES
PO BOX 11000
MONTGOMERY, AL 36191-0001

FEDERATED MUTUAL INSURANCE CO
PO BOX 328
OWATONNA, MN 55060

2400 W DUNLAP AVE, STE 250
PHOENIX, AZ 85021

11050 OLSON DR, STE 100
RANCHO CORDOVA, CA 95670

PO BOX 28477
ATLANTA, GA 30358-0477

121 E PARKS SQ
OWATANNA, MN 55060

PO BOX 390850
EDINA, MN 55439-0850

PO BOX 419444
KANSAS CITY, MO 64141

PO BOX 50487
INDIANAPOLIS, IN 46250-0487

PO BOX 305129
NASHVILLE, TN 37214

FEWELL & ASSOCIATES AMERICAN INVESTORS
PO BOX 8212
LITTLE ROCK, AR 72221-8212

FIC INSURANCE
PO BOX 149138
AUSTIN, TX 78714-9138

FIDELIO INSURANCE CO
2826 MT CARMEL AVE
GLENSIDE, PA 19038-2245

FIDELITY & DEPOSIT CO OF MARYLAND
PO BOX 1227
BALTIMORE, MD 21203-4098

FIDELITY SECURITY LIFE INSURANCE CO
PO BOX 418131
KANSAS CITY, MO 64141-9131

FINANCIAL BENEFIT, INC
PO BOX 13163
KANSAS CITY, MO 64199-3163

FINANCIAL INDEMNITY CO
21650 OXNARD ST, STE 1800
WOODLAND HILLS, CA 91367

FINANCIAL INSURANCE CENTER
UNION FIDELITY OFC PRK
TREVOSE, PA 19049-6511

FIREMAN'S FUND INSURANCE CO
PO BOX 13340
SACRAMENTO, CA 95813-3340

195 SCOTT SWAMP RD
FARMINGTON, CT 06032

PO BOX 26705
GREENSBORO, NC 27407-6705

PO BOX 18025
TAMPA, FL 33679-8025

9690 DEERECO RD
TIMONIUM, MD 21093

PO BOX 419083
SAINT LOUIS, MO 63141-9083

1100 WALNUT, STE 3000- PO BOX 13206
KANSAS CITY, MO 64199-3206

JOHN HANCOCK TOWER
BOSTON, MA 02117

3400 RIVERSIDE DR, STE 300
BURBANK, CA 91510

777 SAN MARIN DR
NOVATO, CA 94998

PO BOX 8217
LITTLE ROCK, AR 72221-8217

PO BOX 50550
ONTARIO, CA 91761-1055

PO BOX 193136
SAN FRANCISCO, CA 94119-3136

PO BOX 1975
SANTA ANA, CA 92702-1975

233 S WACKER DR, STE 2000
CHICAGO, IL 60606-6308

PO BOX 9431
MINNETONKA, MN 55440-9431

538 BROAD HOLLOW RD
MELVILLE, NY 11747

727 CRAIG RD
SAINT LOUIS, MO 63141-7123

101 SW MAINE, STE 710
PORTLAND, OR 97204

PO BOX 650594
DALLAS, TX 75265-0594

PO BOX 13340
SACRAMENTO, CA 95813-3340

PO BOX 26705
GREENSBORO, NC 27407-6705

2101 4TH AVE, STE 1100
SEATTLE, WA 98121

FIREMAN'S INSURANCE CO OF WASHINGTON, DC
7315 WISCONSIN AVE, STE 300 W
BETHESDA, MD 20814

FIRST AMERICAN ADMINISTRATORS
512 MAIN ST, STE 200
RAPID CITY, SD 51709

FIRST AMERICAN INSURANCE CO
3100 BROADWAY, STE 1300
KANSAS CITY, MO 64111

FIRST ASSURANCE LIFE INSURANCE CO
9016 BLUE BONNET BLVD
BATON ROUGE, LA 70884-3480

FIRST CARE
3310 DANVERS
AMARILLO, TX 79106-3504

FIRST HEALTH
3540 WILSHIRE BLVD
LOS ANGELES, CA 90010

PO BOX GG
BOISE, ID 83707

333 ROUSER RD
CORAOPOLIS, PA 15108

14955 HEATHROW FOREST PKY
HOUSTON, TX 77032

2650 DECKER LN
WEST VALLEY CITY, UT 84128

11301 W LAKE PARK DR
MILWAUKEE, WI 53224

FIRST INTEGRATED HEALTH
19191 S VERMONT, STE 700
TORRANCE, CA 90510

FIRST LIFE INSURANCE CO
501 W I-44 SERVICE RD, STE 400
OKLAHOMA CITY, OK 73118

FIRST OPTION HEALTH PLAN
3501 ST HWY 66
NEPTUNE, NJ 07754

FIRST PRIORITY HEALTH
70 N MAIN ST
WILKES-BARRE, PA 18711

PO BOX 3500
WILKES-BARRE, PA 18773-3500

FIRST RELIANCE STANDARD LIFE INSURANCE CO
11 W 42ND ST
NEW YORK, NY 10036

FIRST SECURITY INSURANCE, INC
405 S MAIN, 8TH FL
SALT LAKE CITY, UT 84110

FIRST UNITED AMERICAN LIFE INSURANCE CO
1020 7TH N ST
LIVERPOOL, NY 13088

FIRST UNUM LIFE INSURANCE CO
120 WHITE PLNS RD, STE 300
TARRYTOWN, NY 10591

FIRST VIRGINIA LIFE INSURANCE CO
6402 ARLINGTON BLVD, STE 1120
FALLS CHURCH, VA 22042-2300

FLEX CORP
5700 NW CENTRAL DR, STE 300
HOUSTON, TX 77092-2092

FLORIDA EMPLOYERS INSURANCE SERVICE CORP
2601 CATTLEMEN RD
SARASOTA, FL 34277

FLORIDA HEALTH CARE PLAN, INC
1340 RIDGEWOOD AVE
HOLLY HILL, FL 32117

FORREST T. JONES & CO, INC
3130 BROADWAY ST
KANSAS CITY, MO 64141-9131

FORTIS HEALTH
501 W MICHIGAN
MILWAUKEE, WI 53201

FORTUNE INSURANCE CO
10475 FORTUNE PARKWAY, STE 110
JACKSONVILLE, FL 32241

FRANK M. VACCARO & ASSOCIATES, INC
1 NESHAMINY INTERPLEX, STE 303
TREVOSE, PA 19053

FRANKLIN MUTUAL INSURANCE CO
5 BROAD ST
BRANCHVILLE, NJ 07826

FREE STATE HEALTH PLAN
100 S CHARLES ST- TWR II
BALTIMORE, MD 21201

FREMONT COMPENSATION INSURANCE CO
500 N BRAN BLVD
GLENDALE, CA 91203

520 MARYVILLE CENTER DR, STE 400
SAINT LOUIS, MO 63141

1684 W SHAR AVE
FRESNO, CA 93711

GAB ROBINS NORTH AMERICA
9 CAMPUS DR, STE 7
PARSIPPANY, NY 07054

GATES MCDONALD
3455 MILL RUN DR
HILLIARD, OH 43026

GEORGE N. PEGULA AGENCY
430 PENN AVE
SCRANTON, PA 18503

GEORGE WASHINGTON UNIVERSITY HEALTH PLAN
4550 MONTGOMERY AVE, STE 800
BETHESDA NORTH, MD 20814

GERLING GLOBAL REINSURANCE CORP
110 WILLIAM ST- 7TH FL
NEW YORK, NY 10038

GILBERT-MAGILL CO
920 MAIN ST, STE 1800
KANSAS CITY, MO 64141

GLOBE LIFE & ACCIDENT INSURANCE CO
PO BOX 26400
OKLAHOMA CITY, OK 73126

GRANGE INSURANCE ASSOCIATION
2501 SE COLUMBIA WY #160
VANCOUVER, WA 98661

GRE INSURANCE GROUP
600 COLLEGE RD E
PRINCETON, NJ 08540

6281 TRI-RIDGE BLVD
LOVELAND, OH 45140

600 COLLEGE RD E
PRINCETON, NJ 08540

GREAT AMERICAN INSURANCE COMPANIES
4480 LAKE FORREST DR
CINCINNATI, OH 45242

GREAT WEST CASUALTY CO
1100 W 29TH ST
SOUTH SIOUX CITY, NE 68876-0277

GREAT-WEST LIFE ASSURANCE CO
8515E ORCHARD DR
DENVER, CO 80201

60 OSBOURNE ST N
WINNIPEG, MB R3C-3A5

GREATER GEORGIA LIFE INSURANCE CO
PO BOX 9907
COLUMBUS, GA 31908

GREENBAY HEALTH PROTECTION PLAN
2000 WESTWOOD DR
WAUSAU, WI 54401

GROUP HEALTH NORTHWEST
5615 W SUNSET HWY
SPOKANE, WA 99224-9454

GROUP INSURANCE SERVICE CENTER
1020 PLAIN ST
MARSHFIELD, MA 02050

GUARANTEE RESERVE LIFE INSURANCE CO
530 RIVER OAKS W
CALUMET CITY, IL 60409

GUARANTEE TRUST LIFE INSURANCE CO
1275 MILWAUKEE AVE
GLENVIEW, IL 60025

GUARDIAN LIFE INSURANCE CO OF AMERICA
777 E MAGNESIUM
SPOKANE, WA 99208

GUIDEONE INSURANCE
1111 ASHWORTH RD
WEST DES MOINES, IA 50265

GULF INSURANCE CO
64 PERIMETER CTR E, STE 900
ATLANTA, GA 30302

4600 FULLER DR
IRVING, TX 75038

HANOVER INSURANCE CO
1455 LINCOLN PKY
ATLANTA, GA 30346

10816 EXECUTIVE CTR DR
LITTLE ROCK, AR 72211

100 CENTURY DR
PO BOX 15081
WORCESTER, MA 01615-0081

3740 ST JOHNS BLUFF RD, STE 9
JACKSONVILLE, FL 32224

1455 LINCOLN PKY
ATLANTA, GA 30346

2400 VETERANS BLVD, STE 400
KENNER, LA 70062

27 PEARL ST
PORTLAND, ME 04104-5004

10816 EXECUTIVE CTR DR
LITTLE ROCK, AR 72211

PO BOX 4898
SYRACUSE, NJ 13221

1 HUNTINGTON QUAD, STE 2S04
MELVILLE, NY 11747

103 COMMERCE BLVD
LIVERPOOL, NY 13088

PO BOX 85612
RICHMOND, VA 23285-5612

10816 EXECUTIVE CTR DR
LITTLE ROCK, AR 72211

PO BOX 4898
SYRACUSE, NJ 13221

PO BOX 85612
RICHMOND, VA 23285-5612

2400 VETERANS BLVD, STE 400
KENNER, LA 70062

PO BOX 85612
RICHMOND, VA 23285-5612

HARBISON-FISCHER
PO BOX 2477
FT WORTH, TX 76113

HARCO NATIONAL INSURANCE CO
2850 W GOLF RD
ROLLING MEADOWS, IL 60008

HARLEYSVILLE INSURANCE CO
5250 LOGANS FERRY RD
MURRAYSVILLE, PA 15668

355 MAPLE AVE
HARLEYSVILLE, PA 19438

5250 LOGANS FERRY RD
MURRAYSVILLE, PA 15668

HARRINGTON BENEFIT SERVICES
3501 FRONTAGE RD
TAMPA, FL 33607

HARTFORD INSURANCE CO
2502 ROCKY PT DR, STE 400
TAMPA, FL 33607

8910 PURDUE RD
INDIANAPOLIS, IN 46268-0930

24 NEW ENGLAND EXECUTIVE PARK
BURLINGTON, MA 01803

1 PARK PL- 300 S STATE
SYRACUSE, NY 13202

5832 FARM POND LN
CHARLOTTE, NC 28229

150 S WARNER RD- 3RD FL
KING OF PRUSSIA, PA 19406

720 OLIVE WAY, STE 300
SEATTLE, WA 98101

17855 DALLAS PKY, STE 490
DALLAS, TX 75287

125 S 84 ST, STE 400
MILWAUKEE, WI 53214

HARTFORD LIFE
505 N HWY 169
MINNEAPOLIS, MN 55441-6400

HARVARD PILGRIM HEALTH CARE
HPHC-SNE CLAIMS TEAM
PO BOX 699183
QUINCY, MA 02269

HAWORTH, INC
1 HAWORTH CTR 2-31G
HOLLAND, MI 49423

HEALTH BENEFITS FUND
1233 SHELBY ST
INDIANAPOLIS, IN 46203

HEALTH CARE PLAN
28 CHURCH ST- RM 100
BUFFALO, NY 14202-3998

HEALTH CLAIM SERVICES, INC
PO BOX 9615
DEERFIELD BEACH, FL 33442-9615

HEALTH FIRST
278 BARKS RD W
MARION, OH 43302

HEALTH FIRST, INC
821 E SE LOOP 323, II AMERICAN CTR, STE 200
TYLER, TX 75713

HEALTH FUTURE, INC
825 E MAIN ST, STE D
MEDFORD, OR 97504-7156

HEALTH GUARD SERVICES, INC
322 N COMMERCIAL
BELLINGHAM, WA 98225

HEALTH INSURANCE PLAN OF GREATER NEW YORK
7 W 34TH ST
NEW YORK, NY 10001-8100

HEALTH MANAGEMENT ASSOCIATES
1600 W BROADWAY RD, STE 385
TEMPE, AZ 85282

HEALTH NETWORK AMERICA, INC
187 MONMOUTH PKY
WEST LONG BRANCH, NJ 07764

HEALTH NEW ENGLAND
ONE MONARCH PL
SPRINGFIELD, MA 01144-1006

HEALTH OPTIONS OF SOUTH FLORIDA
4800 BEERWOOD CAMPUS PKY
JACKSONVILLE, FL 32202

HEALTH PARTNERS
TWO PERIMETER PARK S, STE 200 W
BIRMINGHAM, AL 35209

8100 34TH AVE S
BLOOMINGTON, MN 55440

180 E 5TH ST
SAINT PAUL, MN 55101

HEALTH PLAN ADMINISTRATORS, INC
30 SHELTER ROCK RD
DANBURY, CT 06810

HEALTH PLAN SOUTHEAST
3520 THOMASVILLE RD, STE 200
TALLAHASSEE, FL 32317

HEALTH PLUS OF MICHIGAN
2050 S LINDEN RD
FLINT, MI 48501

HEALTH RISK MANAGEMENT
10900 HAMPSHIRE AVE S
MINNEAPOLIS, MN 55430-2306

HEALTH SERVICES BENEFITS ADMINISTRATION
160 AIRWAY BLVD
LIVERMORE, CA 94550

HEALTH SERVICES MEDICAL CORP
8278 WILLETT PKY
BALDWINSVILLE, NY 13024

HEALTH SOURCE NORTH CAROLINA
701 CORPORATE CTR DR
RALEIGH, NC 27607

HEALTH SPECIAL RISK, INC
4001 N JOSEY LN
CARROLLTON, TX 75007

HEALTHCARE AMERICA PLANS, INC
453 S WEBB RD, STE 200
WICHITA, KS 67278

HEALTHNOW
1901 MAIN ST
BUFFALO, NY 14208

HEALTHPLAN MANAGEMENT, INC
101 N WAUKEGAN RD, STE 700
LAKE BLUFF, IL 60044

HEALTHRIGHT, INC
134 STATE ST
MERIDEN, CT 06450

HEALTHSOURCE
CIGNA HEALTHCARE, 900 COTTAGE GROVE RD
BLOOMFIELD, CT 06152

HELLER ASSOCIATES
2755 BRISTOL ST, STE 250
COSTA MESA, CA 92626-5956

HERITAGE MUTUAL INSURANCE CO
10101 W GREENFIELD AVE
WEST ALLIS, WI 53214

HIGHLANDS INSURANCE
4011 W CHASE BLVD
RALEIGH, NC 27607

HIGHLANDS INSURANCE GROUP
4011 WESTCHASE BLVD- 3RD FL
RALEIGH, NC 27611

HIGHLANDS NORTHWESTERN NATIONAL INSURANCE CO
4011 WESTCHASE BLVD
RALEIGH, NC 27607

HINGHAM MUTUAL FIRE INSURANCE CO
230 BEAL ST
HINGHAM, MA 02043

HMA, INC
1600 W BROADWAY RD #385
TEMPE, AZ 85282

HMO BLUE OF EL PASO
4150 PINNACLE ST, STE 203
EL PASO, TX 79902-1035

HMO ILLINOIS
300 E RANDOLPH
CHICAGO, IL 60601-5099

HMO NEBRASKA
2401 S 73RD ST, STE 2
OMAHA, NE 68124

HOMETOWN HEALTH NETWORK
100 LILLIAN GISH BLVD, STE 301
MASSILLON, OH 44647

HUMANA HEALTH CARE PLAN, INC
101 E MAIN
LOUISVILLE, KY 40202

HUMANA/ WISCONSIN HEALTH ORGANIZATION
500 W MAIN ST
LOUISVILLE, KY 40202-1438

IDAHO FARM BUREAU MUTUAL INSURANCE CO
PO BOX 4848
POCATELLO, ID 83205

IFG CO
238 INTERNATIONAL RD
BURLINGTON, NC 27215

IMT INSURANCE CO
4445 CORPORATE DR
WEST DES MOINES, IA 50306

INDEPENDENCE BLUE CROSS
1901 MARKET ST
PHILADELPHIA, PA 19103-1480

INDEPENDENT HEALTH
511 FARBER LAKES DR
BUFFALO, NY 14221

INDIANAPOLIS LIFE
2960 N MERIDIAN ST
INDIANAPOLIS, IN 46208

INSPIRE INSURANCE SOLUTIONS
PO BOX 2269
FT. WORTH, TX 76113-2269

INSURANCE CO OF GREATER NEW YORK
200 MADISON AVE
NEW YORK, NY 10016-6023

INSURANCE & RISK MANAGEMENT
3811 ILLINOIS RD
FT WAYNE, IN 46801-1705

INTER VALLEY HEALTH PLAN
300 S PARK AVE
POMONA, CA 91769

INTERCARE BENEFIT SYSTEMS, INC
5500 GREENWOOD PLZ BLVD, STE 100
ENGLEWOOD, CO 80111

INTERGROUP OF ARIZONA
930 N FINANCE CTR DR
TUCSON, AZ 85710

INTERGROUP OF UTAH, INC
PO BOX 19139
TUCSON, AZ 85731-9139

IOWA MUTUAL INSURANCE GROUP
509 9TH ST
DE WITT, IA 52742

IU MEDICAL GROUP PRIMARY CARE
3901 W 86TH ST, STE 230
PO BOX 78310
INDIANAPOLIS, IN 46278-8310

J.P. FARLEY CORP
22021 BROOKPARK RD, STE 100
CLEVELAND, OH 44126

JARDINE GROUP SERVICES
13 CORNELL RD
LATHAM, NY 12110

JEFFERSON PILOT FINANCIAL
1 GRANITE PL
CONCORD, NH 03301

JENSEN ADMINISTRATIVE SERVICES
4885 S 9TH E, STE 202
SALT LAKE CITY, UT 84117-5725

JFP BENEFIT MANAGEMENT
100 S JACKSON ST, STE 200
JACKSON, MI 49201

JOHN ALDEN LIFE INSURANCE CO
1005 MAIN ST
BOISE, ID 83702

JOHN DEERE HEALTHCARE
3800 23RD AVE, STE 200
MOLINE, IL 61265

JOHNS HOPKINS MEDICAL SERVICES CORPORATION
3100 WYMAN PK DR
BALTIMORE, MD 21211

JOINT WELFARE FUND, LOCAL 164 IBEW
65 W CENTURY RD
PARAMUS, NJ 07652

K & K INSURANCE GROUP
1712 MAGNAVOX WAY
FT WAYNE, IN 46804

KAISER / GROUP HEALTH
521 WALL ST
SEATTLE, WA 98121

KAISER PERMANENTE
393 E WALNUT ST- 3RD FL
PASADENA, CA 91109

3495 PIEDMONT RD NE- BLDG 9
ATLANTA, GA 30305

2101 E JEFFERSON ST
ROCKVILLE, MD 20849

PO BOX 378044
DENVER, CO 80237

ONE CHP PLZ
LATHAM, NY 12110

76 BATTERSON PARK RD
PO BOX 4011
FARMINGTON, CT 06034-4011

PO BOX 40669
RALEIGH, NC 27629

500 NE MULTNOMAH, STE 100
PORTLAND, OR 97232

KANAWHA HEALTHCARE SOLUTIONS, INC
PO BOX 1000
LANCASTER, SC 29720

KANSAS FARM BUREAU & AFFILIATED SERVICES
2627 KFB PLZ
MANHATTAN, KS 66503

KEENAN & ASSOCIATES
2105 S BASCOM AVE, STE 310
CAMPBELL, CA 95008-3271

KEMPER INSURANCE
152 N 3RD ST, STE 710
SAN JOSE, CA 95112

ONE KEMPER DR
LONG GROVE, IL 60049-0001

1861 N ROCK RD, STE 202
WICHITA, KS 67208

KEMPER INSURANCE COMPANIES
16835 W BERNARDO DR, STE 103
SAN DIEGO, CA 92127

5101 UTICA RIDGE RD
DAVENPORT, IA 52805-0520

81 WELBY RD
NEW BEDFORD, MA 02745

1720 LOUISIANA BLVD NE, STE 206
ALBUQUERQUE, NM 87198

KENTUCKY FARM BUREAU MUTUAL INSURANCE CO
9201 BUNSEN PKY
LOUISVILLE, KY 40223

3036 PARRISH AVE
OWENSBORO, KY 42304

KEYSTONE HEALTH PLAN CENTRAL
300 CORPORATE CTR DR
CAMP HILL, PA 17011

KEYSTONE HEALTH PLAN EAST, INC
1901 MARKET ST
PHILADELPHIA, PA 19103

KEYSTONE MERCY HEALTH PLAN
200 STEVENS DR
LESTER, PA 19113-1570

KIRKE-VAN ORSDEL
1 METROPOLITAN SQ, STE 800
SAINT LOUIS, MO 63102-3102

KITSAP PHYSICIANS SERVICE
400 WARREN AVE
BREMERTON, WA 98337

KLAIS & CO
1867 W MARKET ST
AKRON, OH 44313

L.P.C.W.I.F.
5750 15-MILE RD, STE 12
STERLING HEIGHTS, MI 48310

LABORERS LOCAL 190 WELFARE FUND
668 WEMPLE RD
GLENMONT, NY 12077-0339

LAMAR LIFE INSURANCE
222 MERCHANDISE MART PLZ
CHICAGO, IL 60654

LANCER CLAIM SERVICE CORP
333 CITY BLVD W
ORANGE, CA 92868

LANCER CORP
6655 LANCER BLVD
SAN ANTONIO, TX 78219

LANDMARK HEALTH CARE
1750 HOWE AVE, STE 300
SACRAMENTO, CA 95825

LASALLE CLINIC
1165 APPLETON RD
MENASHA, WI 54952

LAWRENCE E. SMITH & ASSOCIATES, INC
1819 CLARKSON RD, STE 300
SAINT LOUIS, MO 63017

LEWER AGENCY, INC
4534 WORNALL RD
KANSAS CITY, MO 64111

LEXINGTON INSURANCE CO
80 PINE ST
NEW YORK CITY, NY 10005

LIBERTY LIFE INSURANCE CO
PO BOX 789, 2000 WADE HAMPTON BLVD
GREENVILLE, SC 29602

1510 NEW TOWN PIKE, STE A
LEXINGTON, KY 40577

2000 WADE HAMPTON BLVD
GREENVILLE, SC 29615

LIBERTY MUTUAL
30200 TELEGRAPH RD
DETROIT, MI 48025

LIBERTY MUTUAL GROUP
10 CORPORATE DR, STE 100
BEDFORD, NH 03110-5954

LIBERTY MUTUAL INSURANCE
3633 E INLAND EMPIRE BLVD- 5TH FL
ONTARIO, CA 91764

175 BERKELEY ST
BOSTON, MA 02116

24651 CENTER RDG RD, STE 400
CLEVELAND, OH 44145

111 CONGRESSIONAL BLVD, STE 200
CARMEL, IN 46032

12250 WEBBER HILL RD
SAINT LOUIS, MO 63127

3333 PL CAVENDISH, STE 105
SAINT LAURENT, PQ H4M-2X6

LIFE & HEALTH INSURANCE CO OF AMERICA
2200 WALNUT ST
PHILADELPHIA, PA 19103

LIFE INSURANCE CO OF NORTH AMERICA
255 EAST AVE
ROCHESTER, NY 14604

LIFE INVESTOR INSURANCE CO OF AMERICA
1020 W 4TH ST
LITTLE ROCK, AR 72203-8063

LIFE INVESTORS INSURANCE CO OF AMERICA
815 TRAILWOOD, STE 205
NORTH RICHLAND HILLS, TX 76182

LIFEGUARD, INC
PO BOX 5506
SAN JOSE, CA 95150-5506

LINCOLN MUTUAL LIFE & CASUALTY INSURANCE CO
203 N 10TH ST
FARGO, ND 58103

LOCAL 365 UAW WELFARE FUND
30-07 39TH AVE
LONG ISLAND CITY, NY 11101

LOCAL UNION 164 IBEW JOINT WELFARE
65 W CENTURY RD
PARAMUS, NJ 07652

LOCAL UNION NO 682 HEALTH & WELFARE
5730 ELIZABETH AVE
SAINT LOUIS, MO 63110

LOCALS 302 & 612 INTERNATIONAL
2815 2ND AVE #300
SEATTLE, WA 98121

LOYAL AMERICAN LIFE INSURANCE CO
2800 DAUEHIN ST
MOBILE, AL 36606

LYNDON INSURANCE CO
520 MARYVILLE CENTER DR, STE 500
SAINT LOUIS, MO 63141

M.S.I. INSURANCE
2 PINE TREE DR
SAINT PAUL, MN 55112

M-CARE ADMINISTRATION
2301 COMMONWEALTH BLVD
ANN ARBOR, MI 48103

MADISON NATIONAL LIFE INSURANCE CO, INC
6120 UNIVERSITY AVE
MADISON, WI 53562

MAINE BONDING & CASUALTY CO
500 ENTERPRISE DR
ROCKY HILLS, CT 06012

MAJESTIC UNDERWRITERS, INC
550 STEPHENSON HWY, STE 407
TROY, MI 48083

MANAGED CARE CONSULTANTS, INC (MCC)
4160 S PECOS RD
LAS VEGAS, NV 89121-5025

MANAGED HEALTH, INC
25 BROADWAY, STE 900
NEW YORK, NY 10004

MANAGED HEALTHCARE CONCEPTS, INC
1100 SPRING ST, STE 610
ATLANTA, GA 30309

MANAGED HEALTHCARE, INC
50 BRIAR HOLLOW, STE 500
HOUSTON, TX 77027

MASSACHUSETTS MUTUAL LIFE INSURANCE CO
1350 MAIN ST
PO BOX 51130
SPRINGFIELD, MA 01151

MAXICARE HEALTH PLANS
PO BOX 861059
LOS ANGELES, CA 90086-1059

MAXICARE OF NORTH CAROLINA, INC
5550-77 CENTER DR, STE 380
CHARLOTTE, NC 28217

MCCREARY CORPORATION
700 CENTRAL PKY
STUART, FL 34994

MEAD CORP
COURTHOUSE PLZ NE
DAYTON, OH 45463

MEADOWBROOK INSURANCE GROUP
PO BOX 5086
SOUTHFIELD, MI 48086-5806

MEDEX ASSISTANCE CORP
9515 DEERECO RD- 4TH FL
PO BOX 5375
TIMONIUM, MD 21093-5375

MEDICAID FISCAL AGENTS
4300 COX RD
PO BOX 3900
GLEN ALLEN, VA 23060

PO BOX 23
BOISE, ID 83707

1720 RANDOLPH RD, STE A
ALBUQUERQUE, NM 87106

MEDICAL ASSOCIATES HEALTH PLANS, INC
700 LOCUST, STE 230
PO BOX 5002
DUBUQUE, IA 52004-5002

MEDICAL CENTER OF OCEAN COUNTY
2121 EDGEWATER PL
POINT PLEASANT, NJ 08742-2212

MEDICAL LIFE INSURANCE CO
1220 HURON RD
CLEVELAND, OH 44115

MEDICAL MUTUAL OF OHIO
PO BOX 6018
CLEVELAND, OH 44101-1355

MEDICAL NETWORK OF COLORADO SPRINGS
555 E PIKES PK AVE
COLORADO SPRINGS, CO 80901

MEDICARE — PART A INTERMEDIARIES
450 RIVERCHASE PKY EAST
BIRMINGHAM, AL 35283-0139

2444 W LAS PAMARITAS DR
PHOENIX, AZ 85002-3466

601 GAINES ST
PO BOX 2181
LITTLE ROCK, AR 72203-2181

21555 OXNARD ST
PO BOX 70000
VAN NUYS, CA 91470

1800 CENTER ST
PO BOX 890089
CAMP HILL, PA 17089-0089

2357 WARM SPGS RD
PO BOX 9048
COLUMBUS, GA 31908-9048

8115 KNUE RD
INDIANAPOLIS, IN 46250-2804

9901 LINN STATION RD
PO BOX 23711
LOUISVILLE, KY 40223-0711

PO BOX 64357
SAINT PAUL, MN 55164-0357

PO BOX 23035
JACKSON, MS 39225-3035

3360 10TH AVE S
PO BOX 5017
GREAT FALLS, MT 59403

3000 GOFFS FALLS RD
MANCHESTER, NH 03111-0001

ONE WORLD TRADE CENTER
PO BOX 1407
NEW YORK, NY 10048

4510 13TH AVE SW
FARGO, ND 58121-0001

1215 S BOULDER AVE
PO BOX 3404
TULSA, OK 74101

1600 SW 4TH AVE
PO BOX 8110
PORTLAND, OR 97207

BOX 71391
SAN JUAN, PR 00936

444 WESTMINSTER ST
PROVIDENCE, RI 02903

730 CHESTNUT ST
CHATTANOOGA, TN 37402-1790

PO BOX 57
COLUMBUS, OH 43216-0057

MEDICARE — PART B CARRIERS
PO BOX 830140
BIRMINGHAM, AL 35283-0140

4510 13TH AVE SW
FARGO, ND 58121-0001

PO BOX 6704
FARGO, ND 58108-6704

450 W EAST AVE
CHICO, CA 95926

PO BOX 6028
FARGO, ND 58108-6028

1800 CENTER ST
PO BOX 890101
CAMP HILL, PA 17089-0101

8115 KNUE RD
INDIANAPOLIS, IN 46250-2804

1901 MAIN ST
PO BOX 80
BUFFALO, NY 14240-0080

622 3RD AVE
NEW YORK, NY 10017

701 NW 63RD
OKLAHOMA CITY, OK 73116

PO BOX 6702
FARGO, ND 58108-6702

PO BOX 71391
SAN JUAN, PR 00936-1391

444 WESTMINSTER ST
PROVIDENCE, RI 02903

PO BOX 100190
COLUMBIA, SC 29202

PO BOX 6707
FARGO, ND 58108-6707

2890 COTTONWOOD PKY
SALT LAKE CITY, UT 84131

PO BOX 6700
FARGO, ND 58108-6700

PO BOX 57
COLUMBUS, OH 43216-0057

PO BOX 1787
MADISON, WI 53701-1787

MEGA LIFE & HEALTH INSURANCE
PO BOX 809096
DALLAS, TX 75380-9096

MEMBER SERVICE LIFE INSURANCE CO
PO BOX 57208
OKLAHOMA, OK 73151-7208

MEMPHIS HOSPITAL SERVICES
PO BOX 98
MEMPHIS, TN 38101-0098

MERCHANTS INSURANCE GROUP
309 FELLOWSHIP RD
MOORESTOWN, NJ 08057-0868

MERCURY CASUALTY CO
PO BOX 54600
LOS ANGELES, CA 90054-0600

PO BOX 49008
SAN JOSE, CA 95161-9008

PO BOX 54600
LOS ANGELES, CA 90054-0600

MERCYCARE HEALTH PLAN, INC
PO BOX 2770
JAMESVILLE, WI 53547-2770

MERIDIAN SECURITY
2955 N MERIDIAN ST
INDIANAPOLIS, IN 46208

MERIT LIFE INSURANCE CO
PO BOX 39
EVANSVILLE, IN 47701-0039

MERRILL BOSTROM ASSOCIATES
PO BOX 651109
SALT LAKE CITY, UT 84124-1109

MET LIFE DISABILITY
PO BOX 3017
UTICA, NY 13504-3017

METRA HEALTHCARE NETWORK OF WISCONSIN, INC
PO BOX 3184
MILWAUKEE, WI 53210-3184

METROPOLITAN LIFE INSURANCE CO
PO BOX 3015
UTICA, NY 13504-3015

177 S COMMONS DR
AURORA, IL 60505

PO BOX 1600
KINGSTON, NY 12401-0600

PO BOX 495
WARWICK, RI 02884-0495

METROPOLITAN LIFE INSURANCE CO/AUTOMOBILE & HOME
PO BOX 48020
DAYTON, OH 45475-8020

METROPOLITAN PROPERTY & CASUALTY INSURANCE CO
700 QUACKER LANE
WARWICK, RI 02887

MGIS COMPANIES
1849 W NORTH TEMPLE - BLDG D
SLC, UT 84116-3067

MICHIGAN FARM BUREAU MUTUAL INSURANCE CO
PO BOX 169
BIRCH RUN, MI 48415-0169

7373 W SAGINOL HWY
LANSING, MI 48089

PO BOX 30960
LANSING, MI 48909-0960

MICHIGAN MILLERS MUTUAL INSURANCE
PO BOX 30060
LANSING, MI 48909-0060

MICHIGAN MUTUAL INSURANCE CO
PO BOX 2060
FARMINGTON HILLS, MI 48333-2060

PO BOX 116
GRAND RAPIDS, MI 49501-0116

PO BOX 419058
SAINT LOUIS, MO 63141-9058

PO BOX 560769
CHARLOTTE, NC 28256-0769

57 GERMAN TOWN CT, STE 100
CORDOVA, TN 38018

PO BOX 569680
DALLAS, TX 75356-9680

MID-ATLANTIC MEDICAL SERVICES, INC
4 TAFT CT
ROCKVILLE, MD 20850

MID-CONTINENT CASUALTY CO
4949 S MEMORIAL
TULSA, OK 74145

MIDDLESEX MUTUAL ASSURANCE CO
PO BOX 891
MIDDLETOWN, CT 06457-0891

MIDLAND CO
PO BOX 5323
CINCINNATI, OH 45210-5323

MIDWEST SECURITY ADMINISTRATORS
PO BOX 19035
GREEN BAY, WI 54307-9035

MILLENNIUM CARE ADMINISTRATORS (DBA MCA ADMINISTRATORS)
820 PARISH ST
PITTSBURGH, PA 15220

MILLETTE ADMINISTRATORS, INC
4619 MAIN ST, STE A
MOSS POINT, MS 39563

MILWAUKEE INSURANCE CO
PO BOX 1450
MILWAUKEE, WI 53201-1450

MINNESOTA MUTUAL LIFE INSURANCE CO
400 ROBERT ST N
SAINT PAUL, MN 55101

MONUMENTAL LIFE INSURANCE CO
PO BOX 61
DURHAM, NC 27702

MOTEL 6 OPERATING LP HEADQUARTERS
PO BOX 809092
DALLAS, TX 75240-9092

MOUNTAIN STATES ADMINISTRATIVE SERVICE
PO BOX 32702
TUCSON, AZ 85710

MOUNTAIN STATES MUTUAL CASUALTY CO
PO BOX 249
ALBUQUERQUE, NM 87103-0249

MOUNTAIN WEST FARM BUREAU MUTUAL INSURANCE CO
PO BOX 1348
LARAMIE, WY 82070-1348

MUTUAL GROUP
PO BOX 65770
WEST DES MOINES, IA 50265-5770

MUTUAL OF OMAHA
PO BOX 9
WOODWARD, OK 73801-0009

NATIONAL AMERICAN INSURANCE CO OF CALIFORNIA
PO BOX 5810
LONG BEACH, CA 90805-5810

NATIONAL AUTOMOBILE & CASUALTY INSURANCE CO
PO BOX 7040
PASADENA, CA 91105-7040

NATIONAL FAMILY CARE LIFE INSURANCE CO
PO BOX 809043
DALLAS, TX 75380-9043

NATIONAL FOUNDATION LIFE INSURANCE CO
110 W 7TH ST STE 300
FT. WORTH, TX 76102

NATIONAL HEALTH INSURANCE CO
PO BOX 61999
DALLAS, TX 75261-9999

NEW AIR LIFE
PO BOX 4884
HOUSTON, TX 77210-4884

NEW YORK CASUALTY INSURANCE CO
120 WASHINGTON ST
WATERTOWN, NY 13601-3330

NOBEL INSURANCE CO
8001 LBJ FWY, STE 300
DALLAS, TX 75251

NOITU INSURANCE TRUST FUND
148-06 HILLSIDE AVE
JAMAICA, NY 11435

NORTH AMERICA ADMINISTRATORS, INC
1212 8TH AVE S
NASHVILLE, TN 37203

NORTH CENTRAL LIFE INSURANCE CO
445 MINNESOTA ST
SAINT PAUL, MN 55101

NRECA
7101 A STREET
LINCOLN, NB 68510

OHIO BUREAU OF WORKERS COMPENSATION
30 W SPRING ST, WILLIAM GREEN BLDG
COLUMBUS, OH 43215

OHIO CASUALTY GROUP
7400 METRO BLVD, STE 350
MINNEAPOLIS, MN 55439

1445 KEMPER MEADOW DR
CINCINNATI, OH 45240

OLD RELIANCE INSURANCE CO
PO BOX 13150
PHOENIX, AZ 85002-3150

OXFORD LIFE INSURANCE CO
2721 N CENTRAL AVE
PHOENIX, AZ 85004-1121

PACIFIC HERITAGE ADMINISTRATORS
111 SW COLUMBIA, STE 600
PORTLAND, OR 97201

PARTNERS NATIONAL HEALTH PLANS
2085 FRONTIS PLZ BLVD
WINSTON-SALEM, NC 27103

PAULA INSURANCE CO
300 NORTHLAKE AVE, STE 300
PASADENA, CA 91101

PHYSICIANS HEALTH PLAN OF SOUTHWEST MICHIGAN
ROUTE 2702
PO BOX 169055
DULUTH, MN 55816-8251

PREFERRED HEALTH NETWORK
153 TECHNOLOGY
IRVINE, CA 92618

PREFERRED RISK GROUP INSURANCE COMPANIES
1111 ASHWORTH
WEST DES MOINES, IA 50265

PRINCIPAL FINANCIAL GROUP
PO BOX 39710
COLORADO SPRINGS, CO 80949

PRINCIPAL HEALTH CARE OF IOWA
PO BOX 15294
WILMINGTON, DE 19850

PROFESSIONAL RISK MANAGEMENT
2101 WEBSTER ST, STE 900
OAKLAND, CA 94612

PROGRESSIVE CASUALTY INSURANCE CO
6300 WILSON MILLS RD
MAYFIELD VILLAGE, OH 44143

PO BOX 6807
CLEVELAND, OH 44101

PROGRESSIVE DIVERSIFIED INSURANCE CO
PO BOX 94950
CLEVELAND, OH 44101

PRUDENTIAL HEALTH CARE PLAN, INC
PO BOX 4711
HOUSTON, TX 77210

PRUDENTIAL HEALTH CARE PLAN OF MID-ATLANTIC
PO BOX 45036
JACKSONVILLE, FL 32232-5036

PRUDENTIAL HEALTHCARE OF CALIFORNIA
PO BOX 60519
LOS ANGELES, CA 90060-0519

PRUDENTIAL INSURANCE CO OF AMERICA
PO BOX 30238
LOS ANGELES, CA 90030-0238

QUAL-MED HEALTH PLAN
PO BOX 640
PUEBLO, CO 81002

REGENCE BLUE SHIELD
1800 9TH AVE
SEATTLE, WA 98101

REGENCE BLUESHIELD
1800 NINTH AVE
SEATTLE, WA 98101-1322

RELIANCE INSURANCE CO
PO BOX 15901
SACRAMENTO, CA 95852

ROYAL & SUNALLIANCE
801 N BRAND BLVD, STE 500
GLENDALE, CA 91203

1600 RIVIERA AVE, STE 210
WALNUT CREEK, CA 94596

7400 E ORCHARD RD, STE 4000
ENGLEWOOD, CO 80111

500 WINDING BRK DR
HARTFORD, CT 06120

80 WOLF RD, STE 606
ALBANY, NY 12211

5 CONCOURSE PKY, STE 500
ATLANTA, GA 30328

255 E 5TH ST, STE 2100
CINCINNATI, OH 45202

100 COMMERCIAL DR
PORTLAND, OR 04101

300 E LOMBARD ST, STE 700
BALTIMORE, MD 21202

NEW ENGLAND WC CTR
PO BOX 2912
HARTFORD, CT 06104

255 PARK AVE, STE 601
WORCESTER, MA 01609

6465 WAYZATA BLVD, STE 810
SAINT LOUIS PARK, MN 55426

2 JERICHO PLZ
JERICHO, NY 11753

25800 NORTHWESTERN HWY, STE 701
SOUTHFIELD, MI 48037

2 COMMERCE DR
BEDFORD, NH 03110

555 TAXTER RD
ELMSFORD, NY 10523

2351 N FOREST RD
GETZVILLE, NY 14068

1393 VETERANS HWY
HAUPPAUGE, NY 11788

1 CHASE MANHATTAN PLZ- 38TH FL
NEW YORK, NY 10005

400 W DIVISION ST
SYRACUSE, NY 13203

PO BOX 1378
BUFFALO, NY 14240

9300 ARROW PT BLVD
CHARLOTTE, NC 28273

1901 ROXBOROUGH RD
CHARLOTTE, NC 28211

1510 VLY CTR PKY, STE 130
BETHLEHEM, PA 18017

501 HOLIDAY DR, FOSTER PLZ 4
PITTSBURGH, PA 15220-2774

107 FLYNN DR, STE 500
MILBANK, SD 57252

12750 MERIT DR, STE 400
DALLAS, TX 75251

720 MOORFIELD PRK DR, STE 300
RICHMOND, VA 23236

999 3RD AVE, STE 2700
SEATTLE, WA 98104-4000

RUSH-PRUDENTIAL HEALTH PLAN
233 S WACKER, STE 3900
CHICAGO, IL 60606

SAFECO INSURANCE CO OF AMERICA
17570 BROOKHURST
FOUNTAIN VALLEY, CA 92708

12499 W COLFAX
LAKEWOOD, CO 80215

1551 JULIET RD
STONE MOUNTAIN, GA 30086

900 E PARIS SE, STE 201
GRAND RAPIDS, MI 49501

3637 S GEYER RD
SAINT LOUIS, MO 63127

3217 FIETCHNER DR
FARGO, ND 58106

5901 E GALBRAITH RD
CINCINNATI, OH 45236

4101 SW KRUSE WAY
LAKE OSWEGO, OR 97035

500 N CENTRAL, STE 300
PLANO, TX 75086

1 PARK W CIR, STE 200
MIDLOTHIAN, VA 23113

14610 E SPRAGUE AVE
SPOKANE, WA 99220

SELF INSURED BENEFIT ADMINISTRATORS
18167 US HWY 19 N, STE 300
CLEARWATER, FL 33764

SELF INSURED SERVICES CO
151 W 8TH ST
DUBUQUE, IA 52001

SELF-INSURED MANAGEMENT SERVICE
9320 SW BARBUR BLVD #350
PORTLAND, OR 97219

SELMAN & CO
6110 PARKLAND BLVD
CLEVELAND, OH 44124

SENTRY INSURANCE A MUTUAL CO
9060 E VIALINDA
SCOTTSDALE, AZ 85258

1800 N POINT DR
STEVENS POINT, WI 54481

SERVICE LIFE & CASUALTY
6907 CAPITOL OF TX HWY, STE 370
AUSTIN, TX 78731

SHAND MORHAN INSURANCE CO
1007 CHURCH ST
EVANSTON, IL 60201

SHELTER INSURANCE COMPANIES
1817 W BROADWAY
COLUMBIA, MO 65218-0001

SIGNA HEALTH CARE HEALTHSOURCE
146 FAIRCHILD ST
DANIEL ISLAND, SC 29492

SIGNA HEALTHCARE
2 COLLEGE PARK DR
HOOKSETT, NH 03106

SOUTHERN BENEFIT ADMINISTRATORS, INC
907 TWO MILE PKY, BLDG C
GOODLETTSVILLE, TN 37072

SOUTHERN RISK SERVICES, INC
2211 7TH AVE S
PO BOX 2408
BIRMINGHAM, AL 35201-2408

ST. PAUL COMPANIES
10777 SUNSET OFFICE DR, STE 200 - PO BOX 8605
SUNSET HILLS, MO 63126-0605

STANDARD INSURANCE CO
900 SW 5TH
PORTLAND, OR 97204

STATE AUTOMOBILE MUTUAL INSURANCE CO
100 STATE AUTO BLVD
GOODLETTSVILLE, TN 37072

STATE COMPENSATION INSURANCE FUND
1504 4TH ST
SAN FRANCISCO, CA 94103

900 CORP CENTER DR
MONTEREY PARK, CA 91754

9801 CAMINO MEDIA
BAKERSFIELD, CA 93310

10 RIVERPARK PLACE E
FRESNO, CA 93720

2955 PERALTA OAKS CT
OAKLAND, CA 94605

2901 N VENTURA RD
OXNARD, CA 93032

364 KNOLLCREST DR
REDDING, CA 96002

2275 GATEWAY OAKS
SACRAMENTO, CA 95815

375 W HOSPITALITY LN
SAN BERNARDINO, CA 92402

9444 WAPLES ST
SAN DIEGO, CA 92186

6203 SANIGNACIO AVE
SAN JOSE, CA 95152

1750 E 4TH ST
SANTA ANA, CA 92705

1450 NEOTOMAS AVE
SANTA ROSA, CA 95405

21300 VICTORY BLVD, STE 500
WOODLAND HILLS, CA 91365

STATE FARM INSURANCE CO
ONE STATE FARM PLZ
BLOOMINGTON, IL 61710-0007

1440 GRANVILLE RD
NEWARK, OH 43055

STATE OF ALASKA WORKERS COMP DIVISION
1111 W 8TH ST
PO BOX 25512
JUNEAU, AK 99802-5512

SURETY LIFE INSURANCE CO
206 S 13TH ST, STE 300
LINCOLN, NE 68501

SWISS RE LIFE & HEALTH AMERICA
969 HIGH RDG RD
STAMFORD, CT 06905

TETON NATIONAL INSURANCE CO
9777 S YOSEMITE
LITTLETON, CO 80124-3115

THE COMMERCE GROUP
PO BOX 900
ELYRIA, OH 44036

THE GUARDIAN
2300 E CAPITAL DR
APPLETON, WI 54911

THE WHEELER COMPANIES
200 CAHABA PARK CIR, STE 250
BIRMINGHAM, AL 35242

TPA
6160 SUMMIT DR, STE 360
BROOKLYN CENTER, MN 55430

TRIGON
2015 STAPLES MILL RD
RICHMOND, VA 23261-6623

TRINITY UNIVERSAL INSURANCE CO
PO BOX 655028
DALLAS, TX 75265-5028

TRUSTMARK INSURANCE
400 FIELD DR
LAKE FOREST, IL 60045

UNICARE
PO BOX 833947
RICHARDSON, TX 75083-3947

UNIGARD SECURITY INSURANCE CO
15805 NE 24TH ST
BELLEVUE, WA 98008-2409

UNITED HEALTH CARE OF LOUISIANA
2431 S ACADIAN THRUWAY, STE 350
BATON ROUGE, LA 70808

WARD NORTH AMERICA, INC
610 W ASH ST #1500
SAN DIEGO, CA 92101-3349

WASATCH CREST INSURANCE CO
PO BOX 27119
SALT LAKE CITY, UT 84127-0008

WAUSAU INSURANCE CO
PO BOX 31312
TAMPA, FL 33631-3312

PO BOX 8017
WAUSAU, WI 54402-8017

WEYERHAEUSER CO
SB-1
PO BOX 2999
TACOMA, WA 98477-2999

WINDSOR GROUP
PO BOX 105091
ATLANTA, GA 30348-5091

ZENITH ADMINISTRATORS, INC
6011 W SAINT JOSEPH, STE 401
LANSING, MI 48917

314 W SUPERIOR ST, STE 750
DULUTH, MN 55802

7645 METRO BLVD
MINNEAPOLIS, MD 55436

4260 SHORELINE DR, STE 170
EARTH CITY, MO 63045

3449 HOLLENBERG DR, STE 150
BRIDGETOWN, MO 63045

3100 BROADWAY, STE 400
KANSAS CITY, MO 64111

33 EASTLAND ST
SPRINGFIELD, MA 01109

3246 HWY 69
NEDERLAND, TX 77705

303 E OHIO ST
CHICAGO, IL 60611

2801 COHO ST, STE 300
MADISON, WI 53713

ZURICH-AMERICAN INSURANCE GROUP
PO BOX 305010
NASHVILLE, TN 37229-5010

1400 AMERICAN LN
SCHAUMBURG, IL 60196

730 HOLIDAY DR, BLDG 8
PITTSBURGH, PA 15017